MW00651563

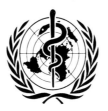

World Health Organization Classification of Tumours

WHO OMS

International Agency for Research on Cancer (IARC)

4th Edition

WHO Classification of Tumours of the Lung, Pleura, Thymus and Heart

Edited by

William D. Travis

Elisabeth Brambilla

Allen P. Burke

Alexander Marx

Andrew G. Nicholson

International Agency for Research on Cancer

Lyon, 2015

World Health Organization Classification of Tumours

Series Editors   Fred T. Bosman, MD PhD
Elaine S. Jaffe, MD
Sunil R. Lakhani, MD FRCPath
Hiroko Ohgaki, PhD

WHO Classification of Tumours of the Lung, Pleura, Thymus and Heart

Editors   William D. Travis, MD
Elisabeth Brambilla, MD
Allen P. Burke, MD
Alexander Marx, MD
Andrew G. Nicholson, DM FRCPath

Project Assistant   Asiedua Asante

Technical Editor   Jessica Cox
Rachel Purcell, PhD

Database   Alberto Machado
Delphine Nicolas

Layout   Stefanie Brottrager

Printed by   Maestro
38330 Saint-Ismier, France

Publisher   International Agency for
Research on Cancer (IARC)
69372 Lyon Cedex 08, France

This volume was produced in collaboration with the

International Association for the Study of Lung Cancer (IASLC)

International Thymic Malignancy Interest Group (ITMIG)

International Mesothelioma Panel

The WHO Classification of Tumours of the Lung, Pleura, Thymus and Heart presented in this book reflects the views of a Working Group that convened for a Consensus and Editorial Meeting at the International Agency for Research on Cancer, Lyon
24–26 April, 2014.

Members of the Working Group are indicated
in the List of Contributors on pages 349–358

Published by the International Agency for Research on Cancer (IARC),
150 cours Albert Thomas, 69372 Lyon Cedex 08, France

© International Agency for Research on Cancer, 2015

Distributed by
WHO Press, World Health Organization, 20 Avenue Appia, 1211 Geneva 27, Switzerland
Tel.: +41 22 791 3264; Fax: +41 22 791 4857; Email: bookorders@who.int

Second print run, with corrections (5000 copies)
See http://publications.iarc.fr/Book-And-Report-Series/Who-Iarc-Classification-Of-Tumours

Format for bibliographic citations:
William D. Travis, Elisabeth Brambilla, Allen P. Burke, Alexander Marx, Andrew G. Nicholson (Eds.):
WHO Classification of Tumours of Lung, Pleura, Thymus and Heart (4th edition).
IARC: Lyon 2015

IARC Library Cataloguing in Publication Data

WHO classification of tumours of the lung, pleura, thymus and heart / edited by William D. Travis, Elisabeth Brambilla,
Allen P. Burke , Alexander Marx, Andrew G. Nicholson. – 4th edition.

(World Health Organization classification of tumours)

1. Lung neoplasms – genetics   2. Lung neoplasms – pathology   3. Pleural neoplasms – genetics
4. Pleural neoplasms – pathology   5. Heart neoplasms – genetics   6. Heart neoplasms – pathology
7. Thymus neoplasms – genetics   8. Thymus neoplasms – pathology

I. Travis, William D. II. Series

ISBN 978 92 832 2436 5   (NLM Classification: WJ 160)

Contents

1 **Tumours of the lung**   **9**
   WHO and TNM classifications   10
   Lymph node stations   12
   Lung cancer staging and grading   14
   Rationale for classification in small biopsies and cytology   16
   Terminology and criteria in non-resection specimens   17
   Molecular testing for treatment selection in lung cancer   22
   Adenocarcinoma   26
      Lepidic adenocarcinoma   34
      Acinar adenocarcinoma   34
      Papillary adenocarcinoma   35
      Micropapillary adenocarcinoma   35
      Solid adenocarcinoma   35
      Invasive mucinous adenocarcinoma   38
         Mixed invasive mucinous and non-mucinous
         adenocarcinoma   38
      Colloid adenocarcinoma   40
      Fetal adenocarcinoma   41
      Enteric adenocarcinoma   42
      Minimally invasive adenocarcinoma   44
      Preinvasive lesions   46
         Atypical adenomatous hyperplasia   46
         Adenocarcinoma in situ   48
   Squamous cell carcinoma   51
      Keratinizing   51
      Non-keratinizing   51
      Basaloid squamous cell carcinoma   56
      Preinvasive lesion   59
         Squamous cell carcinoma in situ   59
   Neuroendocrine tumours   63
      Small cell carcinoma   63
      Large cell neuroendocrine carcinoma   69
      Carcinoid tumour   73
      Diffuse idiopathic pulmonary
      neuroendocrine cell hyperplasia   78
   Large cell carcinoma   80
   Adenosquamous carcinoma   86
   Sarcomatoid carcinoma   88
      Pleomorphic, spindle cell, and giant cell carcinoma   88
      Carcinosarcoma   91
      Pulmonary blastoma   93
   Other and unclassified carcinomas   95
      Lymphoepithelioma-like carcinoma   95
      NUT carcinoma   97
   Salivary gland-type tumours   99
      Mucoepidermoid carcinoma   99
      Adenoid cystic carcinoma   101
      Epithelial-myoepithelial carcinoma   103
      Pleomorphic adenoma   105
   Papillomas   106
      Squamous cell papilloma   106
      Glandular papilloma   108
      Mixed squamous cell and glandular papilloma   108
   Adenomas   110
      Sclerosing pneumocytoma   110
      Alveolar adenoma   112
      Papillary adenoma   113
      Mucinous cystadenoma   114
      Mucous gland adenoma   115
   Mesenchymal tumours   116

      Pulmonary hamartoma   116
      Chondroma   117
      PEComatous tumours   117
      Congenital peribronchial myofibroblastic tumour   119
      Diffuse pulmonary lymphangiomatosis   121
      Inflammatory myofibroblastic tumour   121
      Epithelioid haemangioendothelioma   123
      Pleuropulmonary blastoma   124
      Synovial sarcoma   127
      Pulmonary artery intimal sarcoma   128
      Pulmonary myxoid sarcoma with *EWSR1-CREB1*
      translocation   129
      Myoepithelial tumours / myoepithelial carcinoma   131
      Other mesenchymal tumours   132
   Lymphohistiocytic tumours   134
      Extranodal marginal zone lymphoma of mucosa-
      associated lymphoid tissue (MALT lymphoma)   134
      Diffuse large B-cell lymphoma   136
      Lymphomatoid granulomatosis   138
      Intravascular large B-cell lymphoma   140
      Pulmonary Langerhans cell histiocytosis   141
      Erdheim-Chester disease   142
   Tumours of ectopic origin   144
      Germ cell tumours   144
      Intrapulmonary thymoma   145
      Melanoma   146
      Meningioma   147
   Metastases to the lung   148

2 **Tumours of the pleura**   **153**
   WHO and TNM classifications   154
   Mesothelial tumours   156
      Diffuse malignant mesothelioma   156
         Epithelioid mesothelioma   156
         Sarcomatoid, desmoplastic, and biphasic
         mesothelioma   165
      Localized malignant mesothelioma   169
      Well-differentiated papillary mesothelioma   170
      Adenomatoid tumour   171
   Lymphoproliferative disorders   172
      Primary effusion lymphoma   172
      Diffuse large B-cell lymphoma associated with chronic
      inflammation   174
   Mesenchymal tumours   176
      Epithelioid haemangioendothelioma   176
      Angiosarcoma   177
      Synovial sarcoma   177
      Solitary fibrous tumour   178
      Desmoid-type fibromatosis   179
      Calcifying fibrous tumour   180
      Desmoplastic round cell tumour   180

3 **Tumours of the thymus**   **183**
   WHO classification   184
   TNM classifications   186
   Thymomas   187
      Type A thymoma, including atypical variant   187
      Type AB thymoma   193
      Type B1 thymoma   196
      Type B2 thymoma   199
      Type B3 thymoma   202
      Micronodular thymoma with lymphoid stroma   205

Metaplastic thymoma	207
Other rare thymomas	209
Microscopic thymoma	209
Sclerosing thymoma	210
Lipofibroadenoma	210
Thymic carcinomas	212
Squamous cell carcinoma	212
Basaloid carcinoma	216
Mucoepidermoid carcinoma	218
Lymphoepithelioma-like carcinoma	220
Clear cell carcinoma	222
Sarcomatoid carcinoma	224
Adenocarcinomas	226
NUT carcinoma	229
Undifferentiated carcinoma	232
Other rare thymic carcinomas	233
Thymic neuroendocrine tumours	234
Typical and atypical carcinoids	234
Typical carcinoid	234
Atypical carcinoid	237
Large cell neuroendocrine carcinoma	239
Small cell carcinoma	241
Combined thymic carcinomas	242
Germ cell tumours of the mediastinum	244
Seminoma	244
Embryonal carcinoma	249
Yolk sac tumour	251
Choriocarcinoma	255
Mature and immature teratoma	257
Mixed germ cell tumours	260
Germ cell tumours with somatic-type solid malignancy	263
Germ cell tumours with associated haematological malignancy	265
Lymphomas of the mediastinum	267
Primary mediastinal large B-cell lymphoma	267
Extranodal marginal zone lymphoma of mucosa-associated lymphoid tissue (MALT lymphoma)	270
Other mature B cell lymphomas	272
T lymphoblastic leukaemia / lymphoma	272
Anaplastic large cell lymphoma and other rare mature T- and NK-cell lymphomas	275
Hodgkin lymphoma	277
B-cell lymphoma, unclassifiable, with features intermediate between diffuse large B-cell lymphoma and classical Hodgkin lymphoma	280
Histiocytic and dendritic cell neoplasms of the mediastinum	282
Langerhans cell lesions	282
Histiocytic sarcoma	283
Follicular dendritic cell sarcoma	284
Interdigitating dendritic cell sarcoma	285
Fibroblastic reticular cell tumour	286
Other dendritic cell tumours	287
Myeloid sarcoma and extramedullary acute myeloid leukaemia	288
Soft tissue tumours of the mediastinum	289
Thymolipoma	289
Lipoma	290
Liposarcoma	290
Solitary fibrous tumour	291
Synovial sarcoma	291
Vascular neoplasms	292
Neurogenic tumours	293
Ganglioneuroma, ganglioneuroblastoma, and neuroblastoma	294
Other rare mesenchymal tumours	295
Ectopic tumours of the thymus	296
Ectopic thyroid tumours	296
Ectopic parathyroid tumours	296
Other rare ectopic tumours	297
Metastasis to the thymus or mediastinum	298
4 Tumours of the heart	**299**
WHO classification	300
Introduction	301
Benign tumours and tumour-like lesions	305
Rhabdomyoma	305
Histiocytoid cardiomyopathy	307
Hamartoma of mature cardiac myocytes	309
Adult cellular rhabdomyoma	310
Cardiac myxoma	311
Papillary fibroelastoma	315
Haemangioma	318
Cardiac fibroma	320
Lipoma	322
Cystic tumour of the atrioventricular node	323
Granular cell tumour	324
Schwannoma	325
Tumours of uncertain behaviour	326
Inflammatory myofibroblastic tumour	326
Paraganglioma	326
Germ cell tumours	327
Teratoma, mature	327
Teratoma, immature	327
Yolk sac tumour	327
Malignant tumours	329
Angiosarcoma	329
Undifferentiated pleomorphic sarcoma	331
Osteosarcoma	333
Myxofibrosarcoma	334
Leiomyosarcoma	336
Rhabdomyosarcoma	337
Synovial sarcoma	338
Miscellaneous sarcomas	339
Cardiac lymphomas	340
Metastatic tumours	342
Tumours of the pericardium	344
Solitary fibrous tumour	344
Sarcomas	344
Malignant mesothelioma	345
Germ cell tumours	346
Metastatic tumours	347
Contributors	**349**
IARC/WHO Committee for ICD-O	**359**
Sources of figures and tables	**360**
References	**366**
Subject index	**405**
List of abbreviations	**412**

CHAPTER 1

Tumours of the lung

Adenocarcinoma

Squamous cell carcinoma

Neuroendocrine tumours

Large cell carcinoma

Adenosquamous carcinoma

Sarcomatoid carcinoma

Salivary gland-type tumours

Papillomas

Adenomas

Mesenchymal tumours

Lymphohistiocytic tumours

Tumours of ectopic origin

Metastases to the lung

WHO classification of tumours of the lung[a,b]

Epithelial tumours

Adenocarcinoma	8140/3
Lepidic adenocarcinoma	8250/3*
Acinar adenocarcinoma	8551/3*
Papillary adenocarcinoma	8260/3
Micropapillary adenocarcinoma	8265/3
Solid adenocarcinoma	8230/3
Invasive mucinous adenocarcinoma	8253/3*
Mixed invasive mucinous and non-mucinous adenocarcinoma	8254/3*
Colloid adenocarcinoma	8480/3
Fetal adenocarcinoma	8333/3
Enteric adenocarcinoma	8144/3
Minimally invasive adenocarcinoma	
Non-mucinous	8256/3*
Mucinous	8257/3*
Preinvasive lesions	
Atypical adenomatous hyperplasia	8250/0*
Adenocarcinoma in situ	8140/2
Non-mucinous	8250/2*
Mucinous	8253/2*
Squamous cell carcinoma	8070/3
Keratinizing squamous cell carcinoma	8071/3
Non-keratinizing squamous cell carcinoma	8072/3
Basaloid squamous cell carcinoma	8083/3
Preinvasive lesion	
Squamous cell carcinoma in situ	8070/2
Neuroendocrine tumours	
Small cell carcinoma	8041/3
Combined small cell carcinoma	8045/3
Large cell neuroendocrine carcinoma	8013/3
Combined large cell neuroendocrine carcinoma	8013/3
Carcinoid tumours	
Typical carcinoid	8240/3
Atypical carcinoid	8249/3
Preinvasive lesion	
Diffuse idiopathic pulmonary neuroendocrine cell hyperplasia	8040/0*
Large cell carcinoma	8012/3
Adenosquamous carcinoma	8560/3
Pleomorphic carcinoma	8022/3
Spindle cell carcinoma	8032/3
Giant cell carcinoma	8031/3
Carcinosarcoma	8980/3
Pulmonary blastoma	8972/3
Other and unclassified carcinomas	
Lymphoepithelioma-like carcinoma	8082/3
NUT carcinoma	8023/3*
Salivary gland-type tumours	
Mucoepidermoid carcinoma	8430/3
Adenoid cystic carcinoma	8200/3
Epithelial-myoepithelial carcinoma	8562/3
Pleomorphic adenoma	8940/0

Papillomas	
Squamous cell papilloma	8052/0
Exophytic	8052/0
Inverted	8053/0
Glandular papilloma	8260/0
Mixed squamous cell and glandular papilloma	8560/0
Adenomas	
Sclerosing pneumocytoma	8832/0
Alveolar adenoma	8251/0
Papillary adenoma	8260/0
Mucinous cystadenoma	8470/0
Mucous gland adenoma	8480/0

Mesenchymal tumours

Pulmonary hamartoma	8992/0*
Chondroma	9220/0
PEComatous tumours	
Lymphangioleiomyomatosis	9174/1
PEComa, benign	8714/0
Clear cell tumour	8005/0
PEComa, malignant	8714/3
Congenital peribronchial myofibroblastic tumour	8827/1
Diffuse pulmonary lymphangiomatosis	
Inflammatory myofibroblastic tumour	8825/1
Epithelioid haemangioendothelioma	9133/3
Pleuropulmonary blastoma	8973/3
Synovial sarcoma	9040/3
Pulmonary artery intimal sarcoma	9137/3
Pulmonary myxoid sarcoma with EWSR1-CREB1 translocation	8842/3*
Myoepithelial tumours	
Myoepithelioma	8982/0
Myoepithelial carcinoma	8982/3

Lymphohistiocytic tumours

Extranodal marginal zone lymphoma of mucosa-associated lymphoid tissue (MALT lymphoma)	9699/3
Diffuse large B-cell lymphoma	9680/3
Lymphomatoid granulomatosis	9766/1
Intravascular large B-cell lymphoma	9712/3
Pulmonary Langerhans cell histiocytosis	9751/1
Erdheim-Chester disease	9750/1

Tumours of ectopic origin

Germ cell tumours	
Teratoma, mature	9080/0
Teratoma, immature	9080/1
Intrapulmonary thymoma	8580/3
Melanoma	8720/3
Meningioma, NOS	9530/0

Metastatic tumours

TNM classification of carcinomas of the lung

T – Primary Tumour

TX Primary tumour cannot be assessed, or tumour proven by the presence of malignant cells in sputum or bronchial washings but not visualized by imaging or bronchoscopy

T0 No evidence of primary tumour

Tis Carcinoma in situ

T1 Tumour ≤3 cm in greatest dimension, surrounded by lung or visceral pleura, without bronchoscopic evidence of invasion more proximal than the lobar bronchus, i.e. not in the main bronchus[a]

T1a Tumour ≤ 2 cm in greatest dimension

T1b Tumour > 2 cm but ≤ 3 cm in greatest dimension

T2 Tumour > 3 cm but ≤ 7 cm or tumour with any of the following features (T2 tumours with these features are classified T2a if ≤ 5 cm or if size cannot be determined and T2b if > 5 cm but ≤ 7 cm.):
- Involves main bronchus, ≥ 2 cm distal to the carina
- Invades visceral pleura
- Associated with atelectasis or obstructive pneumonitis that extends to the hilar region but does not involve the entire lung

T2a Tumour > 3 cm but ≤ 5 cm in greatest dimension

T2b Tumour > 5 cm but ≤ 7 cm in greatest dimension

T3 Tumour > 7 cm or one that directly invades any of the following: chest wall (including superior sulcus tumours), diaphragm, phrenic nerve, mediastinal pleura, parietal pericardium; or tumour in the main bronchus < 2 cm distal to the carina[a] but without involvement of the carina[a]; or associated atelectasis or obstructive pneumonitis of the entire lung; or separate tumour nodule(s) in the same lobe as the primary

T4 Tumour of any size that invades any of the following: mediastinum, heart, great vessels, trachea, recurrent laryngeal nerve, oesophagus, vertebral body, carina; separate tumour nodule(s) in a different ipsilateral lobe to that of the primary

N – Regional Lymph Nodes

NX Regional lymph nodes cannot be assessed

N0 No regional lymph node metastasis

N1 Metastasis in ipsilateral peribronchial and/or ipsilateral hilar lymph nodes and intrapulmonary nodes, including involvement by direct extension

N2 Metastasis in ipsilateral mediastinal and/or subcarinal lymph nodes

N3 Metastasis in contralateral mediastinal, contralateral hilar, ipsilateral or contralateral scalene, or supraclavicular lymph node(s)

M – Distant Metastasis

M0 No distant metastasis

M1 Distant metastasis

M1a Separate tumour nodule(s) in a contralateral lobe; tumour with pleural nodules or malignant pleural or pericardial effusion[b]

M1b Distant metastasis

Notes:

a) The uncommon superficial spreading tumour of any size with its invasive component limited to the bronchial wall, which may extend proximal to the main bronchus, is classified as T1a.

b) Most pleural (and pericardial) effusions with lung cancer are due to tumour. In a few patients, however, multiple cytopathological examinations of the pleural (pericardial) fluid are negative for tumour, and the fluid is non-bloody and is not an exudate. Where these elements and clinical judgement dictate that the effusion is not related to the tumour, the effusion should be excluded as a staging element and the patient should be classified as M0.

Stage Grouping

Occult carcinoma	Tx	N0	M0
Stage 0	Tis	N0	M0
Stage IA	T1a	N0	M0
	T1b	N0	M0
Stage IB	T2a	N0	M0
Stage IIA	T1a	N1	M0
	T1b	N1	M0
	T2a	N1	M0
	T2b	N0	M0
Stage IIB	T2b	N1	M0
	T3	N0	M0
Stage IIIA	T1	N2	M0
	T2	N2	M0
	T3	N1	M0
	T3	N2	M0
	T4	N0	M0
	T4	N1	M0
Stage IIIB	T4	N2	M0
	Any T	N3	M0
Stage IV	Any T	Any N	M1a
	Any T	Any N	M1b

Compiled from references {2420,652A}
TNM help desk: http://www.uicc.org/resources/tnm/helpdesk

Lymph node stations

Table 1.01 Anatomical definitions of each lymph node station and station grouping by nodal zones in the map proposed by the International Association for the Study of Lung Cancer (IASLC). Reprinted and adapted from Rusch VW et al. {2225}

Lymph node station number and name	Anatomical limits
Supraclavicular zone	
1. Low cervical, supraclavicular, and sternal notch nodes	• Upper border: the lower margin of cricoid cartilage • Lower border: the clavicles bilaterally, and in the midline, the upper border of the manubrium • Border between 1R and 1L: the midline of the trachea 1R designates right-sided nodes and 1L designates left-sided nodes.
Upper zone	
2. Upper paratracheal nodes	2R • Upper border: the apex of the right lung and pleural space, and in the midline, the upper border of the manubrium • Lower border: the intersection of the caudal margin of the innominate vein with the trachea 2L • Upper border: the apex of the lung and pleural space, and in the midline, the upper border of the manubrium • Lower border: the superior border of the aortic arch Like lymph node station 4R, 2R includes nodes extending to the left lateral border of the trachea.
3. Prevascular and retrotracheal nodes	3a: prevascular • Upper border: the apex of the chest • Lower border: the level of the carina • Anterior border: the posterior aspect of the sternum • Posterior border: the anterior border of the superior vena cava on the right, and the left carotid artery on the left 3p: retrotracheal • Upper border: the apex of the chest • Lower border: the carina
4. Lower paratracheal nodes	4R – includes right paratracheal nodes and pretracheal nodes extending to the left lateral border of the trachea • Upper border: the intersection of the caudal margin of the innominate vein with the trachea • Lower border: the lower border of the azygos vein 4L – includes nodes to the left of the left lateral border of the trachea, medial to the ligamentum arteriosum • Upper border: the upper margin of the aortic arch • Lower border: the upper rim of the left main pulmonary artery
Aortopulmonary zone	
5. Subaortic nodes (aortopulmonary window)	Subaortic lymph nodes lateral to the ligamentum arteriosum • Upper border: the lower border of the aortic arch • Lower border: the upper rim of the left main pulmonary artery
6. Para-aortic nodes (ascending aorta or phrenic)	Lymph nodes anterior and lateral to the ascending aorta and aortic arch • Upper border: a line tangential to the upper border of the aortic arch • Lower border: the lower border of the aortic arch
Subcarinal zone	
7. Subcarinal nodes	• Upper border: the carina of the trachea • Lower border: the upper border of the lower lobe bronchus on the left, and the lower border of the bronchus intermedius on the right
Lower zone	
8. Paraoesophageal nodes (below carina)	Nodes lying adjacent to the wall of the oesophagus and to the right or left of the midline, excluding subcarinal nodes • Upper border: the upper border of the lower lobe bronchus on the left, and the lower border of the bronchus intermedius on the right • Lower border: the diaphragm
9. Pulmonary ligament nodes	Nodes lying within the pulmonary ligament • Upper border: the inferior pulmonary vein • Lower border: the diaphragm

Lymph node station number and name	Anatomical limits
Hilar/interlobar zone	
10. Hilar nodes	Includes nodes immediately adjacent to the mainstem bronchus and hilar vessels, including the proximal portions of the pulmonary veins and main pulmonary artery • Upper border: the lower rim of the azygos vein on the right, and the upper rim of the pulmonary artery on the left • Lower border: the interlobar region bilaterally
11. Interlobar nodes	Between the origin of the lobar bronchi 11s[a]: between the upper lobe bronchus and the bronchus intermedius on the right 11i[a]: between the middle and lower bronchi on the right
Peripheral zone	
12. Lobar nodes	Adjacent to the lobar bronchi
13. Segmental nodes	Adjacent to the segmental bronchi
14. Subsegmental nodes	Adjacent to the subsegmental bronchi
[a] Optional notations for subcategories of station.	

Table 1.02 Lymph node coding of isolated tumour cells (ITCs) or clusters of tumour cells.
Reprinted from Sobin LH et al. {2420}

Code	Type of involvement, and method of identification
pN0	No regional lymph node metastasis histologically, no examination for ITCs
pN0(i−)	No regional lymph node metastasis histologically, negative morphological findings for ITCs
pN0(i+)	No regional lymph node metastasis histologically, positive morphological findings for ITCs
pN0(mol−)	No regional lymph node metastasis histologically, negative non-morphological findings for ITCs
pN0(mol+)	No regional lymph node metastasis histologically, positive non-morphological findings for ITCs
pN0(i−)(sn)	No sentinel lymph node metastasis histologically, negative morphological findings for ITCs
pN0(i+)(sn)	No sentinel lymph node metastasis histologically, positive morphological findings for ITCs
pN0(mol−)(sn)	No sentinel lymph node metastasis histologically, negative non-morphological findings for ITCs
pN0(mol+)(sn)	No sentinel lymph node metastasis histologically, positive non-morphological findings for ITCs
Note: The same coding applies for distant metastasis, in which case pN is replaced by M, e.g. M0(i+).	

Lung cancer staging and grading

K. Geisinger
A.L. Moreira
A.G. Nicholson
R. Rami-Porta
W.D. Travis

Lung cancer staging

In the TNM classification of malignant tumours, staging is determined by assessment of the anatomical extent of three tumour components: the primary tumour (T), the lymph nodes (N), and the metastases (M). The T component has seven categories (Tx, T0, Tis, T1, T2, T3, and T4), defined by tumour size, tumour location, the involved structures, or the effects of tumour growth. In the seventh edition of the TNM classification, the T1 and T2 categories were further subdivided into T1a and T1b, and T2a and T2b, respectively. The N component has five categories (NX, N0, N1, N2, and N3), defined by the absence or the presence and location of the involved nodes. The M component has two categories (M0 and M1), defined by the absence or the presence and location of the metastases. TNM subsets of similar prognosis are grouped in stages {866}. The TNM classification and staging system applies to small and non-small cell carcinomas, and to bronchopulmonary carcinoids {2356,2420,2680,2737}.

Although the TNM classification and staging system is recommended for small cell lung cancer, the revised dichotomous system – limited and extensive disease – is still used {1190}. Limited disease includes tumours with ipsilateral and contralateral hilar, mediastinal, and supraclavicular nodes, and tumours with ipsilateral pleural effusions regardless of cytology. Extensive disease includes tumours spreading beyond the definition of limited disease.

The involvement of the visceral pleura is a T2 descriptor, and this involvement is now defined as tumour invasion through the elastic layer. If invasion is not evident in standard H&E stains, elastic staining is recommended {2677}.

The TNM classification may vary depending on treatment or the natural history of the disease. The pretreatment classification is the clinical TNM classification (cTNM). The classification derived from the histopathological study of the resected specimens, complemented by the cTNM, is the pathological TNM classification (pTNM). The classification defined after or during induction therapy is indicated by the prefix y (ycTNM or ypTNM). The classifications for recurrent tumours, multiple tumours, and tumours first diagnosed at autopsy are indicated by the prefixes r, m, and a (rTNM, mTNM, and aTNM), respectively {2420}.

Lymph node stations

Lymph node involvement has prognostic and therapeutic implications, and must be determined in the most accurate way. For describing the location of involved nodes, the International Association for the Study of Lung Cancer (IASLC) has proposed a new nodal chart for multidisciplinary use (see Tables 1.01 and 1.02, pp. 12–13). One of the chart's advantages is its precise definition of nodal boundaries. Additionally, neighbouring nodal stations are grouped in nodal zones to facilitate nodal staging, especially in patients who will not undergo surgical resection {2225}.

Isolated tumour cells or cellular clusters ≤ 0.2 mm in greatest dimension identified in nodes or bone marrow by morphological techniques (H&E or immunohistochemistry) or non-morphological techniques (flow cytometry or DNA analysis) do not qualify as N1, N2, N3, or M1b disease, but are identified by special coding (see Table 1.02). The presence of micrometastasis (i.e. metastatic lesions ≤ 0.2 mm) is coded with the suffix (mi).

Assessment of anatomical extent is performed using a combination of imaging, metabolic, and invasive techniques. CT and PET have important roles in the assessment of locoregional extent and metastatic spread. Endoscopy and minimally invasive surgical procedures – such as endobronchial ultrasound-guided transbronchial fine-needle aspiration biopsy, oesophageal ultrasound-guided fine-needle aspiration biopsy, mediastinoscopy and its variants, and transcervical mediastinal lymphadenectomy – are key tools for mediastinal nodal staging {66,547,2399}. The intensity with which staging was performed is indicated by the certainty factor (C factor); this value is important for assessing the thoroughness of the staging process and for comparing series {2420}.

Lung cancer grading

Grading is the division of a specific tumour group into two or more prognostically relevant grades based on morphological appearance. Unlike for other tumours, such as breast and prostate cancer, a widely accepted grading system for lung cancer has not yet been established. However, based on recent advances, such a system may be developed in the near future.

In 2011, the IASLC, American Thoracic Society (ATS), and European Respiratory Society (ERS) proposed a new classification for lung adenocarcinoma based on the presence and proportion of five histological patterns {2675}. The predominant histological subtype of a tumour has been shown to be associated with prognostic differences {2699,2983}, and this association may provide the basis for a simple architectural grading system, most applicable to resection specimens, with three grades – grade 1: lepidic predominant, grade 2: acinar or papillary predominant, and grade 3: solid or micropapillary predominant. These grades correspond to well-, moderately, and poorly differentiated tumours, respectively. Other potential grading schemes include classifications based on the two most predominant patterns, the highest-grade pattern, or nuclear features (such as mitotic count) in combination with an architectural approach (such as the predominant subtype). In a study of stage I adenocarcinomas, Sica et al. {2388} proposed a grading system based on a score derived from summing the two most predominant grades, and stratified tumours into a three-tiered classification that also correlated well with prognosis {2388}. The most common (and most heterogeneous) predominant type in adenocarcinoma appears to be the acinar pattern. Several studies have suggested that the acinar subtype can be further divided into prognostically significant subsets. Kadota et al. {1177} and von der Thusen et al. {2789} found that the combination of predominant histological pattern and mitotic activity was helpful in separating the intermediate group into tumours that cluster with well-differentiated tumours and others that cluster with the poorly differentiated group. Other research has shown that the cribriform pattern is a poor-prognosis subset of the acinar subtype, similar to the solid type {1180,1739}. Nakazato et al. {1813} found that nuclear size was a valuable predictor of prognosis. However, this finding has not been confirmed by other investigators {1177,2789}.

Since a definitive grading system for resected lung adenocarcinomas has yet to be established, there is no widely accepted grading system for non-resection specimens either. A recent study in patients with advanced disease evaluated the predominant subtype in core biopsies, and classified tumours with papillary, micropapillary, or solid predominant patterns as high-grade. Patients with these high-grade patterns had better response rates to platinum-based therapy and longer progression-free survival than did patients with lower-grade adenocarcinomas {315,2156}. Another study showed solid and micropapillary subtypes are predictive of survival benefit for adjuvent cisplatinum therapy {2690A}. Further validation is still needed to confirm the clinical relevance of grading in non-resection specimens.

For lung neuroendocrine neoplasms, the clinical relevance of grading is well established in resection samples, and to a lesser extent in tissue biopsies. However, challenges persist with tissue biopsies and cytological specimens. In cytological specimens, it is often possible to distinguish high-grade tumours (such as small cell carcinomas) from carcinoids, but in many lung cancers there is overlap, resulting from the spectrum of differentiation and from sampling errors. Counting mitotic figures in any type of cytological smear is not an established procedure, and has not been validated with concomitantly obtained tissue specimens. Furthermore, it may be impossible

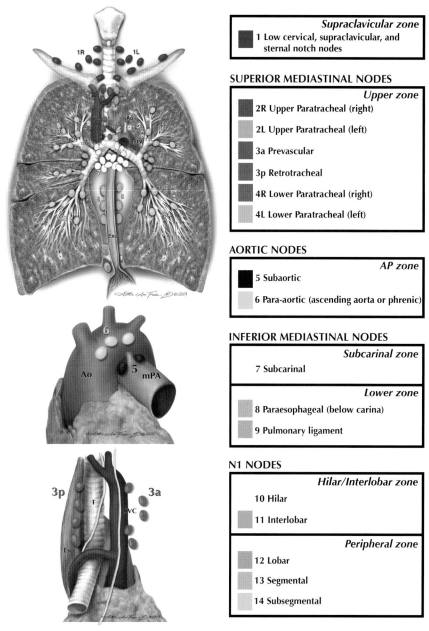

Fig. 1.01 The International Association for the Study of Lung Cancer (IASLC) lymph node map, including the proposed grouping of lymph node stations into zones for the purpose of prognostic analysis. Ao, aorta; AP, aortopulmonary; Eso, oesophagus; mPA, main pulmonary artery; SVC, superior vena cava; T, trachea. Reproduced from Rusch VW et al. {2225}.

to identify small quantities of necrotic debris in smears. It is therefore probably not prudent to distinguish grade 1 and 2 tumours by cytology alone {1042,2391}. Crush artefact in both types of small specimens can make differentiation especially challenging.

There is still insufficient data to determine how to grade carcinomas such as squamous cell carcinoma and adenosquamous carcinoma. Other tumours, such as the sarcomatoid carcinomas (pleomorphic carcinoma, carcinosarcoma, and pulmonary blastoma), are all high-grade tumours.

Rationale for classification in small biopsies and cytology

Y. Yatabe
E. Brambilla
A.G. Nicholson
S. Dacic
R. Dziadziuszko
F.R. Hirsch

M. Ladanyi
M. Meyerson
G. Riely
G. Scagliotti
W.D. Travis

Prior to the 2004 WHO classification, there was no therapeutic implication of distinguishing histological subtypes such as adenocarcinoma and squamous cell carcinoma. Therefore, tumours other than small cell carcinoma were simply lumped together by some pathologists as non-small cell carcinomas (NSCCs), without regard for more specific histological subtyping. However, major therapeutic advances have since taken place in the lung cancer field, with profound implications for pathological diagnosis and molecular testing {1689,1700,2196,2674}. Patients treated with pemetrexed, with adenocarcinoma or NSCC, not otherwise specified fared better than those with squamous cell carcinoma {2290}, and patients with squamous cell carcinoma have a higher risk of life-threatening haemorrhage if treated with bevacizumab {1156}. Also, the publication of the 2004 WHO classification coincided with the publication of the first papers showing significant response to targeted therapy when an *EGFR* gene mutation was present in lung adenocarcinomas {174,647}. This discovery was a major advance, and contributed greatly to the subsequent explosion of knowledge in relation to molecular biology and patient treatment. Epidermal growth factor receptor tyrosine kinase inhibitors are now first-line therapy in patients who have advanced-stage lung adenocarcinoma with *EGFR* mutations {1252}. Furthermore, patients with advanced-stage lung adenocarcinoma that is positive for *ALK* fusion are currently treated with the ALK inhibitor crizotinib, which was clinically developed over a remarkably short period of time, from the initial identification of the *ALK* translocation in lung cancer in 2007 to a phase II clinical trial in non-small cell lung cancer (NSCLC) in 2010, and approval by the United States Food and Drug Administration in 2011 {1373,2421}. Many other drugs related to specific molecular targets, particularly driver mutations associated primarily with either adenocarcinoma or squamous cell carcinoma, are in clinical trials.

The identification of so many new therapeutic targets over the past decade resulted in an urgent need for a classification system for both non-resection specimens (particularly small biopsies) and cytology samples {516}. Such a system was therefore a major new component of the 2011 IASLC/ATS/ERS lung adenocarcinoma classification. Because therapeutic targets are now increasingly being identified outside of adenocarcinoma, a firm diagnosis of squamous cell carcinoma may become just as important.

In light of these developments, tissue samples are no longer managed for diagnosis alone, but also for immunohistochemical staining and molecular testing in relation to potential targeted therapy. This approach is particularly important for small biopsies and cytology, because approximately 70% of lung cancers are inoperable, with presentation at an advanced stage, and molecular targeted therapies that require molecular testing are primarily administered to patients with advanced NSCLC. Therefore, strategic tissue management for ancillary analyses and histological diagnosis is critical {1009}. Although the approach to managing these small specimens varies greatly between laboratories, good clinical practice recommendations have been published for handling small biopsies and cytology preparations, based on a multidisciplinary consensus {2676}. These recommendations are discussed further in the next two sections. Some additional procedures not addressed in the guidelines, such as rapid on-site evaluation of cytology and simultaneous block sectioning for immunohistochemical staining and molecular testing, have also been proposed to facilitate the efficient use of specimens {2638}.

Small biopsy classification should also take into account the fact that certain tumours can only be diagnosed on resection, and histology and cytology reports should reflect this accordingly. For example, adenocarcinoma in situ can only be diagnosed in the setting of

Table 1.03 Guidelines for good practice of small biopsies and cytological preparations {2674,2676}

1. For small biopsies and cytology, NSCC should be further classified into a more specific type, such as adenocarcinoma or squamous cell carcinoma, whenever possible.

2. The term NSCLC-NOS should be used as little as possible, and only when a more specific diagnosis is not possible.

3. When a diagnosis is made in a small biopsy or cytology specimen in conjunction with special stains, it should be clarified whether the diagnosis was established based on light microscopy alone or if special stains were required.

4. The term non-SQCC should not be used by pathologists in diagnostic reports. This categorization is used by clinicians to define groups of patients whose tumours comprise several histological types and who can be treated in a similar manner; in small biopsies/cytology, pathologists should classify NSCLC as ADC, SQCC, NSCLC-NOS, or other terms (Table 1.04, p.18).

5. The above classification of ADC versus other histologies and the terminology in Table 1.04 and Fig. 1.06 should be used in routine diagnosis, future research, and clinical trials, to ensure a uniform classification of disease cohorts in relation to tumour subtypes, stratified according to diagnoses made by light microscopy alone versus diagnoses requiring special stains.

6. When paired cytology and biopsy specimens exist, they should be reviewed together to achieve the most specific and concordant diagnosis.

7. The terms adenocarcinoma in situ (AIS) and minimally invasive adenocarcinoma should not be used for diagnosis of small biopsies or cytology specimens. If a non-invasive pattern is present in a small biopsy, it should be referred to as a lepidic growth pattern. Similarly, if a cytology specimen has the attributes of AIS, then the tumour should be diagnosed as an adenocarcinoma, possibly with a comment that this may represent, AIS, MIA or invasive adenocarcinoma with a lepidic component.

8. The term large cell carcinoma should not be used for diagnosis in small biopsy or cytology specimens and should be restricted to resection specimens where the tumour is thoroughly sampled to exclude a differentiated component.

9. In biopsies of tumours that show sarcomatoid features (marked nuclear pleomorphism, malignant giant cells, or spindle cell morphology), these should be initially classified as above in relation to ADC; NSCC, favour ADC; SQCC; or NSCC, favour SQCC, as this is apt to influence management, with additional statement that giant and/or spindle cell features (depending on what feature) are present. If such features are not present, the term NSCC-NOS should be used, again with comment on the sarcomatoid features.

10. Neuroendocrine immunohistochemical markers should be performed only in cases where there is suspected neuroendocrine morphology.

a resected pure lepidic pattern in conjunction with knowledge of the size of the tumour and an examination of the entire tumour to confirm that there is no invasive component. If this pattern is seen in small samples without confirmation in a resected specimen, it should only be described as adenocarcinoma with a lepidic pattern. With this information, a diagnosis of adenocarcinoma in situ might be suspected based on multidisciplinary review, especially in correlation with CT, but the final diagnosis can be rendered only after review of a resection specimen. Similarly, minimally invasive adenocarcinoma cannot be diagnosed on biopsy. A diagnosis of large cell carcinoma requires analysis of resection specimens to confirm that better-differentiated areas are not present (see *Large cell carcinoma*, p. 80), and a diagnosis of adenosquamous carcinoma requires observation of sufficient percentages of both adenocarcinoma and squamous cell carcinoma on resection, although the diagnosis can be suggested based on biopsy and cytology samples (see the next section for recommended terminology). Similarly, in most cases, large cell neuroendocrine carcinoma can only be suggested on biopsy when there is appropriate morphology and evidence of neuroendocrine differentiation on immunohistochemistry. With the increased use of core biopsies, which provide more tissue than could previously be obtained with bronchoscopic or needle biopsies, this diagnosis may now be made more frequently without resection.

Terminology and criteria in non-resection specimens

A.G. Nicholson
K. Geisinger
S.C. Aisner
F. Al-Dayel
L. Bubendorf
J-H. Chung
K.M. Kerr

M. Meyerson
M. Noguchi
W. Olszewski
N. Rekhtman
G. Riely
G. Scagliotti
W.D. Travis

The above rationale for classification in small biopsies and cytology led to the publication of a proposed classification for non-resection specimens (specifically for biopsies and cytological preparations) in the 2011 IASLC/ATS/ERS lung adenocarcinoma classification {2674,2676}. The proposal was originally developed specifically to update adenocarcinoma classification, but because the WHO classification had never addressed classification in small biopsies, the proposal was extended to address other lung cancer histological types as well. An algorithm for handling biopsy samples was proposed alongside the histological subgroups that addressed the increasing need for distinction between histological types of non-small cell lung cancer (NSCLC) using ancillary techniques such as immunohistochemistry, especially for patients with advanced lung cancer {2676}.

In prior WHO classifications, lung cancer diagnosis was based mainly on light microscopy using routine H&E-stained slides. Immunohistochemistry was introduced for the first time only in the 1999 WHO classification, and even in the 2004 WHO classification, immunohistochemistry was still limited to large cell neuroendocrine carcinomas and sarcomatoid carcinomas only, with no consideration of biopsies {2672}. However, for the reasons given in the previous section, judicious use of immunohistochemistry and/or mucin staining is now recommended (when available) for all cases of non-small cell lung cancer that cannot be classified as adenocarcinoma or squamous cell carcinoma based on morphology alone {2134,2208,2674}.

However, ancillary techniques are not always necessary. In some studies, it was possible to make a diagnosis of adenocarcinoma or squamous cell carcinoma based on morphology alone in biopsy or cytology specimens in 50–70% of patients. Nevertheless, the use of immunohistochemistry increases the refinement of diagnosis, so that a diagnosis of non-small cell carcinoma (NSCC), not otherwise specified (NOS) can be avoided in up to 90% of cases {1504,1841}. It is recommended that the diagnosis non-small cell carcinoma, NOS be used as little as possible, and only when a more specific

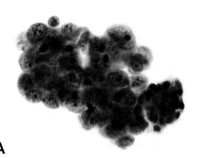
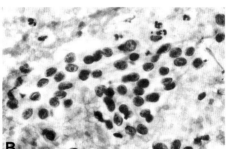
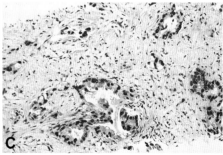

Fig. 1.02 Adenocarcinoma. **A** A three-dimensional aggregate, typical of adenocarcinoma, is dominated by peripherally oriented nuclei appearing to occupy the cluster's very edge. The nuclei are large, with delicate, somewhat smooth membranes. Distinct small nucleoli are present in darkly stained, finely granular chromatin. Faint basophilic cytoplasm extends towards the centre of the aggregate (polarization). **B** Fused acini are formed by central delicate cytoplasm and a peripheral ring of malignant nuclei, demonstrating glandular polarity. The nuclei are large and hyperchromatic, with minor membrane irregularities. Some of the nuclei overlap, indicating the loss of some polarity and high nuclear-to-cytoplasmic ratios. **C** This small biopsy shows fragments of adenocarcinoma with an acinar pattern.

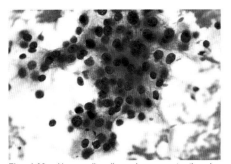

Fig. 1.03 Non-small cell carcinoma, not otherwise specified. A flat sheet of cells is characterized by unevenly spaced, fairly homogeneous, rounded nuclei, many of which have a small but noticeable nucleolus. Their chromatin is hyperchromatic. In many cells, the nuclei are relatively centrally located in the cytoplasm, which is evident at the edge of the sheet in a few foci. The cytoplasm ranges from delicate to fairly dense.

Table 1.04 Terminology and criteria for adenocarcinoma, squamous cell carcinoma, and non-small cell carcinoma, not otherwise specified in small biopsies and cytology compared to terms for resections. Modified from {2674} and {2676}.

New small biopsy/cytology terminology	Morphology/stains	2015 WHO classification
Adenocarcinoma (describe identifiable patterns present)	Morphological adenocarcinoma patterns clearly present	Adenocarcinoma Predominant pattern: Lepidic Acinar Papillary Solid Micropapillary
Adenocarcinoma with lepidic pattern (if pure, add a comment that an invasive component cannot be excluded)		Minimally invasive adenocarcinoma, adenocarcinoma in situ or an invasive adenocarcinoma with a lepidic component.
Invasive mucinous adenocarcinoma (describe patterns present; use the term mucinous adenocarcinoma with lepidic pattern if pure lepidic pattern)		Invasive mucinous adenocarcinoma
Adenocarcinoma with colloid features		Colloid adenocarcinoma
Adenocarcinoma with fetal features		Fetal adenocarcinoma
Adenocarcinoma with enteric features[a]		Enteric adenocarcinoma
Non-small cell carcinoma, favour adenocarcinoma[b]	Morphological adenocarcinoma patterns not present, but supported by special stains (i.e. TTF1-positive)	Adenocarcinoma (solid pattern may be just one component of the tumour)[b]
Squamous cell carcinoma	Morphological squamous cell patterns clearly present	Squamous cell carcinoma
Non-small cell carcinoma, favour squamous cell carcinoma[b]	Morphological squamous cell patterns not present, but supported by stains (i.e. p40-positive)	Squamous cell carcinoma (non-keratinizing pattern may be a component of the tumour)[b]
Non-small cell carcinoma, not otherwise specified[c]	No clear adenocarcinoma, squamous, or neuroendocrine morphology or staining pattern	Large cell carcinoma

[a] Metastatic carcinomas should be carefully excluded with clinical and appropriate but judicious immunohistochemical examination; [b] The categories do not always correspond to solid predominant adenocarcinoma or non-keratinizing squamous cell carcinoma, respectively. Poorly differentiated components in adenocarcinoma or squamous cell carcinoma may be sampled; [c] The non-small cell carcinoma, not otherwise specified pattern can be seen not only in large cell carcinomas, but also when the solid, poorly differentiated component of adenocarcinomas or squamous cell carcinomas is sampled but does not express immunohistochemical markers or mucin.

diagnosis is not possible by morphology and/or special staining {2674,2676}.

Of course, not all laboratories worldwide have access to immunohistochemistry, or even a mucin stain. In these settings, the diagnosis of non-small cell lung cancer, NOS may remain frequent. However, the current classification must encompass all relevant scientific advances. The accepted markers for the identification of differentiation towards adenocarcinoma are TTF1 {1259,1504,1841} and napsin A {2705,2864}, both of which are approximately 80% sensitive, although TTF1 is easier to assess as a nuclear stain. In relation to squamous differentiation, p40 has been reported to be the most specific and sensitive squamous marker {209,2014,2024}. Other antibodies that have been recommended include CK5/6 and p63 {1764,1841,2134,2864}. However, recent data suggest that p63 is less specific than was previously thought {1870}, since p63 expression can also occur in up to a third of adenocarcinomas {1764,1841,2134}. Virtually all tumours that lack squamous cell morphology and show coexpression of p63 and TTF1 are preferably classified as adenocarcinomas. CK7 has also been used as a marker of adenocarcinomatous differentiation by some groups {314}, although this use is not universally accepted. Less used markers for squamous differentiation include desmocollin 3 and desmoglein {22,2287}. Some laboratories have used a cocktail of antibodies to reduce tissue use {266,1157}. When immunohistochemistry is deemed necessary for squamous and glandular differentiation, a reasonable recommendation is to use at least one antibody and no more than two antibodies in each case (e.g. TTF1 and p40 or p63) {2134,2864}. A simple panel of TTF1 and p40 may be sufficient to classify most NSCC, NOS cases.

Whenever immunohistochemistry is used in diagnosis, care must be taken to ensure high-quality staining, and participation in a quality assurance programme is recommended. Care must also be taken with the use of different antibody clones, and in the interpretation of varying degrees of staining.

When squamous or adenocarcinoma differentiation is identified by standard morphological criteria, a tumour can be diagnosed on small biopsies and cytology with the established terms – adenocarcinoma and squamous cell carcinoma {2674,2676}.

Adenocarcinomas may manifest glandular differentiation by displaying one or more architectural features of lepidic (formerly known as bronchioloalveolar carcinoma), acinar, papillary, micropapillary, or solid patterns. If these patterns are present, they should be mentioned in the report. Cytologically, adenocarcinoma differentiation can be expressed in

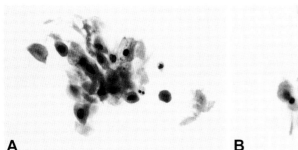 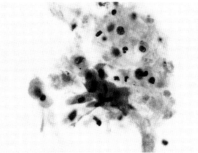 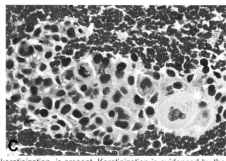

A   B   C

Fig. 1.04 Squamous cell carcinoma. **A** A very loosely arrayed flat aggregate of tumour cells, some with cytoplasmic keratinization, is present. Keratinization is evidenced by the homogeneous, brilliant orange colour and its dense quality. Other cells have opaque cytoplasm, which stains from green to red, typical of non-keratinized squamous cells. The cell edges are distinct. Virtually all the nuclei possess uniform, ink-black chromatin, and are centrally located in the cytoplasm. In the lower-right corner is an anucleated, keratinized squame. **B** A small, flat, multilayered clump of squamous tumour cells with somewhat rectangular configurations is present. Some of their nuclei are boxcar-shaped, with angulated corners and opaque, hyperchromatic, and structureless chromatin. The nuclei are clearly located towards the centres of their cytoplasm, which is dense and eosinophilic, but lacking in obvious keratinization. The malignant cells are surrounded by histiocytes and debris. **C** This poorly differentiated tumour has a focal area showing clear keratinization.

several architectural patterns, including three-dimensional balls of cells, pseudopapillary aggregates or true papillae with central fibrovascular cores, cohesive clusters with acinar structures, or a picket-fence or drunken honeycomb appearance. Individual adenocarcinoma tumour cells typically have basophilic cytoplasm, which may be homogeneous, distinctly granular, or foamy. The cytoplasm is typically translucent, and often has cytoplasmic vacuoles. The nuclei are often situated eccentrically, with chromatin that varies from finely granular and uniform to hyperchromatic, coarse, and irregularly distributed. Most tumour cells have a single macronucleolus.

Squamous differentiation is indicated by three key histological features: keratinization, pearls, and intercellular bridges {2674,2676}. Keratinization is also a distinguishing feature in cytological specimens, because keratinized cytoplasm stains bright yellow, orange, or red with Papanicolaou staining. However, this must be distinguished from cytoplasmic eosinophilia induced by air drying. With Romanowsky staining, keratinized cytoplasm stains a characteristic robin's egg blue. The cytoplasm has an opaque or dense, hard appearance, and is less translucent than that of adenocarcinomas or large cell carcinomas. Cells often have round, ovoid, or elongated contours, with sharply defined cell borders. Cells with long cytoplasmic tails or tadpole configurations may be seen. The nuclei are usually solitary, centrally situated, and hyperchromatic, with rectangular outlines and squared-off edges. The chromatin is typically very dense and homogeneous, with a pyknotic appearance. The nucleoli are not well developed.

When adenocarcinomas or squamous cell carcinomas are poorly differentiated, the defining morphological criteria that would allow for a specific diagnosis may be inconspicuous or absent. In these cases, immunohistochemistry or mucin staining may be necessary to determine a specific diagnosis. The introduction of molecular testing for *EGFR* and *KRAS* mutations, as well as the routine use of immunohistochemistry, has revealed that some adenocarcinomas have a pseudosquamous morphological appearance. So the threshold for morphological evidence of squamous differentiation should be high. If there is any doubt, the diagnosis should be confirmed with immunohistochemistry. In the absence of frank keratinization, pearls, or intercellular bridges, the presence of densely eosinophilic cytoplasm or sharp intercytoplasmic borders is insufficient for a diagnosis of squamous cell carcinoma. In fact, it is likely that many cases of squamous cell carcinoma in which *EGFR* mutation has been reported are actually adenosquamous carcinomas or pseudosquamous adenocarcinomas that could be reclassified using the algorithm of special stains recommended in this volume.

When a specimen shows NSCC lacking either definite squamous or adenocarcinoma morphology, immunohistochemistry may refine the diagnosis. To preserve as much tissue as possible for molecular testing in small biopsies, the work-up should be as limited as possible.

Cases positive for an adenocarcinoma marker (i.e. TTF1) and/or mucin, with a negative squamous marker (i.e. p40 or p63), should be classified as NSCC, favour adenocarcinoma. Cases positive for a squamous marker, with at least moderate, diffuse staining and a negative adenocarcinoma marker and/or mucin stains should be classified as NSCC, favour squamous cell carcinoma. A comment should be included specifying whether the differentiation was detected by light microscopy and/or by special stains.

Table 1.05 Diagnostic terminology for small biopsy/cytology comparing the new IASLC/ATS/ERS terms with 2015 WHO terms in resections {2674,2676}

Small biopsy/cytology: IASLC/ATS/ERS classification	2015 WHO classification
Small cell carcinoma	Small cell carcinoma
Non-small cell carcinoma (NSCC) with neuroendocrine morphology and positive neuroendocrine markers, possible **large cell neuroendocrine carcinoma**	Large cell neuroendocrine carcinoma
Morphological squamous cell and adenocarcinoma patterns both present: **NSCC, not otherwise specified** Comment that adenocarcinoma and squamous components are present, and that this could represent adenosquamous carcinoma.	Adenosquamous carcinoma (if both components ≥ 10%)
Morphological squamous cell or adenocarcinoma patterns not present, but immunohistochemical stains favour separate squamous and adenocarcinoma components: **NSCC, not otherwise specified** Specify the results of the immunohistochemical stains and the interpretation, and comment that this could represent adenosquamous carcinoma	Adenocarcinoma, squamous cell carcinoma, adenosquamous carcinoma or large cell carcinoma with unclear immunohistochemical features.
NSCC with spindle cell and/or giant cell carcinoma Mention if adenocarcinoma or squamous carcinoma is present.	Pleomorphic, spindle cell, and/or giant cell carcinoma

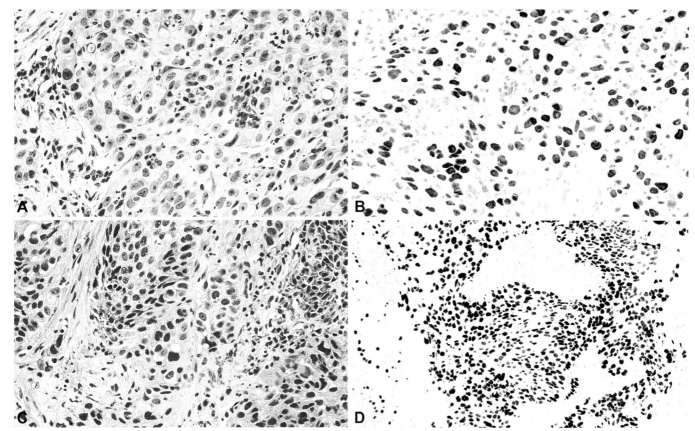

Fig. 1.05 A Non-small cell carcinoma, favour squamous cell carcinoma. This biopsy shows solid nests of tumour cells with no clear glandular or squamous differentiation. **B** Non-small cell carcinoma, favour squamous cell carcinoma. Immunohistochemistry for p40 shows strong nuclear staining. **C** Non-small cell carcinoma, favour adenocarcinoma. This tumour shows a solid pattern of growth, with no clear squamous acinar, papillary, or lepidic growth and no intracytoplasmic mucin. The morphology was pseudosquamous, as the tumour was initially diagnosed as a squamous cell carcinoma. **D** Non-small cell carcinoma. TTF1 immunohistochemical stain is positive, favouring adenocarcinoma.

The markers TTF1 and p40 are generally mutually exclusive. If an adenocarcinoma marker such as TTF1 is positive, the tumour should be classified as NSCC, favour adenocarcinoma, regardless of any expression of squamous markers. If intracytoplasmic mucin can be demonstrated in a poorly differentiated NSCC with a mucin stain in at least two tumour cells in the biopsy (and in the absence of immunohistochemical markers for adenocarcinoma or squamous cell carcinoma), the diagnosis of adenocarcinoma is appropriate {2637}. If TTF1 reactivity is present in one population of tumour cells and another population is positive for squamous markers, this may indicate the possibility of adenosquamous carcinoma, although this diagnosis can only be made based on a resection specimen.

If there is no clear staining for adenocarcinoma or squamous markers, or if the staining pattern is unclear, the tumour should be classified as NSCC, NOS.

Rarely, small samples can show morphological features of both squamous cell carcinoma and adenocarcinoma, either on routine histology or immunohistochemistry. These samples should be classified as NSCC, NOS, with a comment suggesting concurrent glandular and squamous cell differentiation, and specifying the detection method. It is possible that such tumours are adenosquamous carcinomas, but this diagnosis cannot be established without a resection specimen showing ≥ 10% of each component. If TTF1 and p40 or p63 positivity is seen in different populations of tumour cells, this is more suggestive of adenosquamous carcinoma than if the markers are coexpressed in the same tumour cells.

If both TTF1 and p40 are negative in a tumour that lacks clear squamous or glandular morphology, a cytokeratin stain may help to confirm that the tumour is a carcinoma. If a keratin stain is negative, further stains (i.e. S100, CD45, or CD31) may be needed to exclude other tumours that can look epithelioid – such as melanoma, lymphoma, malignant mesothelioma, or epithelioid haemangioendothelioma. Although primary lung adenocarcinomas can be TTF1-negative, additional immunohistochemical studies (i.e. CDX2, CK20, estrogen receptor, or progesterone receptor) or clinical evaluation may help to exclude metastasis from other sites (such as the colon or breast) in this setting.

Additional subgroups have been proposed for non-small cell carcinomas showing morphological evidence of neuroendocrine differentiation. In these cases, immunohistochemical stains are again recommended (such as CD56, chromogranin, and/or synaptophysin), with a final diagnosis of large cell neuroendocrine carcinoma suggested if positive. When there is no morphological evidence of neuroendocrine morphology, routine staining for neuroendocrine markers is not recommended, as the presence of neuroendocrine differentiation on immunohistochemistry in a morphologically confirmed adenocarcinoma or squamous cell carcinoma does not seem to affect prognosis or treatment {1091,2471}.

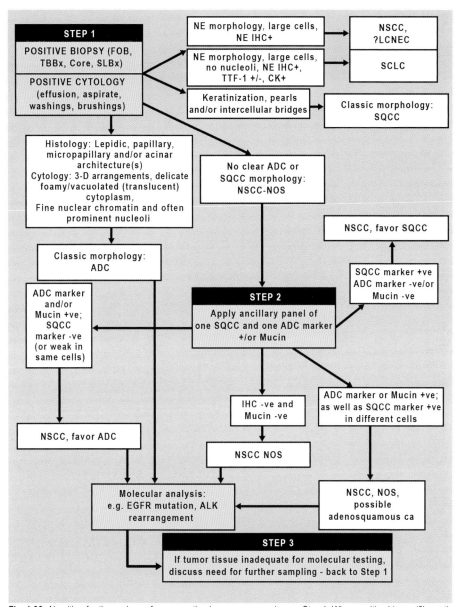

STEP 1

POSITIVE BIOPSY (FOB, TBBx, Core, SLBx)

POSITIVE CYTOLOGY (effusion, aspirate, washings, brushings)

NE morphology, large cells, NE IHC+ → NSCC, ?LCNEC

NE morphology, large cells, no nucleoli, NE IHC+, TTF-1 +/-, CK+ → SCLC

Keratinization, pearls and/or intercellular bridges → Classic morphology: SQCC

Histology: Lepidic, papillary, micropapillary and/or acinar architecture(s)
Cytology: 3-D arrangements, delicate foamy/vacuolated (translucent) cytoplasm,
Fine nuclear chromatin and often prominent nucleoli

No clear ADC or SQCC morphology: NSCC-NOS

Classic morphology: ADC

NSCC, favor SQCC

ADC marker and/or Mucin +ve; SQCC marker -ve (or weak in same cells)

SQCC marker +ve ADC marker -ve/or Mucin -ve

STEP 2
Apply ancillary panel of one SQCC and one ADC marker +/or Mucin

IHC -ve and Mucin -ve

ADC marker or Mucin +ve; as well as SQCC marker +ve in different cells

NSCC, favor ADC

NSCC NOS

NSCC, NOS, possible adenosquamous ca

Molecular analysis: e.g. EGFR mutation, ALK rearrangement

STEP 3
If tumor tissue inadequate for molecular testing, discuss need for further sampling - back to Step 1

Fig. 1.06 Algorithm for the work-up of non-resection lung cancer specimens. Step 1: When positive biopsy (fibreoptic bronchoscopy [FOB], transbronchial biopsy [TBBx], core biopsy, or surgical lung biopsy [SLBx]) or cytology (effusion, aspirate, washings, or brushings) shows clear adenocarcinoma (ADC) or squamous cell carcinoma (SQCC) morphology, the diagnosis can be firmly established. If there is neuroendocrine (NE) morphology, the tumour may be classified as small cell lung carcinoma (SCLC) or non-small cell carcinoma (NSCC), probably large cell neuroendocrine carcinoma according to standard criteria. If there is no clear ADC or SQCC morphology, the tumour is regarded as NSCC, not otherwise specified (NOS) proceed to Step 2 unless IHC stains are not available when the tumour should be classified as NSCC, NOS. Step 2: NSCC, NOS can be further classified based on: 1) IHC stains, 2) mucin (periodic acid–Schiff with diastase or mucicarmine) stains, or 3) molecular data. If the stains all favour ADC – positive ADC marker(s) (i.e. TTF1 and/or mucin) with negative SQCC markers – then the tumour is classified as NSCC, favour ADC. If SQCC markers (i.e. p40, p63, and/or CK5/6) are positive with negative ADC markers, the tumour is classified as NSCC, favour SQCC. If the ADC and SQCC markers are both strongly positive in different populations of tumour cells, the tumour is classified as NSCC, NOS, with a comment that it may be adenosquamous carcinoma. If all markers are negative, the tumour is classified as NSCC, NOS. See the text for recommendations on NSCCs with marked pleomorphic and overlapping ADC/SQCC morphology. *EGFR* mutation testing should be performed in: 1) classical ADC; 2) NSCC, favour ADC; 3) NSCC, NOS; and 4) NSCC, NOS, possible adenosquamous carcinoma. In these cases, if *EGFR* mutation testing is negative, testing for *ALK* rearrangement (*EML4-ALK*) should be performed. In NSCC, NOS, if either *EGFR* mutation or *ALK* rearrangement is positive, the tumour is more likely to be ADC than SQCC. Step 3: If clinical management requires a more specific diagnosis than NSCC, NOS, additional biopsies may be indicated. CK, cytokeratin; IHC, immunohistochemistry. Adapted from Travis WD et al. {2676}.

Similarly, sarcomatoid carcinomas (such as pleomorphic carcinoma) may be suggested if spindle cell and/or giant cell carcinoma components are present, but final diagnosis requires a resection specimen showing ≥ 10% of spindle and/or giant cell components {2674}.

The types of findings discussed in this section should be documented in a structured pathology report including several important components: 1) a pathological or cytopathological diagnosis according to the IASLC/ATS/ERS classification; 2) a report of immunohistochemical and/or mucin stains; 3) a comment about the differential diagnosis (if appropriate); and 4) a comment stating that material has been submitted for molecular testing (if appropriate), specifying which block or slide is optimal for testing. Pathologists should always consider the possibility of metastasis to the lung from other sites, especially in adenocarcinoma cases in which pneumocyte markers or markers suggesting lung origin are negative.

Molecular testing for treatment selection in lung cancer

C.A. Powell
E. Brambilla
L. Bubendorf
S. Dacic
R. Dziadziuszko
K. Geisinger
F.R. Hirsch
M. Ladanyi

M. Meyerson
A.G. Nicholson
G. Riely
G. Scagliotti
I.I. Wistuba
D. Yankelevitz
Y. Yatabe

Oncogenic drivers in non-small cell lung carcinoma

Tumour cells contain many genetic abnormalities, but only certain abnormalities (called driver mutations) are essential for tumour-cell survival. Because tumour cells are dependent on these driver mutations (a phenomenon called oncogene addiction), inactivation of the mutations results in cancer-cell death {2823}.

Driver mutations play a fundamental role in tumorigenesis, so analysis of these mutations can help to reveal the complex molecular pathogenesis of lung cancer. *EGFR, KRAS*, and *ALK* mutations are considered the prototypical driver mutations in lung cancer in general, but these mutations are acquired in a manner almost completely specific to lung adenocarcinoma. Among the adenocarcinomas with these driver mutations, adenocarcinomas with either *EGFR* or *ALK* alterations are preferentially seen in never-smokers, and develop in the lung peripheral parenchyma; while adenocarcinomas with *KRAS* mutation commonly occur in smokers, and frequently in hilar regions – similar to squamous cell carcinoma and small cell carcinoma. The complex relationship is explained well by the anatomical compartment model {2513,2893,2950}. This model is supported by the concept

Table 1.07 Major genetic changes in lung cancer

Alterations	Small cell carcinoma (%)	Adenocarcinoma (%)	Squamous cell carcinoma (%)
Mutation			
BRAF	0	< 5	0
EGFR Caucasian	< 1	10–20	< 1
Asian	< 5	35–45	< 5
ERBB2/HER2	0	< 5	0
KRAS Caucasian	< 1	15–35	< 5
Asian	< 1	5–10	< 5
PIK3CA	< 5	< 5	5–15
RB	> 90	5–15	5–15
TP53	> 90	30–40	50–80
Amplification			
EGFR	< 1	5–10	10
ERBB2/HER2	< 1	< 5	< 1
MET	< 1	< 5	< 5
MYC	20–30	5–10	5–10
FGFR1	< 1	< 5	15–25
Gene rearrangement			
ALK	0	5	< 1
RET	0	1–2	0
ROS1	0	1–2	0
NTRK1	0	< 1	0
NRG1	0	< 1	0

Table 1.06 Guidelines for good practice in the use of tissue for molecular studies

1. Tissue specimens should be managed not only for diagnosis, but also to maximize the amount of tissue available for molecular studies.

2. Cell blocks should be prepared from cytology samples (including pleural fluids) when positive for lung cancer, as it is not possible to predict whether other material is suitable for IHC or molecular analysis.

3. To guide therapy for patients with advanced lung cancer, each institution should have a multidisciplinary team that coordinates the optimal approach to using tissue for molecular studies.

4. The pathology department should ensure that all molecular results become part of the record for each individual specimen.

of region-specific stem cells – basal cells are the putative stem cells of the bronchus for the central airway compartment, and type II pneumocytes {581} are the putative stem cells for the terminal respiratory unit of the peripheral compartment.

Genetic basis for targeted therapies in non-small cell lung carcinoma

Recent advances in our understanding of the complex biology of lung cancer, particularly of the activation of oncogenes by mutations (e.g. *EGFR, KRAS, BRAF*, and *ERBB2*), translocations (e.g. *ALK, ROS1*, and *RET*), and amplifications (e.g. *MET* and *FGFR1*) in adenocarcinomas

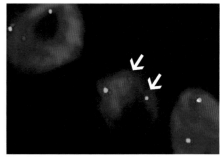

Fig. 1.07 Adenocarcinoma with *ALK* rearrangement. Positive *ALK* FISH in lung adenocarcinoma with *EML4-ALK* gene fusion showing split between green (5') and red (3') signals (indicated by arrows) caused by rearrangement of *ALK*.

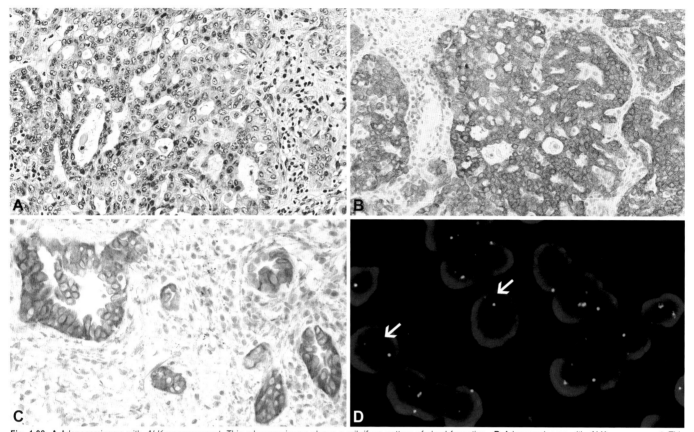

Fig. 1.08 **A** Adenocarcinoma with *ALK* rearrangement. This adenocarcinoma shows a cribriform pattern of gland formation. **B** Adenocarcinoma with *ALK* rearrangement. This adenocarcinoma stains positively with immunohistochemistry for *ALK*. **C** Adenocarcinoma with *ROS1* rearrangement. Immunohistochemistry for *ROS1* shows positive staining in the tumour cells. **D** Adenocarcinoma with *ROS1* rearrangement. This *ROS1* break-apart FISH shows green and red dots, which correspond to the 5' and 3' probes for the *ROS1* gene, respectively. The split of the green and red dots, examples of which are marked by arrows, is consistent with *ROS1* rearrangement.

and squamous cell carcinomas, have provided new treatment targets and faciliated the identification of subsets of tumours with unique molecular profiles that can predict response to therapy {1465,2341,2346}. These discoveries have already resulted in regulatory approval of treatments for lung adenocarcinomas bearing mutations in the *EGFR* gene and activating fusions of the *ALK* gene {637,2348}, and numerous other targeted agents are currently under clinical investigation for the treatment of lung adenocarcinomas and lung squamous cell carcinomas. Broader descriptions of cancer genome alterations can be found in recent next-generation sequencing analyses of lung adenocarcinoma {1076,2626}, squamous cell lung carcinoma {936}, large cell carcinoma {2320}, and small cell lung carcinoma {2012,2219}.

Many of the major receptor tyrosine kinase-targetable driver alterations in lung adenocarcinoma (including *EGFR* mutations and *ALK, RET,* and *ROS1*

translocations) are found mainly in adenocarcinomas from never-smokers and light smokers, while other events (notably *KRAS* and *BRAF* mutations) are found more often in adenocarcinomas from smokers {606,892,2626}. However, these associations are not absolute, so smoking history should not be used to exclude patients from molecular testing for specific alterations {1479}.

Somatic *EGFR* mutations are observed in roughly 10–20% of cases of lung adenocarcinoma from patients of European descent, and in roughly 50% of cases from patients of East Asian descent {1530,1956,1974,2364}. These proportions vary depending on local smoking rates: areas with high smoking rates have lower rates of *EGFR*-mutated cancers and higher rates of *KRAS*-mutated cancers. Randomized trials in patients with advanced *EGFR*-mutant lung adenocarcinomas have shown benefits for first-line treatment with gefitinib {1548,1689,1700}, erlotinib {2196}, and afatinib {2196}. Guidelines for *EGFR* mutation detection

in lung cancer patient samples have recently been published {1480}. Mutation-specific antibodies for epidermal growth factor receptor (EGFR)-L858R and exon 19 are available for detection of these mutations {263A, 410A} and may be useful in the context of molecular testing algorithms but are not currently recommended as sole, stand-alone assays for the selection of patients for EGFR tyrosine kinase inhibitor therapy {1479}.

The sensitivity to small-molecule EGFR inhibitors is greatest with the L858R mutation and the exon 19 deletion mutations {1118,1119}. Most *EGFR* exon 20 insertion mutants are resistant to small-molecule EGFR inhibitors {79,2946,2947}, except for the A763_Y764insFQEA mutant, which is sensitive to erlotinib and gefitinib {2947}.

Secondary resistance to EGFR inhibitors can arise from the acquisition of an additional somatic mutation in *EGFR* (the T790M mutation) {1299,1975}, or from amplification of the *MET* proto-oncogene

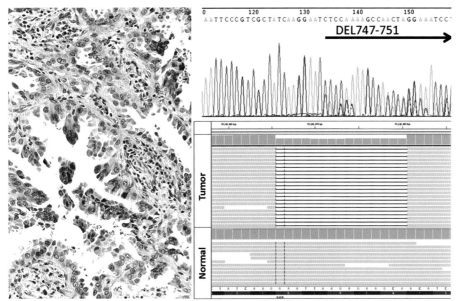

Fig. 1.09 Adenocarcinoma with *EGFR* exon 19 deletion. In a 77-year-old female never-smoker; *EGFR* exon 19 deletion was detected in the tumour by Sanger sequencing (upper-right panel). An example of an *EGFR* exon 19 deletion (an in-frame deletion of the ELREA amino acid sequence – glutamic acid, leucine, arginine, gluctamic acid, alanine) as detected by next-generation sequencing is shown in the lower-right panel, as individual sequencing reads visualized in the Integrative Genomics Viewer.

{157,676} or the *ERBB2* proto-oncogene {2577}. Combinations of small-molecule EGFR inhibitors and EGFR antibodies {2128}, as well as T790M-specific EGFR inhibitors {3025}, are currently under investigation for the treatment of lung cancers with secondary inhibitor resistance arising from *EGFR* T790M mutations.

KRAS mutations are the most common receptor tyrosine kinase/RAS/RAF pathway oncogenic driver alterations in lung adenocarcinomas in Caucasian populations, with a mutation rate of roughly 30% in these populations {1076} and about 10% in East Asian populations {2364,2984}. *KRAS* mutations are associated with lack of response to EGFR-targeted agents in lung adenocarcinoma {665,1573,1976,2171}, but their impact on overall survival remains controversial. Unlike for *EGFR*-mutant lung adenocarcinoma, there are no demonstrably efficacious treatments for *KRAS*-mutant lung adenocarcinomas at this time.

Activating rearrangements of the ALK gene by fusion with the *EML4* gene are seen in 3–7% of lung adenocarcinomas {2158,2421}. Patients whose tumours harbour these translocations respond well to the ALK/MET/ROS1 inhibitor crizotinib {1373,2348,2349} and other ALK inhibitors {2334,2347}; thus, *ALK* fusion detection is now a mainstay of lung adenocarcinoma diagnosis. Clinical testing guidelines for *ALK* fusion detection in lung adenocarcinoma have been published {1479}. Smears may be preferable to histological sections for ALK FISH testing because they eliminate nuclear truncation and any related errors. Immunohistochemistry is a sensitive and specific tool for detection of ALK rearrangements {1425A, 1479, 2917A}.

Activation of the ROS1 and RET genes by fusion with several possible partner genes, including *CD74* and *SLC34A2*, is seen in approximately 1% of lung adenocarcinomas {2158}. Like *ALK*-driven lung adenocarcinomas, *ROS1*-driven lung adenocarcinomas appear to be responsive to crizotinib {186}, although the clinical evidence is less advanced at this point.

RET fusions are another clear driver event in lung adenocarcinomas, found in approximately 1% of cases {1166,1308,1485,2574}, almost exclusively in non-smokers. *RET* fusions have been found to be associated with response to cabozantinib {627}. Other RET inhibitors are under investigation.

Somatic activating ERBB2 mutations – both exon 20 insertions {78,2469} and extracellular domain mutations {900} – occur in about 1–5% of lung adenocarcinomas. Preclinical studies suggest that ERBB2 inhibitors could be effective, but appropriate clinical data are still pending {900}.

Mutations in the BRAF gene are seen in 2–10% of lung adenocarcinomas {265,534,1076,1815,1958}. The proportion of non-V600E mutations is higher in lung adenocarcinoma than in other cancers such as melanoma and colorectal cancer {330,1958}. Although no BRAF inhibitor is currently approved for lung adenocarcinoma, there are reports of responses to vemurafenib {804,2040}.

Predictive testing for immunotherapies in non-small cell lung carcinoma
Immunotherapy has emerged as a major new treatment modality for patients with advanced non-small cell lung carcinoma. The main approach is immune checkpoint blockade with either PD1 or PDL1 antibodies, directed towards PD1 receptors on activated T cells and PDL1 receptors on tumour cells and antigen presenting immune cells, respectively {253}. Preliminary studies that assessed PDL1 expression by immunohistochemistry have shown an encouraging predictive association with response to PD1 antibody therapy {2657}, but further assay validation is needed before recommendations for clinical practice can be made. Additional predictors of response have recently been published {989A}.

Strategic use of small tissue samples and cytology for molecular testing
The development of personalized therapy approaches in advanced lung adenocarcinoma has dramatically changed clinical practice, and has improved clinical outcomes. But there are barriers to the widespread implementation of these approaches, such as the fact that the biopsy and cytology specimens available for molecular testing in advanced metastatic lung tumours are often small – including, in most cases, specimens obtained by core-needle biopsy or fine-needle aspiration biopsy.

The current status of therapy in lung cancer requires the analysis of a panel of molecular abnormalities in tumour specimens {1235}. There is a clear need to adapt current and emerging technologies to the molecular analysis of small tissue specimens obtained from lung cancer patients, but there are several scientific, methodological, and practical challenges associated with widespread molecular testing using lung biopsy and cytology specimens. The ideal specimens for molecular testing are tumour tissues obtained fresh and then immediately frozen. However, samples like these are usually only available for research purposes in academic centres, and used for discovery purposes {2894}. In pathology laboratories, diagnostic clinical tumour tissue specimens (e.g. specimens obtained by core-needle biopsy, bronchoscopy, or surgical resection) are fixed in formalin and embedded in paraffin. Both formalin fixation and paraffin embedding compromise the integrity of nucleic acids for molecular testing. Therefore, specimens should be fixed with buffered formalin (for 6–24 hours) immediately after tissue aquisition. Cytology specimens (e.g. pleural fluids and specimens obtained by bronchial brushing, bronchoalveolar lavage, transbronchial needle aspiration, or fine-needle aspiration biopsy), are usually fixed in alcohol, which is optimal for the preservation of nucleic acids. When a cytology specimen contains abundant material, the sample can be processed as a tissue specimen (cell block) to obtain sections {278,1194}. Although tissue specimens are preferable for molecular testing, cytology samples with abundant malignant cells can also be used successfully for this purpose {2135}.

Pathologists should determine the adequacy of specimens for molecular testing by assessing the malignant cell content and sample quality {1479}. Two important aspects must be addressed when lung cancer biopsy and cytology specimens are received for histological diagnosis. First, the handling of biopsy and cytology specimens for histology and subsequent molecular testing requires thoughtful prioritization of the use of the samples, to avoid using up the tumour material for immunohistochemical studies that may be less critical than the molecular testing required for selection of therapy. Therefore, a limited panel of diagnostic immunohistochemical markers required to make the right histology diagnosis is recommended. Second, the pathologist must determine whether the number of malignant cells available in each specimen is adequate for nucleic acid extraction, as well as for histology section-based molecular tests (e.g. FISH and immunohistochemistry). This requires assessment of the percentage of malignant versus non-malignant cells, as well as the characteristics of the tissue and cells in terms of necrosis and appropriate preservation and fixation. When a specimen

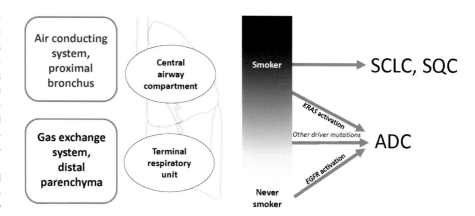

Fig. 1.10 The concept of the two-compartment model in the putative molecular pathogenesis of lung cancer. Anatomically, lung epithelial cells are located in two compartments, which are associated with specific lung functions. The central airway compartment serves mainly as the air conducting system, while respiratory exchange occurs in the terminal respiratory unit of the peripheral compartment. In the individual compartments, different stem cell niches have been identified, and accordingly, different types of lung cancer target different compartments. Carcinogens from tobacco smoke appear to target both the central and peripheral airways, although the magnitude of their effect is greater in the central compartment. In contrast, lung cancers in never-smokers are caused by unidentified factors that appear to specifically target the terminal respiratory unit. *EGFR* activation is associated with never smoking, whereas *KRAS* activation is more frequent in smokers. Other driver mutations also exist. This model illustrates only the major pathways, but other minor pathways may also exist. ADC, adenocarcinoma; SCLC, small cell lung carcinoma; SQC, squamous cell carcinoma.

contains substantial stroma or necrosis, it can be helpful for the pathologist to mark the best tumour area for nucleic acid extraction. In certain tumour specimens with abundant non-malignant cells intermixed with neoplastic cells, tissue microdissection is warranted. Due to our growing understanding of the biology of lung cancer (particularly of the molecular evolution of tumours during local progression and metastasis) and the identification of molecular abnormalities associated with resistance to therapies, it has become extremely important to characterize the molecular abnormalities of the disease at every stage of its progression. For the molecular testing of advanced metastatic lung tumours, it is important to sample and analyse the tumours at each time point of clinical decision-making. If this information affects the further management of the patient, re-biopsy should be considered {1251,2332}. In this scenario, it is important that the pathologist is aware of the purpose of the re-biopsy, both to avoid wasting tissue by performing unnecessary diagnostic immunohistochemical analyses and to direct the sample for the appropriate molecular testing.

Most biomarkers used for clinical applications to date consist of a single genetic mutation, gene amplification, or translocation. But in many patients and cancer types, these single biomarkers are not

sufficient to select patients for targeted therapies. The development of new technologies, such as high-throughput multiplex methodologies, has made it possible to screen whole genomes, proteomes, and transcriptomes for new biomarkers in tumour tissue samples, and to identify specific molecular targets and develop genomic and proteomic profiles or signatures that better reflect the complex molecular aberrations present within a single tumour. The rapid development of technologies for large-scale sequencing (next-generation sequencing) of DNA and RNA has facilitated high-throughput molecular analysis and testing of lung tumour tissue specimens. These technologies provide various advantages over traditional single-gene analyses, including the ability to fully sequence large numbers of genes in a single test, and to simultaneously detect deletions, insertions, copy number alterations, translocations, and exome-wide base substitutions (including known hotspot mutations) in all known cancer-related genes. The amount of starting material (DNA or RNA) needed for the newest next-generation sequencing applications is getting smaller; currently, the analysis of a panel of hundreds of genes for mutations, amplifications, and fusions can be performed even on DNA extracted from small, routine, fixed biopsy and cytology samples.

Adenocarcinoma

W.D. Travis
M. Noguchi
Y. Yatabe
E. Brambilla
A.G. Nicholson
S.C. Aisner
J.H.M. Austin
S.S. Devesa
F.R. Hirsch

M. Ladanyi
M. Meyerson
M. Mino-Kenudson
C.A. Powell
R. Rami-Porta
N. Rekhtman
G. Riely
P. Russell
J. Samet

G. Scagliotti
E. Thunnissen
K-F. To
K. Tsuta
P. van Schil
A. Warth
I.I. Wistuba
D. Yankelevitz

Definition

Invasive adenocarcinoma is a malignant epithelial tumour with glandular differentiation, mucin production, or pneumocyte marker expression. The tumours show an acinar, papillary, micropapillary, lepidic, or solid growth pattern, with either mucin or pneumocyte marker expression. After comprehensive histological subtyping in 5–10% increments, the tumours are classified according to their predominant pattern.

ICD-O codes

Adenocarcinoma   8140/3
Lepidic adenocarcinoma   8250/3
Acinar adenocarcinoma   8551/3
Papillary adenocarcinoma   8260/3
Micropapillary adenocarcinoma   8265/3
Solid adenocarcinoma   8230/3

Synonyms

Lepidic predominant adenocarcinoma; acinar predominant adenocarcinoma; papillary predominant adenocarcinoma; micropapillary predominant adenocarcinoma;

solid predominant adenocarcinoma with mucin and/or pneumocyte marker expression
Obsolete: bronchioloalveolar carcinoma; bronchiolar carcinoma; bronchoalveolar carcinoma

Epidemiology and etiology

Tobacco smoking. Lung cancer is the most common cause of cancer death worldwide, reflecting the global epidemic of the cause of most cases: tobacco smoking {1518}. The spatial and temporal patterns of lung cancer occurrence parallel those of cigarette use. Mortality and incidence rates have generally been highest in high-income countries, particularly the United States and European countries, but are now declining, particularly in younger males and females. Lung cancer has long been more common in men than in women, but in many high-income countries (e.g. the United States), incidence rates in men and women have begun converging {2718}. Around the world, the current pattern of lung cancer occurrence largely reflects historical patterns of cigarette smoking; rates are low

in much of Africa, as well as in Central and South America.

Through decades of research, many causal risk factors for lung cancer have been identified, including smoking combustible tobacco products, radon in indoor environments and mines, other occupational agents, and outdoor air pollution {42}. Cigarette smoking is the leading cause of lung cancer, with 965 500 lung cancer deaths attributable to smoking worldwide in 2010 (http://www.healthdata.org/data-visualization/gbd-cause-patterns). The risks in smokers increase with the duration of smoking and the number of cigarettes smoked daily, and progressively decline following cessation (although never to the level among never-smokers). Lung cancer does occur among never-smokers – at estimated rates as low as 5–10 per 100 000 annually, but at higher rates in some populations based on relatively recent data from cohort studies {2635}; by contrast, the rates in smokers are as much as 20–30 times higher. Possible etiological factors for lung cancer among never-smokers include exposure to secondhand tobacco smoke, radon, various

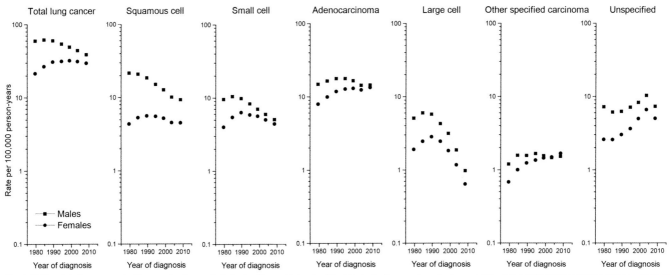

Fig. 1.11 Trends in lung cancer incidence rates (age-adjusted using the world standard) by histological type and sex in nine registries of the United States National Cancer Institute's SEER programme, 1977–1981 through 2006–2010.

occupational agents, and emissions from indoor coal burning, but in most cases, a specific cause cannot be identified and the patterns and types of mutations differ from typical smoking-associated lung cancers {606,2626}.

Histological types. Almost all lung cancers are carcinomas. The predominant histological types are adenocarcinoma, squamous cell carcinoma, small cell carcinoma, and large cell carcinoma. Preinvasive lesions, benign epithelial tumours, lymphoproliferative tumours, and other miscellaneous tumours also occur, but they are relatively rare. With few exceptions, specific risk factors have not been linked to particular histological types of lung cancer. Over the now lengthy course of the tobacco epidemic, there has been a notable shift in the histological types of lung cancer occurring within the population, and in the associations of the various histological types with cigarette smoking. Smoking is associated with all carcinoma types, but the strongest associations are with squamous cell and small cell carcinomas. When the strong association of cigarette smoking with lung cancer was first characterized in the 1950s, squamous cell carcinoma was the predominant histological type in smokers, while adenocarcinoma was the most common type in never-smokers. For non-adenocarcinomas, the relative risk associated with smoking was about 10 in studies carried out in the 1950s and 1960s, while smoking was associated with an approximate doubling of risk for adenocarcinoma.

In the 1960s, a shift began in the major histological types of lung cancer; the relative frequency of adenocarcinoma increased, while squamous cell and small cell carcinomas declined. These trends were first noted in cancer registry data in the United States, and have also been documented in other countries. Illustrative data for the United States are based on the nine registries in the National Cancer Institute's SEER programme, which have contributed data since 1973–1975. Since 1977, histological type has been coded according to the first to third editions of ICD-O, with all codes now converted to the third edition {763,2028,2905}. During 1977–2010, a total of 503 611 cancers of the lung or bronchus were diagnosed in the populations covered by these registries, of which

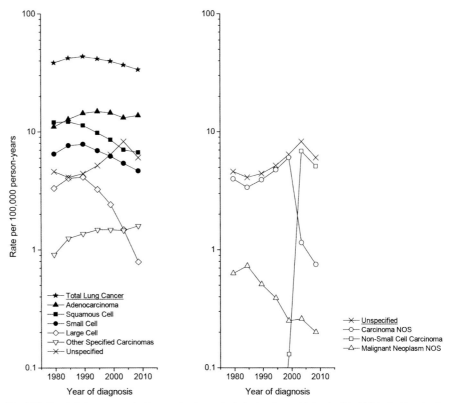

Fig. 1.12 Trends in lung cancer incidence rates (age-adjusted using the world standard) by histological type in nine registries of the United States National Cancer Institute's SEER programme, 1977–1981 through 2006–2010.

90.1% were microscopically confirmed (http://www.seer.cancer.gov/).

After exclusion of cases specified as non-carcinomas or likely to be metastatic carcinoma, 452 714 cases were available for analysis. These were grouped into six major categories: squamous cell carcinoma, small cell carcinoma, adenocarcinoma, large cell carcinoma, other specified carcinomas, and unspecified carcinoma {1459A}. The unspecified category is composed of carcinoma, not otherwise specified; non-small cell carcinoma (a new code introduced in ICD-O-3); and malignant neoplasm, not otherwise specified.

The relative proportions of the histological types have varied considerably over the years. During the earliest period (1977–1981), squamous cell carcinoma accounted for 32% of cases; but by 2006–2010, the proportion had declined to 20%. Adenocarcinoma accounted for < 30% of cases during the earliest years, but the proportion increased to > 40% by 2006–2010. The small cell proportion decreased from 17% to 13%, and the large cell carcinoma proportion from 8% to 2%. The other unspecified carcinoma proportion rose from 2% to 4%. The unspecified

carcinoma proportion of rose from 12% to 23% during 2001–2005, and then dropped to 18%. These recent trends reflect improvements in the determination of histological type over the past decade, especially for large cell carcinoma and adenocarcinoma, such as the introduction of immunohistochemical staining with TTF1 and squamous markers {2676}. This is one likely explanation for the marked decrease in the proportion with large cell carcinoma. There is now an increased emphasis on the accurate determination of histological type, because of treatment and outcome implications.

Lung cancer incidence. The overall lung cancer incidence rate (per 100 000 person-years, age-adjusted using the world standard) increased from 38.4 during 1977–1981 to peak at 43.5 during 1987–1991, and then decreased to 33.6 during 2006–2010. The rates of the various histological types peaked at slightly different times. Squamous cell carcinoma peaked earliest, in 1982–1986; small cell and large cell carcinomas peaked during 1987–1991; and adenocarcinoma peaked during 1992–1996. The rates of unspecified carcinoma and other specified carcinomas did not peak until

2001–2005 and 2006–2010, respectively. It is interesting to note that the adenocarcinoma rate decreased after peaking, but then increased in the most recent time period; the squamous cell carcinoma rate did not continue to decrease as rapidly; and the other specified carcinomas rate increased after having stabilized, whereas the unspecified carcinoma rate dropped substantially after having increased since the mid-1980s. Within the unspecified group, carcinoma, not otherwise specified accounted for the majority of cases until 2000, when non-small cell carcinoma became the dominant group, making consideration of these poorly specified types virtually futile. The differences in the timing of the rate peaks among the histological types likely reflect changes in the construction of cigarettes, the composition of the tobacco, and inhalation patterns.

Lung cancer incidence trends have differed by sex, with overall rates decreasing among males since the mid-1980s and increasing among females through the late 1990s {1459A}.

Among males, squamous cell carcinoma peaked in the late 1970s, small cell and large cell carcinomas in the mid-1980s, adenocarcinoma around 1990, and other specified carcinomas in the mid-1990s. Among females, the peaks were later: in the late 1980s for squamous cell, small cell, and large cell carcinomas; in the late 1990s for adenocarcinoma; and in the late 2000s for other specified carcinomas. The male-to-female incidence rate ratio for lung cancer overall decreased from 2.8 to 1.3 over the study period. The ratio was highest for squamous cell carcinoma, dropping from 5.0 to 2.1, followed by that for large cell carcinoma, which decreased from 2.7 to 1.5. The male-to-female incidence rate ratio for small cell carcinoma decreased from 2.4 to 1.2, that of adenocarcinoma from 1.9 to 1.1, and that of other specified carcinomas from 1.8 to 0.9. Among both males and females, the rate of unspecified carcinoma decreased substantially during the most recent period (2006–2010), in contrast to the increasing rates of adenocarcinoma and other specified carcinomas, and the stabilizing rates of squamous cell carcinoma.

The hypothesized explanations for these time trends in lung cancer histology relate to changes in the design and characteristics of manufactured cigarettes – the

globally dominant cause of lung cancer. Over the course of the decade before this shift began, and continuing during the subsequent decades, cigarettes were changed by the addition of filters, ventilation holes, and other modifications that were intended to reduce the dose of tar and nicotine, as measured by a machine. But as a result of these changes, puff volume may have increased, causing a shift from more central deposition of tobacco smoke to more peripheral deposition. Squamous cell and small cell carcinomas generally arise in the more proximal airways, while adenocarcinomas originate in the peripheral airways. Thus, more peripheral deposition increases the risk for adenocarcinoma. The levels of tobacco-specific nitrosamines in cigarette smoke have also increased as a result of design changes. In animal models, these nitrosamines cause adenocarcinomas specifically.

Table 1.08 Occupational agents and exposure circumstances classified by the IARC Monographs programme (http://monographs.iarc.fr) as carcinogenic to humans, with the lung as a target organ

Agent, mixture, or circumstance	Main industry or use
Arsenic and arsenic compounds	Glass, metals, pesticides
Asbestos	Insulation, filters, textiles
Beryllium and beryllium compounds	Aerospace industry
Bis(chloromethyl)ether and chloromethyl methyl ether	Chemical intermediates
Cadmium and cadmium compounds	Dyes/pigments
Chromium (VI) compounds	Pigments (for textile dyes, paints, inks, plastics), metal industry, chrome plating
Coal – indoor emissions from household combustion	Fuel for heating, cooking
Coal tars	Fuel
Coal-tar pitch	Construction, electrodes
Dioxin (2,3,7,8-tetrachlorodibenzo-p-dioxin)	Chemical industry
Engine exhaust, diesel	Fuel
MOPP chemotherapy (a mixture of vincristine, prednisone, nitrogen mustard, and procarbazine)	Treatment for Hodgkin lymphoma
Nickel compounds	Metallurgy, alloy, catalyst
Outdoor air pollution	
Particulate matter in outdoor air pollution	
Plutonium-239	Nuclear
Radon-222 and its decay products	Mining
Silica, crystalline	Stone cutting, mining, glass, paper
Soot	Pigments
Sulfur mustard	Chemical warfare
Talc containing asbestiform fibres	Paper, paints
Tobacco smoke, secondhand	
Tobacco smoking	
X- and gamma-radiation	Medical, nuclear
Exposure circumstances	
Aluminium production	
Coal gasification	
Coal-tar pitch	
Coke production	
Haematite mining (underground) with exposure to radon	
Iron and steel founding	
Painter (occupational exposure)	
Occupational exposures in the rubber production industry	

The evidence on shifting trends in lung cancer histological types was comprehensively reviewed in the United States Surgeon General's 2014 report {2718}. The report includes four important conclusions related to the changing patterns of lung cancer:

1. The evidence is sufficient to conclude that the risk of developing adenocarcinoma of the lung from cigarette smoking has increased since the 1960s.
2. The evidence is sufficient to conclude that the increased risk of adenocarcinoma of the lung in smokers results from changes in the design and composition of cigarettes since the 1950s.
3. The evidence is not sufficient to specify which design changes are responsible for the increased risk of adenocarcinoma, but there is suggestive evidence that ventilated filters and increased levels of tobacco-specific nitrosamines have played a role.
4. The evidence shows that the decline of squamous cell carcinoma follows the trend of declining smoking prevalence.

Occupational exposure

Smoking is the most important risk factor for lung cancer development; for adenocarcinoma as well as for both small cell carcinoma and squamous cell carcinoma. Lung adenocarcinomas can also develop in never-smokers, among whom they are the most frequent histological subtype. In addition to smoking, other reported causal factors include exposure to secondhand tobacco smoke, radon and other ionizing radiation, asbestos, and indoor air pollution, as well as underlying chronic lung disease (e.g. pulmonary fibrosis, chronic obstructive pulmonary disease, alpha-1 antitrypsin deficiency, and tuberculosis) and family history. There have been rare reports of families with an inherited genetic predisposition to lung cancer associated with germline *EGFR* {173,806,1948,2752} or *ERBB2* {2926} mutation.

Table 1.09 Signs and symptoms of lung carcinoma. Modified from Colby TV et al. {477}

Systemic symptoms
- Weight loss, loss of appetite, malaise, fever

Local/direct effects
- From endobronchial growth and/or invasion of adjacent structures, including chest wall and vertebral column
- Cough, dyspnoea, wheezing, stridor, haemoptysis
- Chest pain/back pain
- Obstructive pneumonia (with or without cavitation)
- Pleural effusion

Extension to mediastinal structures
- Nerve entrapment: recurrent laryngeal nerve (hoarseness), phrenic nerve (diaphragmatic paralysis), sympathetic system (Horner syndrome), brachial plexopathy from superior sulcus tumours
- Vena cava obstruction: superior vena cava syndrome
- Pericardium: effusion, tamponade
- Myocardium: arrythmia, heart failure
- Oesophagus: dysphagia, bronchoesophageal fistula
- Mediastinal lymph nodes: pleural effusion

Metastatic disease
- Direct effects related to the organ(s) involved

Paraneoplastic syndromes
- Dermatomyositis/polymyositis
- Clubbing
- Hypertrophic pulmonary osteoarthropathy
- Encephalopathy
- Peripheral neuropathies
- Myasthenic syndromes (including Lambert-Eaton myasthenic syndrome)
- Transverse myelitis
- Progressive multifocal leukoencephalopathy

Endocrine syndromes
- Parathormone-like substance: hypercalcaemia
- Inappropriate antidiuretic hormone: hyponatraemia
- Adrenocorticotropic hormone: Cushing syndrome, hyperpigmentation
- Serotonin: carcinoid syndrome
- Gonadotropins: gynaecomastia
- Melanocyte-stimulating hormone: increased pigmentation
- Hypoglycaemia, hyperglycaemia
- Hypercalcitonaemia
- Elevated growth hormone
- Prolactinaemia
- Hypersecretion of vasoactive intestinal polypeptide: diarrhoea

Haematological/coagulation defects
- Disseminated intravascular coagulation
- Recurrent venous thromboses
- Non-bacterial thrombotic (marantic) endocarditis
- Anaemia
- Dysproteinaemia
- Granulocytosis
- Eosinophilia
- Hypoalbuminaemia
- Leukoerythroblastosis
- Marrow plasmacytosis
- Thrombocytopenia

Miscellaneous (very rare)
- Henoch-Schönlein purpura
- Glomerulonephritis, nephrotic syndrome
- Hypouricaemia, hyperamylasaemia, amyloidosis
- Lactic acidosis
- Systemic lupus erythematosus

Clinical features

Presenting signs and symptoms

Patients with lung cancer present with a variety of symptoms or no symptoms at all. A wide variety of symptoms can lead to the diagnosis of lung cancer. Some of the more common symptoms include progressive shortness of breath, cough, chest pain/pressure, hoarseness or loss of voice, and haemoptysis. Symptoms related to disseminated disease include weight loss; abdominal pain due to involvement of the liver, adrenals, and pancreas; and pain due to bone (marrow) metastases. Patients with small cell lung cancer are more likely than patients with non-small cell lung cancer to present with symptoms referable to distant metastases. At presentation, brain metastases are identified in many patients with lung cancer, and during the course of illness, ≥ 20% of patients with lung cancer develop central nervous system metastases {142}.

Presenting signs and symptoms often depend on the extent of disease and the sites of metastases. Most patients present with locally advanced or metastatic lung cancer. Of patients whose stage is known, just 16% present with disease confined to the primary site, another 23% have disease involving regional nodes, and > 60% have evidence of distant metastatic disease at the time of diagnosis (http://seer.cancer.gov/statfacts/html/lungb.html).

The presenting findings and stage distribution of lung cancer may change with local implementation of CT screening for lung cancer among high-risk groups. Patients who are diagnosed with lung cancer as part of a programme of low-dose CT screening are less likely to be diagnosed with stage IV disease and more likely to have an adenocarcinoma identified {454,1031}. In the National Lung Cancer Screening Trial study, 50% of the screen-detected cancers were diagnosed at stage I {454}.

Paraneoplastic symptoms
Paraneoplastic symptoms are common in lung cancer. Endocrine and paraneoplastic syndromes are less common in adenocarcinoma than in other histological types of lung cancer. Small cell lung carcinoma is characterized by neuroendocrine activity, and some of the peptides secreted by the tumour mimic the activity of pituitary hormones {1940,2439}.

Cerebrospinal metastases or meningeal seeding may cause neurological symptoms. Neurological symptoms may also be a paraneoplastic phenomena, which might include sensory, sensorimotor, and autoimmune neuropathies and encephalomyelitis. The symptoms may precede the primary diagnosis by many months, and may be the presenting complaint. They may also be the initial sign of

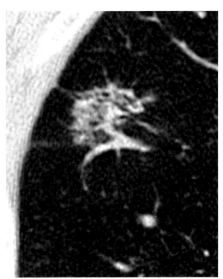

Fig. 1.13 Invasive adenocarcinoma. Showing both solid and non-solid components; two spicules extend to the costal pleura.

relapse from remission. Hypercalcaemia is rare in small cell lung carcinoma, and almost pathognomonic for squamous cell carcinoma.

Initial evaluation of a patient with a possible diagnosis of lung cancer routinely involves imaging and surgical procedures to define the extent of disease; these can include CT, PET, MRI, bronchoscopy, transthoracic needle biopsy, fine-needle aspiration biopsy, mediastinoscopy, and endobronchial ultrasound-guided needle aspiration. These procedures should be tailored to allow accurate staging (i.e. detecting sites of nodal metastases and distant disease) and to procure sufficient material to obtain all required information for treatment (including histological and molecular analysis).

Imaging
As a primary lesion, lung cancer usually manifests as a nodule (i.e. ≤ 3 cm in size), although more complex patterns for the primary lesion do occasionally exist. Intrathoracic manifestations of lung cancer are usually evaluated by plain chest radiography and/or chest CT, and sometimes by PET and MRI. Lung cancer can occur anywhere in the lungs, but is more common in the periphery of the lungs than in the hilar region, and more common in the upper lobes than in other lobes.

Chest radiography, because of its widespread use as the leading imaging tool for assessing chest disease, is by far the most common tool for the imaging

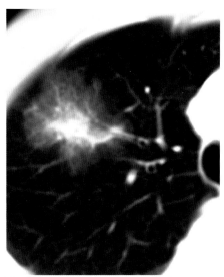

Fig. 1.14 Lepidic adenocarcinoma. CT shows a part-solid tumour in the right upper lobe; the longest diameter of the entire mass is 4.8 cm (T2a), and of the solid portion is 2.2 cm (T1b), approximately.

Imaging characteristics of lung cancer

Invasive adenocarcinoma and squamous cell carcinoma usually present as a solitary peripheral pulmonary nodule or mass.

Cavitation is most commonly seen in squamous cell carcinoma, and is almost never present in small cell carcinoma.

A large carcinomatous hilar mass can be any cell type, but is most commonly squamous cell carcinoma or small cell carcinoma, and less likely invasive adenocarcinoma.

Pneumonia-like consolidation can be seen in invasive mucinous adenocarcinoma and squamous carcinoma with obstructive pneumonia.

A large carcinomatous peripheral mass is most commonly invasive adenocarcinoma, and less commonly squamous cell carcinoma or large cell carcinoma.

Focal calcification, in no characteristic pattern, is occasionally evident in a small portion of all the common cell types of lung cancer. Calcification is more common in central typical carcinoids than in other cell types.

FDG PET yields a numerical standard uptake value for the tumour, the higher that value, the greater the likelihood of distant spread and a fatal outcome. It is also useful for detecting distant metastatic disease.

MRI may be useful for assessing direct invasion of the chest wall, e.g. by Pancoast tumours.

---

detection of lung cancer. However, chest CT provides much better detail than chest radiography in terms of tumour size, shape, and location, as well as in terms of staging. For the screening detection of lung cancer in at-risk individuals, CT is approximately 4 times more sensitive

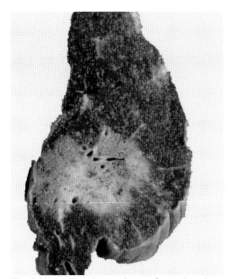

Fig. 1.15 Lepidic adenocarcinoma. Gross view shows a subpleural circumscribed tumour with a solid centre representing the invasive component, surrounded by a poorly defined area that corresponds to the lepidic growth.

than screening chest radiography. The mean size of lung cancers missed by a radiologist at chest X-ray but evident in retrospect is 1.5–2.0 cm. A commonly accepted size at which a peripheral solid lung cancer becomes visible to radiological detection is 0.8–1.0 cm. Lung cancer tumours are usually more or less spherical, and show margins that range from smooth to lobulated, irregular, or spiculated. Generalizations about correlating imaging findings and cell type are approximate at best.

In invasive non-mucinous adenocarcinoma of the lung, the tumour may appear at CT as entirely solid or as mixed solid and non-solid (ground-glass opacity), and very rarely, as non-solid only {2676}. The histological correlate to the solid component typically shows an invasive adenocarcinoma, and the non-solid component is a lepidic pattern. When an early-stage lung cancer (most commonly invasive adenocarcinoma) at CT contains both non-solid elements that correspond with lepidic growth and solid elements that mainly (but not necessarily exclusively) correspond with invasive growth, then postresectional prognosis correlates more closely with size of the solid component on the imaging study than with size of the non-solid component {1796}.

Multiple primary lung cancers are not uncommon, especially multiple adenocarcinomas, including invasive mucinous adenocarcinoma. These must be distinguished from metastatic disease to the lung.

Tumour spread
Tumour spread may occur through the lymphatic or haematogenous route. Lymphatic spread gives rise to involvement of ipsilateral and contralateral hilar and mediastinal lymph nodes, whereas blood-borne metastases are most frequently found in the liver, bone, brain, adrenal glands, and lungs. Metastatic tumour along the pleural surface is another route of metastatic spread, heralding a poor prognosis. Its current descriptor is M1a disease {2078}.

Aerogenous (air-space) tumour spread is also recognized. This includes an increasingly recognized pattern of invasion in lung adenocarcinoma, where tumour cells spread through air spaces (STAS) in the lung parenchyma, surrounding the outer edge of the tumour {1174A,1909,2276,2277}.

Staging
Lung adenocarcinomas are staged according to the standard TNM classification (see p. 11). Tumour size measurement for lepidic predominant tumours may require additional consideration. The Union for International Cancer Control (UICC) TNM Supplement states: "When size is a criterion for the T/pT category, it is a measurement of the invasive component." According to this concept, the lepidic component of lung adenocarcinomas should be excluded, and only the invasive component used for tumour size determination {2420}, although this is not the case with the American Joint Committee on Cancer (AJCC) Staging Manual (seventh edition) {652A}. In early-stage tumours, several studies suggest that invasive tumour size is an independent prognostic factor, and it may be a better predictor of prognosis than overall tumour size in lepidic predominant tumours {2701,2810,2983}.

Localization

The most common localization of invasive adenocarcinoma is in the lung periphery {2378}. Two recently published series of resected lung adenocarcinomas showed that all invasive adenocarcinoma subtypes were most often located in the lung periphery, while 33% of solid predominant, 25% of micropapillary predominant, and 20% of acinar predominant adenocarcinomas were localized centrally {2231,2232}.

Macroscopy

Most invasive adenocarcinomas appear as grey-white nodules with central scarring fibrosis associated with anthracotic pigmentation and pleural puckering {2699}. The peripheral lepidic component may result in a poorly defined border, and individual preserved alveolar spaces may be visible. In fresh unfixed specimens, lepidic tumour components may be difficult to discern.

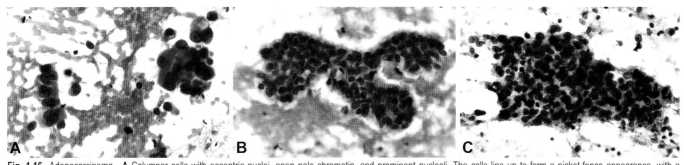

Fig. 1.16 Adenocarcinoma. **A** Columnar cells with eccentric nuclei, open pale chromatin, and prominent nucleoli. The cells line up to form a picket-fence appearance, with a shared luminal edge. Some cells have cytoplasmic mucin. **B** A branching group with a smooth border is a cytological reflection of papillary architecture. **C** Poorly differentiated adenocarcinoma can manifest as groups of overtly malignant cells with no clear morphological features of differentiation; this morphology is indistinguishable from poorly differentiated squamous cell carcinoma in the absence of ancillary studies.

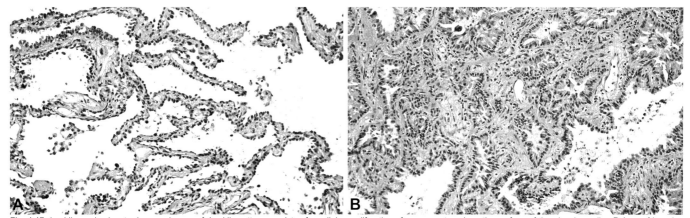

Fig. 1.17 Lepidic predominant adenocarcinoma. **A** Lepidic pattern consists of a cellular proliferation of pneumocytes along the surface of the alveolar walls. **B** Area of invasive acinar adenocarcinoma.

Cytology

In line with the histological heterogeneity of lung adenocarcinoma, the cytological features of these tumours are also highly variable. Glandular morphology may manifest as various arrangements of cells into an anatomical unit, including columnar cells lined up in a picket-fence arrangement, cells arranged in a flat honeycomb structure, and cells organized into three-dimensional cell balls or branching groups with a smooth luminal border (i.e. a community border) {2682}. The nuclei tend to be located in the periphery of the cytoplasm, and tend to have vesicular chromatin with prominent nucleoli. The cytoplasm is usually finely vacuolated, and cytoplasmic mucin may be present. Poorly differentiated adenocarcinomas with solid histology show nondescript, overtly malignant cells, usually in cohesive groups, which may be impossible to distinguish from non-keratinizing squamous cell carcinoma without ancillary studies {2135}. Nuclear grade on cytology has been shown to correlate

with the overall histological grade of lung adenocarcinomas {2396}, but cytological features appear to correlate poorly with individual histological patterns {2221}, particularly a single predominant pattern {2179}.

Histopathology

In 2011, a new IASLC/ATS/ERS classification of lung adenocarcinoma proposed significant changes to the 2004 WHO classification for resected tumours, including: 1) discontinuing the terms bronchioloalveolar carcinoma and mixed subtype adenocarcinoma; 2) adding adenocarcinoma in situ as a preinvasive lesion, to join atypical adenomatous hyperplasia; 3) adding minimally invasive adenocarcinoma; 4) classifying invasive adenocarcinomas according to the predominant subtype after comprehensive histological subtyping by semiquantitatively estimating the percentage of the various subtypes present, in 5% increments; 5) using the term lepidic for a non-invasive component (formerly

classified as bronchioloalveolar carcinoma) present as part of an invasive adenocarcinoma; 6) introducing the term invasive mucinous adenocarcinoma for adenocarcinomas formerly classified as mucinous bronchioloalveolar carcinoma, excluding tumours that meet the criteria for adenocarcinoma in situ or minimally invasive adenocarcinoma; 7) discontinuing the subtypes of clear cell and signet ring adenocarcinoma, and recognizing these as a feature when any amount is present, however small; and 8) discontinuing the term mucinous cystadenocarcinoma, and including these under the category of colloid adenocarcinoma {2672,2673,2676}.

In the current classification, undifferentiated carcinomas formerly classified as large cell carcinoma, but expressing pneumocyte immunohistochemical markers, are included, as are those showing mucin expression, in the category of solid adenocarcinoma (see *Large cell carcinoma*, p. 80).

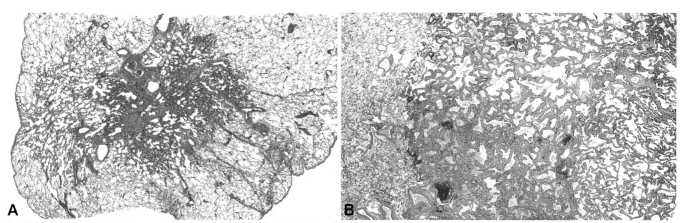

Fig. 1.18 Lepidic predominant adenocarcinoma. **A** and **B** Lepidic predominant pattern with mostly lepidic growth and a smaller area of invasive acinar adenocarcinoma.

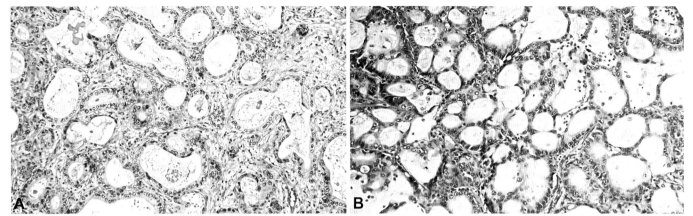

Fig. 1.19 Acinar adenocarcinoma. A Acinar adenocarcinoma consists of round to oval-shaped malignant glands invading a fibrous stroma. B Cribriform pattern of acinar adenocarcinoma.

Invasive adenocarcinomas account for > 70–90% of all surgically resected cases, with the variance reflecting differences in the prevalence of adenocarcinoma in situ and minimally invasive adenocarcinoma. Invasive adenocarcinomas characteristically consist of a complex heterogeneous mixture of histological subtypes, which often represent a morphological continuum rather than discrete compartments. This complexity has presented a great challenge historically, but one of the most important aspects of this classification is that it presents a practical approach to addressing this problem. Because of the continuum of morphology, it can be difficult to distinguish between morphological patterns; for example, lepidic versus acinar or papillary patterns and papillary versus micropapillary patterns. Nevertheless, since the principle of comprehensive histological subtyping was introduced in the 2011 IASLC/ATS/ERS classification, a growing number of studies of resected lung adenocarcinomas have demonstrated the classification's utility in identifying significant prognostic subsets and molecular correlations according to the predominant patterns {2231,2232,2810,2984}.

In the revised classification, the term predominant is appended to all categories of invasive non-mucinous adenocarcinoma, because most of these tumours are heterogeneous, consisting of mixtures of the histological subtypes. This replaces the use of the term adenocarcinoma, mixed subtype. Semiquantitative recording of the patterns in 5% increments encourages observers to identify all patterns that may be present, rather than focusing on a single pattern (e.g. lepidic growth). This comprehensive histological subtyping should be performed based on review of all histological sections of the tumour. Thus, this method provides a basis for determining the predominant pattern. Most previous studies on this topic used 10% increments, but 5% increments allow for greater flexibility in choosing a predominant subtype when tumours have two patterns of relatively similar percentages; it also avoids the need to use 10% for small amounts of components that may be prognostically important, such as micropapillary or solid patterns. Although it is theoretically possible to have equal percentages of two prominent components, in practice, a single predominant component should be chosen. Recording these percentages makes it clear to the reader of a report whether a tumour has relatively even mixtures of several patterns or a clear single predominant pattern.

Spread through air spaces (STAS), which may occur with micropapillary clusters, solid nests, or single cells, probably contributes to the significantly increased recurrence rate for patients with small stage I adenocarcinomas who undergo limited resections {1174A,1859}, and the worse prognosis observed by others {2276}. Because this represents a manifestation of tumour spread, it is not included in the percentage measurement of subtype patterns.

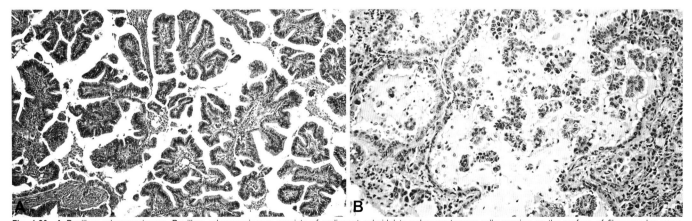

Fig. 1.20 A Papillary adenocarcinoma. Papillary adenocarcinoma consists of malignant cuboidal to columnar tumour cells growing on the surface of fibrovascular cores. B Micropapillary adenocarcinoma. These tumour cells are growing in papillae that lack fibrovascular cores.

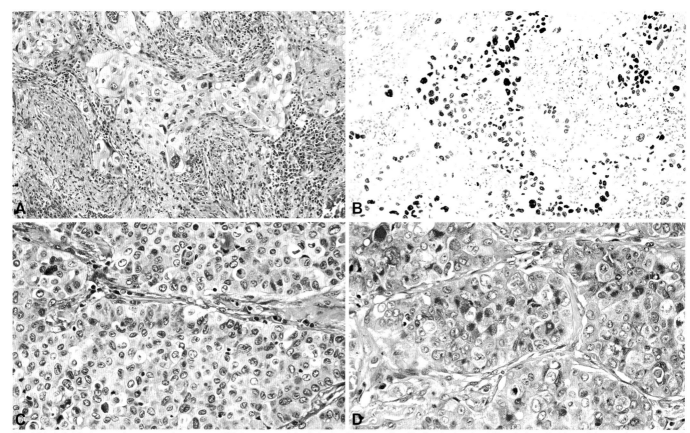

Fig. 1.21 A Solid adenocarcinoma, pseudosquamous. This tumour consists of sheets of tumour cells with abundant eosinophilic cytoplasm that is reminiscent of squamous cell carcinoma. **B** Solid adenocarcinoma, pseudosquamous. This solid adenocarcinoma has a squamous appearance, but is strongly positive for TTF1; p63 was negative. **C** Solid adenocarcinoma. This tumour consists of solid nests of large epithelial cells with abundant cytoplasm and prominent nucleoli; no mucin droplets are seen. **D** Solid adenocarcinoma. Mucin stain highlights numerous droplets of intracytoplasmic mucin, highlighted with mucicarmine stain.

A reproducibility study of selected images of the major lung adenocarcinoma subtypes circulated among a panel of 26 expert lung cancer pathologists documented kappa values of 0.77 ± 0.07 and 0.38 ± 0.14 for classical and difficult images, respectively {2636}. A recent study of reproducibility for predominant pattern showed moderate to good kappa values of 0.44–0.72 for pulmonary pathologists. For untrained pathologists, the kappa values were expectedly lower, ranging from 0.38 to 0.47, but these improved to 0.51–0.66 after a training session, and re-evaluation by the same reviewers led to very high kappa values of 0.79–0.87 {2811}.

Lepidic adenocarcinoma
This variant typically consists of bland pneumocytic cells (type II pneumocytes or Clara cells) growing along the surface of alveolar walls, similar to the morphology defined in the sections on minimally invasive adenocarcinoma and adenocarcinoma in situ. An invasive adenocarcinoma component is present in at least

one focus measuring > 5 mm in greatest dimension. If there are multiple foci of invasion, or invasive size is difficult to measure in a discrete focus, recent data suggest that another way to estimate the invasive size is to sum the percentage of the invasive components and multiply this by the overall tumour diameter {1179}. If the result is > 5 mm, a diagnosis of lepidic predominant adenocarcinoma should be rendered. Invasion is defined as: 1) histological subtypes other than a lepidic pattern (i.e. acinar, papillary, micropapillary and/or solid); 2) myofibroblastic stroma associated with invasive tumour cells; 3) vascular or pleural invasion; and 4) spread through air spaces. The diagnosis of lepidic predominant adenocarcinoma rather than minimally invasive adenocarcinoma is made if the cancer: 1) invades lymphatics, blood vessels, or pleura; 2) exhibits tumour necrosis; 3) contains an invasive component > 5 mm; or 4) shows spread through alveolar spaces in the lung parenchyma surrounding the tumour. It is understood that lepidic growth can

occur in metastatic tumours to the lung as well as in invasive mucinous adenocarcinomas. However, the specific term lepidic predominant adenocarcinoma in this classification defines a non-mucinous adenocarcinoma that has lepidic growth as its predominant component, and these tumours are now distinguished from invasive mucinous adenocarcinoma. The term lepidic predominant adenocarcinoma should not be used in the context of invasive mucinous adenocarcinoma with predominant lepidic growth. Lepidic growth may also be composed of neoplastic cells with nuclear atypia resembling that of the adjacent invasive patterns. Whether there is any clinical difference between these cases and those in which the lepidic tumour cells resemble type II pneumocytes or Clara cells is unknown.

Acinar adenocarcinoma
This variant shows a majority component of glands, which are round to oval-shaped with a central luminal space surrounded by tumour cells {2672,2673,2676}. The

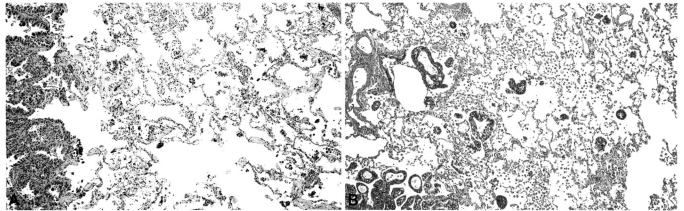

Fig. 1.22 Adenocarcinoma. **A** Spread through air spaces by tumour cells showing a micropapillary pattern in the lung parenchyma surrounding the edge of the tumour (left). **B** Micropapillary and ring patterns. At the edge of this adenocarcinoma, there is spread through air spaces in the form of micropapillary clusters and rings of tumour cells.

neoplastic cells and/or glandular spaces may contain mucin. Acinar structures may also consist of rounded aggregates of tumour cells with peripheral nuclear polarization and central cytoplasm without a clear lumen. When lepidic growth forms nests entrapped by collapse, such gland-like morphology may be difficult to distinguish from the acinar pattern. However, when the alveolar architecture is lost and/or myofibroblastic stroma is present, invasive acinar adenocarcinoma is considered to be present. Cribriform arrangements are regarded as a pattern of acinar adenocarcinoma, although this pattern is associated with poor prognosis {1180}.

Papillary adenocarcinoma
This variant shows a major component of a growth of glandular cells along central fibrovascular cores {2672,2673,2676}. This should be distinguished from tangential sectioning of alveolar walls in an area of lepidic adenocarcinoma. If tumour acini or alveolar spaces are filled with papillary or micropapillary structures, the tumour pattern is classified as papillary or micropapillary adenocarcinoma, respectively. Myofibroblastic stroma is not needed to diagnose this pattern.

Micropapillary adenocarcinoma
This variant has, as a major component, tumour cells growing in papillary tufts forming florets that lack fibrovascular cores {2672,2673,2676}. These may appear detached from and/or connected to alveolar walls. The tumour cells are usually small and cuboidal, with variable nuclear atypia. Ring-like glandular structures may float within alveolar spaces.

Vascular and stromal invasion is common. Psammoma bodies may be seen.

Solid adenocarcinoma
This variant shows a major component of polygonal tumour cells forming sheets that lack recognizable patterns of adenocarcinoma, i.e. acinar, papillary, micropapillary, or lepidic growth {2672,2673,2676}. If the tumour is 100% solid, intracellular mucin should be present in ≥ 5 tumour cells in each of two high-power fields, and confirmed with histochemical stains for mucin {2672,2673,2676}.
Tumours formerly classified as large cell carcinomas that have pneumocyte marker expression (i.e. TTF1 and/or napsin A), even if mucin is absent, are now classified as solid adenocarcinoma (see *Large cell carcinoma,* p. 80). Solid adenocarcinoma must be distinguished from squamous cell carcinomas and large cell carcinomas, both of which may show rare cells with intracellular mucin.

Immunohistochemistry
Currently, the most commonly used pneumocyte markers are TTF1 and napsin A. Approximately 75% of invasive adenocarcinomas are positive for TTF1 {2134,2465}. Among the adenocarcinoma patterns, most lepidic and papillary areas are positive for TTF1, whereas positivity is less common in solid predominant cancer {1174}. A close relationship between the *EGFR* mutation and TTF1 positivity in lung adenocarcinoma has also been reported {2951}. The sensitivity of napsin A is comparable with that of TTF1, although some reports have suggested that the former is superior for differentiating from squamous

cell carcinoma if positive reactions from entrapped pneumocytes are carefully excluded {1920}. p40, which is expressed in a strong, diffuse manner in squamous cell carcinoma, is a more specific squamous marker than p63, as the latter is also positive in up to 30% of lung adenocarcinomas {209,1870,2134}. It is worth noting that TTF1 is also expressed in other tumours, such as small cell lung cancer, large cell neuroendocrine carcinomas, some carcinoid tumours, and thyroid carcinomas. Napsin A is sometimes expressed in other tumours such as renal cell carcinoma.

Differential diagnosis
The differential diagnosis of lung adenocarcinoma involves: 1) distinction from other lung cancer types, 2) distinction of multiple lung primaries from intrapulmonary metastases, and 3) distinction between primary lung adenocarcinoma and metastases from extrapulmonary sites (see *Metastases to the lung,* p. 148).
Squamous cell carcinoma and large cell neuroendocrine carcinoma present the most frequent problems in differential diagnosis. Some solid adenocarcinomas have dense eosinophilic cytoplasm that resembles squamous cell carcinoma. Poorly differentiated resected tumours that may have a suggestion of squamous morphology, but that lack diagnostic squamous features such as keratinization, pearls, or intercellular bridges, may be correctly diagnosed using immunohistochemistry for TTF1 and a squamous marker such as p40 or p63 {209}. Some solid adenocarcinomas must be distinguished from large cell neuroendocrine carcinoma based on the criteria

summarized in *Large cell neuroendocrine carcinoma* (p. 69).

In addition, for multiple lung adenocarcinomas, comprehensive histological subtyping is one tool that can help in distinguishing intrapulmonary metastasis from synchronous or metachronous primaries {842}. However, additional features such as cytological characteristics (e.g. clear cell change and degree of atypia) and tumour stroma (e.g. desmoplasia and inflammation) can help address this problem {842}. The role of molecular testing in this setting is promising, but requires further study {27,453,842,843}.

Genetic profile

Several driver gene alterations are now known in lung adenocarcinomas, including EGFR {1530,1956,1974}, KRAS, BRAF {265,1958}, ERBB2/HER2 {78,2469}, ALK {2421}, ROS1 {2158}, RET {1485,2574,2966}, NTRK1 {2731}, and NRG1 {716}. Among these mutations, EGFR and ALK are the most clinically relevant, because approved molecular targeted drugs are available for patients whose tumours have these molecular abnormalities. HER2, ROS1, and NTRK1 share clinicopathological features with EGFR and ALK in terms of involvement that is nearly specific to adenocarcinoma in lung cancer, particularly frequent in TTF1-positive adenocarcinoma, and preferentially in never-smokers and in women. Because adenocarcinoma in never-smokers has clinical differences from adenocarcinoma in smokers {2505,2513}, the distinct characteristics are supported by unsupervised hierarchical clustering based on expression profiling analyses; adenocarcinomas with EGFR mutation are clustered in one of the branches, which shares the expression profile of the peripheral lung parenchyma {1759,2576}. To explain the distinct group of lung adenocarcinoma, the concept of a terminal respiratory unit has been proposed, because cancer arising from the anatomical unit has unique features in terms of morphology, immune profile, and susceptibility to these gene alterations {2950}. A potential stem cell population in the terminal respiratory unit, which is suggested to develop into a subset of lung adenocarcinoma through transformation, has been identified using a mouse model {830}. TTF1 is amplified in association with progression {2824}. Additional details on the spectrum of genomic alterations in invasive adenocarcinoma can be found in reports from large-scale genomic analyses {1076,2626}.

Unlike the specific genetic alterations seen in other tumours (such as sarcomas, lymphomas, and leukaemias), there are no specific histological–molecular correlations in lung cancer {2673,2676}. The strongest histological–molecular correlation is with invasive mucinous adenocarcinoma (see *Variants of invasive adenocarcinoma,* p. 38), where a high percentage of these tumours have KRAS mutations and lack EGFR mutations. EGFR and KRAS mutations, as well as, ALK rearrangement, can be seen in most of the invasive adenocarcinoma histological subtypes. EGFR mutations are most often seen in association with

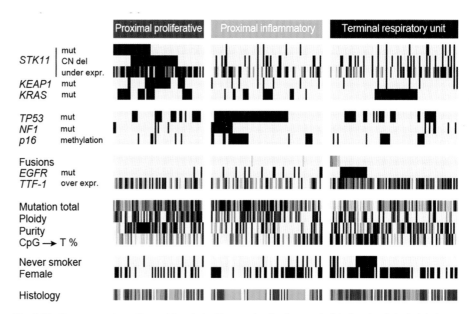

Fig. 1.23 Gene expression subtypes integrated with genomic alterations and clinical and pathological features. To coordinate the naming of the transcriptional subtypes with the histopathological, anatomical, and mutational classifications of lung adenocarcinoma, an updated nomenclature has been proposed: the terminal respiratory unit (formerly bronchioid), the proximal inflammatory (formerly squamoid), and the proximal proliferative (formerly magnoid) transcriptional subtypes. Reprinted from Collisson EA et al. The Cancer Genome Atlas Research Network {2626}.

Table 1.10 Characteristics of *EGFR* mutations in lung adenocarcinoma

The mutations occur in the kinase domain of the receptor tyrosine kinase, and lead to constitutive activation of downstream signalling without ligand.
Females and never-smokers are preferentially affected, but the biological basis for these associations is not well understood.
The two most common mutations – the point mutation at codon 858 (L858R) and the in-frame deletions in exon 19 – account for > 90% of cases, although many other mutations (such as mutations at codon G719 and in-frame insertions in exon 20) are reported in the literature.
These *EGFR* mutations are highly specific for lung adenocarcinoma. Among adenocarcinomas, *EGFR* mutations are frequently detected in cases with lepidic and papillary growth, and are associated with TTF1 positivity.
Genetic alterations of other major lung cancer driver genes such as *KRAS, ALK, ROS1, BRAF, RET,* and *ERBB2,* are mutually exclusive with *EGFR* mutations, presumably because these all converge on the same intracellular signalling pathways, and a single impairment in these pathways is sufficient to drive tumour formation.
Rare families with germline mutations, particularly *EGFR* T790M mutations, have higher risk of lung adenocarcinoma, which can be multifocal.
EGFR mutations in lung adenocarcinoma show ethnic differences, with prevalence ranges of 10–15% in Caucasians and 30–40% in Asians.
EGFR mutation is a prognostic factor as well as a factor predictive of response to *EGFR* tyrosine kinase inhibitor treatment.
Mutations in *EGFR* exon 20, in-frame insertions, and (rarely) T790M mutations, are associated with primary resistance to *EGFR* tyrosine kinase inhibitors, and acquisition of an additional T790M mutation is the most common cause of secondary resistance to *EGFR* tyrosine kinase inhibitors.

non-mucinous adenocarcinomas that are lepidic or papillary predominant, and there have been reports of an association with a micropapillary pattern {553,1759,1759,2951}. *KRAS* mutations are reported most often in tumours with a solid pattern, and can be present in tumours producing extracellular mucin {2133,2231,2984}. *ALK* rearrangement has been mostly associated with an acinar pattern (including a cribriform morphology), and with signet ring cell features {1443,2975}. In The Cancer Genome Atlas project, gene expression subtypes showed correlations between the terminal respiratory unit gene expression subtype and the lepidic subtype, and between the proximal inflammatory gene expression subtype and the solid subtype {2626}.

Prognosis and predictive factors

As for other subtypes of lung cancer, TNM classification and performance status significantly influence the choice of treatment, and strongly predict survival. Never-smoking status and female sex are favourable prognostic factors, independent from the stage of the disease.

Tumour size ≥ 2.5 cm, solid and micropapillary subtypes {357,2232,2810, 2983,2984}, and a maximal standardized uptake value of ≥ 7 are predictors of poor disease-free survival. The presence of the micropapillary subtype is a poor prognostic factor for overall survival {357}, and for recurrence in patients with limited resections {1859}.

Table 1.11 Characteristics of *ALK* gene fusions in lung cancer

Although *ALK* fusions are common in anaplastic large cell lymphoma and inflammatory myofibroblastic tumour, the specific *EML4-ALK* fusion is almost exclusively found in carcinomas of the lung.
ALK rearrangement in lung cancer is strongly associated with adenocarcinoma histology, in particular with acinar and/or solid growth pattern, or with cellular features of signet ring cell carcinoma.
EML4-ALK fusion accounts for > 90% of *ALK* rearrangements in lung adenocarcinomas. Other less common *ALK* fusion partners include *KIF5B*, *LKC1*, *TFG*, and others.
Like *EGFR* mutations, *ALK* rearrangement is frequent in never-smokers, but it is less associated with female sex.
The median age of patients with *ALK*-positive lung cancer is about 10 years younger than that of patients with *ALK*-negative cancer.
ALK-positive lung adenocarcinoma constitutes 4–5% of non-small cell lung carcinomas, and ethnic differences have not been reported, unlike with *EGFR* mutations.
ALK rearrangement is predictive of response to *ALK* inhibitor treatment, but is not a prognostic factor.

The prognosis for stage I lepidic predominant adenocarcinoma is excellent {2232,2699,2810,2983}, and most of the tumours that recur have some high-risk factor, such as a close margin in limited resection and presence of a micropapillary component, or invasion of blood vessels and/or pleura {1179}. In some studies, this prognostic significance is also preserved in more advanced stages {2810}. The relatively good prognosis of CT screen-detected lung cancer is driven by the predominance of early-stage adenocarcinomas with favourable histological features {738}.

Although several other clinical, biological, radiological, and molecular factors pertaining to the tumour or the patient have been investigated in individual studies, few have been demonstrated to be relevant in predicting response to therapy. The probabilities of response to an epidermal growth factor receptor tyrosine kinase inhibitor or to an ALK-inhibiting agent strongly correlate with the presence of an *EGFR* sensitizing mutation or an *ALK* rearrangement, respectively. These are more frequently found in patients with adenocarcinoma, and in never-smokers or former smokers. *EGFR* mutations are more common in Asian patients and women. Conversely, the presence of a *KRAS* mutation is usually associated with resistance to epidermal growth factor receptor tyrosine kinase inhibitors. Individual driver oncogene mutations are generally mutually exclusive; *EGFR* and *ALK*, while they are associated with similar clinical characteristics, do not generally occur in the same tumour {782,1149}. Solid and micropapillary histological subtypes are predictive of responsiveness to cisplatinum therapy {2690A}.

Variants of adenocarcinoma

W.D. Travis
Y. Yatabe
E. Brambilla
Y. Ishikawa
A.G. Nicholson
S.C. Aisner
J.H.M. Austin
M. Meyerson

Y. Nakatani
C.A. Powell
R. Rami-Porta
N. Rekhtman
G. Riely
G. Rossi
P. Russell
J. Samet

G. Scagliotti
E. Thunnissen
K. Tsuta
P. van Schil
A. Warth
I.I. Wistuba
D. Yankelevitz

Invasive mucinous adenocarcinoma

Definition
Invasive mucinous adenocarcinoma is an adenocarcinoma that includes cases formerly classified as mucinous bronchioloalveolar carcinoma, with tumour cells that have a goblet or columnar morphology and abundant intracytoplasmic mucin. Any growth pattern except solid may be seen – acinar, papillary, micropapillary, or lepidic – but the lepidic pattern is most common.

ICD-O codes
Invasive mucinous
  adenocarcinoma   8253/3
Mixed invasive mucinous and non-
  mucinous adenocarcinoma 8254/3

Synonyms
Mucinous bronchioloalveolar carcinoma; mucinous bronchoalveolar carcinoma; mucinous adenocarcinoma (invasive mucinous adenocarcinoma)

Epidemiology
The epidemiology is similar to that of other lung adenocarcinomas (see *Adenocarcinoma*, p. 26).

Clinical features

Signs and symptoms
See *Adenocarcinoma*, p. 26. Some patients with invasive mucinous adenocarcinomas manifest bronchorrhea.

Imaging
The imaging is similar to that for other invasive lung cancers (see *Adenocarcinoma*, p. 26). With invasive mucinous adenocarcinoma of the lung (formerly called mucinous bronchioloalveolar carcinoma), involvement in the lungs may be lobar or multilobar. A spectrum of findings exists, ranging from non-solid to mixed non-solid to solid, and may show consolidation that is either solid or nearly solid {105}. Air bronchograms are common.

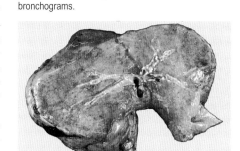

Fig. 1.24 Invasive mucinous adenocarcinoma. This CT shows a large area of consolidation with air bronchograms.

Fig. 1.25 Invasive mucinous adenocarcinoma. This lung is completely replaced by a tumour with a yellow, gelatinous appearance.

Tumour spread
See *Adenocarcinoma*, p. 26. There is a strong tendency for invasive mucinous adenocarcinoma to be multicentric, multilobar, and bilateral, which may reflect aerogenous spread.

Localization
Invasive mucinous adenocarcinoma occurs in the lung periphery {38,336}.

Macroscopy
Invasive mucinous adenocarcinoma appears as a poorly circumscribed, soft, gelatinous tumour without central desmoplastic fibrosis, anthracotic pigmentation, or pleural puckering. Some tumours manifest as widespread disseminated nodules or a diffuse pneumonia-like lobar consolidation.

Table 1.12 The difference between invasive mucinous adenocarcinoma and non-mucinous adenocarcinoma in situ (AIS)/minimally invasive adenocarcinoma (MIA)/lepidic predominant adenocarcinoma (LPA). The numbers given are the proportion of cases that are reported to be positive. Modified from Travis WD et al. {2676}

Characteristics	Invasive mucinous adenocarcinoma (formerly mucinous bronchioloalveolar carcinoma)	Non-mucinous AIS/MIA/LPA (formerly non-mucinous bronchioloalveolar carcinoma)
Female	60%	70%
Smoker	45%	45%
Radiographical appearance	Majority consolidation, air bronchogram, frequent multifocal and multilobar presentation	Majority ground-glass attenuation
Cell type	Mucin-filled, columnar, and/or goblet cells	Type II pneumocytes and/or Clara cells
Immunophenotype		
CK7	90%	95%
CK20	50%	5%
TTF1	15%	65%
Genotype		
KRAS mutation	75%	15%
EGFR mutation	< 5%	45%

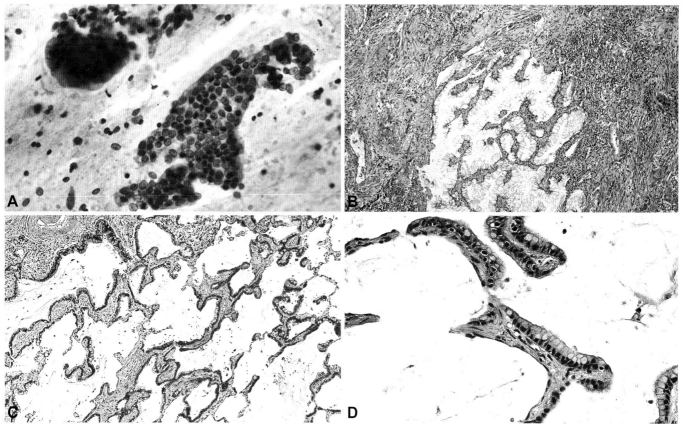

Fig. 1.26 Invasive mucinous adenocarcinoma. A Cytology shows monolayers of bland columnar cells forming a so-called drunken honeycomb, with uneven spacing of nuclei in the background of extracellular mucin. B This area of invasive mucinous adenocarcinoma demonstrates areas with lepidic and acinar patterns; there is also a fibrotic focus, which contains invasive tumour with a desmoplastic stroma. C This area of invasive mucinous adenocarcinoma demonstrates areas with lepidic and papillary patterns. D The tumour cells line alveolar walls and consist of cuboidal to columnar cells with abundant cytoplasmic mucin and small basally oriented nuclei.

Cytology

Invasive mucinous adenocarcinomas demonstrate particular cytological features – monolayers of bland columnar cells forming a so-called drunken honeycomb with uneven spacing of nuclei in a background of extracellular mucin {1740}.

Histopathology

Invasive mucinous adenocarcinoma has been introduced as a new category in the IASLC/ATS/ERS adenocarcinoma classification, because of distinct clinical, radiological, pathological, and genetic characteristics. The tumour was formerly called mucinous bronchioloalveolar carcinoma. Histologically, tumour cells characteristically show a goblet and/or columnar cell morphology with abundant intracytoplasmic mucin and small basally oriented nuclei. Nuclear atypia is usually inconspicuous or absent. Surrounding alveolar spaces often fill with mucin. The tumour may show the same heterogeneous mixture of lepidic, acinar,

papillary, and micropapillary growth as non-mucinous tumours, but it must be distinguished from adenocarcinomas that produce mucin but lack the characteristic goblet cell or columnar cell morphology. Although invasive mucinous adenocarcinoma often shows lepidic predominant growth, extensive sampling usually reveals invasive foci, sometimes with desmoplastic stroma. However, if in a resection specimen, a tumour with the characteristic cellular morphology fulfills the diagnostic criteria of adenocarcinoma in situ or minimally invasive adenocarcinoma, the tumour should be diagnosed as mucinous adenocarcinoma in situ or minimally invasive adenocarcinoma, respectively (see *Minimally invasive adenocarcinoma*, p. 44, and *Adenocarcinoma in situ,* p. 48), although such tumours are extremely rare. If there is ≥ 10% of each component, the tumour should be classified as mixed invasive mucinous and non-mucinous adenocarcinoma, with a description of the various components.

Immunohistochemistry

The immune profile of invasive mucinous adenocarcinoma is quite different from that of other adenocarcinoma subtypes. The tumour is typically positive for CK7 and CK20, and usually negative for TTF1 and napsin A {1414,2698,2910}. HNF4α has been shown to be expressed in this subtype {2508}.

Differential diagnosis

Invasive mucinous adenocarcinoma is distinguished from mucinous adenocarcinoma in situ and minimally invasive adenocarcinoma by the criteria described in *Minimally invasive adenocarcinoma* (p. 44) and *Adenocarcinoma in situ* (p. 48). Metastatic mucinous adenocarcinomas from sites such as the pancreas and ovary can appear morphologically identical to pulmonary invasive mucinous adenocarcinomas, so clinical and radiological correlation should be made to exclude primary tumours in these locations. Pancreatic mucinous adenocarcinomas are more likely to express CK20

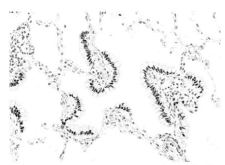

Fig. 1.27 Invasive mucinous adenocarcinoma. Positive immunohistochemical staining for HNF4α.

and MUC2 {447}. Metastatic colorectal adenocarcinomas often express CDX2 and CK20, with lack of CK7. Rarely, TTF1 can also be expressed {2138}.

Genetic profile
Invasive mucinous adenocarcinomas frequently show *KRAS* mutation (in up to 90% of cases) {724,974,1185}. Recent identification of *NRG1* fusions specific to invasive mucinous adenocarcinoma provides further evidence of a distinctive subtype {716,1802}.

Colloid adenocarcinoma

Definition
Colloid adenocarcinoma is an adenocarcinoma in which abundant mucin pools replace air spaces.

ICD-O code   8480/3

Synonyms
Mucinous cystic tumour of borderline malignancy; mucinous cystadenocarcinoma

Epidemiology
The epidemiology is similar to that of other lung adenocarcinomas (see *Adenocarcinoma*, p. 26).

Clinical features
See *Adenocarcinoma*, p. 26.

Imaging
The imaging is similar to that for other invasive lung cancers (see *Adenocarcinoma*, p. 26). Colloid type has a peculiar low-attenuation density at CT, and a mild heterogeneous FDG uptake at PET-CT. Cystic appearance with smooth margins partially bordered by a fibrous wall may occur.

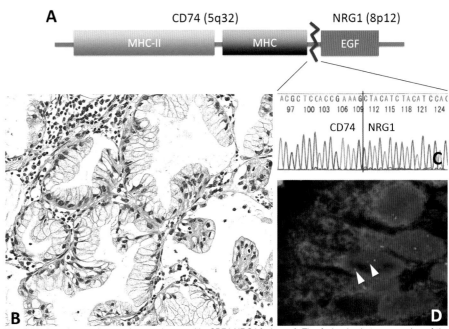

Fig. 1.28 Invasive mucinous adenocarcinoma with *CD74-NRG1* fusion. **A** The fusion leads to expression of the EGF-like domain of *NRG1 III-β3*, thereby providing the ligand for ERBB2/ERBB3 receptor complexes. **B** The fusion is specific to invasive mucinous adenocarcinoma. **C** A direct sequence of reverse transcriptase PCR transcript showed the fusion of *CD74* with *NRG1*. **D** Separate signals with *NRG1* break-apart FISH demonstrate *NRG1* rearrangement.

Tumour spread
See *Adenocarcinoma*, p. 26.

Localization
Colloid adenocarcinoma usually occurs in the lung periphery {2207}.

Macroscopy
Most colloid adenocarcinomas occur as peripheral masses. A soft, gelatinous, well-demarcated nodule with uni- to multilocular formation is observed. Cystic change may be seen.

Cytology
As in other sites, colloid adenocarcinomas manifest with copious pools of extracellular mucin and scant bland tumour cells, appearing either singly or in small clusters floating within mucin pools {1136}.

Histopathology
Colloid adenocarcinoma shows abundant extracellular mucin in pools, which distend alveolar spaces and destroy their walls, showing an overtly invasive growth pattern into the alveolar spaces. Mucin deposits enlarge and dissect the lung parenchyma, creating pools of mucin-rich matrix, while tumour elements consist of foci of tall columnar cells with goblet-like features growing in a lepidic

fashion. Tumour glands may float into the mucoid material. The tumour mucinous cells typically do not completely line the alveoli, and may be extremely well differentiated, resulting in a very challenging diagnosis on small biopsy or intraoperative examination. Epithelial pseudostratification of nuclei and frank cytological atypia may be observed, while the mitotic rate is often low and necrosis absent. Inflammatory infiltrate, with histiocytes and giant cell reaction, may be observed.

Immunohistochemistry
Colloid adenocarcinoma tumour cells generally express intestinal markers (i.e. CDX2, MUC2, and CK20). Weak and focal staining with TTF1 and CK7 may also

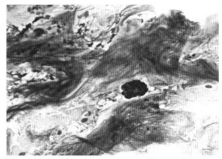

Fig. 1.29 Colloid adenocarcinoma. There are copious pools of extracellular mucin and scant bland tumour cells singly or in small clusters floating within mucin pools.

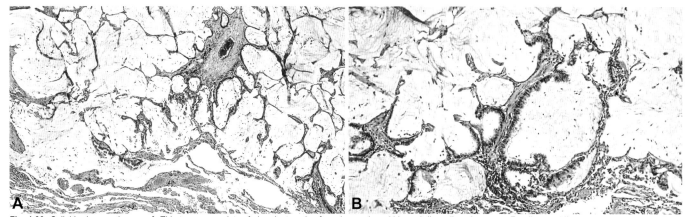

Fig. 1.30 Colloid adenocarcinoma. **A** This tumour consists of abundant pools of mucin growing within and distending air spaces. Focally well-differentiated mucinous glandular epithelium grows along the surface of fibrous septa and within the pools of mucin. **B** Tumour cells are inconspicuous, but line alveolar walls and are floating within pools of mucin.

be observed. Napsin A can be positive {2910}.

Differential diagnosis
Colloid adenocarcinomas differ from invasive mucinous adenocarcinoma in that in the former, mucin pools replace underlying alveolar architecture, and there are scattered clusters of mucinous tumour cells lining air spaces. Clinical correlation is needed to exclude a metastasis from the digestive tract, pancreas, ovary, or breast.

Fetal adenocarcinoma

Definition
Fetal adenocarcinoma is an adenocarcinoma resembling fetal lung. Low-grade tumours are pure in pattern, but high-grade tumours typically have at least 50% fetal morphology.

ICD-O code   8333/3

Synonyms
Pulmonary endodermal tumour resembling fetal lung; former pulmonary blastoma

Epidemiology
The epidemiology is similar to that of other lung adenocarcinomas (see *Adenocarcinoma*, p. 26). Patients with low-grade fetal adenocarcinomas tend to be young smokers. Low-grade fetal adenocarcinomas typically occur in younger patients than do other adenocarcinomas, with the peak incidence in the fourth decade of life, and with a mild female predisposition {1336,1806}. High-grade forms tend to occur in elderly male smokers {1806,2106}.

Clinical features
See *Adenocarcinoma*, p. 26.

Imaging
The imaging is similar to that for other invasive lung cancers (see *Adenocarcinoma*, p. 26).

Tumour spread
See *Adenocarcinoma*, p. 26.

Localization
Low-grade fetal adenocarcinoma tends towards a peripheral location {1806}

Macroscopy
The lesions are solitary, well-demarcated (but unencapsulated) pulmonary masses. The cut surface is bulging and white, tan, or brown, with areas of cystic change and haemorrhage.

Cytology
Fetal adenocarcinoma demonstrates subnuclear glycogen-rich vacuoles on Romanowsky staining, but not on Papanicolaou staining {813}.

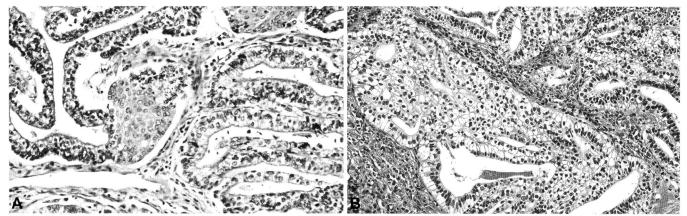

Fig. 1.31 A Low-grade fetal adenocarcinoma. This tumour consists of malignant glandular cells growing in tubules, and papillary structures with endometrioid morphology; some tumour cells have prominent clear cytoplasm, and squamoid morules are present. **B** High-grade fetal adenocarcinoma. This tumour shows complex acinar glands that consist of columnar tumour cells with supranuclear or subnuclear cytoplasmic clearing.

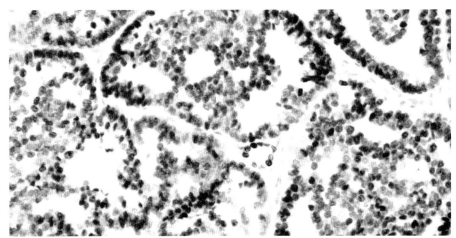

Fig. 1.32 Low-grade fetal adenocarcinoma. This fetal adenocarcinoma stains positively for TTF1.

Histopathology

Fetal adenocarcinoma consists of complex glandular structures composed of glycogen-rich, non-ciliated cells resembling a developing epithelium in the pseudoglandular phase of the fetal lung; low nuclear atypia; and morule formation {1806}.

Low-grade and high-grade fetal adenocarcinomas have been described {1752,1806}. The low-grade form displays low nuclear atypia and morule formation {1806}. The neoplastic glands are typically enveloped by a loose fibromyxoid stroma.

The high-grade form has been found to show more prominent nuclear atypia, a lack of morules, a transition to conventional adenocarcinoma, and necrosis {1806}. Often associated with other conventional types of adenocarcinoma, high-grade fetal adenocarcinoma is rendered as a diagnosis when this histology is predominant. The distinctive nature of the high-grade fetal adenocarcinoa has been questioned {1752}.

Immunohistochemistry

Low-grade fetal adenocarcinomas express TTF1, and aberrant nuclear localization of β-catenin and ERβ can be seen in biotin-rich optically clear nuclei {1807,1808,1809}. More than 90% of low-grade tumours harbour neuroendocrine cells expressing chromogranin A and/or synaptophysin, whereas only about 50% of high-grade tumours show such cells {1752,1806}. High-grade tumours frequently express α-fetoprotein, glypican 3, and SALL4 {1752,1806}.

Differential diagnosis

Fetal adenocarcinomas are distinguished from endometriosis by their malignant cytological features, frequent TTF1 expression, and lack of characteristic stroma that expresses estrogen receptor/progesterone receptor, in addition to the epithelial component. They are distinguished from metastatic endometrial adenocarcinoma by clinical evaluation and lack of estrogen receptor/progesterone receptor and PAX8 expression.

Genetic profile

Uniquely, low-grade fetal adenocarcinomas appear to be driven by mutations in the CTNNB1 gene, and the epithelial cells express aberrant nuclear and cytoplasmic staining for β-catenin by immunohistochemistry {1807,1809,2326}.

Upregulation of components in the Wnt signalling pathway (such as β-catenin) is important in low-grade fetal adenocarcinomas, as well as in biphasic pulmonary blastomas {2326}.

Enteric adenocarcinoma

Definition

Enteric adenocarcinoma is an adenocarcinoma that resembles the adenocarcinomas arising in the colorectum.

ICD-O code   8144/3

Synonyms

Pulmonary intestinal-type adenocarcinoma

Epidemiology

The epidemiology is similar to that of other lung adenocarcinomas (see *Adenocarcinoma*, p. 26).

Clinical features

Signs and symptoms

See *Adenocarcinoma*, p. 26. The diagnosis of primary pulmonary enteric adenocarcinoma requires careful clinical evaluation to exclude a colorectal primary, because the histological and immunohistochemical features can be identical {1410}.

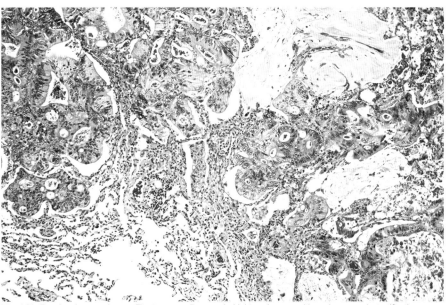

Fig. 1.33 Enteric adenocarcinoma. The tumour cells are cuboidal to columnar, with nuclear pseudostratification.

Imaging
The imaging is similar to that for other invasive lung cancers (see *Adenocarcinoma*, p. 26).

Tumour spread
See *Adenocarcinoma*, p. 26.

Localization
The few reported cases of enteric adenocarcinoma were all located in the lung periphery {1081}.

Macroscopy
Enteric adenocarcinomas are well-demarcated peripheral tumours described as white/grey firm masses with foci of yellow punctate necrosis {2799,2986}.

Cytology
Enteric adenocarcinomas share cytological and immunohistochemical features with colorectal carcinoma.

Histopathology
Primary pulmonary adenocarcinoma with enteric differentiation was first proposed by Tsao et al. {2690}, and a growing number of reports of enteric adenocarcinoma have been published {1081,1410,2799,2986}. The term enteric adenocarcinoma of the lung is now used for a tumour that resembles colorectal adenocarcinoma with acinar and/or cribriform architecture, and papillotubular (or garland-like) structures. Cytologically, there are eosinophilic, tall, columnar cells with a brush border and vesicular nuclei. Central geographical or dotted necrosis, occasional central scarring, and pleural indentation may be present. Since pulmonary adenocarcinoma is heterogeneous,

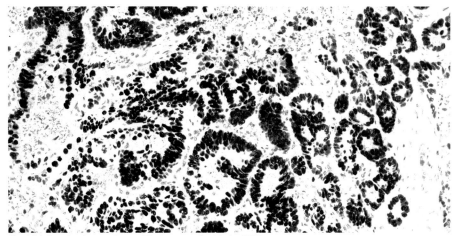

Fig. 1.34 Enteric adenocarcinoma. The tumour cells stain for CDX2.

this diagnosis is applied to tumours with an enteric pattern that is ≥ 50% made up of such histology. Histological resemblance to colorectal cancer is a hallmark of this tumour. Some tumours have enteric differentiation (i.e. positive CDX2 and CK20, and negative CK7), while others have only enteric morphology and an alternative immunoprofile.

Immunohistochemistry
Some enteric adenocarcinoma tumours have enteric differentiation (with expression of CDX2 and/or CK20 and CK7), while others lack this profile and have only enteric morphology. Villin may also be expressed {1475}.

Differential diagnosis
Enteric adenocarcinomas can be regarded as a lung primary only after clinical exclusion of an enteric primary in the gastrointestinal tract, since the immunoprofile may be identical. The differential

with metastatic colorectal adenocarcinoma can be complicated by the rare expression of TTF1 {2589}.

Signet ring and clear cell features
Both clear cell and signet ring features are regarded as cytological features rather than primary histological subtypes {2673,2676}. They both occur most commonly in the solid component of lung adenocarcinomas, but may also be seen in other patterns, such as acinar, papillary, and micropapillary adenocarcinoma. Therefore, these should not be included in predominant subtype or the summary of percentages for comprehensive histological subtyping, but rather can be mentioned at the end of the diagnosis as "with signet ring features" or "with clear cell features", along with the estimated percentage of this cytological change, even if it is very small.

Minimally invasive adenocarcinoma

W.D. Travis
M. Noguchi
Y. Yatabe
E. Brambilla
A.G. Nicholson
S.C. Aisner
J.H.M. Austin
M. Ladanyi

M. Meyerson
M. Mino-Kenudson
C.A. Powell
R. Rami-Porta
N. Rekhtman
G. Riely
G. Rossi
P. Russell

J. Samet
G. Scagliotti
E. Thunnissen
K. Tsuta
P. van Schil
A. Warth
I.I. Wistuba
D. Yankelevitz

Definition

Minimally invasive adenocarcinoma is a small (≤ 3 cm), solitary adenocarcinoma with a predominantly lepidic pattern and ≤ 5 mm invasion in greatest dimension. Minimally invasive adenocarcinoma is usually non-mucinous, but rarely may be mucinous. Minimally invasive adenocarcinoma (MIA) is, by definition, solitary and discrete.

ICD-O codes

Minimally invasive adenocarcinoma
    Non-mucinous   8256/3
    Mucinous   8257/3

Synonyms

Microinvasive adenocarcinoma; bronchioloalveolar carcinoma (obsolete)

Epidemiology

See *Adenocarcinoma*, p. 26.

Table 1.13 Diagnostic criteria for minimally invasive adenocarcinoma. Modified from Travis WD et al. {2673}

A small tumour (≤ 3 cm)
A solitary adenocarcinoma
Predominantly lepidic growth
Invasive component ≤ 0.5 cm in greatest dimension
The invasive component to be measured includes: - any histological subtype other than a lepidic pattern (such as acinar, papillary, micropapillary, solid, colloid, fetal, or invasive mucinous adenocarcinoma) and - tumour cells infiltrating myofibroblastic stroma.
The diagnosis of minimally invasive adenocarcinoma is excluded if the tumour: - invades lymphatics, blood vessels, air spaces, or pleura - contains tumour necrosis - spread through air spaces
The cell type is mostly non-mucinous (type II pneumocytes or Clara cells), but rarely may be mucinous (tall columnar cells with basal nuclei and abundant cytoplasmic mucin, sometimes resembling goblet cells).

Etiology

The factors implicated in the etiology of minimally invasive adenocarcinoma are similar to those involved in the etiology of adenocarcinoma in situ and conventional invasive adenocarcinoma.

Clinical features

Minimally invasive adenocarcinoma are usually discovered as an incidental finding on CT performed for other medical reasons. Minimally invasive adenocarcinoma is variable in its presentations, and more imaging correlative studies are needed, but when the tumour is non-mucinous, a provisional description is a part-solid nodule with a solid component, usually ≤ 5 mm.
If completely resected, these tumours are not expected to recur {232,1179,2962}. Minimally invasive adenocarcinoma is staged as T1a (mi).

Localization

Minimally invasive adenocarcinoma occurs in the lung periphery {2540}.

Macroscopy

Most minimally invasive adenocarcinomas occur at peripheral locations. The lesions show central, collapsed fibrosis and tumour with visible alveolar air spaces. Anthracotic pigmentation and pleural puckering may also be observed. Tumour size may be underestimated on gross examination, so correlation with high-resolution CT findings may be helpful for accurate size determination.

Cytology

It is not possible to cytologically differentiate minimally invasive adenocarcinoma from frankly invasive adenocarcinoma and preinvasive adenocarcinoma, because the cytological criteria for malignancy are the same {2673}. Although there are no studies on the cytological features of minimally invasive adenocarcinoma, features similar to those of

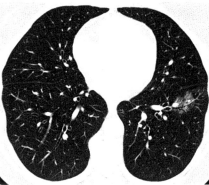

Fig. 1.35 Minimally invasive non-mucinous adenocarcinoma. CT section shows a peripheral, predominantly ground-glass, part-solid nodule in the right upper lobe. It includes a 4 × 3 mm solid component, which corresponded to invasion by pathology.

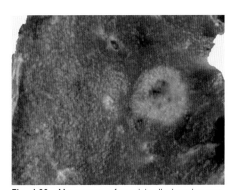

Fig. 1.36 Macroscopy of a minimally invasive non-mucinous adenocarcinoma. This tumour has a small central solid component (< 5 mm) corresponding to the invasive component, surrounded by a poorly defined area that represents the lepidic component.

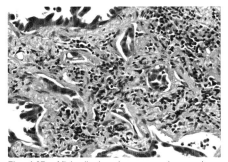

Fig. 1.37 Minimally invasive non-mucinous adenocarcinoma. These acinar glands are invading in the fibrous stroma.

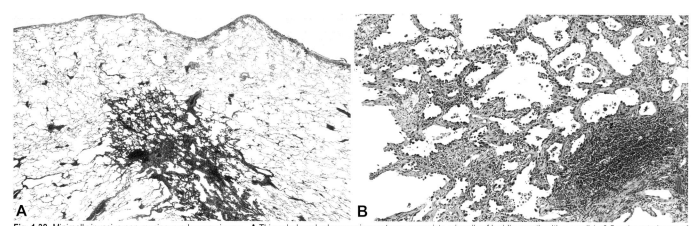

Fig. 1.38 Minimally invasive non-mucinous adenocarcinoma. **A** This subpleural adenocarcinoma tumour consists primarily of lepidic growth with a small (< 0.5 cm) central area of invasion. **B** This is the lepidic area of the tumour.

frankly invasive carcinoma and adenocarcinoma in situ would be expected. Typically, due to the small size and peripheral location of minimally invasive adenocarcinomas, percutaneous fine-needle aspiration biopsy is the most sensitive method for obtaining an adequate cytological and biopsy sample {2166}. As with frankly invasive adenocarcinoma, fine-needle aspiration biopsy of minimally invasive adenocarcinoma typically elucidates small tissue fragments and single cells with malignant features.

Histopathology

Minimally invasive adenocarcinoma is a small, solitary adenocarcinoma (≤ 3 cm), with a predominantly lepidic pattern and ≤ 5 mm invasion {2673,2676}. The size of the invasive area should be measured in the largest dimension {1179,2673}. If there are multiple foci of invasion, or invasive size is difficult to measure, recent data suggest that another way to estimate the invasive size is to sum the percentage of the invasive components and multiply this by the overall tumour diameter {1179}. If the result is ≤ 5 mm, a diagnosis of minimally invasive adenocarcinoma should be rendered.

Like adenocarcinoma in situ, minimally invasive adenocarcinoma is usually non-mucinous, but rarely, may be mucinous or mixed {232,1549,2962,2983}. Non-mucinous minimally invasive adenocarcinoma typically shows type II pneumocyte and/or Clara cell differentiation, and mucinous minimally invasive adenocarcinoma shows columnar cells with abundant apical mucin and small, often basally oriented nuclei, and may show goblet cell morphology. By definition, minimally invasive adenocarcinoma is solitary and

discrete. The invasive component to be measured in minimally invasive adenocarcinoma is defined as histological subtypes other than a lepidic pattern (i.e. acinar, papillary, micropapillary, and/or solid), or tumour cells infiltrating the my-ofibroblastic stroma. Minimally invasive adenocarcinoma is excluded if the tumour invades lymphatics, blood vessels, air spaces, or pleura; contains tumour necrosis; or spread through air spaces.

Immunohistochemistry

Although the number of reported series is limited, non-mucinous minimally invasive adenocarcinoma is known to be positive for pneumocyte markers, including TTF1

and napsin A. The immunoreactions of mucinous minimally invasive adenocarcinoma are similar to those of invasive mucinous adenocarcinoma: pneumocyte markers tend to be negative, whereas CK20 and HNF4A are positive. Mixed patterns associated with existing components are seen in both mucinous and non-mucinous minimally invasive adenocarcinoma.

Differential diagnosis

Minimally invasive adenocarcinoma must be distinguished from invasive adenocarcinomas. The diagnosis of adenocarcinoma in situ or minimally invasive adenocarcinoma should not be made unless

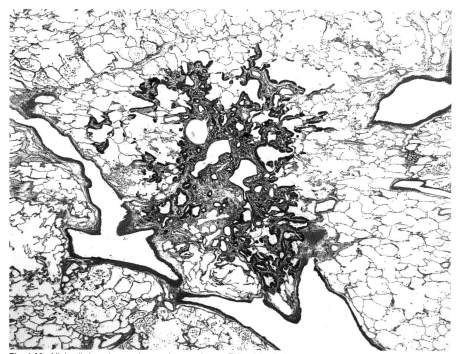

Fig. 1.39 Minimally invasive mucinous adenocarcinoma. This minimally invasive mucinous adenocarcinoma consists of a tumour showing lepidic growth and a small (< 0.5 cm) area of invasion. Reprinted from Travis WD et al. {2676}.

the lesion has a discrete circumscribed border; cases with miliary spread of small foci of tumour into adjacent lung parenchyma and/or with lobar consolidation should be excluded. Mucinous adenocarcinoma in situ and minimally invasive adenocarcinomas are extremely rare, and these diagnoses must be made with caution, because most tumours with this histological appearance are invasive mucinous adenocarcinomas (see *Variants of adenocarcinoma,* p. 38).

Because most of the literature on minimally invasive adenocarcinoma deals with tumours ≤ 2–3 cm, there is insufficient evidence that 100% disease-free survival can occur with minimally invasive adenocarcinoma tumours > 3 cm. These tumours can be classified as lepidic predominant adenocarcinoma, suspect minimally invasive adenocarcinoma.

Genetic profile

A multistep progression of lung adenocarcinoma is presumed, in which atypical adenomatous hyperplasia progresses to adenocarcinoma in situ, followed by invasive adenocarcinoma. Because minimally invasive adenocarcinoma is an early invasive adenocarcinoma, its genetic alterations may reveal early molecular events related to invasion. In addition to repression of *TGFBR2* and amplification of *PDCD6* and *TERT* {107,231}, *EGFR* amplification in association with the *EGFR* mutation is involved in the transition from adenocarcinoma in situ to minimally invasive adenocarcinoma {2384,2426,2952}.

Prognosis and predictive factors

Patients with tumours that meet the criteria for minimally invasive adenocarcinoma should have 100% disease-free and recurrence-free survival if the tumour is completely resected. Multiple successive studies have found that patients with these tumours had 100% disease-free survival {1179,1549,2673,2699}. It remains to be determined whether patients with minimally invasive adenocarcinoma still have 100% disease-free survival if the area of invasion shows a poorly differentiated component (such as solid or micropapillary adenocarcinoma), or if there is a giant cell and spindle cell component that does not meet the criteria for pleomorphic carcinoma.

Preinvasive lesions
Atypical adenomatous hyperplasia
Adenocarcinoma in situ

M. Noguchi
Y. Yatabe
E. Brambilla
A.G. Nicholson
S.C. Aisner
J.H.M. Austin
M. Ladanyi
M. Meyerson

M. Mino-Kenudson
C.A. Powell
R. Rami-Porta
N. Rekhtman
G. Riely
G. Rossi
P. Russell
J. Samet

G. Scagliotti
E. Thunnissen
W.D. Travis
K. Tsuta
P. van Schil
A. Warth
I.I. Wistuba
D. Yankelevitz

Atypical adenomatous hyperplasia

Definition

Atypical adenomatous hyperplasia is a small (usually ≤ 0.5 cm), localized proliferation of mildly to moderately atypical type II pneumocytes and/or Clara cells lining alveolar walls and sometimes respiratory bronchioles. Within the category of preinvasive lesions, atypical adenomatous hyperplasia is the counterpart of squamous dysplasia.

ICD-O code   8250/0

Synonyms

Obsolete: atypical alveolar hyperplasia; bronchial adenoma; atypical bronchioloalveolar hyperplasia; atypical alveolar epithelial hyperplasia; atypical alveolar cell hyperplasia

Epidemiology

See *Adenocarcinoma,* p. 26. *CYP19A1* polymorphisms have been shown to be associated with lung adenocarcinoma with atypical adenomatous hyperplasia, and this may play a role by causing differences in estrogen levels {1309}.

Clinical features

Atypical adenomatous hyperplasia is usually undetectable by imaging techniques. The lesions are typically incidentally found during examination of surgical specimens, most of which bear lung cancer. In autopsy studies, precursor lesions have been reported in 2–4% of patients not bearing cancer {2472,2965}. The rate is higher in surgical specimens from patients with lung cancer (up to 19% in women and 9.3% in men), particularly in cases of pulmonary adenocarcinoma (up to 30.2% in women and 18.8% in men) {395}. This increase has been explained as field cancerization, suggesting that adenocarcinoma and atypical adenomatous hyperplasia share a similar pathogenesis. Atypical adenomatous hyperplasia is usually not evident on CT, but may present as a faint, non-solid, focal nodule, usually ≤ 0.5 cm, but sometimes up to 1.2 cm.

Preinvasive lesions are locally slow-growing tumours without lymphatic/vascular invasion or distant metastases. When the lesions are completely resected, disease-free survival is 100% {1179,2753}. Atypical adenomatous hyperplasia is not included in TNM staging.

Localization

Atypical adenomatous hyperplasia occurs in the peripheral lung – very often close to the pleura {1798,1865}.

Macroscopy

Atypical adenomatous hyperplasia is most often an incidental microscopic finding, but when seen grossly, it is a millimetre-sized, poorly defined, tan-yellow nodule.

Histopathology

Atypical adenomatous hyperplasia is a small localized lesion (usually ≤ 0.5 cm) often arising in the centriacinar region, close to respiratory bronchioles. Mildly to moderately atypical type II pneumocytes and/or Clara cells proliferate along alveolar walls. Inconspicuous pseudopapillae may also be present {1679,2673,2676}. Clara cells are recognized as columnar, with cytoplasmic snouts and pale eosinophilic cytoplasm. Type II pneumocytes are cuboidal or dome-shaped, with fine cytoplasmic vacuoles or clear to foamy cytoplasm. Intranuclear eosinophilic inclusions may be present. There are gaps along the surface of the basement membrane between the cells, which consist of rounded, cuboidal, low columnar or so-called peg cells with round to oval nuclei. Double nuclei are common, and mitoses are extremely rare. There is a continuum of morphological changes between atypical adenomatous hyperplasia and adenocarcinoma in situ {1274,1744,2673,2676}. A spectrum of cellularity and atypia occurs in atypical adenomatous hyperplasia. Although atypical adenomatous hyperplasia has sometimes been classified into low- and high-grade types {1306,1799}, such grading is not recommended {2676}. Distinction between more cellular and cytologically atypical adenomatous hyperplasia and adenocarcinoma in situ can be difficult. The 0.5 cm size is not an absolute

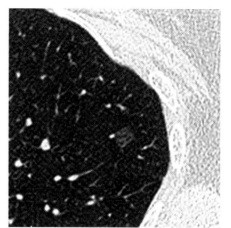

Fig. 1.40 Atypical adenomatous hyperplasia. CT shows 4 mm focal ground-glass opacity.

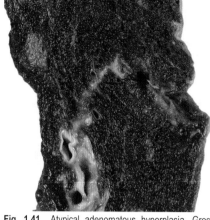

Fig. 1.41 Atypical adenomatous hyperplasia. Gross view shows a 5 mm, poorly defined, tan nodule, in the subpleural lung parenchyma.

criterion, so multiple characteristics in addition to size, including architectural and cytological features, are needed to make this distinction. Atypical adenomatous hyperplasia expresses TTF1 {1275}.

Differential diagnosis

Atypical adenomatous hyperplasia must be distinguished from reactive pneumocyte hyperplasia secondary to parenchymal inflammation or fibrosis in which the alveolar lining cells are not the dominant feature and are more diffusely distributed. It is unusual for atypical adenomatous hyperplasia to occur in the setting of interstitial fibrosis and inflammation. Distinguising atypical adenomatous hyperplasia from non-mucinous adenocarcinoma in situ can be difficult. Adenocarcinoma in situ is usually larger (> 5 mm), with a more cellular, crowded, homogeneous, cuboidal or columnar cell population. There is usually a less graded, more abrupt transition to the adjacent alveolar

lining cells in adenocarcinoma in situ.

Genetic profile

Atypical adenomatous hyperplasia is difficult to distinguish from reactive pneumocyte hyperplasia, although ploidy and clonality studies have shown a clonal/neoplastic nature for this lesion {1811,1855}. Atypical adenomatous hyperplasia has been reported to harbour driver mutations such as *KRAS* and *EGFR*, supporting the notion that atypical adenomatous hyperplasia is a direct precursor lesion of lung adenocarcinoma. *KRAS* and *EGFR* mutations were found in up to 33% and 35%, respectively, of atypical adenomatous hyperplasia specimens, suggesting an early event of peripheral adenocarcinoma {2256,2426,2563,2977}. These rates of *KRAS* and *EGFR* mutations are slightly different than those seen in adenocarcinoma in situ and invasive adenocarcinoma.

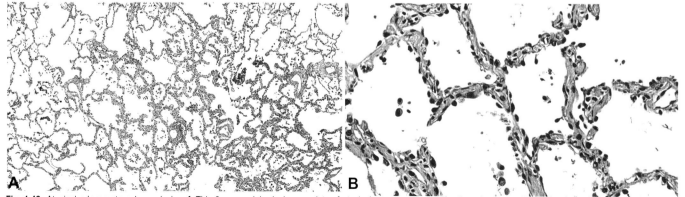

Fig. 1.42 Atypical adenomatous hyperplasia. **A** This 3 mm nodular lesion consists of atypical pneumocytes proliferating along pre-existing alveolar walls; there is no invasive component. **B** The slightly atypical pneumocytes are cuboidal, and show gaps between the cells.

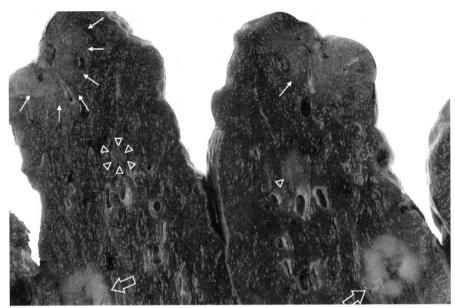

Fig. 1.43 Macroscopic comparison of atypical adenomatous hyperplasia, adenocarcinoma in situ, and invasive adenocarcinoma. The two cut surfaces are arranged as a mirror image. From top to bottom: adenocarcinoma in situ (thin arrows), atypical adenomatous hyperplasia (arrowheads), and invasive adenocarcinoma (bold arrows) are seen.

Prognosis and predictive factors

Patients with resected atypical adenomatous hyperplasia are cured. Since these lesions must be removed before the diagnosis can be established, there are no data demonstrating in vivo progression to adenocarcinoma in situ, minimally invasive adenocarcinoma, or invasive adenocarcinoma. However, since the lesions are frequently found in non-neoplastic lung adjacent to resected lung cancers, and often in patients with multiple adenocarcinomas, it is well accepted that this progression likely occurs in a subset of lung adenocarcinomas {2538}. However, the prognosis for lung adenocarcinomas with atypical adenomatous hyperplasia has not been shown to be different from the prognosis for those without atypical adenomatous hyperplasia {2537}.

Adenocarcinoma in situ

Definition
Adenocarcinoma in situ is a small (≤ 3 cm), localized adenocarcinoma with growth restricted to neoplastic cells along pre-existing alveolar structures (pure lepidic growth), and lacking stromal, vascular, or pleural invasion. Invasive patterns such as acinar, papillary, solid or micropapillary patterns and intra-alveolar tumour cells are absent. Adenocarcinoma in situ is mostly non-mucinous but rare mucinous cases occur.

ICD-O code
Adenocarcinoma in situ	8140/2
Non-mucinous	8250/2
Mucinous	8253/2

Synonym
Bronchioloalveolar carcinoma (obsolete)

Epidemiology and etiology
See *Adenocarcinoma*, p. 26, and *Atypical adenomatous hyperplasia*, p. 46.

Clinical features
Adenocarcinoma in situ is usually an incidental finding on CT performed for other medical reasons.

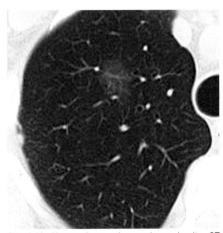

Fig. 1.44 Non-mucinous adenocarcinoma in situ. CT shows a circumscribed ground-glass nodule lacking any solid component.

The tumours are usually ≤ 2 cm, but can be up to 3 cm. By CT they are characteristically non-solid, but may be part-solid or even solid, especially in mucinous adenocarcinoma in situ. Adenocarcinoma in situ may have a so-called bubble-like appearance on CT{105}.

Preinvasive lesions are locally slowly growing tumours without lymphatic/vascular invasion or distant metastases. When the lesions are completely resected, disease-free survival is 100% {1179,2753}.

Although the current TNM classification does not address adenocarcinoma in situ in the lung, if the TNM staging principles for other tumours such as breast cancer were applied, adenocarcinoma in situ would be classified as Tis. Because carcinoma in situ can occur with both lung squamous cell carcinoma and adenocarcinoma, these should be further specified as Tis (squamous) or Tis (adenocarcinoma).

Localization
Adenocarcinoma in situ occurs in the peripheral lung – very often close to the pleura {1798,1865}.

Macroscopy
Adenocarcinoma in situ is a poorly defined nodule measuring up to 3 cm in size, with a tan or pale cut surface. The tumour should be completely sampled and microscopically examined to confirm that there is no invasive component.

Table 1.14 Diagnostic criteria for adenocarcinoma in situ. Reprinted from Travis WD et al. {2673}

A small tumour ≤ 3 cm
A solitary adenocarcinoma
Pure lepidic growth
No stromal, vascular, or pleural invasion
No pattern of invasive adenocarcinoma (such as acinar, papillary, micropapillary, solid, colloid, enteric, fetal, or invasive mucinous adenocarcinoma)
No spread through air spaces
Cell type mostly nonmucinous (type II pneumocytes or Clara cells), rarely may be mucinous (tall columnar cells with basal nuclei and abundant cytoplasmic mucin, sometimes resembling goblet cells)
Nuclear atypia is absent or inconspicuous.
Septal widening with sclerosis/elastosis is common, particularly in non-mucinous adenocarcinoma in situ.

Cytology

The typical cytological features of non-mucinous adenocarcinoma in situ include low-grade (i.e. bland, small, and monomorphous) nuclei, fine chromatin, inconspicuous pinpoint nucleoli, nuclear grooves, nuclear pseudoinclusions, and cell arrangement in orderly strips and small flat monolayers {104,1893,2768}. Overall, the cytological features can closely resemble those of papillary thyroid carcinoma. Tumour cells are often admixed with alveolar macrophages. As with small biopsies, specific diagnosis of adenocarcinoma in situ cannot be made in cytological specimens, because the presence of an unsampled higher-grade invasive component cannot be excluded. Low-grade adenocarcinomas with other patterns, particularly the papillary pattern, can also have overlapping cytological features.

Because of bland cytology, the distinction of adenocarcinoma in situ from benign cellular elements (including reactive pneumocytes and mesothelial cells) is a challenging diagnostic issue {3006}.

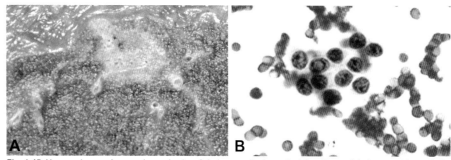

Fig. 1.45 Non-mucinous adenocarcinoma in situ. **A** A circumscribed, poorly defined tan nodule is present beneath the pleura. **B** Papanicolaou staining of percutaneous fine-needle aspirate of a histologically confirmed adenocarcinoma in situ shows a flat group of bland, uniform epithelial cells with minimal cytological atypia. The nuclei have fine, evenly distributed chromatin and pin-point nucleoli. An intranuclear inclusion is seen.

Mucinous adenocarcinoma in situ is extremely rare, but would be expected to show features similar to those of invasive mucinous adenocarcinoma (see *Variants of Adenocarcinoma*, p. 38).

Histopathology

Adenocarcinoma in situ is a localized, small (≤ 3 cm) adenocarcinoma with growth restricted to neoplastic cells along pre-existing alveolar structures (lepidic growth), lacking stromal, vascular, alveolar space, or pleural invasion. Papillary or micropapillary patterns are absent, similar to atypical adenomatous hyperplasia. Intra-alveolar tumour cells, either within the tumour or spread in air spaces in the surrounding parenchyma, are absent. Adenocarcinoma in situ is subdivided into non-mucinous and mucinous variants. Virtually all cases of adenocarcinoma in situ are non-mucinous, typically showing type II pneumocyte and/or Clara cell differentiation.

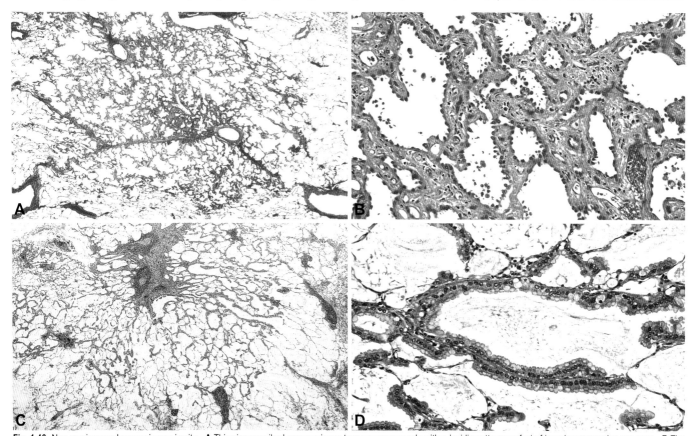

Fig. 1.46 Non-mucinous adenocarcinoma in situ. **A** This circumscribed non-mucinous tumour grows purely with a lepidic pattern; no foci of invasion or scarring are seen. **B** The atypical pneumocytes are crowded, and have slightly hyperchromatic nuclei. **C** This mucinous adenocarcinoma in situ consists of a nodular proliferation of mucinous columnar cells growing in a purely lepidic pattern; although there is a small central scar, no stromal or vascular invasion is seen. **D** The tumour cells consist of cuboidal to columnar cells with abundant apical mucin and small basally oriented nuclei. C and D reprinted from Travis et al. {2676}

However, there is no recognized clinical significance to the distinction between type II pneumocytes and Clara cells, so this morphological distinction is not recommended. The very rare cases of mucinous adenocarcinoma in situ that present as a solitary nodule (≤ 3 cm), consist of tall columnar cells with basal nuclei and abundant cytoplasmic mucin; sometimes they resemble goblet cells. Nuclear atypia is minimal or may be low-grade in non-mucinous adenocarcinoma in situ but is virtually absent in mucinous adenocarcinoma in situ. Alveolar septal widening with sclerosis/elastosis is common in adenocarcinoma in situ, particularly the non-mucinous variant. Lesions that meet the criteria for adenocarcinoma in situ have formerly been classified as bronchioloalveolar carcinoma according to the strict definition of the 1999 and 2004 WHO classifications, and type A and B adenocarcinoma according to the 1995 Noguchi classification {1865,2676}. The criteria for adenocarcinoma in situ can be applied in the setting of multiple tumours only if the other tumours are regarded as synchronous primaries rather than intrapulmonary metastases. Adenocarcinoma in situ expresses TTF1 {1275} and napsin A.

Differential diagnosis
Non-mucinous adenocarcinoma in situ must be distinguished from minimally invasive adenocarcinoma. The distinction between mucinous adenocarcinoma in situ and minimally invasive adenocarcinoma is similar, in that invasive foci should be identified. Clinical correlation is needed to exclude a metastatic mucinous adenocarcinoma from sites such as the pancreas.

Small size (≤ 3 cm) and a discrete circumscribed border is important to exclude cases with miliary spread into adjacent lung parenchyma and/or lobar consolidation, particularly for mucinous adenocarcinoma in situ.

Because most of the literature on adenocarcinoma in situ deals with tumours ≤ 2–3 cm, there is insufficient evidence that 100% disease-free survival can occur with adenocarcinoma in situ tumours > 3 cm. These tumours should be classified as lepidic predominant adenocarcinoma, suspect adenocarcinoma in situ.

Genetic profile
In the multistep progression model, adenocarcinoma in situ is an intermediate step between precursor lesion, atypical adenomatous hyperplasia, and minimally invasive adenocarcinoma. Because driver mutations are involved in early lung cancer development, driver mutations similar to those seen in early invasive adenocarcinoma may be seen in adenocarcinoma in situ. Because the definition of adenocarcinoma in situ was established so recently, there are only sparse data published on the topic, but they show 40–86% and 0–4% of *EGFR* and *KRAS* mutations, respectively, in adenocarcinoma in situ {2699,2984}. In terms of progression-associated genes, the molecular pathogenesis of the progression from atypical adenomatous hyperplasia to adenocarcinoma in situ remains unclear, because atypical adenomatous hyperplasia can be confirmed only with resected specimens, which precludes further progression.

Prognosis and predictive factors
Patients with adenocarcinoma in situ should have 100% disease-free and re-currence-free survival if the lesion is completely resected {1179,1865,2676,2699}. These non-invasive lesions can be carefully observed when detected on chest CT as pure ground-glass opacities < 1 cm {1789}. However, if the size or density increases, surgical resection should be considered. Although results of randomized trials are not yet available, sublobar resections (i.e. anatomical segmentectomy or wide wedge excision) may be valid oncological procedures on the condition that complete resection is achieved {2753}. In the prospective Japan Clinical Oncology Group 0201 study, radiological non-invasive peripheral lung adenocarcinoma could be defined as an adenocarcinoma of ≤ 2 cm with ≤ 25% of the tumour diameter showing consolidation (solid appearance) {2536}.

Squamous cell carcinoma

M-S. Tsao
E. Brambilla
A.G. Nicholson
K.J. Butnor
N.E. Caporaso
G. Chen
T-Y. Chou
S.S. Devesa

P. Hainaut
J. Jen
J. Jett
M. Ladanyi
M. Meyerson
D. Naidich
M. Noguchi
C.A. Powell

R. Rami-Porta
N. Rekhtman
V. Roggli
A. Takano
E. Thunnissen
W.D. Travis
P. van Schil
I.I. Wistuba

Definition
Squamous cell carcinoma is a malignant epithelial tumour that either shows keratinization and/or intercellular bridges, or is a morphologically undifferentiated non-small cell carcinoma that expresses immunohistochemical markers of squamous cell differentiation.

ICD-O codes
Squamous cell carcinoma   8070/3
Keratinizing squamous
   cell carcinoma   8071/3
Non-keratinizing
   squamous cell carcinoma   8072/3

Synonym
Epidermoid carcinoma

Epidemiology
See *Adenocarcinoma*, p. 26. Like all lung cancers (but to a significantly higher degree than adenocarcinoma), squamous cell carcinoma is strongly associated with smoking, and worldwide trends in squamous cell carcinoma incidence closely mirror changes in smoking patterns {1705}.

Etiology
For details, see *Adenocarcinoma*, p. 26. Large-scale epidemiological studies and meta-analyses have shown that squamous cell carcinoma is related to smoking amount, duration, starting age, and tar level, as well as to the fraction smoked {1993}. Although many occupational agents and exposures (including heavy metals and radon) have been associated with lung cancer, greater association of arsenic exposure with squamous cell carcinoma has been reported {921,1044,1591,2553}. There is a large body of literature on the association of lung cancer with HPV infection {1280,2450}, but it remains controversial whether this is actually a significant etiological factor, because several studies with rigorously controlled HPV detection protocols and exclusion of metastases from cervical or

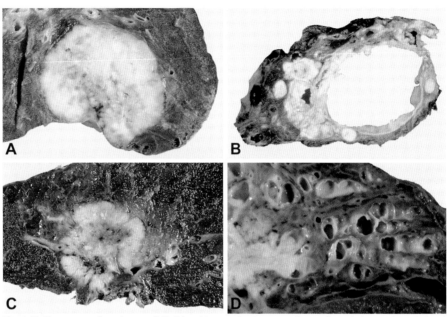

Fig. 1.47 Squamous cell carcinoma. **A** Peripheral tumour showing expansile growth, central necrosis, and pleural puckering. **B** Marked cavitation of a tumour arising in an 18-year-old male with HPV11 infection and papillomatosis. **C** Central tumour arising in a lobar bronchus with bronchial and parenchymal invasion and central necrosis. **D** Central tumour with extensive distal obstructive changes, including bronchiectasis.

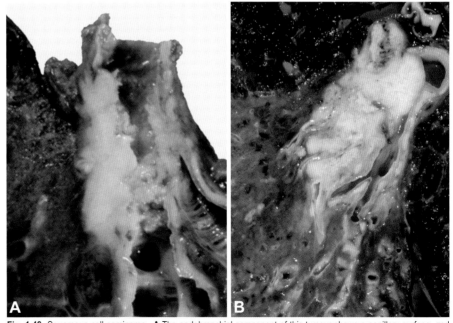

Fig. 1.48 Squamous cell carcinoma. **A** The endobronchial component of this tumour shows a papillary surface, and the tumour has invaded through the bronchial wall superficially into the surrounding lung. Note the postobstructive bronchiectasis. **B** Central tumour arising in the proximal left lower lobe bronchus. Contiguous intralobar lymph node invasion, obstructive lipoid pneumonia, and mucopurulent bronchiectasis in the basal segments.

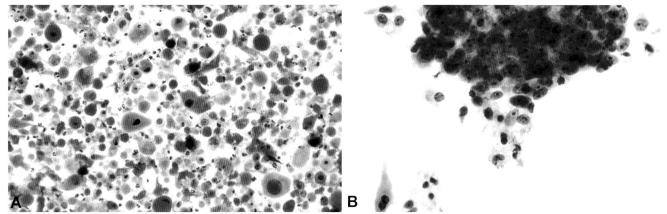

Fig. 1.49 Squamous cell carcinoma. **A** With Papanicolaou staining of keratinizing squamous cell carcinoma, keratinization manifests as dense cytoplasm with bright yellow-orange-red colour. The cells have dark pyknotic nuclei. The dirty background with many anucleated ghost cells is characteristic. **B** Papanicolaou staining of poorly differentiated squamous cell carcinoma with minimal keratinization shows that the majority of tumour cells are non-keratinizing. The cells have open chromatin with prominent nucleoli. This morphology is indistinguishable from that of poorly differentiated adenocarcinoma, except for the focal evidence of cytoplasmic keratinization seen in the lower-left corner. Reprinted from Travis WD, Rekhtman N {2682}.

oropharyngeal cancers have questioned the association, at least in western populations {208,1331,2738,2933}.

Clinical features

The signs, symptoms, and imaging of keratinizing and non-keratinizing squamous cell carcinoma are similar to those of other non-small cell lung carcinomas (see *Adenocarcinoma*, p. 26).

Squamous cell carcinomas are aggressive tumours with spread similar to other non-small cell lung carcinomas (see *Adenocarcinoma*, p. 26). Distant metastases are common.

The tumours are staged according to the TNM classification {866} (see *Staging and grading*, p. 14).

Uncommonly, squamous cell carcinoma manifests as a superficial spreading tumour. As long as the invasive component is limited to the bronchial wall, superficial spreading tumours are classified as T1a, irrespective of size and whether or not they extend to the main bronchus {654}. Squamous cell carcinoma has a tendency to be locally aggressive, involving

adjacent structures through direct invasion. For central tumours, the proximity to the carina is an important element to plan treatment; however, accurate determination of this cannot be established by pathological examination of a pneumonectomy specimen alone, and requires integration of bronchoscopic, operative, and/or imaging data.

Localization

Both keratinizing and non-keratinizing squamous cell carcinomas usually arise in a main or lobar bronchus. Historically, two thirds of the tumours were described as arising in the central portion of the lung, and one third in the periphery. However, one study found that peripheral locations were slightly more common {774}.

Macroscopy

The tumours are usually white or grey, and frequently soft and friable. With increased severity of desmoplasia, they may become firm with focal carbon pigment deposits in the centre and star-like retractions on the periphery. The tumours

may grow to a large size, and may cavitate due to central necrosis. Central tumours form intraluminal polypoid masses and/or infiltrate through the bronchial wall into the surrounding tissues. They may occlude the bronchial lumen, resulting in stasis of bronchial secretions, atelectasis, bronchial dilatation, obstructive lipoid pneumonia, and infective bronchopneumonia {477,494,2445,2672}.

Cytology

The cytological features of pulmonary squamous cell carcinoma are similar to those of squamous cell carcinoma of other sites, and depend on the grade of the tumour {1273}. Well-differentiated squamous cell carcinomas show obvious keratinization, manifesting as dense refractile cytoplasm with red, orange, yellow, or light blue colour in Papanicolaou staining, and robin's egg blue in Romanowsky staining. Unlike squamous cell carcinoma of the cervix or the head and neck, pulmonary squamous cell carcinomas are typically not diffusely keratinized; in most cases, evidence of

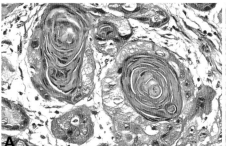
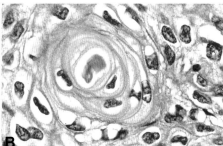
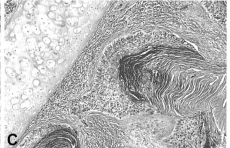

Fig. 1.50 Keratinizing squamous cell carcinoma. Squamous differentiation in these cytologically malignant cells is manifest by: **(A)** squamous pearls, **(B)** distinct intercellular bridges, or **(C)** layers of keratin. Reprinted from Travis WD et al. {2678}.

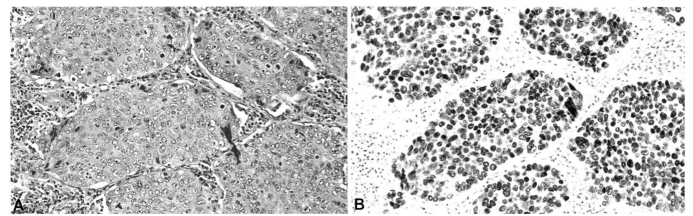

Fig. 1.51 Non-keratinizing squamous cell carcinoma. **A** Non-keratinizing squamous cell carcinoma confirmed by (**B**) diffuse p40 immunostaining. Reprinted from Drilon A et al. {626A}.

cytoplasmic keratinization is only focal The nuclei of well-differentiated squamous cell carcinoma typically have dark, non-transparent chromatin, without obvious nuclear detail and without prominent nucleoli. Spindle cell shapes are common. Extensive necrosis and inflammation is also common, which at low power can closely resemble necrotizing granuloma. Cells are usually present both singly and in large multilayered sheets. Poorly differentiated squamous cell carcinoma has significant morphological overlap with poorly differentiated adenocarcinoma: cytoplasmic keratinization is absent or inapparent, and nuclei may have open chromatin with prominent nucleoli. In this

setting, immunostaining is needed for the distinction from adenocarcinoma.

Histopathology

Squamous cell carcinoma may be keratinizing or non-keratinizing. Keratinizing squamous cell carcinoma is recognized by the presence of keratinization, pearl formation, and/or intercellular bridges. These features vary with degree of differentiation; they are prominent in better-differentiated tumours, where there is typically keratinization and present only focally or are less apparent in those that are more poorly differentiated.

In non-keratinizing squamous cell carcinoma, immunohistochemistry is required

to distinguish tumours from large cell carcinoma with a null phenotype (see *Large cell carcinoma*, p. 80). For such tumours, diffuse positive staining with a squamous marker (i.e. p40, p63, CK5, or CK5/6) and negativity for TTF1 confirm their squamous phenotype and classification. The presence of intracellular mucin in a few cells does not exclude tumours from this category. The issue in small sample diagnosis is addressed in *The new WHO classification: terminology and criteria in non-resection specimens.*

Some non-keratinizing squamous cell carcinomas may morphologically resemble urothelial transitional cell carcinoma.

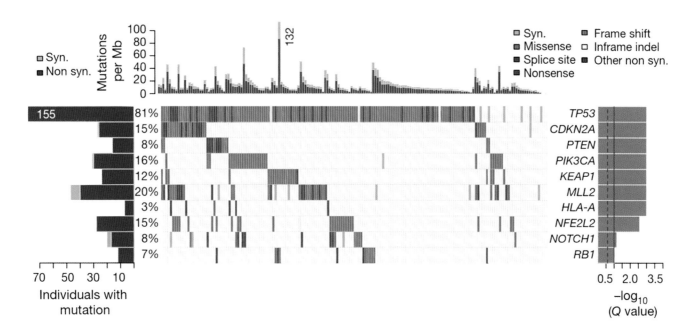

Fig. 1.52 Genetic profile of squamous cell carcinoma. Significantly mutated genes (*Q* value < 0.1) identified by exome sequencing are listed vertically by *Q* value. The percentage of lung squamous cell carcinoma samples with a mutation detected by automated calling is noted at the left. Samples are displayed as columns, with the overall number of mutations plotted at the top, and samples are arranged to emphasize mutual exclusivity among mutations. Syn, synonymous. Reproduced from Hammerman PS et al. The Cancer Genome Atlas Research Network {936}.

Architecturally, some squamous cell carcinomas arising in the proximal airways may show exophytic and papillary endobronchial growth into the lumen, but with invasion into the submucosa of the bronchial wall and surrounding lung tissue {635}. However, architectural and cytological subtyping – used in the 2004 WHO classification {2672} – is no longer recommended, because there is no evidence to suggest that papillary, small cell, and clear cell variants, other than basaloid morphology (see *Basaloid squamous cell carcinoma,* p. 56) have either prognostic or molecular significance. Invasive growth patterns (including single-cell invasion, high-grade tumour budding, and large nuclear size) may have prognostic importance, but validation is needed to confirm these findings {1175}.

Immunohistochemistry
For details, see *Terminology and criteria in non-resection specimens,* p. 17.
Non-keratinizing squamous cell carcinoma should show diffuse positive staining with p40, which is a more specific marker than p63, CK5, or CK5/6. In keratinizing squamous cell tumours, TTF1 should also be negative. In non-keratinizing sqaumous cell carcinoma, p40, p63, CK5, or CK5/6 are diffusely and strongly expressed; there may rarely be weak focal TTF1 expression.

Differential diagnosis
Keratinization is the hallmark of squamous cell carcinoma; thus, differential diagnosis arises mainly in poorly differentiated non-small cell tumours or small biopsy specimens with limited tumour tissue showing no morphological features of squamous cell differentiation, as described above and in *Terminology*

and criteria in non-resection specimens. In these cases, phenotyping by a limited panel of immunomarkers (p40/p63/TTF1) and a mucin stain is necessary, particularly since some adenocarcinomas can show a pseudosquamous appearance {1504,2014,2134,2638A,2676}, although focal intracellular mucin can occasionally be present in tumours that are clearly squamous cell carcinoma. In very well-differentiated central airway squamous carcinoma with papillary features, distinction from a papilloma can be difficult, requiring demonstration of invasion. Metastases from urothelial carcinomas also show positive CK7/p63/p40, but compared to lung squamous cell carcinomas, they are more often GATA3, uroplakin 3 and CK20 positive {904A}. Massive involvement of the anterior mediastinal tissue by a primary pulmonary squamous cell carcinoma can make differentiation from thymic squamous cell

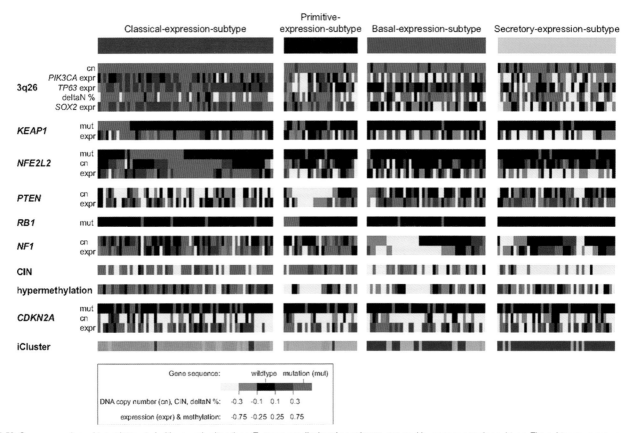

Fig. 1.53 Gene expression subtypes integrated with genomic alterations. Tumours are displayed as columns, grouped by gene expression subtype. The subtypes were compared by Kruskal-Wallis tests for continuous features, and by Fisher exact tests for categorical features. The features displayed showed significant association with gene expression subtype ($P < 0.05$), except for *CDKN2A* alterations. DeltaN expression percentage represents transcript isoform use between the *TP63* isoforms deltaN and TAp63, as determined by RNA sequencing. Chromosomal instability (CIN) is defined as the mean of the absolute values of chromosome arm copy numbers from the GISTIC output. Absolute values are used so that amplification and deletion alterations are counted equally. CIN, methylation, gene expression, and deltaN values were standardized for display using z-score transformation. Reproduced from Hammerman PS et al. The Cancer Genome Atlas Research Network {936}.

carcinoma difficult, and requires careful correlation with operative and radiological findings. Distinguishing primary lung squamous cell carcinoma from a metastasis in patients with prior history of squamous cell carcinoma of other sites, such as the head and neck, oesophagus, or cervix, can be challenging. This may require comparing the TP53 mutation/p53 immunostaining status between the lung and prior tumour of other sites, loss of heterozygosity involving microsatellite markers {823,824,1454,2745,2818}, or HPV testing/genotyping {208,2933} and p16 immunohistochemistry.

In the lung parenchyma, squamous cell carcinoma may entrap alveolar pneumocytes, which sometimes results in histological misinterpretation as adenosquamous carcinoma. Squamous metaplasia with cytological atypia in diffuse alveolar damage may also raise concern for squamous carcinoma. The presence of overall features of diffuse alveolar damage, such as hyaline membranes, diffuse alveolar septal connective tissue proliferation with pneumocyte hyperplasia, and bronchiolocentricity of the squamous changes, favours a metaplastic process.

Genetic profile

A comprehensive analysis of the genome of squamous cell carcinoma identified a very high rate of mutations per megabase (3–10 times higher than in other common cancers {936}), reflecting the mutagenic effects of cigarette smoke in this strongly smoking-associated lung cancer subtype.

Squamous cell carcinomas are characterized by gene copy number alterations, including gain/amplification of chromosomes 3q (SOX2, TP63) {147,2655}, 7p (EGFR), and 8p (FGFR1), as well as frequent deletion of chromosome 9p (CDKN2A), which occurs in 72% of cases {1006,2320}. Common gene mutations include TP53 (being the most frequent), CDKN2A, PTEN, PIK3CA, KEAP1, MLL2, HLA-A, NFE2L2, NOTCH1, and RB1 {936}. Two pathways appear to be preferentially involved by genetic alterations. The first, involving the oxidative stress response pathway, includes mutations in NFE2L2, KEAP1, or CUL3 (a partner of NEF2L2). The second commonly genetically altered pathway is implicated in squamous differentiation, and includes overexpression and amplification of SOX2 and TP63, and loss-of-function mutations in NOTCH1, NOTCH2, and ASCL4, and focal deletions in FOXP1 {936}. With only rare exceptions, pure squamous carcinomas, as diagnosed in resection specimens, do not harbour EGFR and KRAS mutations {936,2136}. In The Cancer Genome Atlas project, four gene expression subtypes were identified. However, no correlation was seen between the basal gene expression subtype and the basaloid histological subtype {936}.

Prognosis and predictive factors

The prognosis of squamous cell carcinoma is mainly dependent on the patient's performance score and the clinical/tumour stage, with the highest stages having the worst prognosis. To date, no validated clinical factors or biomarkers have been identified that are predictive of tumour response to local or systemic therapies.

Basaloid squamous cell carcinoma

E. Brambilla
S. Lantuejoul
A.G. Nicholson
K.J. Butnor
N.E. Caporaso
G. Chen
T-Y. Chou
S.S. Devesa

K. Geisinger
P. Hainaut
J. Jen
J. Jett
M. Ladanyi
M. Meyerson
D. Naidich
C.A. Powell

R. Rami-Porta
V. Roggli
A. Takano
M-S. Tsao
P. van Schil
I.I. Wistuba

Definition
Basaloid squamous cell carcinoma is a poorly differentiated malignant epithelial tumour that presents in its pure form as a proliferation of small cells with lobular architecture and peripheral palisading. These cells lack squamous morphology, but show immunohistochemical expression of squamous markers. Tumours with a keratinizing or non-keratinizing squamous cell component, but a basaloid component of > 50%, are also classified as basaloid squamous cell carcinoma. This tumour was previously considered a variant of large cell carcinoma, but was recognized as a distinct entity in the 1999 and 2004 WHO classifications {258}.

ICD-O code   8083/3

Synonyms
Basaloid carcinoma

Epidemiology
See *Adenocarcinoma*, p. 26.

Etiology
See *Adenocarcinoma*, p. 26.

Clinical features
The signs, symptoms, and imaging of this cell type are similar to those of other non-small cell lung carcinomas (see *Adenocarcinoma*, p. 26).
Tumour spread is similar to that of keratinizing and non-keratizing squamous cell carcinoma and other types of non-small cell lung carcinoma (see *Adenocarcinoma*, p. 26, and *Squamous cell carcinoma*, p. 51).
Basaloid squamous cell carcinoma is staged according to the TNM system {654,2420} (see *Staging and grading*, p. 14). The same caveats apply as for staging non-basaloid squamous cell carcinoma, including the importance of integrating clinicoradiographical data (e.g. distance from the carina) to accurately determine the T category of resected tumours that are centrally located {548, 866,2225,2399}.

Localization
The localization of basaloid squamous cell carcinoma is predominantly central/endobronchial {258,1755}.

Macroscopy
The tumours have a similar appearance to conventional squamous cell carcinoma of the lung, with a grey to white colour, solid parenchymal or exophytic endobronchial growth, and occasional central necrosis {258,2672,2920}. The tumours vary in size, and may grow quite large.

Cytology
The cytomorphological description of basaloid squamous cell carcinoma has been reported only infrequently, and these tumours may be misdiagnosed as small cell carcinoma {633,747,1557,2920}. Smears are generally cellular, with a large proportion of the malignant cells in flat to three-dimensional cohesive aggregates, which may demonstrate well-developed nuclear palisading at their peripheries. Tumour cells are small and homogeneous, with solitary hyperchromatic nuclei and very high nuclear-to-cytoplasmic ratios. Their chromatin is finely granular and evenly dispersed; the nucleoli are characteristically inconspicuous. Mitoses may be evident. Rosettes and/or moulding may be present. Uncommon keratinized squamous cells are occasionally noted.

Histopathology
This tumour shows a solid nodular or anastomotic trabecular invasive growth pattern, with peripheral palisading of multiple cell layers. The tumour cells are relatively small, monomorphic, cuboidal, or fusiform, with moderately hyperchromatic nuclei, finely granular to vesicular chromatin, and absent or focal nucleoli. Cytoplasm is scant but well defined, and nuclear moulding is absent. The mitotic rate is high (15–50 mitoses per 2 mm^2).

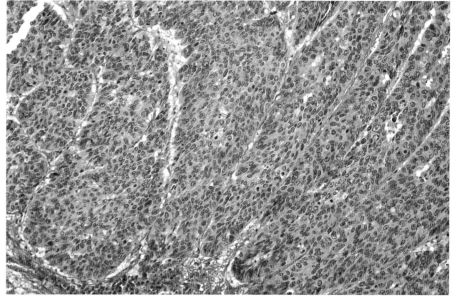

Fig. 1.54 Basaloid squamous cell carcinoma showing tightly packed nests of epithelial tumour cells with peripheral palisading, relatively small nuclei with coarse chromatin and visible nucleoli, and a high rate of mitoses.

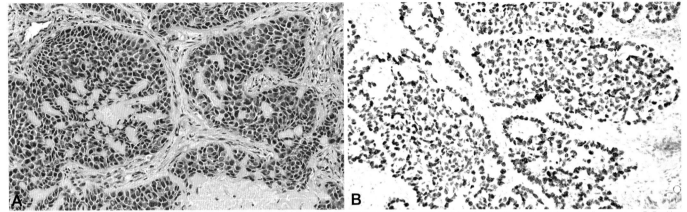

Fig. 1.55 Basaloid squamous cell carcinoma. **A** H&E staining shows the typical histological appearance, with peripheral palisading and prominent hyaline stroma. **B** Positive immunohistochemical nuclear staining for p40.

The proliferative index, as indicated by Ki-67, ranges from 50% to 80%. Progressive squamous differentiation is absent, but keratin pearl formation may be seen. Comedo-type necrosis is common. Rosettes are seen in one third of cases. Extensive carcinoma in situ is often observed in adjacent bronchial epithelium. Most basaloid squamous cell carcinomas have hyaline or mucoid stroma {258}.

Tumours that show a clear keratinizing and/or non-keratinizing squamous cell carcinoma (as defined in *Keratinizing and non-keratinizing squamous cell carcinoma*), but that have a major basaloid component (constituting > 50% of the tumour), are also classified as basaloid squamous cell carcinomas.

Immunohistochemistry

Basaloid squamous cell carcinoma consistently expresses (diffusely and strongly) p40 and p63. Cytokeratins (CK5/6, CK1, CK5, CK10, and CK14) are also expressed in all cases, sometimes in a less diffuse fashion. TTF1 is never expressed {2499}. Neuroendocrine markers (CD56, chromogranin, and synaptophysin) are usually negative, but occasionally one is focally positive (in 10% of cases).

Differential diagnosis

The main differential diagnoses are large cell neuroendocrine carcinoma (LC-NEC), small cell carcinoma, adenoid cystic carcinoma, NUT carcinoma, and poorly differentiated squamous cell or adenocarcinoma {258,301}. Palisading and rosette-like structures can be seen in basaloid squamous cell carcinoma, mimicking LCNEC. Some basaloid squamous cell carcinomas have very small tumour cells that can closely resemble those of small cell lung carcinoma (SCLC), particularly if crush artefact is present.

Distinguishing poorly differentiated squamous cell carcinoma from basaloid squamous cell carcinoma in biopsy samples can be particularly problematic, as defining foci of squamous differentiation may not be represented {2638A}. In poorly preserved or crushed specimens, the peripheral palisading that facilitates the distinction of basaloid squamous cell carcinoma from squamous cell carcinoma may be obscured. Similarly, nuclear features that aid in distinguishing small cell carcinoma, with its fine granular chromatin and nuclear moulding from the few basaloid squamous cell carcinomas that show tumour cells with more vesicular chromatin and visible nucleoli. In cytology, the features helpful in distinguishing basaloid squamous cell carcinoma from SCLC include greater intercellular cohesion, less karyorrhectic debris, focal squamous differentiation, a lack of pyknotic-like chromatin, and less obvious rosettes and moulding. Smaller cell size, higher nuclear-to-cytoplasmic ratios, and a lack of nucleoli favour basaloid squamous cell carcinoma over LCNEC.

Immunohistochemistry is essential in assessing the differential diagnosis. The diffuse, strong keratin, p40, or p63 positivity

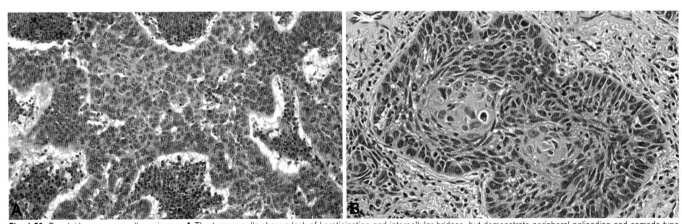

Fig. 1.56 Basaloid squamous cell carcinoma. **A** The tumour cells show a lack of keratinization and intercellular bridges, but demonstrate peripheral palisading and comedo-type necrosis. **B** This tumour shows abrupt keratinization, with typical basaloid squamous cell carcinoma morphology, abruptly merging with a focus of keratinizing squamous cell carcinoma.

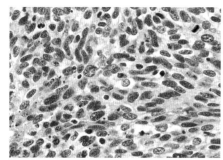

Fig. 1.57 Basaloid squamous cell carcinoma. This area of a basaloid squamous cell carcinoma shows morphology overlapping with that of small cell carcinoma, with small tumour cells, scant cytoplasm, finely granular nuclear chromatin, and inconspicuous nucleoli.

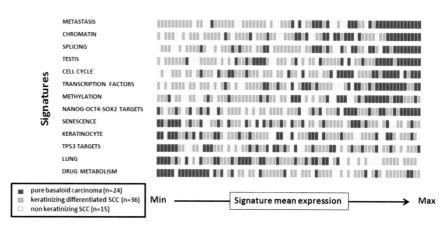

Fig. 1.58 Basaloid squamous cell carcinoma genetics. Basaloid squamous cell carcinomas are characterized by their expression signature pathways relative to keratinizing and non-keratinizing squamous cell carcinoma. This figure shows the 13 most deregulated signature pathways found in basaloid squamous cell carcinomas as compared with non-basaloid squamous cell carcinoma. Samples (N = 75) are independently ordered for each signature, on the mean expression of the corresponding signature. Reproduced from Brambilla C et al. {256A}, with permission.

that characterizes basaloid squamous cell carcinoma is absent in LCNEC and SCLC. Conversely, the diffuse staining for multiple neuroendocrine markers and TTF1 characteristic of most LCNECs and SCLCs is not seen in basaloid squamous cell carcinomas, although CD56 can uncommonly be positive {301,2499}. Staining for CD117 or myoepithelial markers such as smooth muscle actin, or demonstration of translocation involving the *MYB* gene by FISH (see *Adenoid cystic carcinoma,* p. 101) helps to distinguish adenoid cystic carcinoma from basaloid squamous cell carcinoma. Distinguishing from NUT carcinoma is challenging, as both share squamous differentiation and immunophenotype; the distinction can thus only be made using a highly specific monoclonal nuclear protein in testis (NUT) antibody (see *NUT carcinoma,* p. 97). Basaloid squamous cell carcinoma of the lung must also be distinguished from metastases, particularly from the head and neck, which requires careful integration of clinical and radiographical data.

Genetic profile
Basaloid squamous cell carcinoma shares most of the genetic features and alterations of other classical squamous cell carcinomas {936}, with *TP53* mutations occurring at a similarly high frequency as in squamous cell carcinoma in general (> 90%). However, a recent genomic and expression profiling study revealed some specific features {256A}. Although no copy number aberrations were significantly different from other subtypes of squamous cell carcinoma, transcriptomic analyses found significantly upregulated genes in basaloid squamous cell carcinoma compared to other squamous cell carcinoma, including genes related to *TP53* mutation signatures, transcription factor targets (*SOX* and *E2F* families, and *MYB*), embryonic development (*FGF3* and *FGF19*), DNA methylation regulation (*TET1*, *DNMT1*, and *DNMT3A*), cell cycle (*MKI67* and *BUB1*), splicing, and cell survival (*BCL2*), while the most downregulated genes were related to epithelial and keratinocytic differentiation {256A}. An ectopic male germ cell/placenta-specific gene expression signature has being linked to aggressive behaviour in lung tumours {2212}, and was found to be highly correlated with pure basaloid pattern. Upregulation of signatures associated with testis and embryonic stem cells and poorly differentiated tumour markers (NANOG, OCT4, SOX2, and MYC targets), and the downregulation of signatures related to the Polycomb gene silencing system are in line with the aggressiveness and the poor differentiation of basaloid squamous cell carcinoma {256A}.

Prognosis and predictive factors
Although these tumours are rare and data are limited, the prognosis of basaloid squamous cell carcinomas is considered to be poorer than that of other non-small cell lung cancers {1755,1757}. To date, no significant markers have been identified that are predictive of therapy response for basaloid squamous cell carcinomas.

I.I. Wistuba   S. Lam
W.A. Franklin   S. Lantuejoul
N.E. Caporaso   R. Rami-Porta
K. Geisinger

Preinvasive lesion
Squamous cell carcinoma in situ

Definition

Squamous dysplasia is a precursor lesion of squamous cell carcinoma, arising in the bronchial epithelium. Squamous dysplasia and carcinoma in situ are part of a continuum of recognizable histological changes in the large airways. Dysplasia can occur as single or multifocal lesions throughout the tracheobronchial tree.

ICD-O code

Squamous cell carcinoma in situ   8070/2

Synonyms

Squamous atypia; angiogenic squamous dysplasia; bronchial premalignancy; preinvasive squamous lesion; high-grade intraepithelial neoplasia; early non-invasive cancer

Epidemiology and etiology

See *Adenocarcinoma*, p. 26, and *Squamous cell carcinoma*, p. 51.

Clinical features

Signs and symptoms

Squamous dysplasia is nearly always asymptomatic, but occurs in individuals with heavy tobacco exposure (> 30 pack-years of cigarette smoking) and obstructive airway disease {1008,1756}. Preinvasive squamous bronchial lesions are found more frequently in men than in women {1390}. Dysplastic foci may persist in the airways for many years, but progression of individual lesions to malignancy is rarely observed.

White-light bronchoscopy

Approximately 40% of cases of carcinoma in situ can be detected by white-light reflectance bronchoscopy. About 75% of detected carcinoma in situ lesions appear as superficial or flat lesions; the remaining 25% have a nodular or polypoid appearance {1219,1786}. Because nodular/polypoid lesions are elevated from the adjacent normal mucosa, lesions as small as 1–2 mm in diameter can be seen. Flat or superficially spreading lesions > 1–2 cm in surface diameter are generally visible as areas of focal thickening, increase in vascularity, or marked irregularity of the mucosa. Flat lesions 5–10 mm in diameter usually produce non-specific thickening, redness, fine roughening, loss of lustre, or a slight increase in granularity, which are difficult to distinguish from inflammation or squamous metaplasia {2723}.

Autofluorescence bronchoscopy

Preinvasive lesions that have subtle or no visible findings on white-light bronchoscopy can be localized by autofluorescence bronchoscopy using a violet or blue light for illumination instead of white light. As the bronchial epithelium changes from normal to dysplasia, and then to carcinoma in situ and invasive cancer, there is a progressive decrease in green autofluorescence, but a proportionately smaller decrease in the red fluorescence intensity. Therefore, when a combination of reflected blue/violet light and autofluorescence is used, preinvasive and invasive lesions appear brownish red, red, purple, or magenta, while normal areas appear green or light blue. Lesions as small as 0.5 mm can be localized by this method {1638}.

Narrow-band imaging (image-enhanced endoscopy)

To highlight the vasculature, narrow-band imaging using blue light centred at 415 nm (400–430 nm) and green light centred at 540 nm (530–550 nm), corresponding to the maximal haemoglobin absorption peaks, is used. Preinvasive lesions and invasive cancers can be highlighted by their increase in angiogenesis. Dotted vessels, increased vessel growth, and complex networks of tortuous vessels of various sizes are observed with angiogenic squamous dysplasia. With carcinoma in situ, dotted vessels and small spiral- or corkscrew-type tumour

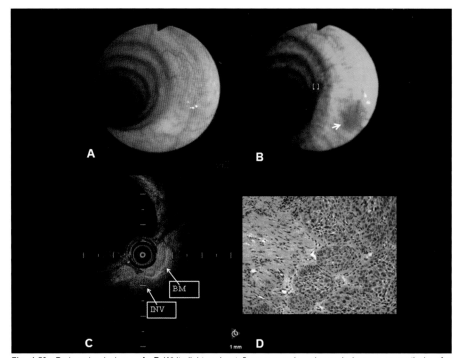

Fig. 1.59 Preinvasive lesions. **A, B** White-light and autofluorescence bronchoscopic images, respectively, of a squamous cell carcinoma in situ with microinvasion in the trachea. There was no abnormality on white-light examination. An area of abnormal fluorescence (arrow) was observed. **C** Optical coherence tomography showed invasion of the tumour (INV) through the basement membrane (BM). **D** Biopsy confirmed squamous cell carcinoma.

Table 1.15 Microscopic features of squamous dysplasia and carcinoma in situ. Reprinted from Travis WD et al. {2672}

Abnormality	Thickness	Cell size	Maturation/orientation	Nuclei
Mild dysplasia	Mildly increased	Mildly increased Mild anisocytosis and pleomorphism	Continuous progression of maturation from base to luminal surface Basilar zone expanded, with cellular crowding in the lower third of epithelium Distinct intermediate (prickle cell) zone present Superficial flattening of epithelial cells	Mild variation of nuclear-to-cytoplasmic ratio Finely granular chromatin Minimal angulation Nucleoli inconspicuous or absent Nuclei vertically oriented in lower third Mitoses absent or very rare
Moderate dysplasia	Moderately increased	Mildly increased Cells often small May have moderate anisocytosis and pleomorphism	Partial progression of maturation from base to luminal surface Basilar zone expanded, with cellular crowding in the lower two thirds of epithelium Intermediate zone confined to upper third of epithelium Superficial flattening of epithelial cells	Moderate variation of nuclear-to-cytoplasmic ratio Finely granular chromatin Angulations, grooves, and lobulations present Nucleoli inconspicuous or absent Nuclei vertically oriented in lower two thirds Mitotic figures present in lower third
Severe dysplasia	Markedly increased	Markedly increased May have marked anisocytosis and pleomorphism	Little progression of maturation from base to luminal surface Basilar zone expanded, with cellular crowding well into the upper third of epithelium Intermediate zone greatly attenuated Superficial flattening of epithelial cells	Nuclear-to-cytoplasmic ratio often high and variable Chromatin coarse and uneven Nuclear angulations and folding prominent Nucleoli frequently present and conspicuous Nuclei vertically oriented in lower two thirds Mitotic figures present in lower two thirds
Carcinoma in situ	May or may not be increased	May be markedly increased May have marked anisocytosis and pleomorphism	No progression of maturation from base to luminal surface; epithelium can be inverted, with little change in appearance Basilar zone expanded, with cellular crowding throughout the epithelium Intermediate zone absent Surface flattening confined to the most superficial cells	Nuclear-to-cytoplasmic ratio often high and variable Chromatin coarse and uneven Nuclear angulations and folding prominent Nucleoli may be present or inconspicuous No consistent orientation of nuclei in relation to epithelial surface Mitotic figures present through full thickness

vessels are observed. Prominent spiral- or corkscrew-type tumour vessels of various sizes and grades are visible in invasive lung cancer {2362}. Narrow-band imaging can localize preinvasive lesions and early lung cancer with high specificity {992}.

Optical coherence tomography
Illumination of the bronchial surface with an infrared light via a fibreoptic probe inserted through the biopsy channel of bronchoscopes, and analysis of the back-scattered light by optical interferometry allows visualization of cellular and extracellular bronchial structures at and below the tissue surface, with near histological resolution {951,1391,2609}. Optical coherence tomography can differentiate between carcinoma in situ and invasive tumour, and guide endobronchial therapy.

Distribution and spread
Since the entire central airway is exposed to tobacco smoke, squamous dysplasia and carcinoma in situ may occur anywhere in airways, a phenomenon referred to as field carcinogenesis, and first described in the head and neck {590,980}. Lesions are typically multiple, but may also occur at a single site. Whether dysplastic lesions are the product of the spread of a single clone of genetically altered precursor cells or of local clonal expansion is unknown {590}.

Staging
Dysplasia has no staging system, but carcinoma in situ is classified as Tis according to the TNM classification (see *Staging and grading*, p. 14).

Macroscopy and localization
Foci of carcinoma in situ usually arise near bifurcations in the segmental bronchi, subsequently extending proximally into the adjacent lobar bronchus and distally into subsegmental branches. The lesions are less common in the trachea. Grossly focal or multifocal plaque-like greyish lesions resembling leukoplakia, non-specific erythema, and even nodular or polypoid lesions may be seen.

Cytology
Cytomorphologically, the cells of these lesions are defined largely on the basis of progressive nuclear abnormalities: size, membrane irregularities, granularity and distribution of chromatin, and chromatin staining intensity. As the dysplasia increases in severity, the enlarged nuclei have more membrane contour irregularities, more darkly stained chromatin, and more coarsely granular and irregularly distributed chromatin granules, or a homogeneous (pyknotic-like) appearance {112,2240,2241}. Cytoplasmic keratinization may be present, especially in more severe lesions. With the Papanicolaou stain, this appears a brilliant, dense orange hue. The nuclear-to-cytoplasmic ratio also increases progressively. It is not possible to reliably distinguish squamous cell carcinoma in situ from invasive squamous cell carcinoma based on cytological preparations.

Histopathology
In response to irritants, including carcinogens, the bronchial epithelium may show basal cell hyperplasia, or squamous metaplasia with loss of the normal goblet and ciliated bronchial cell types. Exposure to tobacco smoke in particular is associated with further cellular changes (atypia {2710} or dysplasia), which

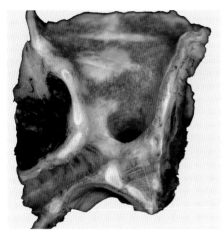

Fig. 1.60 Squamous carcinoma in situ at bronchial bifurcation. Note the plaque-like greyish lesions.

can be graded for severity (Table 1.15). By definition, preinvasive bronchial lesions include dysplasia of various degrees (mild, moderate, and severe) and carcinoma in situ; distinction between these four lesions is based on cell size and maturation, nuclear features, cell orientation, and epithelial thickness. This grading system imposes a somewhat arbitrary order on changes that in realty are a continuum, but the reproducibility of histological criteria among trained observers has been good {1843}.

Immunohistochemistry
Immunohistochemical changes in dysplasia reflect the biological properties of dysplastic epithelium. The increased proliferative activity at dysplastic sites is indicated by overexpression of Ki-67 {1640,1657,2051}, cyclin D1 {256,1140,2123}, cyclin E {1140}, PCNA {271}, and MCM2 {1657,2587}, all increasing with increasing grade of dysplasia. Immunohistochemical evidence of increased proliferative activity is associated with an increase in cell signalling proteins, including epidermal growth factor receptor {751,1365,2222}, HER2/neu {751,1450,1657}, and VEGF {744,1398}. Possible alteration in DNA repair mechanisms and apoptotic pathways is indicated by increased expression of p53 protein {179,255,1589,2594} and Bcl2 {255}. Nuclear p53 accumulation is usually focal, and dysplastic cells rarely express the robust signal present in tumours with missense mutation. Changes in the in situ expression of several structural proteins have been described, such as overexpression of CK5/6 {60} and fatty acid synthase {2623}, defects in

basement membrane visible in collagen IV stains {788}, maldistribution of MUC1, and changes in matrix metalloproteinase and TIMP expression {788} that correlate with the severity of dysplasia. Finally, the loss of expression of several key proteins, many of which have been regarded as tumour suppressors, has been documented in dysplastic epithelium, including loss of FHIT {820,2441}, p16 {256,1394}, folate binding protein {752}, RARB {1590}.

Differential diagnosis
Differential diagnosis with mild dysplasia includes basal cell (reserve cell) hyperplasia and squamous metaplasia; all considered to be reactive lesions resulting from chronic irritation or injury. Squamous metaplasia and dysplasia may be angiogenic and papillary {1767}, but angiogenic or papillary features have no prognostic influence by themselves. The distinction between carcinoma in situ and invasive carcinoma may be difficult on small fragments as far as they can coexist on a biopsy. Carcinoma in situ can extend to the bronchial gland ducts, mimicking invasion; however, necrosis and the presence of an endoscopic mass favour an invasive process {1236}. Dysplasia and carcinoma in situ may be associated with small cell carcinoma, sometimes with pagetoid migration of small cells within the dysplastic epithelium. Dysplasia and carcinoma in situ are independent findings, and must be

distinguished from extension of invasive carcinoma onto the bronchial surface, as this may have implications for staging and assessing resection margins.

Genetic profile
Squamous dysplastic lesions are thought to result from sequential genetic and epigenetic changes that begin with cigarette carcinogen exposure. Precise microdissection of epithelial cells followed by molecular genetic analysis of such lesions has revealed a sequence of molecular changes similar to that observed in other epithelial cancers {1007,2892}. These studies also indicated similarities and differences between the sequential changes leading to central and peripheral lung tumours. DNA aneuploidy is common in dysplastic lesions, particularly in high-grade lesions. Small foci of allelic loss are common at multiple sites in the bronchial epithelium, and persist long after smoking cessation {1986}.
Loss of heterozygosity occurs at 3p and 9p21 early in neoplastic development, starting in histologically normal epithelium. Later changes include 8p21-23, 13q14 (*RB*), and 17p13 (*TP53*), which can be detected in histologically normal epithelium {1574,2889,2890,2895}. Allelic loss at 5q21 (*APC* region) has been detected in carcinoma in situ, and *TP53* mutations appear at variable times {2509,2889,2895}. Chromosome 3p losses in normal epithelium, basal cell hyperplasia, and squamous metaplasia

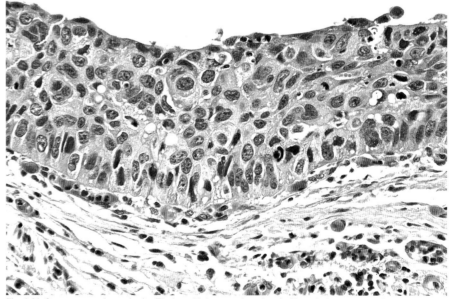

Fig. 1.61 Squamous carcinoma in situ. The bronchial mucosa is replaced with atypical squamous cells extending from the surface to the base of the epithelium. Note the severe nuclear polymorphism, hyperchromasia, and enlarged nuclei.

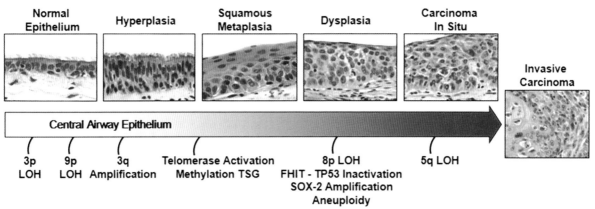

Fig. 1.62 Molecular multistage pathogenesis of squamous cell carcinoma of the lung. Several sequential molecular abnormalities have been recognized in the multistep pathogenesis of squamous cell carcinoma of the lung, starting at the normal epithelium stage. LOH, loss of heterozygosity; TSG, tumour suppressor gene. Modified from Kadara H, Wistuba II {1172}.

are small and multifocal, starting at the central (3p21) region of the chromosomal arm. In later lesions, such as carcinoma in situ, allelic loss is present along nearly all of the short arm of chromosome 3p {2889,2890}. The clonal patches of bronchial epithelium displaying molecular changes are usually small, and have been estimated to contain approximately 40,000–360,000 cells {1986}. *p16INK4a* methylation has also been detected at early stages of squamous preinvasive lesions, increasing in frequency during progression from basal cell hyperplasia to squamous metaplasia to carcinoma in situ {170}. Detection of aberrant gene methylation in sputum may be of predictive value in identifying smokers at increased risk of developing lung cancer {171,1449,2664}. Similar changes have been detected in telomerase activation {2945}. Weak telomerase RNA expression is detected in basal layers of normal and hyperplastic epithelium, but dysregulation of telomerase expression increases with histological tumour progression. Amplification of the oncogene *SOX2*, located in 3q26.3, has been detected in invasive squamous cell carcinomas and

high-grade squamous bronchial dysplasias, suggesting that this lineage-specific gene could play a role in the pathogenesis of this tumour type {1621}.

Prognosis and predictive factors

Carcinoma in situ, being a preinvasive lesion, is classified as stage 0 disease. Resection of specific lesions at this stage results in 100% curability, although frequent multifocality means that other foci are liable to present elsewhere in the airways. In general, higher grades of dysplasia are more closely associated with synchronous invasive carcinomas, although the prognostic significance of identifying dysplasia in isolation is uncertain. Genetic alterations such as loss of heterozygosity in chromosome 3p or chromosomal aneusomy {1792,2412,2890}, as well as host factors such as the inflammatory load and levels of anti-inflammatory proteins in the lung, influence the progression or regression of preneoplastic lesions {262,1104}. The progression rate of mild dysplasia was almost 10 times higher in patients who developed squamous cell carcinoma compared with those who developed

adenocarcinoma {1104}. The underlying mechanism has not yet been identified. Some lesions appear to progress rapidly from hyperplasia/metaplasia to carcinoma in situ/invasive cancer (within 2 years) {262,1104}, which is much shorter than the traditional 10- to 20-year evolution {2895}. Array comparative genomic hybridization studies have revealed that the presence of many copy number alterations with acquired gains and losses (i.e. genomic instability) is the hallmark of progressive squamous dysplasia {2739,2740}. A model based on copy number alterations at 3p26.3–11.1, 3q26.229, and 6p25.324.3 predicted cancer development with 97% accuracy. p53, p63, and Ki-67 immunostaining was not predictive for a differential clinical outcome of the lesions. The presence of high-grade dysplasia or carcinoma in situ is a risk marker for lung cancer both in the central airways and the peripheral lung {1104,1143}. Close follow-up with bronchoscopy and radiological imaging should be considered in patients with these lesions {2888}.

Neuroendocrine tumours
Small cell carcinoma

E. Brambilla
M.B. Beasley
J.H.M. Austin
V.L. Capelozzi
L.R. Chirieac
S.S. Devesa
G.A. Frank

A. Gazdar
Y. Ishikawa
J. Jen
J. Jett
A.M. Marchevsky
S. Nicholson
G. Pelosi

C.A. Powell
R. Rami-Porta
G. Scagliotti
E. Thunnissen
W.D. Travis
P. van Schil
P. Yang

Definition

Small cell carcinoma is a malignant epithelial tumour that consists of small cells with scant cytoplasm, poorly defined cell borders, finely dispersed granular nuclear chromatin, and absent or inconspicuous nucleoli. The cells are round, oval, or spindle-shaped. Nuclear moulding is prominent. Necrosis is typically extensive, and the mitotic count is high. Most small cell carcinomas express neuroendocrine markers.

Combined small cell carcinoma has an additional component that consists of any of the histological types of non-small cell carcinoma (NSCC); usually adenocarcinoma, squamous cell carcinoma, large cell carcinoma, or large cell neuroendocrine carcinoma (LCNEC), or less commonly spindle cell carcinoma or giant cell carcinoma.

ICD-O codes

Small cell carcinoma   8041/3
Combined small cell carcinoma 8045/3

Synonyms

Obsolete: oat cell carcinoma; intermediate cell type carcinoma; small cell anaplastic carcinoma; undifferentiated small cell carcinoma; mixed small cell/large cell carcinoma

Epidemiology

Small cell lung carcinoma (SCLC) accounts for about 13% of all newly diagnosed lung cancer cases worldwide, and virtually all patients with SCLC were heavy smokers {591}. In the USA, the incidences of SCLC in men and women peaked in the mid-1980s (at about 15.5/100 000) and early 1990s (at about 9.4/100 000), respectively, and decreased to 11.3/100 000 in men and 6.7/100 000 in women in 2010 {1036} (see *Adenocarcinoma*, p. 26, for a review of epithelial cancer). The same trend was observed in South East England from 1970 to 2007 {2148}. Increased incidence is expected in countries where smoking prevalence remains high, such as those in Asia and eastern Europe. Among

the major lung cancer subtypes, SCLC shows the strongest association with cigarette smoking; the odds ratio (or risk) is estimated to be 111 in current smokers with a > 30 pack-year history compared to never-smokers {2039}. Additional risk factors include the presence of chronic obstructive pulmonary disease {1035} or asthma (odds ratio = 1.71) {2199}. Use of hormone replacement therapy is a protective factor (odds ratio = 0.37) {2037}. Continued smoking multiplies the risk of a second primary cancer by up to 4 times in people who survive SCLC {449,1997}. CT screening can shift the SCLC diagnosis towards an early stage (by 30%), and decreased mortality {106}.

Etiology

Neuroendocrine tumours of the lung are a distinct family of tumours with shared morphological, ultrastructural, immunohistochemical, and molecular characteristics. The four major categories of neuroendocrine tumours of the lung are small cell carcinoma and LCNEC (which are high-grade neuroendocrine tumours) and typical carcinoid and atypical carcinoid (which are considered to be low- and intermediate-grade malignant tumours, respectively) {2157,2160,2683}. There is increasing evidence that typical and atypical carcinoids are morphologically associated more closely with each other than with LCNEC and small cell carcinoma. Clinically, approximately 40% of patients with either typical or atypical carcinoids are non-smokers, while virtually all patients with SCLC or LCNEC are heavy smokers. Unlike SCLC and LCNEC, both typical and atypical carcinoids can occur in patients with multiple endocrine neoplasia type 1 (8%), and contain *MEN1* mutations in sporadic cases (40%) {560,561}. In addition, diffuse idiopathic pulmonary neuroendocrine cell hyperplasia, with or without tumourlets, may be present in both typical and atypical carcinoids, for which it is considered a preoplastic lesion (see *Preinvasive lesion – Diffuse idiopathic pulmonary neuroendocrine cell hyperplasia,* p. 78),

but it is not an established preinvasive lesion for LCNEC or SCLC. Preneoplastic lesions have not been identified in SCLC or LCNEC, but genetic alterations in the normal-appearing contiguous bronchial epithelium are common {2891}. Histological heterogeneity with other major histological types of lung carcinoma (e.g. squamous cell carcinoma and adenocarcinoma) occurs with both SCLC and LCNEC, but usually not with typical or atypical carcinoids {113,1848}. This suggests that the cell of origin of SCLC has the same endodermal origin as rest of respiratory epithelium, and that the cells arise from a multipotent precursor cell as indicated by mouse models {1630,1660,1988,2531}.

The neuroendocrine properties of small cell carcinoma are thought to be driven by the key transcription factor ASCL1 {1672}, possibly aided by the transcription factor NeuroD1 {1935}. Although SCLC is often considered to be a poorly differentiated tumour (based on its morphology and paucity of dense core granules), most neuroendocrine cell features are expressed in relative abundance in most cases. Small cell carcinoma cells produce a wide range of neuroendocrine and non-neuroendocrine cell products, accounting for the large number of associated paraneoplastic syndromes {2749}. In addition to having general neuroendocrine properties, small cell carcinoma cells may also express many cell-specific neuroendocrine products present in normal respiratory neuroendocrine cells (including gastrin-releasing peptide and calcitonin), as well as ectopic hormones such as antidiuretic hormone and adrenocorticotropic hormone, which is rare in LCNEC.

Consistent with their dependency on tobacco consumption, both types of high-grade neuroendocrine tumours contain the characteristic tobacco carcinogen-associated molecular signature (i.e. abundant numbers of mutations and a high fraction of G→T transversions caused by polycyclic aromatic hydrocarbons and often occurring at methylated CpG dinucleotides)

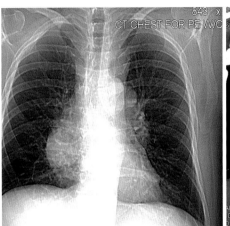
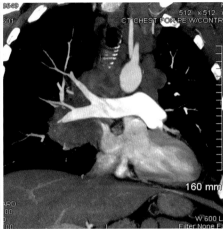
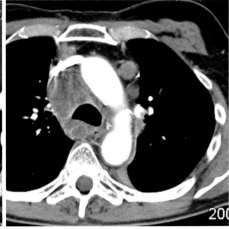

Fig. 1.63 Small cell carcinoma. Right perihilar pulmonary mass invading hilar and mediastinal lymph nodes on CT.

{2012,2065}. The most potent carcinogens leading to SCLC development are polycyclic aromatic hydrocarbons, such as benzo[a]pyrene and the tobacco-specific nitrosamine called nicotine-derived nitrosoaminoketone {2849}. In small cell carcinoma cells, nicotine or nitrosoaminoketone binds to the membrane receptor alpha7 nAChR, which results in cation influx and activation of the mitogenic signal transduction pathway {2310,2317}.

Clinical features

Signs and symptoms

SCLC is commonly located centrally in the major airways, but may occur peripherally in the lungs in about 5% of cases. Patients often present with rapid-onset signs or symptoms due to local intrathoracic tumour growth, extrapulmonary distant spread, paraneoplastic syndromes, or a combination of these features. The symptoms of small cell carcinoma are similar to those of other lung cancers (see *Adenocarcinoma*, p. 26, for a review of common epithelial cancers). Paraneoplastic signs or symptoms are more frequently documented in SCLC than in other histological types of lung cancer. Hyponatraemia (due to inappropriate secretion of antidiuretic hormone), Cushing syndrome, Lambert-Eaton myasthenic syndrome, peripheral neuropathy, or limbic encephalopathy may portend the cancer. Rarely, SCLC can develop in patients with *EGFR*-mutated lung adenocarcinomas, and sometimes the morphological transition develops following tyrosine kinase inhibitor therapy as a mechanism of resistance {1876}.

Imaging

SCLC presents with the full spectrum of imaging findings of lung cancer, but because of rapid growth compared to most NSCCs of the lung, the tumour at presentation tends to be larger and to show more advanced stage than the NSCCs {2356}. A characteristic presentation is as a large hilar mass and bulky mediastinal lymph nodes. The mass is often lobulated, and occasionally endobronchial {1848}. However, when detection is by CT screening, presentation as a node-negative small peripheral nodule is not a rarity {106}. Cavitation of SCLC is exceedingly rare. Invasion of hilar vessels and the superior vena cava is more common in SCLC than in NSCC.

Tumour spread

SCLC can spread to virtually every part of the body, and metastatic spread is a common finding at clinical presentation. The most common sites of local spread are intrathoracic lymph nodes (often as bulky disease potentially leading to superior vena cava syndrome) and supraclavicular lymph nodes. Commonly involved distant sites of spread include the liver, bone, brain, ipsilateral and contralateral lung, and adrenal glands. Malignant pleural and pericardial effusions are also common, and are associated, according to the seventh edition of the TNM classification of malignant tumours, with a similar prognosis as cases with nodules in the contralateral lung (M1a category), and intermediate between locally advanced (stage IIIB) and metastatic (M1b category – extrathoracic) disease {2078}.

Staging

Staging is based on the TNM classification, which parallels the anatomical extent of the disease {2356,2737}. The revised dichotomous staging system of limited versus extended disease can also be used, although the TNM classification is preferred, because it distinguishes between different prognostic groups otherwise grouped as limited disease (see *Staging and grading*, p. 14).

Macroscopy and localization

Grossly, SCLC is typically a large perihilar mass, with subsequent peribronchial compression and obstruction, and nodal involvement. It is frequently identified

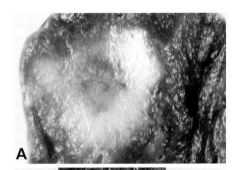
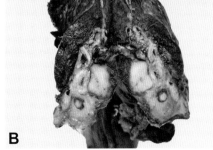

Fig. 1.64 Small cell carcinoma. **A** Small cell carcinoma presenting as a peripheral coin lesion. **B** Bronchial tumour with lymph node metastases.

on chest imaging. In lung parenchyma, the tumour may spread along bronchi in a subepithelial and radial pattern, also involving lymphatic vessels. SCLC presents as a solitary peripheral nodule in about 5% of cases {2669}. In resected cases, the tumour is usually a circumscribed peripheral lung nodule measuring 2–4 cm in size, with a tan, sometimes necrotic cut surface {2669}.

Cytology

Giemsa-stained aspiration smears show loosely branching sheets of piled-up cells and singly dispersed bare nuclei. Necrosis and foamy histiocyte debris may feature in the background. In sheets and cell aggregates, rosette shapes may be seen. Individual cells are small with round, oval, or spindle-shaped nuclei, where chromatin is uniformly finely divided and nucleoli are not prominent, although chromocentres are visible. Scant, if any, cytoplasm surrounds the nuclei, and nuclear moulding is prominent {2671}. Dense dark apoptotic bodies may be seen over and around viable cells. Giant tumour nuclei may also be seen. Necrosis or chromatin streaking is variable and sample-dependent {2142}. Mitotic figures are not as common as might be expected in such proliferative tumours.

With liquid-based cytology preparations such as brushings and washings, alcohol fixation reduces the already small size of the nucleus to a size similar to that of a bronchial epithelial cell nucleus. With these preparation methods, the nuclear diameter is usually no greater than three small resting lymphocytes. The nuclear shapes are round or spindled. Nuclear outlines are irregular. Singly dispersed nuclei and nuclear clusters are seen. With Papanicolaou staining, the nuclear chromatin ranges from a rich blue/black to almost vesicular when chromatin is very fine. Nucleoli are not prominent, but small chromocentres are visible. The cytoplasm is usually stripped away. Necrosis is variable {156}, but dense black apoptotic debris is a constant feature.

Histopathology

Small cell carcinoma

Densely packed small tumour cells commonly form a sheet-like diffuse growth pattern, without obvious neuroendocrine morphology apart from nuclear

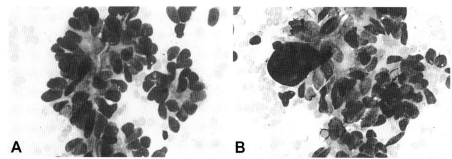
Fig. 1.65 Small cell carcinoma. **A** Rosette formation, scant cytoplasm, and nuclear moulding. **B** An occasional giant malignant nucleus is seen amid small moulded nuclei. Nucleoli are absent.

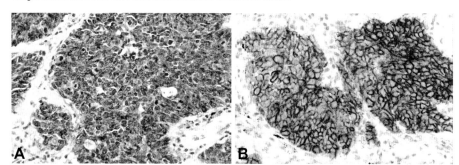
Fig. 1.66 Small cell carcinoma. **A** Many tumour cells show cytoplasmic staining with an antibody to chromogranin. **B** CD56 immunoreactivity with a membranous staining pattern.

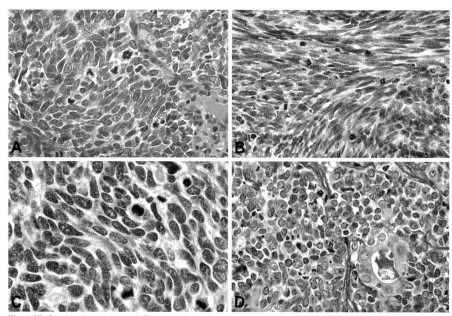
Fig. 1.67 Small cell carcinoma. **A** Tumour cells are densely packed and small, with scant cytoplasm, finely granular nuclear chromatin, and an absence of nucleoli. Mitoses are frequent. **B** The fusiform (spindle cell) shape is a prominent feature. The nuclear chromatin is finely granular and nucleoli are absent. **C** In this example, the cells are somewhat larger and show some cytoplasm, as well as a few inconspicuous nucleoli. **D** Combined small cell carcinoma and adenocarcinoma. A malignant gland is present within the small cell carcinoma.

characteristics. Architectural patterns such as nesting, trabeculae, peripheral palisading, and rosette formation (as seen in other neuroendocrine tumours) are less common. Tumour cells are usually less than the diameter of 3 small resting lymphocytes, and have round, ovoid, or spindled nuclei and scant cytoplasm.

Nuclear chromatin is finely granular and nucleoli are absent or inconspicuous. Cell borders are rarely seen, and nuclear moulding is common. There is a high mitotic rate (at least 10 mitoses per 2 mm², but averaging over 60 mitoses per 2 mm²). The proliferative index as evaluated by Ki-67 antigen immunohistochemistry is

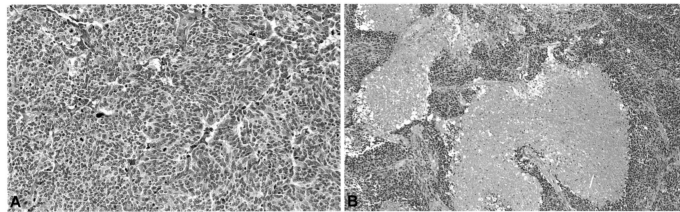

Fig. 1.68 Small cell carcinoma. **A** Overview of a small cell lung carcinoma showing sheets of small cells. **B** Small cell carcinoma with extensive necrosis.

> 50%, averaging ≥ 80%. SCLC is by definition a high-grade tumour, so grading is implied in the diagnosis. No in situ phase is recognized. In larger specimens, the cell size may be larger, with more abundant cytoplasm. Scattered pleomorphic giant tumour cells, prominent nucleoli, extensive necrosis, brisk apoptotic activity, and crush artefacts with encrustation of basophilic nuclear DNA around blood vessels (the Azzopardi effect) may all be seen {1848}.

Combined small cell carcinoma
Combined SCLC refers to the admixture of NSCLC elements including squamous cell carcinoma, adenocarcinoma, large cell carcinoma, LCNEC, and (less commonly) spindle cell carcinoma or giant cell carcinoma. Because of the morphological continuum between SCLC and LCNEC, at least 10% of the tumour should show large cells to be subclassified as combined SCLC and large cell carcinoma (or LCNEC). There is no percentage requirement for components of adenocarcinoma, squamous cell carcinoma, or sarcomatoid carcinoma, as they are easily recognized {1848}.

Immunohistochemistry
The diagnosis of SCLC can be reliably made based on routine histological and cytological preparations, but immunohistochemistry may be required for confirmation of the neuroendocrine and epithelial nature of the tumour cells. Broadly reactive cytokeratin antibody mixtures, including AE1/AE3 cocktail, CAM5.2, and MNF116, highlight epithelial differentiation in nearly all cases of SCLC, with either dot-like, paranuclear, or diffuse cytoplasmic staining pattern {1598,1848,2867}. A high-molecular weight cytokeratin cocktail (recognizing CK1, CK5, CK10, and CK14) is always negative in pure SCLC {2500}. A panel of neuroendocrine markers is useful, including NCAM/CD56 (mostly decorating the cell membrane) {1401,1402}. Dense core granule-associated protein chromogranin A, and the synaptic vesicle protein synaptophysin (both with cytoplasmic labelling) are regularly expressed in SCLC {915,1848}. NCAM/CD56 is the most sensitive marker, but it is also less specific, and should be interpreted in the appropriate morphological context. Synaptophysin and NCAM/CD56 can diffusely and strongly stain SCLC, while chromogranin A can be more focal and weak. However, < 10% of SCLC can be completely unreactive or only very focally reactive for neuroendocrine markers, probably due to the lack of overt neuroendocrine differentiation {2867}. SCLC is also positive for TTF1 in up to 90–95% of instances {1224,1598,1918,2501}, especially when a less specific clone is used {1377}, whereas napsin A, a marker of adenocarcinoma differentiation, is consistently unreactive {266}. More than 60% of SCLCs express CD117 (KIT) also in phosphorylated form {316,2018,2582}, but there is no known significant correlation with survival {1511} or responsiveness to targeted therapy {646}. The G1 arrest pathway is consistently altered in SCLC, with loss of the retinoblastoma protein and cyclin D1 at variance with carcinoids {158,618}, so these markers may serve in the relevant differential diagnosis. Whenever possible, particularly

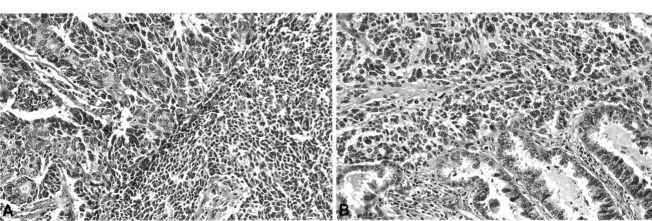

Fig. 1.69 A Combined small cell (right side) and large cell neuroendocrine carcinoma. **B** Combined small cell carcinoma and adenocarcinoma.

in small biopsies, the proliferation activity of SCLC as assessed by Ki-67 antigen immunostaining should be performed to avoid misdiagnosing carcinoid tumours in the presence of crush artefact. In SCLC, it ranges from 64.5% to 77.5%, and may reach 100% {2020,2021}.

Differential diagnosis

The differential diagnoses of small cell carcinoma include LCNEC, typical and atypical carcinoids (especially in small biopsy specimens with crush artefact), lymphoid infiltrates, the Ewing family of tumours (EFTs), primary non-small cell lung carcinoma, and metastatic carcinomas {2671}.

The distinction between SCLC and LCNEC is made on H&E-stained slides, based on cytological criteria. The diagnosis of SCLC is often more evident on corresponding cytology specimens than in biopsies. The most useful discriminatory features between SCLC and LCNEC are the nuclear-to-cytoplasmic ratio and the nucleoli {1034,2671}. In small biopsies with crush artefact or during intraoperative diagnosis, SCLC should be distinguished from carcinoid tumours (typical or atypical), reactive or neoplastic lymphocytic proliferations, and EFTs. Cytokeratin, neuroendocrine markers (synaptophysin, chromogranin, and NCAM/CD56), leukocyte common antigen (CD45RB), and CD99 are useful immunohistochemical markers in this scenario. SCLCs have nuclear moulding with finely dispersed nuclear chromatin, necrosis, numerous apoptotic bodies, and mitoses. The Ki-67 proliferative index in SCLC is typically > 50%, approaching 100% in most cases {2020,2021,2160}. Typical carcinoids have < 2 mitoses per 2 mm^2, and no necrosis; whereas atypical carcinoids have 2–10 mitoses per 2 mm^2 and/or the presence of punctate necrosis {159,1848}. TTF1 expression is usually absent in typical carcinoids, particularly central tumours, but present in SCLC and LCNEC. EFTs are less mitotically active than SCLC, with a lower Ki-67 labelling index. The majority of EFTs have diffuse membranous expression of CD99 and usually lack keratin expression. The diagnosis can be confirmed by FISH for the *EWSR1* gene {932,1523}. Approximately 20% of EFTs can focally express any of the epithelial markers {1535}. Positive staining for CK20 or neurofilaments, but not for CK7 or TTF1,

distinguishes Merkel cell carcinoma from SCLC {380,418}. SCLC must be distinguished from basaloid squamous cell carcinoma, especially on small biopsies. The diffuse, strong immunoreactivity for p40, p63, and/or high molecular weight cytokeratins CK1, CK5, CK10, CK14 (CK34beta E12 antibody) characterize basaloid squamous cell carcinoma and are absent in SCLC. Conversely, the diffuse staining of multiple neuroendocrine

markers and TTF1 characteristic of most SCLCs is not seen in basaloid squamous cell carcinomas, although uncommonly CD56 can be positive {301,2499}.

Genetic profile

The neuroendocrine tumours of the lung do not form a continuous pathogenetic spectrum. Rather, they account for low- to intermediate-grade malignant tumours (typical carcinoid and atypical carcinoid)

Table 1.16 Differential diagnosis of neuroendocrine tumours based on clinicopathological characteristics.

	Typical carcinoid	Atypical carcinoid	Large cell neuroendocrine carcinoma	Small cell lung carcinoma
Average age	Sixth decade	Sixth decade	Seventh decade	Seventh decade
Sex predominance	Female	Female	Male	Male
Smoking association	No	Variable*	Yes	Yes
Diagnostic criteria				
Mitoses per 2 mm^2	< 2	2–10	> 10 (median of 70)	> 10 (median of 80)
Necrosis	No	Focal, if any	Yes	Yes
Neuroendocrine morphology	Yes	Yes	Yes	Yes
Ki-67 proliferation index	Up to 5%	Up to 20%	40–80%	50–100%
TTF1 expression	Mostly negative	Mostly negative	Positive 50%	Positive 85%
Synaptophysin / chromogranin	Positive	Positive	Positive 80–90%	Positive 80–90%
CD56	Positive	Positive	Positive 80–90%	Positive 80–90%
Combined with a non-small cell lung carcinoma component	No	No	Sometimes	Sometimes

* The majority of carcinoid patients are never-smokers or light smokers, although atypical carcinoid is more associated with current or former smokers than typical carcinoid patients.

Table 1.17 Criteria for diagnosis of neuroendocrine tumours. Reprinted from Travis WD et al. {2678}

Typical carcinoid
A tumour with carcinoid morphology and < 2 mitoses per 2 mm^2, lacking necrosis, and ≥ 0.5 cm

Atypical carcinoid
A tumour with carcinoid morphology and 2–10 mitoses per 2 mm^2 and/or necrosis (often punctuate) or both

Large cell neuroendocrine carcinoma
1. A tumour with a neuroendocrine morphology (organoid nesting, palisading, rosettes, trabeculae)
2. High mitotic rate: > 10 mitoses per 2 mm^2, median of 70 mitoses per 2 mm^2
3. Necrosis (often in large zones)
4. Cytological features of a non-small cell carcinoma: large cell size, low nuclear-to-cytoplasmic ratio, vesicular, coarse or fine chromatin, and/or frequent nucleoli; some tumours have fine nuclear chromatin and lack nucleoli, but qualify as non-small cell lung carcinoma because of large cell size and abundant cytoplasm
5. Positive immunohistochemical staining for one or more neuroendocrine markers (other than neuron-specific enolase) and/or neuroendocrine granules by electron microscopy.

Small cell carcinoma
Small size (generally less than the diameter of 3 small resting lymphocytes)
1. Scant cytoplasm
2. Nuclei: finely granular nuclear chromatin, absent or faint nucleoli
3. High mitotic rate: > 10 mitoses per 2 mm^2, median of 80 mitoses per 2 mm^2
4. Frequent necrosis (often in large zones)

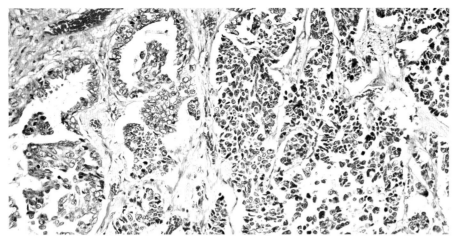

Fig. 1.70 Combined small cell carcinoma and adenocarcinoma in patient with previous lung adenocarcinoma and *EGFR* exon L858R mutation that initially responded to erlotinib. The tumour then recurred and was resected, revealing a component of small cell carcinoma, a known manifestation of tyrosine kinase inhibitor resistance.

driven by *MEN1* and related chromatin modifier gene mutations, and high-grade neuroendocrine tumours (LCNEC and SCLC) driven by inactivating mutations in the *RB* and *TP53* genes. The high-grade tumours (but not the lower grade ones) contain the characteristic tobacco carcinogen-associated molecular signature (abundant numbers of mutations and a high fraction of G→T transversions caused by polycyclic aromatic hydrocarbons, often occurring at methylated CpG dinucleotides) {2012,2065}. The early inactivation of *TP53* results in genomic instability, with multiple frequent sites of allelic imbalance {465}, including losses as chromosomes 3p, 4q, 5q, 13q, and 15q. Extensive and multiple site deletions at

chromosome 3p were the first cytogenetic finding {2858}, and are also frequent in non-small cell lung carcinoma. These 3p sites contain several known or suspected tumour suppressor genes {3003}, including *FHIT, RASSF1* {2016}, *FUS1, VHL,* and *DUTT1,* as well as *FRA3B,* the most active fragile site in the human genome. Amplification of the *MYC* gene family (especially after therapy) {808,1154,1269} and the *MAD1L1* gene on chromosome 7p are frequent with 7p22.3 gain {465}.

Two reports that used integrated multi-platform genome-wide approaches provided new insights {2012,2219}. A small number of molecular changes, in particular *TP53* mutations and high total numbers of so-called smoking signature mutations, are common to all lung cancers, but inactivating *RB1* mutations are a hallmark of SCLC. *PTEN* mutations and *FGFR1* amplifications occur in important subsets of SCLC (10% and 6%, respectively), as do *SOX2* amplification and mutations in *SLIT2, EPHA7,* and multiple histone modifier genes (*CREBBP, EP300,* and *MLL*). Recurrent *RLF-MYCL* fusions are also present. Several of these changes are also present in other lung cancers, and are the subject of current clinical trials.

Many genomic and epigenomic aberrations have been identified (although clinical therapeutic targets have yet to be achieved) {514,1189,2451}, such as KIT overexpression {2018,2185,2582}; telomerase activation {1404,2916}; *RASSF1* inactivation upon hypermethylation {2016}; and TTF1, BAI3, and BRN2 expression {139,2250}. Cell cycle regulators are severely affected in SCLC and LCNEC,

with overexpression of E2F1 {691}, loss of *p14ARF* {809}, and cyclin E and SKP2 upregulation {2264}. Apoptosis-related factors are also severely affected, with constant Bcl2 upregulation {259} and loss of retinoblastoma protein expression and related retinoblastoma pathway disruption {158,889}. PARP1 is a promising novel therapeutic target for SCLC, identified through proteomic profiling {304}. Another promising novel therapeutic target is activation of the Hedgehog signalling pathway {1989}.

Prognosis and predictive factors

SCLC has a dismal prognosis, with a 2 year survival rate of only 10% with metastatic disease and a 5 year survival rate of approximately of 25% when there is no metastatic involvement {2063,2543}. The median overall survival time was only 12.7 months {1145}. No differences in survival have been described between SCLC and LCNEC {2157,2160,2683}. In a recent series, the seventh edition of the TNM staging system was found useful for determining prognosis. Younger age, female sex, and surgery for limited disease are favourable features {800,2543}, whereas continued smoking is a strong adverse prognostic factor {2778}. A higer number of metastatic sites, especially in the central nervous system and bone marrow, is associated with a poorer prognosis, as are elevated lactate dehydrogenase, low haemoglobin, and endocrine paraneoplastic syndromes. Ectopic activation of genetically altered prolactin messenger RNA is suggested to be a poor prognostic factor in both resected SCLC and LCNEC {1423}.

Table 1.18 Distribution of significantly altered drivers in small cell lung carcinoma. Reprinted from Brambilla E et al. {259A}

Significantly altered (≥ alleles) genes (drivers)	Mode	Percentage
TP53	Inactivation	100
RB1	Inactivation	100
CREBBP	Mutation	18
EP300	Mutation	18
MLL	Mutation	10
PTEN	Mutation	10
SLIT2	Mutation	10
EPHA7	Mutation	5
FGFR1	Amplification	6
MYCL	Amplification	16
E2F2	Amplification	5
CCN2	Amplification	5

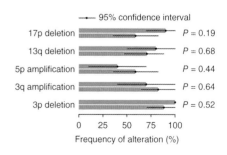

Fig. 1.71 Small cell lung cancer. Frequency of mutations in autopsy and resection specimens. Reprinted from Peifer M et al. {2012}.

Large cell neuroendocrine carcinoma

E. Brambilla
M.B. Beasley
L.R. Chirieac
J.H.M. Austin
V.L. Capelozzi
S.S. Devesa
A. Gazdar

Y. Ishikawa
J. Jett
S. Nicholson
G. Pelosi
C.A. Powell
R. Rami-Porta
G. Riely

G. Scagliotti
W.D. Travis
P. van Schil
P. Yang
D. Yankelevitz

Definition

Large cell neuroendocrine carcinoma (LCNEC) is a NSCLC that shows histological features of neuroendocrine morphology (including rosettes and peripheral palisading) and expresses immunohistochemical neuroendocrine markers. Combined LCNEC is LCNEC with components of adenocarcinoma, squamous cell carcinoma, or spindle cell carcinoma, and/or giant cell carcinoma.

ICD-O codes

Large cell neuroendocrine
    carcinoma   8013/3
Combined large cell neuroendocrine
    carcinoma   8013/3

Synonyms

LCNEC was classified as a variant of large cell carcinoma in the second and third editions of the WHO classification. Obsolete terms include large cell neuroendocrine tumour and atypical endocrine tumours of the lung. Large cell carcinoma with neuroendocrine differentiation lacks NE morphology and does not have distinct clinical characteristics.

Epidemiology

See *Adenocarcinoma*, p. 26, for a review of common epithelial tumours and *Small cell carcinoma*, p. 63.

Etiology

Like small cell lung carcinoma (SCLC), LCNEC is highly related to smoking; > 90% of these tumours occur in heavy smokers. The molecular etiology, carcinogenesis, tumour suppressor gene inactivation, and oncogene drivers are the same as those for SCLC (see *Small cell carcinoma*, p. 63). The progenitor cell of origin has not been fully characterized, but a pluripotent epithelial cell like Clara (club) cell with neuroendocrine differentiation potential has been suggested from animal models, giving rise to SCLC {1988,2531}. Combined LCNEC associated with non-neuroendocrine components occurs with the same frequency as in SCLC, supporting the theory of a common stem cell progenitor.

Clinical features

Signs and symptoms

LCNEC is generally considered to be a high-grade neuroendocrine lung tumour. The signs and symptoms are similar to those of other non-small cell lung carcinomas (NSCLCs) (see *Adenocarcinoma*, p. 26, for a review of common epithelial tumours). It is most commonly located in the peripheral lung and may be asymptomatic. A central location occurs in 20% of cases, and can be associated with postobstructive findings such as atelectasis and pneumonia. Cough, haemoptysis, dyspnoea, pneumonia, and chest pain are common symptoms at presentation. Hoarseness due to vocal cord paralysis or superior vena cava syndrome may be present with mediastinal metastases. Weight loss, fatigue, or signs and symptoms due to distant metastatic disease may be the initial presentation. Unlike SCLC, paraneoplastic syndromes are uncommon.

Imaging

This tumour presents in the full range of sizes and stages, but bulky enlargement of intrathoracic lymph nodes is rare {36}. Although the tumour is usually peripheral, an associated pleural effusion is rare. Irregular margins are common and intratumoural calcification may be seen {36}. When the tumour is large, CT examination using intravenous contrast medium commonly shows central inhomogeneous enhancement {1938}. Cavitation may occur, but is uncommon {36}.

Tumour spread

LCNEC tends to share some, if not all, of the biologically aggressive properties that are exhibited by SCLC {867} (see *Small cell carcinoma*, p. 63). It has the potential to spread to many sites, mainly to

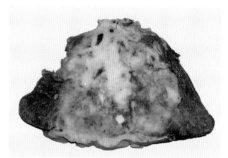
Fig. 1.72 Large cell neuroendocrine carcinoma. Macroscopic view of a pulmonary mass invading bronchi and vessels of the left lower lobe.

regional and extraregional lymph nodes, ipsilateral and contralateral lung parenchyma, liver, brain, and bones. However, metastatic sites are less frequently reported than in SCLC.

Staging

Staging is similar to other NSCLCs (see *Staging and grading*, p. 14).

Macroscopy and localization

LCNECs are usually large masses, frequently occurring in the lung periphery (84%) and the upper lobes (63%). They may also involve subsegmental or large bronchi {1938}. Their size averages 3–4 cm (ranging from 0.9 to 12 cm) {574,1114,2669,2957}. Grossly, the tumour is circumscribed, with a necrotic, tan-red cut surface {1938}. The tumour often invades the pleura, chest wall, and adjacent structures {1}. Haemorrhage is

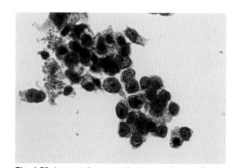
Fig. 1.73 Large cell neuroendocrine carcinoma. Cluster of cells with hyperchromatic nuclear chromatin but visible nucleoli.

occasionally present, but cavitation is rare.

Cytology

Although cytological criteria for LCNEC have been proposed {1151,1186,2865}, in practice its cytological features overlap with those of other neuroendocrine tumours and adenocarcinoma, making this diagnosis difficult {1849}. In liquid-based preparations, loose syncytial aggregates are present. Both tumour cell and nucleus size may be small. The appearance is monotonous, which suggests a low-grade neoplasm; but necrosis, if present, suggests a high-grade tumour, and apoptotic debris may be seen. Nuclei are round or ovoid. Nuclear membranes are irregular. Nuclear chromatin is finely divided, but more hyperchromatic than vesicular. Nuclear hyperchromatism might suggest small cell carcinoma, but nucleoli are easily seen in many (if not all) cells. The preservation of delicate cytoplasmic tails results in some columnar cell shapes, and a resemblance to adenocarcinoma. Overall, the cytological features of LCNEC are similar to those of SCLC, but the visible nucleoli and more abundant cytoplasm indicate a non-small cell carcinoma.

Histopathology

Large cell neuroendocrine carcinoma
LCNEC shows neuroendocrine morphology such as organoid nesting, trabecular growth, rosette-like structures, and peripheral palisading patterns. Solid nests with multiple rosette-like structures forming cribriform patterns are common. The tumour cells are generally large, with moderate to abundant cytoplasm. Nucleoli are frequent, often prominent, and their presence facilitates distinction from small cell carcinoma. Mitotic counts should be > 10 mitoses per 2 mm² (with an average of 75) of viable tumour, and they are rarely < 30 mitoses per 2 mm². The proliferation index as evaluated by Ki-67 index ranges from 40% to 80%. Necrosis usually consists of large zones, but it may be punctate. Rarely, tumours look like atypical carcinoid, but the mitotic rate exceeds the 10 mitoses per 2 mm² criterion, so these tumours are classified as LCNEC. Confirmation of neuroendocrine differentiation is required, using immunohistochemical markers such as chromogranin, synaptophysin, and

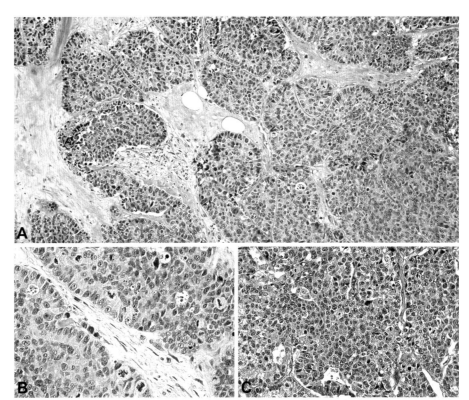

Fig. 1.74 Large cell neuroendocrine carcinoma. **A** Overview of a large cell neuroendocrine carcinoma with lobular pattern, peripheral palisading, and large areas of necrosis. **B** A high-magnification view shows details of palisading, rosettes, nuclei with vesicular chromatin, and brisk mitotic activity. **C** Lobular pattern and rosettes are prominent.

NCAM (CD56). A panel of markers is useful, but one positive marker is enough if the staining is clearcut in more than 10% of the tumour cells. The diagnosis is difficult in small biopsy specimens unless all morphological and immunohistochemical criteria are met; although with the recent trend towards core biopsies, diagnosis may be made more readily. In some cases, the diagnosis of non-small cell carcinoma, suspect LCNEC is the best diagnosis in this setting (see *Terminology and criteria in non-resection specimens*, p. 17).

Combined large cell neuroendocrine carcinoma
Combined LCNEC is a LCNEC with components of adenocarcinoma, squamous cell carcinoma, giant cell carcinoma, or spindle cell carcinoma. If these components are well recognized, any amount qualifies the tumours as combined LCNEC. Each component should be mentioned in the diagnosis. In view of the many shared clinical, epidemiological, survival, and neuroendocrine properties between LCNEC and small cell carcinoma, these tumours are classified as combined LCNEC with specification about

the additional histological subtypes present. Combinations with SCLC also occur, but such tumours are classified as combined SCLC.

Immunohistochemistry
The diagnosis of LCNEC requires immunohistochemistry for confirmation of neuroendocrine differentiation {2669,2681,2683}. In decreasing order of frequency, NCAM/CD56 stains 92–100% of LCNEC cases, followed by chromogranin A in 80–85%, and synaptophysin in 50–60% {2205,2206,2669,2681}. NCAM/CD56 needs a note of caution because of its lower specificity for neuroendocrine differentiation in lung cancer, but it is the most sensitive marker in the appropriate morphological context of a neuroendocrine neoplasm {1401}. Chromogranin A and synaptophysin are the most reliable stains for diagnostic accuracy in distinguishing LCNEC from non-neuroendocrine tumours, and one positive marker is enough if the staining is clear-cut {1115,2205,2206,2683}. LCNEC also produces amine-peptide hormones {1148}, albeit at a lower level than carcinoid tumours {227}. About half of all LCNECs express TTF1, a figure

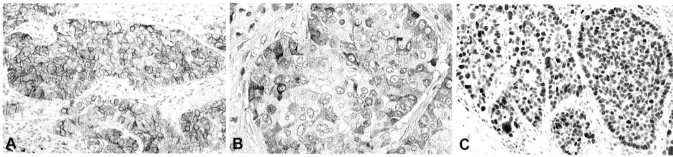

Fig. 1.75 Large cell neuroendocrine carcinoma. **A** NCAM (CD56) immunostaining in the large cell neuroendocrine component of combined large cell neuroendocrine carcinoma; note the typical cell membrane pattern. **B** This combined large cell neuroendocrine carcinoma associated with adenocarcinoma is immunostained with chromogranin antibody. **C** TTF1 immunoreactivity with a typical nuclear pattern.

that is generally lower than that for SCLC {2205,2206,2499,2501}, but all LCNECs demonstrate pancytokeratin, low-molecular weight cytokeratin, or CK7 reactivity, with either a dot-like or diffuse cytoplasmic pattern {2206,2681,2683}. Expression of squamous cell-related markers, such as CK5/6 {1860}, CK1, CK5, CK10, CK14, {2499,2500} and p40 {2024}, is usually lacking in pure forms of LCNEC {1818,2546}. Positive staining with napsin A {2206} has rarely been described in LCNEC, and p63 may be detected even with no overt squamous cell differentiation {2019}. More than 70% of LCNECs also demonstrate CD117 immunoreactivity {337,2018}, which may be associated with reduced survival and increased recurrence rate {337}.

Differential diagnosis
The primary differential diagnoses for LCNEC include SCLC, atypical carcinoid, basaloid squamous cell carcinoma, adenocarcinoma, and other large cell carcinomas with neuroendocrine morphology or staining. Distinction from atypical carcinoid and LCNEC is based on mitotic count, (> 10 mitoses per 2 mm², more extensive necrosis, and to some extent cytological features {1848,2679}. Discrimination between LCNEC and SCLC is based on a constellation of features including prominent nucleoli, vesicular to clumped versus finely granular chromatin, cell size (greater than the diameter of 3 resting lymphocytes), and more abundant cytoplasm in LCNEC {575,1576}. Adenocarcinoma with a solid or cribriform pattern lacks neuroendocrine markers, whereas basaloid squamous cell carcinoma lacks TTF1 and neuroendocrine markers, and is positive for p40 {209,2024} and CK5/6 {2500}. Metastatic carcinomas from the endometrium, ovary, breast, prostate, pancreas, or large

bowel may enter differential diagnosis with LCNEC when showing neuroendocrine differentiation. Endometrial {2586} and ovarian {636} carcinomas are differentially positive for PAX8 {1924} and/or WT1 {136}, whereas breast cancer {1832}, is more consistently positive for estrogen and progesterone receptors.

About 10–20% of lung squamous cell carcinomas, adenocarcinomas, and large cell carcinomas, which do not show neuroendocrine morphology by light microscopy, do demonstrate neuroendocrine differentiation on immunohistochemistry and/or electron microscopy, and are collectively referred to as NSCLC with neuroendocrine differentiation; however, they should be classified as squamous, adenocarcinoma, or large cell carcinoma, with a comment about positive neuroendocrine markers. The clinical inference of this tumour category on survival and chemotherapy response is still

unclear, so they are not recognized as specific entities. Neuroendocrine stains are not recommended for routine use on tumours lacking neuroendocrine morphology. Large cell carcinomas with neuroendocrine morphology and negative neuroendocrine markers may be called large cell carcinomas with neuroendocrine morphology. Such tumours should be regarded as large cell carcinoma with unclear immunophenotype (see *Large cell carcinoma*, p. 80).

Genetic profile
The genetic profile of some LCNEC is very similar to that of SCLC (see *Small cell carcinoma*, p. 63), but very different from that of carcinoid tumours {715,2012} (see *Carcinoid tumour*, p. 73). Like small cell carcinoma, LCNEC exhibits an extremely high mutation rate (of more than 7.4 protein-changing mutations per million base pairs) as compared to other lung tumour

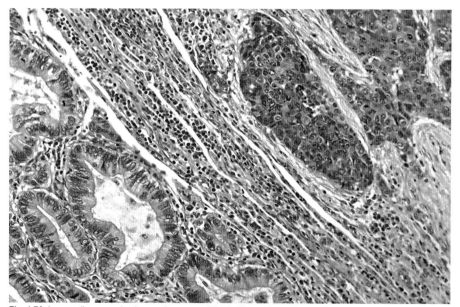

Fig. 1.76 Large cell neuroendocrine carcinoma, combined with an acinar adenocarcinoma. Reprinted from Travis WD et al. {2678}.

types, likely linked to tobacco carcinogens (see *Small cell carcinoma,* p. 63). *TP53* and *RB* mutational inactivation are frequent, as are recurrent mutations of *CREBBP/EP300* and *MLL* genes encoding histone modifiers, which are observed in 18% of SCLCs and are characteristic of a so-called LCNEC/SCLC genetic subtype of LCNECs. Whole-exome, genome, and transcriptome sequencing of a large series of LCNECs identified additional mutations compatible with adenocarcinoma genotype: *TTF1* amplification and *CDKN2A* deletions, and frequent mutations of *STK11* and *KEAP1*, evocative of the genetic profile of adenocarcinoma or squamous carcinoma. These findings are compatible with LCNEC representing an evolutionary trunk branching to SCLC, adenocarcinoma, or squamous cell carcinoma {714}. This was already suggest-ed by the frequency of combined LCNEC and SCLC tumours, and by the occurrence of resistance in tyrosine kinase inhibitor-treated adenocarcinoma recurring as SCLC {2332}, as well as by the observation of recurrence of chemotherapy-treated SCLC in the form of NSCLC {257}. *FGFR1* amplifications occur in a significant subset of LCNECs {714}.

TP53 and *RB* double genetic inactivation, which is universal in SCLC, occurs in most LCNECs. This is illustrated by the difference in loss of RB1 protein expression in only 70% of LCNECs versus 95% of SCLCs {158,890}. Apoptotic pathways with a high level of Bcl2 relative to Bax (i.e. with a Bcl2-to-Bax ratio > 1) are characteristic of both high-grade neuroendocrine tumours {259}.

Prognosis and predictive factors
Patients with LCNEC are more likely to develop recurrence and have shorter actuarial survival than patients with other histological types of NSCLC, even in those with stage I disease {713}. In two series, 5-year survival rates as low as 32.1% and 33%, respectively, have been reported for patients with stage I disease {153,2202}. The role of multimodality treatment in early disease is not yet established. Because of the limited incidence of this subtype, no definitive data are available about specific prognostic or predictive markers. The clinical efficacy of chemotherapy for unresectable LCNEC has been shown to be comparable with that for extensive small cell lung cancer, and patients may benefit from a SCLC-based chemotherapy {2202}.

Carcinoid tumour

M.B. Beasley
E. Brambilla
L.R. Chirieac
J.H.M. Austin
S.S. Devesa
P. Hasleton

J. Jett
A.M. Marchevsky
S. Nicholson
M. Papotti
G. Pelosi
R. Rami-Porta

G. Scagliotti
E. Thunnissen
W.D. Travis
P. van Schil
P. Yang

Definition
Carcinoid tumours are neuroendocrine epithelial malignancies, and can be divided into two subcategories: Typical carcinoids are carcinoid tumours with < 2 mitoses per 2 mm^2, and lacking necrosis. They measure ≥ 0.5 cm in size. Atypical carcinoids are carcinoid tumours with 2–10 mitoses per 2 mm^2, and/or foci of necrosis.

ICD-O codes
Typical carcinoid   8240/3
Atypical carcinoid   8249/3

Synonyms
Typical carcinoid:
Not recommended: well-differentiated neuroendocrine carcinoma, grade 1 neuroendocrine carcinoma
Atypical carcinoid:
Not recommended: moderately differentiated neuroendocrine carcinoma, grade 2 neuroendocrine carcinoma

Epidemiology
Lung carcinoid tumours include typical carcinoids and atypical carcinoids. Typical carcinoids and atypical carcinoids are low- and intermediate-grade subtypes of lung neuroendocrine tumours, respectively, relative to the high-grade large cell neuroendocrine carcinoma (LCNEC) and small cell carcinoma (see *Small cell carcinoma,* p. 63). The estimated age-adjusted incidence of carcinoid tumours ranges from < 0.1 per 100 000 to 1.5 per 100 000, with 70–90% being typical carcinoids. Carcinoid tumours account for < 1% of all lung cancers {987,1782,2105,2942}. Carcinoids occur more often in people who are aged < 60 years, female, or White than in people who are older, male, or non-White {726}. Other reported risk factors include having a family history of carcinoid tumours and carrying the *MEN1* gene {464,987,2942}. Typical carcinoids are not related to tobacco smoking, although atypical carcinoids have been reported more frequently in smokers. A population-based study of 1882 women

and men showed significantly increased risks of breast and prostate cancers in the first 5 years after carcinoid tumour diagnosis, with risk ratios of 1.7 and 2.8, respectively {497}.

Etiology
The mechanisms of carcinoid tumour development and progression are not clear, although some cases are postulated to develop in the setting of proliferating pulmonary neuroendocrine cells via diffuse idiopathic pulmonary neuroendocrine cell hyperplasia (DIPNECH) and tumourlets (see *Preinvasive lesion – Diffuse idiopathic pulmonary neuroendocrine cell hyperplasia,* p. 78), involving aberrations of specific genetic events such as menin or its targets and interaction partners {2546} (see *Small cell carcinoma,* p. 63). The cell of origin is unknown, although it was historically thought to arise from pulmonary neuroendocrine (Kulchitsky) cells.

Clinical features

Signs and symptoms
Lung carcinoid tumours most commonly arise in the central airways. Approximately a third of pulmonary carcinoid tumours occur peripherally, and may be asymptomatic at the time of detection by an incidental radiograph. Clinical syndromes due to peptide production are uncommon, but include carcinoid syndrome, Cushing syndrome, and acromegaly.

Imaging
Bronchial involvement, a lobulated contour, and considerable enhancement on CT using intravenous contrast medium are common {1647}. Calcification can occur in central carcinoid tumours {3034}. When bronchial involvement is present, secondary distal effects include atelectasis, bronchiectasis, and hyperlucency on CT {1647}.

Tumour spread
For bronchopulmonary carcinoid tumours, the seventh edition of the TNM classification is applied {2680}. As with

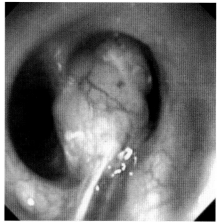

Fig. 1.77 Bronchoscopic image of a typical carcinoid presenting as a polypoid endobronchial mass.

other types of non-small cell lung carcinomas, tumour spread may occur through the lymphatic or haematogenous route. Metastatic disease may involve ipsilateral and contralateral hilar and mediastinal lymph nodes, as well as the liver and bones. However, lymph node and distant metastases are more frequently encountered with atypical carcinoid than typical carcinoid.

Staging
Since 2009, with the seventh edition of the TNM classification, staging has been based on the tumour, node, and metastasis classification, which determines the anatomical extent of the disease {2680} (see *Staging and grading,* p. 14). In the setting of DIPNECH, multiple carcinoid tumours should not be regarded as intrapulmonary metastases, but as separate primaries.

Localization
Carcinoid tumours can be found from the trachea to the bronchioles. In the trachea they are rare, but their precise prevalence at this site cannot be established, because of inconsistencies in the nomenclature and the inconsistent distinction between tracheal versus bronchial location. Carcinoids are rarely associated with DIPNECH, and may rarely produce a miliary pattern in the lung {121}.

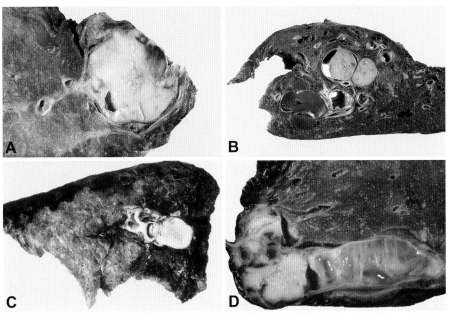

Fig. 1.78 A Central bronchial carcinoid in a 26-year-old woman. B More peripherally located carcinoid with bronchiectasis. C Typical carcinoid presenting as round, partially endobronchial mass. Note the poststenotic pneumonia. D Carcinoid. A circumscribed tan mass forming a tan endobronchial mass causing complete obstruction of the bronchus. There is postobstructive dilation of the distal bronchus.

Most central carcinoids are seen in main stem or lobar bronchi {971}. Peripheral carcinoid tumours are described in 40% of cases {2669}, and they are more likely to be atypical {880}.

Macroscopy
Central carcinoid tumours are well circumscribed, round to ovoid, and sessile or pedunculated. They often fill the bronchial lumen. The tumours may grow between the cartilaginous plates into adjacent tissues. An obvious airway association may not be observable in peripheral tumours. In a large series of neuroendocrine tumours, an endobronchial component was seen in 54% and 31% of typical carcinoids and atypical carcinoids, respectively. Nodular neuroendocrine proliferations measuring < 0.5 cm are classified as tumourlets. Carcinoids

range in size from 0.5 to 9.5 cm. Atypical carcinoids are on average larger than typical carcinoids {2736}; however, size is not a reliable determinant of histological type {878}. Central tumours may cause postobstructive pneumonia, abscesses, and bronchiectasis.

Cytology
Carcinoid tumour cells are discohesive, but Giemsa-stained direct smears may show loosely branching clusters, single-cell dispersal, and bare nuclei. Fragments of capillaries are a helpful clue if present. Necrosis is absent and the background is clean. Rosette shapes may be seen. Individual cells are small and have round, oval, or spindle-shaped nuclei. Nuclear outlines are smooth. Chromatin is finely granular and nucleoli are not prominent {478}. Scant, if any, cytoplasm

surrounds the nuclei. The discohesive nature may suggest a haematolymphoid population. Mitotic figures are not seen. In liquid-based Papanicolaou-stained preparations, the small size and bland appearance of the often bare round and ovoid nuclei is subtle. If small amounts of granular cytoplasm are preserved, then low columnar or cuboidal cell shapes may be present and recognized as a tumour cell population.

Histopathology

Typical carcinoid
Carcinoid tumours are characterized by growth patterns suggesting neuroendocrine differentiation. Organoid and trabecular patterns are most common; however, rosette formation, papillary growth, pseudoglandular growth, and follicular growth may also be seen. Spindle cell growth is also commonly encountered, more so in peripheral tumours. A mix of patterns may be seen in an individual tumour. The tumour cells are usually uniform in appearance, with polygonal shape, finely granular nuclear chromatin, inconspicuous nucleoli, and moderate to abundant eosinophilic cytoplasm. Oncocytic, clear cell, and melanin-laden variants have been reported. Typical carcinoids may contain cells with pronounced pleomorphism or prominent nucleoli, which should not be taken as criteria for atypical carcinoid. The background stroma is classically highly vascularized, but extensive hyalinization, cartilage, or bone formation may be encountered. Stromal amyloid has also been reported, as well as prominent mucinous stroma. Peripheral tumours in particular may be associated with multiple tumourlets, with or without DIPNECH (*Preinvasive lesion – Diffuse idiopathic pulmonary neuroendocrine cell hyperplasia,* p. 78). Central carcinoids may extend through the bronchial cartilage plates.

Atypical carcinoid
Atypical carcinoid generally shows the same range of histological features as typical carcinoid. The defining features are the presence of 2–10 mitoses per 2 mm^2 and/or the presence of necrosis. Necrosis is usually punctate, although larger zones may be seen. These findings may be present only focally, so careful examination of a resected tumour is necessary for accurate subtyping.

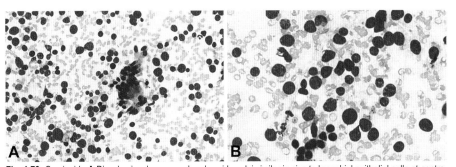

Fig. 1.79 Carcinoid. A Discohesive, bare, round and ovoid nuclei similar in size to bronchial epithelial cells at centre. B Smooth, bare, ovoid nuclei next to bronchial epithelial cells.

Mitoses should be counted in the area of highest mitotic activity in the fields filled with as many viable tumour cells as possible. Mitoses should be counted per 2 mm², rather than 10 high-power fields. Due to differences in microscope models, adjustments need to be made in the number of high-power fields reviewed to assess a 2 mm² area of tumour {2683}. In tumours that are near the cutoffs of 2 or 10 mitoses per 2 mm², at least three sets of 2 mm² should be counted and the mean used for determining the mitotic rate, rather than the single highest rate. Mitotic rate and necrosis status should be included in pathology reports.

Immunohistochemistry
Immunohistochemistry may be required to confirm neuroendocrine and epithelial differentiation, especially in small biopsy or cytology specimens. An antibody panel including chromogranin A and synaptophysin (both with cytoplasmic labelling), and CD56 (mostly decorating cell membranes) {1401,2132,2821} is recommended. However, none of these markers distinguish typical carcinoid from atypical carcinoid. Most carcinoids are also reactive for pancytokeratin antibodies, with reported negative cases limited to a few peripheral tumours {1678}. High-molecular weight cytokeratins are typically negative in carcinoids and normal and hyperplastic bronchial neuroendocrine cells {2500}. Some peripheral tumours also stain with TTF1, which is less specific (see *Rationale for classification in small biopsies and cytology,* p. 16, and *Small cell carcinoma,* p. 63) but carcinoids are mostly negative for TTF1 {375,629,1377,2275,2501}. Pulmonary carcinoids may express several types of polypeptides, such as calcitonin, gastrin-related peptide/bombesin, and adrenocorticotropic hormone, similar to

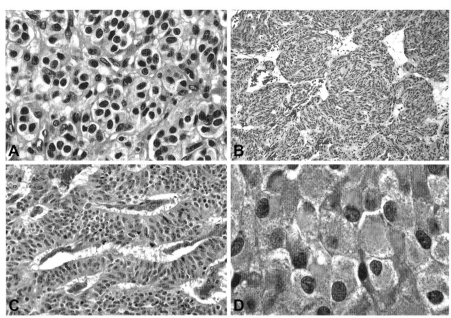

Fig. 1.80 Typical carcinoid. **A** Tumour cells grow in an organoid nesting arrangement, with a fine vascular stroma; the moderate amount of cytoplasm is eosinophilic and the nuclear chromatin finely granular. **B** Prominent spindle cell pattern. **C** Trabecular pattern. **D** Oncocytic features with abundant eosinophilic cytoplasm. Reprinted from Travis WD et al. {2678}.

gastroenteropancreatic neuroendocrine tumours {227,886} but they are not recommended for diagnosis, although they are sometimes associated with an endocrine syndrome {217,659}. The Ki-67 labelling index is valuable in biopsy or cytology samples, particularly with crush artefact, where mitotic index is difficult to assess, to avoid misdiagnosing carcinoid tumours as high-grade neuroendocrine carcinomas {2021}. However, the utility of this marker to discriminate typical carcinoid from atypical carcinoid or to predict prognosis (with cut-off values ranging from 2.5 to 5.8%) within individual carcinoid tumour categories is not established {2020}.

Differential diagnosis
The differential diagnosis of pulmonary carcinoids includes metastatic carcinoids from elsewhere, especially those originating in the gastrointestinal tract {574}. Glandular structures are unusual in pulmonary carcinoids, but a frequent finding in gastrointestinal carcinoids. In crushed biopsies, carcinoid may be mistaken for small cell lung carcinoma (SCLC). Ki-67 plays an important role in this setting, because SCLC has a high labelling index (> 50%) contrasting with a low labelling index (< 10–20%) in carcinoids {2021}.
Rarely, a tumour with carcinoid-like morphology has a mitotic rate of > 10 mitoses per 2 mm², and because it is likely to be aggressive, it is best classified as an LCNEC.
The monotonous nuclear appearance of carcinoids may also be seen in salivary

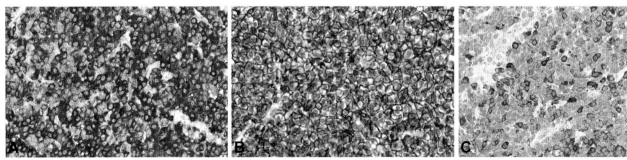

Fig. 1.81 Typical carcinoid. **A** Strong cytoplasmic chromogranin staining. **B** The tumour cells show strong membranous staining for CD56. **C** Scattered tumour cells show strong cytoplasmic adrenocorticotropic hormone staining in a patient presenting with Cushing syndrome, due to ectopic adrenocorticotropic hormone production. Reprinted from Travis WD et al. {2678}.

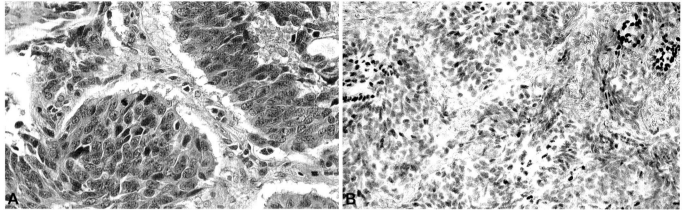

Fig. 1.82 Atypical carcinoid. **A** Haematoxylin-eosin-saffron staining section showing two mitoses in the same high-power field. **B** Faint or negative TTF1 immunostaining on tumour cells, in contrast with strong positive TTF1 staining on entrapped pneumocytes.

gland-type tumours, metastases of lobular breast carcinoma, paraganglioma, and glomangioma. Carcinoids, salivary gland-type tumours, and lobular carcinoma of the breast show cytokeratin (CK8/18 and AE1/AE3) positivity, and lack vimentin expression. This contrasts with the opposite staining pattern in paraganglioma and glomangioma {83,1334,2408,2708}. Paraganglioma usually shows neuroendocrine staining, but cytokeratin staining is negative. Glomus tumours express desmin, but not neuroendocrine markers. Metastases of breast carcinoma may be positive for estrogen and/or progesterone receptors, and are usually negative for neuroendocrine markers {2111}. However, positive staining for estrogen or progesterone receptors has been reported in some carcinoid tumours {2387}. Metastases from thyroid carcinoma are TTF1- and thyroglobulin-positive. Mucoepidermoid carcinomas may show more than one cell type (e.g. goblet cells and squamoid cells), and often express p63, cytokeratin, CK4/14, and or mucin, with negative neuroendocrine markers {2101,2266} (see *Salivary gland-type tumours*, p. 99).

Genetic profile

Lung carcinoids display the lowest somatic mutation rate (0.4 per million base pairs) among lung and other tumours, in contrast with the high-grade SCLC and LCNEC, which have the highest rates (> 7 per million base pairs) in human tumours. *TP53* and *RB1* mutation and inactivation with loss of RB1 protein expression are rare in typical carcinoids (< 5%) but more frequent in atypical carcinoids (20%) {259,807,889,890}. The disruption of p16/retinoblastoma pathways is seen in a low proportion of atypical carcinoids (20%) but not in typical carcinoids {158,1910}. The only significant mutations affect the chromatin remodelling gene family *MEN1* (13% of cases) in mutual exclusion with *PSP1* {716}. *MEN1* is a tumour suppressor gene interacting with H3K4 methyl transferases. *MEN1* somatic mutations were previously reported in 40% of sporadic carcinoids in patients without multiple endocrine neoplasia type 1 familial disease {560}, more frequently in atypical carcinoids than typical carcinoids, but never in SCLC or LCNEC {561}. With other mutations in genes of the methylation complex, *CBX6* of Polycomb repressive complex 1 and

EZH2 of Polycomb repressive complex 2, the methylation complex is mutated in 34% of carcinoids. In addition, 25% of cases exhibit mutations that affect the chromatin remodelling SWI/SNF complex gene pathway *ARID1A*, *SMARCC1*, *SMARCC2*, *SMARCA4*. With sister chromatid cohesion genes mutation (*NIPBL*, *DICER1*), 52.3% of carcinoids show alterations of chromatin remodelling genes. Other significant mutations of *EIF1AX* and trafficking and E3 ubiquitin ligase mutations occur in 9% and 18%, respectively. Mutations in these gene families are mostly mutually exclusive, consistent with their role as driver genes. Altogether, a candidate driver mutation was identified and validated in 72.7% of carcinoids. No genetic segregation was observed between typical and atypical carcinoids, which appear to derive from the same clonal proliferation {715}.

These data strongly support a pathogenetic model, which would indicate that carcinoid tumours are not early progenitors of the high-grade neuroendocrine tumours, SCLC, or LCNEC, but are genetically and phenotypically independent proliferations. Finally, they show that mutations in chromatin remodelling genes

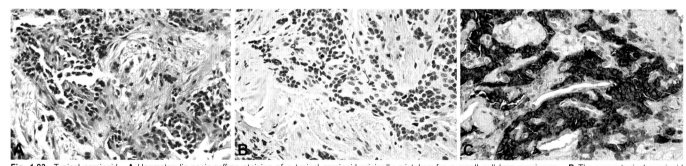

Fig. 1.83 Typical carcinoid. **A** Haematoxylin-eosin-saffron staining of a typical carcinoid originally mistaken for a small cell lung carcinoma. **B** The same typical carcinoid immunostained with Ki-67 antibody, showing < 1% Ki-67-positive cells, but (**C**) strong immunostaining with synaptophysin antibody.

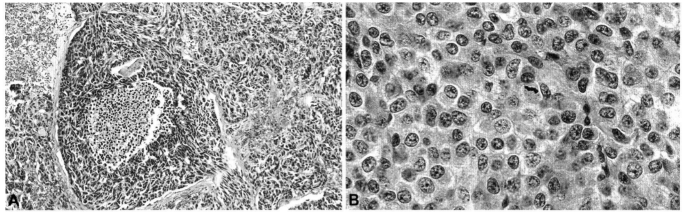

Fig. 1.84 Atypical carcinoid. **A** A small necrotic focus. **B** A single mitosis is present in this high-power field. The tumour cells show carcinoid morphology, with moderate eosinophilic cytoplasm and finely granular nuclear chromatin. Reprinted from Travis WD et al. {2678}.

are sufficient to drive the early steps of tumorigenesis in carcinoids {715,716}. Molecular genetic abnormalities in cell cycle arrest and DNA repair genes such as *E2F1* {691}, *p14ARF* {809}, and cyclin E {2263} are seen in < 5% of typical carcinoids, but in 20–30% of atypical carcinoids.

Prognosis and predictive factors
Distinction between typical carcinoid and atypical carcinoid is the most important prognostic factor. Atypical carcinoid has a worse prognosis than typical carcinoid {319,522}. Atypical carcinoids are more likely to metastasize than typical carcinoids; 5 year survival rates for patients with typical carcinoids and atypical carcinoids are approximately 90% and 60%, respectively, and higher for those with resectable tumours {1867,2409,2422}. Prognosis in each group mainly depends on the TNM classification, either clinical or pathological, with the highest stages carrying the worst prognosis. In a series of 247 atypical carcinoids, age, smoking habits, and lymph node involvement were significant prognostic factors in multivariate analysis {522}. The mitotic index also appears to be prognostic in atypical carcinoids {159,522}. For resectable cases, prognosis depends on complete resection. For correct pathological staging, a systematic nodal dissection is recommended for tumours undergoing surgical resection, which is also valid for typical carcinoids {1623}.

No significant markers have yet been identified that are predictive of response to systemic therapy for carcinoid tumours.

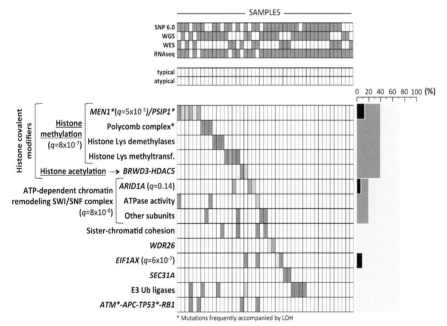

Fig. 1.85 Whole genomic analysis of 45 cases of carcinoid tumours. Significantly mutated genes (*Q* value < 0.2) and frequently mutated pathways identified by genome, exome, and transcriptome sequencing. Samples are displayed as columns and arranged to emphasize mutually exclusive mutations. A total of 72% of carcinoids were found to have driver mutations. LOH, loss of heterozygosity. Reprinted from Fernandez-Cuesta L et al. {715}.

J.R. Gosney   S. Nicholson
J.H.M. Austin   R. Rami-Porta
J. Jett   W.D. Travis
A.G. Nicholson   P. van Schil

Preinvasive lesion

Diffuse idiopathic pulmonary neuroendocrine cell hyperplasia

Definition

Diffuse idiopathic pulmonary neuroendocrine cell hyperplasia (DIPNECH) is a generalized proliferation of pulmonary neuroendocrine cells (PNCs) that may be confined to the mucosa of airways (with or without luminal protrusion), may invade locally to form tumourlets, or may develop into carcinoid tumours {26,535,1819}. DIPNECH is often accompanied by mild, chronic lymphocytic inflammation and fibrosis of involved airways (specifically, constrictive bronchiolitis).

ICD-O code   8040/0

Synonyms

DIPNECH was not recognized and named until 1992 {26}, but unidentified cases with clinical and pathological features identical to those of DIPNECH appear earlier in the literature.

Epidemiology

DIPNECH typically presents in the fifth or sixth decade, and is more common in women than in men {26,535,819}.

Etiology

Though idiopathic by definition, DIPNECH may be a consequence of unrecognized pulmonary injury, of which the mild inflammatory and fibrotic changes in airways that often accompany this hyperplasia are a legacy. However, it is more likely that these changes are secondary to a local effect of amines and peptides released by the proliferating PNCs {535,563,1819}.

Clinical features

Signs and symptoms

There are two major presentations. Most symptomatic patients present with a long history of cough, breathlessness, and wheezing, often misdiagnosed as asthma. Other cases are identified incidentally, typically during high-resolution CT for other conditions {26,535,1326,1819}. Rarely, DIPNECH is a component of multiple endocrine neoplasia type 1 {535}.

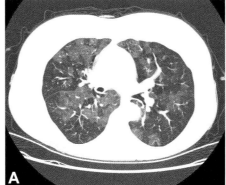 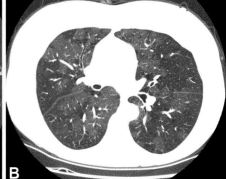

Fig. 1.86 Diffuse idiopathic pulmonary neuroendocrine cell hyperplasia, manifesting as multifocal air-trapping and mosaic perfusion, both in inspiration (**A**) and especially in expiration (**B**).

Imaging

Findings on chest radiography are of diffuse reticulonodularity {26}. High-resolution CT shows nodular bronchial wall thickening caused by intraluminal protrusion of proliferating cells and mosaic attenuation caused by mucus plugging, airway obstruction, air-trapping, and sometimes bronchiectasis {1326}. Detection of air-trapping may require expiration high-resolution CT. Pulmonary nodules due to tumourlets or carcinoids may be seen.

Tumour spread

DIPNECH probably arises in terminal bronchioles as proliferation of single cells or clusters of neuroendocrine cells. When tumourlets develop, they extend locally into and through the bronchiolar wall, sometimes into adjacent parenchyma. It is unknown what proportion of patients with DIPNECH eventually develop carcinoid tumours, but it is probably the minority. Most of the carcinoids that develop in this context are typical, but occasional atypical carcinoids with more aggressive behaviour have also been described {535,1819}. The most aggressive pulmonary neuroendocrine tumours, large cell neuroendocrine carcinoma and small cell carcinoma, have never been described in association with DIPNECH.

Staging

DIPNECH is a preinvasive condition. Car-

cinoid tumours that may develop from DIPNECH are staged using the TNM scheme.

Macroscopy

Intramucosal lesions of DIPNECH are not apparent macroscopically, but tumourlets are sometimes discernible as grey-white nodules, a few millimetres in diameter, intimately associated with small airways.

Histopathology

The proliferating PNCs in DIPNECH may remain confined to the mucosa as small groups or a monolayer, may form aggregates that protrude into the lumen as nodular or papillary growths, or may invade across the basal lamina to form tumourlets {535,1819}. The PNCs are round to oval or spindle-shaped and have

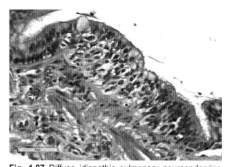

Fig. 1.87 Diffuse idiopathic pulmonary neuroendocrine cell hyperplasia. An early intramucosal aggregate of pulmonary neuroendocrine cells elevating the epithelium in a terminal bronchiole.

a moderate amount of eosinophilic cytoplasm with round to oval nuclei that have a salt-and-pepper chromatin. Although early intramucosal proliferation may not be obvious in H&E-stained sections, the later stages are readily apparent. Immunolabelling for neuroendocrine antigens, the full range of which is almost always expressed in DIPNECH, usually reveals more extensive involvement than is apparent in H&E-stained sections {881}.

Reactive proliferation of PNCs in chronically inflamed or otherwise damaged lungs is distinguished from DIPNECH by the presence of the causative pathology and absence of carcinoid tumours. The relationship between DIPNECH and the peritumoural proliferation of PNCs seen in the vicinity of many pulmonary carcinoids {2167} is unclear, but it is limited, in the latter, to the immediate vicinity of the tumour. If widespread PNC proliferation is seen in the non-neoplastic lung surrounding a carcinoid tumour but the diagnosis of DIPNECH is not certain morphologically, high-resolution CT may be useful to look for the characteristic findings. The distinction between tumourlets and small carcinoid tumours in DIPNECH is usually clear from their size and histological characteristics. Tumourlets are poorly defined, with irregular, infiltrative margins and a conspicuously fibrotic stroma. They are also intimately related to an airway and are ≤ 5 mm in diameter.

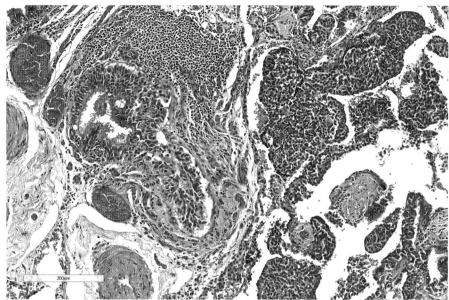

Fig. 1.89 Diffuse idiopathic pulmonary neuroendocrine cell hyperplasia. Florid proliferation of pulmonary neuroendocrine cells within and around a terminal bronchiole (left), spreading into the surrounding parenchyma and forming a tumourlet. A chronic lymphocytic infiltrate is evident adjacent to the airway, and there is mild peribronchiolar fibrosis.

Genetic profile

Little is known about the genetic pathology of DIPNECH, although it is occasionally associated with multiple endocrine neoplasia type 1 {535}. The proliferating PNCs in DIPNECH, unlike those proliferating as a reaction to pulmonary injury, express Ki-67 at all stages and show earlier expression of p16 {881}.

Prognosis and predictive factors

DIPNECH is a chronic, slowly progressive disease, usually treated by steroids. The carcinoid tumours that may develop are usually typical and indolent. Occasionally, patients develop a progressive, obliterative bronchiolitis that has been treated by transplantation {26,535,1819}.

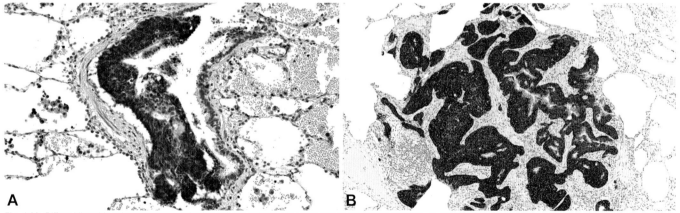

A **B**

Fig. 1.88 Diffuse idiopathic pulmonary neuroendocrine cell hyperplasia, observed with chromogranin staining. **A** A large, irregular aggregate of pulmonary neuroendocrine cells encroaching into the lumen of a terminal bronchiole, although not invading the submucosa. **B** A typical tumourlet with its characteristic infiltrative edge and conspicuous stroma.

Large cell carcinoma

A.G. Nicholson
E. Brambilla
M.B. Beasley
N.E. Caporaso
L. Carvalho
M.L. Dalurzo
S.S. Devesa
K. Geisinger

J. Jett
K.M. Kerr
M. Ladanyi
M. Meyerson
D. Naidich
M. Noguchi
I. Petersen
C.A. Powell

R. Rami-Porta
N. Rekhtman
G. Riely
L. Sholl
E. Thunnissen
W.D. Travis
P. van Schil
Y. Yatabe

Definition
Large cell carcinoma is an undifferentiated non-small cell carcinoma (NSCC) that lacks the cytological, architectural, and immunohistochemical features of small cell carcinoma, adenocarcinoma, or squamous cell carcinoma. The diagnosis requires a thoroughly sampled resected tumour, and cannot be made on non-resection or cytology specimens.

Historical perspective
Many tumours previously classified as large cell carcinoma according to the 2004 WHO classification are now classified as solid adenocarcinoma or non-keratinizing squamous cell carcinoma, based on immunohistochemistry and mucin stains. The diagnosis of large cell carcinoma is only made when additional staining is negative, unclear, or not available.

The 2004 WHO classification included several large cell carcinoma subtypes that have now been moved to other tumour categories, such as basaloid carcinoma (under squamous cell carcinoma), large cell neuroendocrine carcinoma (LCNEC) (under neuroendocrine tumours), and lymphoepithelioma-like carcinoma (under other and unclassified carcinomas). Clear cell and rhabdoid variants are no longer considered histological subtypes, but should be recorded as cytological features even when only small proportions are present.

ICD-O code
Large cell carcinoma   8012/3

Based on their immunohistochemical profiles, three subtypes of large cell carcinoma can be distinguished (see Table 1.19):
- Large cell carcinoma with null immunohistochemical features
- Large cell carcinoma with unclear immunohistochemical features
- Large cell carcinoma with no additional stains

Synonyms
Large cell anaplastic carcinoma; large cell undifferentiated carcinoma

Epidemiology
In the 1990s, large cell carcinoma accounted for approximately 10% of all lung cancers {2684}. However, more recent data from the National Cancer Institute's SEER programme in the United States show that age-adjusted rates have decreased over the past three decades, from 9.4% to 2.3% (see Adenocarcinoma, p. 26). This decrease likely reflects changes in pathologists' diagnostic approach due to the introduction of immunohistochemistry for glandular and squamous markers. The average age at diagnosis is about 60 years, and most patients are male.

Etiology
The etiology of large cell carcinoma is similar to that of other lung cancers (see Adenocarcinoma, p. 26). Most patients are smokers.

Clinical features
The symptoms, imaging, tumour spread {2078}, and staging of large cell carcinoma are similar to those of other non-small cell lung carcinomas (NSCLCs) (see Adenocarcinoma, p. 26, and Staging and grading, p. 14).

Localization
Large cell carcinomas are typically peripheral masses.

Macroscopy
Large cell carcinomas are usually large, circumscribed, solid masses, often with necrosis and rarely with cavitation.

Cytology
As with small tissue biopsies, the diagnosis of large cell carcinoma should not be rendered in cytological specimens. Rather, an interpretation of NSCC, not otherwise specified is preferred if neither distinguishing morphological nor immunohistochemical characteristics of other tumour types can be identified: by definition, keratinization, cytoplasmic secretory products, and other evidence of glandular differentiation are absent. Cytological samples may provide evidence of subtle morphological differentiation that is not

Table 1.19 Subtyping of resected, morphologically undifferentiated non-small cell carcinomas (formerly large cell carcinoma)

Adenocarcinoma, solid subtype[a]	Positive for TTF1 and/or napsin A and/or mucin Negative (or focal staining in scattered tumour cells) for p40, p63[b], and/or CK5/6
Non-keratinizing squamous cell carcinoma[a]	Negative for TTF1, napsin A, and mucin Diffusely positive for p40, p63[b], and/or CK5/6
Adenosquamous carcinoma[a]	Positive for adenocarcinoma and squamous markers in geographically distinct cell populations, each accounting for > 10% of tumour cells
Large cell carcinoma with null immunohistochemical features	Positive for cytokeratins Negative for lineage-specific markers and mucin
Large cell carcinoma with unclear immunohistochemical features (see Table 1.20)	Positive for cytokeratins Unclear immunoprofiles and negative for mucin
Large cell carcinoma with no stains available	No immunohistochemical or mucin staining available

[a] In cases where there is morphological evidence of either squamous cell carcinoma or adenocarcinoma, immunohistochemistry is not required to assess undifferentiated areas.
[b] p63 (4A4) can rarely be more diffusely positive in some TTF1-positive tumours. These should be classified as adenocarcinomas.

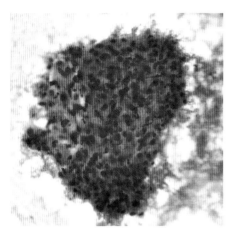

Fig. 1.90 Large cell carcinoma. A percutaneous fine-needle aspirate shows large cohesive aggregates of overtly malignant epithelioid cells with no distinctive features of squamous or glandular differentiation. This was classified as non-small cell carcinoma, not otherwise specified on cytology, and proven to be a large cell carcinoma on resection.

apparent in resection specimens in the absence of immunostains {2135}. Typically, the tumour cells are cohesive and have high-grade, overtly malignant cytological features, similar to those of other poorly differentiated NSCCs. Malignant cells with rhabdoid cytology show voluminous cytoplasm with eccentrically placed nuclei and massive nucleoli. Especially with Romanowsky staining, ovoid perinuclear inclusions may be evident, as may small irregular and brightly eosinophilic structures, possibly megamitochondria. Cohesion is less marked in tumours with rhabdoid cytology {294,812,1159,2398}.

Histopathology

Large cell carcinomas consist of sheets or nests of large polygonal cells with vesicular nuclei, prominent nucleoli, and moderate amounts of cytoplasm. By definition, large cell carcinomas are resected undifferentiated NSCCs. It is a diagnosis of exclusion made after ruling out the presence of a morphological component of squamous cell carcinoma, adenocarcinoma, or small cell carcinoma, and clear-cut evidence of squamous and adenocarcinomatous differentiation on immunohistochemistry and/or mucin stains {1983,2137,2206}.
Exclusion of LCNEC is based on a combination of morphology and expression of neuroendocrine markers by immunohistochemistry.
The clear cell and rhabdoid phenotypes, the latter characterized by eosinophilic

cytoplasmic globules {344,415,2369}, are no longer regarded as subtypes of large cell carcinoma, but are cytological features that can occur in any histological type of NSCLC. Rhabdoid cytology should be documented as a percentage of the total tumour, as its extent is prognostically significant (see below).
Large cell carcinoma must only be diagnosed in resection specimens, and immunohistochemistry should be used to reclassify tumours according to their line of differentiation whenever possible (see below and *Rationale for classification in small biopsies and cytology*, p. 16), as this may affect the type of adjuvant therapy in resections of more advanced stage, and if there is recurrence.

Immunohistochemistry

Similar data to those that led to the reclassification of NSCLC, not otherwise specified in biopsies using immunohistochemistry (see *Rationale for classification in small biopsies and cytology*, p. 16) have emerged for assessing resections that are morphologically undifferentiated. Based on analysis of sensitivity and specificity of markers in conventional adenocarcinomas and squamous cell carcinomas, the markers that have emerged as preferred classifiers of morphologically undifferentiated NSCLC include TTF1 and napsin A for identification of adenocarcinoma, and p40 – or p63 (4A4) – and CK5/6 (or CK5) for identification of squamous cell carcinoma {209,1764,1870,2014,2023,2134}. Of these, TTF1 and p40 are viewed as the most useful {1058, 1870,2137,2137,2206,2637}. Both p63 (4A4) and to a lesser extent p40 can be seen focally in TTF1-positive tumours; in this situation, the tumours should be

regarded as adenocarcinomas, solid subtype.
Of note, TTF1 is also expressed in small cell lung carcinoma and LCNEC, and therefore positive TTF1 can be regarded as evidence of glandular differentiation only after exclusion of small cell lung carcinoma and LCNEC by morphology and, if needed, immunohistochemistry for neuroendocrine markers (synaptophysin, chromogranin, and CD56).
Only cases that are either negative using these immunohistochemical markers or show unclear patterns should be classified as large cell carcinoma, other than when there is no facility to use immunohistochemistry in which a diagnosis of large cell carcinoma should be made, noting that further testing cannot be undertaken.
Rare cases of large cell carcinoma with neuroendocrine morphology but an absence of neuroendocrine differentiation on immunohistochemistry may be found. These are discussed under neuroendocrine tumours (see *Neuroendocrine tumours*, pp. 63–79). Neuroendocrine markers need not be undertaken routinely in morphologically undifferentiated NSCCs.
Other markers with differential reactivity in adenocarcinomas and squamous cell carcinomas may also be expressed in resected morphologically undifferentiated NSCLCs, but are of lower specificity and/or sensitivity compared to those discussed above. These markers are not recommended for subtyping. CK7 is positive in nearly all resected morphologically undifferentiated NSCLCs with adenocarcinomatous profiles (high sensitivity) based on TTF1-positive and p40, or p63-negative staining, but is also frequently positive in p40-positive and

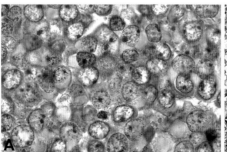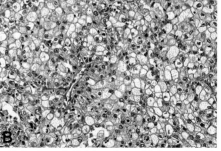

Fig. 1.91 Large cell carcinoma. **A** Rhabdoid cytology, with tumour cells that have large globular eosinophilic cytoplasmic inclusions; the nuclear chromatin is vesicular and nucleoli are prominent. Reprinted from Travis et al. {2678}. **B** Clear cell cytology, with numerous tumour cells showing clear cytoplasm; the cytological features should be noted. Classification as a large cell carcinoma requires morphological and immunohistochemical exclusion of other tumour types, as both cytological appearances can occur in other types of NSCLC.

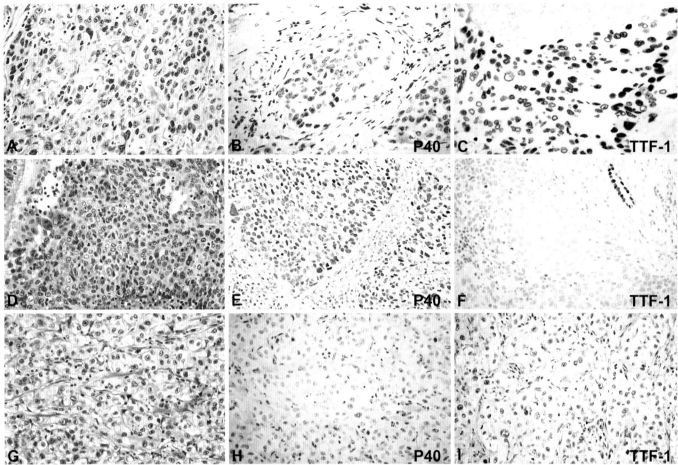

Fig. 1.92 A H&E staining of a resected morphologically undifferentiated non-small cell carcinoma, which would hitherto have been classified as large cell carcinoma, but stains negative for p40 (**B**) and positive for TTF1 (**C**), with subsequent classification as an adenocarcinoma, solid subtype. **D** H&E staining of a resected morphologically undifferentiated non-small cell carcinoma, which would hitherto have been classified as large cell carcinoma, but stains positive for p40 (**E**) and negative for TTF1 (**F**), with subsequent classification as a non-keratinizing squamous cell carcinoma. **G** H&E staining of a resected morphologically undifferentiated non-small cell carcinoma that does not stain for p40 (**H**) or TTF1 (**I**); the tumour cells also did not contain mucin, with subsequent classification as a large cell carcinoma, null phenotype.

TTF1-negative tumours {134}, consistent with frequent (up to 30%) positivity of CK7 in pulmonary squamous cell carcinomas (low specificity). 34βE12 (CK903) frequently stains squamous cell carcinomas (high sensitivity), but is frequently diffuse in solid pattern adenocarcinomas (low specificity), and such reactivity should not be regarded as evidence of squamous differentiation. Desmocollin 3 is a fairly specific squamous marker, but it has lower sensitivity for squamous differentiation than p40 {2206}.

Differential diagnosis
The differential diagnosis of large cell carcinoma primarily includes:
- Adenocarcinomas with a wholly solid pattern lacking pneumocyte markers and ≥ 5 intracytoplasmic droplets present in at least two high-power fields,
- Adenocarcinoma with a wholly solid pattern based solely on immunohistochemical evidence of adenocarcinoma differentiation (see *Adenocarcinoma*, p. 26),
- Non-keratinizing squamous cell carcinoma in which intercellular bridges are sparse,
- Non-keratinizing squamous cell carcinoma based solely on immunohistochemical evidence of squamous differentiation (see *Squamous cell carcinoma*, p. 51), and
- Adenosquamous carcinoma (see *Adenosquamous carcinoma*, p. 86).
As discussed above, immunohistochemistry should be used in addition to morphology to reassign cases suspected to be large cell carcinoma. This is based on several studies on large cell carcinomas diagnosed on morphology alone, which show positive staining for TTF1, napsin A, p40 (or p63), and CK5/6 (or CK5) in 30–60%, 35–45%, 20–35%, and 17–43% of cases, respec-

tively {134,1709,1983,2137,2206,2637}. When assessing immunohistochemistry in this context, markers of adenocarcinomatous and squamous differentiation are largely mutually exclusive, except for occasional focal reactivity for p40 in scattered tumour cells (accounting for < 10% of the tumour cells), similar to observations in conventional adenocarcinomas {209,1870,2014}. Coexpression of markers of adenocarcinomatous and squamous differentiation in different tumour cell populations, suggesting adenosquamous differentiation, has been reported in only a minority (2%) of resected morphologically undifferentiated NSCCs {2137} (see *Adenosquamous carcinoma*, p. 86).

Following immunohistochemical analysis and mucin stains, 18–41% of tumours with large cell morphology remain negative or cannot be reclassified, and are therefore currently classified as large cell carcinoma. It is hypothesized that large cell carcinomas with a null immunophenotype by the above markers represent variants of TTF1- (and napsin A-) negative adenocarcinoma, because an absence of TTF1 (and napsin A) is known to occur in 15–20% of morphological adenocarcinomas, whereas complete absence of p40 is uncommon in squamous cell carcinoma. Therefore, TTF1/p40 double-negative tumours are more likely to be adenocarcinomas, solid subtype, than non-keratinizing squamous cell carcinomas. This is supported by studies of microRNAs that proposed reclassification of TTF1/p40 double-negative large cell carcinomas as adenocarcinomas {134}, and the fact that large cell carcinomas with null immunophenotype tend to have molecular features similar to those of solid pattern adenocarcinomas, such as a high frequency of KRAS mutations {1058,2137}. Rhabdoid cells sometimes raise the possibility of a carcinosarcoma showing areas of rhabdomyosarcomatous differentiation, although are positive for cytokeratins and negative for desmin and myogenin {344,415,2369}.

Cytokeratin positivity and other markers, as well as clinicoradiological correlation, are also essential to exclude the possibility of unsuspected poorly differentiated tumours other than NSCLC, such as metastatic carcinoma or melanoma. For example, clear cell cytology raises the possibility of metastatic clear cell carcinomas arising in organs such as the kidney, thyroid, and salivary gland. Lymphoepithelioma-like carcinomas also consist of sheets of undifferentiated cells, although the extent of lymphocytes is usually far greater than in large cell carcinoma, and EBV will normally be present {342,388,938}. If ≥ 10% of the tumour shows pleomorphic features (spindle and/ or giant cells), then the tumour should be classified as a pleomorphic carcinoma.

Genetic profile

Genomic analyses have provided a basis for the refinement of large cell carcinoma classification, leading to major revisions in the current classification for tumours formerly classified as large cell carcinoma in the 2004 WHO classification. Historically, large cell carcinomas have been classified as poorly differentiated carcinomas that lack any morphological squamous carcinoma or adenocarcinoma differentiation. Two studies have provided

Table 1.20 Immunohistochemical typing of cytokeratin-positive, morphologically undifferentiated non-small cell lung carcinoma (NSCLC), with mucin stains already undertaken to exclude solid pattern adenocarcinoma[a]. Focal: 1–10% of cells positive; diffuse: > 10% of cells positive

TTF1[b]	p63	p40	CK5/6	Diagnosis (resection)	Diagnosis (biopsy / cytology)
Positive (focal or diffuse)	Negative	Negative	Negative	Adenocarcinoma	NSCLC, favour adenocarcinoma
Positive (focal or diffuse)	Positive (focal or diffuse)	Negative	Negative	Adenocarcinoma	NSCLC, favour adenocarcinoma
Positive (focal or diffuse)	Positive (focal or diffuse)	Positive (focal)	Negative	Adenocarcinoma	NSCLC, favour adenocarcinoma
Positive (focal or diffuse)	Negative	Negative	Positive (focal)	Adenocarcinoma	NSCLC, favour adenocarcinoma
Negative	Any one of the above diffusely positive			Squamous cell carcinoma	NSCLC, favour squamous cell carcinoma
Negative	Any one of the above focally positive			Large cell carcinoma, unclear[c]	NSCLC, not otherwise specified
Negative	Negative	Negative	Negative	Large cell carcinoma-null[d]	NSCLC, not otherwise specified
No stains available	No stains available	No stains available	No stains available	Large cell carcinoma with no additional stains	NSCLC, not otherwise specified (no stains available)

[a] Positive for mucin is defined as (≥ 5 intracytoplasmic droplets in two high-power fields in resections {2672} and mucin droplets in two or more cells within a biopsy); fewer positive cells are regarded as negative.
[b] Napsin may be used as an alternative to TTF1, CK7 is not recommended as a marker of adenocarcinomatous differentiation due to a lack of specificity.
[c] Negativity for TTF1 and focal positivity for p63/p40/CK5/6 point to adenocarcinoma cell lineage once neuroendocrine tumours are excluded.
[d] Sarcomatoid carcinoma and neuroendocrine tumours should be excluded (i.e. undifferentiated morphology with no spindle/giant cells).

important evidence for the biologically heterogeneous nature of large cell carcinoma. In a study of 102 large cell carcinomas, immunohistochemistry for TTF1 and ΔNp63/p40 as classifiers for adenocarcinoma and squamous cell carcinoma, respectively, correlated with therapeutically relevant genetic alterations of adenocarcinoma or squamous cell carcinoma {2137}. Thus, molecular alterations characteristic of adenocarcinoma (EGFR, KRAS, BRAF, and ALK fusions) occurred only in large cell carcinoma with immunoprofiles of adenocarcinoma or markernull, but not in large cell carcinoma with a squamous immunoprofile {2137}.

These observations were further extended in a recent comprehensive analysis of lung cancer genome alterations, where investigators first defined specific differences between and among histological types {2320}. The co-occurrence of patterns of gene copy number changes and driver mutations in individual lung cancer

types suggested that they were specific markers of these subtypes. However, according to the previous classification, large cell carcinoma did not exhibit a specific pattern of genomic copy number alterations or specific mutation, but shared many of the characteristics of adenocarcinoma, squamous cell carcinoma, or even small cell carcinoma. As in the previous, more limited, study {2137}, this suggested that the existing large cell carcinoma classification included tumours that more properly could be reassigned to other histological classes to which they had more biological similarity. An independent immunohistochemistry-based pathology review indicated that most large cell carcinoma cases could be reassigned based on their immunoprofile of lineage-specific transcription factor expression p63 (or p40)/TTF1 to other subtypes that shared similar immunohistochemical and genetic features. Combined immunohistochemical and genomic analysis is

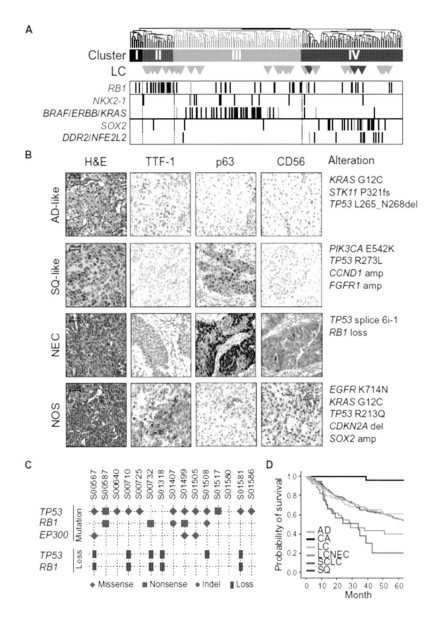

Fig. 1.93 Genetic features typical of other lung cancer subtypes in large cell carcinoma (LC). **A** Unsupervised hierarchical clustering using 294 highly variable (standard deviation/mean > 2.1) expressed genes identified four gene expression subgroups containing mainly carcinoid (CA; I), small cell lung cancer (SCLC; II), adenocarcinoma (AD; III), and squamous cell carcinoma (SQ; IV). LC samples are indicated as triangles at corresponding positions below the cluster dendrogram. They are coloured orange if they have AD-specific alterations, blue if they have SQ-specific alterations, grey if the case was initially diagnosed as a large cell neuroendocrine carcinoma, and green if they have no known alteration. Genetic alterations (label: red, amplified; blue, deleted; black, mutated; *ERBB* includes mutation in *EGFR* or *ERBB2*) are given for selected genes per sample as vertical lines (LC cases in green; others in black). **B** Typical immunohistochemistry is shown for LC specimens with immunohistochemical and genetic characteristics of AD (AD-like), SQ (SQ-like), and neuroendocrine differentiation (NEC), as well as LC lacking features of other lung cancer subtypes (not otherwise specified – NOS). The corresponding genetic alterations are indicated on the right. **C** Distribution of mutations (in red, symbols according to type of mutation: diamond for missense, square for nonsense, and circle for indel) and copy number loss (in blue) of *TP53*, *RB1*, and *EP300* across all whole-exome-sequenced large cell neuroendocrine carcinomas. **D** Overall survival corresponding to each histological lung cancer subtype, with LC separated into LCs with neuroendocrine features – i.e. large cell neuroendocrine carcinoma (LCNEC; grey) – and LCs without neuroendocrine features (green).
Reprinted from Seidel D, et al. Clinical Lung Cancer Genome Project (CLCGP), Network Genomic Medicine (NGM) (2013). A genomics-based classification of human lung tumours. Sci Transl Med. 5(209):209ra153. {2320} With permission from AAAS.

therefore able to reassign large cell carcinoma cases to adenocarcinoma, squamous cell carcinoma, or neuroendocrine tumour {1058,2137,2206,2320}. This justifies the reassignment of most large cell carcinoma cases to other histological types in this new classification, leaving as large cell carcinoma the few cases with either a null or unclear phenotype.

After the exclusion of large cell carcinomas that are now viewed as being related to adenocarcinoma or squamous cell carcinoma based on immunohistochemistry, data specific to large cell carcinoma with null or unclear phenotype are sparse. Thus, when limited to marker-null large cell carcinomas, the few tumours that harboured mutations showed some associated with adenocarcinomas {1058,2137,2206,2320}, including *KRAS* and occasional *EGFR* mutations. *TP53* mutations, *CDKN2A* deletions, and *MYC* and *CCNE1* amplifications occur with the same frequency as in other histological types. Based on these data, molecular testing is recommended in this subgroup when there is advanced disease and targeted therapy is to be considered.

Gene expression profiling has also shown evidence of epithelial-mesenchymal transition as a frequent finding in large cell carcinomas, reflecting their poor differentiation compared to other NSCCs {793}.

Prognosis and predictive factors

The clinical prognostic criteria are similar to those of other NSCLCs. The major criteria are performance status at diagnosis and the disease extension reflected by the TNM stage.

Histopathological marker-null large cell carcinomas may be associated with inferior disease-free and overall survival compared to solid predominant adenocarcinomas and non-keratinizing squamous cell carcinomas that would previously have been classified as large cell carcinoma {2137}. Large cell carcinomas that show rhabdoid cytology have a poorer prognosis than large cell carcinomas in which rhabdoid cytology is absent {344,415,2369}.

Prediction of response to targeted therapy in large cell carcinoma is based on the presence of the same genetic abnormalities found in other adenocarcinomas or squamous cell carcinomas {2137,2206}.

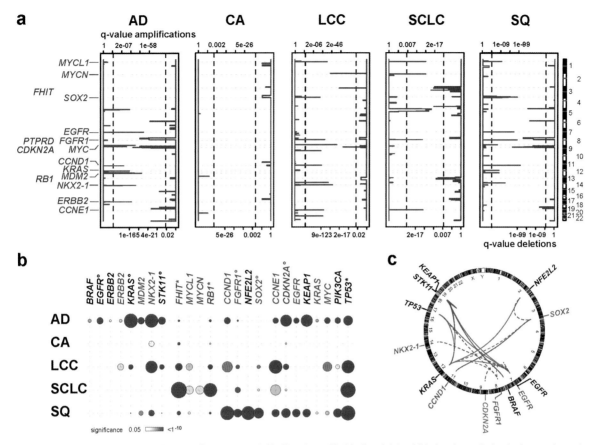

Fig. 1.94 Genomic alterations in histological subgroups of lung cancer. **A** Significantly amplified (red) and deleted (blue) regions calculated using a rank-sum-based algorithm are plotted along the genome (y-axis) for the five major lung cancer subtypes: AD, adenocarcinoma (n = 421); CA, carcinoid (n = 69); LC, large cell carcinoma (n = 101); SCLC, small cell lung cancer (n = 63), and SQ, squamous cell carcinoma (n = 338). Statistical significance, expressed by Q values (x-axes: amplification, upper scale; deletion, lower scale), was computed for each genomic location. Known or potential oncogenes (red) or tumour suppressor genes (blue) are given at respective locations. Vertical lines indicate a level of significance of $Q = 0.01$. **B** Frequencies of significant genomic alterations are given per gene per histological subtype. The colours of gene names are encoded as follows: red, amplified; blue, deleted; and black, mutated. The frequencies of alterations correspond to circle size. The frequencies of deletions of *FHIT* and *RB1* and mutations in *TP53* were adapted by dividing the values by 3 (asterisks). The frequencies of mutations in *EGFR*, *KRAS*, and *STK11*; of deletions in *CDKN2A*; and of amplifications in *FGFR1* and *SOX2* were adapted by dividing the values by 2 (circles). Significant mutations were determined using a binomial test with a background mutation rate of 0.5%. *P* values were adjusted for multiple hypothesis testing using the Benjamini-Hochberg method across each histological subtype. The Q values of significant results ($Q < 0.05$) are indicated by the colour code of the symbols (colour key provided below the chart). **C** Associations of copy number alterations and mutations calculated using the Fisher exact test followed by Benjamini-Hochberg adjustment are represented with a Circos plot. The involved genes are named at corresponding genomic locations (copy number gains in red, copy number deletions in blue, and mutations in black) outside the ring representing the genome. The internal lines show significant co-occurring (red) and mutually exclusive (blue) events (Q < 0.05) between two copy number alterations or two frequently mutated genes (solid lines), or between a copy number alteration and a mutation (dashed lines) found in lung cancer.
Reprinted from Seidel D, et al. Clinical Lung Cancer Genome Project (CLCGP), Network Genomic Medicine (NGM) (2013). A genomics-based classification of human lung tumours. Sci Transl Med. 5(209):209ra153. {2320} With permission from AAAS.

Adenosquamous carcinoma

Y. Yatabe
E. Brambilla
N. Rekhtman
S.C. Aisner
N.E. Caporaso
S. Gonzalez

A.G. Nicholson
C.A. Powell
G. Riely
S. Seiwerth
W.D. Travis
P. van Schil

Definition

Adenosquamous carcinoma is a carcinoma showing components of both squamous cell carcinoma and adenocarcinoma, with each components constituting at least 10% of the tumour. Definitive diagnosis requires a resection specimen, although it may be suggested based on findings in small biopsies, cytology or excisional biopsies.

ICD-O code   8560/3

Epidemiology

Although the incidence varies between studies due to diverse histological criteria and variable tumour sampling, adenosquamous carcinoma is estimated to account for 0.4–4% of all lung cancers {805,1037,1546,2371}.

Etiology

Adenosquamous carcinoma is associated with smoking (see *Adenocarcinoma*, p. 26).

Clinical features

Adenosquamous carcinoma has a male predominance, and the median age is similar to those seen with other histological subtypes {2564,2813}. More than half of all patients with adenosquamous carcinoma have abnormal findings on chest X-ray without symptoms, although some patients were reported to show haemoptysis, cough, shoulder pain, and clubbed fingers {2813}. Radiographical features are similar to those of other non-small cell lung carcinoma (see *Adenocarcinoma*, p. 26); peripheral tumours may show central scarring and spiculation or pleural indentation. Some may display a peripheral ground-glass opacity and air bronchogram {1227,2813}. In resections, adenosquamous carcinomas tend to present with higher pathological T stage, although the frequency of nodal spread and overall pathological stage are not different from those of adenocarcinoma and squamous cell carcinoma {2371,2382}.

Macroscopy and localization

Adenosquamous carcinomas typically arise in the peripheral pulmonary parenchyma {2564,2813}, but they have also been reported to arise centrally {1456}. Their gross pathological features are similar to those of other non-small cell lung cancers {2564}.

Cytology

Cytological specimens have the same limitation in the diagnosis of adenosquamous carcinomas as small biopsies, due to sampling issues. Either the adenocarcinomatous or the squamous component may predominate diffusely or focally in adenosquamous carcinomas; and sampling of only a single component by cytology sample (or small biopsy) leads to common underdiagnosis of adenosquamous carcinoma in small samples {516,2135,2136}. If both adenocarcinomatous and squamous components are represented, the possibility of adenosquamous carcinoma can be suggested on cytology (see *Terminology and criteria in non-resection specimens,* p. 17).

Histopathology

Because there is a continuum of histological heterogeneity with both squamous cell and adenocarcinoma, the criterion of 10% for each component is arbitrary. However, a minor component of the

different histological subtype constituting < 10% should be reported, because recent molecular analyses have suggested that tumours with mixed features can reflect the genetic status of either component regardless of the proportion {2136}. Well-defined components of squamous cell carcinoma (see *Squamous cell carcinoma,* p. 51) and adenocarcinoma (see *Adenocarcinoma,* p. 26, and *Variants of invasive adenocarcinoma,* p. 38) are evident on light microscopy. The two components may be separate, or merged and mingled, and the degree of differentiation of each can vary. Diagnosis is more difficult if the tumour has a partly solid adenocarcinoma component or a non-keratinizing squamous cell carcinoma component, in addition to a clearly differentiated component.

Immunohistochemistry

Just as light microscopy shows a dual population of adenocarcinoma and squamous cell carcinoma components, the immunophenotype should support the presence of a dual population of tumour cells with adenocarcinoma and squamous cell differentiation. For differentiation of a morphologically unclear component, including solid adenocarcinoma and non-keratinizing squamous cell carcinoma components, immunohistochemistry as well as mucin histochemistry

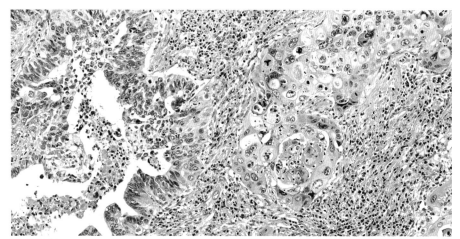

Fig. 1.95 Adenosquamous carcinoma, with adenocarcinoma (left) and squamous cell carcinoma (right).

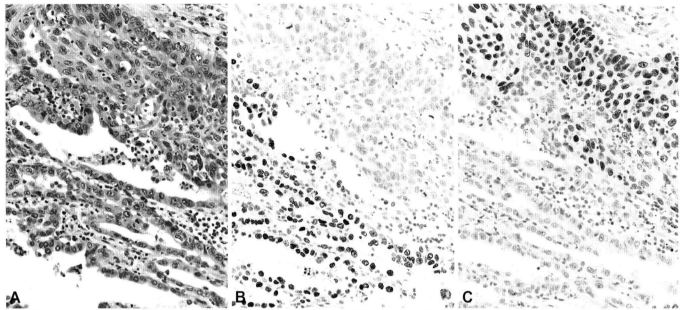

Fig. 1.96 Adenosquamous carcinoma. H&E staining (**A**), TTF1 staining (**B**), and p40 staining (**C**) using serial sections. Geographically distinct components of adenocarcinoma (at the lower left) and squamous cell carcinoma (at the upper right) are positive for TTF1 and p40, respectively. Note the diffuse and clearly positive staining of the individual components.

should be performed, with a panel of adenocarcinoma and squamous markers (TTF1 and p40 are currently the best options, respectively). When applying immunohistochemistry in this setting, only diffuse and clearly positive staining for the relevant component has significance. Reactivity for p63 (4A4) or cytokeratins CK1,CK5, CK10, CK14 (34βE12) in TTF1-positive cells should not be taken as evidence of an adenosquamous phenotype {1870,2621} (see also *Terminology and criteria in non-resection specimens*, p. 17). Also, squamous differentiation is only supported by diffuse (sheet-like) labelling for p40, whereas focal labelling in scattered tumour cells can be seen in adenocarcinomas. Although a partly solid component with a null immunoprofile may exist, its presence does not change the diagnosis.

Differential diagnosis

Non-neoplastic components, such as entrapped TTF1-positive pneumocytes, should be differentiated from an adenocarcinomatous component. Similarly, squamous metaplasia of entrapped bronchiolar structures can occasionally resemble the squamous component.

Low-grade mucoepidermoid carcinoma is centrally located, and can be distinguished by histological features identical to the salivary gland counterpart, including a mixture of mucinous glands, intermediate and/or squamoid cells, and no

more than mild atypia. A high-grade mucoepidermoid carcinoma is more difficult to differentiate from an adenosquamous carcinoma. However, a mucoepidermoid carcinoma more often presents with 1) a characteristic admixture of mucinous and squamoid cells; 2) a proximal exophytic endobronchial location; 3) areas of classical low-grade mucoepidermoid carcinoma; 4) a lack of keratinization or squamous pearl formation; 5) no overlying squamous cell carcinoma in situ {2991}; and 6) a tubular, acinar, and papillary growth pattern. A lack of TTF1 in a mucoepidermoid carcinoma may also be useful for differential diagnosis {2366}. *MAML2* rearrangement is exclusively seen in mucoepidermoid carcinoma {14}. However, these two types of lung tumours cannot be reliably distinguished in all cases {1399}.

Clinical clues that a cytology or a small biopsy sample showing only squamous carcinoma may be derived from adenosquamous carcinoma include younger patient age, never or light smoking history, and the presence of a ground-glass component on imaging {361,2136}. This situation may influence decisions to perform genetic testing.

Genetic profile

The genetic profile of adenosquamous carcinoma shows both squamous and adenocarcinoma characteristics. Although the number of cases reported

is limited, *EGFR* mutations tend to be detected in women and non-smokers, even with adenosquamous carcinoma, whereas the *KRAS* mutation has been noted in smokers. Identification of identical mutations of *EGFR* and *KRAS* in both components shown by microdissection analyses revealed a morphologically divergent but clonally related tumour {1203,2648,2665}. Adenosquamous carcinoma may also harbour *ALK* rearrangement {313,361}, *HER2* mutations {2652}, *LKB1* mutations {1311}, *ROS1* rearrangement {2972}, *RET* rearrangement {2806}, and *FGFR1* amplification {2084}.

Prognosis and predictive factors

Adenosquamous carcinoma behaves aggressively. A poor prognosis is reported compared to other non-small cell lung carcinomas, even after multivariate adjustment {894,1794,2564}. The 5-year survival rate after resection is about 40% in large cohorts {90,894}. The predominant component within individual tumours has not been shown to have an impact on prognosis {2371,2813}.

Pleomorphic, spindle cell, and giant cell carcinoma

K.M. Kerr   J. Jett   W.D. Travis
G. Pelosi   M.N. Koss   K. Tsuta
J.H.M. Austin   A.G. Nicholson   P. van Schil
E. Brambilla   C.A. Powell   P. Yang
K. Geisinger   G. Riely
N.A. Jambhekar   G. Rossi

Definition

Pleomorphic carcinoma is a poorly differentiated non-small cell lung carcinoma namely a squamous cell carcinoma, adenocarcinoma, or undifferentiated non-small cell carcinoma that contains at least 10% spindle and/or giant cells or a carcinoma consisting only of spindle and giant cells. Spindle cell carcinoma consists of an almost pure population of epithelial spindle cells, with no differentiated carcinomatous elements.

Giant cell carcinoma consists almost entirely of tumour giant cells (including multinucleated cells), with no differentiated carcinomatous elements.

Definite diagnosis may only be made on a resected tumour. The specific histological components should be mentioned in the diagnosis.

ICD-O codes

Pleomorphic carcinoma	8022/3
Spindle cell carcinoma	8032/3
Giant cell carcinoma	8031/3

Synonyms

These carcinomas were previously classified as monophasic or biphasic, with the latter group further subtyped as either homologous or heterologous, but this terminology is no longer recommended {2869}. Sarcomatoid carcinoma is a general term that includes pleomorphic carcinoma, carcinosarcoma and pulmonary blastoma.

Epidemiology

Together, these tumours account for 2–3% of all cancer cases in surgical series, but for < 1% in epidemiological studies {2960}. Otherwise, their epidemiology is similar to that of other non-small cell lung cancers (see *Adenocarcinoma*, p. 26).

Pure spindle cell and giant cell carcinomas are very rare {731,1695,2026,2203}.

Etiology

Most cases of these carcinomas arise in tobacco smokers {731,1695,2026,2203}, although cases in never-smokers have also been documented {362,1045}. Other possible etiological factors (although uncommon) include asbestos, chemicals, and immunosuppression {1045,1949}. No precursor lesion has been identified, but carcinoma in situ may be found close to pleomorphic elements {2015}.

Clinical features

The signs and symptoms of these tumours are similar to those of other non-small cell lung carcinomas (see *Adenocarcinoma, Clinical features*, p. 29).

The most common presentation on imaging is as a large peripheral mass, usually in an upper lobe {2126}, showing low central attenuation at CT, and frequently invading adjacent pleura {1262}. Otherwise, the imaging of these tumours is similar to that of other lung carcinomas (see *Adenocarcinoma, Clinical features*, p. 29).

These are aggressive tumours, with spread similar to that of other non-small cell lung carcinomas (see see *Adenocarcinoma, Clinical features*, p. 29). Distant metastases are commonly found, including in unusual locations (e.g. the gastrointestinal tract and the retroperitoneal space).

The tumours are staged according to the TNM classification {866} (see *Staging and grading*, p. 14).

Localization

Pleomorphic carcinomas are often peripherally located {2203}, favouring the upper lobes {2126}.

Macroscopy

Pleomorphic carcinomas are usually well-circumscribed grey/tan masses measuring > 5 cm in diameter, with necrosis and/or cavitation. They often invade the chest wall or mediastinum {386}. The cut surface may have a grayish-gelatinous appearance.

Cytology

By definition, definitive diagnosis of these tumours is not possible on cytology specimens, but the features may be recognized and described.

Smears may contain both malignant epithelial and mesenchymal-like elements (i.e. spindle and/or giant neoplastic cells) {435,3004}. The neoplastic epithelial cells fully resemble their usual counterparts. Elongated spindle cells show

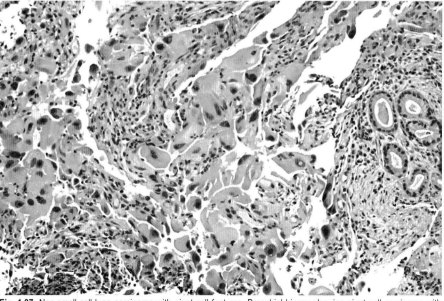

Fig. 1.97 Non-small cell lung carcinoma with giant cell features. Bronchial biopsy showing giant cell carcinoma with huge tumour cells; TTF1, p63, and CK5/6 were all negative; the tumour had a *BRAF* mutation.

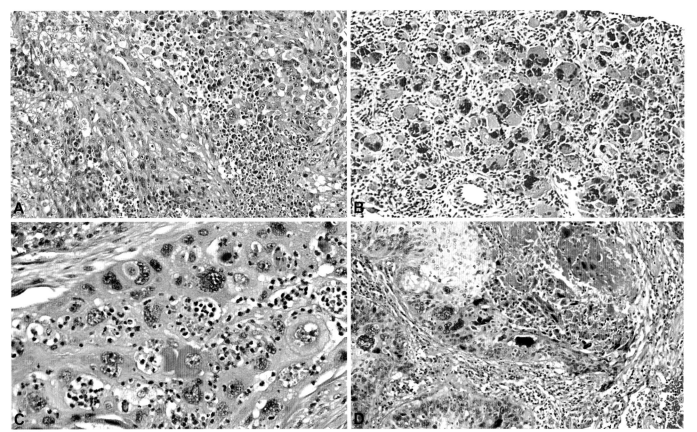

Fig. 1.98 A Pleomorphic carcinoma. Undifferentiated carcinoma with some spindle cells. **B** Possible giant cell carcinoma. Core biopsy shows giant cell features in undifferentiated carcinoma. **C** Pleomorphic carcinoma. Histology shows tumour giant cells and neutrophil emperipolesis. **D** Pleomorphic carcinoma with squamous cell carcinoma. The tumour shows keratinizing squamous cell carcinoma (top right), but also foci of bizarre tumour giant cells.

eosinophilic homogeneous cytoplasm, spindle-shaped nuclei with thick nuclear membranes, and well-developed nucleoli, all arranged singly or in bundles. Discohesive, round to oval tumour giant cells with abundant eosinophilic cytoplasm, and single/multiple large, irregularly lobulated, hyperchromatic nuclei occur. Collagen or myxoid stroma, mitotic figures, necrotic debris, lymphocytes, and often neutrophils may also feature.

Histopathology

In pleomorphic carcinoma, the giant and/ or spindle cell elements comprising at least 10% of the tumour are admixed with components such as adenocarcinoma (in 31–72% of cases), squamous cell carcinoma (in 12–26% of cases), or undifferentiated non-small cell carcinoma (in up to 43% of cases) {731,1182,1441,1695}. Carcinomas composed of a mixture of spindle and giant cell carcinoma qualify as pleomorphic carcinoma. Squamous cell or adenocarcinoma components should be reported (e.g. pleomorphic carcinoma with adenocarcinoma). By

definition, in small biopsy samples, sarcomatoid elements may be described, but definitive diagnosis is not possible. Giant and/or spindle cell elements may be diffusely admixed with differentiated tumour. Giant tumour cells show abundant, often eosinophilic, sometimes granular cytoplasm, and may contain eosinophilic globules. The nuclei are large, irregular, and multilobated or multiple, with coarse or vesicular chromatin and prominent nucleoli. The stroma may be fibrous, myxoid, or minimal. Neutrophil emperipolesis, necrosis, haemorrhage, and vascular invasion are common.

Spindle cell carcinoma consists almost entirely of malignant spindle cells in fascicular or storiform patterns, and differentiated elements are absent. Nuclei are often hyperchromatic, with nucleoli and granular chromatin. Inflammation is common.

Giant cell carcinoma is composed almost entirely of pleomorphic tumour giant cells, which may be multinucleated. Cells show eosinophilic cytoplasm, bizarre shapes, discohesive growth, and other

features described above. Neutrophilic infiltration and emperipolesis can occur.

Immunohistochemistry

Although these tumours are diagnosed by morphology, immunohistochemistry may highlight the different cell components. The differentiated epithelial elements show the expected immunophenotype. Keratin expression is not required in the spindle/giant cell component if non-pleomorphic carcinomatous elements are clearly present. The pleomorphic, spindle, or giant cell components express vimentin and fascin {731,2015,2026,2203}. Cytokeratins and differentiation-associated markers such as napsin A {2570,2620}, TTF1 {2203}, p63 {1460}, CK5/6, and desmocollin 3 are variably expressed in pleomorphic elements.

Differential diagnosis

The differential diagnoses include metastatic sarcomatoid carcinoma, primary or metastatic sarcoma or melanoma, and (in an appropriate context) malignant

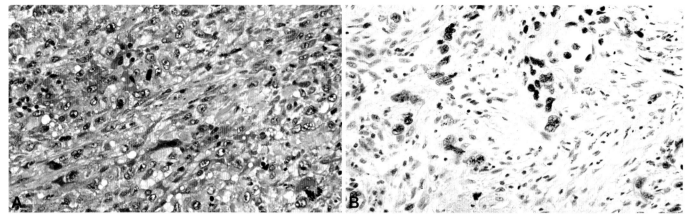

Fig. 1.99 Spindle cell carcinoma. **A** Malignant spindle tumour cells with enlarged hyperchromatic nuclei. **B** Positive staining for TTF1.

pleural mesothelioma. Generous tumour sampling and adequate, contextually interpreted immunohistochemistry are required to determine the correct diagnosis.

Cytokeratins, TTF1, p63, or similar markers in pleomorphic elements help in the distinction from sarcoma or cellular stroma {1816,2026,2670,2869}. Distinction from synovial sarcoma may be difficult, but can be assisted by the identification of *SS18-SSX* gene fusion/X;18 translocation in synovial sarcoma {686} (see *Synovial sarcoma*, p. 127).

Vasoformative morphology and immunohistochemistry (CD31 and CD34) help identify epithelioid haemangioendothelioma (see *Epithelioid haemangioendothelioma*, p. 123) and angiosarcoma. Inflammatory myofibroblastic tumour or localized organizing pneumonia show bland neoplastic cells. Biphasic or sarcomatoid mesothelioma, spindle cell melanoma, follicular dendritic cell sarcoma, and reactive fibrotic and inflammatory processes may be distinguished by

clinical history, imaging data, and appropriate immunohistochemistry {474}. Giant cell carcinoma should be distinguished from pleomorphic rhabdomyosarcoma (desmin-positive and MyoD1-positive), metastatic adrenocortical carcinoma (inhibin alpha-positive and melan A/MART1-positive), metastatic choriocarcinoma, and other pleomorphic malignant tumours by morphology, immunohistochemistry, and clinicopathological correlation.

Genetic profile

Genetic studies provide evidence that this subtype of lung cancer represents sarcomatoid, spindle cell, or pleomorphic change in a carcinoma {1024,2017,2025}. Gains at chromosomes 8q, 7, 1q, 3q, and 19 have been reported in sarcomatoid carcinomas, with additional gains at 5p, 11q, 12p, 9q, 17q, and 13q in pleomorphic/spindle cell carcinomas, and at 13p and 15p in giant cell carcinoma {215}. *TP53* mutations are described in spindle cell carcinoma

{1024,1325} and pleomorphic carcinoma {389,2017,2094}. The prevalence of *KRAS* (in up to 38% of cases) {1106,2025} and *EGFR* mutations (in up to 25% of cases) {389,1182,1452} partially reflects the tumour components (i.e. adenocarcinoma), patient ethnicity, and smoking habits {1441}. *MET* or *FGFR2* gene copy number gain have also been reported {1441,2700}. A sarcomatoid carcinoma with *EML4-ALK* rearrangement has been reported as a transformation from a conventional adenocarcinoma with acquired crizotinib resistance {1302}. Molecular testing is recommended according to known genetic abnormalities associated with histological components that may determine therapy (i.e. tumours with an adenocarcinoma component should be tested for *EGFR* mutation and ALK rearrangement).

Prognosis and predictive factors

These tumours have a poor prognosis, even in early-stage disease.

Carcinosarcoma

M.N. Koss
K.M. Kerr
G. Pelosi
J.H.M. Austin
E. Brambilla
K. Geisinger

A.G. Nicholson
C.A. Powell
R. Rami-Porta
G. Riely
G. Rossi
G. Scagliotti

W.D. Travis
K. Tsuta
P. van Schil
P. Yang
D. Yankelevitz

Definition

Carcinosarcoma is a malignant tumour that consists of a mixture of non-small cell lung carcinoma (NSCLC) (typically squamous cell carcinoma or adenocarcinoma) and sarcoma-containing heterologous elements such as rhabdomyosarcoma, chondrosarcoma, and osteosarcoma.

ICD-O code   8980/3

Synonyms

The terms heterologous sarcomatoid carcinoma (for carcinosarcoma), and homologous sarcomatoid carcinoma (for pleomorphic carcinoma) have been suggested {2869}, but are not recommended.

Epidemiology

It has been estimated that sarcomatoid carcinomas account for only 0.1–0.4% of all lung cancers; and of these, only 4% are carcinosarcomas {2203}. Men are affected 7–8 times more commonly than women. Patients range from 38 to 81 years of age, with a median age of 65 years {1332,1805}.

Etiology

Most patients are heavy smokers {1332,2427}, or (rarely) report asbestos exposure {701}.

Clinical features

The clinical features are similar to those of other NSCLCs (see *Adenocarcinoma*, p. 26).
Imaging is also similar to that of other lung cancers (see *Adenocarcinoma*, p. 26), including possible calcification {1258}. Endobronchial location can occur {277}.
These highly invasive tumours are characterized by an aggressive clinical behaviour. Spread is similar to that of other NSCLCs. Distant metastases are commonly found.
These tumours are staged like other lung cancers, according to the TNM classification (see *Staging and grading*, p. 14).

Localization

Carcinosarcomas are centrally located relatively frequently compared with other sarcomatoid carcinomas.

Macroscopy

The tumours usually present as greywhite, necrotic, haemorrhagic masses.

Cytology

This diagnosis is rarely possible in cytology specimens. Representative smears of carcinosarcoma must contain both clearly malignant epithelial and mesenchymal components. Most often, the former is squamous cell carcinoma, which may be heavily keratinized. In addition, nondescript spindle cells resembling those of a synovial sarcoma or leiomyosarcoma are present, along with malignant heterologous tissue cells of chondrosarcoma, osteosarcoma, and rhabdomyosarcoma.

Histopathology

Carcinosarcomas are tumours with intimately admixed non-small cell carcinoma and sarcoma. Pathological diagnoses should list all of the histological types of carcinoma and sarcoma present. The carcinomas are of conventional non-small cell type, most often squamous cell carcinoma, followed by adenocarcinoma, adenosquamous carcinoma, and large cell carcinoma {1332}. The frequencies of squamous cell carcinoma and adenosquamous carcinoma are significantly higher than in pleomorphic carcinomas, where adenocarcinoma predominates. The rare occurrence of neuroendocrine components in the form of small cell lung carcinoma and/or large cell neuroendocrine carcinoma is better classified as combined small cell lung carcinoma or combined large cell neuroendocrine carcinoma with associated sarcoma elements {2026,2869}. The epithelial component often governs location, in that tumours containing squamous cell carcinoma are more often central, endobronchial growths, while tumours

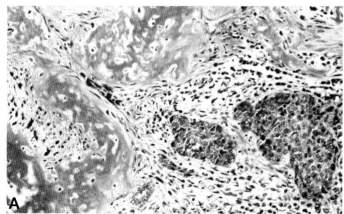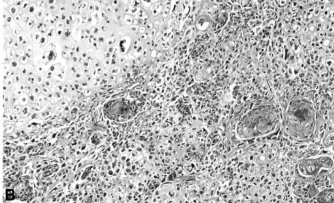

Fig. 1.100 Carcinosarcoma. **A** The sarcomatous element has osteoid formation (osteosarcoma) (top and left), while the carcinoma in this image is undifferentiated (right). **B** Chondrosarcoma is juxtaposed with squamous cell carcinoma.

containing adenocarcinoma are more often peripheral.

The sarcomatous elements include, in descending order of frequency, rhabdomyosarcoma, chondrosarcoma, and osteosarcoma; and combinations of these tumour types are common {1332}. Rare cases contain liposarcoma or angiosarcoma {277,1276}. Less differentiated areas are composed of malignant spindle cells arranged in fascicular, storiform, or haemangiopericytomatous patterns.

The diagnosis of carcinosarcoma is difficult in small biopsies or cytology, and usually requires a larger specimen to show both components. Most carcinosarcomas contain conventional non-small cell carcinomas, but a component of high-grade fetal adenocarcinoma/ clear cell adenocarcinoma may occur in up to 18% of cases {1332}. This finding has been referred to as the blastomatoid variant of carcinosarcoma; but to avoid confusion, these tumours should be called carcinosarcoma, and the presence of high-grade fetal adenocarcinoma mentioned {1809,2292,2670}. Metastases can contain carcinoma, sarcoma, or both.

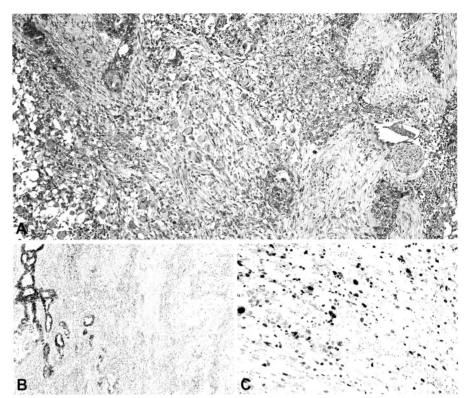

Fig. 1.101 Carcinosarcoma. **A** Adenocarcinoma and rhabdomyosarcoma components. **B** The adenocarcinoma component stains positively for TTF1, and the rhabdomyosarcoma component is negative. **C** The rhabdomyosarcoma component stains tumour cell nuclei for myogenin.

Immunohistochemistry
Immunohistochemistry may be helpful to highlight epithelial and sarcomatous differentiation {2026,2203,2670}. The NSCLC component recapitulates the immunoprofile usually seen in conventional counterparts (i.e. TTF1, napsin, and CK7 in adenocarcinoma and p63, p40, and CK5/6 or other high-molecular weight cytokeratin cocktails in squamous cell carcinoma) {1565,2023}. S100 or desmin and myogenin may highlight chondrosarcoma or rhabdomyosarcomatous elements, respectively.

If a high-grade fetal adenocarcinoma component is present, it may show β-catenin immunoreactivity strikingly restricted to the membrane of the epithelial component, unlike classical pulmonary blastoma, in which nuclear β-catenin decorates nuclei in both glandular and blastematous parts {1809}.

Differential diagnosis
The differential diagnoses include pleomorphic carcinoma, pulmonary blastoma, sarcoma, and mesothelioma. Pleomorphic carcinomas (see *Pleomorphic, spindle cell, and giant cell carcinoma,* p. 88) differ in that they lack heterologous differentiation, a feature that may require extensive sampling to be uncovered (at least one tissue block per cm of resected tumour).

Carcinosarcoma lacks the low-grade fetal adenocarcinoma component and primitive stroma of pulmonary blastoma (see *Pulmonary blastoma,* p. 93).

Sarcomas such as rhabdomyosarcoma or chondrosarcoma occur rarely, as primaries in the lung or as metastatic tumours, but they lack a carcinomatous component. Sarcomas may entrap benign, TTF1-positive pneumocytes, which may mimic carcinoma. Biphasic synovial sarcomas have glandular elements that lack TTF1 staining and manifest less uniform keratin staining, and the *SS18-SSX* fusion gene is present.

Malignant mesothelioma usually presents as diffuse pleural thickening rather than a localized intrapulmonary mass, and the epithelioid elements typically stain for mesothelial markers.

Genetic profile
Carcinosarcomas are clonal tumours {519,1024,1982,2634} developing through sarcomatoid change in a carcinoma {519,1982}. *TP53* mutations are often present in carcinosarcoma {1024, 2017}, whereas *KRAS* mutations occur less frequently {1024,2017}, and *EGFR* mutations are very uncommon {2017,2663}.

Prognosis and predictive factors
Prognosis is poor, and dependent on TNM factors {1045}.

Pulmonary blastoma

Y. Nakatani
M.N. Koss
K.M. Kerr
J.H.M. Austin
E. Brambilla
K. Geisinger

A.G. Nicholson
G. Pelosi
C.A. Powell
R. Rami-Porta
G. Riely
G. Rossi

G. Scagliotti
W.D. Travis
K. Tsuta
P. van Schil
P. Yang
D. Yankelevitz

Definition

Pulmonary blastoma is a biphasic tumour that consists of fetal adenocarcinoma (typically low-grade) and primitive mesenchymal stroma. Foci of specific mesenchymal differentiation (osteosarcoma, chondrosarcoma, or rhabdomyosarcoma) may also be present, but are not required for the diagnosis.

ICD-O code   8972/3

Epidemiology

Pulmonary blastoma is very rare, accounting for < 0.1% of all resected lung cancers {2203}. They are most common in the fifth decade, and there is no sex predominance {1336,1805}. These tumours are completely different from pleuropulmonary blastomas (see *Pleuropulmonary blastoma*, p. 124).

Etiology

Most patients are smokers {1805}.

Clinical features

The signs, symptoms, and imaging of these tumours are similar to those of other non-small cell lung carcinomas (see *Adenocarcinoma*, p. 26).
These uncommon tumours are characterized by an aggressive clinical behaviour and spread like other non-small cell lung cancers. Distant metastases are common and overall prognosis is poor. These tumours are staged like other lung cancers (see *Staging and grading*, p. 14).

Localization

Pulmonary blastomas are usually large, solitary, peripherally located masses.

Macroscopy

Pulmonary blastomas are usually well circumscribed and unencapsulated. They may show lobulation, haemorrhage, and necrosis {1336}.

Cytology

In smears, pulmonary blastoma may present a very distinctive cytological picture {1552,2340}. The glandular elements resemble those of fetal adenocarcinoma: uniform, small columnar cells with relatively small nuclei. Their cytoplasm has clear vacuoles in both supra- and subnuclear locations. The nuclear-to-cytoplasmic ratios vary. The nucleoli are generally inconspicuous. Immediately adjacent to the glands, the smear background may have a reticulated, bubbly appearance due to the rupture of the vacuoles with release of glycogen (i.e. tigroid background). The stromal component typically consists of small homogeneous cells with ovoid to somewhat more elongated contours, single nuclei without obvious nucleoli, and high nuclear-to-cytoplasmic ratios. These blastematous cells are often individually dispersed or present in loose arrays; however, they may also be embedded in myxoid tissue fragments.

Histopathology

Pulmonary blastoma shows areas of epithelial and mesenchymal differentiation in various proportions. The epithelial component is essentially low-grade fetal adenocarcinoma/well-differentiated fetal adenocarcinoma (see *Variants of adenocarcinoma*, p. 38), consisting of branching tubules lined by pseudostratified columnar cells with relatively small, uniform, rounded nuclei and clear to weakly eosinophilic cytoplasm {1336,1806}. The columnar cells are rich in glycogen, and resemble the airway epithelium of fetal lung in the pseudoglandular period, although focally they may demonstrate pleomorphism, resembling either high-grade fetal or conventional adenocarcinoma {967,1336}. Morules are seen in 43–60% of blastoma cases {967,1336}. Scattered neuroendocrine cells are present in two thirds of cases, and combined small cell carcinoma has rarely been described {254}. The mesenchymal component typically shows tightly packed primitive oval cells with a high nuclear-to-cytoplasmic ratio, and a tendency to differentiate towards more mature fibroblast-like cells in the myxoid or fibrous background. Occasional bizarre giant cells may be seen. Heterologous elements such as osteosarcoma, chondrosarcoma, and rhabdomyosarcoma are noted in up to 25% of cases. Components of unusual differentiation have rarely been described in pulmonary blastoma, including yolk sac tumour {2394}, teratoma, seminoma, embryonal carcinoma {77}, and melanoma {472}.

Immunohistochemistry

The epithelial cell component (including the morules) is diffusely positive for CK7 {2203}, cytokeratin AE1/AE3 {1336,2994}, 34βE12 {1570}, carcinoembryonic antigen {1336,2994}, epithelial membrane antigen, TTF1 {795,1766,2203}, and milk fat globulin {1336}, and is focally positive for chromogranin A {2326,2994}, synaptophysin {795}, Clara cell antigen {2994}, vimentin {1336,2994}, and polypeptide hormones (calcitonin, adrenocorticotropic hormone, serotonin, and L-enkephalin) {1336}. Surfactant has been reported as

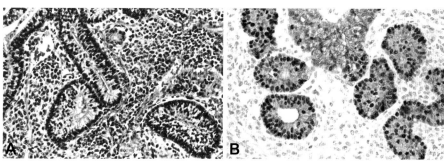

Fig. 1.102 Pulmonary blastoma. **A** Showing fetal-type glandular structures mixed with primitive blastematous stroma. **B** Tumour cells of both glandular and blastematous stromal components show nuclear positivity for β-catenin. The glandular cells also show cytoplasmic staining.

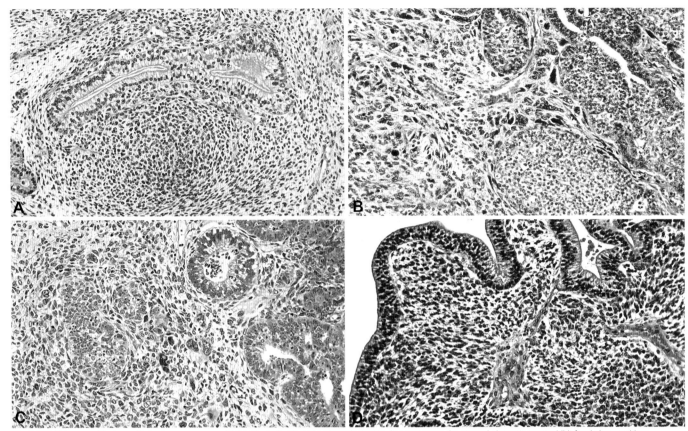

Fig. 1.103 Pulmonary blastoma. Biphasic appearance, with fetal-type glands and embryonic stroma. In some cases the stromal elements may exhibit focal pleomorphism. C and D reprinted from Travis WD et al. {2678}.

either negative {2203} or focally positive {1804,2994}.

Mesenchymal blastematous cells show diffuse immunoreactivity for vimentin and muscle-specific actin {2994}, and only focal reactivity for cytokeratin AE1/AE3 {2994}. Desmin and/or myogenin as well as S100 are found in heterologous rhabdomyosarcomatous and chondrosarcomatous elements, respectively {2869}.

Both glandular elements (including morules) and blastematous elements show nuclear/cytoplasmic accumulation of β-catenin. Rarely, pulmonary blastoma shows a germ cell tumour component, such as yolk sac tumour and seminoma, accordingly staining for α-fetoprotein or placental alkaline phosphatase {77,2394}.

Differential diagnosis

The main differential diagnoses include fetal-type adenocarcinoma, pleuropulmonary blastoma, biphasic sarcomas such as biphasic-type synovial sarcoma, and metastatic tumours – particularly malignant mixed Müllerian tumour from the gynaecological tract {2026,2670}. Fetal-type adenocarcinoma lacks a blastematous component. Pleuropulmonary blastoma occurs in a young (paediatric) group, typically appears cystic, and has a peripheral location (see *Pleuropulmonary blastoma*, p. 124). Virtually all synovial sarcomas are monophasic and lack a glandular component and typically demonstrate the X:18 SS18-SSX translocation {167}. The glandular component of biphasic synovial sarcomas lacks a fetal adenocarcinoma morphology.

Carcinosarcomas can have high-grade fetal adenocarcinoma as the epithelial component {1332,1809}, but this should be distinguished from pulmonary blastoma. In these cases, β-catenin is solely membrane-localized in the epithelial component {1807,1809,2326}.

A history of uterine tumour assists recognition of metastatic mixed Müllerian tumour. Immunohistochemistry (for hormonal receptors in uterine Müllerian tumour) may be of value.

Genetic profile

Pulmonary blastoma and well-differentiated fetal adenocarcinoma (a putative precursor lesion) are frequently associated with missense mutations in exon 3 of *CTNNB1*, responsible for activation of the Wnt pathway through aberrant nuclear/cytoplasmic localization of β-catenin protein {1536,1807,2017,2326}. *TP53* mutation and both p53 and MDM2 protein accumulation are occasionally detected in pulmonary blastoma {219,1024,2017}.

Prognosis and predictive factors

Prognosis is very poor, and correlates with stage. Other negative prognostic factors are biphasic type and tumour recurrence {40,2748}. No significant predictive markers have been identified.

L.R. Chirieac
Y-L. Chang
Y. Yatabe

Other and unclassified carcinomas
Lymphoepithelioma-like carcinoma

Definition
Lymphoepithelioma-like carcinoma is a rare and distinctive type of carcinoma characterized by poorly differentiated morphology admixed with marked lymphocyte infiltrate (similar to undifferentiated nasopharyngeal carcinoma) and the presence of EBV in the nuclei of neoplastic cells.

ICD-O code   8082/3

Synonyms
Obsolete: lymphoepithelial carcinoma; lymphoepithelioma

Epidemiology
Lymphoepithelioma-like carcinoma is rare (accounting for only 0.92% of all lung cancer cases), and is more common in South-East Asia. Fewer than 200 cases have been reported. It affects non-smoking, younger patients (with a median age of 51 years), and mostly women {166,388,390,1470}.

Etiology
The presence of EBER1 in the nuclei of tumour cells, the expression of LMP1 and BCL2, and the presence of CD8+ T lymphocytes suggest a role for EBV in the pathogenesis of this unique type of tumour {388,993,1470}. There is a direct correlation between EBV serology titre and tumour burden in lymphoepithelioma-like carcinoma {388}.

Clinical features
Up to a third of all lymphoepithelioma-like carcinomas are identified as incidental radiographical findings {1470}.
Cough (with or without blood-tinged sputum) is the most common presenting symptom {388}. Other symptoms are similar to those observed in other lung cancers, such as chest pain, body weight loss, and haemoptysis {388,1470}.
Imaging. On imaging, lymphoepithelioma-like carcinoma usually presents as a discrete coin lesion that is indistinguishable from ordinary non-small cell lung carcinomas. The presence of a cavitary lesion with a smooth inner surface is rare {1038}, and pleural effusions are uncommon {388}.
Spread. The pattern of spread of lymphoepithelioma-like carcinoma is similar to that of other non-small cell lung carcinomas. Metastases occur most frequently to hilar or mediastinal lymph nodes, followed by the pericardium, liver, bone, and brain {388}.
Therapy. Complete resection is the primary approach to obtain a cure for early resectable lesions {1016,1470}. Patients with locally advanced disease can receive neoadjuvant or adjuvant chemotherapy or chemoradiation {388,1470}.

Localization
Lymphoepithelioma-like carcinomas are often peripheral, but a minority of cases have an endobronchial component {388}.

Macroscopy
The tumours are usually solitary, circumscribed, and round to ovoid. They range in size from 1 to 11 cm. The cut surfaces are pink-white and rubbery, with a fish-flesh appearance {388}.

Cytology
Typically, lymphoepithelioma-like carcinomas show cohesive sheets and clusters of uniform large tumour cells associated with heavy lymphocytic infiltration. Round or oval vesicular nuclei with syncytial appearance, conspicuous nucleoli, occasional spindle growth, prominent mitotic figures, and finely granular to flocculent cytoplasm are present.
In situ hybridization for EBER1 reveals localization of EBV genomes within the nuclei of tumour cells {977}.

Histopathology
The typical pulmonary lymphoepithelioma-like carcinoma is characterized by a seemingly syncytial pattern of growth, large vesicular nuclei with prominent eosinophilic nucleoli, and a marked lymphocytic infiltrate. Focal squamous and spindle cell differentiation can occur {378,1016}. It has predominantly pushing borders and a permeative interface with the adjacent lung parenchyma. The tumour has anastomosing smooth-contoured borders with irregular islands or diffuse sheets of tumour cells {388,1016,1470}.

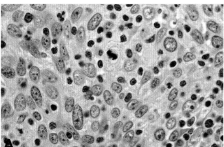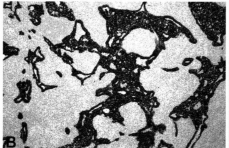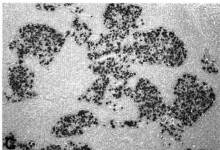

Fig. 1.104 Lymphoepithelioma-like carcinoma. **A** Lymphoepithelioma-like carcinoma cells have a characteristic syncytial pattern of growth, large vesicular nuclei with prominent eosinophilic nucleoli, and a marked lymphocytic infiltrate. **B** The tumour cells express cytokeratin (AE1/AE3). **C** Chromogenic in situ hybridization for EBER1 demonstrates positivity confined to the nuclei of large undifferentiated neoplastic cells, but is absent in the surrounding lymphocytic infiltrate.

The stroma may occasionally show non-necrotizing granulomatous reaction {939}, or intratumoural amyloid deposition {378,388}. Some of the tumour islands show central necrosis. The mitotic count is variable, with a median of 10 mitoses per 2 mm² {378}. The tumour cells typically express cytokeratin (AE1/AE3), CK5/6, p40, and p63, which suggests squamous cell lineage. The accompanying lymphoid infiltrate reveals a mixture of CD3+ T cells and CD20+ B cells. The presence of EBV in the epithelial tumour nuclei is detected by chromogenic in situ hybridization for EBER1. No EBER1 signal is identified in the surrounding lymphoid cells.

The major differential diagnoses for lymphoepithelioma-like carcinoma are non-Hodgkin lymphoma and metastatic nasopharyngeal carcinoma {388,977,1470}.

Genetic profile

KRAS and *EGFR* mutations are uncommon in lymphoepithelioma-like carcinoma, indicating that these genes are not important events in the development of this type of tumour {1470,2581}.

Prognosis and predictive factors

The survival is better in patients with lymphoepithelioma-like carcinoma (the 2-year and 5-year overall survival rates are 88% and 62%, respectively) than in patients with typical non-small cell lung carcinomas {378,388,1016,1470}. Tumour recurrence and necrosis are poor prognostic factors for survival. Factors that may account for a better prognosis are the presence of abundant CD8+

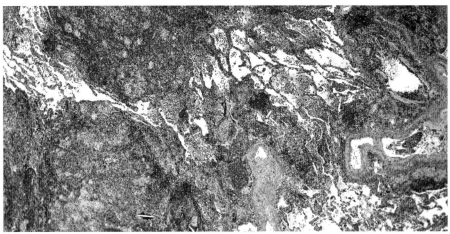

Fig. 1.105 Lymphoepithelioma-like carcinoma. Lymphoepithelioma-like carcinoma has irregular islands with predominantly smooth, pushing borders, and a permeative interface with the adjacent lung parenchyma.

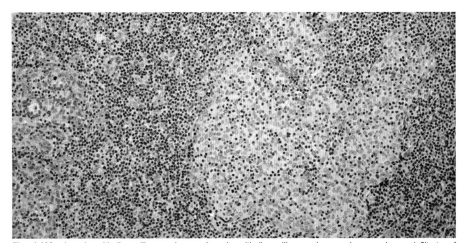

Fig. 1.106 Lymphoepithelioma-like carcinoma. Lymphoepithelioma-like carcinoma shows a heavy infiltrate of lymphocytes surrounding an island of neoplastic epithelial cells.

cytotoxic T lymphocytes adjacent to lymphoepithelioma-like carcinoma cells, and the absence of both p53 and epidermal growth factor receptor oncoproteins in tumour cells {388,1016,1470}.

NUT carcinoma

L.R. Chirieac
C.A. French
L. Sholl
Y. Yatabe

Definition

NUT carcinoma is an aggressive, poorly differentiated carcinoma defined by the presence of *NUT* (nuclear protein in testis, i.e. *NUTM1*) gene rearrangement.

ICD-O code   8023/3

Synonyms

NUT midline carcinoma; t(15;19) carcinoma; carcinoma with t(15;19) translocation; aggressive t(15;19) positive carcinoma; midline lethal carcinoma; midline carcinoma of children and young adults with *NUT* rearrangement; *BET*-rearranged carcinoma

Epidemiology

Fewer than 100 cases of NUT carcinoma have been reported. NUT carcinoma affects males and females equally. Although it was originally reported in children and younger adults {154,758}, NUT carcinoma can affect people of any age {756,2353,2463}. At sites outside of the lung, NUT carcinoma may account for 4–18% of tumours diagnosed as poorly differentiated carcinomas or undifferentiated malignant neoplasms {689,758,2463}. Its true prevalence in the lung is unknown. There is no known racial predisposition.

Etiology

The etiology of NUT carcinoma is unknown. Smoking, HPV infection, and EBV infection are not known risk factors.

Clinical features

Thoracic NUT carcinoma usually presents at an advanced stage, with pleural effusions, pleuritic chest pain, non-productive cough, weight loss, and shortness of breath {1428,1824}.
Chest X-rays usually demonstrate extremely rapid tumour progression, with complete opacification of the thorax within 2–8 weeks from initial presentation {2068}. On CT, NUT carcinoma appears as a hypoattenuating, heterogeneously enhancing, often extensively necrotic mass, with poorly defined, infiltrative

borders {1824,2068,2464}. High FDG uptake by NUT carcinoma is characteristic, so PET-CT is the modality of choice to determine the systemic disease burden and monitor the response to treatment {2197,2315,2353}.
NUT carcinoma is characterized by aggressive local invasion and by lymphatic and haematogenous spread {758}. Thoracic NUT carcinoma may disseminate to the bone, ovaries, liver, and brain {154, 680,2068,2097,2353,2590,2759}.

Macroscopy

Thoracic NUT carcinomas often present at advanced stages, and are therefore not amenable to surgical resection. NUT carcinoma typically grows as a large mass extending into hilar structures or along the pleura and chest wall {2590}. The tumours have a fleshy, tan-white cut surface, and geographic necrosis may be prominent.

Cytology

Aspirates yield cellular smears composed of discohesive clusters and solitary monomorphic cells with irregular nuclear contours, variable granular to coarse chromatin, and discrete nucleoli. Mitoses, necrotic debris, and crush artefact are common {175,3028}. The cytological characteristics are non-specific, and similar to those of other undifferentiated carcinomas.

Histopathology

NUT carcinoma typically consists of sheets and nests of small to intermediate-sized undifferentiated cells with a monomorphic appearance. The nuclei have irregular contours and granular to coarse chromatin. NUT carcinomas commonly and characteristically demonstrate abrupt foci of keratinization {572,1428,2462}. Tumour cells infiltrate and expand the interstitium, and may appear contiguous with bronchial epithelium {2590}; however, convincing in situ lesions have never been described. Tumour cells may be associated with a reactive pneumocyte proliferation. This

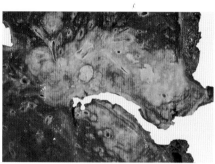

Fig. 1.107 NUT carcinoma. Cross-section of lung showing tumour infiltrating the lung parenchyma, with compression of bronchovascular structures and extension to the pleural surface; multifocal geographical necrosis is evident.

should not be misinterpreted as an adenocarcinomatous component.

Immunohistochemistry

NUT carcinoma consistently shows speckled nuclear positivity in more than 50% of tumour cells, using a highly specific monoclonal nuclear NUT antibody {925}. Seminomas may have weak and focal NUT staining. Broad-spectrum cytokeratins are positive in the majority of cases, although in rare cases are negative {689,3028}. Variable results are obtained with other epithelial markers such as epithelial membrane antigen, BerEP4, and carcinoembryonic (CEA) antigen. Most cases have positive nuclear staining for p63/p40, indicating squamous lineage. Occasionally, NUT carcinomas can stain for chromogranin, synaptophysin, or even TTF1 {2590}. NUT carcinomas

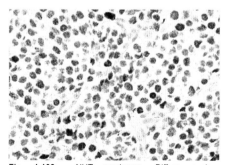

Fig. 1.108 NUT carcinoma. Diffuse nuclear immunohistochemical staining with nuclear protein in testis (NUT) antibody is diagnostic of NUT carcinoma. The speckled pattern of staining is characteristic.

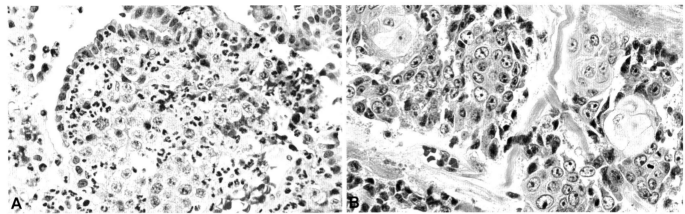

Fig. 1.109 NUT carcinoma. **A** NUT midline carcinoma. Monomorphic, primitive-appearing tumour cells with pale eosinophilic to basophilic cytoplasm, irregular nuclei, and distinct nucleoli infiltrating in lung tissue. The tumour cells appear to be undermining reactive epithelium. Infiltrating neutrophils are a prominent feature. **B** Focal squamous differentiation is characteristic, but not present in all cases. Also apparent are clear spaces between cells, which are also frequently seen in NUT carcinoma.

are often positive for CD34, which may lead to a misdiagnosis of acute leukaemia {758}. Germ cell, lymphoid, and myeloid markers are negative.

Differential diagnosis
The differential diagnosis includes any poorly differentiated malignant neoplasm {757} (see also *Thymomas,* p. 187). NUT carcinoma may be mistaken for squamous cell carcinoma (especially basaloid squamous cell carcinoma), undifferentiated carcinoma, small cell carcinoma, adenosquamous carcinoma, Ewing sarcoma, metastatic germ cell tumour, or acute leukaemia {2048,2463}. Testing for NUT expression by immunohistochemistry should be considered in all poorly differentiated carcinomas that

lack glandular differentiation or specific etiology, particularly in non-smokers and patients presenting at a young age.

Genetic profile
NUT carcinoma is characterized by a chromosomal translocation between the *NUT* gene (*NUTM1*) on chromosome 15q14 (in essentially 100% of cases) and other genes: *BRD4* on chromosome 19p13.1 (70%), *BRD3* on chromosome 9q34.2 (6%), or an unknown partner gene (24%) {154,758,759,760}. Among previously unknown partner genes to *NUT* is *NSD3* on chromosome 8p11.23 {759A}. Unlike pulmonary squamous carcinomas, NUT carcinoma may show few cytogenetic alterations by classical karyotype, with the chromosomal

translocation sometimes being the only abnormality. Demonstration of *NUT* rearrangement by molecular or cytogenetic analyses or NUT protein overexpression by immunohistochemistry is diagnostic of NUT carcinoma {689}.

Prognosis and predictive factors
NUT carcinoma is extremely aggressive, with a median survival of 7 months {2315}. Survival is not correlated with age, translocation type, sex, or tumour location. No specific chemotherapeutic regimen has demonstrated efficacy in treating NUT carcinoma, but trials investigating the treatment of NUT carcinoma with bromodomain inhibitors are ongoing (http://www.clinicaltrials.gov/).

Salivary gland-type tumours
Mucoepidermoid carcinoma

Y. Ishikawa   S. Dacic
E. Alvarez-Fernandez A.G. Nicholson
M.C. Aubry

Definition
Mucoepidermoid carcinoma is a salivary gland-type tumour that consists of mucin-secreting cells, squamous or squamoid cells, and intermediate-type cells.

ICD-O code   8430/3

Synonym
Mucoepidermoid tumour

Epidemiology
Mucoepidermoid carcinoma accounts for < 1% of lung carcinomas, with no sex predominance. It occurs between the first and eighth decade, with a mean age between 30 and 40 years. About 50% of the tumours occur in patients aged < 30 years.

Etiology
There is no association with smoking.

Clinical features
The signs and symptoms are wheezing, cough, haemoptysis, and obstructive pneumonia, although some patients are asymptomatic {1704,2991}.
CT shows a well-defined, centrally located endobronchial mass {1466}. Mucoepidermoid carcinoma is usually PET-positive {1466}.
Both low-grade and high-grade mucoepidermoid carcinomas may involve lymph nodes, either remotely or by direct extension, with this being more common in high-grade lesions {1704,2991}. TNM staging should be applied.

Localization
Mucoepidermoid carcinomas are usually endobronchial, and typically arise in the central airways.

Macroscopy
Mucoepidermoid carcinomas are well-demarcated soft tumours, measuring 3 cm on average. They show a grey-white to pink-tan, sometimes mucinous, and varyingly cystic cut surface {983,2990}. High-grade tumours are more infiltrative.

Cytology
Three cell types are present, all intermingled {2319}: glandular cells with eccentric nuclei, delicate cytoplasm, and indistinct cell borders; small, round, uniform intermediate cells with even chromatin, in sheet-like arrangements; and squamoid cells with dense cytoplasm and distinct cell borders.

Histopathology
Subclassification into low-grade and high-grade types has been proposed. Low-grade tumours are composed of three cell types: mucin-secreting, squamous (or squamoid), and intermediate cells, and often show cystic patterns with solid areas. Tumour islands contain both cystic and solid patterns. Cystic components consist of cytologically bland columnar cells with mucin and rare mitoses. Solid components, consisting of squamoid and/or intermediate cells, typically surround the cystic areas. Intermediate cells are oval or polygonal, with round nuclei, eosinophilic or clear cytoplasm, and rare necrosis. Stromal calcification and ossification, often with a granulomatous reaction, are seen around areas of mucous extravasation. High-grade mucoepidermoid carcinoma is mainly composed of atypical squamoid and intermediate cells, with frequent mitosis and necrosis, accompanied by variable numbers of mucin-secreting cells.
High-grade tumours are rare, and the diagnosis should be determined after careful exclusion of adenosquamous carcinoma. Criteria more typical of high-grade mucoepidermoid carcinoma include: 1) exophytic endobronchial growth, 2) surface epithelium lacking the changes of carcinoma in situ, 3) absence of individual cell keratinization and squamous pearl formation, and 4) transitional areas to low-grade mucoepidermoid carcinoma. A lack of TTF1 and napsin A in a mucoepidermoid carcinoma may also be useful for differential diagnosis {2175,2366}. *MAML2* rearrangement is exclusively seen in mucoepidermoid carcinoma {14}. However, these two types of lung tumours cannot be reliably distinguished in all cases {1399}.

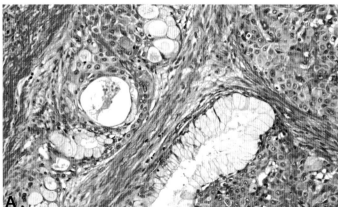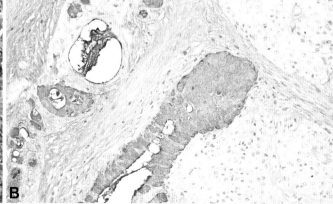

Fig. 1.110 Mucoepidermoid carcinoma. **A** This tumour consists of mucinous glands and squamoid cells. **B** Alcian blue staining.

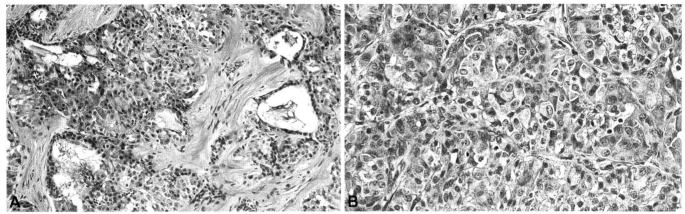

Fig. 1.111 High-grade mucoepidermoid carcinoma. **A** This area consists of a mixture of mucin-producing glands and nests of squamoid cells. **B** This higher-grade area shows tumour cells with more atypical nuclei, some prominent conspicuous nucleoli, and a mitotic figure.

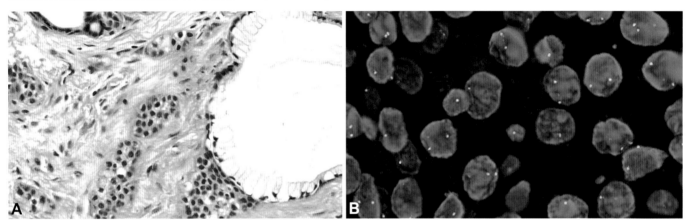

Fig. 1.112 A Low-grade mucoepidermoid carcinoma. Glands with mucinous cells and surrounding intermediate/squamoid cells. **B** Mucoepidermoid carcinoma. A FISH break-apart *MAML2* probe shows split signals indicative of translocation.

Genetic profile

A fusion gene *CRTC1-MAML2* occurs in both low-grade and high-grade mucoepidermoid carcinoma {14}, more frequently in low-grade tumours, as is also seen in the salivary gland counterpart {2654}. This fusion gene has potential as a diagnostic marker. *EGFR* mutations have been reported in some cases, but their significance is unclear {941,1884,3000}.

Prognosis and predictive factors

Low-grade mucoepidermoid carcinoma has a good prognosis, whereas high-grade tumours behave similarly to other non-small cell carcinomas {484, 1704,2991}. Poor prognostic factors include positive resection margins and lymph node metastasis {484,1704,2991}.

Adenoid cystic carcinoma

Y. Ishikawa
S. Dacic
A.G. Nicholson

Definition
Adenoid cystic carcinoma is a malignant salivary gland-type tumour that consists of epithelial and myoepithelial cells. It shows variable morphological configurations, including tubular, cribriform, and solid patterns.

ICD-O code   8200/3

Synonyms
Cylindroma; adenocystic carcinoma

Epidemiology
Adenoid cystic carcinoma accounts for < 1% of all lung tumours {178}, with no sex predominance. The average age at presentation is 50 years {1704,1735}.

Etiology
There is no evidence of an association with smoking.

Clinical features
Common symptoms include shortness of breath, cough, wheezing, and haemoptysis due to airway obstruction {1618}. Imaging typically shows a centrally located mass that may have an endobronchial component. Adenoid cystic carcinomas are larger, more frequently involve the central airways, and have a higher median FDG uptake than mucoepidermoid carcinomas {667}.Adenoid cystic carcinoma grows insidiously and infiltratively, sometimes extending to the lung parenchyma and mediastinum. Perineural invasion makes complete surgical resection

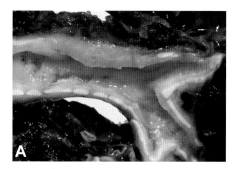

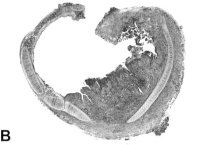

Fig. 1.114 Adenoid cystic carcinoma. **A** Macroscopy of an adenoid cystic carcinoma arising within the bronchus. **B** This whole-mount section shows a tumour growing in an endobronchial manner, with infiltration of the peribronchial soft tissues.

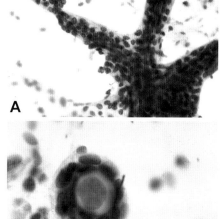

Fig. 1.115 Adenoid cystic carcinoma. **A** Papanicolaou staining of a bronchial brushing shows a finger-like stromal structure, with cohesive cells containing oval nuclei and little cytoplasm. **B** Papanicolaou staining of a bronchial brushing shows a translucent hyaline globule surrounded by small uniform epithelial cells.

difficult, and local recurrence is common. Metastases to remote organs are uncommon. TNM staging should be used.

Localization
Adenoid cystic carcinoma typically arises as an endobronchial tumour.

Macroscopy
The tumours may show a well-delineated, greyish-white, homogeneous cut surface, but frequently infiltrate beyond the visible macroscopic margins. Sampling of peribronchial soft tissue is therefore worthwhile.

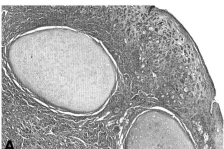
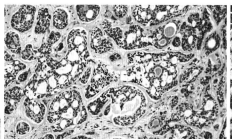
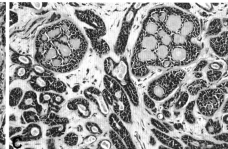

Fig. 1.113 Adenoid cystic carcinoma. **A** Adenoid cystic carcinoma growing diffusely within the airway wall, both above and below cartilage plates. **B** A cribriform pattern is common in adenoid cystic carcinoma; note that materials within the gland-like structure actually connect to the outside stroma, and that the tumour cells have no glandular polarity. **C** The tumour consists of nests and tubules, many of which show eosinophilic hyaline cores forming cylindrical structures.

Cytology

Three-dimensional microacinar patterns are seen, with pink to pale opaque globules corresponding to intraluminal hyalinized or myxoid materials.

Histopathology

Adenoid cystic carcinoma is composed of small-sized cells with scant cytoplasm and usually homogeneous hyperchromatic nuclei, showing frequent perineural invasion and infrequent mitosis. Architecturally, it shows characteristic features including cribriform, tubular, and solid patterns. The most characteristic cribriform array shows cells surrounding connective tissue cylinders with myxoid and hyalinized material, from which the name cylindroma was derived. When forming tubules with two-layered cells, the luminal cells show a cuboidal appearance and the peripheral cells form a myoepithelial layer. Immunohistochemistry demonstrates both ductal and myoepithelial phenotypes, including cytokeratin, vimentin, actin, S100, and KIT. The matrix recapitulates basement membrane-like characters such as collagen IV, laminin, and heparin sulfate. The differential diagnoses include carcinoid tumours, basaloid squamous cell carcinoma, and small cell carcinoma – all of which can be typically distinguished by immunohistochemical staining. Additionally, basaloid squamous cell carcinoma has a high proliferation rate, unlike most adenoid cystic carcinomas. Pleomorphic adenoma with a focally cribriform architecture may resemble adenoid cystic carcinoma. Metastasis from other organs should be carefully ruled out {1618}.

Genetic profile

A fusion of the *MYB* oncogene and *NFIB* transcription factor has been reported in 30–100% of adenoid cystic carcinomas of the head and neck and breast {1685,2035}, but there are no reports for bronchopulmonary counterparts. Loss of heterozygosity of chromosomes 3p14

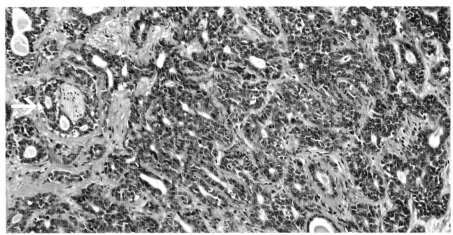

Fig. 1.116 Adenoid cystic carcinoma. Showing predominantly tubular growth of small hyperchromatic epithelial cells; perineural invasion is present (arrow).

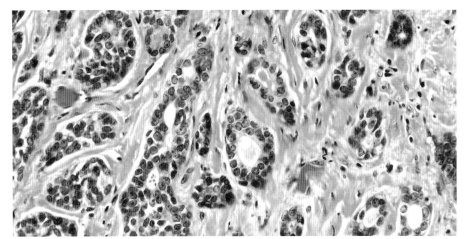

Fig. 1.117 High-power view of the tubular area of the adenoid cystic carcinoma.

and 9p has been reported rarely in bronchial adenoid cystic carcinoma {2510}. High-resolution comparative genomic hybridization analysis showed losses at 3p, 4p, and 15q, and gains at 12q15 (the *MDM2* site) {191}. *EGFR* and *RAS* mutations were not identified {1534,2856}. Despite immunoreactivity for KIT, *KIT* mutations are absent {102,2856}. Although whole-exome sequencing of head and neck adenoid cystic carcinoma identified mutations in *PIK3CA*, *ATM*, *CDKN2A*, *SF3B1*, *SUFU*, *TSC1*, *CYLD*, *NOTCH1/2*, *SPEN*, and *FGFR2* {2470}, there are no similar studies for bronchopulmonary adenoid cystic carcinoma.

Prognosis and predictive factors

Tumours behave in an indolent fashion, and local recurrence (often multiple) may occur over a 10 to 15 year period following resection. Distant metastases may eventually occur. Poor prognosis relates to stage of the tumour at diagnosis, positive margins at surgery, and a solid growth pattern.

Epithelial-myoepithelial carcinoma

Y. Ishikawa
S. Dacic
A.N. Husain
A.G. Nicholson

Definition
Epithelial-myoepithelial carcinoma is a low-grade malignant epithelial tumour with biphasic morphology, consisting of an inner layer of duct-like structures made up of epithelial cells, and a surrounding layer of myoepithelial cells with spindle, clear cell, or plasmacytoid features.

ICD-O code   8562/3

Synonyms
Adenomyoepithelioma; pneumocytic adenomyoepithelioma; epithelial-myoepithelial tumour; epimyoepithelial carcinoma; epithelial-myoepithelial tumour of unproven malignant potential; malignant mixed tumour comprising epithelial and myoepithelial cells

Epidemiology
Epithelial-myoepithelial carcinoma occurs in patients aged from 30 to 70 years, with an average age of 50 years. There is no sex predominance {82,1831}.

Etiology
There is no association with smoking.

Clinical features
Epithelial-myoepithelial carcinomas typically present with symptoms such as productive cough, fever, voice change, and dyspnoea. TNM staging should be used.

Localization
Epithelial-myoepithelial carcinoma typically arises in the central region of the lung, and shows endobronchial localization.

Macroscopy
Epithelial-myoepithelial carcinoma is typically a well-demarcated, homogeneous, solid endobronchial tumour, with a greyish-white to tan cut surface {1831}.

Histopathology
Epithelial-myoepithelial carcinoma consists variably of two types of cells: epithelial cells and myoepithelial cells. The epithelial cells are cuboidal, have bland nuclei and eosinophilic cytoplasm, and form a duct-like structure surrounded by myoepithelial cells with usually clear cytoplasm. The myoepithelial cells sometimes become spindle-shaped and grow in a solid fashion, which may predominate, sometimes to the exclusion of the epithelial component. Mitoses are usually rare, and no necrosis is observed. The tumour may extend to the lung parenchyma or metastasize to lymph nodes and even the chest wall {2431}. The epithelial cells are positive for keratin and negative for vimentin and S100, whereas the myoepithelial cells are weakly positive for cytokeratins, CD117 (KIT), and glial fibrillary acidic protein, strongly positive for S100 and actin, and negative for carcinoembryonic antigen and HMB45. Rarely, epithelial-myoepithelial tumours have an epithelial component showing pneumocytic differentiation (with positive staining for TTF1 and surfactant protein A in the epithelial component), and a myoepithelial component without any distinct clear cells. Tubules and glands with an inner epithelial lining and an outer myoepithelial layer are prominent. This variant, called pneumocytic adenomyoepithelioma by some, has to date shown no recurrence or metastasis, although the cases are very few {385,1771}.

The differential diagnoses include mucoepidermoid carcinoma, adenoid cystic carcinoma, pleomorphic adenoma, and PEComatous tumours (clear cell tumour of the lung). These are particularly important for small biopsy specimens. Metastases of tumours with clear cells, such as renal clear cell carcinoma, should be carefully ruled out.

Genetic profile
The molecular studies of primary pulmonary epithelial-myoepithelial carcinoma are limited to a single case report. No mutations were found in *KRAS* or *EGFR* genes {1902}. The *HRAS* exon 3 (codon 61) mutations p.Q61R and p.Q61K have been reported in head and neck epithelial-myoepithelial carcinoma {429}. Similarly, loss of heterozygosity was demonstrated at the D13S217 (13q12), D18S58 (18q21), D9S162 (9p22–21), D10S251,

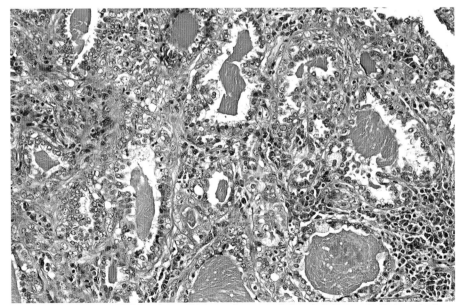

Fig. 1.118 Epithelial-myoepithelial carcinoma. This tumour is composed of glands that have a double layer of cells: an inner layer of eosinophilic epithelial cells and an outer layer of myoepithelial clear cells.

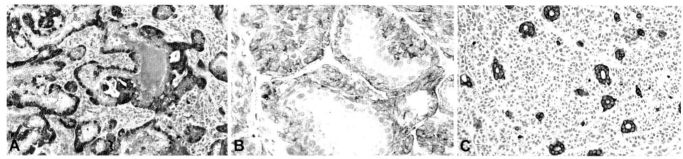

Fig. 1.119 Epithelial-myoepithelial carcinoma. **A** The outer layer of myoepithelial cells stains with S100. **B** The outer layer of myoepithelial cells stains with smooth muscle actin. **C** The inner layer of ductal cells stains positively with pancytokeratin.

and D10S541 loci surrounding the *PTEN* gene. No mutation or methylation of the *p16* gene or alteration of the *PTEN* gene could be found {1284}. No similar studies have been reported for bronchopulmonary epithelial-myoepithelial carcinoma.

Prognosis and predictive factors
Although there are insufficient data with long-term follow-up available, epithelial-myoepithelial carcinoma typically behaves in an indolent fashion, with rare cases reported to metastasize {1831, 2431}. Epithelial-myoepithelial carcinoma is usually treated surgically, which is typically curative, although recurrence may occur, sometimes after several years.

Pleomorphic adenoma

E. Alvarez-Fernandez
S. Dacic
Y. Ishikawa
A.G. Nicholson

Definition
Pleomorphic adenoma is a benign tumour that consists of epithelial cells and modified myoepithelial cells intermingled with myxoid or chondroid stroma.

ICD-O code   8940/0

Synonym
Benign mixed tumour

Epidemiology
Pleomorphic adenoma occurs within an age range of 8–74 years {120}, but usually in adults. There is no sex predominance. One third of all cases are found incidentally.

Clinical features
Endobronchial tumours may present with dyspnoea or haemoptysis. Peripheral parenchymal tumours are frequently asymptomatic. Chest X-rays and CT show well-circumscribed solid masses {334,946}. The heterogeneity of CT and MRI corresponds to different histological elements of pleomorphic adenoma. Tumours may be PET-positive {946}.

Localization
Most pleomorphic adenomas arise in the proximal bronchi or the trachea.

Macroscopy
Pleomorphic adenoma ranges in diameter from 1 to 16 cm {1733}. Endobronchial pleomorphic adenoma is polypoid, while peripheral parenchymal tumours are well-circumscribed nodules. The cut surface is white-grey, myxoid, and soft to rubbery.

Histopathology
Pulmonary pleomorphic adenomas are histologically similar to those seen in the salivary glands. They have prominent glandular or ductal components embedded in chondromyxoid stroma. A cartilaginous stroma is not prominent {1733}. Solid islands of epithelial cells with a focal myxoid stroma can be seen.

Immunohistochemically, epithelial, myoepithelial, and stromal cells are positive for cytokeratin and S100 protein. Myoepithelial cells are positive for calponin, α-SMA, and smooth muscle myosin heavy chain, and are variably immunoreactive for vimentin and glial fibrillary acidic protein {1733}.

The most important differential diagnosis is metastatic salivary gland tumour of the head and neck. Other differential diagnoses include hamartoma and carcinosarcoma. Hamartomas typically have well-developed chondroid elements. Pulmonary blastomas and carcinosarcomas have sarcomatous elements. Exceptionally, a malignancy may arise within a pleomorphic adenoma, which should be called carcinoma ex pleomorphic adenoma. Tumours with malignant features in both components – such as prominent necrosis, cellular atypia, ≥ 5 mitoses per 2 mm^2, and vascular invasion – should be called malignant mixed tumour {1733}.

Genetic profile
Unlike with salivary gland pleomorphic adenoma, molecular studies are rare {2571}. There are no reports yet of pulmonary pleomorphic adenomas studied for the PLAG1 and HMGA2 fusions, known to occur in their much more common salivary gland counterparts {2466}.

Prognosis and predictive factors
Small, well-circumscribed tumours are usually benign. Tumours with infiltrative borders may recur and metastasize, and usually behave as low-grade malignancies {2834}. The most reliable prognostic factors include tumour size, local infiltration, and mitoses {1733}.

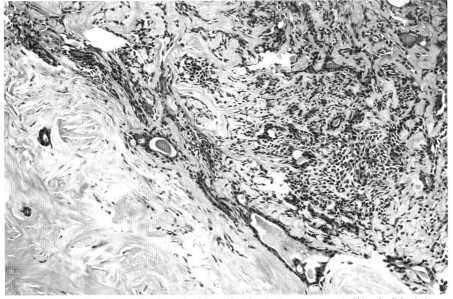

Fig. 1.120 Pleomorphic adenoma. Prominent glandular or ductular structures are present within a hyalinized stroma; areas consisting of small spindled myoepithelial cells are also present.

Papillomas

D.B. Flieder
A.G. Nicholson
W.D. Travis
Y. Yatabe

Squamous cell papilloma

Definition
Squamous cell papilloma is a papillary tumour that consists of delicate connective tissue fronds lined with squamous epithelium. Squamous cell papillomas can be either solitary or multiple, and either exophytic or inverted.

ICD-O codes
Squamous cell papilloma	8052/0
Exophytic	8052/0
Inverted	8053/0

Synonym
Squamous papilloma

Epidemiology
Solitary squamous cell papillomas are exceedingly rare, accounting for < 1% of all lung neoplasms, but are the most common subtype of benign papillomas {739,2688}. These tumours are three times as common in men as in women, and patients are usually in their sixth decade of life {2688}. Papillomatosis involving the bronchial tree or lung parenchyma is related to laryngotracheal papillomatosis {947,1409}.

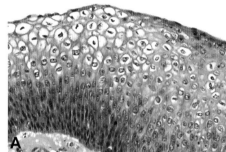
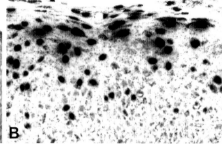

Fig. 1.122 Exophytic squamous cell papilloma. **A** Koilocytosis is obvious in the upper epithelial layers. **B** In situ hybridization staining for HPV subtypes 6 and 11.

Etiology
HPV plays a pathogenetic role in less than half of all solitary lesions, but virtually all papillomatosis lesions {739,947, 1409,1635}. Serotypes 6 and 11 are reported in simple papillomas, while subtypes 16, 18, and 31/33/35 may play a role in malignant transformation {2075, 2076}. The majority of patients with solitary papillomas are tobacco smokers, but an etiological role of smoking has not been established {739,2688}.

Clinical features
Most patients present with obstructive symptoms or haemoptysis, but up to 25% may be asymptomatic, with incidental radiographical detection. High-resolution CT findings demonstrate endobronchial plaques, nodules, or airway thickening in addition to air-trapping, atelectasis, consolidation, and bronchiectasis {1296}. Lung involvement with papillomatosis demonstrates diffuse, poorly defined, non-calcified parenchymal centrilobular opacities, and cavitated thick-walled nodules {2217}.

Localization
Papillomas are usually central and endobronchial, or in rare cases peripheral and endobronchiolar.

Macroscopy
Solitary squamous cell papillomas arise from the wall of mainstem, secondary, or tertiary bronchi. They range from 0.7 to > 9 cm, with a median size of 1.5 cm {739}. Almost all are exophytic. The lesions are polypoid, tan-white, and

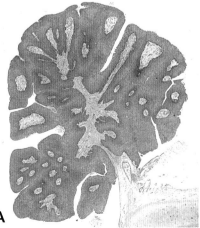
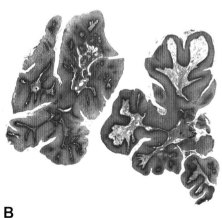
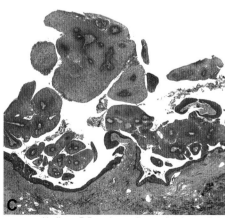

Fig. 1.121 Exophytic squamous cell papilloma. **A** This endobronchial lesion features papillary fronds lined by mature squamous epithelium. **B** Bronchoscopic samples demonstrate the papillary nature of the tumour and vascular nature of the stromal stalks; the epithelium is acanthotic. **C** Laryngotracheal papillomatosis involving the lung. Papillary fronds fill a bronchiectatic cavity; parenchymal invasion is not seen.

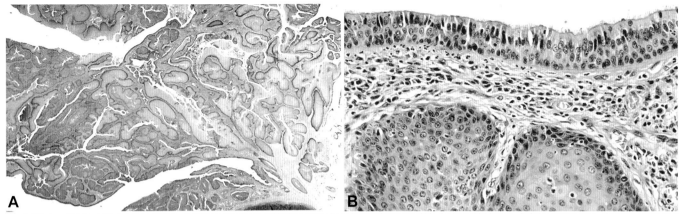

Fig. 1.123 Inverted squamous cell papilloma. **A** Mature squamous epithelium grows in an inverted pattern within the bronchial lumen. **B** Submucosal nests of mature sqaumous epithelium are present. Reprinted from Flieder DB et al. {739} and Travis WD et al. {2689}.

friable, and protrude into airway lumens. Distal and sometimes proximal airways may be bronchiectatic. The distal lung may show secondary obstructive effects such as atelectasis, consolidation, or honeycomb change. Multiple lesions may impart a velvety appearance to the bronchial mucosa. Involved lung is bronchiectatic, with cavities filled with white-tan friable papillary fronds {579}.

Cytology

Exfoliated samples demonstrate sheets and single squamous cells with sharp cellular borders and dense, glassy cytoplasm. Cells may be multinucleated, and nuclei vary from small and pyknotic to large with uneven chromatin. Perinuclear haloes and degenerative vacuoles may be seen. Smaller basal cells featuring scant basophilic cytoplasm and round regular nuclei mix with neutrophils in the background. Fine-needle aspiration biopsy samples feature well-developed three-dimensional branching papillae lined by crowded, non-keratinized, round to oval cells with scant, dense cytoplasm. Single cells are also seen. Irregular nuclear contours, enlarged nuclei, anisonucleosis, and/or prominent nucleoli may be seen, but keratinization, mitoses, karyorrhexis, and necrosis are absent {1396,2000}.

Histopathology

Squamous cell papillomas feature arborizing loose fibrovascular cores covered by stratified squamous epithelium. Exophytic tumours have orderly epithelial maturation, and often keratinized surface cells. Acanthosis, parakeratosis, and intraepithelial neutrophils are common. Less than 25% of solitary papillomas feature typical HPV viral cytopathic effect, including binucleate forms, wrinkled nuclei, and perinuclear haloes. Occasional dyskeratotic cells, large atypical cells, and mitotic figures above the basal layer can be seen. Dysplasia is graded according to the current WHO classification (see *Preinvasive lesion – Squamous cell carcinoma in situ*, p. 59).

Inverted papillomas are also exophytic, but have squamous epithelial invaginations. Cells may extend into seromucinous glands, but basal lamina invests the endophytic nests. Cells are usually non-keratinizing, and demonstrate orderly maturation.

Parenchymal involvement can feature either solid intra-alveolar nests of cytologically bland non-keratinizing cells or large cysts lined by similar cells. Reactive type II pneumocytes lining alveolar walls may be prominent. Surrounding lung may be inflamed or fibrotic. Viral cytopathic effect is usually seen in instances of pulmonary laryngotracheal papillomatosis. Immunohistochemical or in situ DNA hybridization studies correlate with the morphological finding of koilocytosis.

The differential diagnoses include inflammatory polyp and squamous cell carcinoma. Endobronchial inflammatory polyps, despite focal squamous metaplasia, lack true papillary architecture, stromal cores, and proliferative epithelium. Squamous cell carcinoma, which can be endobronchial and papillary, shows malignant cytological features even when stromal invasion and desmoplasia are not apparent. Inverted papillomas can be indistinguishable from invasive squamous cell carcinoma; however, parenchymal destruction and overt cytological atypia favour a diagnosis of malignancy. Recognizing even focal carcinoma within a papilloma warrants a diagnosis of carcinoma.

Genetic profile

Malignant transformation to squamous cell carcinoma may occur in association with *TP53* mutations {853,2112}.

Prognosis and predictive factors

Surgically resected solitary squamous cell papillomas do not recur, but up to 20% of patients treated with endoscopic removal have local tumour recurrence {739,1635}. Transformation into squamous cell carcinoma is uncertain, and most reported cases represent poorly sampled or misdiagnosed carcinoma; however, HPV-associated papillomas (particularly subtypes 16, 18, and 31/33/35) are recognized as having malignant potential {2075,2076}. Laryngotracheal papillomatosis can spread into the lower respiratory tract in up to 5% of patients, and into the alveolar parenchyma in < 5% of juvenile cases {815,1220}. Bronchial and pulmonary involvement may be related to prior treatments or reflux disease. These lesions may develop into abscesses and eventually bronchiectasis. Malignant transformation does not exceed 2% {853}. This disease is incurable, although HPV vaccines are promising.

Glandular papilloma

Definition
Glandular papilloma is a benign papillary tumour lined by ciliated or non-ciliated columnar cells, with varying numbers of cuboidal and goblet cells.

ICD-O code
8260/0

Synonym
Columnar cell papilloma

Epidemiology
Glandular papillomas are rare, accounting for < 20% of all solitary papillomas {739,2446,2688}. Men and women are equally affected, and most patients are in their sixth or seventh decade of life {2688}.

Clinical features
Patients often present with obstructive symptoms including productive or paroxysmal cough, wheezing, or mild haemoptysis {33}. Lesions may be incidentally detected on high-resolution CT {33,670}. Endobronchial protuberances, nodules, masses, airspace consolidation. and atelectasis are noted on scans and at bronchoscopy {1795}. PET avidity has been reported {2591}.

Localization
Most glandular papillomas arise from central lobar or segmental bronchi, but peripheral endobronchiolar lesions also occur.

Macroscopy
Glandular papilloma manifests as pale grey-white, semifirm endobronchial or endobronchiolar tumours measuring 0.7 to 4 cm. The tumours may demonstrate obvious papillary fronds, and may extend into the surrounding lung parenchyma {33,670,739,2688}.

Histopathology
Both central and peripheral tumours feature broad epithelial-lined fronds with vascular or hyalinized stromal cores. Stratified or pseudostratified columnar epithelium may form micropapillary tufts.

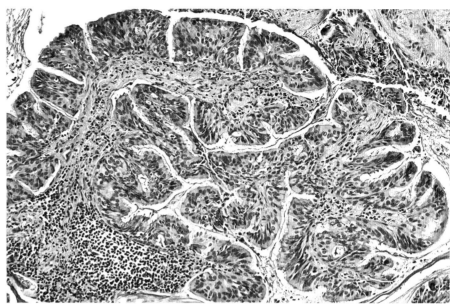

Fig. 1.124 Glandular papilloma. Cytologically bland pseudostratified columnar cells with cilia are admixed with occasional mucous cells.

Uniform columnar cells have eosinophilic cytoplasm and round regular nuclei, and interspersed ciliated and mucinous cells may be seen. The cytoplasm can be clear, but nuclear atypia, mitoses, and necrosis are absent. Stromal cores often contain sheets of plasma cells, and mucopurulent debris surrounds arborizing stromal stalks. Peripheral lesions may extend into alveoli, with minimal lepidic growth {33,670}.

The differential diagnoses include primary and metastatic adenocarcinoma and other adenomas. Complete excision is necessary for definitive diagnosis. Carcinomas feature epithelial crowding and malignant cytological features, but lack basal, ciliated, and mucinous cells. Mucous gland adenoma is composed of mucus-filled cysts and tubules, while papillary adenoma is a parenchymal tumour without an attachment to an airway. This tumour also features a single layer of tumour cells with pneumocytic differentiation.

Prognosis and predictive factors
Complete excision should be curative. Tumours may recur if not completely removed {739}. Malignant transformation has not been reported.

Mixed squamous cell and glandular papilloma

Definition
Mixed squamous cell and glandular papilloma is an endobronchial papillary tumour showing a mixture of squamous and glandular epithelium, with the glandular type constituting at least one third.

ICD-O code
8560/0

Synonyms
Mixed papilloma; transitional cell papilloma

Epidemiology
Mixed squamous cell and glandular papillomas are extremely rare, with fewer than 20 reported cases. The male-to-female ratio is 3:1, and the median age is in the sixth decade {739,1342,1474,2688}.

Clinical features
Patients present with obstructive symptoms or haemoptysis; tumours are also identified on radiographical studies {1384}. CT shows smooth-edged and partially cystic nodules. Peripheral lesions may pucker overlying visceral pleura {1342,1474}. PET avidity is reported

{9,1342}. Bronchoscopic findings may be very subtle, with only mucosal oedema {1957}.

Localization
Mixed papillomas are usually central and endobronchial, or in rare cases peripheral and endobronchiolar.

Macroscopy
Mixed squamous cell and glandular papilloma manifests as endobronchial polypoid lesions measuring 0.2 to 2.5 cm. The lesions are typically tan to red. Lesions with peripheral grey to yellow colouring may be partially cystic, and measure up to 6 cm {1384}.

Cytology
Bronchial brushing shows a mixture of keratinized and/or non-keratinized squamous and glandular cells. Mild nuclear atypia may be seen. Scattered single columnar cells may be ciliated or non-ciliated without atypia {1173}.

Histopathology
Histology mirrors the findings in pure squamous cell and glandular papillomas; however, most of the epithelium lining fibrovascular cores is glandular, with interspersed squamous islands. The pseudostratified ciliated and non-ciliated cuboidal to columnar cells with scattered mucin-filled cells are distinct from the acanthotic and focally keratinizing squamous epithelium. Glandular atypia and necrosis are not seen, but squamous atypia ranges from mild to severe. Viral cytopathic effect is not present, and studied cases are HPV-negative. There are rare reports of both glandular

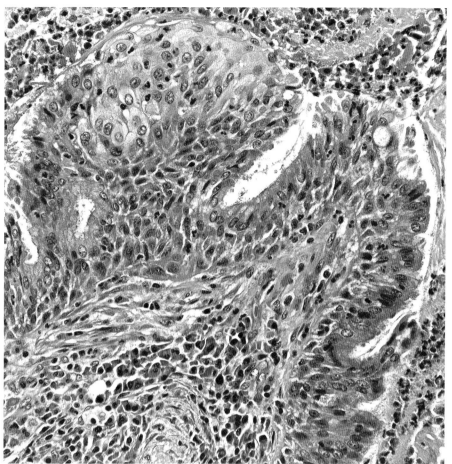

Fig. 1.125 Mixed squamous cell and glandular papilloma. The papillary frond is lined with discrete foci of glandular and squamous epithelium; the fibrovascular core is inflamed.

and squamous components staining with antibodies directed against CK19, CAM5.2, CK5/6, CK903, and MUC1 {1080}. A definitive diagnosis can only be rendered on a completely resected tumour. The differential diagnosis mirrors that of pure squamous cell and glandular papillomas.

Prognosis and predictive factors
Surgical resection appears to be curative {739,1080,1342}. Squamous cell carcinoma arising in a mixed papilloma has been reported {1384}.

Adenomas

Sclerosing pneumocytoma

M.B. Beasley
W.D. Travis

Definition
Sclerosing pneumocytoma is a tumour of pneumocytic origin with a combination of histological findings, including solid, papillary, sclerotic, and haemorrhagic regions. The tumour consists of a dual population of surface cells resembling type II pneumocytes and round cells, with slightly different histogenetic profiles.

ICD-O code   8832/0

Synonym
Sclerosing haemangioma

Epidemiology
Sclerosing pneumocytoma has a striking female predominance, with 80% of cases occuring in females. It has a wide age range (11–80 years), but is most commonly seen in middle-aged adults. The incidence is higher in East Asian populations, and sclerosing pneumocytoma is rare in Western countries {399,593,1191,1355}.

Etiology
The postulation of the cell of origin for this tumour has changed over time. The tumour was previously widely considered to be a vascular neoplasm (based on morphology), and was therefore called sclerosing haemangioma. Other origins have also been postulated, including mesothelial, neuroendocrine, and mesenchymal origins.

Currently, based primarily on immunohistochemical data, the tumour is thought to derive from primitive respiratory epithelium {370,399,593,1191}. This is the basis for the proposed new term sclerosing pneumocytoma.

Clinical features
Patients are typically asymptomatic, with the lesion discovered incidentally.

Chest X-ray shows a solitary circumscribed mass. The tumours are rarely calcified, and may occasionally be cystic. CT may show marked contrast enhancement and foci of sharply marginated low attenuation. MRI may demonstrate a haemorrhagic component {945,1814, 2102,2257,2805}.

Regional lymph node metastases have been reported in a small number of cases {381,1257,1692,2728,2941}.

Localization
Sclerosing pneumocytomas are classically solitary and peripheral. Rare cases are multiple, involve the visceral pleura or mediastinum, or occur as an endobronchial polyp.

There is no preferential lobe distribution, although one study suggested a higher frequency in the right middle lobe {399,592,2535}.

Macroscopy
The tumours are well-circumscribed masses that are solid and grey-tan to yellow on cut section, with foci of haemorrhage. Cystic degeneration and calcification may be evident.

Cytology
Fine-needle aspiration biopsy may show a dual cell population, as well as hyalinized stromal fragments. The round cells are small, round to spindle-shaped, and arranged in cohesive papillary clusters or flat sheets. Discrimination from adenocarcinoma may be difficult if nuclear atypia is present, but the cells of sclerosing pneumocytoma typically lack nucleoli, which may be a useful discriminating feature. Cytology may be a useful adjunct to frozen section in intraoperative evaluation {214,588,784}.

Histopathology
The key feature of sclerosing pneumocytoma is the presence of two cell types: cuboidal surface cells and stromal round cells, both of which are considered to be neoplastic. The surface cells are cuboidal and morphologically similar to type II pneumocytes. Occasionally, they may be multinucleated or have clear, vacuolated, or foamy cytoplasm. As in type II pneumocytes and intranuclear inclusions may be seen. The round cells are small, with well-defined borders, central bland nuclei with fine chromatin and absent nucleoli. The cytoplasm is typically

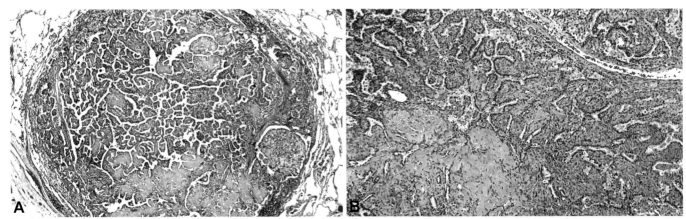

Fig. 1.126 Sclerosing pneumocytoma. **A** A well-circumscribed unencapsulated nodule, with a mixture of papillary, solid, and sclerotic patterns. **B** Sclerotic, solid, and papillary patterns are present. Reprinted from Travis WD et al. {2678}.

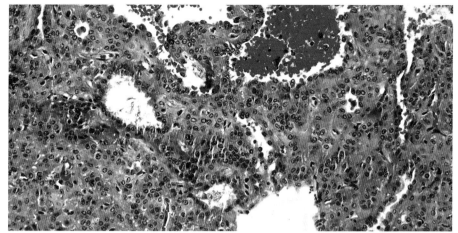

Fig. 1.127 Sclerosing pneumocytoma. In this haemorrhagic pattern, the tumour forms ectatic spaces filled with red blood cells that are surrounded by type II pneumocytes. Reprinted from Travis WD et al. {2678}.

eosinophilic, but may be vacuolated, which may impart a signet ring appearance. Lamellar bodies may be seen, and mature fat and calcifications may occasionally be encountered. Most tumours have at least three of the four primary growth patterns in varying proportions. In the papillary pattern, complex papillary structures are covered by surface cells overlying a core of round cells as opposed to true fibrovascular cores. In the sclerotic pattern, dense areas of stromal collagen may be present at the periphery of haemorrhagic areas, within papillary stalks, or in solid areas. The solid pattern is composed of sheets of round cells, and surface cells may be present as small tubules. In the haemorrhagic pattern, large blood-filled spaces may be present, which may be lined by epithelial cells and/or contain haemosiderin deposits, foamy macrophages, or cholesterol clefts {399,593,1355}.

Immunohistochemistry
The two cell types have slightly different immunohistochemical profiles.
The surface cells are positive for pancytokeratin, epithelial membrane antigen, CAM5.2, CK7, TTF1, surfactant markers, Clara cell antigen, vimentin, and napsin A. They are negative for CK20, CK5/6, CK903, S100, smooth muscle actin, factor VIII antigen, calretinin, estrogen receptor, progesterone receptor, and neuroendocrine markers.
Unlike the surface cells, the round cells are usually negative for pancytokeratin, and are only focally positive for CAM5.2 and CK7. They are positive for epithelial membrane antigen, TTF1, and vimentin, but negative for surfactant markers and Clara cell antigen. They may rarely be weakly positive for napsin A.
The remainder of the markers that are listed as negative in the surface cells are also negative in the round cells, with the

notable exceptions of estrogen receptor and progesterone receptor, which are positive in the round cells of 7% and 61% of cases, respectively {370,593,1070,1192, 2201,2284,2298,2932}.

Differential diagnosis
The differential diagnoses consist primarily of carcinoid tumours and papillary adenocarcinoma. Tumours with clear cytoplasm may need to be distinguished from carcinomas with clear cell features, both primary and metastatic, as well as clear cell tumour of the lung. In general, the presence of bland cytological features, a dual-cell population, and the characteristic immunostaining profile of sclerosing pneumocytoma discriminate this tumour from other entities. However, accurate diagnosis on small biopsy, cytology, or frozen section may be difficult, especially in the absence of appropriate clinical and radiographical information {371,1554}.

Genetic profile
Molecular data have demonstrated the same monoclonal pattern in both the round and surface cells, consistent with a true neoplasm. Aberrant mTOR signalling may play a role in tumour development {57}. Frequent allelic loss on 5q and 10q can be found by loss of heterozygosity analysis, as can aberrations in microsatellite marker D5S615 {521}.

Prognosis and predictive factors
There have been reports of lymph node metastases in a very small percentage of cases, but these do not appear to adversely affect prognosis, and the tumour clinically behaves in a benign fashion {1446,1692}.

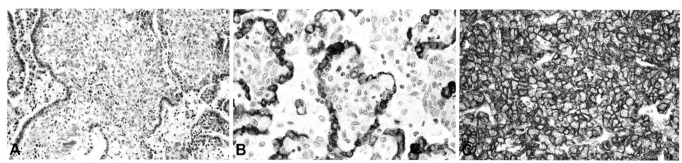

Fig. 1.128 Sclerosing pneumocytoma. **A** Papillary growth showing a population of cuboidal surface cells overlying a core of round cells; a true fibrovascular core is lacking. **B** Cytokeratin (AE1/AE3) staining shows positive staining of the surface cells, but negative staining of the round cells. **C** Epithelial membrane antigen shows membranous staining of round and surface cells.

Alveolar adenoma

M.B. Beasley
A.N. Husain
W.D. Travis

Definition
Alveolar adenoma is a solitary, well-circumscribed, peripheral lung tumour that consists of a network of cystic spaces lined with a simple layer of type II pneumocytes overlying a spindle-rich stroma of variable thickness, sometimes with a myxoid matrix.

ICD-O code   8251/0

Epidemiology
Alveolar adenoma is very rare, and has a slight female predominance. The age range is 39–74 years.

Etiology
The etiology of alveolar adenoma is controversial. Chromosomal aberrations suggest a neoplastic origin for the lesion, but it is unclear whether both the epithelial and mesenchymal components are neoplastic {345}.

Clinical features
Patients are usually asymptomatic and the tumour is usually an incidental finding. Radiographs demonstrate a well-circumscribed, homogeneous, non-calcified solitary mass. Contrast enhancement on CT and MRI may show cystic spaces with central fluid and rim enhancement {1320}. Low-level PET positivity has been reported {1877}.

Localization
Alveolar adenoma has been reported in all five lobes, with a predilection for the left lower lobe. Most tumours are peripheral, although hilar tumours have also been reported.

Macroscopy
The tumours measure 0.7–6.0 cm; are well demarcated; and have smooth, lobulated, multicystic, pale yellow to tan cut surfaces of variable firmness.

Cytology
The cytological features of alveolar adenoma are poorly described. Smear preparations taken from a resected specimen demonstrated a proteinaceous background and small cohesive monolayered epithelial clusters. The findings were determined to be useful for the exclusion of a malignant lesion, but were acknowledged to be non-specific for diagnosis {871}.

Histopathology
Alveolar adenomas are well-circumscribed multicystic masses featuring cystic spaces that often resemble alveolar spaces. They may be empty or filled with eosinophilic granular material. The spaces are lined by cytologically bland, flattened to cuboidal cells, which correspond to type II pneumocytes by immunohistochemical and electron microscopy. The cystic

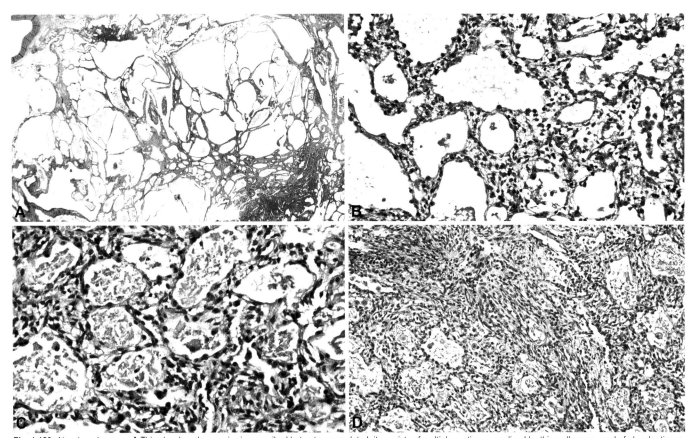

Fig. 1.129 Alveolar adenoma. A This alveolar adenoma is circumscribed but not encapsulated; it consists of multiple cystic spaces lined by thin walls composed of alveolar tissue. B Multiple small cysts resemble normal alveolar walls, with hyperplastic pneumocytes and a few alveolar macrophages within the alveolar lumens. C The alveolar spaces in this tumour are filled with proteinaceous material; they are lined by thin alveolar walls lined by hyperplastic pneumocytes. D Focally, there is prominent stroma in this alveolar adenoma, consisting of bland spindle cells.

spaces tend to be larger towards the centre of the lesion. Squamous metaplasia may be seen. The associated stroma may be myxoid or collagenous, and contains variable numbers of cytologically bland spindle cells {291,2989}. One case with mature adipocytes in the stroma has been reported {345}.

The cyst-lining cells are positive for cytokeratin, TTF1, carcinoembryonic antigen, and surfactant protein. The stromal cells are negative for these markers, and may show focal staining for smooth muscle actin and muscle-specific actin {291}. S100 and CD34 staining have also been reported. The proliferation index of both components is low {345,556}.

Alveolar adenoma may be confused with lymphangioma, which many early alveolar adenoma cases were mistakenly called. The cytokeratin staining in the lining cells of alveolar adenoma aids in distinguishing between these two lesions. Sclerosing pneumocytoma has solid, papillary, sclerosing, and/or haemorrhagic growth patterns, and lacks diffuse cystic spaces. The stromal cores of sclerosing pneumocytoma are positive for TTF1, while the stroma of alveolar adenoma is negative. Alveolar adenoma is generally distinguished from adenocarcinoma by the greater cytological and architectural complexity of the latter, as well as its infiltrative growth pattern. Metastatic tumours, especially spindle cell sarcomas, may become cystic when metastatic to the lung, and may also mimic alveolar adenoma.

Genetic profile
Alveolar adenoma appears to represent a combined proliferation of alveolar pneumocytes and septal mesenchyme. Microsatellite abnormalities have been demonstrated in the epithelial component, but not the mesenchymal component, although this does not prove whether one or both components are truly neoplastic {345}. A diploid DNA pattern has been reported {2249}. An unbalanced translocation (10;16) has been reported in some cases {2188}.

Prognosis and predictive factors
Alveolar adenomas are benign tumours, and surgical excision is curative.

Papillary adenoma

M.B. Beasley
W.D. Travis

Definition
Papillary adenoma is a circumscribed papillary neoplasm that consists of cytologically bland, cuboidal to columnar cells lining the surface of a fibrovascular stroma.

ICD-O code   8260/0

Synonyms
Bronchial adenoma; papillary adenoma of type II pneumocytes; type II pneumocyte adenoma; peripheral papillary tumour of type II pneumocytes; Clara cell adenoma

Epidemiology
Papillary adenoma is rare, with fewer than 25 cases reported. The age range is from 2 months to 70 years, with a mean age of 34 years. There is a male predominance {493,2446}.

Etiology
Based on electron microscopy, the tumour appears to be derived from a combination of type II pneumocytes and Clara (club) cells, and it has been hypothesized that they are derived from stem cells with bidirectional differentiation {699}. The etiology in humans is unknown, although a possible relationship with FGFR2-IIIb has been proposed {1602}.

Clinical features
Patients are usually asymptomatic, and the tumour is typically incidentally noted. Radiology typically demonstrates a well-defined pulmonary nodule, usually in the periphery.

The tumours are generally regarded as benign, and metastatic disease has not been reported.

Localization
Papillary adenoma is typically peripheral and solitary. No lobar predilection has been reported {2446}.

Macroscopy
Grossly, papillary adenomas are well-circumscribed, unencapsulated masses with a reported size range of 0.2 to 6 cm. The cut surface is white-tan or yellow, and contains granular material but lacks grossly evident papillae or necrosis. Haemorrhage may be present {493}.

Cytology
The cytological features of papillary adenoma are not well characterized, and may be misinterpreted as those of papillary carcinoma {1680}.

Histopathology
The tumour consists of papillary structures containing fibrovascular cores lined by a single layer of cuboidal epithelium. Nuclear atypia and mitoses are absent, and evaluation by Ki-67 has demonstrated a low proliferative index {243,982,1372,1864,1979,2446}.

The surface epithelial cells are positive for TTF1. CK7, pancytokeratin, surfactant protein, and epithelial membrane antigen positivity have also been reported in most cases. No staining for these markers should be present in the

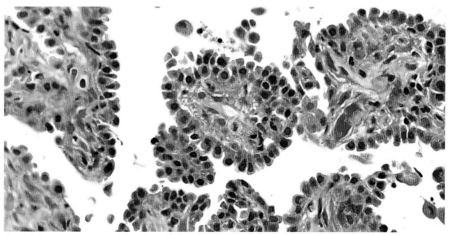

Fig. 1.130 Papillary adenoma. Cuboidal epithelial cells line the surface of fibrovascular cores. Reprinted from Travis WD et al. {2678}.

underlying stroma {2357}. *Sclerosing pneumocytoma* (haemangioma) typically demonstrates a more varied growth pattern consisting of papillary, sclerotic, and solid growth as well as comprising two cell types. The papillary structures contain a cellular core rather than a fibrovascular core, and the cells are positive for TTF1 and epithelial membrane antigen {493,1842}.

Alveolar adenomas typically form multiple cysts (often filled with proteinaceous material), which are lined by type II pneumocytes. A spindle and inflammatory stroma is characteristically present, and the tumours are usually encapsulated. Papillary morphology is not a feature {291,2249}.

Papillary adenocarcinomas generally show a greater degree of cellular proliferation, nuclear atypia, and complex branching architecture. Mitotic activity and necrosis may be present. *Carcinoid tumours* may have papillary architecture, but are positive for neuroendocrine markers, which are negative in papillary adenoma.

Genetic profile
A specific genetic profile has not been reported. No *EGFR*, *KRAS*, or *BRAF* mutations have been reported {493,1801}.

Prognosis and predictive factors
Some papillary adenomas with infiltrative growth have been described, raising the issue of whether they should be categorized as tumours of low malignant potential. However, there are no reported cases of metastatic disease or recurrence, and the tumour is generally considered to be benign and is cured by resection {493,582,174}.

Mucinous cystadenoma

M.B. Beasley

Definition
Mucinous cystadenoma is a localized cystic mass filled with mucin and surrounded by a fibrous wall lined by well-differentiated columnar mucinous epithelium.

ICD-O code   8470/0

Epidemiology
Mucinous cystadenoma is exceedingly rare. It has been reported in both males and females, primarily in the sixth and seventh decades. Although most reported cases have occurred in smokers, no specific etiology has been identified {912,1343,2214,2265,2666}.

Clinical features
Patients are typically asymptomatic, and lesions are usually found incidentally.
Tumours are typically well-demarcated masses on CT {912}.

Localization
Mucinous cystadenomas tend to involve the periphery of the lung.

Macroscopy
Grossly, the lesion consists of a localized mucin-filled cyst not associated with an airway. Reported tumours range in size from 1 to 5 cm. The cyst wall is thin and lacks mural nodules {2214,2265,2666}.

Cytology
Fine-needle aspirates may contain mucin and/or goblet cells, but a definitive diagnosis requires surgical excision and thorough sampling {2214,2265}.

Histopathology
The tumour consists of a localized cyst filled with mucin. The cyst wall consists of fibrous tissue lined by a discontinuous layer of low-cuboidal to tall columnar mucin-secreting epithelium. Micropapillary fronds, necrosis, and overt cytological atypia are absent. A foreign body giant cell reaction may be associated with extravasated mucin, and associated chronic inflammation may be present {912,2214,2265,2666}.

The lining cells are positive for pancytokeratin and CK7, and are rarely positive for carcinoembryonic antigen, TTF1, and surfactant protein {2214,2265,2666}. The primary entity in the differential diagnosis is colloid carcinoma of the lung, which now includes tumours previously classified as mucinous cystadenocarcinoma {2676}. The spread of the tumour beyond the wall of the cyst in either a lepidic or invasive fashion, significant cytological atypia, and necrosis are indicators of malignancy {792,2214}. Developmental and postinfectious bronchogenic cysts may also be a consideration.

Genetic profile
Genetic abnormalities of this very rare tumour have not been reported.

Prognosis and predictive factors
Mucinous cystadenoma is benign, and surgical excision is curative.

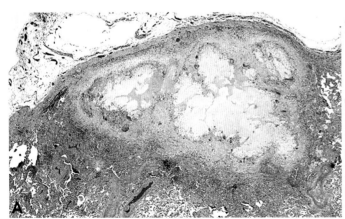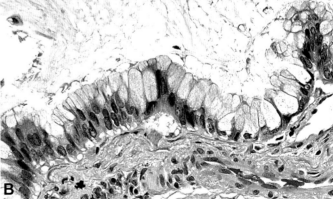

Fig. 1.131 Mucinous cystadenoma. **A** A subpleural cystic tumour is surrounded by a fibrous wall and contains abundant mucus. **B** Columnar epithelial cells line the wall of the cyst. Most of the nuclei are basally oriented, but there is focal nuclear pseudostratification. The apical cytoplasm is filled with abundant mucin. Reprinted from Travis WD et al. {2678}.

Mucous gland adenoma

A.G. Nicholson
M.B. Beasley
W.D. Travis

Definition
Mucous gland adenoma is a benign, predominantly exophytic tumour of the tracheobronchial seromucinous glands and ducts. It features mucus-filled cysts, tubules, glands, and papillary formations lined by an epithelium composed of cells such as tall columnar cells, flattened cuboidal cells, goblet cells, oncocytic cells, and clear cells.

ICD-O code   8480/0

Synonyms
Bronchial cystadenoma; mucous cell adenoma; polyadenoma; bronchial adenoma arising in mucous glands

Epidemiology
Mucous gland adenoma is extremely rare, with no sex predominance. Tumours have been reported in both children and the elderly, with a mean age of 52 years in one series {678} and 26 years in another {979}.

Etiology
The etiology of mucous gland adenoma is unknown, but it is presumed to arise from bronchial seromucinous glands.

Clinical features
Patients present with signs and symptoms of obstruction. Excision is usually required for definitive diagnosis {569}.
Radiographical studies demonstrate a coin lesion. CT may show a well-defined intraluminal mass with the air meniscus sign {1374}.
Mucous gland adenomas are benign, and are usually limited to the airway wall.

Localization
Most mucous gland adenomas are central and limited to the airways {678}. Rare cases are unrelated to the airways {1214}.

Macroscopy
Grossly, mucous gland adenomas are white-pink to tan, smooth, shiny tumours with gelatinous, mucoid, solid and cystic cut surfaces. They measure 0.7–7.5 cm, with a mean size of 2.3 cm {678}.

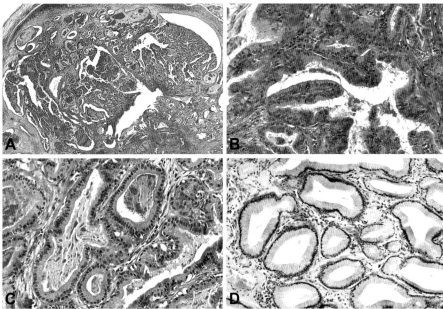

Fig. 1.132 Mucous gland adenoma. **A** An endobronchial mass contains numerous mucin-filled cystic spaces, microacini, glands, tubules, and papillae. **B** Papillary fronds are a minor architectural pattern. **C** Neutral and acid mucin-filled cysts are lined by cytologically bland columnar, cuboidal, or flattened mucus-secreting cells. **D** Glands lined by columnar epithelium with small basally oriented nuclei and abundant apical mucinous cytoplasm. Reprinted from Travis WD et al. {2678}.

Cytology
Very rare cases have been diagnosed on cytology {569}.

Histopathology
Mucous gland adenomas are well-circumscribed, predominantly exophytic nodules above the cartilaginous plates of the bronchial wall. The tumours contain numerous mucin-filled cystic spaces. Non-dilated microacini, glands, tubules, and papillae may also be seen. Neutral and acid mucin-filled cysts are lined by cytologically bland columnar, cuboidal, or flattened mucus-secreting cells. Oncocytic and clear cell change can also be seen, as can focal ciliated epithelium. Hyperchromasia, pleomorphism, and mitoses are rare, while squamous metaplasia only involves overlying surface respiratory epithelium. Bands of spindle cell-rich stroma may be hyalinized or occur with prominent lymphocytes and/or plasma cells.
Immunohistochemistry demonstrates similar staining to non-neoplastic bronchial glands, with epithelial cells positive for epithelial membrane antigen, broadspectrum cytokeratins, and carcinoembryonic antigen. Focal stromal cell positivity for broad-spectrum cytokeratins, smooth muscle actin, and S100 protein indicates a myoepithelial component.

Proliferating cell nuclear antigen and Ki-67 staining performed in several cases have demonstrated rare tumour cell positivity {678}. Mucinous and myoepithelial cell types have been identified by electron microscopy {678,979,1214}.
Low-grade mucoepidermoid carcinomas (including the papillary and cystic variants) may closely mimic mucous gland adenoma. Despite architectural similarities, the lack of squamous and intermediate cells distinguishes mucous gland adenoma from mucoepidermoid carcinoma. Adenocarcinomas of the lung may have a prominent or exclusively acinar pattern, but are usually infiltrative and show malignant features such as nuclear pleomorphism, mitotic activity, and necrosis.

Prognosis and predictive factors
Mucous gland adenomas are benign. Conservative lung-sparing bronchoscopic or sleeve resection is recommended when feasible {678,1612}.

Mesenchymal tumours

Pulmonary hamartoma

J.F. Tomashefski
S. Dacic

Definition
Pulmonary hamartomas are benign neoplasms composed of varying amounts of at least two mesenchymal elements (such as cartilage, fat, connective tissue, and smooth muscle), combined with entrapped respiratory epithelium.

ICD-O code   8992/0

Synonyms
Chondroid hamartoma; chondromatous hamartoma; mixed mesenchymoma; hamartochondroma; adenochondroma

Epidemiology
Pulmonary hamartomas are the most common benign pulmonary neoplasms.

They account for 8% of so-called coin lesions on chest radiographs {2656}. Pulmonary hamartomas are more common in men than in women, with incidence peaking in the sixth decade {2742}. They are rare in children.

Etiology
The etiology of pulmonary hamartoma is unknown, but molecular and cytogenetic data suggest a neoplastic origin.

Clinical features
Peripheral pulmonary hamartomas present radiographically as asymptomatic, solitary, well-circumscribed nodules. Multifocal pulmonary hamartomas are rare. So-called popcorn calcification is an important diagnostic feature infrequently seen in imaging studies. The detection of adipose tissue on CT also adds diagnostic specificity {851}. Endobronchial lesions produce symptoms and radiographical signs of bronchial obstruction {495}.

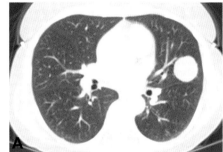

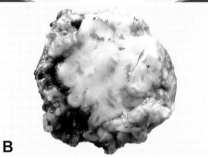

Fig. 1.134 Pulmonary hamartoma. A Soft-tissue windows from a contrast-enhanced CT demonstrate a round, 4 cm, circumscribed mass in the lingula. B A hamartoma that has shelled out of the lung at operation.

Localization
Most pulmonary hamartomas are peripheral, and approximately 10% are endobronchial. Pulmonary hamartomas are distributed fairly uniformly throughout the lungs {2742}.

Macroscopy
Pulmonary hamartomas are firm, round to multilobulated, pale, well-circumscribed nodules that shell out from the lung. Most are < 4 cm in diameter. Large size and/or cavitation are uncommon. Endobronchial pulmonary hamartomas manifest as yellow to grey sessile polyps of large airways.

Cytology
The cytological features are fibromyxoid tissue, fat, and/or cartilage associated with benign reactive epithelial cells. Mesenchymal elements may be subtle in Papanicolaou-stained slides, and epithelial cells may be abundant – leading to false-positive diagnoses of malignancy {1049}.

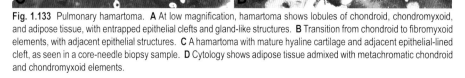

Fig. 1.133 Pulmonary hamartoma. A At low magnification, hamartoma shows lobules of chondroid, chondromyxoid, and adipose tissue, with entrapped epithelial clefts and gland-like structures. B Transition from chondroid to fibromyxoid elements, with adjacent epithelial structures. C A hamartoma with mature hyaline cartilage and adjacent epithelial-lined cleft, as seen in a core-needle biopsy sample. D Cytology shows adipose tissue admixed with metachromatic chondroid and chondromyxoid elements.

Histopathology

Pulmonary hamartomas are composed predominantly of chondroid or chondromyxoid tissue intermixed with variable proportions of other mesenchymal components, including fat, connective tissue, smooth muscle, and bone. Clefts of respiratory epithelial cells represent entrapment by expanding mesenchymal growth. Endobronchial pulmonary hamartomas may have a prominent adipose tissue component, while epithelial inclusions tend to be inconspicuous. Immunohistochemical stains show reactivity for mesenchymal markers and sex steroid receptors, but immunohistochemistry is not usually necessary for diagnosis {2022}.

Pulmonary hamartomas differ from benign monomorphic soft tissue tumours by the presence of two or more mesenchymal components. Pulmonary chondromas in patients with Carney triad (i.e. gastric stromal sarcoma, pulmonary chondroma, and extra-adrenal paragangliomas) are parenchymal cartilaginous nodules that lack entrapped epithelium, frequently show osseous metaplasia, and are bordered by a thin fibrous pseudocapsule. Sporadic chondromas (not associated with Carney triad) are infrequent, and usually endobronchial {2180}. The lack of atypia distinguishes pulmonary hamartomas from primary or metastatic sarcomas in the lung. So-called fibroleiomyomatous hamartomas usually represent lung metastases from low-grade leiomyosarcomas, frequently of uterine origin.

Genetic profile

Pulmonary hamartomas have a high frequency of the translocation t(3;12)(q27–28;q14–15), resulting in gene fusion of the high mobility group protein gene *HMGA2* and the *LPP* gene. The *HMGA2-LPP* fusion gene usually consists of exons 1–3 of *HMGA2* and exons 9–11 of *LPP*, and seems to be expressed in all tumours with this translocation {526,737,1228,2788}.

Prognosis and predictive factors

Pulmonary hamartomas are slowly growing neoplasms with an excellent prognosis. Surgical resection is the optimal treatment for endobronchial lesions and symptomatic or expanding parenchymal tumours. Recurrence and malignant transformation are very rare {146}.

Chondroma

M.C. Aubry

Definition

Chondroma is defined as benign neoplasm composed of hyaline or myxohyaline cartilage.

ICD-O code   9220/0

Synonym
Osteochondroma

Epidemiology

Chondromas are typically found in young women (usually aged < 30 years) who are affected by Carney triad {2180}.

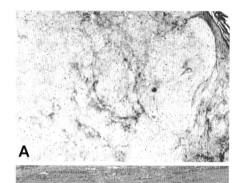

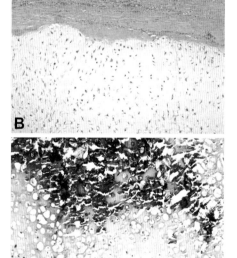

Fig. 1.135 Chondroma. **A** At low power, chondromas appear lobulated and well delineated, and are predominantly composed of cartilage. No adipose tissue or smooth muscle is identified. **B** Chondromas are separated from adjacent normal lung by a fibrous pseudocapsule. There is no invagination or entrapment of benign respiratory mucosa. In this case, the cartilage is mostly hyaline. **C** This chondroma is composed of focally calcified, hyaline-type cartilage.

Rarely, they are sporadic – mostly in men (with a mean age of 53 years) {333}.

Clinical features

Patients are usually asymptomatic. Reported symptoms include cough, chest pain, and dyspnoea {2180}.

Nodules which are multiple (averaging 3) in Carney triad and solitary in sporadic cases are peripheral and random in all lobes.

Localization

Chondromas usually occur in the peripheral lung parenchyma, or they may be endobronchial.

Macroscopy and localization

Chondromas are well circumscribed and lobulated.

Histopathology

Chondromas consist of hyaline or myxoid, moderately cellular cartilage without atypia, and are surrounded by a pseudocapsule. Calcification and ossification is common.

The differential diagnoses include pulmonary hamartoma and chondrosarcoma. Pulmonary hamartomas have entrapped respiratory epithelium between lobulated cartilage and frequently contain other mesenchymal elements {2180}. Chondrosarcomas show increased cellularity and cytological atypia.

Genetic profile

Gain of chromosome 6 and loss of 1q have been reported {2478}.

Prognosis and predictive factors

No metastasis or death has been reported.

PEComatous tumours

A.G. Nicholson
E. Henske
W.D. Travis

Definition

PEComatous tumours are thought to arise from perivascular epithelioid cells (PECs). In the lung, they can take several forms: 1) a diffuse multicystic proliferation termed lymphangioleiomyomatosis; 2) more rarely, a benign localized mass termed PEComa, of which clear cell tumour is the major subset, and 3) exceptionally, a diffuse proliferation with overlapping features between lymphangioleiomyomatosis and clear cell tumour.

ICD-O codes

Lymphangioleiomyomatosis	9174/1
PEComa, benign	8714/0
Clear cell tumour	8005/0
PEComa, malignant	8714/3

Synonyms
Clear cell tumour has been called sugar tumour in the lung and myomelanocytoma at other sites.

Epidemiology
Lymphangioleiomyomatos is is a disorder occurring almost exclusively in women {978,1158,1915,2720}, although rare cases have been reported in men with tuberous sclerosis {2237}. It was originally believed that lymphangioleiomyomatosis occurred primarily in women of reproductive age, but lymphangioleiomyomatosis is now increasingly recognized in postmenopausal women, in whom there appears to be a slower rate of disease progression. Lymphangioleiomyomatosis can occur sporadically or in women with tuberous sclerosis. Most women with sporadic lymphangioleiomyomatosis have renal angiomyolipomas, many have retroperitoneal and abdominal lymphadenopathy, and some have chylous pleural effusions. PEComas, of which clear cell tumour is the major subset, show a slight male predominance, with an age range of 8–73 years {409,780,2672}.

Etiology
Historically considered an interstitial lung disease, lymphangioleiomyomatosis is now considered to be a low-grade destructive metastasizing neoplasm, as the lesional cells usually have growth-promoting biallelic mutations in the tuberous sclerosis gene *TSC2*. Lymphangioleiomyomatosis cells also show evidence of clonal origin, as well as invasive and metastatic potential, further supporting the theory of a neoplastic underpinning {335,515,1588,1625,1956A}. There is a very rare association between clear cell tumours and tuberous sclerosis {741}. Isolated cases with more diffuse features that overlap with lymphangioleiomyomatosis have also been described {780}, called diffuse PEComatosis {1419}.

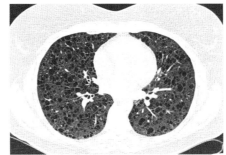

Fig. 1.136 Lymphangioleiomyomatosis. High-resolution CT shows abundant cysts of similar sizes evenly distributed throughout both lungs.

Clinical features
Patients with lymphangioleiomyomatosis present most commonly with exertional dyspnoea and pneumothorax, with chylous effusions occurring less frequently {978,1158,1915,2720}. PEComas are generally asymptomatic, and discovered incidentally {409,780}.

Localization and macroscopy
Lymphangioleiomyomatosis presents with thin-walled cysts uniformly distributed throughout the lungs. Most PEComas are solitary, peripheral and usually 2–3 cm in diameter (ranging from 1 mm to 6.5 cm) {409,780}. They are well circumscribed and solitary, with red-tan cut surfaces.

Histopathology
Lymphangioleiomyomatosis consists of a proliferation of plump spindle-shaped myoid cells with typically pale eosinophilic cytoplasm. These are usually found in the walls of the cystic air spaces, where their growth may be overt and nodular, although some cases may be very subtly infiltrated, to the extent that multiple levels are required to identify the lesional cells. Lesional cells may infiltrate blood vessels and lymphatics, causing secondary pulmonary haemorrhage. Lymphangioleiomyomatosis can be associated with micronodular type II pneumocyte hyperplasia, particularly in individuals with tuberous sclerosis {1593}. PEComas comprise rounded or oval cells with distinct cell borders and abundant clear or eosinophilic cytoplasm. There is mild variation in nuclear size, and nucleoli may be prominent, but mitoses are usually absent {409,780}. Necrosis is extremely rare, and should lead to consideration of malignancy {780,2261A}, as should significant mitotic activity and an infiltrative growth pattern. Thin-walled sinusoidal vessels are characteristic. Due to the glycogen-rich cytoplasm, there is usually strong periodic acid–Schiff positivity that is removed with diastase digestion {1400}. Cases with diffuse PEComatosis show features overlapping between lymphangioleiomyomatosis and clear cell tumour {1419}. Angiomyolipomas may rarely occur in the lung and are also part of the PEComa spectrum {917A}.

Immunohistochemistry and electron microscopy
Both lymphangioleiomyomatosis and PEComas stain most consistently for

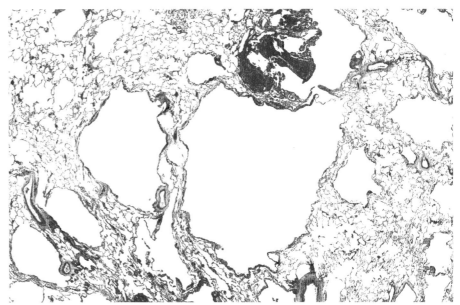

Fig. 1.137 Lymphangioleiomyomatosis. The lung architecture is replaced by cystic air spaces, within which lesional cells either form overt nodules (upper right) or more subtly infiltrate the edges of the cystic airspaces.

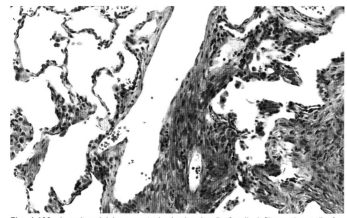
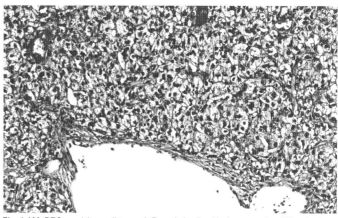

Fig. 1.138 Lymphangioleiomyomatosis. Lesional cells focally infiltrate the wall of a pulmonary vein.

Fig. 1.139 PEComa (clear cell tumour). Rounded cells with clear or eosinophilic cytoplasm form solid sheets around sinusoidal blood vessels.

HMB45, melan A, and micropthalmia transcription factor. PEComas may also stain for S100. Lymphangioleiomyomatosis stains for smooth muscle actin and is S100-negative; some cases also stain for estrogen receptor and progesterone receptor. Lymphangioleiomyomatosis also stains for β-catenin {734}. Electron microscopy shows abundant free and membrane-bound glycogen.

Differential diagnosis
The diagnosis of lymphangioleiomyomatosis, per the current European Respiratory Society (ERS) guidelines, requires a characteristic high-resolution CT plus a diagnosis of tuberous sclerosis, a renal angiomyolipoma, a chylous pleural effusion, or an elevated plasma VEGF-D level. Plasma VEGF-D levels are elevated in approximately 60% of women with biopsy-proven lymphangioleiomyomatosis. However, a normal VEGF-D level does not exclude a diagnosis of lymphangioleiomyomatosis, and the implications of an elevated VEGF-D level in the absence of the characteristic multiple thin-walled pulmonary cystic lesions is unknown. In the absence of one or more of these diagnostic criteria, a biopsy is required if it is clinically necessary to distinguish lymphangioleiomyomatosis from Langerhans cell histiocytosis, Birt-Hogg-Dubé syndrome, or extensive centrilobular emphysema. Establishing a tissue diagnosis is most important if lymphangioleiomyomatosis-specific therapy, such as sirolimus, is under consideration. Other multifocal smooth muscle proliferations include benign metastasizing leiomyomas – although these are normally solid nodules, the tumours can be extensively cystic {11}. Other low-grade metastatic tumours (such as metastatic cellular fibrous histiocytoma) may also enter the differential diagnosis {1934}.

PEComas are distinguished from clear cell carcinomas, both primary and metastatic, on the basis of a lack of cytological atypia, the presence of thin-walled sinusoidal vessels within the tumour, positive staining for S100 and HMB45 (melanocytic markers), and negative staining for cytokeratins. Metastatic renal cell carcinomas may contain intracytoplasmic glycogen, but show necrosis and stain for epithelial markers. Granular cell tumours stain for S100 but not HMB45, and do not contain abundant glycogen in their cytoplasm. Metastatic melanomas and clear cell sarcomas have a similar immunophenotype and ultrastructure, but the tumour cells do not show significant atypia, and there is usually a history of a previous neoplasm.

Genetic profile
Both PEComas and lymphangioleiomyomatosis are part of the spectrum of PEComatous tumours that arise at several sites throughout the body, originating from the perivascular epithelioid cells, although no counterpart in normal tissue has yet been identified. The *TSC* mutations that occur in lymphangioleiomyomatosis result in abnormal signalling through the mTOR pathway {1085}. TFE3 fusions are seen in a distinct subset of PEComas arising at other sites {79A,2305A}.

Prognosis and predictive factors
Over the past decade, studies have shown that lymphangioleiomyomatosis has a better prognosis than was first thought, with mortality being 10–20% {978,1158,1915,2720}. Patients may undergo transplantation {1915}, although there are very rare reports of recurrence {1212}. Sirolimus therapy has been shown in a double-blind randomized clinical trial to improve quality of life and diminish the rate of lung function decline in women with lymphangioleiomyomatosis {1624}. Serum VEGF-D has recently been shown to correlate with disease severity in lymphangioleiomyomatosis {2985}. Virtually all PEComas of the lung have been cured by excision. Diffuse PEComatosis has also been successfully treated with sirolimus {1419}.

Congenital peribronchial myofibroblastic tumour

W.D. Travis

Definition
Congenital peribronchial myofibroblastic tumour is an interstitial, peribronchovascular proliferation of uniform, plump to more fusiform cells arranged in broad, interlacing fascicles. Cellularity and mitotic activity may be marked. This spindle cell neoplasm is reminiscent of congenital infantile fibrosarcoma.

ICD-O code   8827/1

Synonyms
Congenital fibrosarcoma; congenital leiomyosarcoma; congenital bronchopulmonary leiomyosarcoma; congenital pulmonary myofibroblastic tumour; congenital mesenchymal malformation of lung; neonatal pulmonary hamartoma

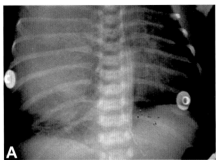

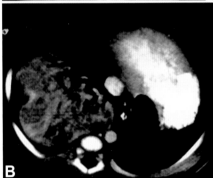

Fig. 1.140 Congenital peribronchial myofibroblastic tumour. A Plain chest radiograph shows opacification of the right hemithorax of a 7-week-old female infant who presented with respiratory distress. B CT reveals a well-circumscribed mass lesion with a collage of high- and low-density foci, representing areas of tumour and compressed uninvolved parenchyma.

Epidemiology

Congenital peribronchial myofibroblastic tumour is a rare neoplasm that occurs in the intrauterine and perinatal period. Only 16 case studies have been published {1267,1631}.

Etiology

This tumour occurs sporadically, and has neither syndromic association nor relevant maternal history.

Clinical features

As a congenital tumour, it is recognized shortly after birth, although the pregnancy may be complicated by polydramnios and non-immune hydrops fetalis. However, its detection by prenatal ultrasonography can be anticipated {53,1267,1631}.
A mass partially or totally opacifying the haemithorax is the usual appearance on a plain chest radiograph {53}. CT reveals a well-circumscribed heterogeneous mass {309,1267,1631}.

Macroscopy

The tumours are well circumscribed and unencapsulated, and have a smooth or multinodular surface, with or without fine trabeculations. The cut surface has a fleshy, tan-grey to yellow-tan appearance. Haemorrhage and necrosis are variable features. The largest dimension ranges from 5 to 10 cm, and the tumour may weigh in excess of 100 g. The bronchus is often distorted or totally obliterated.

Histopathology

The lung parenchyma is replaced by uniform spindle cells {1267,1631} arranged in intersecting fascicles with or without a herringbone pattern. The nuclei are elongated and have finely dispersed chromatin, no pleomorphism or anaplasia, and variable mitotic activity. Atypical mitotic figures are not present. Bronchial invasion is often seen, and the peribronchial distribution is implicit in the name. The growth may diffusely obliterate the parenchyma or form islands and nodules of spindle cells with interspersed foci of uninvolved parenchyma {53,1267,1631}. Tumour growth in septa or on the pleural surface may occur. In less cellular perivascular areas, the tumour cells appear less sarcomatous, with a more fibromyxoid or myofibroblastic proliferation. Cystic foci of haemorrhage may be present.

Immunohistochemistry

A myofibroblastic immunophenotype is not demonstrable in all cases. The spindle cells are consistently positive for vimentin, whereas staining for desmin and smooth muscle actin is absent or restricted to isolated cells {1267,1631}. Muscle-specific actin immunoreactivity is present in < 5% of the cells, and desmin reactivity may be observed rarely.
This tumour is considered to be identical (or at least related) to the lesions reported as congenital leiomyosarcoma, fibrosarcoma, and fibroleiomyosarcoma. These tumours have non-specific immunoprofiles, and have been reported to express α-SMA, HHF35, and muscle-specific actin {309,468}. Desmin, S100 protein, CD34, CD57, CD68, factor XIIIa, and CAM5.2 are also occasionally expressed. Ultrastructural studies suggest myofibroblastic differentiation {1267}.

Genetic profile

One case has been reported with a complex karyotype, which included a t(8;10)(p11.2;p15) translocation {53}. Although these tumours resemble congenital infantile fibrosarcoma and congenital mesoblastic nephroma in their gross and microscopic features, there are no reports to date of the detection of t(12;15)(p13;q2526) translocation in a congenital peribronchial myofibroblastic tumour {2268}.

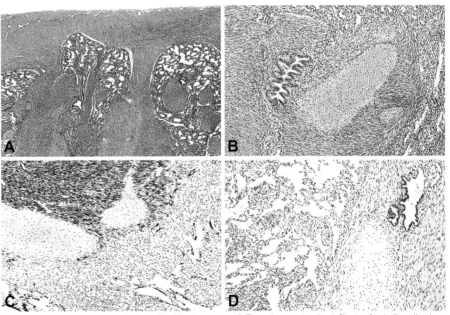

Fig. 1.141 Congenital peribronchial myofibroblastic tumour. A There is an extensive infiltrate of spindle cells along lymphatic routes: pleura, septa, and bronchovascular bundles. B The spindle cells resemble smooth muscle cells and infiltrate around bronchial cartilage, epithelium, and vessels. C There is focal positive actin staining in the spindle cells, supporting myofibroblastic differentiation. D A spindle cell infiltrate surrounds bronchial cartilage and mucosa with extension into surrounding interstitium of alveolar walls. A and B reprinted from Travis WD et al. {2678}.

Prognosis and predictive factors

Surgical resection of the involved lobe or lung is the treatment of choice. However, the presence of fetal hydrops, with its own associated morbidity and mortality, may complicate the clinical outcome.

Diffuse pulmonary lymphangiomatosis

E.S. Yi

Definition

Diffuse pulmonary lymphangiomatosis is a diffuse proliferation of lymphatic spaces and smooth muscle along otherwise normal lymphatic vessels of the lungs, pleura, and mediastinum.

Synonyms

Lymphangiomatosis; lymphatic dysplasia

Epidemiology

Diffuse pulmonary lymphangiomatosis is typically diagnosed shortly after birth or during childhood, and rarely during adulthood. It affects both sexes equally.

Clinical features

In paediatric patients the disease has an aggressive course, with progressive respiratory failure and death. Adult patients may present with mild wheezing, non-productive cough, recurrent chylous pleural effusions, or respiratory failure {1171}.

Imaging

Chest radiographs may show increased interstitial markings and pleural effusions. CT shows mediastinal soft tissue infiltration, pleural thickening with effusions, thickening of peribronchovascular bundles, and interlobular septa {660, 1529,2958}.

Localization

Lymphangiomatosis frequently involves the mediastinum, or may be limited to the lung and pleura.

Macroscopy

Lymphatic distribution manifests as prominence of visceral pleura, interlobular septa, and bronchovascular bundles {2607}. Cysts or mass lesions are absent.

Histopathology

Anastomosing, variable-sized, endothelial-lined spaces containing acellular eosinophilic material are distributed along the lymphatic routes and lined by a layer of flattened lymphatic endothelial cells. Collagen layers or spindle cells resembling smooth muscle cells are present between channels. The adjacent lung parenchyma shows variable haemosiderin-laden macrophages {225,2607}.
The lining cells are positive for D2-40, CD31, factor VIII-related antigen, and ulex europaeus agglutinin. Spindle cells express vimentin, desmin, actin, and progesterone receptor, but not estrogen receptor, keratin, or HMB45 {225,2607}.
The differential diagnoses include lymphangioleiomyomatosis, lymphangiectasis, haemangiomatosis, and Kaposi sarcoma. Lymphangioleiomyomatosis contains HMB45-positive cells. Lymphangiectasis does not show an increased number of anastomosing lymphatic vessels. Kaposi sarcoma does not show the complex anastomosing lymphatic channels. In haemangiomatosis, vascular spaces are blood-filled.

Prognosis and predictive factors

Prognosis is poor, and there is no curative treatment.

Inflammatory myofibroblastic tumour

A. Borczuk
C. Coffin
C.D.M. Fletcher

Definition

Inflammatory myofibroblastic tumour is a distinctive lesion composed of myofibroblastic spindle cells accompanied by an inflammatory infiltrate usually composed mainly of plasma cells and lymphocytes.

ICD-O code   8825/1

Synonyms

Not recommended: inflammatory pseudotumour; plasma cell granuloma; fibroxanthoma; fibrous histiocytoma; pseudosarcomatous myofibroblastic tumour; invasive fibrous tumour of the tracheobronchial tree

Epidemiology

Inflammatory myofibroblastic tumour occurs in adult and paediatric populations. In adults, it accounts for substantially less than 1% of all tumours {1650,2629}. Inflammatory myofibroblastic tumour has a wide age distribution, with an average age in paediatric patients of 8 years, and an average age in adults of 44 years.

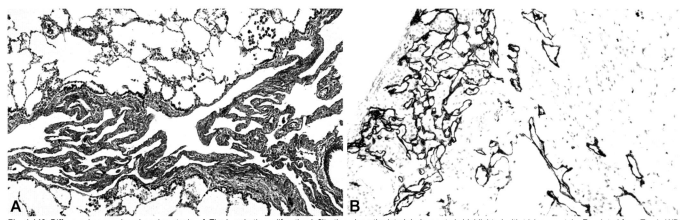

Fig. 1.142 Diffuse pulmonary lymphangiomatosis. **A** The lymphatic proliferation infiltrating along the interlobular septa is highlighted with trichrome stain. Reprinted from Travis WD et al. {2678}. **B** Expression of D2-40 by lining cells supports their lymphatic endothelial phenotype.

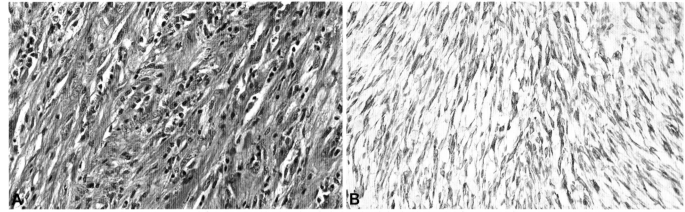

Fig. 1.143 Inflammatory myofibroblastic tumour. **A** Spindle cells with minimal cytological atypia admixed with chronic inflammatory infiltrate composed of lymphocytes and plasma cells. **B** Spindle cells with cytoplasmic immunohistochemical reactivity for ALK.

The male-to-female ratio is about 1:1 {124,1605,2444}.

Clinical features

About 50–60% of patients are asymptomatic. When present, symptoms include cough, chest pain, fever, and pneumonia, and less commonly haemoptysis, dyspnoea, fatigue, stridor, or weight loss {350,693,1253,1650,2629}. Elevated erythrocyte sedimentation rate, thrombocytosis, and hypergammaglobulinaemia can also be seen {451}.

Inflammatory myofibroblastic tumours are usually peripheral circumscribed lesions; however, irregular nodules or pneumonia-like patterns are also reported. Tumours can be bronchial or tracheal, with 10–20% in a central location {25,1253}. Necrosis or calcification is seen in 10–15% of cases.

Inflammatory myofibroblastic tumour is usually localized. Involvement of the chest wall, mediastinum, or pleura is rare.

Localization

The intrapulmonary mass is typically solitary, but multiple masses or extrapulmonary involvement can also occur {846, 1605,2050}.

Macroscopy

Inflammatory myofibroblastic tumour manifests as a firm, circumscribed mass with a fleshy white, tan, or grey cut surface, which may display necrosis or gritty calcifications {846,2050,2260}. The diameter ranges from 1 to 15 cm, with an average of 4 cm.

Cytology

Fine-needle aspiration biopsy smears are moderately to poorly cellular, and contain a combination of plasma cells, lymphocytes, and spindle cells {943,2639}. Although these findings are non-specific, the diagnosis of inflammatory myofibroblastic tumour may be suggested by the combination of clinical, radiological, and cytological findings.

Histopathology

Inflammatory myofibroblastic tumour is composed of spindle cells with pale eosinophilic cytoplasm, indistinct borders, and variably tapering or plump ovoid vesicular nuclei {467,849}. Nuclear atypia is generally absent or only minimal. The spindle cells are arranged in an orderly fascicular pattern. A storiform arrangement is less common. The mitotic rate is variable, but does not correlate with clinical behaviour. The lesional cells are associated with a mainly chronic inflammatory infiltrate, within which plasma cells are characteristically predominant. Occasionally, the inflammatory component may include prominent foamy histiocytes, multinucleated giant cells, or neutrophils.

The immunophenotype of inflammatory myofibroblastic tumour in the lung is comparable to that in soft tissue locations. There is variable positivity for smooth muscle actin, muscle-specific actin, and desmin, and up to 30% of cases may be keratin-positive. These findings are consistent with myofibroblastic differentiation. About 50% of cases, particularly those in children and young adults, show immunopositivity for ALK1, and this usually correlates with *ALK* gene rearrangement {355,469,849}. With the advent of ALK inhibitor therapy, there may be a role for more sensitive immunohistochemical testing {2573}.

Genetic profile

Particularly in cases arising in children and young adults, inflammatory myofibroblastic tumour commonly shows clonal rearrangement of the *ALK* gene at 2p23, resulting in fusion of the 3′ kinase region of *ALK* with a variety of genes, including most often *TPM3*, *TPM4*, *CLTC*, and *RANBP2*, but the list continues to expand {901,1418,2003}. The same gene fusions are also found in some examples of anaplastic large cell lymphoma and ALK-positive B-cell lymphoma. Such rearrangements are readily detected by break-apart FISH. *ALK* rearrangement is very uncommon in inflammatory myofibroblastic tumours diagnosed in older adults. The nosological status of some ALK-negative cases, particularly in adults, remains controversial. It has been recently found that cases lacking ALK fusions harbor ROS1 and PDGFR β fusions {1517}.

Prognosis and predictive factors

Although inflammatory myofibroblastic tumour is indolent, complete resection is advocated to avoid recurrence and metastasis. Recurrence and poorer outcome are seen with larger tumour size {467}, incomplete resection {693,1650}, and non-surgical treatments {350}. ALK protein expression may be inversely related to metastasis {467}; poorer outcome after incomplete resection has been seen in ALK-negative tumours {451}. Tumours harbouring *ALK* chromosomal rearrangement may show response to crizotinib {303}; this therapy may be useful in reducing tumour size before surgery {1517}.

Epithelioid haemangioendothelioma

P. Cagle
S. Dacic

Definition

Epithelioid haemangioendothelioma is a low- to intermediate-grade malignant vascular tumour composed of solid nests and short cords of epithelioid endothelial cells in a myxohyaline stroma.

ICD-O code   9133/3

Synonym

Intravascular bronchioloalveolar tumour (obsolete)

Epidemiology

About 60–80% of patients with epithelioid haemangioendothelioma are women. Patient ages range from 7 to 81 years, with a median age of 38 years.

Etiology

Epithelioid haemangioendothelioma is a rare neoplasm of endothelial cells, associated with a specific fusion gene (see *Genetic profile*).

Clinical features

Lung involvement alone accounts for 12% of cases of epithelioid haemangioendothelioma (the third most common presentation), and lung with liver involvement accounts for 18% of cases (the second most common presentation). About 50–70% of patients are symptomatic at presentation, with pain as the most common symptom in the majority of symptomatic patients. Less frequent symptoms include cough, dyspnoea, haemoptysis, pleural effusion, and systemic symptoms {1413}.

In > 60% of cases, epithelioid haemangioendothelioma presents as multiple bilateral perivascular nodules (< 2 cm in size), with well- or poorly defined borders on CT, that mimic metastatic cancer or granulomas. In 10–19% of cases, epithelioid haemangioendothelioma presents as a solitary lung nodule up to 5 cm in diameter. Cavitary or calcified nodules have also been reported.

Since epithelioid haemangioendothelioma may arise in more than one site (e.g. liver, lung, bone, and soft tissue) simultaneously or sequentially, it is not always easy to determine whether a second lesion is a metastasis. As with other sarcomas, metastases are haematogeneous, and are generally considered rare. Reported sites of metastases include mostly liver, as well as skin, serosa, spleen, tonsils, retroperitoneum, kidney, bone, and soft tissue {2954}.

There is no standardized staging for epithelioid haemangioendothelioma.

Localization

Most epithelioid haemangioendothelioma nodules are intraparenchymal.

Macroscopy

Epithelioid haemangioendothelioma presents with multiple circumscribed nodules with a grey-white cut surface and a chondroid appearance. Tumours extending to the pleura may show diffuse pleural thickening, mimicking the gross appearance of malignant mesothelioma {125,3017} (see pleural *Epithelioid haemangioendothelioma*, p. 176).

Cytology

Cytology shows round and polygonal cells with pale cytoplasm. Nuclear pleomorphism correlates with the grade of the neoplasm. Intracytoplasmic vacuoles are a characteristic feature.

Histopathology

Epithelioid haemangioendothelioma is often associated with arterioles, venules, or lymphatic vessels. At low-power magnification, epithelioid haemangioendothelioma forms round to oval nodules with increased cellularity at the periphery, and an abundant hypocellular, eosinophilic, sclerotic centre with focal necrosis. Tumours are composed of strands and solid nests of rounded to slightly spindled endothelial cells, with intracytoplasmic lumina containing red blood cells. Intracytoplasmic vacuoles may create a signet ring appearance. The cells are usually cytologically bland, appearing with low grade tumours showing no or rare mitotic activity. Stroma may be chondroid, hyaline, mucinous, or myxomatous. Calcification and ossification may occur. Tumours frequently show an intra-alveolar growth pattern. They may be low or intermediate grade with the latter distinguished by the presence of necrosis, increased mitotic activity (mean 2/2 mm2) and greater nuclear atypia {61A}.

The vascular markers CD31, CD34, and FLI1 are more sensitive than factor VIII, and most epithelioid haemangioendothelioma expresses these markers. Focal cytokeratin expression is present in 25–30% of cases. Up to 50% of cases may show positivity for CK7 {2831}.

Differential diagnosis

The differential diagnosis of epithelioid haemangioendothelioma is broad. Several benign non-neoplastic processes should be considered in the differential diagnosis, including old granulomatous disease, organizing infarcts, and amyloidoma. Benign neoplasms such as hamartoma and sclerosing pneumocytoma (formerly called sclerosing haemangioma), and malignant neoplasms including

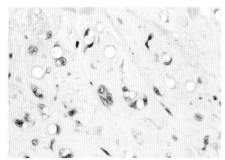

Fig. 1.144 Epithelioid haemangioendothelioma. A solid nest of tumour cells with central, round to ovoid nuclei and intracytoplasmic lumina.

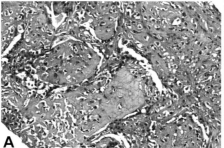
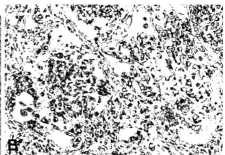

Fig. 1.145 Epithelioid haemangioendothelioma. **A** An intra-alveolar solid nest of tumour cells embedded in a prominent hyaline stroma. **B** The tumour cells show strong and diffuse positivity for CD31.

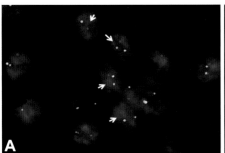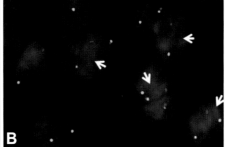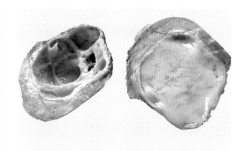

Fig. 1.146 Epithelioid haemangioendothelioma. FISH analysis using custom BAC probes shows break-apart signals (arrows) in *CAMTA1* (**A**) and *WWTR1* (**B**). Red, centromeric; green, telomeric.

Fig. 1.148 Type I pleuropulmonary blastoma showing a typical loculated cystic architecture (left) after removal of purulent fluid due to superimposed infection (right).

mesothelioma, adenocarcinoma, angiosarcoma, and other sarcomas should be excluded. Identification of *WWTR1-CAMTA1* fusion genes is helpful in establishing the diagnosis of epithelioid haemangioendothelioma {61A}. Compared to the high-grade angiosarcomas, epithelioid haemangioendotheliomas are low- to intermediate-grade tumours, and are more likely to show intracytoplasmic vacuoles, nuclear cytoplasmic inclusions, and stroma that is myxoid, hyaline or chondroid. In contrast, angiosarcomas are more likely to have capillary vessels, vascular lakes, papillary growth, prominent nucleoli, and marked nuclear atypia {61A}. In addition, *WWTR1-CAMTA1* fusion genes are not characteristic of angiosarcomas {61A}.

Genetic profile

A recurrent t(1;3)(p36.3;q25) chromosomal translocation is characteristic of epithelioid haemangioendothelioma {61A,1652}. The translocation involves two genes, *WWTR1* (3q25), which encodes a transcriptional coactivator that is highly expressed in endothelial cells, and *CAMTA1* (1p36), a DNA-binding transcriptional regulatory protein that is normally expressed during brain development {683,2592}. A subset of epithelioid haemangioendothelioma occurring in young adults shows recently described *YAP1-TFE3* fusions {69}.

Prognosis and predictive factors

Epithelioid haemangioendothelioma is a low- to intermediate-grade malignant tumour with metastatic potential and a 5year survival rate of 60%. Prognosis is worse for intermediate grade compared to low grade tumours and can be as low as 20% {61A}. Negative prognostic indicators include extensive intrapulmonary and pleural spread, weight loss, anaemia, and haemorrhagic pleural effusions {119}. Although partial regression has been rarely reported, most patients with intermediate grade tumours eventually die of respiratory failure due to replacement of the pulmonary parenchyma by tumour.

Pleuropulmonary blastoma

P. Cagle
C.D.M. Fletcher
A.G. Nicholson
W.D. Travis

Definition

Pleuropulmonary blastoma is a malignant tumour of infancy and early childhood arising as a cystic and/or solid sarcomatous neoplasm in the lung or (rarely) the pleura {2088}. The cystic component is lined by native epithelium, which may be ciliated. This embryonic or dysontogenetic neoplasm of the lung and/or pleura is the nosological counterpart of other neoplasms of childhood, including Wilms tumour, neuroblastoma, hepatoblastoma, and retinoblastoma.

ICD-O code 8973/3

Synonyms

Rhabdomyosarcoma arising in congenital cystic adenomatoid malformation; pulmonary blastoma of childhood; pulmonary sarcoma arising in mesenchymal cystic hamartoma; embryonal rhabdomyosarcoma arising within congenital bronchogenic cyst; pulmonary blastoma associated with cystic lung disease; pleuropulmonary blastoma in congenital cystic adenomatoid malformation

Epidemiology

Pleuropulmonary blastoma was first recognized as a distinct clinicopathological entity in 1988 {1567}, and the International Pleuropulmonary Blastoma Registry was subsequently created to register cases (http://www.ppbregistry.org/). Pleuropulmonary blastomas are very rare

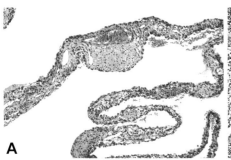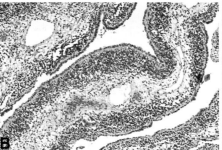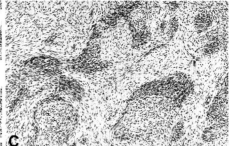

Fig. 1.147 Pleuropulmonary blastoma. **A** A nodule of immature cartilage is present in a cyst wall. **B** A cellular cambium layer is present beneath the hyperplastic mesothelial cells lining the cyst wall. **C** The alternating hypercellular and paucicellular pattern is distinctive for this tumour.

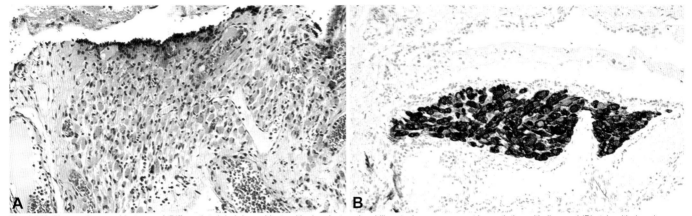

Fig. 1.149 Pleuropulmonary blastoma. **A** Differentiated rhabdomyoblasts with abundant eosinophilic cytoplasm are present beneath the epithelium and (**B**) stain with desmin.

tumours – rarer than their counterparts at other sites (such as Wilms tumour), although several hundred cases have now been registered and/or published in the literature worldwide.

Pleuropulmonary blastoma tumours are subgrouped as type I (purely cystic), type II (cystic and solid), and type III (purely solid), although these types are considered to represent a biological continuum. In a given patient, the aggressiveness of pleuropulmonary blastoma appears to increase over time. Types I, II, and III occur, on average, in progressively older cohorts of children. Type I pleuropulmonary blastoma typically occurs in children < 2 years of age, with a median age of 10 months. Type II pleuropulmonary blastoma occurs at a median age of 35 months. And type III pleuropulmonary blastoma occurs at a median age of 41 months (http://www.ppbregistry.org/). Overall, most cases are diagnosed at or before 4 years of age {2088}. The male-to-female ratio is approximately 1:1.

Etiology

Understanding of the etiology of pleuropulmonary blastoma has increased substantially over the past decade. About 40% of cases are estimated to have a genetic basis, called the pleuropulmonary blastoma family tumour and dysplasia syndrome {226} or *DICER1* syndrome {2410}. Patients typically suffer from neoplastic and dysplastic disease, usually presenting in the first 5–6 years of life, although some disorders appear in adolescence or early adulthood. Bilateral and multifocal disease occurs in 15% of patients, with the most common non-pulmonary tumour being cystic nephroma (occurring in about 10% of

patients with pleuropulmonary blastoma or their relatives). Other tumours include Sertoli-Leydig cell ovarian tumours, embryonal rhabdomyosarcoma, multinodular goitre, Wilms tumour, primitive neuroectodermal tumour, juvenile intestinal polyps, intraocular medulloepithelioma, and nasal chondromesenchymal hamartoma {504,617,989,2312,2410}. Germline loss-of-function mutations in *DICER1* have been identified in some families with the above syndrome, with loss of *DICER1* staining in epithelial cells, yet normal staining in malignant mesenchyme, suggesting that autocrine dysregulation plays a role in tumour development {995}. However, most mutation carriers are unaffected, indicating that the tumour risk is modest {2410}.

Clinical features

Signs and symptoms
The clinical manifestations depend on patient age and pathological type. Respiratory distress due to air-filled cysts, with or without pneumothorax, is the most common presentation of the cystic type I pleuropulmonary blastoma in the first 12–18 months of life {2087,2088,2089}, although some cases present without symptoms and are incidental findings {1977,2088,2089}. Dyspnoea, fever, chest pain, and cough are more common in patients with types II and III pleuropulmonary blastomas, as are pleural effusions, although pneumothoraces may still occur with cases that are partially cystic {1682}.

Imaging
CT may show either a mass or consolidation. There may also be multiloculated

cystic or cystic/solid changes {902,1353, 1779,1785,1917,2088,2089}. Typically, pleuropulmonary blastomas involve the lung parenchyma and pleura, but the chest wall peripherally or the mediastinum may rarely be involved. Because of the potential for multifocal disease, bilateral disease should always be looked for {1978}.

Tumour spread
In type I pleuropulmonary blastoma, 50–60% of tumours are limited to the lungs, although 40% recur – usually with type II or III morphology {2087}. Spread beyond the lung is more common in patients presenting with type II or III pleuropulmonary blastomas. Approximately 3% of cases with type II or III tumours show vascular and/or cardiac extension, mainly to the left side {2086}.

Staging
There is no formal staging system for pleuropulmonary blastoma, but it is recommended that patients with type I pleuropulmonary blastoma undergo chest and abdominal CT, to help exclude associated cystic nephromas. For patients with type II or III pleuropulmonary blastoma, chest and abdominal CT, head MRI, and bone scan are recommended.

Localization
Pleuropulmonary blastoma occurs mainly within the lung, with no obvious zonal distribution. A minority of cases arise from the visceral or parietal pleura, the mediastinum {118}, or the dome of the diaphragm.

Macroscopy
Cystic type I pleuropulmonary blastomas consist of thin-walled, often loculated

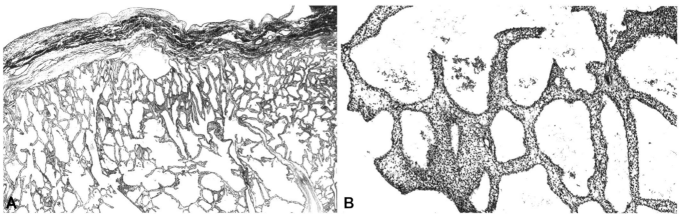

Fig. 1.150 Fetal lung interstitial tumour. **A** A localized mass shows spongiform alveoli-like structures resembling lung of 20–24 weeks' gestation. Note the thick capsule. **B** Interstitial cells are monotonous and uniformly distributed, with the walls covered by native epithelium.

structures, which may collapse after resection. Rarely, cysts may become infected and appear solid. Solid type III pleuropulmonary blastomas can occupy an entire lobe or lung, with a variegated cut surface that may be haemorrhagic and/or necrotic. Type II pleuropulmonary blastomas contain a mixture of solid and cystic elements.

Cytology
Fine-needle aspiration biopsy has been used to diagnose pleuropulmonary blastomas with varying success, with the findings reflecting the heterogeneous nature of the malignant mesenchymal and small ovoid blastemal elements {628,1850,2379}.

Histopathology
Cystic type I pleuropulmonary blastomas consist of multicystic structures lined by respiratory-type epithelium, beneath which is a population of small primitive malignant cells that can lie as a continuous or discontinuous cambium layer-like zone. However, blastematous cells can be difficult to identify. Areas of rhabdomyoblastic differentiation may be present, as may immature cartilage. In some cases, blastematous elements are wholly lacking, and some recommend that these cystic lesions be classified as regressed type I pleuropulmonary blastomas (so-called type Ir) {996}. In these, there is only hyalinized stroma within the septa, morphologically identical to that of type 4 congenital cystic adenomatoid malformations, first described by Stocker {1543}. Type II pleuropulmonary blastomas may show partial or complete overgrowth of the septal stroma by sheets of primitive small cells, without apparent

differentiation, areas of embryonal rhabdomysarcoma, or fascicles of a spindle cell sarcoma. Other type II pleuropulmonary blastomas show a grossly visible solid component and microscopically identifiable type I foci. Type III tumours show solid mixed sheets of blastematous and sarcomatous areas; the latter may contain nodules of chondrosarcoma-like areas, fibrosarcoma-like areas, rhabdomyosarcomatous foci, or anaplastic areas. Foci of necrosis, haemorrhage, and fibrosis are variably present. Neoplastic epithelial elements have not been seen in pleuropulmonary blastomas, although native epithelium is often entrapped.

Immunohistochemistry
Most of the neoplastic cells are reactive for vimentin. Desmin is expressed in identifiable rhabdomyoblastic cells, and is often helpful in their identification in type I pleuropulmonary blastomas. Desmin staining is less consistent in the primitive small cells in the cambium layer. Areas of chondroid differentiation may express S100 protein. Cytokeratins and TTF1 highlight the native respiratory-type cells, both entrapped and lining the cysts.

Differential diagnosis
Immunohistochemistry is useful in the differential diagnosis of cystic synovial sarcomas of the lung and chest wall {509}. When the latter is a consideration, epithelial membrane antigen, cytokeratin, and CD99 are useful, since these three markers are not expressed in pleuropulmonary blastoma. Molecular analyses for relevant molecular abnormalities (*DICER1* mutation and X;18 translocation) are also of value in this situation. Imaging

features overlap with those of congenital cystic adenomatoid malformations {902}, as do the histological features of type 4 congenital cystic adenomatoid malformations and so-called regressed type 1 pleuropulmonary blastoma, although the presence of any blastematous area warrants classification as pleuropulmonary blastoma. The immunohistochemical differences in the epithelial cells in congenital cystic adenomatoid malformations and pleuropulmonary blastoma have been described in relation to the FGF10 signaling pathway, being weak or absent in pleuropulmonary blastomas {1461}. An additional pattern of fetal lung interstitial tumour with features resembling lung of 20–24 weeks' gestation has been described, with no recurrences after resection. It remains uncertain whether this is a neoplasm or is related to pleuropulmonary blastoma, but it enters the differential diagnosis {604}.

Genetic profile
Several reports have documented gains in chromosome 8, usually trisomy {544,1881,2603}, with losses in 9p21–24 and 11p14 {544}. The *DICER1* gene is located on chromosome 14q, and patients with pleuropulmonary blastomas should undergo surveillance in relation to the possibility of other related tumours (see above). Surveillance of siblings or family members is more controversial, due to the need to balance the modest risk of tumour development against the potential of causing anxiety rather than providing reassurance.

Prognosis and predictive factors
Patients with cystic type I pleuropulmonary blastomas have an 80–90% 5-year

disease-free survival, although 40% of cases may recur {211,996}, whereas types II and III are associated with a 5-year disease-free survival of < 50% {211,2088}. Most patients with type I tumours have surgery as a diagnostic procedure {211}, although some authors advocate adjuvant chemotherapy {2087}. For type II and III pleuropulmonary blastomas, surgery is recommended if feasible, followed by chemotherapy and/or radiotherapy. Unresectable disease should be marked for possible radiotherapy targeting. Intracavitary chemotherapy has occasionally been used, with apparent success {250}. Recurrence is often local, and there is a predilection for metastasis to the brain, spinal cord, and skeletal system {2088}, although pleuropulmonary blastomas can metastasize widely. Favourable prognostic factors for pleuropulmonary blastoma are complete tumour resection at diagnosis and absence of invasion. There is a benefit of doxorubicin-based regimens in type II and III pleuropulmonary blastomas {211}.

Synovial sarcoma

S. Dacic
T.J. Franks
M. Ladanyi

Definition
Synovial sarcoma is a distinct soft tissue sarcoma with variable mesenchymal and epithelial differentiation. It is characterized by a specific chromosomal translocation: t(X;18)(p11.2;q11.2).

ICD-O codes
Synovial sarcoma	9040/3
Synovial sarcoma, spindle cell	9041/3
Synovial sarcoma, epithelioid cell	9042/3
Synovial sarcoma, biphasic	9043/3

Synonyms
Obsolete: synovial cell sarcoma; malignant synovioma; synovioblastic sarcoma

Epidemiology
Lung is the most common organ-based site for primary synovial sarcoma {1666}. It manifests in older patients, with a mean age of 42 years. There is no sex predominance {957}.

Etiology
The name synovial sarcoma is a misnomer, because these tumours lack evidence of synovial differentiation {1669, 2416}. Synovial sarcoma is thought to be derived from multipotent stem cells capable of differentiating into both mesenchymal and epithelial cells {2267}.

Clinical features
As with other lung tumours, the common presenting signs and symptoms include dyspnoea, chest pain, cough, haemoptysis, and incidental radiographical findings {957}.

On chest radiographs, pulmonary synovial sarcomas are homogeneous, with sharply marginated borders. Cavitation, calcification, and lymphadenopathy are typically absent. By CT, tumours show homogeneous or heterogeneous enhancement, and are often pleural-based, without bone destruction, chest wall invasion, or calcification. Ipsilateral pleural effusion is common {754,957}.

Pulmonary synovial sarcomas spread primarily by direct extension into adjacent structures, and recurrence is typically local. Regional lymph nodes may be involved at diagnosis. Metastases to the lung, regional lymph nodes, bone, liver, skin, central nervous system, omentum, and spleen can occur {957,1897,3010}.

Localization
Pulmonary synovial sarcoma usually presents as a peripheral, parenchymal tumour nodule, and may occasionally infiltrate the chest wall or mediastinum. Cases involving the tracheobronchial tree and presenting as an endobronchial mass are rare.

Macroscopy
The tumours are well circumscribed, soft, and tan, with foci of necrosis, haemorrhage, and cystic change. They range from 0.6 to 17 cm, with a mean size of 7.5 cm {167,686,957}.

Cytology
Pulmonary synovial sarcoma may be suggested by cytology when a biphasic pattern of spindle and epithelioid cells is present. Monophasic synovial sarcoma is a diagnostic possibility for a uniform population of spindle cells {690}.

Histopathology
The histological features of pulmonary synovial sarcoma are identical to those of its soft tissue counterpart {686,779,957,2524}. Monophasic synovial sarcoma is the most common pulmonary subtype. It consists of sheets or fascicles of uniform, elongated spindle cells with scant cytoplasm and indistinct cell borders. Biphasic synovial sarcoma has variable proportions of spindle and epithelial cells. The epithelial component contains gland- and/or slit-like structures with mucin or papillary structures with single or multiple layers of uniform cells. The epithelial cells may form solid nests or cords. The cells are cuboidal with round nuclei, occasional nucleoli, and a moderate amount of eosinophilic cytoplasm. Other features include haemangiopericytoma-like vasculature, hyalinized or eosinophilic stroma, and focal myxoid change {957}. Benign entrapped pneumocytes are common. The mitotic count is variable (from 2 to > 20 mitoses per 2 mm^2). Necrosis is present in most tumours. Calcification and mast cell infiltration are less common than in soft tissue synovial sarcoma {957}. Rarely, tumours can be predominantly cystic {509}.

At least one epithelial marker (such as epithelial membrane antigen) and cytokeratin (pancytokeratin, CK7, and CK5/6) should be positive, and coexpressed with vimentin. CD99 and BCL2. S100, smooth muscle actin, CD56, and calretinin can also be seen {167,686,957,1897}. TLE1 is another marker with high specificity for synovial sarcoma {1483,2622}.

Differential diagnosis
Before the diagnosis of primary pulmonary synovial sarcoma is made, a soft tissue primary must be excluded. Otherwise, the differential diagnosis is wide, and includes a large number of epithelial and mesenchymal neoplasms such as spindle cell carcinoma, malignant mesothelioma, pleuropulmonary blastoma, solitary fibrous tumour, small cell carcinoma, smooth muscle sarcomas, malignant peripheral nerve sheet tumour, and Ewing sarcoma. A combination of clinical, histological, immunohistochemical, and cytogenetic findings can easily differentiate synovial sarcoma from these entities. The diagnostic translocation t(X;18)(p11.2;q11.2) is valuable in the differential diagnosis of synovial sarcoma.

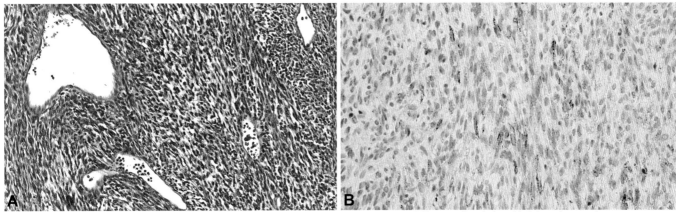

Fig. 1.151 Synovial sarcoma. **A** Cellular monomorphic spindle cells with a pericytomatous vascular pattern. **B** Tumour cells stain for epithelial membrane antigen.

Genetic profile

Synovial sarcoma tumour cells, including primary intrathoracic synovial sarcoma {167,1897}, contain the translocation t(X;18)(p11.2;q11.2), which fuses the *SS18* (also called *SYT*) gene on chromosome 18 to either *SSX1* or *SSX2*, both located at Xp11.2. Very rare variants include *SS18-SSX4*, which appears cytogenetically identical, and *SS18L1-SSX1*, resulting from a t(X;20) translocation, but these have not yet been described in primary pulmonary synovial sarcoma. Cases with *SS18-SSX1* are much more likely to show glandular epithelial differentiation than cases with *SS18-SSX2* {68,1379}.

Prognosis and predictive factors

The prognosis of pulmonary synovial sarcoma is worse than that of its soft tissue counterpart: 5-year disease-specific survival is about 30% {167,686,688}, and the 2-year local recurrence rate ranges from 27% to 75% {167,686,1897}. Negative prognostic factors such as larger tumour size (≥ 5 cm), high mitotic rate (≥ 10 mitoses per 2 mm^2), high histological grade, and poorly differentiated histology have been reported in synovial sarcoma {957}.

Pulmonary artery intimal sarcoma

A.P. Burke
E.S. Yi

Definition

Pulmonary artery intimal sarcoma originates from the arterial intima of elastic pulmonary arteries. It may be completely undifferentiated or show heterologous components, such as osteosarcoma and chondrosarcoma. The preferred designation is the histological subtype, followed by the presumed site of origin (e.g. undifferentiated pleomorphic sarcoma of intimal origin).

ICD-O code   9137/3

Synonym

The term pulmonary artery sarcoma has been used interchangeably with pulmonary artery intimal sarcoma, but the term pulmonary artery sarcoma also encompasses exceedingly rare mural sarcoma, which is distinct from intimal sarcoma.

Epidemiology

Pulmonary artery intimal sarcoma is a rare tumour. Its incidence is unknown, and probably underestimated {1777}. Patients are typically misdiagnosed on clinical grounds as having acute or chronic pulmonary embolism. Pulmonary artery intimal sarcoma is present in 1-4% of pulmonary thromboendarterectomy specimens from patients with chronic thromboembolic pulmonary hypertension {61,190}. The average age is 56 years (with a range of 26–78 years), and the sex distribution is equal {1777}.

Clinical features

The most common presenting symptom is dyspnoea, followed by (in decreasing order) chest or back pain, cough, haemoptysis, weight loss, malaise, syncope, fever, and (rarely) sudden death. These clinical manifestations mimic acute or chronic thromboembolism and pulmonary hypertension {1984}. Progressive weight loss, anaemia, and fever should raise suspicion for malignancy {1984}. Other clinical manifestations include pulmonary artery aneurysm, right heart failure, symptoms mimicking Takayasu disease, and cauda equina syndrome due to spinal metastasis {169,1527,2120,2619}. Systolic ejection murmur, cyanosis, peripheral oedema, jugular venous distension, hepatomegaly, and clubbing are common {1984}. On CT, intimal sarcomas present as a lobulated enhancing mass in the central arteries, causing filling defects, with occlusion and expansion of the entire lumen {100,2876}. A patchy or delayed contrast enhancement has been described on CT angiography, which is more evident in the venous phase {100}. Avid uptake of FDG on PET-CT may be useful in distinguishing pulmonary artery intimal sarcoma from pulmonary embolism {100,1432}. MRI can be used in equivocal cases by PET-CT. Extravascular extension into the surrounding lung parenchyma or mediastinal structures can be a diagnostic finding of intimal sarcoma {2876}. Endobronchial ultrasound is useful for producing real-time images of the interior of pulmonary arteries adjacent to bronchi {1711,2380}.

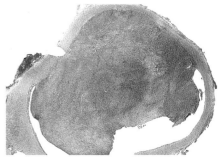

Fig. 1.152 Pulmonary artery intimal sarcoma. In this resection, the tumour is entirely intraluminal.

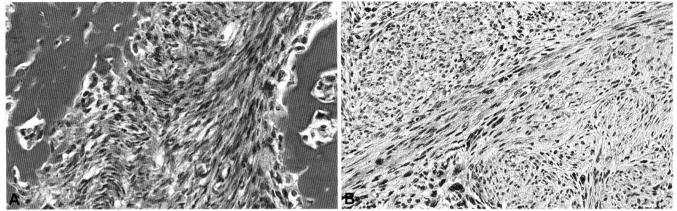
Fig. 1.153 A Osteosarcoma of pulmonary arterial intima. There is a pleomorphic spindle cell tumour with a malignant osteoid matrix. This tumour arose just distal to the pulmonary valve. **B** Leiomyosarcoma of pulmonary intimal origin. There are interlacing fascicles of tumour cells.

Localization
Pulmonary artery intimal sarcoma occurs in the proximal elastic arteries, from the level of the pulmonary valve to the lobar branches. Most cases have bilateral involvement, although one side is usually dominant. Conversely, a unilateral mass lesion within the pulmonary artery is more likely to be intimal sarcoma, since unilateral involvement by chronic pulmonary thromboemboli is quite unusual {2876}.

Macroscopy
Pulmonary artery intimal sarcoma has an intraluminal polypoid growth pattern. Intimal sarcomas resemble mucoid or gelatinous clots filling vascular lumens. Distal extension may show smooth tapering of the mass. The cut surface may show firm fibrotic areas and bony/gritty or chondroid foci if the tumour has an osteosarcomatous or chondrosarcomatous component. Haemorrhage and necrosis are common in high-grade intimal sarcomas. The entire tumour is often intraluminal, and can be shelled out by endarterectomy. Limited tumour extension into the surrounding adventitia and periarterial soft tissue may occur.

Histopathology
The histological patterns are heterogeneous {1054,2604}. The largest group is undifferentiated pleomorphic sarcomas, followed by low-grade spindle cell sarcomas with a myxoid background. Such myxofibrosarcomas may demonstrate areas containing bland spindle cells in a dense fibrous background, resembling fibrosarcoma. About 1 in 6 pulmonary artery intimal sarcomas show heterologous elements in the form of osteosarcoma or chondrosarcoma, in which case the term extraskeletal osteosarcoma is applied. Less common histological patterns include rhabdomyosarcoma, leiomyosarcoma, undifferentiated sarcoma with epithelioid or round cell features, synovial sarcoma, epithelioid haemangioendothelioma, and angiosarcoma {1054,1230}. A rare histological subtype is low-grade inflammatory myofibroblastic tumour, which is characterized by a relative lack of cellularity, a variable inflammatory and myxoid background, a lack of pleomorphism or significant mitotic activity, and a myofibroblastic cellular appearance (so-called tissue culture growth). The immunohistochemical profile of pulmonary artery intimal sarcoma is that of the differentiated areas. Undifferentiated tumours express vimentin and (focally) actin. Leiomyosarcomas and rhabdomyosarcomas both express desmin, and rhabdomyosarcomas express myogenin. Angiosarcomas are positive for endothelial markers (v-ets avian erythroblastosis virus E26 oncogene homologue protein and CD31).

Genetic profile
In a series of undifferentiated intimal sarcomas of the pulmonary artery, *MDM2* amplification was observed in most tumours {218}, often coexisting with amplification of *PDGFRA* {594}

Prognosis and predictive factors
One study found that survival was approximately 70% at 3 years after surgical treatment {1230}. In another study, the median survival was 3 years for patients undergoing an attempt at curative resection versus < 1 year for those undergoing incomplete resection {114}. Factors associated with a favourable outcome include low-grade tumours such as leiomyosarcomas and especially low-grade inflammatory myofibroblastic tumour {2604}. There is disagreement as to whether multimodality treatment with chemotherapy and radiation therapy improves survival. Some data show an increased survival after multimodality treatment {114}, others show no clear benefit {1777}.

Pulmonary myxoid sarcoma with EWSR1-CREB1 translocation
A.G. Nicholson

Definition
Primary pulmonary myxoid sarcoma is a malignant tumour that typically arises in the airways. It predominantly consists of lobules made up of delicate, lace-like strands and cords of mildly atypical round and spindle cells within a prominent myxoid stroma. The tumours contain an *EWSR1-CREB1* fusion gene.

ICD-O code   8842/3

Synonym
Low-grade malignant myxoid endobronchial tumour {1840}

Epidemiology
Primary pulmonary myxoid sarcoma was first described in 1999 {1840}. It is seen most often in young adult females, but fewer than 15 cases have been published {1608,2642}. The tumour is characterized by distinct histological features and an *EWSR1-CREB1* fusion gene. Although *EWSR1-CREB1* is also found in

other tumours (such as angiomatoid fibrous histiocytoma {2643} and clear cell sarcomas {2641}), primary pulmonary myxoid sarcomas are morphologically different from these entities.

Etiology

Most patients are smokers {2642}, but there are no known etiological factors such as inherited cancer-predisposing syndromes.

Clinical features

Patients may present with cough, haemoptysis, systemic symptoms such as weight loss, or symptoms from metastases, or the tumour may be detected incidentally {2642}.

Most cases present with a hilar mass either on chest radiograph or CT. Obstructive changes may be present {2642}.

Most patients underwent resection and remained free of disease, although metastatic spread to the brain and kidney have been reported {2642}.

Localization

Primary pulmonary myxoid sarcomas are nearly always related to a bronchus, and are often predominantly endobronchial, although they may also spread into the surrounding alveolar parenchyma.

Macroscopy

The tumours generally measure < 4 cm and are well circumscribed or nodular, pale, and glistening or gelatinous on cut surface, ranging in colour from white/grey to yellow {2642}.

Histopathology

At low power, pulmonary myxoid sarcomas have a lobulated architecture, with endobronchial location. A fibrous pseudocapsule may be present. Tumours are typically composed of spindle cells and stellate to polygonal cells, with a predominant reticular network of delicate lacelike strands and cords within a prominent myxoid stroma that may be lightly basophilic, although more solid areas may be found. A minority have a predominantly solid architecture with a more patternless distribution of cells within the myxoid stroma. In one case, cells showed focal multinucleation. Cellular atypia is generally mild to moderate in extent, although rare cases have shown focal marked atypia and multinucleation. Mitotic rates of up to 32 mitoses per 2 mm² with

atypical forms are described, although the majority show < 5 mitoses per 2 mm². Necrosis is seen in about 50% of tumours, and tends to be focal. The stroma is myxoid in all cases, but may be focally collagenous. No chondroid differentiation is seen. Most cases have a patchy background chronic inflammatory cell infiltrate of mainly lymphocytes and plasma cells. Vascular invasion is rare {2642}.

All tumours express vimentin, and 60% show weak and focal staining for epithelial membrane antigen. Other common markers are negative, in particular cytokeratins, S100, smooth muscle actin, desmin, CD34, and neuroendocrine markers. The myxoid stroma is positive for Alcian blue, with staining sensitive to treatment with hyaluronidase {1840}.

Differential diagnosis

The main differential diagnosis on morphology is extraskeletal myxoid chondrosarcoma, although these are tumours mainly of the proximal extremities and limb girdles, with only rare cases reported in the lung {3024} and pleura

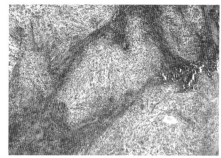

Fig. 1.155 Primary pulmonary myxoid sarcoma. At low-power magnification, the tumour has a nodular architecture.

{858}. They are also more common in males and present at an older age. On histology, the distinguishing features are that the myxoid stroma in extraskeletal myxoid chondrosarcoma is positive for Alcian blue, but resistant to hyaluronidase; and stromal haemorrhage, a characteristic feature of extraskeletal myxoid chondrosarcoma, is not seen in primary pulmonary myxoid sarcomas. Extraskeletal myxoid chondrosarcomas are also characterized by recurrent chromosomal translocations

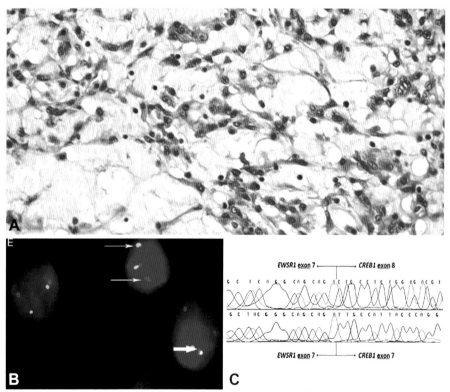

Fig. 1.154 Primary pulmonary myxoid sarcoma. **A** Spindle and rounded cells with typically bland nuclei show a lacelike or reticular architecture within sparsely cellular myxoid stroma, with a mixed chronic inflammatory infiltrate. **B** FISH shows split red and green signals (thin arrows) with *EWSR1* break-apart probes in tumour nuclei, consistent with the presence of rearrangements of this gene, contrasting with the fusion signal in a non-rearranged gene (thick arrow). **C** Direct sequencing confirms the presence of *EWSR1-CREB1* fusions, which predominantly involve exon 7 of each gene (lower diagram), or more rarely occur between exon 7 of *EWSR1* and exon 8 of *CREB1* (upper diagram). B and C reprinted from Thway K et al. {2642}.

that fuse *NR4A3* (also called *CHN* or *TEC*) on chromosome 9q22 to a variety of partners.

Other tumours in the morphological differential diagnosis include epithelial-myoepithelial carcinomas and myoepithelioma {773}, but these tumours typically have ductular elements and express cytokeratin and S100 protein, and are also variably positive for calponin, epithelial membrane antigen, and smooth muscle actin. Myoepitheliomas have been reported to show rearrangements involving the *EWSR1* gene, but none have been partnered with *CREB1* {70,261}. Other myxoid tumours described in the lung are pulmonary myxoma {202}, primary myxoid liposarcoma {2430}, aggressive angiomyxoma {440}, and so-called microcystic fibromyxoma {2367}. However, these are different histologically, and are not known to carry the specific *EWSR1-CREB1* translocation.

The *EWSR1-CREB1* fusion is also seen in angiomatoid fibrous histiocytoma {2643} and clear cell sarcomas {2641}, but the clinicopathological features of these two tumours differ significantly.

Genetic profile
EWSR1 rearrangements are detectable by FISH, with real-time reverse transcriptase PCR analysis showing *EWSR1-CREB1* fusion transcripts that have been confirmed with direct sequencing. In assessable cases, the break point in *EWSR1* involved exon 7, whereas for the *CREB1* gene, exon 7 was involved in 6 cases and exon 8 in 1. Cases have been assessed for the fusion transcripts *EWSR1-NR4A3* and *TAF15-NR4A3*, but neither were detected {2642}.

Prognosis and predictive factors
If localized to the lung, the majority of cases remain free of disease. However, some patients progress to (or present with) metastatic disease, with poor prognosis. The rare cases that showed metastatic spread did not correlate with the histological features typically associated with aggressive behaviour, such as necrosis and pleomorphism {2642}.

Myoepithelial tumours / myoepithelial carcinoma

W.D. Travis
C.D.M. Fletcher

Definition
Myoepithelial tumours of the lung are rare, showing predominantly or exclusively myoepithelial differentiation. Malignant myoepithelial tumours are classified as myoepithelial carcinomas. Myoepithelial tumours differ from mixed tumours in that mixed tumours also show ductal differentiation.

ICD-O codes
Myoepithelioma   8982/0
Myoepithelial carcinoma   8982/3

Synonyms
Myoepithelial tumour; malignant myoepithelial tumour; salivary gland myoepithelial tumour

Epidemiology
Pulmonary myoepithelial tumours are very rare, with fewer than 15 case reports published. They occur in adults, with most benign cases occurring in females and most malignant cases occurring in males.

Clinical features
Tumours presenting as endobronchial masses present with symptoms of airway obstruction, such as cough or dyspnoea. Patients with peripheral lung tumours may be asymptomatic. CT shows a circumscribed mass either in the lung periphery or as a central endobronchial mass.

Localization
These tumours may present as an endobronchial mass or as a peripheral nodule.

Macroscopy
The tumours consist of circumscribed masses with a yellow-tan cut surface. Malignant tumours may show locally invasive growth, necrosis, and/or haemorrhage. Tumour size ranges from 1.5 to 13 cm, with larger size seen in malignant tumours.

Histopathology
Histologically, the tumours show a spectrum of trabecular or reticular

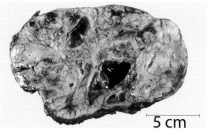

Fig. 1.156 Myoepithelial carcinoma. This 13 cm right lower lobe mass involved the visceral pleura. It shows a yellow, soft cut surface with areas of haemorrhage and necrosis. Reprinted from Sarkaria IS et al. {2279}.

patterns, with abundant myxoid stroma {1032,1061,1339,1603,2279}. The tumour cells are epithelioid or spindled, and the nuclei are uniform, with eosinophilic or clear cell cytoplasm. Cells with a plasmacytoid appearance and cytoplasmic hyaline inclusions can be present {735}. Myoepithelial carcinomas also show malignant features such as a high mitotic rate, necrosis, or nuclear atypia {1061,2279}.

Immunohistochemistry shows that most tumours stain positively for keratin, S100, and calponin. Most are also positive for glial fibrillary acidic protein. Smooth muscle actin and p63 may also be positive. Staining for desmin and CD34 is negative {735,1032}.

Differential diagnosis
The differential diagnoses include other salivary gland tumours, such as mixed tumour and epithelial-myoepithelial carcinoma; other lung carcinomas, such as large cell carcinoma and basaloid squamous cell carcinoma; and metastatic tumours from the salivary gland or soft tissue. Mixed tumours have a ductal component (see *Pleomorphic adenoma*, p. 105). Epithelial-myoepithelial carcinoma has distinctive morphological and immunohistochemical characteristics (see *Epithelial-myoepithelial carcinoma*, p. 103). To date, epithelial-myoepithelial

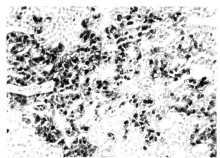

Fig. 1.157 Myoepithelioma. The tumour stains strongly for S100.

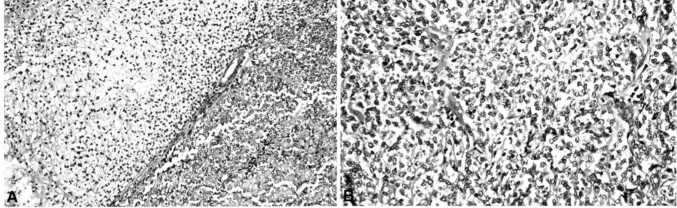

Fig. 1.158 Myoepithelioma. **A** This tumour shows an area of clear cells and myxoid stroma adjacent to sheets of small round cells with focal hyaline stroma. **B** This tumour consists of sheets of round to spindle-shaped cells with small nucleoli and vesicular chromatin. The cytoplasm is eosinophilic to clear.

carcinomas have not been shown to carry the *EWSR1* gene rearrangement. Basaloid squamous cell carcinomas (see *Basaloid squamous cell carcinoma*, p. 56) can have areas of hyaline stroma and express keratins and p63/p40, but they lack the characteristic myoepithelioma morphology, and are typically negative for S100, calponin, and smooth muscle actin. Large cell carcinomas typically lack myxoid stroma and prominent trabecular or reticular pattern, as well as S100 and calponin.

Genetic profile
EWSR1 gene rearrangement can be found in pulmonary myoepithelial tumours. *EWSR1-ZNF444* and *FUS* gene rearrangements were found in two malignant tumours that showed clear cell and spindle cell morphology {70}.

Prognosis and predictive factors
Benign tumours are cured by surgical resection {1339}. Malignant tumours can metastasize to the soft tissue, liver, brain, and contralateral lung. A lower mitotic rate may be more favourable for malignant tumours, although data are limited {1061}.

Other mesenchymal tumours

S. Dacic
G. Elmberger

Definition
Primary bronchopulmonary mesenchymal tumours are rare, and resemble their counterparts elsewhere in the body. They

should be classified according to the current criteria for soft tissue tumours, independent of their origin in the lung.

Epidemiology
Sarcomas of the lung affect middle-aged and elderly patients, with a slight male predominance. They account for < 0.5% of all lung neoplasms.

Etiology
Most pulmonary sarcomas derive from smooth muscle or fibrous tissue. Rare cases of bronchopulmonary sarcomas have developed in bronchial cysts {192} or arteriovenous fistulas {2804}, or after radiation therapy {1856}. Leiomyosarcomas have been reported in association with EBV in patients with AIDS {1622} and following solid organ transplantation {2539}.

Clinical features
The symptoms are essentially similar to those seen with epithelial tumours, and depend on the tumour location rather than histological type. Intrapulmonary parenchymal tumours most frequently present with chest pain and cough {688,1230}. Endobronchial tumours present earlier, with symptoms of pulmonary obstruction such as chest pain, cough, fever, wheezing, haemoptysis, dyspnoea, and even expectoration of tumour fragments. Patients may also be asymptomatic, although rarely {688}.
All radiographical appearances resemble bronchogenic carcinoma. Primary pulmonary sarcomas usually present as a large peripheral or perihilar, well-circumscribed mass {688}. They tend to occur more frequently in the upper lobes {688}. Endobronchial lesions frequently

show atelectasis. Tumours usually show local invasion into contiguous thoracic structures such as the pericardium, blood vessels, and chest wall. Tumours should be staged according to the TNM classification of soft tissue sarcomas.

Localization
Mesenchymal tumours may present as a solitary lesion in the lung parenchyma, or (less often) as bilateral lesions {688,1230}. They may also present as endobronchial lesions {767}.

Macroscopy
The tumours are well circumscribed, grey-tan, and firm, frequently with necrosis and haemorrhage. The median reported size is 6 cm, ranging from 2.5 to 16 cm {688}.

Cytology
The cytological characteristics of primary pulmonary mesenchymal tumours resemble those of their soft tissue counterparts; but descriptions are limited to case reports {688,767}.

Histopathology
Common types of primary pulmonary sarcomas not covered as specific entities in this book include Kaposi sarcoma, fibrosarcoma, leiomyosarcoma, and undifferentiated pleomorphic sarcoma. Morphological features of primary pulmonary leiomyosarcomas recapitulate those seen in soft tissue; namely, a fascicular proliferation of spindle cells with moderate amounts of eosinophilic cytoplasm, cigar-shaped nuclei, and inconspicuous nucleoli. Pulmonary leiomyosarcoma can show a wide spectrum of differentiation, with a variable amount of

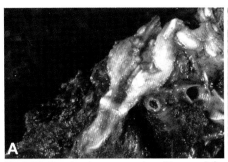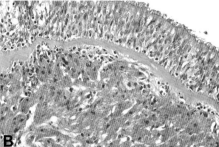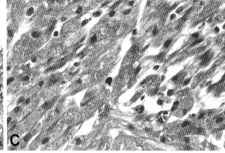

Fig. 1.159 Bronchopulmonary granular cell tumour. **A** Gross appearance of the bronchial granular cell tumour, showing endobronchial nodules. **B** A bronchial polyp composed of polygonal cells with abundant eosinophilic cytoplasm. **C** High-power magnification showing abundant, coarsely granular cytoplasm.

necrosis and cytological atypia, and a variable number of mitoses {668}. Pulmonary undifferentiated pleomorphic sarcoma (formerly called malignant fibrous histiocytoma) may present as storiform-pleomorphic, giant cell, and inflammatory subtypes. Five cases of angiomatoid fibrous histiocytoma have been reported {401,2643}, showing the typical histological features such as a peritumoural cuff of lymphoplasmacytic infiltrate, multinodular aggregates of dendritic-like tumour cells, blood-filled spaces, and abundant admixed plasma cells. The tumour cells are predominantly short and spindly, with indistinct cell borders, a moderate amount of eosinophilic cytoplasm, and oval or elongated nuclei with fine chromatin. Cells with scant cytoplasm resembling Ewing sarcoma, or clear cytoplasm, can also be seen {401}. Mitotic figures are rare. Unlike at other intrathoracic sites, malignant nerve sheath tumours of the lung are extremely rare {1083,1376}. They may occur as a manifestation of neurofibromatosis type I, or may be sporadic. Other rare cases of sarcomas reported in the lung include liposarcoma myxoid variant {2430}, angiosarcoma, rhabdomyosarcoma {436}, chondrosarcoma {1642, 3024}, ganglioneuroblastoma, osteosarcoma {2130}, giant cell tumour {1366}, and alveolar soft part sarcoma {1268}. Benign mesenchymal pulmonary tumours are rare, and the described variants include lipoma, chondroma (as part of Carney's triad), fibroma, haemangioma, lymphangioma, haemangiomatosis, lymphangiomatosis,

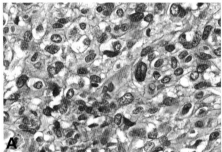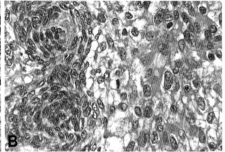

Fig. 1.160 Angiomatoid fibrous histiocytoma. **A** Tumour composed of oval cells with fine chromatin, admixed with occasional cells with larger and hyperchromatic nuclei. **B** A cluster of small tumour cells admixed with typical larger cells. Reprinted from Chen G et al. {401}.

glomus tumours, chemodectoma, granular cell tumours, and meningioma. The immunophenotype of mesenchymal tumours in the lung is comparable to that in soft tissue locations.

Differential diagnosis
The most important differential diagnosis is the more common occurrence of metastatic mesenchymal tumours, usually originating in deep soft tissue sites or the female genital tract. Otherwise, the differential diagnosis is wide, and includes a large number of epithelial and mesenchymal neoplasms, including sarcomatoid carcinomas, mesotheliomas, malignant melanomas, and different types of sarcomas. Uncommonly, various types of pseudotumours with a spindle cell pattern (such as mycobacterial spindle cell pseudotumour) can enter the differential diagnosis. The combination of clinical, histological, and immunohistochemical findings is helpful. The specific translocations can differentiate between the various types of sarcomas.

Genetic profile
The genetic profile of primary pulmonary mesenchymal tumours is identical to that of their soft tissue counterparts. For example, angiomatoid fibrous histiocytoma is characterized by *EWS* gene translocation, with partner genes being *CREB1* and *ATF1* {401,2643}. Myxoid liposarcoma has a reciprocal translocation involving *DDIT3* and *FUS*.

Prognosis and predictive factors
Treatment and prognosis do not differ from those of other soft tissue sarcomas. The prognosis appears to correlate with tumour grade and degree of differentiation. Low-grade tumours generally follow a less aggressive course than high-grade tumours. Malignant peripheral nerve sheet tumours occurring in patients with neurofibromatosis type I generally have a poorer prognosis than sporadic types.

Lymphohistiocytic tumours

A.G. Nicholson
E.S. Jaffe
D. Guinee

Extranodal marginal zone lymphoma of mucosa-associated lymphoid tissue (MALT lymphoma)

Definition
Pulmonary extranodal marginal zone lymphoma of mucosa-associated lymphoid tissue (MALT) origin (MALT lymphoma) is an extranodal lymphoma composed of a morphologically heterogeneous infiltrate made up of small B cells, monocytoid B cells, scattered immunoblasts, and centroblast-like cells. Plasma cell differentiation occurs in some cases. Neoplastic B cells predominate in the marginal zone of reactive follicles, and extend into the interfollicular region. The cells often infiltrate the bronchiolar mucosal epithelium, forming lymphoepithelial lesions.

ICD-O code   9699/3

Synonyms
Pseudolymphoma (obsolete); bronchus-associated lymphoid tissue (BALT) lymphoma; BALTOMA

Epidemiology
MALT lymphomas make up approximately 70–90% of all primary pulmonary lymphomas, but they account for < 0.5% of all primary lung neoplasms, and a similarly low proportion of all lymphomas. Patients tend to be in their fifth, sixth, or seventh decades, and there is a slight female predominance {168,1368,1844,2454}.

Etiology
Pulmonary MALT lymphomas are thought to arise in acquired MALT secondary to inflammatory or autoimmune processes. MALT is not thought to be a normal constituent of the human bronchus, and likely develops in this site as a response to various antigenic stimuli (e.g. smoking, autoimmune disease {1847}, and particularly Sjögren syndrome {1074,1107}). A common association (as is seen between gastric lymphomas of MALT origin and *Helicobacter pylori* infection) has not

been found, although the incidence of individual chlamydiae was higher in MALT lymphomas than in tissue without lymphoproliferative disease {34,391}. Rare cases are seen in patients with common variable immunodeficiency syndrome {510}, but lymphoid hyperplasia is much more common in this setting {2269}. The etiology of most cases of pulmonary MALT lymphoma is unknown.

Clinical features

Signs and symptoms
The most common presentation is a mass discovered on a chest radiograph in an asymptomatic patient. Symptomatic patients present with cough, dyspnoea, chest pain, and haemoptysis. Previous or synchronous MALT lymphomas at other extranodal sites are not uncommon. Monoclonal gammopathy is rarely evident; its presence warrants clinical evaluation and genetic studies (e.g. *MYD88* mutation analysis) to rule out pulmonary involvement by lymphoplasmacytic lymphoma associated with Waldenstrom macroglobulinaemia {1673}. Rarely, patients manifest systemic or so-called B symptoms {235,1043,1368,1890}.

Imaging
Chest radiographs and high-resolution CT show multiple solitary masses or alveolar opacities with associated air bronchograms. High-resolution CT may also show airway dilatation, positive angiogram signs, and haloes of ground-glass shadowing at lesion margins {1272,2454}. A diffuse interstitial pattern may rarely be seen {117}. Most lesions demonstrate homogeneous increased uptake on FDG PET {2971,3018}.

Tumour spread
When distant spread occurs, there is preferential spread to other mucosal sites rather than to lymph nodes (just as other lymphomas of MALT origin may spread to the lung), although the incidence of nodal involvement varies considerably between series {1844,1890,2454}.

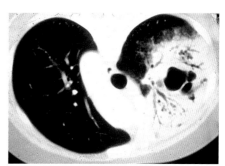

Fig. 1.161 Extranodal marginal zone lymphoma of mucosa-associated lymphoid tissue. High-resolution CT shows a localized area of consolidation, with ground-glass changes at the periphery. Air bronchograms and focal cystic air spaces are also present.

Pulmonary MALT lymphomas not infrequently co-involve ocular and gastrointestinal sites {1101,1891}. However, immunoglobulin sequences may be distinct in different sites, suggesting that tumours may arise in a background of chronic antigenic stimulation leading to oligoclonal and eventually monoclonal expansion {1323}. Rarely, disease may present in the pleura {1686}.

Staging
Cases with unilateral pulmonary involvement are stage IE, and cases with regional lymph node (hilar/mediastinal) involvement are stage IIE. Bilateral pulmonary involvement, even in the absence of nodal disease, is stage IV {2454}.

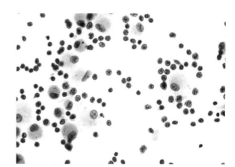

Fig. 1.162 Extranodal marginal zone lymphoma of mucosa-associated lymphoid tissue. Cells in a bronchoalveolar lavage show a homogeneous population of small lymphocytes, mixed with alveolar macrophages, that showed B-cell phenotype on immunohistochemistry.

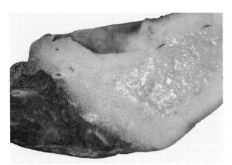

Fig. 1.163 Extranodal marginal zone lymphoma of mucosa-associated lymphoid tissue. The tumour consists of a localized area of consolidation with a solid, cream-coloured cut surface that is similar in texture to the cut surface of a lymph node involved by lymphoma.

Localization

These tumours have no zonal or lobar predisposition. They are typically peripheral, and range from solitary nodules {235,1043,1368,1844,1890} to diffuse bilateral disease (the pattern that mimics lymphoid interstitial pneumonia) {117}. Rare cases may be predominantly endobronchial {2971}.

Macroscopy

Nodular areas of pulmonary involvement by pulmonary MALT lymphomas typically show a consolidative mass that is yellow to cream in colour and similar in texture to the cut surface of a lymph node involved by lymphoma {1272}. Rarely, tumours are focally cystic – often those with coexistent amyloidosis {1403}.

Cytology

Primary diagnosis of MALT lymphoma based only on cytological specimens is not advised, due to the tumours' polymorphous cellular composition. Cells may be obtained for examination from both bronchoalveolar lavage {234} and aspiration biopsy {1295}. Aspiration samples are usually cellular, and include generally numerous, closely aggregated (but not cohesive) populations of small lymphoid cells, sometimes called lymphoid tangles {1295}. The individual cells are small and have solitary nuclei, which tend to be relatively smooth and round with even dark chromatin and inconspicuous nucleoli. A proportion of the cells may show plasmacytoid features.

Viable cells derived from fine-needle aspiration biopsies may be studied by flow cytometry for surface markers and immunoglobulin expression. In cell block preparations, immunohistochemistry and/or PCR are necessary to confirm monoclonality {1295}. Distinction from other B-cell lymphomas in the lung is difficult on cytological grounds alone. FISH may provide further confirmation of the diagnosis in limited samples, by identifying MALT-associated translocations.

Histopathology

Pulmonary MALT lymphomas generally appear as a diffuse infiltrate of small lymphoid cells, which surround reactive follicles. Follicles, best seen when highlighted with a CD21 stain, may be overrun by tumour cells (follicular colonization). Tumours are composed of small lymphocytes, plasmacytoid lymphocytes, so-called centrocyte-like B cells, and monocytoid B cells, which are all thought to be variations of the same neoplastic cell {1093,1368}. Infiltration of bronchial, bronchiolar, and alveolar epithelium (lymphoepithelial lesions) is characteristic but not pathognomonic, since this phenomenon can be seen in non-neoplastic pulmonary lymphoid infiltrates. Scattered transformed large cells (centroblasts and immunoblasts) are typically seen, but are in the minority. Lymphoid cells often track along bronchovascular bundles and interlobular septa at the periphery of masses, but alveolar parenchyma is destroyed towards their centres. Airways are often left intact, correlating with the presence of air bronchograms on high-resolution CT. Central sclerosis may also be a feature. Giant lamellar bodies are seen in about 20% of cases, most likely reflecting the indolent nature of the neoplasm {2034}. Vascular infiltration, pleural involvement, and granuloma formation are not uncommon, but have no prognostic significance. Necrosis is very rare. Coexistent amyloidosis may be present {904}; it may also be seen in association with crystal-storing histiocytosis of the lung {2204,3012}, and may rarely be obscured by organizing pneumonia {529} (see *Diffuse large B-cell lymphoma*, p. 136).

Immunohistochemistry

The neoplastic cells are monoclonal B cells, and may be identified by CD20 or CD79a staining, with a variable reactive T-cell population in the background. Flow cytometry identifies light chain restriction on viable cells in suspension, but due to the presence of reactive germinal centres, a prominent polyclonal background may be present.

Cells with plasmacytoid differentiation show monotypic cytoplasmic immunoglobulin, most often of the IgM class. Rare cases may be CD5-positive {1135}. The neoplastic B-cells are negative for CD10, CD23 and Bcl6. CD43 is expressed in some cases, but is not specific. The tumour cells are usually positive for BCL2. Stains for follicular dendritic cells, such as CD21, CD23, and CD35, highlight reactive follicles, which may be disrupted and overrun. The proliferation fraction (Ki-67) is usually low (< 20%);

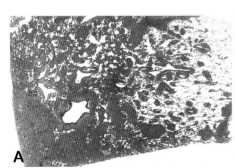
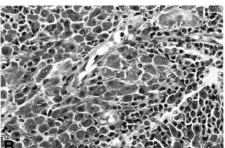
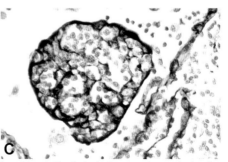

Fig. 1.164 Extranodal marginal zone lymphoma of mucosa-associated lymphoid tissue. **A** A monotonous population of small lymphoid cells track along bronchovascular bundles and interlobular septa at the periphery of the mass, with increased filling and destruction of alveolar parenchyma towards their centre. **B** The lymphoma is associated with a crystal-storing histiocytosis, with a monomorphous population of plasmacytoid cells mixed with histiocytes filled with crystalloid structures. **C** Lymphoepithelial lesions are highlighted by this MNF116 cytokeratin stain.

residual follicles show numerous Ki-67positive cells. Stains for cytokeratin highlight lymphoepithelial lesions.

Differential diagnosis
Based on clinical and imaging aspects, the differential diagnoses include sarcoidosis, invasive mucinous adenocarcinoma, organizing pneumonia, infections, and rarer alveolar filling disorders. The histological differential diagnoses include both non-neoplastic conditions (lymphoid interstitial pneumonia, nodular lymphoid hyperplasia, IgG4-related disease, and hypersensitivity pneumonitis) and neoplastic conditions. Lymphoid hyperplasia affecting the lung is common in a variety of immune conditions, including common variable immunodeficiency disorder {2269} and Sjögren's syndrome {1616}. For both of the above conditions, distinction from MALT lymphoma may be difficult with limited biopsy material {517}. In relation to lymphoid interstitial pneumonia, pulmonary MALT lymphomas tend to infiltrate and destroy the alveolar architecture, with greater widening of alveolar septa by the lymphoid infiltrate. Lymphoepithelial lesions are more prominent in lymphoma, but are not specific. The presence of expanded infiltrates of B cells outside of follicles is characteristic of MALT lymphoma, while in reactive infiltrates, CD20-positive B cells are present mainly within primary or secondary follicles.
Histologically, nodular lymphoid hyperplasia consists of numerous reactive germinal centres with well-preserved mantle zones and interfollicular sheets of mature plasma cells, with varying degrees of interfollicular fibrosis {4}. Increased numbers of IgG4 plasma cells may be present {916}, and nodular lymphoid hyperplasia may be part of the spectrum of IgG4-related disease. PCR shows no rearrangements of the immunoglobulin genes, and there is no light chain restriction in reactive conditions {4,1845}.
The differential diagnoses, particularly on small biopsy specimens, also include other small B-cell lymphomas, such as follicular lymphoma, mantle cell lymphoma, small lymphocytic lymphoma, and lymphoplasmacytic lymphoma. A lack of cyclin D1 and a lack of CD10 and Bcl6 help to exclude mantle cell lymphoma and follicular lymphoma, respectively. Lymphoplasmacytic lymphoma, typically associated with Waldenstrom

macroglobulinaemia, has a more monomorphic cytology, and is associated with the L265P mutation in *MYD88* in a high proproportion of cases {1053}.
MALT lymphoma has a polymorphous cellular composition, and may contain large cells resembling centroblasts or immunoblasts. Sheets of large cells should raise suspicion for diffuse large B-cell lymphoma (see *Diffuse large B-cell lymphoma*, p. 136).

Genetic profile
Immunoglobulin genes are clonally rearranged. The most common genetic aberration in pulmonary MALT lymphomas is t(11;18)(q21;q21) {432,1079,1770,1942,2955}, followed by t(14;18)(q32;q21) {432,2485} – both involve the *MALT1* gene at locus 18q21 {2139,2140}. The translocation frequency in pulmonary MALT lymphoma ranges from 14% to 57%. The t(11;18)(q21;q21) translocation results in a functional fusion protein containing the N terminus of *API2* {1773}. The t(14;18)(q32;q21) translocation occurs in approximately 5% of MALT lymphomas, and brings the *MALT1* gene under the control of the *IGH* enhancer on chromosome 14, resulting in the deregulated expression of *MALT1*. These translocations lead to activation of the NF-κB signalling pathways, implicated in tumour growth {1263}. *A20* deletion (6q23.3) and *TNFa/b/c* gain (6p.21.222.1) are seen in translocation-negative MALT lymphomas at other sites (particularly ocular), but are not seen in the lung {392}. Trisomies involving chromosomes 3, 7, 12, and 18 are also frequently found.

Prognosis and predictive factors
In patients with resectable disease, surgery has resulted in prolonged remission, but for those with either bilateral or unresectable unilateral disease, treatment (such as with chlorambucil {235}) has been governed by the principles that apply to more advanced nodal lymphomas {3029}. Fludarabine and mitoxantrone regimes have been associated with an 80% complete response {3030}. The addition of rituximab, or rituximab alone, is also of value in some patients {1889,2454}, although this may lead to pure plasma cell histology {1281}.
The 5-year survival rate for MALT lymphoma is reported at 84–94% {85,235,2454}, and 10-year survival at 70% {235,1368}. Prognostic data are variable. One study

showed a median time to progression of 5.6 years, with extrapulmonary involvement and lymph node involvement being poor prognostic factors {1890}. In a review of 326 cases from the SEER database, 55% were stage IE, 10% were stage IIE, 3% were stage IIIE, and 22% were stage IV; after a median follow-up of 35 months, the median overall survival was 112 months, with the disease-specific median survival not reached. At 90 months, disease-specific survival was 85%, with no significant differences in outcome between patients presenting with different stages {2454}.

Diffuse large B-cell lymphoma

Definition
Diffuse large B-cell lymphoma (DLBCL) is a lymphoma that consists of a diffuse proliferation of large B cells (i.e. B cells with a nuclear size equal to or exceeding that of a normal macrophage nucleus, or more than twice the size of a normal lymphocyte). Primary pulmonary DLBCL tumours are those that are localized to the lungs at presentation. DLBCL is not a single disease; it includes DLBCL, not otherwise specified, as well as other aggressive B-cell lymphomas with differing morphologies and etiologies. Among these, EBV-positive large B-cell lymphoma in the elderly also occurs with some frequency in the lung.

ICD-O code   9680/3

Synonyms
Diffuse large B-cell non-Hodgkin lymphoma; high-grade mucosa-associated lymphoid tissue lymphoma (not recommended)

Epidemiology
DLBCL accounts for about 5–20% of all primary pulmonary lymphomas {1254,1335,1674,1844}. Patients are usually aged between 50 and 70 years at presentation (similar to pulmonary extranodal marginal zone lymphoma of mucosa-associated lymphoid tissue). There is no sex predisposition. EBV-positive large B-cell lymphomas are predominantly seen in elderly patients, with median age of > 70 years.

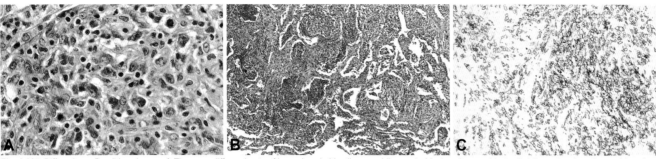

Fig. 1.165 Diffuse large B-cell lymphoma. **A** There are diffuse sheets of large, lymphoid cells resembling centroblasts or immunoblasts, 2–4 times the size of normal lymphocytes. **B** The tumour cells are partly obscured by coexistent organizing pneumonia. **C** CD20 staining highlights the diffuse infiltration of the organizing pneumonia by neoplastic large B cells.

Etiology

The etiology of most DLBCLs is unknown. An association between diffuse large B-cell non-Hodgkin lymphomas arising in the lung and collagen vascular diseases (both with and without associated pulmonary fibrosis) has been described {1847}. Iatrogenic immunosuppression may lead to EBV-associated pulmonary lymphoma, which cannot be excluded in previous cases. Both congenital immunodeficiency disorders and AIDS may be predisposing factors for EBV-positive large B-cell lymphomas presenting in the lung. Age-related EBV-positive large B-cell lymphoma is a provisional entity {2548} associated with decreased immune surveillance {610,1950}. A large proportion of cases occur in extranodal sites, including the lung.

Clinical features

Patients are nearly always symptomatic, and present with cough, haemoptysis, and dyspnoea. Some patients report systemic (so-called B) symptoms. Imaging shows solid and often multiple masses. DLBCL may present, with single or multiple nodules, or consolidation {1254}. Extranodal DLBCL can be limited to the lungs, involve other extranodal sites, or involve hilar and mediastinal lymph nodes.

Cases with unilateral pulmonary involvement are considered stage IE, and cases with regional lymph node (hilar/mediastinal) involvement are IIE. Bilateral pulmonary involvement constitutes stage IV disease.

Localization

DLBCLs have no zonal or lobar predisposition, and are typically peripheral.

Macroscopy

The nodules are typically solid and cream-coloured. They may also exhibit paler and softer areas that correlate with necrosis.

Cytology

Smears may be prepared from both exfoliative material and fine-needle aspirates. They are dominated by a largely monotonous population of individual neoplastic lymphocytes. The malignant cells have distinct and variably irregular nuclear membranes. Chromatin tends to be vesicular, with nucleoli. Cytoplasm tends to be scant, resulting in high nuclear-to-cytoplasmic ratios. A consistent feature of aspirates is fragments of lymphoid cell cytoplasm (so-called lymphoglandular bodies) in the smear background. Fine-needle aspiration biopsy is useful for triage and the differential diagnosis of lymphoma versus other neoplasms; however, primary diagnosis of DLBCL is not advised on cytological specimens alone.

Histopathology

DLBCLs of the lung are morphologically similar to those in other sites. The tumours consist of diffuse sheets of large, lymphoid cells resembling centroblasts or immunoblasts, 2–4 times the size of normal lymphocytes, infiltrating and destroying the lung parenchyma. Vascular infiltration and pleural involvement are commonly seen, but lymphoepithelial lesions are rare. Necrosis is common. Superimposed pneumonia may mask the lymphoma.

The neoplastic cells are of B-cell phenotype, expressing pan-B-cell antigens (CD20 and CD79a), with a variable reactive T-cell population in the background. However, the CD20 phenotype may be lost after treatment with rituximab {1281}. Light chain restriction usually cannot be detected by immunohistochemistry, but may be observed by flow cytometry. Subclassification into germinal centre B-cell and activated B-cell subtypes of DLBCL may be accomplished through the use of gene expression profiling or immunohistochemical algorithms {439,1060,1092}. The presence of EBV should be investigated by in situ hybridization for EBV-encoded small RNA.

Differential diagnosis

The differential diagnoses include undifferentiated carcinoma of either large cell or small cell type, some variants of Hodgkin lymphoma, anaplastic large cell lymphoma, and (rarely) germ cell tumours. The diagnosis can usually be made using an immunohistochemical panel including cytokeratins, placental alkaline phosphatase, CD20, CD3, CD30, ALK1, CD15, CD45, and epithelial membrane antigen. Primary pulmonary DLBCL must be distinguished from primary mediastinal large B-cell lymphoma, which is frequently associated with extension to lung (see *Primary mediastinal large B-cell lymphoma,* p. 267). Knowledge of the clinical features, including the age and sex of the patient and the presence of a mediastinal mass, is important in establishing the correct diagnosis. Distinction from EBV-positive DLBCL and pulmonary lymphomatoid granulomatosis may be difficult. In lymphomatoid granulomatosis, the T-cell infiltrate is usually more prominent, with the EBV-positive cells showing a greater range in size than in EBV-positive DLBCL.

Genetic profile

Immunoglobulin genes are clonally rearranged. Based on patterns obtained with gene expression profiling, DLBCL, not otherwise specified, is divided into germinal centre B-cell and activated B-cell subtypes {1124}. Little is known about genetic abnormalities in primary pulmonary DLBCL.

Prognosis and predictive factors

Patients may inadvertently undergo resection for localized disease, but are usually treated with combination immunochemotherapy as employed for DLBCL in other sites. Patients with involvement of extranodal sites, such as the lung, generally have a poorer prognosis {340,2559}. The International Prognostic Index, with more recent modifications, is most widely applied as a prognostic guide {3027}.

Lymphomatoid granulomatosis

Definition

Lymphomatoid granulomatosis is a rare disorder characterized by pulmonary nodules composed of an angiocentric/ angiodestructive polymorphous lymphoid infiltrate containing EBV-positive B cells and a large number of reactive T cells, which usually predominate. The EBV-positive B cells vary in number and cytological atypia. The number of EBV-positive B cells and their cytological atypia determine histological grade, and correlate with prognosis.

ICD-O code   9766/1

Synonym

Angiocentric immunoproliferative lesion (obsolete)

Epidemiology

The median age at the time of lymphomatoid granulomatosis diagnosis is in the sixth decade, although the disorder may occur at any age. The male-to-female ratio is 2:1. Lymphomatoid granulomatosis is more common in

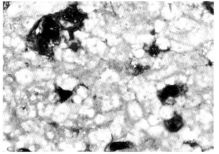
Fig. 1.166 Grade 2 lymphomatoid granulomatosis. Double labelling in situ hybridization for EBV with immunohistochemical staining for CD20 shows that CD20 (brown) decorates cells that are also positive for EBV by in situ hybridization (black). Reprinted from Guinee D Jr et al. {914}.

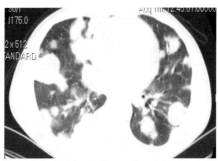
Fig. 1.167 Lymphomatoid granulomatosis. Chest CT shows multiple cavitary masses.

immunocompromised patients – such as those with AIDS or congenital immunodeficiencies such as X-linked lymphoproliferative disease or Wiskott-Aldrich syndrome {944,1073,1690} (see below). Lymphomatoid granulomatosis appears to be more common in western countries than in Asia.

Etiology

Based on multiple studies using double labelling/in situ hybridization, lymphomatoid granulomatosis is considered to be an EBV-associated B-cell lymphoproliferative disorder, with prominent background T-cell reaction {914,917,1780,1846}. Diminished immunity is an important factor in the development of lymphomatoid granulomatosis. The incidence of lymphomatoid granulomatosis is higher in patients with congenital or acquired immunodeficiency (e.g. Wiskott-Aldrich syndrome and AIDS) {944,1073,1125}. Previously healthy patients with lymphomatoid granulomatosis have been shown to have various defects in cell-mediated and/or humoral immunity {2436,2887}. Although lymphomatoid granulomatosis has been reported in recipients of solid organ transplants, such cases would now be classified as post-transplant lymphoproliferative disorder (PTLD) {935,1663,2797}.

Clinical features

Presenting symptoms include cough, chest pain, and dyspnoea. Extrapulmonary symptoms reflect the sites involved. Symptoms of central nervous system involvement (present in 30% of cases) include confusion, dementia, ataxia, and cranial nerve palsies. Cutaneous symptoms include macular rashes, nodules and plaques {705,1221,1333,1472}.
On routine chest X-ray, well to poorly defined pulmonary nodules or masses are present throughout both lungs,

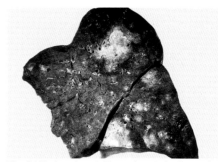
Fig. 1.168 Lymphomatoid granulomatosis. Gross view shows multiple yellow-white necrotic masses.

predominantly involving the lower lobes. Hilar adenopathy is usually absent {1221,1333,1472}. On high-resolution CT, nodules are located along bronchovascular structures or interlobular septa, sometimes accompanied by thin-walled cystic lesions representing cavitation within pre-existing nodules {1437}. Rare cases may present with interstitial infiltrates and ground-glass opacities, mimicking interstitial lung disease {1100}.

Localization

Lymphomatoid granulomatosis involves the lung in nearly all cases. Involvement of extrapulmonary sites is also common – including the central nervous system (30%), kidney (30%), skin (> 40%), gastrointestinal tract, and other organs. Involvement of lymph nodes or bone marrow is rare {1221,1333,1472}.

Macroscopy

Gross examination of resected specimens from the lung shows single or multiple nodules or masses of variable size, with or without central necrosis. The nodules are often bilateral in distribution. Nodular lesions from the kidney and brain often contain central necrosis {1221,1333,1472}.

Cytology

Diagnosis of lymphomatoid granulomatosis should not be made on cytological specimens.

Histopathology

Histologically, lymphomatoid granulomatosis is characterized by nodules containing a polymorphous lymphoid infiltrate with an angiocentric distribution. The majority of cells are lymphocytes, admixed with variable numbers of histiocytes, plasma cells, and immunoblasts. Marked central necrosis is often (although variably) present. Lymphomatoid

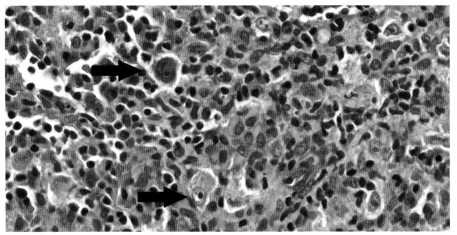

Fig. 1.169 Lymphomatoid granulomatosis. A grade 2 lesion shows large atypical immunoblasts (arrows) with variably prominent nucleoli present in a mixed polymorphous background of small lymphocytes and macrophages.

granulomatosis is further distinguished by two key features: 1) the infiltrate is strikingly angiocentric, with transmural involvement by lymphocytes of small and medium-sized arteries; and 2) there are variable numbers of large B cells that are positive for EBV by in situ hybridization {914,1221,1223,1333,1472}. The EBV-positive cells vary in size and may show cytological atypia. They may have an appearance of immunoblasts or superficially resemble Reed-Sternberg (RS) cells with multinucleate forms. Nonetheless, classical RS cells are usually not identified, and if present, should lead to consideration of Hodgkin lymphoma. Despite the name, well-formed granulomas are typically absent in lesions of the lung and other extranodal sites {1484}. However, a granulomatous reaction may be present in the subcutaneous tissue of cutaneous lesions {161}. The inflammatory infiltrate affecting the vessels is polymorphous, and usually dominated by T cells {1222}.

Lymphomatoid granulomatosis is graded by comparing the proportion of EBV-positive B cells and their degree of cytological atypia to the background population of reactive T lymphocytes. Distinction of grade 3 lesions from either grade 1 or grade 2 lesions is most important. Cases with a uniform population of large atypical EBV-positive B cells are outside the spectrum of lymphomatoid granulomatosis, and are best classified as EBV-positive large B-cell lymphoma (see *Diffuse large B-cell lymphoma*, p. 136).

Some authors have questioned the validity of grading based on the number of EBV-positive cells present, contending that there is little evidence to support the value of this approach, and that there is considerable diversity of grading in the sampling from one nodule of lymphomatoid granulomatosis to another in the same biopsy {476,1222}. Nonetheless, despite these limitations, grading is conceptually reasonable, and although imperfect, does provide prognostic and therapeutic information.

Grade 1 lesions are composed of a polymorphous lymphoid infiltrate without significant atypia. Necrosis may be absent or focal. Large transformed lymphocytes are absent or rare. EBV-positive cells are

rare and may be absent. In grade 2 lesions, occasional large lymphoid cells are present. Necrosis is more common. The number of EBV-positive cells is variable, but ranges from 5 to 50 per high-power field. Grade 3 lesions are characterized by a greater number of large atypical B cells. These are readily identified by CD20, and may occur in clusters. The atypical B cells show striking pleomorphism, and may superficially resemble Hodgkin cells. Necrosis is common and often extensive. EBV-positive cells are numerous (> 50 per high-power field) and may form confluent aggregates. In the presence of extensive necrosis, due to poor RNA preservation, in situ hybridization for EBV may be unreliable. In this case, additional molecular studies for EBV (e.g. PCR) may be helpful in supporting the diagnosis.

Immunohistochemistry
On immunohistochemistry, the scattered large atypical lymphoid cells stain positively for the pan-B-cell marker CD20. EBV-encoded small RNA can be identified within the atypical cells by in situ hybridization. On double labelling studies with CD20, staining is restricted to the cytologically atypical B cells {914,917,1780,1846}. The cells may stain positively for LMP1, are variably positive for CD30, and are negative for CD15. Immunohistochemical stains for kappa and lambda are of limited utility, although rare cases may show monoclonal light chain expression in admixed plasma cells {2887}. The smaller background reactive lymphocytes, which constitute the majority of cells, stain positively for the pan-T-cell marker CD3, with the number of CD4+ cells usually exceeding that of CD8+ cells. Many of the lymphocytes infiltrating the vascular walls are of T-cell derivation.

Differential diagnosis
The differential diagnoses of lymphomatoid granulomatosis include pulmonary involvement by peripheral T-cell lymphoma, PTLD, nasal-type extranodal T/NK-cell lymphoma, Wegener's granulomatosis, and several other conditions that occasionally may superficially resemble lymphomatoid granulomatosis.

Pulmonary involvement by T-cell lymphomas may resemble lymphomatoid granulomatosis. However, the large atypical cells do not stain with B-cell markers, but

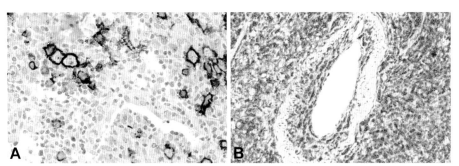

Fig. 1.170 Lymphomatoid granulomatosis. **A** Immunohistochemical staining shows that CD20 decorates the scattered large cytologically atypical cells. **B** Immunohistochemical staining for CD3 highlights the background majority of small lymphocytes, which permeate the wall and intima of a small artery.

instead stain with T-cell markers such as CD3. EBV is generally not identified in these cases by in situ hybridization techniques. The histological features of PTLD in the lung overlap with those of lymphomatoid granulomatosis. Consideration of the clinical history is of critical importance. Pulmonary lesions resembling lymphomatoid granulomatosis in transplant recipients are best considered variants of PTLD {1222}.

Similar to lymphomatoid granulomatosis, the cells of extranodal T/NK-cell lymphoma contain EBV by in situ hybridization. However, unlike in lymphomatoid granulomatosis, most of the large atypical cells express CD3 and NK-associated antigens (CD56). Scattered, cytologically atypical B cells are not identified. Clinical history is also important, because extranodal/NK-cell lymphomas usually present as aggressive destructive lesions in the nasal cavity {1123}.

Wegener's granulomatosis is easily differentiated based on its clinical and histological features. Despite its name, lymphomatoid granulomatosis lacks the granulomatous inflammation typically present in Wegener's granulomatosis. Likewise, large atypical EBV-positive B cells are not seen in Wegener's granulomatosis.

Several other conditions may superficially resemble lymphomatoid granulomatosis. Cases of acute pulmonary histoplasmosis may show a nodular infiltrate with vasculitis and necrosis resembling grade 1 lymphomatoid granulomatosis {1763}. Pulmonary involvement of IgG4-related sclerosing disease may also show striking vascular infiltration and resemble grade 1 lymphomatoid granulomatosis {2929}. Primary or secondary involvement by Hodgkin lymphoma is distinguished by the finding of classical RS cells or their variants in the appropriate cellular milieu {2992}. RS cells and variants stain positively for CD15 and CD30, but are negative for CD3 and CD45. CD20 is focally and variably positive.

Genetic profile

Clonal immunoglobulin heavy chain gene rearrangements may be identified by PCR analysis in most grade 2 and grade 3 lesions {914,1637,1780}. Different clonal rearrangements may occasionally be identified in different lesions or from different sites of involvement from the same patient {1690,2887}.

Clonal rearrangements of the T-cell receptor gene are typically not present {914,1637,1780}. Clonality of EBV may be identified on Southern blot analysis {1639}. Unlike in grade 2 and grade 3 lesions, clonality in grade 1 lesions is often difficult to demonstrate, presumably due to the paucity of EBV-positive cells. Alternatively, some cases of lymphomatoid granulomatosis may be polyclonal.

Prognosis and predictive factors

The prognosis of lymphomatoid granulomatosis is variable. Up to 63% of patients die with a median overall survival of 14 months. However, approximately 14–27% undergo spontaneous remission without treatment {1221}. Death usually occurs due to extensive destruction of the lung and other affected organs.

Treatment depends on the grade of the lesion. IFN-alpha 2b was used in the treatment of grade 1 and grade 2 lesions in one series {2887}. Grade 3 lesions should be considered, for clinical purposes, as similar to diffuse large B-cell lymphoma. Accordingly, treatment for these patients consists of combination chemotherapy with rituximab {1041,2170,2194}.

Intravascular large B-cell lymphoma

Definition

Intravascular lymphoma is a very rare, aggressive subtype of extranodal diffuse large B-cell lymphoma. It is characterized by the presence of lymphoma cells within small vessels, particularly capillaries {2071}.

ICD-O code   9712/3

Synonyms

Malignant angioendotheliomatosis; angioendotheliomatosis proliferans syndrome; intravascular lymphomatosis; angioendotheliotropic lymphoma

Epidemiology

Intravascular lymphoma occurs in adults, with no known sex predisposition.

Etiology

The neoplastic cells have been shown to lack CD29 (integrin beta-1) and CD54 (ICAM1) – a molecule integral to lymphocyte trafficking {2070}. Other tumour types may rarely show a similar pattern of intravascular dissemination, such as lymphomas positive for human herpesvirus 8 {720} or EBV {1199}.

Clinical features

Intravascular lymphoma is a systemic disorder, but it may enter the differential diagnosis of interstitial lung disease at presentation {1297}, and may also cause pulmonary hypertension {1338}, hypoxaemia {1592}, and pulmonary embolism {819}. Associated haemophagocytosis has been reported in Asian patients, particularly Japanese patients, but not in patients from western countries {719}.

Diffuse ground-glass and centrilobular opacities may be seen on CT {2103,2440}, although CT may also be normal {1188}. Recent cases have shown diffuse pulmonary uptake on FDG PET {2928}, sometimes with normal CT {2793,2928}.

In most cases, the disease is disseminated at presentation.

Localization

When the lungs are involved, the disease is generally disseminated, with extensive systemic disease (including involvement of the central nervous system).

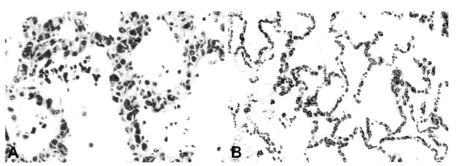
Fig. 1.171 Intravascular large B-cell lymphoma. A Large lymphoma cells fill the alveolar capillaries, with no involvement of the alveolar spaces. B The tumour cells stain for CD20.

Histopathology

The neoplastic lymphoid cells are usually identified solely within the lumens of small arteries, veins, and capillaries, with fibrin thrombi sometimes seen. The tumour cells are large with vesicular nuclei and prominent nucleoli, often with mitotic activity. Rarely, tumours can be anaplastic.

Tumour cells are usually positive for B-cell markers (CD20 and CD79a). CD5 expression is often seen {1241}.

Rare aggressive T-cell lymphomas may show intravascular involvement as well, although these should be identifiable through their different immunohistochemical profile {352,1199}.

Genetic profile

Most cases analysed show immunoglobulin gene rearrangements. An accumulation of structural aberrations in chromosomes 1, 6, and 18, especially 1p and trisomy 18, has been identified {2695}. A t(14;19)(q32;q13) translocation was described in one case {1300}.

Prognosis and predictive factors

Prognosis has historically been poor, although cases of successful treatment with the addition of rituximab have been described {718,1027,2259,2559}.

Pulmonary Langerhans cell histiocytosis

Definition

Pulmonary Langerhans cell histiocytosis (PLCH) is caused by a proliferation of Langerhans cells with associated interstitial changes in the lung. Some cases have a mutation in the *BRAF* gene, and are thus thought to be neoplastic, although clonality is ambiguous in most pulmonary cases.

ICD-O code   9751/1

Synonyms

Pulmonary eosinophilic granuloma; pulmonary Langerhans cell granulomatosis; pulmonary histiocytosis X (obsolete)

Epidemiology

PLCH is an uncommon histiocytic proliferation that presents as interstitial lung disease. Its sex predominance has varied across series; although the incidence in males and females is probably roughly equal. Most patients are adults, and the lung is the sole site of involvement in most cases. The mean age at diagnosis is approximately 40 years, with a wide range of 18–70 years (excluding children with disseminated Langerhans cell histiocytosis) {2762,2763}.

Etiology

More than 95% of patients are current or former cigarette smokers {2762,2763}, and V600E mutations in the *BRAF* gene have been found in 38–57% of cases {115,953,2243,2988}.

Clinical features

Patients may be asymptomatic (in 15–25% of cases), or may present with pulmonary symptoms (e.g. cough, dyspnoea, or chest pain) or systemic complaints (e.g. malaise, weight loss, or fever) {2762,2763}. Approximately 15% of adults with PLCH have extrapulmonary involvement, with features such as diabetes insipidus being a clue to the diagnosis of PLCH {771}.

Pulmonary function studies are abnormal in most patients (≥ 85%), and include (in order of decreasing frequency) restrictive deficits, obstructive deficits, isolated decreased diffusing capacity, and mixed restrictive/obstructive deficits {2763}. The systemic form of Langerhans cell

histiocytosis may involve the lung secondarily {1126}.

Chest radiographs show interstitial lung disease with predilection for the mid- and upper lung zones {2763}. High-resolution CT is distinctive, most typically showing nodules or nodules and cystic change with mid- and upper lung zone predilection {2763}. Diffuse metabolic activity on FDG PET-CT has recently been used to measure disease activity in the lungs {2552}.

Localization

PLCH occurs predominantly in the upper and middle zones, with sparing of the costophrenic angles.

Macroscopy

The lungs may appear cystic and contain stellate localized fibrous scars, depending on the extent and activity of disease.

Cytology

Lesional cells can be identified in bronchoalveolar lavage fluid, which may assist in the diagnosis of Langerhans cell histiocytosis {948}.

Histopathology

Histologically, most cases of PLCH show concomitant changes of smoking, including emphysema and respiratory bronchiolitis {2762,2763}. The lesions of PLCH begin as cellular proliferations of Langerhans cells along small airways, primarily bronchioles and alveolar ducts. As the lesions enlarge, rounded or stellate nodules develop and the bronchiolocentricity is less easy to discern. The nodules undergo a natural history progression from cellular lesions rich in Langerhans cells to fibrotic (often stellate) scars, which in their end stage are entirely devoid of identifiable Langerhans cells. In healed PLCH cases, the diagnosis is possible

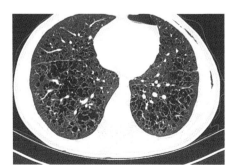

Fig. 1.172 Langerhans cell histiocytosis. CT shows a combination of thin-walled cysts and a few poorly defined nodules.

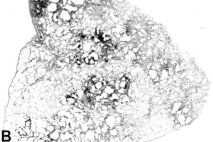

Fig. 1.173 Langerhans cell histiocytosis. **A** Lesional cells have pale cytoplasm, with indistinct cell borders and delicate infolded nuclei. A few eosinophils and lymphocytes are present. **B** Cellular lesions of Langerhans cells stain for S100.

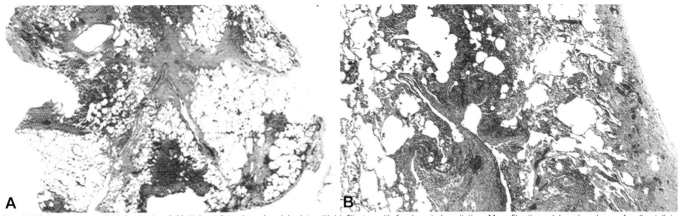

Fig. 1.174 Langerhans cell histiocytosis. **A** Multiple stellate-shaped nodular interstitial infiltrates with focal central cavitation. More fibrotic nodules also show a focally stellate architecture. **B** Early lesions are bronchocentric and show focal central cavitation.

based on the presence of stellate centri-lobular scarring in the setting of typical high-resolution CT changes. Cyst formation is also commonly seen as lesions develop.

Langerhans cells are recognized by their distinctive morphology, with pale eosinophilic cytoplasm and delicate nuclei with prominent folding of the nuclear membranes {1471,2762,2763}.

Immunohistochemistry, genetics, and ultrastructure

Langerhans cells are positive for S100, CD1a, and langerin, typically showing aggregation into nodules, although cells can rarely be intra-alveolar. Classical cases can be diagnosed on morphology alone. Conversely, burnt-out cases may be totally lacking in the lesional cells. Birbeck granules are seen on ultrastructural analysis within the Langerhans cells. V600E mutations in the *BRAF* gene have been described in 38–57% of patients with Langerhans cell histiocytosis, although relatively few of the tested cases

were of lung origin {115,953,2243}. A lower incidence, approximately 30%, has been reported in PLCH {2176}. Concurrent nodules in 2 of 5 patients with PLCH showed *BRAF* V600E mutations {2988}. It is speculated that smoking may generate transversion of this allele within multiple clones in the lung, producing polyclonal disease with the same mutation {115}. Cases with the mutation stain positively with a monoclonal antibody to the mutant protein, whether primary in the lung or not {2176}.

Prognosis and predictive factors

Approximately 15% of patients have progressive respiratory disease that may be fatal or lead to lung transplantation {2763}. Progression may be slow (spanning decades), and may be dominated by clinical features of obstructive lung disease. Predictors of shorter survival include older age, lower forced expiratory volume in 1 second (FEV1), higher residual volume, lower ratio of FEV1 to forced vital capacity, and reduced carbon monoxide

diffusing capacity {2763}. Development of pulmonary hypertension is also associated with increased mortality {1425}.Steroids are the mainstay therapy for PLCH {2762,2763}. Smoking cessation is also important, although a prospective study showed no difference in survival between those who stopped smoking and those who continued {2305}. Refractory cases may respond to immunosuppressive therapy, while other cases of PLCH clear spontaneously.

Erdheim-Chester disease

Definition

Erdheim-Chester disease is a rare xan-thogranulomatous histiocytosis characterized by infiltration of the skeleton and viscera by lipid-laden histiocytes. In the lung, this leads to interstitial fibrosis with a perilymphatic distribution.

ICD-O code   9750/1

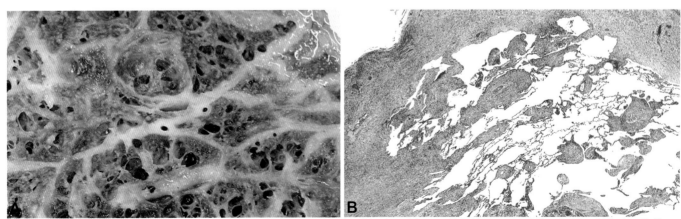

Fig. 1.175 Erdheim-Chester disease. **A** The cut surface of the lung shows fibrous thickening of the visceral pleura and interlobular septa. **B** There is diffuse thickening with fibrous tissue and cellular histiocytic infiltration predominantly involving the visceral pleura, interlobular septa, and bronchovascular bundles, with relative sparing of the alveolar interstitium.

Synonyms

Lipogranulomatosis; lipoidgranulomatosis; lipid (cholesterol) granulomatosis; polyostotic sclerosing histiocytosis

Epidemiology

Erdheim-Chester disease involves the lungs in 20–30% of patients {343}, and there is a slight male predominance. Peak incidence occurs within the fifth to seventh decade, with a range of 4–87 years and a mean age at diagnosis of 53 years {86,87,343}.

Etiology

Erdheim-Chester disease is believed to be a clonal disorder, with a V600E mutation in the *BRAF* gene present in more than half of all cases. The proliferation may be associated with an intense helper T cell type 1 immune response {2476}.

Clinical features

Pulmonary symptoms are typically cough and dyspnoea, although pulmonary involvement may also be asymptomatic {343}. Pleural effusions occur in about 20% of patients {87}. General symptoms consist of mild bone pain (occasionally associated with soft tissue swelling), fever, weight loss, and weakness. Other manifestations include exophthalmos, diabetes insipidus, kidney failure, and cardiac or neurological symptoms. The serum lipid profile is relatively normal.

The lung is involved in more than half of all cases with thoracic involvement, with septal and subpleural thickening, poorly defined centrilobular nodular opacities, ground-glass opacities, and lung cysts being reported {270,2898}. Mediastinal infiltration, pleural thickening, and effusions are also commonly seen {270}.

Localization

The lung is involved in 20–30% of cases, and the skeleton is nearly always involved {343}. Other extraskeletal manifestations (e.g. in the kidney/retroperitoneum, the heart/pericardium, or the central nervous system) occur in > 50% of cases.

Macroscopy

The lung is firm, with pleural and interlobular septa often visible due to thickening.

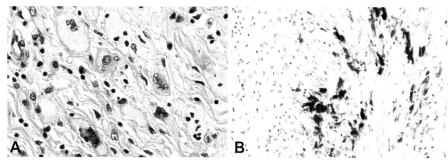

Fig. 1.176 Erdheim-Chester disease. **A** Diffuse infiltration by histiocytic cells including a few Touton giant cells. **B** The histiocytes stain for S100.

Cytology

Patients may undergo bronchoalveolar lavage as part of investigations for interstitial lung disease, and these show a predominance of histiocytes that are often foamy in morphology. Occasional cases have been shown to be S100-positive and CD1a-negative {87}.

Histopathology

Architecturally, histiocytic infiltration and fibrosis predominate along the distribution of the pulmonary lymphatics (visceral pleura, bronchovascular bundles, and interlobular septa). Histiocytes are often foamy, with Touton giant cells often seen. This is associated with variably dense fibrosis, lymphocytes, plasma cells, and eosinophils.

Immunohistochemistry

This confirms the monocyte/macrophage lineage of the lipid-laden foamy histiocytes and giant cells by their expression of Factor XIIIa, lysozyme, MAC387, CD68 (KP1), CD4, alpha-1 antichymotrypsin, alpha-1 antitrypsin, and S100 protein (variable) {2229}. They are negative for CD1a. Electron microscopy shows a predominance of histiocytes with indented nuclei; abundant intracytoplasmic lipid vacuoles; and sparse mitochondria, lysosomes, and endoplasmic reticulum. Birbeck granules are absent {656}.

Differential diagnosis

Due to its presentation with bony lesions and the involvement of various viscera, Erdheim-Chester disease may clinically mimic malignancy, especially other lymphoproliferative diseases, lymphangitis carcinomatosis {2919}, and even mesothelioma (due to its prominent pleural involvement) {1839,2092}. In the lungs, because of the lymphatic distribution, interstitial lung diseases may enter the differential diagnosis {656}. Cytologically, the main differential diagnosis is Langerhans cell histiocytosis, although the lesional cells are more foamy in nature, do not stain for CD1a, are variably positive for S100, and lack Birbeck granules on ultrastructural analysis. Furthermore, Langerhans cell histiocytosis typically forms nodules, cysts, and stellate scars that are bronchocentric in distribution.

Genetic profile

BRAF V600E mutations have been detected in 54% of patients {953}, and the histiocytic proliferation has been shown to be clonal in some studies {413,2770}, but not in others {869}.

Prognosis and predictive factors

Involvement of the lungs is a poor prognostic factor, with the majority of patients dying within 3 years, of either pulmonary complications or complications related to other viscera {2229,2777}. However, one study showed no survival difference between patients with pulmonary involvement and those without {87}. Targeted therapy with vemurafenib has been shown to provide rapid clinical and biological response, although with persistence of disease {954}. Patients may also respond to IFN-alpha therapy, and this has been shown to be an independent predictor of survival {86}. Rare response to steroids and cyclophosphamide has also been reported in a case with lung involvement {247}.

Tumours of ectopic origin

E. Duhig
A.G. Nicholson

Germ cell tumours

Definition
Germ cell tumours are a heterogeneous group of neoplasms arising from germ cells. Most germ cell tumours in the lung are teratomas, and consist of tissues derived from more than one embryonic germ layer. The criteria for pulmonary origin are exclusion of a gonadal or other extragonadal primary site, and origin entirely within the lung.

ICD-O codes
Teratoma, mature   9080/0
Teratoma, immature   9080/1

Synonym
Germ cell neoplasms

Epidemiology
The majority of cases occur in the second to fourth decade (with a range of 10 months to 68 years). There is a slight female predisposition.

Etiology
Pulmonary teratomas are thought to arise from ectopic tissues derived from the third pharyngeal pouch.

Clinical features
Patients may present with chest pain, haemoptysis, cough, or pyothorax {91,1741,2593}. Expectoration of hair (trichoptysis) is the most specific symptom of teratoma {1741,2596,2722}.
On imaging, lesions are typically well-circumscribed heterogeneous masses, often cystic with focal calcification {1741}. Mature teratomas remain localized but may rupture. Malignant germ cell tumours may be locally invasive or show distant metastasis {764}.

Localization
Teratomas are more common in the upper lobes, principally on the left side {91,1741,2541}. Cysts are often in continuity with the bronchi, and may have an endobronchial component {1741}.

Macroscopy
The tumours range from 2.8 to 30 cm in diameter. They are generally cystic and multiloculated. Rarely, the tumours may be predominantly solid, and these tend to be immature.

Cytology
Polymorphic constituents may be identified, including hair shafts as well as mesenchymal and epithelial components {2390}.

Histopathology
In teratomas, mesodermal, ectodermal, and endodermal elements are seen in varying proportions {91}, and include bone, cartilage, thymic, and pancreatic elements, as well as hair-bearing squamous-lined cysts. Rupture may cause bronchopleural fistulas and a marked inflammatory and fibrotic reaction. Malignant elements may consist of sarcoma and carcinoma. Immature elements, such as neural tissue, infrequently occur. Rarely, intrapulmonary teratomas may have other germ cell tumour components, including seminoma and yolk sac tumour {764,1187}.
Germ cell malignancies other than immature teratomas are extremely rare, and require exclusion of an extrapulmonary primary tumour.
Immunohistochemistry may be used to delineate components of non-pulmonary origin and non-teratomatous germ cell tumour elements.

Differential diagnosis
Metastatic teratoma requires exclusion via thorough clinical investigation. Trichoptysis is not a specific sign of a lung origin, because it may follow rupture of a mediastinal teratoma into the lung {2533}. Also, teratomas treated by chemotherapy often consist of wholly mature elements in their metastases {305}. Rarely, teratoma may mimic a hamartoma. Glial heterotopia in the lung is usually seen in infants with neural tube defects, and should be distinguished from teratoma {587}. Carcinosarcomas, pleuropulmonary blastomas, and pulmonary

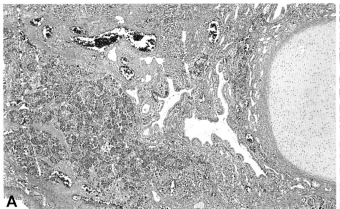
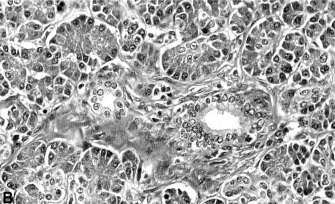

Fig. 1.177 Mature teratoma. **A** Mature cartilage, glands, and pancreatic tissue. **B** Pancreatic tissue with acinar and ductal epithelium.
Reprinted from Colby TV et al. {477} and Travis WD et al. {2678}.

blastomas do not recapitulate specific organ structures.

Non-teratomatous germ cell tumours should be distinguished from carcinomas of the lung (including pleomorphic and giant cell carcinomas), which may produce alpha-fetoprotein, chorionic gonadotropins, or placental lactogen. Most cases reported as choriocarcinoma of the lung are pleomorphic carcinomas with ectopic production of the β-subunit of human chorionic gonadotropin. Instead of the dual population of cytotrophoblasts and syncytiotrophoblasts typical of choriocarcinoma, there is a continuous spectrum of morphology from large to pleomorphic tumour cells.

Prognosis and predictive factors

About 80% of pulmonary teratomas are mature and follow a benign course, unlike immature teratomas in adults, which are aggressive and have a poor prognosis {1538}. Surgery is the treatment of choice, with all mature teratomas being cured {1741}. Resection of malignant teratomas has also led to prolonged disease remission, although most cases were unresectable and the patients died within 6 months of diagnosis.

Intrapulmonary thymoma

Definition
Intrapulmonary thymomas are epithelial neoplasms within the lung that are histologically identical to mediastinal thymoma, and are thought to arise from ectopic thymic rests {1734,1781}.

ICD-O code   8580/3

Epidemiology
Sex distribution differs between series. One series showed a female predisposition {1734}, but others have shown greater equality {1781}. Ages range from 14 to 77 years, with a median age of about 50 years.

Etiology
Intrapulmonary thymoma probably derives from thymic epithelial rests.

Clinical features
Symptoms include cough, weight loss, chest pain, fever, and dyspnoea. Incidental asymptomatic cases have also been reported. Associated paraneoplastic syndromes include myasthenia gravis and Good's syndrome with hypogammaglobulinaemia {1781,2235}.

Most intrapulmonary thymomas are solitary, but multifocal cases involving the same lung have been described. Tumours may show FDG PET positivity {919,3023}.

Most intrapulmonary thymomas remain confined to the lung, but isolated cases have invaded beyond the pleura {1098,3023} or have subsequently recurred in the pleura {1734}. Although nodal involvement has not been described in primary lung tumours, this should be considered, because it is known to occur in primary mediastinal tumours.

Some authors have modified the Masaoka staging system for an intrapulmonary location {1781}.

Localization
Intrapulmonary thymomas may be hilar or peripheral.

Macroscopy
The tumours range in size from 0.5 to 12 cm. They are usually solitary, circumscribed, encapsulated masses, although cases with multiple lesions have also been described. The cut surface is often lobulated, and may be focally cystic, with variable coloration.

Cytology
Preoperative cytology has generally failed to correctly identify these tumours, with some specimens reported as nondiagnostic {3023} and others suggesting the possibility of other tumours {870}.

Histopathology
Intrapulmonary thymomas have the same features as those arising in the mediastinum (see *Thymomas,* p. 187).

Immunohistochemical staining is identical to that of tumours of thymic origin {770,2069} (see *Thymomas,* p. 187).

Radiographical studies and/or surgical inspection must exclude primary mediastinal thymomas infiltrating the lung. Predominantly epithelial thymomas may be mistaken for carcinomas or spindle cell carcinoids, and lymphocyte-rich variants for lymphoma or small cell carcinoma {1734}. Thymomas usually lack cytological atypia and have a more lobulated architecture than small and non-small cell carcinomas.

Prognosis and predictive factors
Surgical resection is the treatment of choice, with disease-free survival in most patients when the tumour is confined to the lung. Early death has been reported in association with respiratory failure secondary to myasthenia gravis {919,1354}.

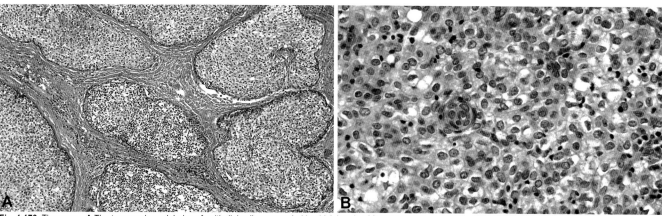

Fig. 1.178 Thymoma. **A** The tumour shows lobules of epithelial cells surrounded by thick bands of fibrous stroma. **B** The tumour consists of a mixture of thymic epithelial cells with a few lymphocytes. Reprinted from Travis WD et al. {2678}.

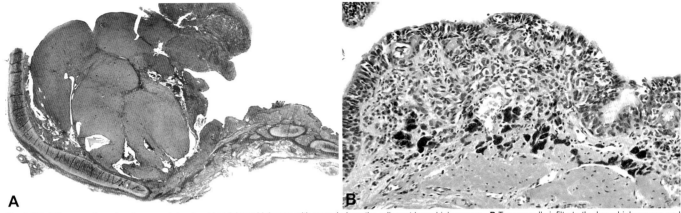

Fig. 1.179 Primary malignant melanoma. A A polypoid endobronchial mass with spread along the adjacent bronchial mucosa. B Tumour cells infiltrate the bronchial mucosa and involve the epithelium in a pagetoid fashion. Reprinted from Colby TV et al. {477} and Travis WD et al. {2678}.

Melanoma

Definition
Melanomas are malignant tumours derived from melanocytes. The criteria for primary pulmonary origin are best based on clinical criteria {2318}, and include exclusion of previous and contemporaneous cutaneous, ocular, or other mucosal origin {702}. Follow-up is also required, to exclude occult metastasis {2318,2374}.

ICD-O code   8720/3

Synonym
Melanoma of unknown primary

Epidemiology
Metastatic melanoma to the lungs is common, but primary pulmonary melanoma is extremely rare. Sex distribution differs between series; some have shown equal sex distribution {43,1939}, and others report male predominance {558,2885}. The median age is between 51 and 59 years, with a range of 29–80 years {43,558,1939}.

Etiology
No precursor lesion is known. Adjacent naevus-like proliferations of melanocytic cells have been reported, but benign naevi are not known to occur in the bronchus, and these may represent cytologically bland tumour spread rather than a precursor. Alternative hypotheses include an origin from melanocytic metaplasia or from cells that have migrated during embryogenesis {2885}.

Clinical features
Presentation is typically with obstructive symptoms.
Site varies between series, with predominance in the lower lobes {558} and the left upper lobe {2885} reported.
Metastasis to various sites, including the lung, lymph node, liver, bowel, brain, adrenal glands, and bone, has been reported {558,2885}.
Melanomas are generally isolated lesions with a median size of 3.75 cm {2885}. In one series, no patient who underwent mediastinal dissection was found to have lymph node metastasis at surgery {558}.

Localization
Most cases are endobronchial, but tracheal origin has also been described {43, 630}. Solitary peripheral melanomas are usually metastatic.

Macroscopy
Most melanoma tumours are solitary and polypoid, with variable pigmentation {43,2885}, although cases of so-called flat melanomas in the trachea have also been described {1742}.

Cytology
These tumours can rarely be diagnosed by fine-needle aspiration biopsy or direct smear.

Histopathology
The tumour is typically lobulated. Architecturally and cytologically, the tumour cells are similar to those of melanoma at other sites. The tumour may show pagetoid spread within the adjacent bronchial mucosa, and rarely benign naevus-like lesions can also be seen {43,2885}.
Immunohistochemistry shows positivity for S100 protein, melan A, HMB45, and SOX10. Ultrastructural analysis shows melanosomes within the cytoplasm {2885}.
Metastatic melanoma requires exclusion, and it may be impossible to prove a primary pulmonary origin with absolute certainty, since a junctional component may be seen in association with cutaneous metastases {981}. Bronchial carcinoids may contain melanin pigment, but will stain for cytokeratin and neuroendocrine markers.

Prognosis and predictive factors
Whether these are considered of pulmonary origin or malignant melanoma

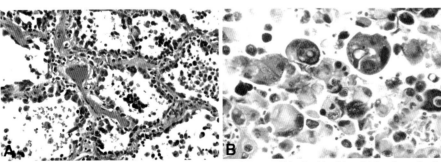

Fig. 1.180 Metastatic malignant melanoma. A A lepidic growth pattern. This should not be mistaken for an in situ component of a primary melanoma. B Cytology of an aspirate of metastatic malignant melanoma, showing highly pleomorphic and dissociated malignant cells. Note the presence of nuclear pleomorphism, massive nucleoli, and occasional nuclear pseudoinclusion.

of unknown primary, superior 5-year survival has been reported when compared to known metastatic disease. Treatment by surgical resection is recommended {558,2318}. However, prognosis varies between series; some have shown generally poor survival {2885}, but a subset of patients remained free of disease for up to 11 years {43,558}.

Meningioma

Definition
Pulmonary meningiomas are identical to the respective intracranial meningothelial (arachnoidal) cell neoplasms which are typically attached to the inner surface of the dura mater. They occur primarily in the lung without CNS involvement.

ICD-O code
Meningioma, NOS   9530/0

Epidemiology
Metastatic meningioma to the lungs is very uncommon, but primary pulmonary meningioma is even rarer. There is a slight female predominance, and the median age is 57 years {1082}, with a range of 18–108 years {1116,2816}.

Etiology
The origin of meningioma remains speculative, with hypotheses including origin

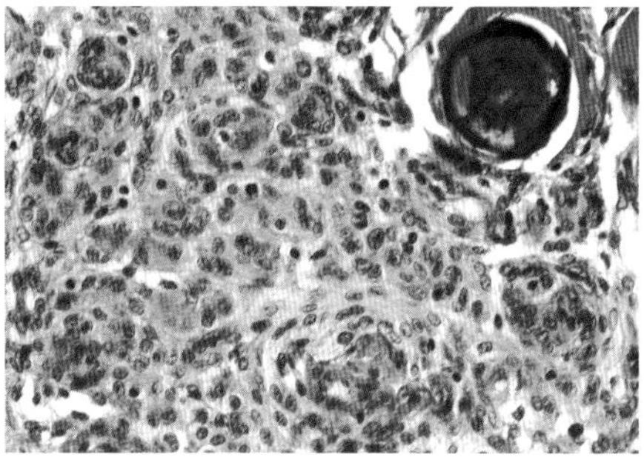

Fig. 1.181 Intrapulmonary meningioma. An intrapulmonary mass shows classical features of a meningioma, with whorls of spindle cells interspersed with abundant psammoma bodies.

from pluripotent cells, heterotopic embryonic rests, and meningothelioid nodules {1082,1715}. Although isolated meningothelioid nodules lack mutational damage {1090}, multiple meningothelial nodules have shown increased genetic alterations, and may represent a transition to a neoplastic proliferation. Occasional cases occur in the setting of multiple meningothelioid nodules {868}.

Clinical features
Most cases are incidental, although some present with respiratory symptoms including haemoptysis {1082}. Most meningiomas are peripheral, with no predilection for any lobe {1715}. Lesions are well circumscribed and often show slow growth. FDG PET has demonstrated metabolically active lesions that may be

suspicious for malignancy {1082}. Most tumours behave in a benign manner, but rare examples have recurred in the lung, lymph nodes, and liver, one after a 40-year history {2083,2283,2816}. Most meningiomas are localized to the lung, but a rare central example was reported to have invaded the mediastinum {2744}.

Macroscopy
Most pulmonary meningiomas are solitary, well circumscribed, and firm, with a yellow-tan to grey cut surface. They range from 4 to 60 mm, with a median size of 18 mm {1082}.

Cytology
In rare cases, these tumours can be diagnosed by fine-needle aspiration biopsy {868}, using criteria identical to those of meningiomas arising at other sites.

Histopathology
The tumour is typically well demarcated. Most tumours are reported to have transitional or psammomatous patterns, but rare examples of anaplastic meningioma {2816} and chordoid meningiomas characterized by cords and trabeculae of cells in an abundant mucoid matrix have been described {2049,2215}. The cells are positive for vimentin, epithelial membrane antigen, and occasionally and focally for S100 protein. Cytokeratin, other melanoma markers, and neuroendocrine markers are negative. An increased Ki-67 proliferative index may be seen in anaplastic meningiomas {2816}. On electron microscopy, features typical of meningioma arising in the central nervous system have been documented, with long interdigitating processes, intercellular desmosomes, and abundant intracytoplasmic intermediate filaments {868}. Metastatic meningioma requires exclusion, as do spindle cell thymoma, solitary fibrous tumour, and monophasic synovial sarcoma, using appropriate immunohistochemistry {1715} (see *Mesenchymal tumours*, p. 116).

Prognosis and predictive factors
The rare tumours with aggressive behaviour show features of atypical or anaplastic meningioma (WHO grades II–III), with pleomorphism, increased mitotic activity and proliferative indices {2083,2816}. Infiltrative behaviour and tumour recurrence may be associated with prolonged survival if the tumour is of WHO grade I and is completely resected {2283,2744}.

Table 1.21 Meningiomas grouped by likelihood of recurrence and grade {1516A}

Meningiomas with low risk of recurrence and aggressive growth:		ICD-O code
Meningothelial meningioma	WHO grade I	9531/0
Fibrous (fibroblastic) meningioma	WHO grade I	9532/0
Transitional (mixed) meningioma	WHO grade I	9537/0
Psammomatous meningioma	WHO grade I	9533/0
Angiomatous meningioma	WHO grade I	9534/0
Microcystic meningioma	WHO grade I	9530/0
Secretory meningioma	WHO grade I	9530/0
Lymphoplasmacyte-rich meningioma	WHO grade I	9530/0
Metaplastic meningioma	WHO grade I	9530/0
Meningiomas with greater likelihood of recurrence and/or aggressive behaviour:		
Chordoid meningioma	WHO grade II	9538/1
Clear cell meningioma (intracranial)	WHO grade II	9538/1
Atypical meningioma	WHO grade II	9539/1
Papillary meningioma	WHO grade III	9538/3
Rhabdoid meningioma	WHO grade III	9538/3
Anaplastic (malignant) meningioma	WHO grade III	9530/3
CNS meningiomas of any subtype or grade with high proliferation index and/or brain invasion		

Metastases to the lung

G. Pelosi
J. Fukuoka
K. Hiroshima
A.M. Marchevsky

Definition

Metastatic tumours in the lung result from tumour cells spreading to the lung from extrapulmonary sites. Discontinuous growth from primary lung carcinomas presenting as separate nodules is discussed in *Staging and grading*, p. 14. Pulmonary metastases may present as clinically evident tumour masses during the course of an underlying malignancy, or they may be discovered as incidental findings on bronchoscopy {789}, in surgically resected lung specimens {1544,2345,2496}, or on autopsy {426,825}.

ICD-O codes

The behaviour code /6 (malignant, metastatic site) is included in the ICD-O codes of the relevant tumours.

Synonym

Secondary tumours in the lung

Epidemiology

Carcinomas are the major source of metastases (especially from the gastrointestinal tract, gynaecological tract, breast, urothelium, head and neck, prostate, and other sites), followed by sarcomas, melanomas, and germ cell tumours {338,2001}. Sex and age distribution depend on the varying incidence of malignancies in various patient populations. For example, colorectal cancer affects mainly elderly patients of both sexes, with 11% synchronous and 5.8% metachronous metastases {1688}. Breast cancer and melanoma prevail in somewhat younger adults {762,1451}. Germ cell tumours and sarcomas are usually found in young adults or children {338}.

Etiology

The lung is one of the most common metastatic sites {605,643,1375,2437,2812}. A large autopsy study showed that pulmonary metastases were present in 10.7% of autopsy cases, ranking fourth after local and regional lymph nodes and the liver {605}. Carcinomas, sarcomas, and other neoplasms usually metastasize to the lungs through the pulmonary circulation, although primary lung carcinoma metastases may arise from the lymphatic or aerogenous route {1152,2812}.

Metastases can be single or multiple, and usually involve the parenchyma and the pleura, although carcinomas of the breast, kidney, colon, endometrium, and other tumours can present even as an isolated endobronchial mass {643,1375,2812}. Isolated tumour cells in the lungs do not necessarily lead to metastasis formation, which requires a complex and coordinated series of events {2032}.

Clinical features

Signs and symptoms

Most patients with metastatic lung disease do not present with pulmonary symptoms, even in the presence of fulminant metastases occupying almost an entire lung {1131,1861}. When present, pulmonary symptoms depend on the anatomical location within the lung, and can simulate primary tumours. For example, endobronchial metastases may cause cough, haemoptysis, wheezing, dyspnoea, fever, and postobstructive pneumonia {2863}.

Pleural spread usually results in chest pain and dyspnoea, whereas the symptoms of vascular/thromboembolic or lymphatic spread may mimic those of interstitial pneumonia, tuberculosis, and/or cor pulmonale, leading to delayed diagnostic recognition.

Table 1.22 Tissue-restricted gene products involved in tissue development and maintenance that can be used in metastasis characterization

Bladder	Uroplakin 2, uroplakin 3
Breast	Mammoglobin 1, lipophilin B
Colon	Mucin 2, A33 antigen, glutathione peroxidase 2
Ovary	Lipophilin B
Pancreas	TTF2, prostate stem cell antigen, metallothionein, glutathione peroxidase 2
Prostate	Prostate-specific antigen, lipophilin B
Stomach	Pepsinogen C

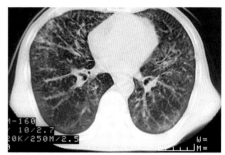

Fig. 1.182 Metastasis to the lung. CT shows diffuse thickening of bronchovascular bundles and interlobular septa, suggesting lymphatic involvement (lymphangitic carcinomatosis). Discrete nodules may represent foci of haematogenous metastasis.

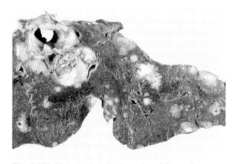

Fig. 1.183 Metastasis to the lung. A nodular coalescence of metastatic cholangiocarcinoma with synchronous lung hilar lymph node involvement on autopsy.

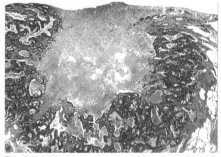

Fig. 1.184 Metastasis to the lung. Metastasis of colonic adenocarcinomas with abundant dirty necrosis, garland-like architecture with tall columnar cells, and visceral pleura involvement.

Imaging

CT (often with simultaneous PET) is the most sensitive imaging modality for detecting pulmonary metastases {2329}. Typical radiological findings include multiple, peripherally located, round, variable-sized nodules (haematogenous metastases) or diffuse thickening of the

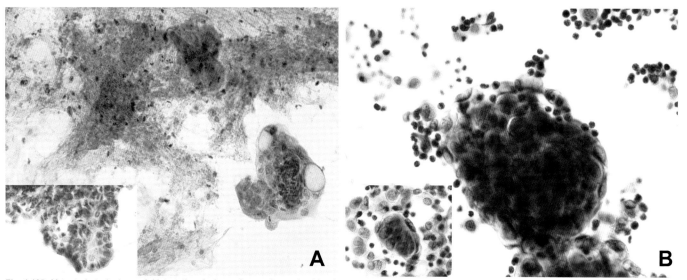

Fig. 1.185 Metastasis to the lung. **A** Metastatic colonic carcinoma shows gland-forming aggregates of cohesive columnar cells with palisading nuclei (inset) and abundant dirty necrosis. **B** Metastatic breast ductal carcinoma forming so-called cannonball clusters in the pleural effusion, with variably bland-appearing cancer cells (inset).

interstitium (lymphangitic carcinomatosis) {537,1002,2329}. Metastases are usually well circumscribed, with expanding growth and smooth margins, but irregular contours can occur {776,1002}. Peritumoural haemorrhage causes nodular attenuation surrounded by a halo of ground-glass opacity (the CT halo sign) or poorly defined, blurry margins {1002,1265,2329}. Squamous cell carcinoma metastases are mostly cavitating lesions {1002,2329}. Chest X-ray is normal in 50% of lymphangitic carcinomatosis cases, but CT shows beaded or nodular septal thickening {1002}. Endobronchial metastases may lead to atelectasis of a lobe or the entire lung, and can occasionally be seen on chest CT {2329}. Rarely, metastases to the lung from indolent tumours, such as endometrial stromal sarcoma, benign metastasizing leiomyoma, and cellular fibrous histiocytoma, can present with prominent cystic spaces {11,103,1934}

Tumour spread
There are six major spreading modalities for lung metastases: intrapulmonary aerogenic, haematogenous, lymphangitic, endobronchial, pleural, and direct invasion from adjacent organs. Haematogenous spread is the most common form, resulting in micronodular (miliary), macronodular, solitary, cavitary, and thromboembolic lesions. The latter spread may be bland and associated with marked angiopathy (so-called pulmonary tumour thrombotic microangiopathy) {2721}.

Staging
Based on the current pathological TNM system and the American Joint Committee on Cancer (AJCC) manual, metastatic tumours are generally considered stage IV disease (see *Staging and grading,* p. 14).

Localization
Pulmonary metastases usually occur as multiple, bilateral parenchymal nodules, and less commonly as solitary nodules. They mainly involve the middle and lower peripheral lung fields {537,1002,2329}.

Macroscopy
Metastatic tumour nodules are usually round, circumscribed, and variably sized {1577}. Large masses may be found. Brown to black nodules may correspond to metastatic melanoma. Golden-yellow nodules raise the possibility of metastatic renal cell carcinoma. Endobronchial metastases can occur anywhere in the bronchial tree.

Cytology
The cytological features of metastatic carcinomas vary according to the type of lesion. Metastatic colonic carcinomas present as gland-forming cohesive clusters, with columnar cells, palisading nuclei, and abundant necrosis {1312}. Breast cancer cells of ductal type often cause pleural effusion with rounded diagnostic arrangement (so-called cannonballs), whereas linear arrays of uniform small tumour cells may suggest metastasizing breast lobular carcinoma. The distinction

between metastatic and primary squamous cell carcinoma is unreliable in cytology. Pancreas or biliary adenocarcinoma is often especially challenging, as it closely resembles pulmonary mucinous adenocarcinoma. Melanoma shows discohesive tumour cells with cytoplasmic melanin, whereas primary lung melanoma is extremely rare {2885} (see *Melanoma,* p. 146). Both liquid-based cytology and cell block preparations can be used for immunohistochemical, cytogenetic, and molecular tests {1337}.

Histopathology
The histopathological features of lung metastases are similar to those of the primary lesions, and there is often growth inside or along blood or lymphatic vessels. Tumour patterns can be interstitial, lepidic, infiltrating/destructive, or alveolar-filling. For example, metastatic colonic adenocarcinomas typically exhibit a garland-like architecture, with tall columnar cells and elongated nuclei (so-called cigar nuclei) and dirty necrosis. Metastatic breast tumours can exhibit trabecular, single-file, or solid features, with comedo-type necrosis and growth along pleural serosa. Renal cell carcinomas may show clear cells with prominent vascularity. Pancreatobiliary adenocarcinoma may growth in a lepidic fashion, simulating primary mucinous adenocarcinoma. Metastatic uterine leiomyosarcoma may colonize the interstitium to enclose bronchioles, whereas melanoma

and germ cell tumours replace the lung parenchyma destructively.

Immunohistochemistry

Immunohistochemistry is valuable in differential diagnosis, and can suggest the primary sites. Most primary adenocarcinomas (except mucinous carcinomas) are positive for TTF1, napsin A, and CK7, whereas most non-lung adenocarcinomas are negative for TTF1 and napsin A, and variably positive for CK7 {446,1127,1764,2910}. Colonic adenocarcinomas are positive for CK20 and CDX2, but usually negative for CK7, TTF1, and napsin A {135,446}. Breast carcinoma exhibits estrogen/progesterone nuclear receptors, GCDFP15, GATA3, and/or mammaglobin, but not TTF1 {1127,2036,2937}. Prostatic adenocarcinomas are positive for prostate-specific membrane antigen, prostate-specific antigen, and/or androgen receptors {620,2358,2908}. Merkel cell carcinomas are positive for CK20, neurofilaments, and polyomavirus, and negative for TTF1 {295,1127,2751}. Melanomas are positive for S100 protein, HMB45, and melan A, but negative for cytokeratins and TTF1 {1127}. Thymic carcinomas are positive for CD5, PAX8, and CD117, but negative for TTF1 {1127,1965,1966,2832}. There is no immunohistochemical marker that helps in the differentiation between primary and metastatic squamous cell carcinoma {904A,1017A,1127}. Metastases from urothelial bladder cancer may be positive for CK7 and p40, but unlike lung cancer staining with these antibodies, urothelial carcinomas may also be positive for GATA3 and/or uroplakin 2 and uroplakin 3 {383, 904A,918, 1017A}. Germ cell tumours are variably positive for CD30, α-fetoprotein, cytokeratins, SALL4, PLAP, and the β-subunit of human chorionic gonadotropin {1127,1643,1853,1962}, whereas metastatic sarcomas are either immunophenotypically uncommitted or show varying cell differentiation lineages.

Differential diagnosis

The differential diagnoses of multiple metastatic nodules include synchronous primary tumours of the lung, vasculitis, diffuse idiopathic pulmonary neuroendocrine cell hyperplasia {535}, and granulomatous diseases. Lymphangitic carcinomatosis must be distinguished from sarcoidosis, pulmonary fibrosis, and malignant lymphoma. A halo of

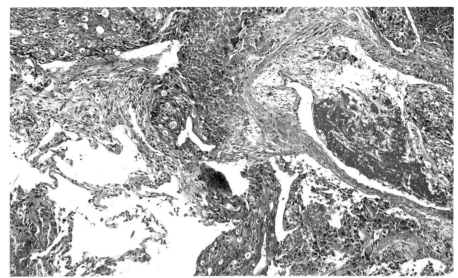

Fig. 1.186 Metastasis to the lung. Vascular invasion with neoplastic thromboembolism of a poorly differentiated gastric adenocarcinoma with extensive necrosis (same case as shown in Fig. 1.182).

ground-glass opacity may be seen in invasive aspergillosis, candidiasis, Wegener granulomatosis, tuberculoma associated with haemoptysis, and lymphoma {1002,2329}. Angiosarcoma and choriocarcinoma are the most representative causes of haemorrhagic metastases.

Genetic profile

Many of the same molecular genetic alterations of tumour suppressor genes and oncogenes can be found in both pulmonary primary and metastatic carcinomas. Organ-specific or relatively restricted markers for certain metastatic carcinomas are candidates for the identification of primary sites. Tissue-restricted markers are produced by regulatory genes dealing with nuclear transcription factors (such as homeobox genes), controlling tissue development and maintenance. Loss of heterozygosity and

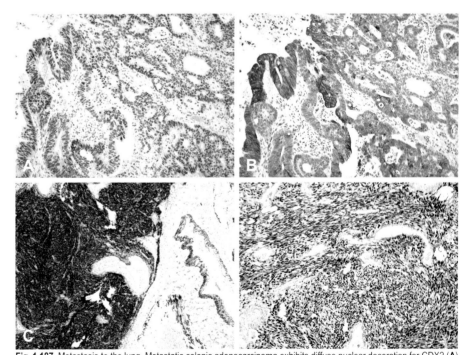

Fig. 1.187 Metastasis to the lung. Metastatic colonic adenocarcinoma exhibits diffuse nuclear decoration for CDX2 (**A**) and cytoplasmic expression for CK20 (**B**). The same case of metastatic well-differentiated uterine leiomyosarcoma as shown in panel B of Fig. 1.188 presents with strong desmin (**C**) and estrogen receptor (**D**) immunoreactivity.

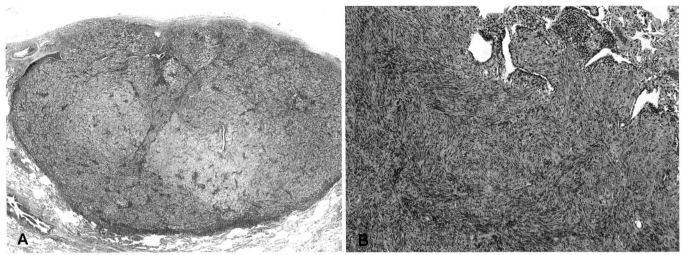

Fig. 1.188 Metastasis to the lung. **A** Renal cell carcinoma pulmonary metastasis with prominent vascularity and visceral pleura involvement. **B** Metastatic well-differentiated uterine leiomyosarcoma growths in the interstitium entrapping normal bronchiolar structures.

TP53 mutation analysis may help in distinguishing primary versus metastasis for squamous cell carcinoma {824}. The presence of HPV in a squamous cell carcinoma is suggestive of a metastasis {2933}, although this requires correlation with the clinical history. Many next-generation molecular techniques are feasible on formalin-fixed paraffin-embedded tissues, and can detect the primary site of tumours more accurately than more traditional methods {681,1645,2059}. High-throughput analyses using microarray on hundreds of tumours of different types have been generated, compared, and used to develop diagnostic algorithms. Microarray-based large-scale molecular profiles have been achieved at the messenger RNA, microRNA, DNA, and epigenetic levels.

Prognosis and predictive factors

Lung metastases from extrapulmonary malignancies usually have a dismal prognosis, but some patients with a solitary metastasis or a small number of metastases confined to the lung experience long survival after resection of the primary lesion and the pulmonary metastases. The International Registry of Lung Metastases indicates that complete metastasectomy is curative for a variety of tumours, with a disease-free interval ≤ 36 months and a higher number of metastases being unfavourable prognostic factors {305,762,1981,2001}. Germ cell tumours are associated with the best prognosis after metastasectomy {305,338}, whereas the prognoses of carcinomas (colonic, renal, and others), sarcomas (osteosarcoma, leiomyosarcoma, and others),

and melanoma {338} are less favourable. Although metastatic sarcomas and melanoma usually have a dismal prognosis, the more prolonged survival of these patients supports metastasectomy in selected cases. Preoperative staging and time to pulmonary metastases to exclude synchronous extrapulmonary metastases are fundamental for proper patient selection for surgery {845,2002}, whereas concurrent regional lymph node involvement seems not to affect long-term survival {338}. Predictive factors of response to therapy also depend on the type of metastatic cancer, including mutation assessment (e.g. *EGFR*, *KRAS*, *BRAF*, and *KIT*), gene copy evaluation (e.g. *ALK*, *ROS1*, and *HER2*), and immunohistochemical characterization (e.g. estrogen and progesterone receptors).

CHAPTER 2

Tumours of the pleura

Mesothelial tumours

Lymphoproliferative disorders

Mesenchymal tumours

WHO classification of tumours of the pleura[a,b]

Mesothelial tumours
Diffuse malignant mesothelioma
    Epithelioid mesothelioma 9052/3
    Sarcomatoid mesothelioma 9051/3
       Desmoplastic mesothelioma 9051/3
    Biphasic mesothelioma 9053/3
Localized malignant mesothelioma
    Epithelioid mesothelioma 9052/3
    Sarcomatoid mesothelioma 9051/3
    Biphasic mesothelioma 9053/3
Well-differentiated papillary mesothelioma 9052/1*
Adenomatoid tumour 9054/0

Lymphoproliferative disorders
Primary effusion lymphoma 9678/3
Diffuse large B-cell lymphoma associated
    with chronic inflammation 9680/3

Mesenchymal tumours
Epithelioid hemangioendothelioma 9133/3
Angiosarcoma 9120/3
Synovial sarcoma 9040/3
Solitary fibrous tumour 8815/1
    Malignant solitary fibrous tumour 8815/3
Desmoid-type fibromatosis 8821/1
Calcifying fibrous tumour 8817/0
Desmoplastic round cell tumour 8806/3

[a] The morphology codes are from the International Classification of Diseases for Oncology (ICD-O) {763}. Behaviour is coded /0 for benign tumours; /1 for unspecified, borderline, or uncertain behaviour; /2 for carcinoma in situ and grade III intraepithelial neoplasia; and /3 for malignant tumours. [b] The classification is modified from the previous WHO classification {2672}, taking into account changes in our understanding of these lesions. * This new code was approved by the IARC/WHO Committee for ICD-O.

TNM classification of pleural mesothelioma

T – Primary Tumour

TX	Primary tumour cannot be assessed
T0	No evidence of primary tumour
T1	Tumour involves ipsilateral parietal pleura, with or without focal involvement of visceral pleura
T1a	Tumour involves ipsilateral parietal (mediastinal, diaphragmatic) pleura; no involvement of visceral pleura
T1b	Tumour involves ipsilateral parietal (mediastinal, diaphragmatic) pleura, with focal involvement of the visceral pleura
T2	Tumour involves any ipsilateral pleural surfaces, with at least one of the following:

- confluent visceral pleural tumour (including the fissure)
- invasion of diaphragmatic muscle
- invasion of lung parenchyma

T3*	Tumour involves any ipsilateral pleural surfaces, with at least one of the following:

- invasion of endothoracic fascia
- invasion into mediastinal fat
- solitary focus of tumour invading soft tissues of the chest wall
- non-transmural involvement of the pericardium

T4**	Tumour involves any ipsilateral pleural surfaces, with at least one of the following:

- diffuse or multifocal invasion of soft tissues of chest wall
- any involvement of rib
- invasion through diaphragm to peritoneum
- invasion of any mediastinal organ(s)
- direct extension to contralateral pleura
- invasion into the spine
- extension to internal surface of pericardium
- pericardial effusion with positive cytology
- invasion of myocardium
- invasion of brachial plexus

Notes:

* T3 describes locally advanced, but potentially resectable tumour.

** T4 describes locally advanced, technically unresectable tumour.

N – Regional Lymph Nodes

NX	Regional lymph nodes cannot be assessed
N0	No regional lymph node metastasis
N1	Metastasis in ipsilateral bronchopulmonary and/or hilar lymph node(s)
N2	Metastasis in subcarinal lymph node(s) and/or ipsilateral internal mammary or mediastinal lymph node(s)
N3	Metastasis in contralateral mediastinal, internal mammary, or hilar node(s) and/or ipsilateral or contralateral supraclavicular or scalene lymph node(s)

M – Distant Metastasis

M0	No distant metastasis
M1	Distant metastasis

Stage Grouping

Stage IA	T1a	N0	M0
Stage IB	T1b	N0	M0
Stage II	T2	N0	M0
Stage III	T1, T2	N1	M0
	T1, T2	N2	M0
	T3	N0, N1, N2	M0
Stage IV	T4	Any N	M0
	Any T	N3	M0
	Any T	Any N	M1

Compiled from references {2420,652A}

TNM help desk: http://www.uicc.org/resources/tnm/helpdesk

Mesothelial tumours
Diffuse malignant mesothelioma
Epithelioid mesothelioma

F. Galateau-Salle
A. Churg
V. Roggli
L.R. Chirieac
R. Attanoos
A. Borczuk
P. Cagle

S. Dacic
S. Hammar
A.N. Husain
K. Inai
M. Ladanyi
A.M. Marchevsky
D. Naidich

N.G. Ordóñez
D.C. Rice
M.T. Sheaff
W.D. Travis
J. van Meerbeeck

Definition

Diffuse epithelioid malignant mesothelioma of the pleura is a malignant tumour originating from mesothelial cells and showing epithelioid morphology and a diffuse pattern of growth over the pleural surfaces. Diffuse malignant mesotheliomas must be differentiated from localized malignant mesotheliomas, which have different clinical behaviours.

ICD-O code   9052/3

Synonyms

Epithelioid malignant mesothelioma; epithelial-type mesothelioma (not recommended)

Epidemiology

Malignant mesotheliomas occur over a very wide age range. They occasionally occur in children, but the vast majority of tumours are seen in patients aged ≥ 60 years. Patients with the pleomorphic variant tend to be older. The male-to-female ratio is on average 4:1, but varies by geographical location based on the proportion of cases attributable to occupational asbestos exposure {746,1426}.

In North America, the rate in men increased steadily from the 1970s to the early 1990s, peaking at about 23 cases per million per year. Subsequently, there has been a slow but steady decline. In 2009, the rate was about 17 per million men per year. In women, the rate over this same time period remained essentially constant at 2–3 cases per million per year. Mathematical projections suggest that steady decline in the number of cases in males will lead to the convergence of the male and female incidence rates at some time between 2040 and 2050, reflecting the disease's long latency period (about 30 years) and the increased restrictions on the use of asbestos in the 1970s {1426,2085}. In countries that used large amounts of amosite or crocidolite (such as Australia), the incidence rates are considerably higher, but are also starting to show a similar decrease {1020,1710,2042}.

Approximately 60–80% of malignant mesotheliomas are of the epithelioid type.

Etiology

The most common cause of mesothelioma is asbestos exposure. Other

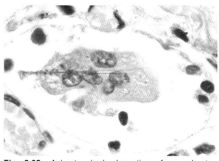

Fig. 2.02 Asbestos body. Ingestion of an asbestos fibre by a multinucliated macrophage. Note the iron-rich deposits on the surface of the fibre.

established causes include therapeutic radiation for other malignant neoplasms and (in a localized area of Turkey) the mineral fibre erionite. Some mesotheliomas do not have an identifiable cause.

Asbestos

The relationship between asbestos exposure and mesothelioma is complex, and highly dependent on fibre type and dose. In North America and France, up to 80–90% of mesotheliomas in men are related to asbestos exposure, but only about 20% of cases in women {862,2447}. In western Europe and Australia, a higher proportion of cases in women are asbestos-induced, but the attributable asbestos fraction is < 50% {312}. The latency (time from first exposure to disease) is long, averaging 30–40 years, and few (if any) mesotheliomas are seen with latencies < 15 years {1397}.

Mathematical modelling suggests that mesothelioma incidence is a linear function of amphibole asbestos dose, and a power function of time since first exposure {188,1019,2043}. There are marked differences in the potency of different fibre types in inducing mesothelioma: commercial amphibole asbestos (amosite and crocidolite) is 2–3 orders of magnitude more carcinogenic than chrysotile {188,1019}. Some argue that the mesothelial carcinogenicity of chrysotile depends on the level of contamination by the amphibole fibre tremolite, and that pure chrysotile may not be mesotheliogenic in humans {188,832,1626,1628}.

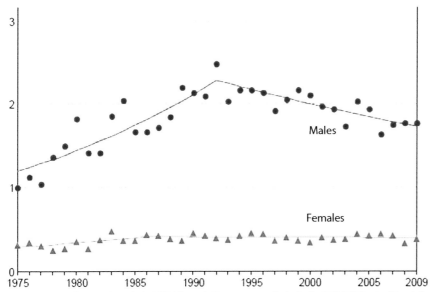

Fig. 2.01 Incidence of mesothelioma in the USA (all races). Rates are age-adjusted to the 2000 US Standard Population. Source: SEER 9 areas. United States National Cancer Institute.

However, in sufficiently high doses, chrysotile appears to cause lung cancer, and at very high doses causes mesotheliomas in experimental animals. There are a few places in the world where other forms of amphibole fibres with dimensions similar to amosite or crocidolite are found, and a high mesothelioma incidence is seen in these locations. An example is Libby, Montana, USA, where the fibre winchite is present in mined vermiculite deposits {832,1627,2862}. There have also been reports that pleural plaques may be an independent risk factor for pleural mesothelioma. In a follow-up study of 5287 male subjects, pleural plaques confirmed on CT were significantly associated with a high risk of mesothelioma, after adjustment for time since first asbestos exposure and cumulative asbestos exposure {1959}.

Erionite

In the Cappadocia region of Turkey, there are outcrops of rock containing erionite fibres of the same size and durability of commercial amphibole asbestos. The incidence of mesothelioma in this region is extraordinarily high {140,602,1134}. Similar fibres have been found in other regions, such as North Dakota, USA (in road surfacing material) {329} and Mexico {1287}.

Therapeutic radiation

There is an increased incidence of pleural mesothelioma after therapeutic radiation for breast cancer, Hodgkin lymphoma, and testicular cancer {430,539,589,2668}. The mesotheliomas typically develop years after the radiation {2625,2896}.

Inherited predisposition

Germline mutations in BAP1 define a new familial cancer syndrome, which includes malignant mesothelioma, uveal melanoma, clear cell renal cell carcinoma, intrahepatic cholangiocarcinoma, atypical cutaneous melanocytic lesions, and possibly other cancers {700,2053,2074,2624}. More studies are needed to define the lifetime risk of mesothelioma in carriers of germline mutations, but awareness of this syndrome is necessary to ensure that patients with other cancers in the syndrome (especially ocular melanoma) are screened for mesothelioma. Although the interaction with other risk factors such as asbestos

exposure remains unclear, some patients with pleural malignant mesothelioma with germline mutation do not have a clear history of asbestos exposure {420,2624,2875}.

Other putative etiological agents

Simian virus 40 (SV40) causes malignancies, including mesothelioma, in experimental animals, in part by inactivating the TP53 and RB genes {2337}. However, neither epidemiological nor molecular data support a role for SV40 in human pleural malignant mesothelioma {811,1513,1562,2337}.

Clinical features

Signs and symptoms

Patients with pleural mesothelioma typically present with insidious onset of chest pain and/or dyspnoea {666,997,2294}. The chest pain is usually dull, unilateral, and non-pleuritic. It sometimes has neuropathic components because of the entrapment of intercostal, autonomic, or brachial plexus nerves. In the early stages, dyspnoea is usually caused by a pleural effusion, but later may occur due to the restrictive effects of pleural thickening. A chest wall mass, weight loss, abdominal pain, and ascites (due to peritoneal involvement) are less common presentations. Cervical adenopathy, haemoptysis, paraneoplastic syndromes, and symptoms due to distant metastases are unusual. Irregular episodes of low-grade fever, profuse sweating, weight loss, and declining performance status are common presenting complaints, although these tend to indicate more advanced disease or the pleomorphic variant of mesothelioma {1178}. Some patients present with acute pleuritic chest pain and a small effusion, but initial investigations may fail to provide a diagnosis. The patient may then remain symptom-free for many months until recurrence of the fluid or development of chest pain leads to further investigation. Other uncommon presentations include pneumothorax, mass lesions, segmental or lobar pulmonary collapse, mediastinal invasion with laryngeal nerve palsy, and superior vena caval obstruction {1407}.

Imaging

Imaging findings in patients with mesothelioma exhibit a wide range of abnormalities. Most classical is the finding of

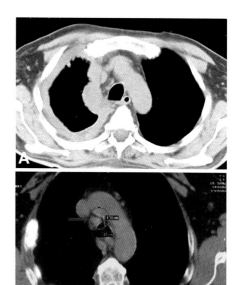

Fig. 2.03 Diffuse malignant mesothelioma. **A** CT shows diffuse right unilateral pleural thickening, with no intraparenchymal lung mass. **B** PET shows increased avidity in the tumour, which is causing right pleural nodularity and thickening.

a diffuse circumferential rind of nodular pleura, usually associated with ipsilateral volume loss and an effusion. Less commonly, malignant mesothelioma appears as a pleural effusion without obvious pleural nodularity, which may be associated with acute pleuritic chest pain. Rarely, tumours appear as an isolated nodular pleural density, with or without an accompanying effusion. The presence of pleural plaques, especially when calcified, is suggestive of asbestos exposure; however, they are often absent. The involved haemithorax is sometimes reduced in size, and there may be retraction of the intercostal spaces. CT and MRI are important for evaluation of

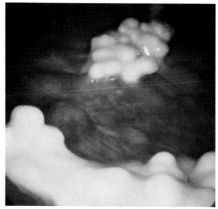

Fig. 2.04 Diffuse malignant mesothelioma. The surface of the pleura is covered by white fibrous plaques and small tumour nodules with a pink surface.

tumour volume and invasion of contiguous anatomical structures (e.g. mediastinal and pericardial involvement).

Tumour spread

Disease progression is variable. Some patients have periods of apparent stability, while others have relentless, rapid deterioration. The disease is more likely to progress by local extension in chest wall and lung than by haematogenous spread. Direct involvement of mediastinal structures is common. Lymphangitic involvement of the lung parenchyma is more common in epithelioid type, and particularly in the predominant micropapillary subtype {1178}. Lymphatic spread gives rise to ipsilateral or contralateral mediastinal lymph node involvement. Ascites may develop at any time during the disease course due to abdominal spread with peritoneal involvement. Distant metastases are common; their presence is reported in more than half of all cases, although usually late in the clinical course or at autopsy {2953}. None of the clinical symptoms or imaging findings described above is specific for pleural mesothelioma; they may be representative of other pleural tumours, or metastasis to the pleura as well.

Staging

The current staging system for malignant pleural mesothelioma is based on the classification proposed in 1995 by the International Mesothelioma Interest Group and adopted by the American Joint Committee on Cancer (AJCC) and the Union for International Cancer Control (UICC) {2223}. The system applies to both clinical and pathological staging. Clinical staging is inaccurate for early stages, due to the low accuracy of CT and MRI {622}. Integrated FDG PET-CT is expected to improve the accuracy {2064}. In clinical series, patients most commonly presented with disease that was locally advanced (stage III, 40%), followed by advanced (stage IV, 35%) and local (stage I–II, 25%). A modified TNM-based classification is currently under revision, based on the retrospective analysis of a large series of incident cases accumulated by the International Association for the Study of Lung Cancer (IASLC) {2227}. A prospective database has been created by the IASLC to obtain more meaningful long-term data.

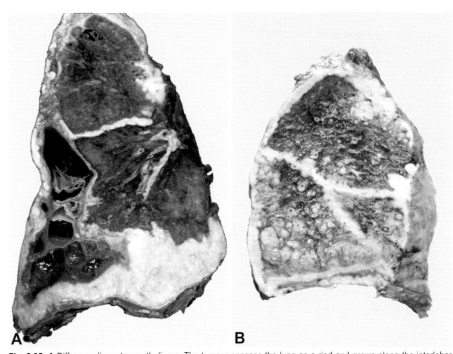

Fig. 2.05 A Diffuse malignant mesothelioma. The tumour encases the lung as a rind and grows along the interlobar septa, compressing the lung parenchyma. Reprinted from Galateau-Salle F {785}. **B** Pseudomesotheliomatous adenocarcinoma. The tumour encases the lung, mimicking a malignant mesothelioma. Unlike malignant mesothelioma, the adenocarcinoma shows multiple nodules that infiltrate the lung parenchyma.

The current T descriptors are only qualitative, and best applicable for invasive staging procedures, as is the case for T1a and T1b, which require thoracoscopic assessment of the pleural cavity. They account insufficiently for invasion, extent, thickness, and volume of the circumferential pleural rind. The regional lymph node map and nomenclature are the same as those used for lung cancer, with the addition of lymph nodes in the anterior peridiaphragmatic region and around the internal mammary artery as N2 nodes. This empirical assumption discounts the possible prognostic role of lymph nodes in the extrapleural space and pericardial fat, and associates a better prognosis with intrapulmonary nodes. It may not be possible to perform a thorough N classification, particularly in unresectable tumours. With regard to stage definition, the absence of significant survival differences between stages I and II reflects the above-mentioned inaccuracy of staging, while stages III and IV define broad categories of disease, including locally advanced tumours (T3 and T4), regionally advanced disease (N1 and N2), and metastatic disease (M1). It is expected that substages will be defined in the new classification {653,2418}.

Localization

There is no significant difference in location between the different histological types of mesothelioma. Right-sided involvement is more common than left-sided involvement by a ratio of 3:2. Bilateral involvement at diagnosis is unusual {2953}. Spread occurs along the interlobar fissures and into the underlying lung, and can extend through the diaphragm and into the chest wall. Mediastinal involvement, with direct invasion of the pericardium and other mediastinal structures, is common. The unusual occurence of direct extension into the peritoneum is more common with the epithelioid type.

Macroscopy

The gross findings depend on when mesothelioma is observed during its natural history. Early mesothelioma presents as small nodules distributed on the parietal and (less commonly) on the visceral pleura. As mesothelioma progresses, the nodules coalesce to form a rind of tumour encasing the lung. They typically grow along the interlobular fissures. In late stages, the pleura may be several centimetres thick. The tumour is grey-white and soft. There may be cystic areas containing mucoid-like material.

Cytology

In industrialized countries, about 1% of malignant pleural effusions are caused by diffuse malignant mesothelioma. Malignant mesothelial cells in effusions are nearly always epithelioid morphologically, since sarcomatoid mesotheliomas seldom shed cells into the fluid {1941}. Mesothelioma cells in effusions may be arranged in sheets, clusters, morules, or papillae. Psammoma bodies may be present. These cells show a range of cytological appearances, from bland to pleomorphic, but often lack the degree of atypia associated with carcinoma. In contrast, benign mesothelial cells may exhibit features most often associated with malignancy, such as increased cellularity, nuclear pleomorphism, and mitotic activity. Therefore, differentiation of mesothelioma from benign mesothelial reactions may be very difficult or even impossible in cytological specimens. Similarly, tissue invasion (an important histological feature of malignancy) cannot be evaluated in effusion specimens. Overall, the accuracy of purely cytological diagnoses of malignant mesothelioma is fairly low compared to that of tissue diagnoses {1056}.

Histopathology

Most epithelioid mesotheliomas are cytologically bland, but more anaplastic forms may be observed {457}. Epithelioid mesotheliomas show a wide range of histological patterns. Several different patterns are often observed in the same tumour, although one pattern may predominate. In most tumours, the cells have eosinophilic cytoplasm with bland vesicular chromatin. Mitoses

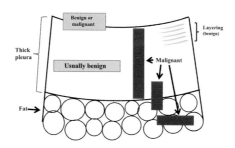

Fig. 2.06 Schematic diagram showing benign versus malignant processes as a function of the distribution of mesothelial cells in a thickened pleura. Reprinted from Churg A et al. {459}.

are infrequent. In the more poorly differentiated forms, the nuclei tend to have coarse chromatin with prominent nucleoli and frequent mitoses; however, these tumours are uncommon, and may be difficult to distinguish from carcinomas {1056}.

The most commonly encountered patterns are solid, tubulopapillary, and trabecular. Less common patterns include micropapillary, adenomatoid (microcystic), clear cell, transitional, decidoid, and small cell. The tubulopapillary form exhibits varying combinations of tubules and papillae, with connective tissue cores and clefts. The morphology of the cells lining the tubules and papillae ranges from low cuboidal and relatively bland to larger and more atypical. The trabecular pattern consists of relatively small, uniform cells arranged in thin cords, sometimes with a single-file appearance. Psammoma bodies may be observed. The micropapillary pattern consists of papillary structures lacking fibrovascular cores. The adenomatoid form shows microcystic structures, with lace-like or

signet ring appearances. Sheets and nests of cells are often seen in association with other patterns. Solid, monotonous, relatively non-cohesive sheets of polygonal cells uncommonly occur, simulating large cell carcinoma or lymphoma. Tumours with anaplastic or prominent giant cells, often multinucleated, are designated pleomorphic {1178,1923}.

Malignant mesothelioma with a heavy lymphoid infiltrate obscuring the polygonal neoplastic cells can mimic malignant lymphoma or lymphoepithelioma-like carcinoma, and these tumours are called lymphohistiocytoid mesothelioma {786}. When there are prominent large cells with clear cytoplasm, these mesotheliomas must be distinguished from renal cell carcinoma and other metastatic clear cell carcinomas. Small foci of cells with abundant eosinophilic cytoplasm resembling the deciduoid cells of pregnancy can be observed in epithelioid mesothelioma, but it is very uncommon in the pleura for this to be a predominant feature (so-called deciduoid mesothelioma) {1921,2342}. A pattern with small cell tumour cells mimicking small cell carcinoma is seen in some cases, but usually lacks the karyorrhexis and haematoxyphylic staining of blood vessels typical of small cell carcinoma. The term small cell mesothelioma is discouraged in diagnostic reports, to avoid confusion with small cell carcinoma {1617,1922}. The term transitional pattern has been used to describe tumours with a sheet-like growth pattern in which the cells are cohesive but have elongated morphology.

The fibrous stroma of epithelioid mesotheliomas can vary from scant to prominent, and can show varying degrees

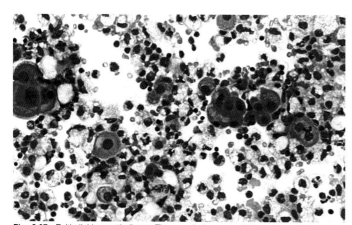

Fig. 2.07 Epithelioid mesothelioma. The sample is very cellular, with multiple atypical mesothelial cells arranged in three-dimensional structures with morules.

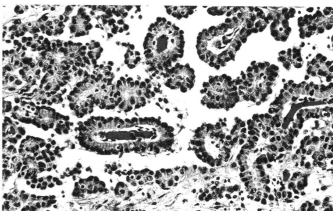

Fig. 2.08 Epithelioid malignant mesothelioma. This mesothelioma consists of sheets of epithelioid tumour cells with a moderate amount of eosinophilic cytoplasm and uniform nuclei with conspicuous nucleoli. Reprinted from Travis WD et al. {2678}.

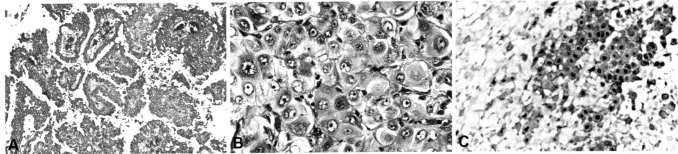

Fig. 2.09 Epithelioid malignant mesothelioma. **A** Papillary pattern. **B** This mesothelioma consists of sheets of epithelioid tumour cells with a moderate amount of eosinophilic cytoplasm and uniform nuclei with conspicuous nucleoli. Reprinted from Travis WD et al. {2678}. **C** Immunohistochemistry shows a diffuse, strong nuclear and weak cytoplasmic staining for calretinin.

of cellularity (from hyalinized acellular to highly cellular), which may make it difficult to distinguish from a true sarcomatoid component. Such tumours may be easily confused with biphasic mesothelioma. Myxoid change may be conspicuous in 5–10% of cases, with nests of cytologically bland, often vacuolated epithelioid cells floating in the matrix. The matrix in such tumours is typically hyaluronate, showing hyaluronidase-sensitive staining with Alcian blue {2361}. Malignant mesotheliomas are generally negative for neutral mucin (with periodic acid–Schiff with diastase or mucicarmine stains); but exceptions occur, limiting diagnostic utility.

Immunohistochemistry
Immunohistochemistry plays an important role in distinguishing epithelioid malignant mesotheliomas from other tumours involving the pleura, particularly lung adenocarcinoma. This distinction can be greatly facilitated by the combined use of a minimum of two mesothelial markers and two carcinoma markers. Based on their specificity and sensitivity, calretinin, CK5/6, WT1, and D2-40 are the best positive markers to support a diagnosis of mesothelioma, and BerEP4 or MOC31, B72.3, carcinoembryonic antigen, and BG8 are the are most commonly used to diagnose carcinoma {1056,1925,1926}. A pancytokeratin such as AE1/AE3 is also useful, as a negative result suggests the possibility of other tumours. Other markers can be helpful in the differential diagnosis between mesothelioma and metastatic carcinoma, and also help determine tumour origin. Examples include markers for lung adenocarcinoma (TTF1 and napsin A), breast carcinoma (ERα, progesterone receptor, GCDFP15, and mammaglobin) {1929}, renal cell carcinoma (PAX8), papillary serous carcinoma (PAX8, PAX2, and estrogen receptor), and adenocarcinomas of the gastrointestinal tract (CDX2) and prostate (prostate-specific antigen) {1056,1925,1927,1928}. GATA3 is expressed in more than half of all mesotheliomas, including both epithelial and sarcomatoid types {1668}.

Table 2.01 Immunohistochemistry of epithelioid malignant mesothelioma vs. metastatic carcinomas {1925,2569}

Mesothelial markers		
Markers	**Sensitivity**	**Specificity versus lung adenocarcinoma**
Calretinin	> 90%	90–95%
CK5/6	75–100%	80–90%
WT1	70–95%	~100%
D2-40	90–100%	85%
Adenocarcinoma (positive epithelial markers)		
Markers	**Sensitivity**	**Specificity versus malignant mesothelioma**
MOC31	95–100%	85–98%
BerEP4	95–100%	74–87%
BG8 (Lewis Y)	90–100%	93–97%
B72.3	25–85%	> 95%
Monoclonal carcinoembryonic antigen	80–100%	> 95%
Organ specific – lung		
Markers	**Sensitivity**	**Specificity versus malignant mesothelioma**
TTF1 (8G7G3/1)	~80%	High
Napsin A	~80%	High
Organ specific – breast		
Markers	**Sensitivity**	**Specificity versus malignant mesothelioma**
Estrogen receptor α	NA (not available)	NA
Progesterone receptor	NA	NA
GCDFP15	30–40%	High
Mammaglobin	50–85%	High
Organ specific – renal		
Markers	**Sensitivity**	**Specificity versus malignant mesothelioma**
PAX8	70–100%	Unknown
PAX2	80%	Unknown
RCC	Up to 85%	75–90%
CD15 (LeuM1)	60%[a]	High
[a] Variable by subtype.		

Additionally, p40 (or p63) is helpful for distinguishing epithelioid mesotheliomas with pseudosquamous morphology from squamous cell carcinomas {1919}. CK5/6 is not helpful in this differential diagnosis, as it stains both tumours. Some non-epithelial tumours that are usually keratin-negative (including epithelioid haemangioendotheliomas and angiosarcomas, melanomas, and large cell lymphomas) can occasionally mimic epithelioid mesothelioma. In such cases, endothelial-associated markers (i.e. CD31, CD34, ERG (v-ets avian erythroblastosis virus E26 oncogene homologue protein, and FLI1), melanoma markers (i.e. HMB45, melan A, and SOX10), and haematopoietic markers (i.e. CD20 and CD45) can be used. All of these markers are negative in mesothelioma. Keratin can occasionally be positive in epithelioid vascular tumours, although it is usually focal. A relatively large number of immunohistochemical markers for distinguishing between malignant mesotheliomas and reactive mesothelial proliferations have been investigated, but the results of these studies remain controversial. No marker or combination of markers has yet been identified that can be used with confidence for routine diagnostic work in this differential diagnosis. As a general recommendation, whenever immunohistochemistry is used in diagnosis, high-quality staining must be ensured, and participation in a quality assurance programme is encouraged.

Differential diagnosis
The primary differential diagnosis is between epithelioid mesothelioma and metastatic adenocarcinoma. The presence of an intrapulmonary mass favours lung cancer, as the distribution of mesothelioma is typically limited to the pleura. Pseudomesotheliomatous adenocarcinoma with diffuse pleural spread is uncommon, but it can mimic epithelioid mesothelioma clinically, macroscopically, and microscopically. Immunohistochemistry is often helpful in resolving this differential diagnosis. Other epithelioid tumours that can have a pseudomesotheliomatous appearance include epithelioid haemangioendothelioma (see *Epithelioid haemangioendothelioma,* p. 176, and *Angiosarcoma,* p. 177), intrapleural thymoma (see *Thymomas,* p. 187), melanoma, lymphoma, and synovial sarcoma with scant spindle cells (see *Synovial*

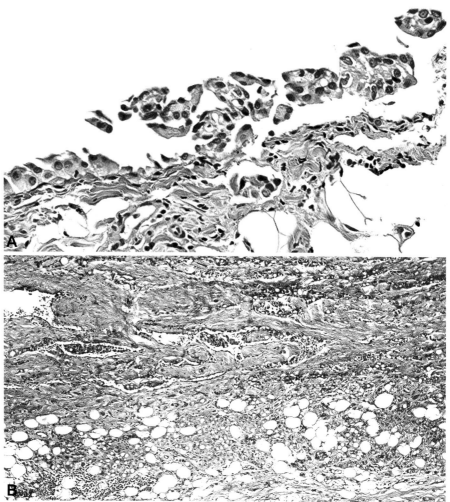

Fig. 2.10 Atypical mesothelial hyperplasia versus invasive epithelioid malignant mesothelioma. **A** Atypical mesothelial hyperplasia of the parietal pleura. The epithelial proliferation on the surface is suspicious for malignancy; however, in the absence of invasion, this is best diagnosed as atypical mesothelial hyperplasia. **B** This proliferation of atypical epithelioid mesothelial cells shows invasion into chest wall fat, supporting the diagnosis of malignant mesothelioma.

Table 2.02 Reactive atypical mesothelial hyperplasia versus malignant mesothelioma {458}

Histological features	Atypical mesothelial hyperplasia	Malignant mesothelioma
Major criteria		
Stromal invasion	Absent	Present (the deeper, the more definitive)
Cellularity	Confined to the pleural surface	Dense, with stromal reaction
Papillae	Simple, lined by single-cell layer	Complex, with cellular stratification
Growth pattern	Surface growth	Expansile nodules, complex and disorganized pattern
Zonation	Process becomes less cellular towards chest wall	No zonation of process, often more cellular away from effusion
Vascularity	Capillaries are perpendicular to the surface	Irregular and haphazard
Minor criteria		
Cytological atypia	Confined to areas of organizing effusion	Present in any area, but many cells are deceptively bland and relatively monotonous
Necrosis	Rare (necrosis may be within pleural exudate)	Necrosis of tumour area is usually a sign of malignancy
Mitoses	Mitoses may be plentiful	Many mesotheliomas show very few mitoses (but atypical mitoses favour malignancy)

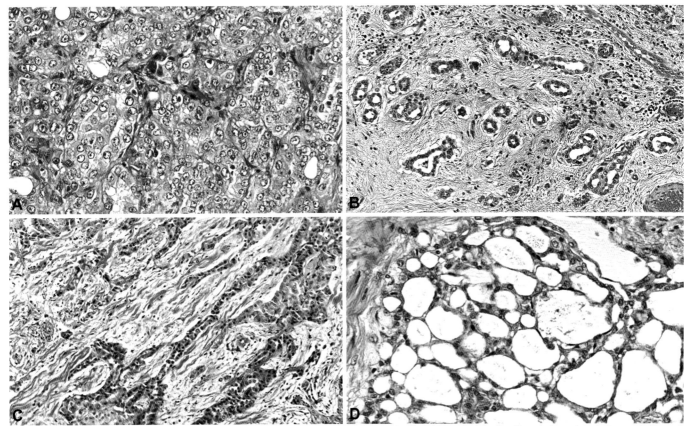

Fig. 2.11 Epithelioid malignant mesothelioma. **A** High-power view showing sheets of large, polygonal epithelioid mesothelial cells with central, round, vesicular nuclei with small nucleoli. Reprinted from Galateau-Salle F {785}. **B** Tubular pattern. **C** Trabecular patterns. **D** Microcystic pattern.

sarcoma, p. 177). Synovial sarcoma can be excluded by negative testing for the translocation t(X;18) {2822}. In the differential diagnosis with synovial sarcoma, TLE1 nuclear immunostaining may not be helpful {1613}. Proximal variant epithelioid sarcoma can involve the pleura and chest wall, mimicking epithelioid mesothelioma {35,966}; however, staining for cytokeratins is typically patchier than would be expected with an epithelioid mesothelioma, and other mesothelial markers (e.g. calretinin, D2-40, and WT1 nuclear staining) are typically negative. In contrast, epithelioid sarcomas stain strongly positive for fascin and vimentin. *SMARCB1* homozygous deletion can be reliably detected by FISH in epithelioid sarcoma.

Reactive mesothelial hyperplasia may be extremely florid, and mimic mesothelioma in the context of a wide variety of diseases, particularly infection. To avoid misdiagnosis on a pleural tissue sample, in the absence of unequivocal malignant tumour fragments, the presence of invasion in the chest wall soft tissue or in the underlying lung parenchyma by the mesothelial cells is the only robust criterion

for malignancy. In the case of pleural effusion, the diagnostic utility of FISH for *p16* homozygous deletion for the diagnosis of malignant mesothelioma is promising, but validation studies are needed {1069A,1708}.

In cases with superficial mesothelial proliferation, the diagnostic term mesothelioma in situ should be avoided. In such proliferations, the presence of *p16* deletion in the context of strong clinical and/ or radiological evidence of tumour may support a diagnosis of malignant mesothelioma, but this approach needs further validation {1059}.

Florid mesothelial proliferations have also been reported in lymph nodes of patients with recurrent pleuritis without evidence of malignant mesothelioma. They typically involve the subcapsular sinuses without destruction of lymph node architecture {475}.

Genetic profile

Cytogenetic and genomic molecular studies have demonstrated that most malignant pleural mesotheliomas have multiple chromosomal alterations. Chromosomal losses are more common than

gains in malignant pleural mesothelioma. The most common losses are on chromosomal arms 1p, 3p, 4q, 6q, 9p, 13q, 14q, and 22q. The most common gains are on chromosomal arms 1q, 5p, 7p, 8q, and 17q {1348,1481,1778}. Several tumour suppressor genes, including *NF2*, *CDKN2A* (*p16INK4a*), *CDKN2B* (*p15INK4b*), and *BAP1*, are frequently altered in malignant pleural mesothelioma.

The *NF2* gene located on 22q12.1 was one of the first tumour suppressor genes shown to be inactivated in malignant mesothelioma {198,2324}. *NF2* is inactivated by some combination of heterozygous deletions, nonsense mutations, and missense mutations in up to two thirds of cases; mutations account for 20% of these alterations {240}. *NF2* inactivation has not been associated with a specific histological subtype of malignant mesothelioma or prognosis. The neurofibromin 2 protein (merlin) is a membrane cytoskeleton-associated protein downstream of integrin-like kinase. It regulates several downstream pathways (including mTOR and the Hippo pathway), and is a key molecule determining invasion, cell growth, and survival of malignant

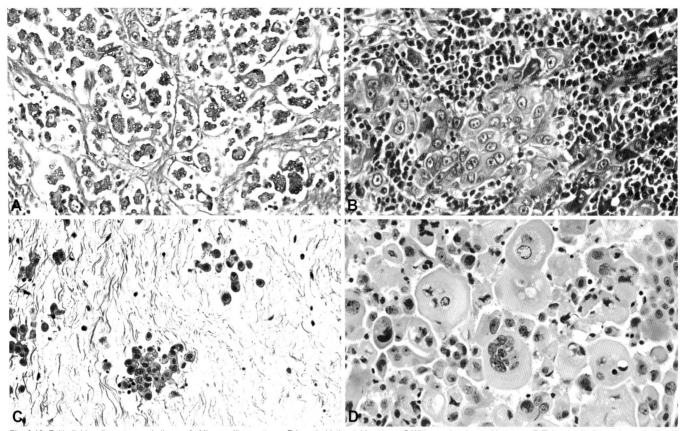

Fig. 2.12 Epithelioid malignant mesothelioma. **A** Micropapillary pattern. **B** Lymphohistiocytoid pattern. **C** With prominent myxoid stroma. **D** This mesothelioma shows deciduoid features and is composed of numerous large tumour cells with abundant eosinophilic cytoplasm. Some tumour cells show multinucleation.

mesothelial cells {934,1382,2640}. *NF2* inactivation is associated with increased mTOR signalling and Hippo pathway activation {1510,2967}. Deletion of the 9p21 locus is the most common genetic abnormality in malignant pleural mesothelioma {1004,1071,1512,2090}, resulting in loss of *CDKN2A* (*p16INK4a*), and p53 regulator *CDKN2A/p14ARF*, as well as the frequent loss of *CDKN2B* (*p15INK4b*) and *MTAP*. *CDKN2A* (*p16INK4a*) and *CDKN2B* (*p15INK4b*) are tumour suppressor genes that encode cyclin-dependent kinase inhibitor proteins that function in the retinoblastoma pathway, regulating the cell cycle during the G1/S phase. The loss of *p14ARF* leads to destabilization of p53. Since *TP53* is rarely mutated in malignant pleural mesothelioma, loss of *p14ARF* is a mechanism for functional loss of p53 in malignant pleural mesothelioma.

Loss of *p16/CDKN2A* in malignant pleural mesothelioma is a result of deletion, promoter hypermethylation, or point mutation, with homozygous deletion being the most common {2322,2909}. Deletion of *p16/CDKN2A* has been reported in 67–83% of malignant pleural

mesotheliomas. The reported frequency of deletion varies depending on the histological subtype; rates are highest in sarcomatoid mesothelioma – approaching 100% {240,428,1512,2918}.

Between 42% and 60% of malignant pleural mesotheliomas harbour some form of *BAP1* loss (with a combination of large deletions, point mutations, and insertions). The rate may be higher in epithelioid malignant mesothelioma than other histological subtypes {2981,3009}. The rate of somatic mutations is about 20–30% {2981,3009}. Patients with *BAP1* somatic mutations are more commonly smokers, but no other distinct clinical feature has been reported {3009}. It is estimated that < 5% of patients with a newly diagnosed malignant mesothelioma have *BAP1* germline mutations {240,420,2624,2875}. No association has been found between *BAP1* mutations and the other common alterations in malignant pleural mesothelioma (i.e. *CDKN2A* deletion and *NF2* deletion/mutation) {240}. BAP1 is a nuclear protein that functions as a deubiquitinase that regulates multiple cellular functions, including the activity of specific transcription

factors, the presence of specific chromatin modifications, and the activity of double-stranded DNA repair mechanisms {1382}. It is currently unclear which of these functions are important in malignant mesotheliomas.

Other tumour suppressor genes that are occassionally mutated include *LATS1* and *LATS2*.

LATS2 kinase is a key member of the Hippo signalling pathway, which regulates transcriptional targets through YAP1. Approximately 10% of malignant mesotheliomas harbour mutations in *LATS2* and the closely related *LATS1* {240,1772,2323}. There is no clear association with histological subtype or prognosis. Loss of LATS2 results in activation of Hippo signalling through YAP1 {1693,2967}.

Although activating mutations in RTKs have been described as oncogenic drivers in a variety of malignancies, these do not appear to be a common mechanism in pleural malignant mesothelioma. Even in the absence of activating mutations, many studies have confirmed the importance of receptor tyrosine kinase signalling pathways, including

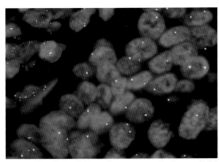

Fig. 2.13 Epithelioid malignant mesothelioma. 9p21 (*p16*) FISH: Malignant mesothelial cells with homozygous deletion of 9p21 show centromere 9p only (green signal) and lack the *p16* gene (red signal). Normal cells (as a positive control) show both red and green signals.

Table 2.03 Genes of potential interest for malignant pleural mesothelioma characterization and predictive prognostic value {1138}

Genes	Significance	Sources
p16/CDKN2A	Gene loss or no protein expression is associated with poor survival	{411,1378A, 520,1345,1512}
KIAA0977/GDIA1, L6/CTHBP, L6/GDIA1	Gene ratios predict outcome	{875}
CD9/KIAA1199, CD9/THBD, DLG5/KIAA1199, DLG5/THBD	Gene ratios predict outcome	{876}
TM4SF1/PKM2, TM4SF1/ARHDDIA, COBLL1/ARHDDIA	Gene ratios discriminate high-risk from low-risk patients	{874}
Gbx2, KI67, CCNB1, BUB1, KNTC2, USP22, HCFC1, RNF2, ANK3, FGFR2, CES1	Expression associated with poor prognosis	{852}
CDH2	Overexpressed in the short-term recurrence group	{1109}
DNAJA1	Underexpressed in the short-term recurrence group	{1109}
AURKA, AURKB	Expression associated with poor outcome	{502}
MELK	Upregulation associated with poor survival	{1512}
BIRC5, KIF4A, SEPT9	Upregulation associated with poor prognosis	{501}
HAPLN1	Expression negatively correlated with survival	{1110}
DNAJA1	Underexpressed in the short-term recurrence group	{1109}
MMP14	High expression associated with poor survival	{501}
LELK1	Upregulation associated with poor survival	{1512}
13 genes involved in extracellular matrix, regulators of extracellular matrix assembly, angiogenesis	High expression associated with poor survival	{2939}

epidermal growth factor receptor, MET (the hepatocyte growth factor receptor), VEGFR, platelet-derived growth factor receptor, and insulin-like growth factor pathways {1138,1944}. Overexpression of VEGF/VEGFR, hepatocyte growth factor/MET, and insulin-like growth factor receptor and ligands suggests the possibility of distinct autocrine loops driving cell growth in malignant pleural mesothelioma {1017,1600,1765,2486}. Activation of p38 MAPK and PI3K/Akt kinase, which are the downstream effectors of receptor tyrosine kinase activation, is well described in pleural malignant mesothelioma {263,1138,1914,1944}.

Gene expression profiling has identified specific gene expression changes in malignant mesothelioma compared with normal mesothelium, effects of fibre/asbestos exposure, and several new candidate oncogenes and tumour suppressor genes {897,1138}. Patient prognosis and response to therapy have been shown to correlate with specific gene expression profiles {1138}. However, published expression microarray studies show only limited overlap in predictive or prognostic expression profiles {1512}. MicroRNA profiling has shown multiple microRNAs to be implicated in

the biology, prognosis, and diagnosis of malignant mesothelioma {177,2686}. Gene expression changes due to promoter methylation have been reported, and affect many genes (e.g. *APC, p16, p14, RASSF1,* and *RARB*) {443,730} and pathways, including the Wnt pathway {152,1307,1429,2757}.

Prognosis and predictive factors

The long-term survival rate of patients with malignant mesothelioma is poor {2227,2228,2750}. Younger age, epithelioid type (versus sarcomatoid or biphasic type), and early TNM staging are indicators of longer median survival, and strongly influence the therapeutic

strategy {742,2226}. Although the evidence is sparse, multimodality therapy is indicated in patients with a good performance status and early-stage disease {2754}. Additionally, a histological subtype of epithelioid mesothelioma, such as mesothelioma with abundant myxoid changes, is a more favourable prognostic factor {2361}. In contrast, the presence of pleomorphic features strongly predicts poor survival {1178}. A histological grading system has not been established for malignant mesothelioma, but preliminary data suggest that nuclear grade (including nuclear atypia) and mitotic count are independent poor prognostic factors {1176}.

Sarcomatoid, desmoplastic, and biphasic mesothelioma

V. Roggli
A. Churg
L.R. Chirieac
F. Galateau-Salle
A. Borczuk
S. Dacic

S. Hammar
A.N. Husain
K. Inai
M. Ladanyi
A.M. Marchevsky
D. Naidich

N.G. Ordóñez
D.C. Rice
M.T. Sheaff
W.D. Travis
J. van Meerbeeck

Definition

Diffuse sarcomatoid malignant mesothelioma of the pleura is a malignant tumour arising from mesothelial cells and showing a diffuse pattern of growth over the pleural surfaces and a mesenchymal or spindle cell morphological appearance.

Diffuse desmoplastic malignant mesothelioma is characterized by dense collagenized tissue separated by malignant mesothelial cells arranged in a storiform or so-called patternless pattern, which must be present in at least 50% of the tumour.

Diffuse biphasic malignant mesothelioma is a mesothelioma showing at least 10% each of epithelioid and sarcomatoid patterns.

Diffuse malignant mesotheliomas must be differentiated from localized malignant mesotheliomas, which have different clinical behaviours.

ICD-O codes

Sarcomatoid mesothelioma   9051/3
Desmoplastic mesothelioma   9051/3
Biphasic mesothelioma   9053/3

Synonyms

Sarcomatoid mesothelioma: sarcomatous mesothelioma

Biphasic mesothelioma: mixed mesothelioma; mixed epithelioid and sarcomatoid mesothelioma; mixed epithelial and sarcomatous mesothelioma

Epidemiology

Among the mesotheliomas, these tumours are rare. Sarcomatoid type accounts for < 10%, biphasic for 10–15%, and desmoplastic for < 2% of all mesotheliomas. The epidemiology for all histological types of mesothelioma is similar (see *Epithelioid mesothelioma*, p. 156).

Etiology

See *Epithelioid mesothelioma*, p. 156.

Clinical features

The signs, symptoms, and staging of these tumours are similar to those of the epithelioid histological type (see *Epithelioid mesothelioma*, p. 156). Desmoplastic mesothelioma progresses more rapidly than epithelioid mesothelioma, and there is a trend towards older patient age and greater pain, weight loss, and loss of performance status {1278}. Sarcomatoid mesotheliomas are associated with frequent distant metastases and little or no effusion. Desmoplastic mesothelioma can metastasize to bone {1537}.

Localization

See *Epithelioid mesothelioma*, p. 156.

Macroscopy

See *Epithelioid mesothelioma*, p. 156. Sarcomatoid mesothelioma typically presents with diffuse pleural thickening or as a pleural-based mass.

Cytology

For information about effusion cytology, see *Epithelioid mesothelioma*, p. 156. In fine-needle aspiration biopsy specimens, sarcomatoid mesotheliomas may have features similar to those of other soft tissue sarcomas or sarcomatoid carcinoma, with spindle morphology and varying degrees of atypical nuclear features. Biphasic mesotheliomas can also have an epithelial component {457}.

Histopathology

Sarcomatoid mesothelioma

Sarcomatoid mesothelioma is characterized by a proliferation of spindle cells arranged in fascicles or with a haphazard pattern, and involves the adipose tissue of the parietal pleura or the adjacent lung parenchyma. Sarcomatoid mesotheliomas may present a wide range of morphologies – from plump cells to thin, long cells with scant cytoplasm. Nuclear atypia and mitotic activity vary from minimal to moderate or marked. In the latter setting, there is also marked pleomorphism. The presence of necrosis and the degree of atypia and mitoses parallel the aggressiveness of the tumour {457}.

The term mesothelioma with heterologous elements is applied when a mesothelioma shows rhabdomyosarcomatous, osteosarcomatous, or chondrosarcomatous elements {1279}. These elements must be differentiated from osteoid and chondroid metaplasia.

Some sarcomatoid mesotheliomas are characterized by atypical giant cells with large, multilobulated, bizarre, hyperchromatic nuclei with a high mitotic count and atypical mitoses {1178}. These may morphologically mimic undifferentiated high-grade pleomorphic sarcoma.

Table 2.04 Immunochemistry and molecular findings in the differential diagnosis between sarcomatoid malignant mesothelioma and selected other neoplasms {167,957,2025,2670,2973}

Sarcomatoid malignant mesothelioma	Sarcomatoid carcinoma	Monophasic synovial sarcoma	Solitary fibrous tumour	Angiosarcoma
Immunochemistry				
- Keratin positive - Low expression of mesothelial markers	- Keratin positive - TTF1 or p63/p40 may be positive - Positive carcinoma markers (see Table 2.01)	- Keratin usually weak and/or focal	- CD34 positive - STAT6 positive - Bcl2 positive - Keratin usually negative; rarely focally positive	- Keratin usually negative; can be focal/weak; rarely strong - CD31, CD34 - ERG, FLI1
Molecular findings				
	- *KRAS* mutation (20–30%) - Rare *EGFR* mutations	- Translocation - t(X;18) (p11.2;q11.2) - SYT-SSX fusion protein	- Translocation - *NAB2-STAT6*	

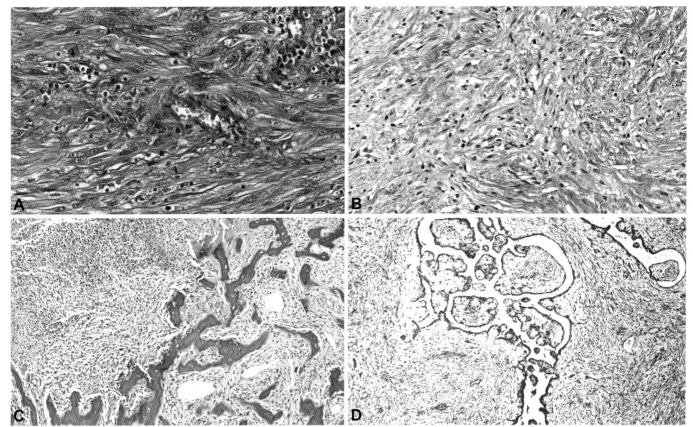

Fig. 2.14 A Diffuse sarcomatoid malignant mesothelioma showing high cellularity, with plump spindle cells with elongated nuclei and mitoses. B Diffuse sarcomatoid malignant mesothelioma showing low cellularity, with long, thin spindle cells, bland nuclei, and sparse cytoplasm. C Diffuse sarcomatoid malignant mesothelioma with a heterologous element (osteosarcoma). Reprinted from Galateau-Salle F {785}. D Biphasic malignant mesothelioma. This mesothelioma consists of an epithelial component (which is mostly papillary) and a sarcomatoid component.

Desmoplastic mesothelioma

Desmoplastic mesothelioma is characterized by areas of atypical spindle cells arranged in a so-called patternless pattern {1563} within a dense, hyalinized, fibrous stroma constituting at least 50% of the tumour. Invasion of adipose tissue is the most reliable criterion to distinguish desmoplastic mesothelioma from organizing pleuritis. In small biopsy, the diagnosis of desmoplastic mesothelioma is very difficult. In addition to invasion, other helpful criteria that favour malignancy include the presence of bland necrosis, cellular stromal nodules, and other areas of clear epithelioid or sarcomatoid mesothelioma.

Biphasic mesothelioma

Diffuse biphasic malignant mesothelioma is a mesothelioma showing at least 10% each of epithelioid and sarcomatoid patterns. Reporting the amount of the sarcomatoid component is recommended, because of its potential impact on prognosis and the therapeutic management of the patient.

Immunohistochemistry

Sarcomatoid mesotheliomas almost invariably stain, at least focally, with the AE1/AE3 broad-spectrum antikeratin antibody cocktail and the pancytokeratin antibodies OSCAR and KL1, as well as with the CAM5.2 antibody, which reacts primarily with CK8 {431,1056,2570}. CK18 may be positive in tumours where other keratins are negative. However, keratin negativity may be encountered in 5% of sarcomatoid malignant mesotheliomas, and in 10% of tumours with heterologous elements {1279}. About 30% of these tumours express calretinin {98,998,1278}, and these tumours are more often positive for D2-40 {431,998,1955}. Other mesothelial markers, including CK5/6 and WT1, are relatively insensitive {1056}. Sarcomatoid mesotheliomas are often vimentin-positive and occasionally express actin, desmin, or S100 protein.

Immunohistochemistry must be applied to rule out a sarcomatoid carcinoma; TTF1, napsin A, and p63/p40 expression support a diagnosis of sarcomatoid carcinoma. Myogenin and MyoD1 nuclear staining is useful for recognizing a rhabdomyosarcomatous component in mesothelioma with heterologous elements.

In desmoplastic mesothelioma, keratin immunostaining can be very useful for highlighting the tumour cells and for demonstrating invasion into adjacent soft tissues, particularly adipose tissue.

Differential diagnosis

The major differential diagnoses for sarcomatoid mesothelioma are soft tissue sarcoma metastatic to the pleura and primary chest wall sarcoma that has reached the pleura. Unlike sarcomatoid mesotheliomas, most sarcomas are keratin-negative. However, keratin-positive sarcomas (such as primary angiosarcomas of the pleura and monophasic synovial sarcomas) can present a diagnostic problem. Most sarcomas also show specific lineage markers and characteristic genetic changes {2670,2822}.

Primary pleural tumours causing diffuse pleural thickening with

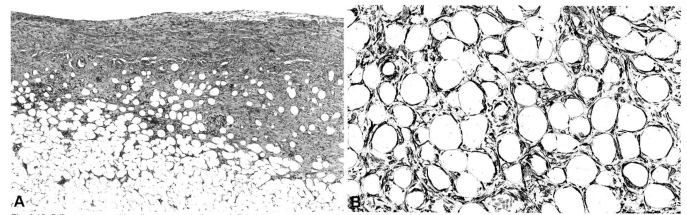

Fig. 2.15 Diffuse sarcomatoid malignant mesothelioma. **A** Full-thickness cellularity and invasion into true chest wall adipose tissue. **B** Cytokeratin-positive cells of desmoplastic mesothelioma in the chest wall fat.

osteosarcomatous or chondrosarcomas differentiation are probably all mesotheliomas. In most cases, pankeratin staining is positive, but keratin expression is sometimes difficult to demonstrate {1279}. Cases have been reported of osteosarcomas and chondrosarcomas growing diffusely in the pleural cavity with a gross distribution mimicking that of malignant mesothelioma {828,1132,1215}. *IDH1/2* mutation can differentiate chondrosarcoma from chondroblastic osteosarcoma or mesothelioma with a heterologous component.

Inflammatory myofibroblastic tumours can involve the pleura, but it is very unusual for these tumours to show diffuse pleural thickening. The myofibroblastic spindle cells with bland nuclei admixed with inflammatory cells and collagen may be difficult to distinguish from cells of mesothelioma with a dense inflammatory component {1279,1499}. The spindle cells may show ALK expression

and *ALK* chromosomal rearrangement {303,467,828}.

Finally, there are some chest wall sarcomas, formerly classified as malignant fibrous histiocytomas, that are pleomorphic (undifferentiated), with anaplastic multinucleated giant cells and bizarre mitotic figures {565}. They typically stain positive for vimentin but negative for broad-spectrum cytokeratins and mesothelial markers.

Desmoplastic mesotheliomas must be distinguished from organizing pleuritis {458,1563}. In organizing pleuritis, there is typically zonation, with a more cellular infiltrate immediately under the effusion, and increasing degrees of fibrosis towards the chest wall. Desmoplastic mesotheliomas do not show zonation. In organizing pleuritis, there are often small capillaries perpendicular to the pleural surface, whereas in desmoplastic mesotheliomas, capillaries are generally inconspicuous. Desmoplastic mesotheliomas may also form cellular

stromal nodules, which are not seen in organizing pleuritis. Desmoplastic mesotheliomas often invade the chest wall fat, and in such cases keratin-positive cells can be found infiltrating fat. Care should be taken not to confuse so-called fake fat (a traction artefact within markedly thickened and fibrotic pleura) with true invasion of fat in desmoplastic mesotheliomas. In true invasion, spindle cells course at some angle downwards from the pleura, whereas in fake fat, the spindle cells are all parallel to the pleural surface {456}. Organizing pleuritis may extend into the fat, but the cells in the fat are not keratin-positive {458}. The presence of bland tumour necrosis or focal areas of frankly malignant sarcomatoid or epithelioid mesothelioma also favours desmoplastic mesothelioma.

Biphasic mesotheliomas must be distinguished from pleomorphic carcinomas and synovial sarcomas. Pleomorphic carcinomas usually form a localized peripheral lung mass, which can invade

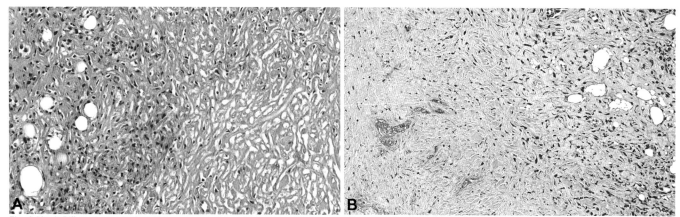

Fig. 2.16 **A** Diffuse desmoplastic malignant mesothelioma. Note the paucicellular spindle cell proliferation with bland necrosis, hyalinized stroma, and chest wall invasion. **B** Desmoplastic malignant mesothelioma. This mesothelioma shows bland necrosis and atypical spindle cells surrounded by a wire-like arrangement of hyaline stroma. The tumour also invades fat.

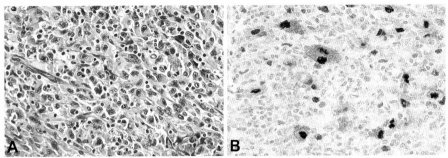

Fig. 2.17 Sarcomatoid malignant mesothelioma with rhabdomyosarcoma differentiation. **A** This mesothelioma shows some pleomorphic tumour cells with abundant eosinophilic cytoplasm, which suggests the possibility of rhabdomyosarcoma. **B** Scattered tumour cells show positive staining for myogenin.

the chest wall, and they frequently show areas of conventional adenocarcinoma or squamous cell carcinoma. They may stain for typical broad-spectrum carcinoma markers such as MOC31/BerEP4 or monoclonal carcinoembryonic antigen; however, these markers may be negative in some tumours, and it may be impossible to morphologically distinguish pleomorphic carcinoma from sarcomatoid mesothelioma. Most synovial sarcomas in the pleura are monophasic, but biphasic tumours also occur {779,2822}. Primary pleural synovial sarcomas can show a mixture of epithelial and spindle cells. Synovial sarcomas show a characteristic t(X;18)(p11.2;q11.2) translocation {1293,2822,2822}.

Genetic profile

The karyotypic and genomic characteristics of sarcomatoid malignant mesothelioma overlap with those of epithelioid malignant mesothelioma (see *Epithelioid mesothelioma*, p. 156). However, there are several differences in the frequency of somatic alterations. For example, homozygous deletion in the region of 9p21 (*p16*) is seen in most sarcomatoid pleural malignant mesotheliomas, approaching 100% of cases in some series {1071,2647,2909,2918}. This higher rate may also be true of biphasic tumours, although reported rates of deletion vary between studies {240,1071}.

In one series, losses at 14q32 and gains in 8q24 were seen at a significantly higher rate in sarcomatoid malignant mesothelioma {2565}. In another series, lower rates of 3p and 17p losses, and higher rates of 15q gain were reported {1348}. *TERT* promoter mutations are more common in sarcomatoid malignant mesothelioma (40%) than in the biphasic (19%) or epithelioid (11%) subtypes {2579} (see *Epithelioid mesothelioma*, p. 156).

Prognosis and predictive factors

In most series, sarcomatoid and desmoplastic variants have poorer prognoses than epithelioid mesothelioma {2224,2227}. Biphasic tumours have an intermediate survival. Desmoplastic mesothelioma has a dismal prognosis; most patients die within 6 months after diagnosis. No patient with sarcomatoid mesothelioma has been known to survive for 5 years. TNM staging is a significant predictor of prognosis.

Localized malignant mesothelioma

A. Churg
V. Roggli
L.R. Chirieac
F. Galateau-Salle
A. Borczuk
S. Dacic

A. Gibbs
S. Hammar
A.N. Husain
K. Inai
A.M. Marchevsky
D. Naidich

N.G. Ordóñez
D.C. Rice
M.T. Sheaff
W.D. Travis
J. van Meerbeeck

Definition
Localized malignant mesothelioma is a rare tumour that grossly appears as a distinctly localized nodular lesion. It shows no gross or microscopic evidence of diffuse pleural spread, but has the microscopic, immunohistochemical, and ultrastructural features of diffuse malignant mesothelioma.

ICD-O codes
Localized malignant mesothelioma should be coded according to the histological type of analogous mesothelioma.
Epithelioid mesothelioma   9052/3
Sarcomatoid mesothelioma   9051/3
Biphasic mesothelioma   9053/3

Synonyms
Localized mesothelioma; solitary malignant mesothelioma

Epidemiology
This tumour is very rare; fewer than 50 cases have been reported. There is a slight male predisposition, and the mean age is between 60 and 65 years {52,1803}.

Etiology
The etiological role of asbestos exposure in localized malignant mesothelioma is unclear.

Clinical features
Localized mesothelioma can be an incidental finding. Patients may present with chest pain, dyspnoea, malaise, fever, or night sweats.

Localization
Localized malignant mesotheliomas usually grow into the chest wall or the adjacent lung parenchyma.

Macroscopy
Localized mesothelioma is a solitary, circumscribed, pleural-based mass attached to the visceral or parietal pleura. The tumours can be pedunculated or sessile.

Cytology
Pleural effusions are uncommon, so cytological examination of these tumours is mostly conducted on fine-needle aspirates. The cytological features resemble those of diffuse malignant mesothelioma (see *Epithelioid mesothelioma*, p. 156, and *Sarcomatoid, desmoplastic, and biphasic mesothelioma*, p. 165).

Histopathology
Localized malignant mesotheliomas have morphological, immunohistochemical, and ultrastructural features indistinguishable from those of diffuse malignant

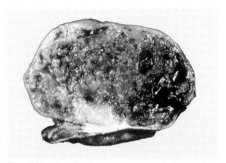

Fig. 2.18 Localized malignant mesothelioma. This mesothelioma consists of a circumscribed pleural-based mass. The cut surface is tan-brown, with focal haemorrhage and cystic changes.

mesotheliomas. The tumours can show epithelioid, sarcomatoid, or biphasic morphologies {52,507} (see *Epithelioid mesothelioma*, p. 156, and *Sarcomatoid, desmoplastic, and biphasic mesothelioma*, p. 165).
The differential diagnoses include solitary fibrous tumour (see *Solitary fibrous tumour*, p. 178), carcinoma (see *Epithelioid mesothelioma*, p. 156 and *Sarcomatoid, desmoplastic, and biphasic mesothelioma*, p. 165), and synovial sarcoma (see *Synovial sarcoma*, p. 177).

Prognosis and predictive factors
Localized mesotheliomas have a better prognosis than diffuse mesotheliomas, and may be cured by surgical excision {52}.

Well-differentiated papillary mesothelioma

V. Roggli
A. Borczuk
L.R. Chirieac
A. Churg
S. Dacic
F. Galateau-Salle

A. Gibbs
S. Hammar
A.N. Husain
K. Inai
D. Naidich
N.G. Ordóñez

D.C. Rice
M.T. Sheaff
W.D. Travis
J. van Meerbeeck

Definition

Well-differentiated papillary mesothelioma (WDPM) of the pleura is a rare, distinct tumour of mesothelial origin, with papillary architecture, bland cytological features, and a tendency towards superficial spread without invasion. This is a clinically, morphologically, and prognostically separate entity from diffuse epithelioid malignant mesothelioma with papillary pattern.

ICD-O code   9052/1

Epidemiology

This tumour is much rarer in the pleura than in the peritoneum, with fewer than 50 cases reported {302,787}. It has occurred over a wide age range, with a mean of about 60 years. There is no sex predominance.

Etiology

The histogenesis of WDPM remains poorly understood. When it occurs in the peritoneum of women, it appears to be unrelated to asbestos exposure. The reports of pleural cases have suggested a link with asbestos exposure, but this has not been established in a formal epidemiological study.

Clinical features

Most patients present with a history of dyspnoea and recurrent pleural effusion without chest pain. Chest radiography and CT show unilateral pleural effusions, without nodularity.

Localization

These mesothelial lesions may be localized or multifocal.

Macroscopy

WDPM may present with a granular pleural surface or as multiple millimeter sized nodules on the parietal and/or visceral pleura, resulting in a velvety appearance {787}.

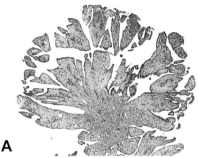
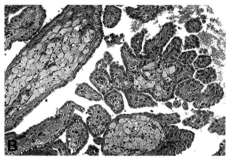

Fig. 2.19 Well-differentiated papillary mesothelioma. **A** Solitary, with exophytic growth. **B** Showing macrophages filling the papillae.

Cytology

In cytological specimens, WDPM demonstrates stout papillary cores lined by a single layer of flattened to cuboidal mesothelial cells. These cells have bland nuclear features and inconspicuous nucleoli. Mitotic figures are typically absent. The finding of significant nuclear atypia, architectural complexity, or solid areas tends to suggest malignant epithelioid mesothelioma with papillary pattern. Since cytological specimens may fail to reveal an invasive component, cytological diagnosis of WDPM is not recommended.

Histopathology

Histologically, the proliferation arises from the mesothelial surface of the pleura, and is characterized by a prominent papillary architecture composed of papillae with more-or-less myxoid cores covered by a single layer of flattened or cuboidal bland epithelioid cells. Macrophages may be present in the cores of the papillae. The nuclei are round, small, and devoid of atypia and mitoses. Invasion is generally not seen. Rare cases with superficial invasion should be called WDPM with invasive foci {455}.

The immunohistochemical pattern of WDPM is that of mesothelial origin {787} (see *Diffuse malignant mesothelioma*, p. 156).

The most important differential diagnosis is epithelioid diffuse malignant mesothelioma with a papillary pattern. Such foci may be extremely difficult to distinguish

Table 2.05 Differential diagnosis between epithelioid malignant mesothelioma with papillary pattern and well-differentiated papillary mesothelioma

Characteristic	Epithelioid malignant mesothelioma with papillary pattrn	Well-differentiated papillary mesothelioma
Growth feature - bulk of disease	Diffuse or multinodular, grossly apparent	Often incidental, solitary, focal area of velvety appearance
Morphology of papillae	Fibrous cores, lined by cells with stratification	Fibrous and stout cores, single-cell layer
Cytology	Cuboidal cells with nucleoli and variable anisocytosis	Flat cuboidal, no anisocytosis
Mitoses	Low	Low
Other growth patterns	Tubular, solid, cribriform, complex papillae	Absent
Stromal invasion	Present	Predominantly exophytic growth, usually absent; when present, only very focal and superficial
Prognosis	Poor	Good, with local recurrence

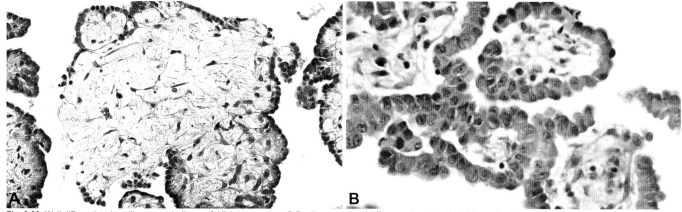

Fig. 2.20 Well-differentiated papillary mesothelioma. **A** High-power view. **B** Papillary pattern of diffuse malignant epithelioid mesothelioma.

morphologically from a WDPM in a small biopsy. Areas of solid tumour favour a diagnosis of malignant mesothelioma. Reference to the operative or radiological findings can be extremely helpful. WDPM should appear as small translucent nodules, whereas diffuse malignant mesothelioma typically looks like diffuse carcinomatosis or a rind of tumour.

Genetic profile
The molecular pathogenesis of WDPM is largely unstudied, so its relation to diffuse malignant epithelioid mesothelioma is unknown. A single pleural WDPM was reported to have a germline *BAP1* mutation {2149}. Single cases of peritoneal WDPM with *NF2* heterozygous deletion {1826} and *E2F1* point mutation {2999} have also been reported.

Prognosis and predictive factors
WDPMs of the pleura are indolent tumours (and in most cases probably clinically benign if completely resected), and are associated with a very long survival.

Whether WDPMs give rise to malignant mesotheliomas remains uncertain. Their clinical behaviour and the results of molecular analyses are suggestive of a neoplastic process {302,787} Follow-up of patients presenting with WDPM with focal invasion is recommended on the basis of possible recurrence {455}.

Adenomatoid tumour

K. Inai
A. Churg
H. Minato

Definition
Pleural adenomatoid tumour is a mesothelial tumour histologically identical to adenomatoid tumours in other locations (especially the female genital tract), but located in the visceral or parietal pleura {1681}. Very few examples of pleural adenomatoid tumours have been reported.

ICD-O code   9054/0

Clinical features
The tumour is found incidentally on gross examination of the pleura {196,1208}.

Localization
Adenomatoid tumours can occur on the visceral or parietal pleura {196,1208}.

Macroscopy
The tumours are solitary, whitish, firm nodules measuring 0.5–2.5 cm.

Histopathology
Irregularly shaped, gland-like spaces are composed of flattened or cuboidal cells, and associated with a fibrous stroma {196,1208}. The tumour cells have a bland nucleus and scant eosinophilic cytoplasm. Intracytoplasmic vacuoles can sometimes be seen, and the spaces may contain basophilic material.

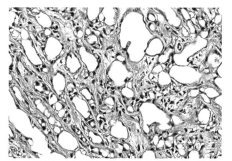

Fig. 2.21 Adenomatoid tumour. Irregularly shaped tubular and microcystic spaces lined by flattened endothelial-like cells within a fibrous stroma.

Immunohistochemically, the tumour cells stain identically to those of epithelioid malignant mesothelioma (see *Diffuse malignant mesothelioma*, p. 156).
The crucial distinction is from epithelial malignant mesotheliomas that have adenomatoid-appearing areas. Epithelial malignant mesotheliomas always show diffuse spread along the pleura and invasion of the underlying stroma, whereas adenomatoid tumours (by definition) are solitary localized lesions. Similar to adenomatoid tumours in the genitourinary tract, they only show localized infiltration of tissue adjacent to the tumour.

Prognosis and predictive factors
Like adenomatoid tumours in other locations, this tumour is benign. Complete removal should be curative.

Lymphoproliferative disorders

C. Bacon
E.S. Jaffe
A.G. Nicholson

Primary effusion lymphoma

Definition
Primary effusion lymphoma (PEL) is a rare neoplasm of large, atypical B cells that are positive for human herpesvirus 8 (HHV8) – also called Kaposi sarcoma-associated herpesvirus (KSHV). The neoplasm presents as an effusion in serous body cavities. Solid tumour masses are not usually present at diagnosis, but may develop during the course of the disease. Clinical presentation as a tissue mass without detectable effusions has been termed extracavitary primary effusion lymphoma. Most patients are immunocompromised.

ICD-O code   9678/3

Synonym
Body cavity-based lymphoma (obsolete)

Epidemiology
Most cases of primary effusion lymphoma occur in HIV-positive patients. The majority of HIV-positive patients with primary effusion lymphoma are men in their fourth to sixth decade, who have sex with men, and are severely immunocompromised (with < 200 CD4+ T cells per μL) {244,359,1783,2400}. Primary effusion lymphoma accounts for approximately 3–4% of HIV-associated lymphomas {328,2400}. Primary effusion lymphoma develops rarely in immunosuppressed organ transplant recipients {84}. It may also arise in the absence of overt immunodeficiency in elderly patients, often individuals from areas of high HHV8 seroprevalence, such as the Mediterranean. Immunosenescence and possibly chronic liver disease are contributing factors {92,245,790,1659,2961}.

Etiology
All cases of primary effusion lymphoma are HHV8-positive. Most neoplastic cells contain 40–80 mono-/oligoclonal episomal viral genomes and display a latency-associated gene expression pattern {354, 359,1216,1995}.

Latency-associated nuclear protein (LANA) and viral microRNAs play diverse roles in lymphomagenesis, cooperatively subverting normal cellular signalling pathways and proliferation and survival controls {353,834,1658}. Among other functions, LANA maintains latency, mediates episomal persistence, and inhibits p53 and β-catenin signalling; vFLIP activates NF-κB; viral cyclin acts as a D-type cyclin and perturbs p21/p27-mediated cell cycle controls and checkpoints; kaposins A and B modulate MAPK signalling and cytokine messenger RNA stability; and vIRF3 contributes to transformation and promotes immune evasion by inhibiting IFN production and HLA class II expression {131,138,909,2545}. A small minority of tumour cells express lytic-phase genes such as *vIL6* and *vG-PCR*, which may also have important oncogenic roles, perhaps partly in a paracrine manner {359,1784,2252}.

Approximately 80% of HIV-associated primary effusion lymphomas show monoclonal coinfection with EBV, but primary effusion lymphoma in HIV-negative patients is usually EBV-negative {359,1301,1783,2432}. EBV exhibits a restricted type I latency-like gene expression pattern, with expression of EBNA1 and EBV-encoded small RNA, but little or no expression of LMP1 or LMP2A; its role in tumour development is unclear {1030}. Gene expression profiling studies have shown either few or no significant differences between EBV-positive and EBV-negative primary effusion lymphoma

{698,1283}. EBV and HHV8 may cooperate in the infection and initial transformation of B cells, and a role for EBNA1 in the proliferation of dually infected primary effusion lymphoma cells has been reported {1286,1539}.

Clinical features
Patients typically present with signs and symptoms of effusions, and with constitutional symptoms. Kaposi sarcoma or (less often) HHV8-associated multicentric Castleman disease may coexist {244,2400}.

Localization
The pleural cavity is the most common site of effusion, followed by the peritoneal and pericardial cavities. More than one body cavity may be simultaneously involved {58,339,1301}. Most patients lack solid tumour masses at first presentation, but contiguous or distal lymph node involvement or extranodal solid tissue involvement is seen in up to approximately 30–40% of patients {58,244,1301,2400}. Effusions may be absent in extracavitary primary effusion lymphoma {327,359,577,1266}.

Cytology
The neoplastic cells are large and pleomorphic, with large nuclei, one or more prominent nucleoli, and abundant amphophilic (sometimes vacuolated) cytoplasm. There is a morphological spectrum within and between cases. Immunoblast-like forms have round nuclei,

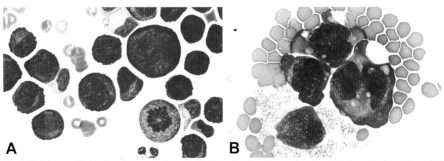

Fig. 2.22 Primary effusion lymphoma. **A** Pleural effusion cytospin shows cells of varied size with deeply basophilic cytoplasm and plasmacytoid features. Even the smaller cells are more than twice the size of a normal lymphocyte. **B** This example shows greater nuclear pleomorphism.

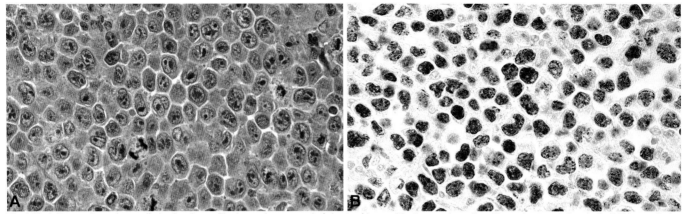

Fig. 2.23 **A** Extracavitary primary effusion lymphoma. The tumour is composed of sheets of immunoblastic-appearing cells, with prominent central nucleoli. **B** Primary effusion lymphoma. This section has been stained for LANA. All the tumour cells show nuclear reactivity.

while anaplastic forms have polylobated nuclei and are typically very large. Cells with plasmablastic morphology have basophilic cytoplasm, eccentric nuclei, and a prominent Golgi zone. Reed-Sternberg-like cells may be present. Mitoses may be frequent. The appearances in tissues sections are generally similar to those in cytological preparations, but the cells may appear less pleomorphic {328,1783}.

Histopathology

In solid tissue, primary effusion lymphoma cells often have an immunoblastic appearance. They almost always express CD45, but usually lack pan-B-cell antigens such as CD19, CD20, CD79a, and PAX5. IRF4/MUM1 and PRDM1/BLIMP1 are expressed, and CD138 is usually positive, consistent with a plasma cell-like phenotype, but surface and cytoplasmic immunoglobulin are rarely present. CD30, CD38, and epithelial membrane antigen are expressed in most cases. Bcl6 is absent {359,360,1301,1971}. A small number of cases express pan-T-cell antigens, either with or without immunophenotypic or molecular evidence of B-cell lineage {245,359,1023,2244}. Although lineage assignment may therefore be difficult, diagnosis is facilitated by demonstrating nuclear expression of LANA, present in all cases {642}. EBV may be detected by in situ hybridization for EBV-encoded small RNA, but LMP1 is immunohistochemically undetectable.

Differential diagnosis
Primary effusion lymphoma is readily distinguished from most other lymphoid neoplasms by its HHV8 positivity. In

particular, primary effusion lymphoma should be distinguished from HHV8-negative effusion-based diffuse large B-cell lymphomas (often mistermed primary effusion lymphoma-like or HHV8-negative primary effusion lymphoma), which are morphologically similar to primary effusion lymphoma but typically express pan-B-cell antigens. They occur mostly in elderly HIV-negative individuals and may be associated with fluid overload states {44,1301,2915}.
Body cavity effusions lacking sufficient atypical cells for a diagnosis of primary effusion lymphoma may occur in patients with HHV8-associated multicentric Castleman disease or the Kaposi sarcoma-associated herpesvirus inflammatory cytokine syndrome associated with severe Kaposi sarcoma and high viral loads {249,2067}.
Primary effusion lymphoma must also be distinguished from effusion-based Burkitt lymphoma and malignant effusions secondary to solid lymphomas or plasma cell neoplasms, in particular from diffuse large B-cell lymphoma associated with chronic inflammation, the prototypical form of which is pyothorax-associated lymphoma. Pyothorax-associated lymphoma presents as a mass in the pleura or peripheral lung with infrequent effusions. It is typically EBV-positive but always HHV8-negative {72}.

Genetic profile
Immunoglobulin genes are clonally rearranged {359,1783}. The somatic mutation pattern suggests derivation from antigen-selected postgerminal centre B cells; rare EBV-negative primary effusion lymphomas with germline immunoglobulin genes have been reported

{695,781,937,1604}. Regardless of immunoglobulin mutation and EBV status, gene expression profiling suggests plasmablastic/incomplete plasma cell differentiation {1141,1283}. Occasional cases carry both immunoglobulin and T-cell receptor gene rearrangements {359,1023,2244}. Rare HHV8-positive cases with a T-cell immunoprofile and only T-cell receptor gene rearrangement, but otherwise within the spectrum of primary effusion lymphoma, have been reported {498,1427,1812}.
Somatic genetic alterations cooperating with viral oncogenes are poorly characterized. Rearrangements of *MYC*, *BCL2*, and *BCL6* have not been identified, and *TP53* mutations or deletions are found in only occasional cases {246,328,781,1783}. Primary effusion lymphomas typically have complex karyotypes with evidence of clonal cytogenetic heterogeneity. Recurrent numerical abnormalities include trisomies of chromosomes 7, 8, and 12 {2883}. Array-based analyses have revealed numerous regions and several discrete genes showing recurrent genomic copy number gain or loss, including frequent loss of fragile site candidate tumour suppressor genes in primary effusion lymphoma cell lines and amplification of the migration-associated genes *SELPG* and *CORO1C* at 12q24.11 {1520,2216}. EBV-positive primary effusion lymphoma cell lines showed fewer copy number changes than EBV-negative lines, consistent with a cooperative role for EBV in lymphomagenesis {2216}.

Prognosis and predictive factors
Patients are often treated with anthracycline-containing chemotherapy, and

if HIV-positive, with highly active antiretroviral therapy (HAART). The overall prognosis of primary effusion lymphoma is poor in all epidemiological groups. The median overall survival is approximately 6 months, although complete response rates of 25–50% and 1 to 2 year overall survival rates of 20–40% are reported, and some patients achieve durable remission {58,244,339,410,2400}. Occasional responses to HAART alone, or in HIV-negative patients, to chemical pleurodesis or intracavitary cidofovir have been reported {1525,2162,2961}. Poor performance status, absence of HAART before primary effusion lymphoma diagnosis (in HIV-positive patients), and multicavity disease are reported adverse prognostic factors {244,339}. Ann Arbor stage is generally not relevant in patients with effusions.

Diffuse large B-cell lymphoma associated with chronic inflammation

Definition
Diffuse large B-cell lymphoma (DLBCL) associated with chronic inflammation (DLBCL-CI) is an EBV-associated B-cell neoplasm that occurs in the context of long-standing chronic inflammation, usually presenting in body cavities or other anatomical sites that are enclosed spaces with limited vascularization. The most common site is the pleural cavity.

ICD-O code   9680/3

Synonym
Pyothorax-associated lymphoma

Epidemiology
DLBCL-CI occurs in patients with long-standing pyothorax or other chronic inflammatory processes {73}. The interval between the initial inflammatory event and the presentation of lymphoma is usually > 10 years. Most cases have occurred in the context of artificial pneumothorax and chronic tuberculosis {1810}. The majority of cases have been reported from Japan, but the disease has also been reported in the west, and there is no definite evidence of racial or ethnic predisposition {2041}. DLBCL-CI is more common in males than in females (with a male-to-female ratio of at least 10:1). It

presents in adults, with a median age of approximately 65 years.

Etiology
DLBCL-CI has been universally associated with EBV. Most cases exhibit a type III latency pattern of infection. Some cases exhibit type II latency or have not been fully characterized {2281}. The tumour develops in an anatomical site, such as the pleural cavity, that may be protected from immune surveillance due to restricted access by immune cells. It is believed that the chronic inflammatory reaction may produce cytokines (such as IL6 and IL10) that promote B-cell proliferation, and may also exert an immunosuppressive effect. Other clinical settings include chronic osteomyelitis, long-standing metallic implants, long-standing hydrocele, and chronic skin ulcer {236,416,1509}.

Clinical features

Signs and symptoms
Patients with pleural involvement may present with signs and symptoms related to the tumour mass, including chest pain, cough, fever, and other respiratory symptoms {1810}. In other sites, the symptoms are related to the local mass lesion, and there may be evidence of an inflammatory reaction with swelling and erythema. There may also be evidence of pleural effusion, but effusions generally do not contain readily identified tumour cells.

Imaging
Radiography shows evidence of a mass lesion. Pyothorax-associated cases show a pleural mass, which may show involvement of the chest wall and compression of the adjacent lung. In approximately 10% of cases, there is infiltration of the adjacent lung parenchyma {1810}. Cases with involvement of bone show evidence of a lytic lesion.

Tumour spread
The tumour shows less evidence of systemic spread than do other forms of DLBCL, either positive or negative for EBV. Local spread and invasion around the primary lesion is common, but distant spread is less often seen. Lymph node involvement is not common.

Staging
Staging is based on the Ann Arbor sta-

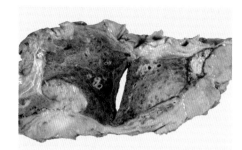

Fig. 2.24 Diffuse large B-cell lymphoma with chronic inflammation involving the pleural cavity. At autopsy, a dense, tan-coloured mass compresses the adjacent lung.

ging system employed for other forms of lymphoma. Since nearly all cases arise in extranodal sites, tumours are at least stage IE. Distant spread is considered stage IV, with or without symptoms (A, B).

Localization
The most common site is the pleural cavity, with other extranodal sites less commonly involved.

Macroscopy
The tumour masses are firm and tan, with or without areas of haemorrhage. Necrosis is common, with a cheesy white to light-tan appearance. The tumour may appear surrounded and walled-off by a dense fibrous pseudocapsule.

Cytology
Cytological specimens show a predominance of large blastic lymphoid cells. Cellular debris and evidence of necrosis and apoptosis are common.

Histopathology
Morphologically, the tumours resemble other forms of DLBCL. The cells resemble centroblasts or immunoblasts, with large vesicular nuclei and prominent nucleoli. Cellular apoptosis may be prominent, often with large areas of tumour necrosis. Although the process arises in the context of chronic inflammation, a prominent inflammatory reaction within the tumour is not seen. Marked fibrosis may be present, especially at the periphery of the tumour mass.
The cells express a mature B-cell phenotype, with positivity for CD20, CD19, and CD79a. Some cases may show evidence of plasmacytic differentiation, with loss of CD20. IRF4/MUM1 is positive in nearly all cases. CD30 is often expressed, but CD15 is negative. CD138 may be expressed in tumours with marked

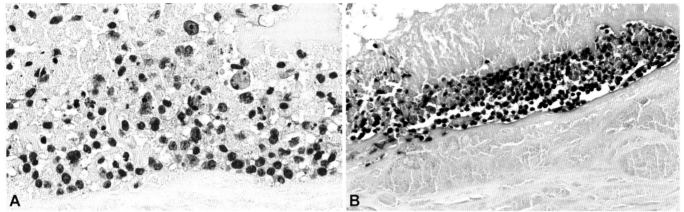

Fig. 2.25 Diffuse large B-cell lymphoma with chronic inflammation involving the pleural cavity. **A** Large blastic tumour cells are surrounded by a dense fibrous pseudocapsule. **B** Tumour cells are positive for EBV with in situ hybridization for EBV-encoded small RNA.

plasmacytic differentiation. Aberrant expression of T cell-associated antigens may be seen; CD2, CD3, CD4, and/or CD7 are most commonly seen, but a complete T-cell phenotype is absent. The cells express a type III latency phenotype with positivity for LMP1, EBNA1, and EBNA2. Downregulation of HLA class I may contribute to escape from immune surveillance {2041,2281}.

Differential diagnosis
The differential diagnosis includes primary effusion lymphoma, which is associated with both human herpesvirus 8/Kaposi sarcoma-associated herpesvirus and EBV. In primary effusion lymphoma, a tumour mass lesion is absent, and the tumour cells are found in the effusion fluid. The neoplastic cells in primary effusion lymphoma generally lack B cell-associated

antigens, and are negative for CD20 and CD79. The differential diagnosis also includes DLBCL, not otherwise specified, negative for EBV. The morphological appearance in such cases may be similar. For cases with pulmonary involvement, the differential diagnosis includes lymphomatoid granulomatosis and DLBCL in the elderly {2062}. These latter conditions usually show preferential involvement of the lung parenchyma, with only incidental pleural involvement {640}.

Genetic profile
The immunoglobulin genes are clonally rearranged. EBV sequences are detected by PCR, and in situ hybridization for EBV-encoded small RNA is positive. The tumour cells show a complex karyotype, but specific genetic alterations or translocations have not been reported. The gene expression profile shows an

activated B-cell (postgerminal centre) pattern {1691,1858,2597,2597}.

Prognosis and predictive factors
DLBCL-CI is an aggressive lymphoma. For pyothorax-associated lymphoma, the 5-year overall survival ranges from 20% to 35%. For patients who achieve complete remission with chemotherapy and/or radiotherapy, the 5-year survival is 50%. Complete tumour resection (pleuropneumonectomy with or without resection of adjacent involved tissues) has also been reported to provide good results. Poor performance status, high serum levels of lactate dehydrogenase, and advanced clinical stage are unfavourable prognostic factors. The advanced age of many patients with pyothorax-associated lymphoma may contribute to the poor prognosis.

Mesenchymal tumours

Epithelioid haemangioendothelioma

C.D.M. Fletcher
W.D. Travis

Definition
Epithelioid haemangioendothelioma is a malignant endothelial neoplasm composed of cords of epithelioid endothelial cells and characterized in most cases by *WWTR1-CAMTA1* gene fusion. It is often angiocentric.

ICD-O code   9133/3

Synonym
Intravascular bronchioloalveolar tumour (obsolete)

Epidemiology
Pleural epithelioid haemangioendothelioma is rare. It affects mainly adults, with a wide age range. Unlike epithelioid haemangioendothelioma at other sites, pleural epithelioid haemangioendothelioma appears to have a marked male predominance {506,1473}.

Clinical features
Patients most often present with pleural thickening (which may be diffuse), pleural effusion, and/or pleuritic pain. There may be coexistent lung involvement. Imaging may show nodular or diffuse pleural involvement. Progressive local pleural spread is common. Metastases to lung, liver, and locoregional nodes may be seen {506}.

Macroscopy and localization
Pleural epithelioid haemangioendothelioma often shows diffuse involvement of the pleura, and may mimic mesothelioma {99,506}.

Histopathology
Epithelioid haemangioendothelioma consists of cords, strands, or small nests of epithelioid endothelial cells, having somewhat glassy eosinophilic cytoplasm and relatively uniform ovoid vesicular nuclei. Cytoplasmic vacuoles (lumina) are a common finding. These cells are typically distributed in a myxohyaline stroma {2828}. Lesions often have an infiltrative growth pattern. A subset of cases show greater nuclear atypia and hyperchromasia, sometimes associated with more sheet-like growth. These lesions may be labelled malignant epithelioid haemangioendothelioma, and more consistently pursue an aggressive clinical course {1655}.
Epithelioid haemangioendothelioma is quite consistently positive for the most sensitive endothelial markers: CD31, ERG, and CD34. In about a third of cases, keratins may also be positive {1655}. Epithelioid angiosarcoma differs in that is composed of larger cells with more copious cytoplasm and irregular vesicular nuclei, typically growing in sheets. Metastatic carcinoma or (less likely) mesothelioma can be excluded by immunopositivity for endothelial antigens. When a suspected carcinoma or mesothelioma is keratin-negative, vascular markers should be considered.

Genetic profile
Most examples of epithelioid haemangioendothelioma have a specific translocation: (1;3)(p36;q2325), which results in *WWTR1-CAMTA1* gene fusion {683,2592}. A much smaller subset of cases, often with more vasoformative architecture, show a distinct *YAP1-TFE3* gene fusion, resulting in overexpression of TFE3 protein {69}. Recent data suggest that multicentric lesions (at least in the liver) are in fact monoclonal (i.e. locally metastatic) rather than separate primaries {682}.

Prognosis and predictive factors
Epithelioid haemangioendothelioma arising in the pleura is almost invariably aggressive, with most patients surviving < 1 year, usually due to uncontrolled local spread as well as metastasis {506}.

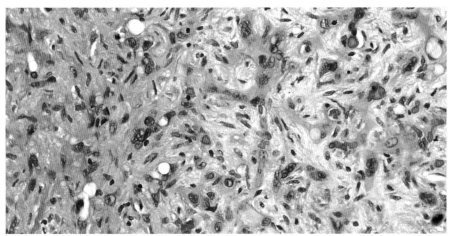
Fig. 2.26 Epithelioid haemangioendothelioma. Cords and strands of epithelioid endothelial cells, some with cytoplasmic vacuoles, infiltrate fibrous tissue.

Angiosarcoma

C.D.M. Fletcher
W.D. Travis

Definition
Angiosarcoma is a malignant neoplasm showing endothelial differentiation, and often having a vasoformative architecture.

ICD-O code   9120/3

Synonyms
Obsolete: haemangiosarcoma; malignant haemangioendothelioma

Epidemiology
Primary angiosarcoma of the pleura is extremely rare. It most often affects adult males {523,1369,1514,3017}.

Etiology
Rare cases from Japan have been reported to be associated with asbestos exposure or tuberculous pyothorax {3017}.

Clinical features
Most patients present with dyspnoea, pleural effusion or haemothorax, and pleural thickening. Extensive and rapid pleural spread is typical.

Macroscopy and localization
Diffuse pleural thickening, often with associated haemorrhage, is usual.

Histopathology
The large majority of primary pleural angiosarcomas have epithelioid morphology, being composed of sheets of large cells with copious eosinophilic cytoplasm, large vesicular nuclei, and prominent nucleoli. Intracytoplasmic vacuoles (lumina) may be focally evident.
These tumours express endothelial antigens (CD31, ERG, or CD34), and are very often keratin-positive, at least focally {3017}.
Epithelioid angiosarcoma in the pleura may be morphologically indistinguishable from metastatic carcinoma or mesothelioma. The occasional expression of cytokeratins can further confound this differential diagnosis. Detection of endothelial antigens is often the key discriminant.

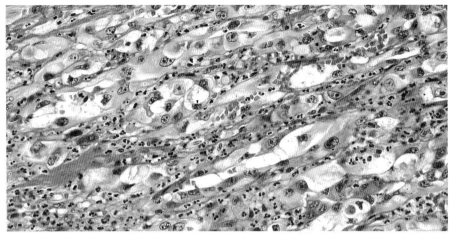

Fig. 2.27 Pleural angiosarcoma. Pleural angiosarcoma most often has epithelioid morphology, and may closely mimic carcinoma or mesothelioma.

Prognosis and predictive factors
Almost all patients with primary pleural angiosarcoma die very rapidly, usually within just days or weeks after first presentation.

Synovial sarcoma

C.D.M. Fletcher
S. Dacic
M. Ladanyi

Definition
Synovial sarcoma is a distinct soft tissue sarcoma with variable mesenchymal and epithelial differentiation. It is characterized by a specific chromosomal translocation: t(X;18)(p11.2;q11.2).

ICD-O codes
Synovial sarcoma	9040/3
Synovial sarcoma, spindle cell	9041/3
Synovial sarcoma, epithelioid cell	9042/3
Synovial sarcoma, biphasic	9043/3

Synonyms
Obsolete: malignant synovioma; tenosynovial sarcoma

Epidemiology
Pleural synovial sarcoma is rare, and often also involves the lung. Most patients are adults, with a median age of 40 years. Sex distribution is equal {101,167,779}.

Clinical features
Patients most often present with chest pain, pleural effusion, dyspnoea, or haemothorax.

Localization
Pleural synovial sarcomas are usually localized solid tumours, but can also present with diffuse pleural thickening.

Macroscopy
Pleural synovial sarcomas are usually large, with a mean size of 13 cm (ranging from 4 to 21 cm). Some tumours may have a pseudocapsule or grow on a pedicle. The cut surface is tan-grey, and may show cystic changes and necrosis.

Cytology
Aspirate smears are cellular, with loosely cohesive tissue fragments composed of spindle cells with stripped nuclei and indistinct cytoplasm. The epithelial cells are reminiscent of mesothelial cells, but appear plumper. They may form gland-like clusters, papillary aggregates, or solid cords and nests {479,2605}.

Histopathology
The histological features of pleural synovial sarcoma are exactly the same as those described in the lung (see *Synovial sarcoma*, p. 177). Most pleural synovial sarcomas are monophasic {167}.
At least one epithelial marker (such as epithelial membrane antigen or cytokeratin) is positive, and often coexpressed with vimentin, CD99, and Bcl2 (all of which are non-specific). Calretinin and S100 may be focally positive. TLE1 staining is somewhat more specific and useful {1483}. Smooth muscle actin, desmin, and CD34 are negative.
The most important differential diagnosis is malignant mesothelioma, followed by sarcomatoid carcinoma, solitary fibrous tumour, and metastatic synovial

sarcoma. The combination of clinical, histological, immunohistochemical, and cytogenetic findings can easily differentiate these entities. The diagnostic translocation t(X;18)(p11;q11), and the resulting fusion oncogene(s) are helpful in the differential diagnosis of synovial sarcoma {167,2822}.

Genetic profile
Synovial sarcoma, including intrathoracic cases {167}, is characterized by the translocation t(X;18)(p11.2;q11.2), which fuses the *SS18* (also called *SYT*) gene on chromosome 18 with either *SSX1* or *SSX2*, both located at Xp11.2. Cases with *SS18-SSX1* fusion are much more likely to show a glandular (biphasic) appearance {68,1379}. Cases with *SS18-SSX4* or *SS18L1-SSX1* fusion have not yet been described in the pleura.

Prognosis and predictive factors
These tumours are aggressive, and the median survival is approximately 2 years. For intrathoracic synovial sarcoma, there are no well-defined factors that predict outcome, unlike for their counterparts in somatic soft tissue.

Solitary fibrous tumour

C.D.M. Fletcher
A. Gibbs

Definition
Solitary fibrous tumours of the pleura are uncommon fibroblastic neoplasms that very often show a prominent branching vascular pattern and exhibit varied biological behaviour. Morphologically similar tumours can occur in the lung and mediastinum, and at extrathoracic sites.

ICD-O codes
Solitary fibrous tumour   8815/1
Malignant solitary fibrous tumour 8815/3

Synonyms
Obsolete: localized fibrous tumour; pleural fibroma; localized mesothelioma; fibrous mesothelioma; benign mesothelioma

Epidemiology
Solitary fibrous tumour can occur at any age, but is most common in the sixth and seventh decades of life, with no sex

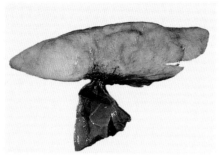

Fig. 2.28 Solitary fibrous tumour. A typical pedunculated lesion arising from the visceral pleura.

predisposition. Solitary fibrous tumour accounts for < 5% of primary pleural tumours, and has been estimated to occur with a frequency of 2.8 cases per 100 000 individuals {423}.

Etiology
No etiological agent has been established. There is no link with asbestos exposure.

Clinical features
These tumours are most often slow-growing, relatively benign neoplasms, but up to 10% are malignant. Many lesions are asymptomatic and discovered incidentally, but they may present with cough, dyspnoea, chest pain, general malaise, finger clubbing, or hypoglycaemia (related to production of an insulin-like growth factor) {2173}.
On imaging, they are usually sharply demarcated pleural-based soft tissue masses with no chest wall abnormality.

Localization
Solitary fibrous tumours of the pleura most often arise in the visceral pleura, but are widely distributed throughout the pleural cavity.

Macroscopy
The tumours are usually solitary, but may be multiple. They are typically

well-circumscribed, solid grey, whorled masses, frequently pedunculated and of variable size (often large: > 10 cm). Cysts, haemorrhage, calcification, and necrosis may be present.

Cytology
Fine-needle aspiration biopsy may yield diagnostic material with the use of cell blocks for immunohistochemistry, but core-needle biopsy samples are preferable {2857}. Solitary fibrous tumours show a wide range of cellularity, usually with small, bland, oval to spindle cells.

Histopathology
Solitary fibrous tumour typically shows uniform fibroblastic spindle cell morphology, varying cellularity, a patternless architecture, variably prominent stromal hyalinization, and branching haemangiopericytoma-like vessels of varying size and number {679}. Perivascular hyalinization is common. Lesional cells have tapering nuclei and limited amounts of pale, indistinct cytoplasm. Focally, there may be a storiform or fascicular growth pattern. Rarely, the stroma is predominantly myxoid. Usually, there are < 3 mitoses per 2 mm². Malignant examples are usually hypercellular, and exhibit > 4 mitoses per 2 mm². Cytological atypia is often limited, and necrosis is infrequent. Rare examples of malignant solitary fibrous tumour show dedifferentiation.
The large majority of lesions are CD34-positive, but this is non-specific. Positive staining for Bcl2 and CD99 is very non-specific, and not helpful. Much more specific is STAT6, which is positive in > 95% of cases {624,2973}. Some cases are smooth muscle actin-positive and occasional cases may stain for epithelial membrane antigen, keratin, S100, or desmin {1455}.
Solitary fibrous tumour may be confused with synovial sarcoma, sarcomatoid

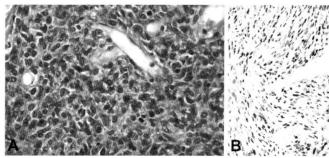

Fig. 2.29 Solitary fibrous tumour. **A** Showing hypercellularity and mitoses. Cytological atypia is minimal. **B** Diffuse nuclear positivity for STAT6 is characteristic.

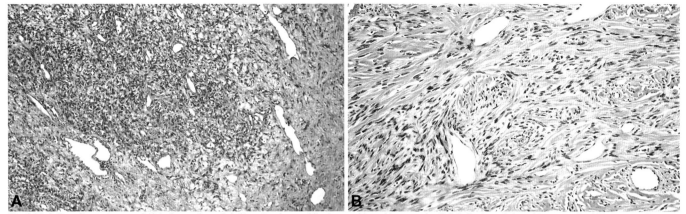

Fig. 2.30 Solitary fibrous tumour. **A** Note the varying cellularity, patternless architecture, and branching vessels. **B** Spindle- to oval-shaped tumour cells within a ropy collagenous stroma are growing in fascicles, with some storiform and perivascular arrangements.

mesothelioma, nerve sheath tumours, or type A thymoma. Immunohistochemistry is very helpful in the distinction.

Genetic profile
Solitary fibrous tumour harbours the characteristic (and to date specific) gene fusion *NAB2-STAT6*, which results from the intrachromosomal inversion inv(12)(q13q13), not detectable by conventional karyotyping {2172}, and leads to overexpression of STAT6, which is diagnostically useful (see above). IGF2 overexpression in some cases appears to be due to loss of *IGF2* imprinting {930}.

Prognosis and predictive factors
Local recurrence occurs in about 10% of cases, and the rate of metastasis is in the range of 5–10%. A mitotic rate of > 4 mitoses per 2 mm² is the most reliable indicator of aggressive behaviour. Tumour size, cytological atypia, and necrosis are much less predictive {623}. It is well recognized that isolated cases with benign morphology may give rise to metastasis.

Desmoid-type fibromatosis

C.D.M. Fletcher
P. Cagle

Definition
Desmoid-type fibromatosis is a locally aggressive but non-metastasizing myofibroblastic neoplasm, typically arising in deep soft tissue and often exhibiting *CTNNB1* gene mutation.

ICD-O code   8821/1

Synonyms
Aggressive fibromatosis; desmoid tumour

Epidemiology
Desmoid-type fibromatosis arising primarily in the pleura is rare. It most often affect adults, with no sex predominance {62,2884}.

Etiology
As at other sites, some cases may be associated with prior trauma. An association with familial adenomatous polyposis (Gardner syndrome) would not be unexpected, but has not been well documented in pleural lesions to date.

Clinical features
Pleural desmoid-type fibromatosis presents with chest pain or dyspnoea. Some may be an incidental radiological finding; however, the radiological features are non-distinctive.

Macroscopy
These are deep-seated, usually large masses, often extending into the chest wall soft tissue. Some are polypoid. As elsewhere, the cut surface is firm, trabeculated, and white, and often has a gritty consistency. The margins are poorly defined. Necrosis is absent.

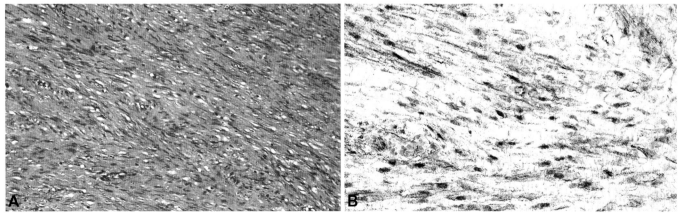

Fig. 2.31 Desmoid-type fibromatosis. **A** The lesion consists of long fascicles of cytologically uniform fibroblastic/myofibroblastic cells. **B** The tumour cells show distinct nuclear positivity for β-catenin, in addition to non-specific cytoplasmic staining.

Histopathology

As at other locations, desmoid-type fibromatosis consists of cytologically uniform fibroblastic/myofibroblastic cells arranged in long fascicles. The tumour cells have palely eosinophilic cytoplasm and ovoid or more tapering nuclei. The mitotic rate is extremely variable. The cells are distributed in a collagenous (sometimes hyalinized) matrix. Myxoid stroma is much less common. Stromal vessels are variably prominent.

Most cases stain focally or more diffusely for smooth muscle actin or muscle-specific actin. Desmin and CD34 are generally negative. About 70–75% of cases show nuclear positivity for β-catenin {332,1829}.

Orderly fascicular architecture and negativity for STAT6 distinguish desmoid-type fibromatosis from solitary fibrous tumour. The absence of nuclear atypia, cytological pleomorphism, and necrosis helps to distinguish desmoid-type fibromatosis from any type of spindle cell sarcoma.

Genetic profile

Mutations of *CTNNB1* are present in about 85% of cases {613}. Cases associated with familial adenomatous polyposis demonstrate inactivating mutations of the *APC* gene. The prognostic significance of *CTNNB1* mutations, with regard to recurrence, is uncertain {481,613}.

Prognosis and predictive factors

Approximately 20–25% of desmoid tumours recur locally, but local recurrence cannot be predicted based on histological findings. In particular, it has become clear that there is no good correlation with status of excision margins. Consensus about the prognostic role of mutational analysis may emerge in the near future.

Calcifying fibrous tumour

C.D.M. Fletcher
S. Dacic
W.D. Travis

Definition

Calcifying fibrous tumour is a rare, benign tumour occurring in visceral pleura, composed of paucicellular collagenized fibrous tissue with associated chronic inflammation and psammomatous and/or dystrophic calcification.

ICD-O code   8817/0

Synonyms

Calcifying fibrous pseudotumour; childhood fibrous tumour with psammoma bodies

Epidemiology

Pleural calcifying fibrous tumours occur mainly in women, with a median age of 39 years (and a range of 23–54 years) {1687,2061,2511}, whereas extrathoracic tumours are predominantly reported in children and young adults. Multiple (i.e. disseminated) pleural calcifying fibrous tumours are mostly reported in Asian patients {1095,1687}.

Etiology

The etiology is unknown. Rare extrathoracic cases are familial.

Clinical features

Patients may be asymptomatic or they may present with chest pain and non-productive cough.

Imaging studies show either a single pleural mass or multiple pleural-based nodular masses. Radiographs show well-marginated, non-calcified tumours, and CT shows pleural-based tumours with central areas of increased attenuation due to calcification.

Calcifying fibrous tumour is confined to the pleura, and does not involve the underlying lung parenchyma. So-called disseminated (more likely multiple/multicentric) bilateral pleural lesions have been reported {1146,2511}.

Localization

Calcifying fibrous tumour is typically limited to the pleura and does not involve the underlying lung parenchyma.

Macroscopy

The tumours are well circumscribed, unencapsulated, solid, and firm, with a gritty texture. The average size is 5 cm (ranging from 1.5 to 12.5 cm).

Histopathology

Calcifying fibrous tumour is usually circumscribed but unencapsulated, and may entrap adjacent structures. These lesions are diffusely hyalinized and hypocellular, consisting of bland

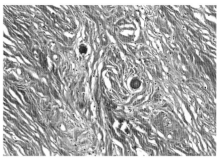

Fig. 2.32 Calcifying fibrous tumour. Note the scattered chronic inflammatory cells and calcospherites.

fibroblasts in a prominent collagenous stroma, which also contains a scattered lymphoplasmacytic infiltrate. There are usually dystrophic or psammomatous calcifications, which vary in number {1817,2061}. By immunohistochemistry, lesional cells may be CD34-positive, while β-catenin and ALK1 are negative. In the differential diagnosis, both inflammatory myofibroblastic tumour and solitary fibrous tumour are more cellular, the former being fascicular and the latter more patternless, with branching vessels.

Genetic profile

Although rare cases are familial, there are no molecular genetic data regarding calcifying fibrous tumour.

Prognosis and predictive factors

At least 10–15% of these lesions recur locally (sometimes repeatedly), but not destructively. Local recurrence is not predictable on morphological grounds. There is no potential for metastasis.

Desmoplastic round cell tumour

C.D.M. Fletcher
S. Dacic
M. Ladanyi

Definition

Desmoplastic small round cell tumour (DSRCT) is a malignant mesenchymal neoplasm with round cell morphology, polyphenotypic differentiation, and consistent *EWSR1-WT1* gene fusion.

ICD-O code   8806/3

Synonym

Polyphenotypic small round cell tumour

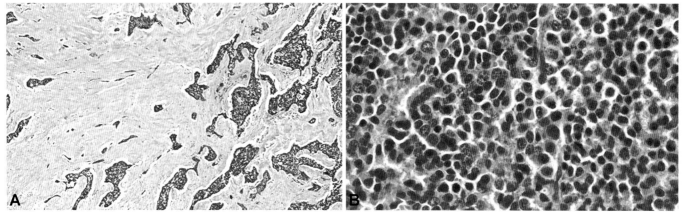

Fig. 2.33 Desmoplastic small round cell tumour. **A** Characteristic morphology with irregularly shaped islands of tumour cells in a desmoplastic stroma. **B** Histological appearance of small round cells with minimal nuclear pleomorphism, admixed with occasional cells that have rhabdoid inclusions.

Epidemiology

Primary pleural DSRCT is exceedingly rare. It usually affects teenagers and young adults, with a male predominance {1211,1994}.

Clinical features

Like other pleural malignancies, DSRCT usually presents with chest pain and effusion.

Macroscopy and localization

The cut surface is firm and grey-white, with foci of necrosis and haemorrhage {1994}. DSRCT forms multiple pleural-based nodules, with lung encasement and spread into the mediastinum. Bilateral pleural involvement and pulmonary parenchymal metastases may also occur.

Cytology

Effusion cytology shows tightly cohesive clusters of small, round, poorly differentiated malignant cells with accompanying desmoplastic stromal cells {197}.

Histopathology

The tumour is composed of variably sized and shaped, sharply demarcated islands of small, round, uniform tumour cells in a desmoplastic stroma, which often contains numerous vessels. The tumour cells have hyperchromatic nuclei, scant cytoplasm, and indistinct cytoplasmic borders. Intracytoplasmic eosinophilic rhabdoid inclusions may be present. Mitoses and individual cell necrosis are common {1994,2550}. The typical immunophenotype includes expression of cytokeratins, epithelial membrane antigen, desmin (with a perinuclear dot-like pattern), WT1 (antibodies to the C terminus), and neuron-specific enolase. Myogenin and MyoD1 are negative {1994,2550}.

A major clinical differential diagnosis based on imaging and gross characteristics may be mesothelioma. The morphological differential diagnosis also includes lymphoma, neuroblastoma, rhabdomyosarcoma, and Ewing sarcoma/primitive neuroectodermal tumour.

Genetic profile

Essentially all cases of DSRCT are characterized by diagnostic *EWSR1-WT1* gene fusion {821,2550}.

Prognosis and predictive factors

Like their counterparts in abdominal locations, these tumours may initially be chemosensitive, but most patients succumb within 2 years.

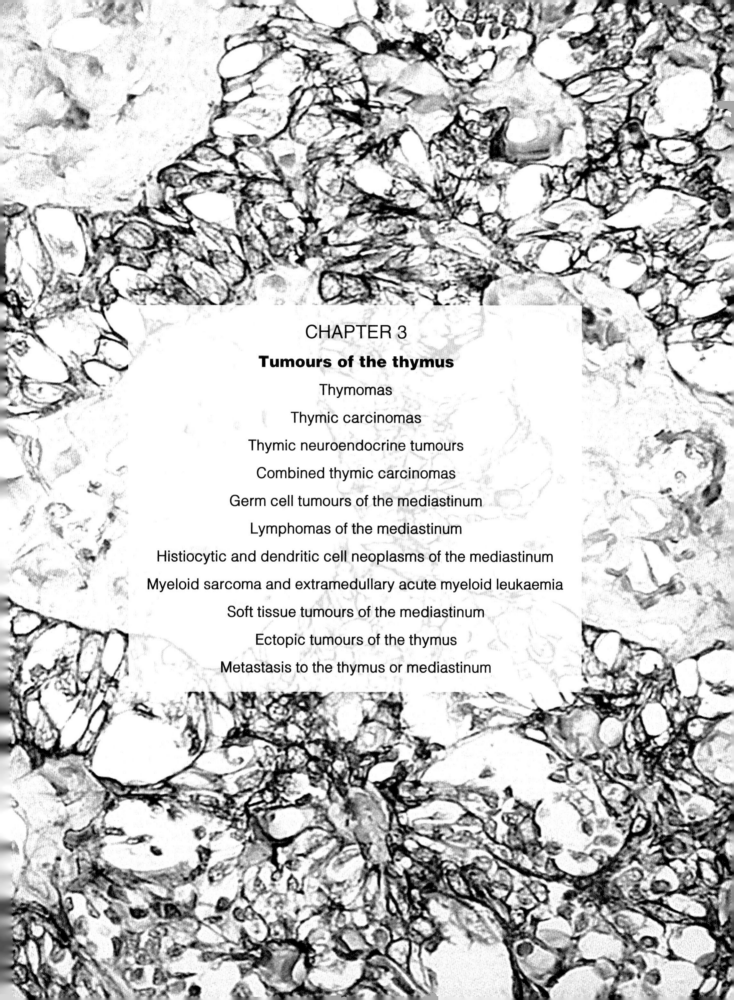

CHAPTER 3

Tumours of the thymus

Thymomas

Thymic carcinomas

Thymic neuroendocrine tumours

Combined thymic carcinomas

Germ cell tumours of the mediastinum

Lymphomas of the mediastinum

Histiocytic and dendritic cell neoplasms of the mediastinum

Myeloid sarcoma and extramedullary acute myeloid leukaemia

Soft tissue tumours of the mediastinum

Ectopic tumours of the thymus

Metastasis to the thymus or mediastinum

WHO classification of tumours of the thymus[a,b]

Epithelial tumours
Thymoma
- Type A thymoma, including atypical variant   8581/3*
- Type AB thymoma   8582/3*
- Type B1 thymoma   8583/3*
- Type B2 thymoma   8584/3*
- Type B3 thymoma   8585/3*
- Micronodular thymoma with lymphoid stroma   8580/1*
- Metaplastic thymoma   8580/3
- Other rare thymomas
  - Microscopic thymoma   8580/0
  - Sclerosing thymoma   8580/3
  - Lipofibroadenoma   9010/0*

Thymic carcinoma
- Squamous cell carcinoma   8070/3
- Basaloid carcinoma   8123/3
- Mucoepidermoid carcinoma   8430/3
- Lymphoepithelioma-like carcinoma   8082/3
- Clear cell carcinoma   8310/3
- Sarcomatoid carcinoma   8033/3
- Adenocarcinomas
  - Papillary adenocarcinoma   8260/3
  - Thymic carcinoma with adenoid cystic carcinoma-like features   8200/3*
  - Mucinous adenocarcinoma   8480/3
  - Adenocarcinoma, NOS   8140/3
- NUT carcinoma   8023/3*
- Undifferentiated carcinoma   8020/3
- Other rare thymic carcinomas
  - Adenosquamous carcinoma   8560/3
  - Hepatoid carcinoma   8576/3
  - Thymic carcinoma, NOS   8586/3

Thymic neuroendocrine tumours
- Carcinoid tumours
  - Typical carcinoid   8240/3
  - Atypical carcinoid   8249/3
- Large cell neuroendocrine carcinoma   8013/3
  - Combined large cell neuroendocrine carcinoma   8013/3
- Small cell carcinoma   8041/3
  - Combined small cell carcinoma   8045/3
Combined thymic carcinomas

Germ cell tumours of the mediastinum
Seminoma   9061/3
Embryonal carcinoma   9070/3
Yolk sac tumour   9071/3
Choriocarcinoma   9100/3
Teratoma
- Teratoma, mature   9080/0
- Teratoma, immature   9080/1
Mixed germ cell tumours   9085/3

Germ cell tumours with somatic-type solid malignancy   9084/3
Germ cell tumours with associated haematological malignancy   9086/3*

Lymphomas of the mediastinum
Primary mediastinal large B-cell lymphoma   9679/3
Extranodal marginal zone lymphoma of mucosa-associated lymphoid tissue (MALT lymphoma)   9699/3
Other mature B-cell lymphomas
T lymphoblastic leukaemia / lymphoma   9837/3
Anaplastic large cell lymphoma (ALCL) and other rare mature T- and NK-cell lymphomas
- ALCL, ALK-positive (ALK+)   9714/3
- ALCL, ALK-negative (ALK−)   9702/3
Hodgkin lymphoma   9650/3
B-cell lymphoma, unclassifiable, with features intermediate between diffuse large B-cell and classical Hodgkin lymphoma   9596/3

Histiocytic and dendritic cell neoplasms of the mediastinum
Langerhans cell lesions
- Thymic Langerhans cell histiocytosis   9751/1
- Langerhans cell sarcoma   9756/3
Histiocytic sarcoma   9755/3
Follicular dendritic cell sarcoma   9758/3
Interdigitating dendritic cell sarcoma   9757/3
Fibroblastic reticular cell tumour   9759/3
Indeterminate dendritic cell tumour   9757/3

Myeloid sarcoma and extramedullary acute myeloid leukaemia   9930/3

Soft tissue tumours of the mediastinum
Thymolipoma   8850/0
Lipoma   8850/0
Liposarcoma
- Well-differentiated   8850/3
- Dedifferentiated   8858/3
- Myxoid   8852/3
- Pleomorphic   8854/3
Solitary fibrous tumour   8815/1
- Malignant   8815/3
Synovial sarcoma
- Synovial sarcoma, NOS   9040/3
- Synovial sarcoma, spindle cell   9041/3
- Synovial sarcoma, epithelioid cell   9042/3
- Synovial sarcoma, biphasic   9043/3
Vascular neoplasms
- Lymphangioma   9170/0
- Haemangioma   9120/0
- Epithelioid hemangioendothelioma   9133/3
- Angiosarcoma   9120/3

Neurogenic tumours
   Tumours of peripheral nerves
   Ganglioneuroma   9490/0
   Ganglioneuroblastoma   9490/3
   Neuroblastoma   9500/3

Ectopic tumours of the thymus
Ectopic thyroid tumours
Ectopic parathyroid tumours
Other rare ectopic tumours

[a] The morphology codes are from the International Classification of Diseases for Oncology (ICD-O) {763}. Behaviour is coded /0 for benign tumours; /1 for unspecified, borderline, or uncertain behaviour; /2 for carcinoma in situ and grade III intraepithelial neoplasia; and /3 for malignant tumours. [b] The classification is modified from the previous WHO classification {2672}, taking into account changes in our understanding of these lesions. * These new codes were approved by the IARC/WHO Committee for ICD-O.

TNM classification of malignant thymic epithelial tumours[a]

TNM classification[1,2,3]

T – Primary Tumour

TX	Primary tumour cannot be assessed
T0	No evidence of primary tumour
T1	Tumour completely encapsulated
T2	Tumour invades pericapsular connective tissue
T3	Tumour invades into neighbouring structures, such as pericardium, mediastinal pleura, thoracic wall, great vessels, and lung
T4	Tumour with pleural or pericardial dissemination

N – Regional Lymph Nodes

NX	Regional lymph nodes cannot be assessed
N0	No regional lymph node metastasis
N1	Metastasis in anterior mediastinal lymph nodes
N2	Metastasis in other intrathoracic lymph nodes excluding anterior mediastinal lymph nodes
N3	Metastasis in scalene and/or supraclavicular lymph nodes

M – Distant Metastasis

M0	No distant metastasis
M1	Distant metastasis

Stage Grouping

Stage I	T1	N0	M0
Stage II	T2	N0	M0
Stage III	T1	N1	M0
	T2	N1	M0
	T3	N0, N1	M0
Stage IV	T4	Any N	M0
	Any T	N2, N3	M0
	Any T	Any N	M1

[1] From Wittekind Ch et al. {2897A}.

[2] TNM help desk: http://www.uicc.org/resources/tnm/helpdesk

[3] This is not an official UICC TNM classification.

[a] It has been proposed to modify the TNM table {586A,1840A,1319A} in order to increase its usefulness, e.g. for thymic carcinomas {2630,1317A,2176A}.

TNM classification of thymic germ cell tumours

TNM classification[1,2,3]

T – Primary Tumour

TX	Primary tumour cannot be assessed
T0	No evidence of primary tumour
T1	Tumour confined to the organ of origin (thymus and mediastinal fat)
T1a	Tumour ≤ 5 cm
T1b	Tumour > 5 cm
T2	Tumour infiltrating contiguous organs or accompanied by malignant effusion
T2a	Tumour ≤ 5 cm
T2b	Tumour > 5 cm
T3	Tumour invades into neighbouring structures, such as pericardium, mediastinal pleura, thoracic wall, great vessels and lung
T4	Tumour with pleural or pericardial dissemination

N – Regional Lymph Nodes

NX	Regional lymph nodes cannot be assessed
N0	No regional lymph node metastasis
N1	Metastasis in regional lymph nodes
N2	Metastasis in other intrathoracic lymph nodes excluding anterior mediastinal lymph nodes
N3	Metastasis in scalene and/or supraclavicular lymph nodes

M – Distant Metastasis

M0	No distant metastasis
M1	Distant metastasis

Stage Grouping of the Paediatric Study Group[1,3]

Stage I	Locoregional tumour, non-metastatic, complete resection
Stage II	Locoregional tumour, non-metastatic, macroscopic complete resection but microscopic residual tumour
Stage III	Locoregional tumour, regional lymph nodes negative or positive; no distant metastasis; biopsy only or gross residual tumour after primary resection
Stage IV	Tumour with distant metastasis

[1] From Billmire D et al. {203}.

[2] TNM help desk: http://www.uicc.org/resources/tnm/helpdesk

[3] This is not an official UICC TNM classification.

Thymomas
Type A thymoma, including atypical variant

P. Ströbel
A. Marx
S. Badve
J.K.C. Chan
G. Chen
F. Detterbeck
N. Girard

M.O. Kurrer
A.M. Marchevsky
E.M. Marom
Y. Matsuno
A.G. Nicholson
D. Nonaka
R.J. Rieker

Definition

Type A thymoma is a thymic epithelial neoplasm composed of usually bland spindle/oval tumour cells, with few or no admixed immature lymphocytes. It can show a wide variety of histological patterns, which may cause diagnostic problems.

ICD-O code   8581/3

Synonyms

Spindle cell thymoma; medullary thymoma (not recommended)

Epidemiology

Thymoma is a rare malignancy overall, but it is the most common mediastinal tumour in adults. Incidence rates reported in population studies have ranged from 2.2 to 2.6 per million per year (compared with 0.3–0.6 per million per year for thymic carcinomas) {543,675,778,1584}. The average thymoma incidence rates derived from SEER (Survival, Epidemiology and End Results) data range from 1.3 to 1.5 per million per year, but are about 3 times higher in Asians and Pacific Islanders in the USA {677}.

Type A thymoma is a relatively uncommon subtype. In a review of more than 2400 thymomas reported in multiple international studies, type A accounted for 11.5% (ranging from 3.1% to 26.2%) of all thymomas {584,922,1578,1579,1580}. This proportion is in line with data from the International Thymic Malignancy Interest Group (ITMIG) database {2826}. Patient ages range from 8 to 88 years, with a mean age of 64 years {584,1469}, which is older than the mean age of about 50 years for all thymomas {402,1360}. Although there is no consistent sex predominance in thymoma overall, a slight female predominance has been reported for type A thymoma in most studies {584,1129}.

Etiology

No environmental, viral, or nutritional factors appear to play an etiological role in thymomas {405,674,1462}. Reports of the

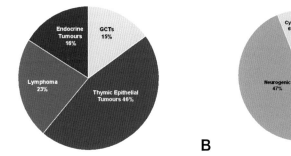

Fig. 3.01 A Frequency distribution of various groups of mediastinal tumours in adults. **B** Frequency distribution of various groups of tumours of the mediastinum (anterior and posterior compartment) in children. GCTs, germ cell tumours. Modified from Williamson SR, Ulbright TM {1581}.

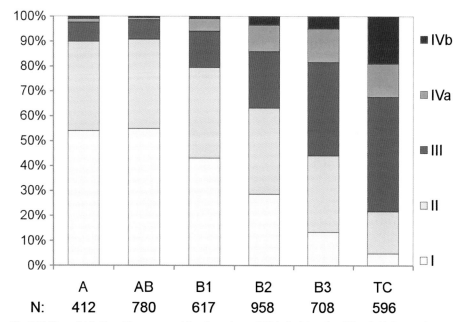

Fig. 3.02 Stage distribution of thymomas and thymic carcinoma (TC) in the International Thymic Malignancy Interest Group (ITMIG) retrospective database.

Table 3.01 Masaoka-Koga staging system {1305}, combining histological criteria and the corresponding (tentative) TNM classification. For details see {585}

Masaoka-Koga stage	Criteria {585}	TNM classification (T, N, M)
I	Grossly and microscopically completely encapsulated tumour	1, 0, 0
IIa	Microscopic transcapsular invasion	2, 0, 0
IIb	Macroscopic invasion into thymic or surrounding fatty tissue, or grossly adherent to (but not breaking through) mediastinal pleura or pericardium	2, 0, 0
III	Macroscopic invasion into neighbouring organs (i.e. pericardium, great vessels, or lung)	3, 0, 0
IVa	Pleural or pericardial metastases	4, 0, 0
IVb	Lymphogenous or haematogenous metastasis	Any T > N0 or > M0

Table 3.02 Selected autoimmune and paraneoplastic disorders associated with thymoma {1282,1596}

Neuromuscular disorders:
- Myasthenia gravis
- Limbic encephalopathy
- Peripheral neuropathy
- Neuromyotonia
- Stiff person syndrome
- Polymyositis

Haematological disorders:
- Pure cell aplasia
- Pernicious anaemia
- Pancytopenia
- Haemolytic anaemia

Collagen and autoimmune disorders:
- Systemic lupus erythematosus
- Rheumatoid arthritis
- Sjögren syndrome
- Scleroderma
- Interstitial pneumonitis

Immune deficiency disorders:
- Hypogammaglobulinaemia (Good syndrome)
- T-cell deficiency syndrome

Endocrine disorders:
- Autoimmune polyglandular syndrome
- Addison syndrome
- Thyroiditis

Dermatological disorders:
- Pemphigus
- Lichen planus
- Chronic mucocutaneous candidiasis
- Alopecia areata

Miscellaneous disorders:
- Giant cell myocarditis
- Glomerulonephritis/nephrotic syndrome
- Ulcerative colitis
- Hypertrophic osteoarthropathy

development of thymoma after radiation {865,1142}, solid organ transplantation {911}, or HIV infection {728} are so rare that coincidence is likely. A minor role of genetic risk factors appears possible, based on the rare occurrence of histologically diverse thymomas (including type A thymoma) with familial background {251,2211,2614} or in association with cancer susceptibility syndromes (e.g. Lynch syndrome {1972,2585}, myotonic dystrophy type 1 {722,1000,1698,1762}, and multiple endocrine neoplasia type 1 {1315}). Non-thymic haematopoietic and solid cancers occur with increased frequency in thymoma patients, irrespective of familial predisposition, myasthenia gravis status, or thymoma histotype {460, 723,778,1946,2848}. Since these second cancers are observed both before and after thymoma diagnosis, it is unclear whether an unknown shared oncogenic trigger or thymoma-associated immune compromise underlies this risk.

An origin of type A thymomas from a putative thymic epithelial cell precursor with minimal potential for corticomedullary differentiation has been proposed {2489}.

Clinical features

On average, 17% of patients with type A thymomas present with myasthenia gravis {358,584,1129,1469}. Others present with symptoms related to the mass lesion, or are incidentally discovered to have a mediastinal tumour on imaging examination. Association with pure red cell aplasia may occur, but this phenomenon is not restricted to this thymoma type, as was claimed in earlier reports {1357}. In the ITMIG database, 26% of patients with type A thymoma had myasthenia gravis {2826}. Other autoimmune diseases are rare.

Imaging

On imaging, type A thymomas are more likely to be smooth, to have a distinct border, and to be smaller at presentation than other thymic epithelial tumours {181,1086,2651}. On FDG PET-CT images, type A thymomas show low FDG uptake, only slightly greater than the background activity of the liver.

Staging

Thymomas are currently staged according to the Masaoka-Koga classification system {585,1305}. This staging system is currently under revision by the International Association for the Study of Lung Cancer (IASLC) and the International Thymic Malignancy Interest Group (IT-MIG) {586A,1840A,1319A}.

Older publications used the original Masaoka staging system. Most type A thymomas in the anterior mediastinum are in stage I (60%); stage II is the next most common (31%), while stage III is rare (8%) {402,1129,1249,1905,1991}. Stage IV type A thymoma is also rare {543,1129,2488}.

Localization

Type A thymoma occurs in the anterior mediastinum. Ectopic localization is rare.

Macroscopy

Type A thymoma is generally well circumscribed or encapsulated. The cut surface is homogeneous and light tan to white, and shows vague lobulation. Focal cystic change can be seen in some tumours. Mean tumour size ranges from 5.9 to 7.4 cm {369,1129,1967}.

Cytology

Cytological diagnosis of thymoma is feasible, with acceptable sensitivity and specificity, although reliable classification is generally not possible {45,422,2795}. Smears of type A thymoma may contain only epithelial cells, and thus can mimic other spindle cell lesions such as carcinoid tumour, low-grade sarcoma,

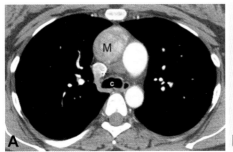
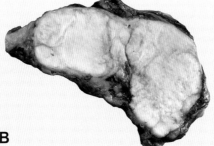
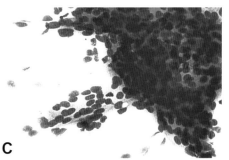

Fig. 3.03 Type A thymoma. **A** Contrast-enhanced chest CT at the level of the carina (C) demonstrates uniform enhancement of a smooth, homogeneous, well-demarcated anterior mediastinal mass (M). There is fat separating the mass from the abutting mediastinal structures. **B** An encapsulated tumour showing a cut surface with vague lobulation and slight septation. **C** Fine-needle aspirate showing fragments of loosely packed bland spindle cells with oval nuclei, with almost no accompanying lymphocytes.

Table 3.03 Proportion of thymoma types in relation to all thymomas, as well as epidemiological and clinicopathological features

Type	Relative frequency[a] (range)	Age range (years) (average[b])	Male-to-female ratio[b]	Proportion with myasthenia gravis[b] (mean)	Masaoka stage[c]				
					I	II	III	IVa	IVb
Type A	11.5% (3.1–26.2)	8–88 (64)	1:1.4	0–33% (17)	60%	31%	8%	0.5%	0.5%
Type AB	27.5% (15–43.0)	11–89 (57)	1:1.4	6–42% (18)	67%	26%	6%	1%	–
Type B1	17.5% (5.9–52.8)	6–83 (50)	1:1.6	7–70% (44)	50%	37%	9%	3%	1%
Type B2	26.0% (8.0–41.1)	4–83 (49)	1:1	24–71% (54)	32%	29%	28%	8%	3% (range: 0–5%)
Type B3	16.0% (3.4–35.1)	8–87 (55)	1:0.8	25–65% (50)	19%	36%	27%	15%	3% (range: 0–15%)
Micronodular	1.0%	41–80 (65)	1.5:1	Rare[d]	62%	36%	–	2%	–
Metaplastic[e]	< 1.0%	28–71 (50)	1:1	Very rare[f]	75%	17%	8%	–	–

[a] {584,922,1578,1579,1580}; [b] {358,584,1129,1469}; [c] {402,1249,1319,1905,2488}; [d] {1967}; [e] See *Metaplastic thymoma*, p. 207; [f] {1202}.

mesothelioma, and stromal cells in lymphoma {2795,3005}.

Histopathology

The tumours are typically surrounded by a complete or incomplete fibrous capsule, and may display coarse lobulation with thick fibrous bands. Microcystic change can occur, but is often more pronounced in subcapsular areas. Other characteristic growth patterns include rosettes (with or without a central lumen), glandular or glomeruloid structures, Masson haemangioma-like papillary projections in cystic spaces, meningioma-like whorls, fascicular growth, and storiform growth {1193,1360,1768,1967}. Multiple patterns can occur in the same tumour. A haemangiopericytoma-like vascular pattern is common {1967}. Perivascular spaces are less commonly seen than in other types of thymoma {369}. Hassall corpuscles are absent.

The tumour cells are spindly and/or oval-shaped, with bland nuclei, finely dispersed powdery chromatin, and inconspicuous nucleoli. In some cases, subpopulations of tumour cells are polygonal, with uniform round nuclei exhibiting a similar chromatin pattern. Mitotic activity is low, with counts usually < 4 mitoses per 2 mm². Type A thymomas are tumours with no or only very few (easily countable) immature lymphocytes throughout. The determination of immature T cells may require immunohistochemistry, such as terminal deoxynucleotidyl transferase (TdT) staining. Tumours with any lymphocyte-dense areas (TdT+ T cells impossible to count) or in > 10% of the tumour area with moderate infiltrate of TdT+ T cells (exemplified in Fig. 3.14B) are classified as type AB thymoma {1595}. Two distinctive features of type A thymomas versus other thymomas are a high content of bland spindly and oval (and rarely polygonal)

epithelial cells, and paucity or absence of immature TdT+ T cells throughout the tumour. The recommended reporting of heterogeneous thymic epithelial tumours is described below. Type A thymomas show foci of micronodular thymoma with lymphoid stroma in about 5–10% of cases, while type A thymoma areas occur in up to 30% of micronodular thymomas with lymphoid stroma {2492}. In contrast, the presence of areas resembling type B1 and B2 thymoma in a tumour that otherwise looks like a type A thymoma should lead to a diagnosis of type AB thymoma (see *Differential diagnosis*). Type A thymoma combined with a thymic carcinoma is very rare (see *Combined thymic carcinomas*, p. 242).

Atypical type A thymoma variant

It is now accepted that rare type A thymomas can display some degree of atypia (such as hypercellularity, increased

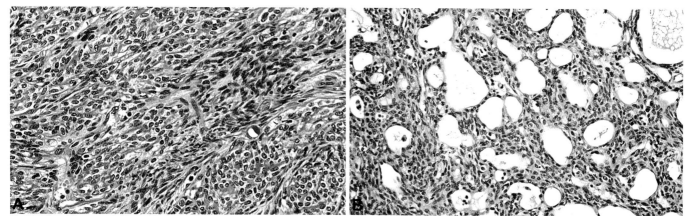

Fig. 3.04 Type A thymoma. **A** Classical fascicular spindle cell pattern and paucity of interspersed lymphocytes. **B** Common growth pattern: microcystic. Reprinted from Marx A et al. {1595}.

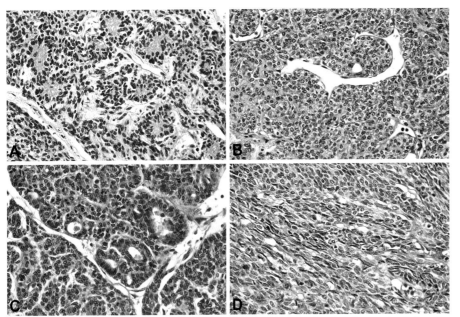

Fig. 3.05 Type A thymoma. **A** Common growth pattern: rosetting. **B** Common growth pattern: haemangiopericytoma-like. **C** Common growth pattern: adenoid. **D** Common growth pattern: synovial sarcoma-like. Reprinted from Marx A et al. {1595}.

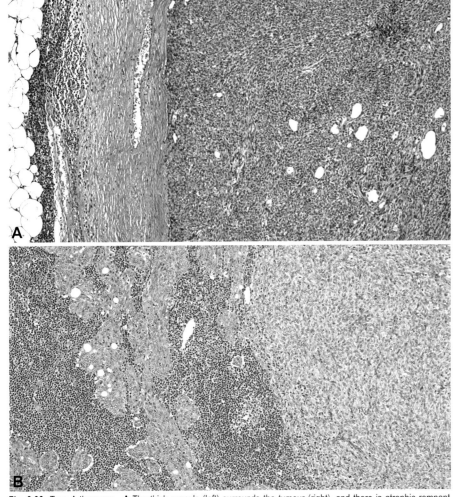

Fig. 3.06 Type A thymoma. **A** The thick capsule (left) surrounds the tumour (right), and there is atrophic remnant thymus adjacent to the capsule (left). **B** Tumour heterogeneity: type A thymoma (right) in continuity with micronodular thymoma with lymphoid stroma (left).

mitotic counts, and focal necrosis), but the significance of such features remains to be determined {899A,1595,1874,2782} (http://www.itmig.org/).

Diagnostic labels for tumours with more than one histological pattern

Thymomas that show different histological types in the same tumour are so common {1738,2488} that we propose to abandon the previously recommended term combined thymoma {2672}. Instead, the diagnosis should list all the histological types that are present, starting with the predominant component; minor components should be quantified in 10% increments {1595}. Type AB thymoma is a distinct entity by definition {1088,2489}, to which this rule does not apply. Thus, for cases of type AB thymoma, it is not correct to render a diagnosis of type A thymoma with admixed type B1, B2, or B3 components.

In contrast, heterogeneous tumours that consist of a thymic carcinoma component of any size/percentage together with a thymoma should be labelled thymic carcinoma (specifying the percentage and histological type), and the accompanying thymoma component(s) and their relative size should be listed, as detailed above (see *Combined thymic carcinomas*, p. 242), particularly for tumours that consist of more than one carcinoma component.

The heterogeneity of thymic epithelial tumours implies the need for extensive sampling of resection specimens {1738} (following the general rule of one block per centimetre) and cautious interpretation of small biopsies in terms of definitive thymoma typing {1712}. Nevertheless, distinction of thymoma from other mediastinal tumours (e.g. lymphoma) is possible even in small biopsies, and is clinically relevant {67,2091,3007}.

Immunohistochemistry

Most thymic epithelial tumours do not require immunohistochemical analysis for definitive diagnosis. However, less prototypical thymic epithelial tumours can raise differential diagnostic questions that may be answered by immunohistochemistry. Typical situations are the distinction of type A thymoma from other spindle cell tumours, or the distinction of type B1 thymoma from lymphoblastic lymphoma. Furthermore, the definitions of some thymic epithelial tumours depend

Table 3.04 Routine immunohistochemical markers that are helpful for distinguishing thymoma subtypes from each other, thymomas from thymic carcinomas, and thymic carcinomas from other cancers. Compartment-specific antibody targets label subsets of cortical and medullary thymic epithelial cells of normal thymus and thymoma {2489}

Marker	Reactivity
Routine immunohistochemical markers	
Cytokeratins	- Cortical and medullary thymic epithelial cells
CK19	- Cortical and medullary thymic epithelial cells
CK10	- Terminally mature medullary thymic epithelial cells, Hassall corpuscles, and squamous epithelial cells - Focally positive in type B thymoma and thymic squamous cell carcinoma - Negative in type A and AB thymomas (with rare exceptions)
CK20	- Negative in normal and neoplastic thymic epithelial cells - May be positive in rare thymic adenocarcinomas (differential diagnosis: metastases to the mediastinum)
p63	- Cortical and medullary thymic epithelial cells - Cross-reacts with tumour cells of primary mediastinal large B-cell lymphoma {424}
CD5	- T cells - Epithelial cells in ~70% of thymic squamous cell carcinomas - Variably positive in thymic (and other) adenocarcinomas
CD20	- B cells - Epithelial cells in ~50% of type A and AB thymomas
CD117	- Epithelial cells in ~80% of thymic squamous cell carcinomas
PAX8	- Positive in thymomas and most thymic carcinomas {2845}
Terminal deoxynucleotidyl transferase	- Immature T cells in thymus and thymoma - Lymphoblastic lymphoma
Desmin	- Myoid cells of thymic medulla, type B1 thymoma, rare type B2 and B3 thymomas, and thymic carcinomas
Ki-67	- Any proliferating cells (immature T cells in normal thymic cortex, most thymomas, T lymphoblastic lymphoma, etc.)
Compartment-specific antibody targets	
Beta5t {2489}	- Thymic epithelial cells with cortical differentiation (thymus and thymoma)
PRSS16	- Thymic epithelial cells with cortical differentiation (thymus and thymoma)
Cathepsin V	- Thymic epithelial cells with cortical differentiation (thymus and thymoma)
Claudin 4	- Subset of thymic epithelial cells with medullary differentiation
CD40	- Subset of thymic epithelial cells with medullary differentiation
Autoimmune regulator AIRE	- Subset of thymic epithelial cells with medullary differentiation
Involucrin	- Like CK10, but focally positive in type AB thymoma

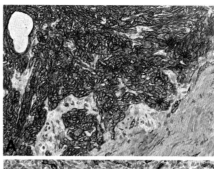
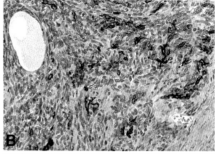
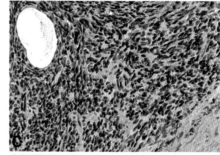
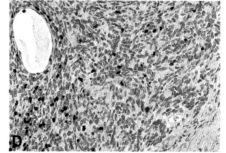

Fig. 3.07 Type A thymoma. Serial immunohistochemistry sections showing expression of (**A**) CK19, (**B**) CD20 in spindle cells, (**C**) p63 in tumour cell nuclei and, (**D**) paucity of terminal deoxynucleotidyl transferase-positive T cells.

on quantitative features, like the content of immature TdT+ T cells that may be impossible to distinguish from mature TdT– T cells by H&E histology alone. Type A thymoma tumour cells are strongly positive for AE1-defined acidic keratins and p63 {424,619}, and negative for AE3-defined basic keratins. They show variable expression of other keratins of various molecular weights, but are always negative for CK20 {1361}. In general, keratin expression is stronger in the cystic and glandular structures. Epithelial membrane antigen is variably and only focally expressed. Tumours are positive for thymic epithelial markers PAX8, FOXN1, and CD205 {1871,2832}, while CD5 and CD117 are negative {1011,1793}.

A useful and frequent feature is ectopic expression of CD20 in the neoplastic epithelial cells, although the staining is often focal, and may be missed in small biopsies. In rare cases, single desmin-positive myoid cells may be seen. TdT+ immature T cells by definition are completely absent or make up only a minority of the CD3+ T cells. CD20+ B cells are usually absent.

The epithelial cells of type A thymomas are mostly negative for markers of medullary and cortical differentiation (such as CD40, claudin 4, the autoimmune regulator (AIRE), HLA class II, and thymoproteasome) {2489,2923}. Some cases show evidence of terminal epithelial

differentiation, such as focal expression of involucrin and CK10 {2489}.

Differential diagnosis

Type A thymoma should be distinguished from type AB thymomas based on morphology and the number of immature TdT+ T cells. A more critical distinction is from a spindle cell variant of type B3 thymoma, or even spindle cell thymic carcinoma. Distinction from spindle cell type B3 thymoma can be difficult

Table 3.05 Summary of genetic findings reported for the different WHO thymoma subtypes and thymic squamous cell carcinoma; the recurrent loss of chromosome 6q25.2–25.3 that is observed across the spectrum of thymomas and in thymic squamous cell carcinoma is shown in bold

WHO type	Chromosomal gains	Chromosomal losses	Other mutations	Sources
Type A thymoma	–	2, 4, 6p21, 6q, **6q25.2–25.3**, 13	• Activating *HRAS* mutation (rare) • t(15;22)(p11;q11) • GTF2I missense mutation in 82%	{525,844,1088, 2044A,3011}
Type AB thymoma	–	2, 4, 5q21-22, 6p21, **6q25.2–25.3**, 7p15.3, 8p, 13q14.3, 16q, 18	• Ring chromosome 6 • XX,+del(X)(q24),+i(5p), +?del(7)(q22),der(11) t(1;11)(q23;q25),t(11;?) (p15;?),-18,+r • 46,XX,del(6)(p22p25) • 46,XY,r(6),der(21)t(6;21) (p25;q22) • GTF2I missense mutation in 74%	{1088,1349,1683, 2741,2044A}
Type B1 thymoma	9q	1p, 2q, 3q, 4, 5, 6q, 8, 13, 18	• GTF2I missense mutation in 32%	{1434} (only one study) {2044A}
Type B2 thymoma	1q	1p, 3p, **6q25.2–25.3**	• Activating *KRAS* mutation (rare) • 44,XY,+X,inv(2) (p25q13),del(6)(q15),-8, -16,-17 • 57,X,2Y,+i(1) (q10),+add(4)(q12),+7,+8, +9,+14,+15,+16,der(17) t(9;17)(q13;p13),+20,+22 • GTF2I missense mutation in 22%	{1088,1349,2027, 2044A,2435}
Type B3 thymoma	1q, 4[a], 5, 7, 8, 9q, 17q, X	3p, 6, **6q25.2–25.3**, 9p, 11q42. qter, 13q, 16q, 17p	• *BCL2* copy number gains (18q21.33) • *CDKN2A/B* copy number losses (9p21.3) • Translocation t(11;X) • GTF2I missense mutation in 21%	{844,1088,2044A, 2046,3011}
Thymic squamous cell carcinoma	1q, 4, 5, 7, 8, 9q, 12, 15, 17q, 18, 20	3p, 6, **6q25.2–25.3**, 9p, 13q, 14, 16q, 17p	• Activating *KIT* mutations (2–11%) • Activating *KRAS* mutation (rare) • *BCL2* copy number gains (18q21.33) • *CDKN2A/B* copy number losses (9p21.3) • 52,XY,+4,+5,+8,+12, +16,der(16)t(1;16)(q12; q12.1) x2,+17 • GTF2I missense mutation in 8%	{844,2044A,2045, 2490,3011}

[a] Single cases {844,3011}.

in the absence of CD20 expression, and is currently mainly based on histological features such as prominent perivascular spaces in type B3 thymoma or the focal presence of glands, rosettes, or the pericytomatous vascular pattern seen in type A thymoma. Expression of CD117 and especially CD5 aids in the diagnosis of thymic carcinoma. Moreover, type A thymoma with a spindle or trabecular growth pattern or rosetting may resemble thymic carcinoid tumour. Finally, type A thymomas can resemble mesenchymal neoplasms, especially solitary fibrous tumour and synovial sarcoma, both of which can occur in the mediastinum.

A panel of immunohistochemistry including p63, CD34, STAT6, CD56, and TLE1 {2622} and appropriate molecular tests are helpful.

Genetic profile

Type A thymomas harbour few genetic alterations {844}, although exceptions have been reported {1434,2027}. Rare cases with t(15;22)(p11;q11) {525} or a partial loss of the short arm of chromosome 6 {3011} have been described. Consistent loss of heterozygosity has been found only in 6q25.2–25.3, which is common to type A, AB, and B3 thymomas, as well as squamous cell thymic carcinomas {1088}. Recently, the tumour suppressor gene FOXC1 was identified as a potential target of this commonly deleted region {2046A}. Unlike type B3 thymomas and squamous cell thymic carcinoma, type A thymoma contains no aberrations in the *APC*, *RB1*, or *TP53* gene loci, or in regions 3p14.2 and 8p11.21 {1088}. *EGFR* and *KIT* mutations are also absent. Recently, a recurrent missense mutation of the *GTF2I* transcription factor gene has been detected in type A and AB thymomas (in 82% and 75% of cases, respectively), but rarely in type B1, B2 and B3 thymomas (in 21–32%) and thymic carcinomas (8%) {2044A}.

Prognosis and predictive factors

The overall survival of patients with type A thymoma has been reported to be as high as 100% at 5 years and 10 years {1905,2488}. In the ITMIG database, the overall survival rates of R0 resected type A thymoma at 5 and 10 years were 90% and 80%, respectively {2826}. The risk of recurrence is low if the tumour can be completely removed surgically {1360,1905,2488}. However, exceptional cases with local recurrence or distant metastasis have been documented {1129,1305,1967}. In the ITMIG database, the rates of recurrence at 5 and 10 years after an R0 resection are about 5% and 9%, respectively {2826}. Association with myasthenia gravis has been reported to either improve or have no effect on prognosis {369,1905,2107}.

Type AB thymoma

P. Ströbel   A.M. Marchevsky
A. Marx   E.M. Marom
S. Badve   Y. Matsuno
G. Chen   A.G. Nicholson
F. Detterbeck   D. Nonaka
N. Girard   R.J. Rieker
M.O. Kurrer

Definition

Type AB thymoma is a thymic epithelial neoplasm composed of a lymphocyte-poor spindle cell (type A) component and a lymphocyte-rich (type B-like) component, with a significant population of immature T cells. The relative proportion of the two components is highly variable.

ICD-O code   8582/3

Synonym

Mixed thymoma (not recommended)

Epidemiology

Type AB thymoma accounts for 27.5% (ranging from 15% to 43%) of the more than 2400 thymomas reported in multiple studies {543,584,922,1578,1579,1580}. Patient ages range from 11 to 89 years, with a younger mean age (of 57 years) than that in type A thymoma {358,584,1129,1469}. A slight female predominance has been noted. In the International Thymic Malignancy Interest Group (ITMIG) database, 23% of thymomas are coded as type AB (with an average patient age of 57 years) {2826}.

Etiology

The etiology is unknown. A putative thymic epithelial cell precursor with the potential for bilineage corticomedullary differentiation and restricted terminal medullary maturation is hypothesized to be the cell of origin {2489}.

Clinical features

On average, 18% of type AB thymomas are associated with myasthenia gravis. Pure red cell aplasia has also been reported {1357}. Other patients present with symptoms related to the mass lesion or are asymptomatic.

The imaging features of type AB thymoma have not been studied individually; when grouped, the morphological imaging features of types A, AB, and B1 thymoma (as compared to B2 and B3 thymoma) overlap {2191}.

Most type AB thymomas are in stage I (67%); stage II is the next most common

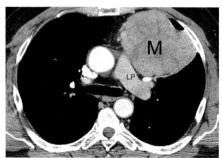

Fig. 3.08   Type AB thymoma. In a 52-year-old man; contrast-enhanced chest CT at the level of the left pulmonary artery (LP) shows a lobular anterior mediastinal mass (M) with a fat plane separating the tumour from the mediastinum. There is homogeneous enhancement of the mass without low-attenuation necrotic regions within it. These imaging features are suggestive of thymoma rather than thymic cancer, as they lack aggressive features such as calcifications, necrotic low-attenuation regions, and infiltration into surrounding organs; however, these imaging features overlap between the different histological types of thymoma.

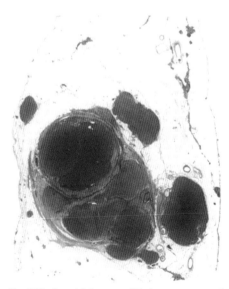

Fig. 3.09   Type AB thymoma. This low-power scan of a histological slide shows a small type AB thymoma with infiltration of the mediastinal fat and small thymic remnants (right margin). The dark blue nodules represent a lymphocyte-rich type B-like component, separated by pale spindle cell areas.

(26%), followed by stage III (6%). Stage IV is rare {524,1129,1683,1903,1905}. More advanced stage has been associated with atypical histological features {2783}.

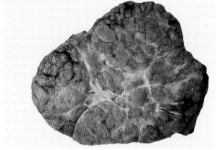

Fig. 3.10   Type AB thymoma. A well-circumscribed tumour showing multiple nodules separated by white septa.

Localization

Type AB thymoma occurs in the anterior mediastinum. Ectopic localization is rare.

Macroscopy

The tumours are usually encapsulated. The cut surface shows multiple tan-coloured nodules of various sizes, separated by white fibrous bands. The average tumour size ranges from 7.3 to 7.9 cm {369,1129,1967}.

Histopathology

Type AB thymoma is usually well demarcated. It shows a lobulated growth pattern, and is composed of a highly variable mixture of a lymphocyte-poor type A component and a more lymphocyte-rich type B-like component. These components either form discrete, separate nodules, or are intricately intermingled {1768}. The type B-like component includes a prominent infiltrate of immature, terminal deoxynucleotidyl transferase (TdT)+ T cells. Immature T cells are often found in dense clusters (T cells impossible to count), which when present (irrespective of size) qualify an otherwise typical type A thymoma as type AB. Sometimes the immature T cells are more scattered, and such tumours can be distinguished from type A thymomas by the presence of a moderate infiltrate of TdT+ lymphocytes (difficult to count) in > 10% of the tumour area {1595}.

All histological features of type A thymoma can also be seen in the type A component. Type A components may

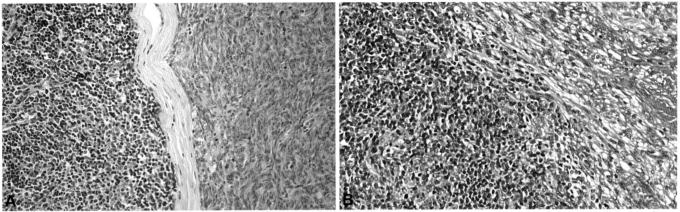

Fig. 3.11 Type AB thymoma. **A** Classical biphasic tumour with delineation of a spindle cell-rich type A area (right) and a lymphocyte-rich type B-like area (left) through a fibrous septum. **B** Biphasic tumour with sharp separation of type A and type B-like areas, but no fibrous septum.

consist of spindle cell fascicles that course around and among lymphocyte-rich nodules (the type B-like component) like cellular fibrous septa. The type B-like areas are different from type B1, B2, or B3 thymoma. The tumour cells are small and oval, plump spindly, or polygonal in shape, with round to oval pale-staining nuclei showing dispersed chromatin and inconspicuous nucleoli {1361,1768}. The large, vesicular nuclei with distinct nucleoli that are characteristic of the neoplastic cells in type B2 thymoma are only rarely seen {1361}. Medullary islands are very rare, and Hassall corpuscles are generally absent.

Three distinctive features of type AB thymoma versus other thymomas are: 1) an admixed spindle cell-predominant, lymphocyte-poor component and lymphocyte-rich component; 2) bland, spindly, oval, and focally polygonal thymic epithelial cells; and 3) a focal or diffuse abundance of immature T cells.

Areas of micronodular thymoma with lymphoid stroma can rarely occur in type AB

thymomas {1967,2492}, while associated thymic carcinoma is exceptional {1787}. The reporting of such tumours is described in *Type A thymoma*.

Immunohistochemistry

The patterns of keratin and consistent p63 expression {619} are essentially similar to those of type A thymoma. However, the epithelial cells in type B-like areas are usually CK14-positive {1361}. CD20-positive epithelial tumour cells can be seen in both type A and type B-like areas, and the associated lymphocytes are CD3+ T cells that are mainly immature (TdT+). CD20+ B cells and desmin-positive myoid cells are usually absent. Areas with fibroblast-like elongated spindle cells are strongly positive for vimentin and epithelial membrane antigen, and may show weak keratin staining. There is no epithelial expression of CD5. The Ki-67 proliferation index is usually low in the neoplastic epithelium, but interpretation can be difficult due to a high number of admixed proliferating immature T cells.

Type AB thymoma shows complex mixtures of epithelial cells with cortical and medullary differentiation (expressing markers such as CD40, claudin 4, the autoimmune regulator, HLA class II, or thymoproteasome) down to the single-cell level {2489,2922}. The epithelial cells usually lack markers of terminal differentiation, such as involucrin and CK10.

Differential diagnosis

Type A thymoma (see above and *Type A thymoma*, p. 187) and micronodular thymoma with lymphoid stroma must be distinguished from type AB thymoma. Type AB thymoma and micronodular thymoma with lymphoid stroma can occur in the same tumour. The distinction is usually straightforward: type AB thymomas do not contain large numbers of CD20+ B cells and the lymphocytes are always intimately admixed with keratin-positive neoplastic epithelial cells, while the epithelial cells in micronodular thymoma with lymphoid stroma are arranged in nodules, and most of the lymphocytes

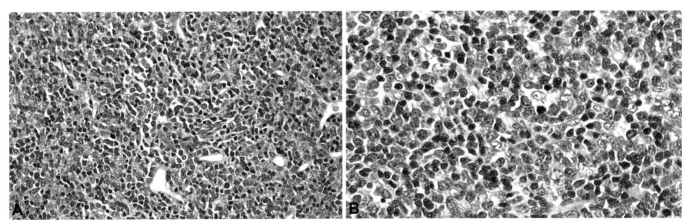

Fig. 3.12 Type AB thymoma lacking a lymphocyte-poor component, i.e. without biphasic architecture. **A** Low-power view of a monophasic tumour with high lymphocyte content among spindle tumour cells. **B** High-power view of a type B-like area featuring small polygonal tumour cells with inconspicuous nucleoli.

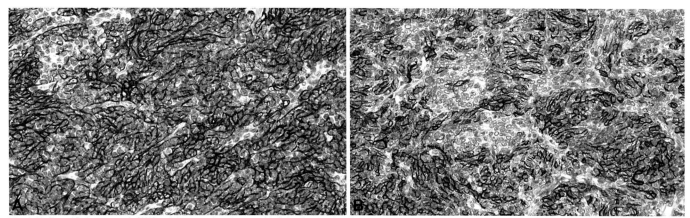

Fig. 3.13 Type AB thymoma. **A** CK19 staining reveals a dense epithelial cell network, without conspicuous perivascular spaces. Both features are typical of type AB thymoma as opposed to type B1 thymoma. **B** The extensive, strong expression of CD20 shown here is less common in type AB thymoma.

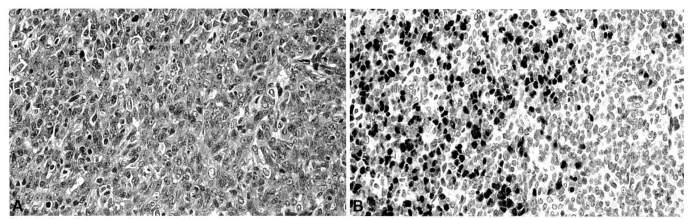

Fig. 3.14 Type AB thymoma. **A** A histological section illustrating a moderate number of immature T cells in a relatively lymphocyte-poor spindle cell thymoma. **B** A serial section illustrating a moderate number of immature T cells by terminal deoxynucleotidyl transferase staining; spindle cell thymomas showing this number of terminal deoxynucleotidyl transferase-positive T cells in > 10% of the investigated tumour material should be called type AB thymoma, while spindle cell thymomas with moderate numbers of immature T cells in smaller areas should be labelled type A thymoma; spindle cell thymomas showing areas of any size with a higher number of terminal deoxynucleotidyl transferase-positive T cells (impossible to count) should be considered type AB thymomas. Reprinted from Marx A et al. {1595}.

occur outside these nodules in an epithelial-free stroma.

Unlike type AB thymomas, type B1 thymomas resemble the normal thymus, with highly organized, TdT-positive cortical areas and medullary structures that often contain Hassall corpuscles. Type AB thymoma typically shows a dense and often CD20-positive epithelial cell network, while the epithelial cell network in type B1 thymoma is always delicate and consistently CD20-negative.

Genetic profile
The genetic alterations are more frequent and more complex than in type A thymoma {1088,1434}. Loss of heterozygosity at 5q2122 (*APC*), which is usually found

in type B thymoma, has been detected in a minority of type AB thymomas {1088}. The type A areas in type AB thymomas appear to be genetically distinct from type A thymomas {1088}. On the other hand, a close relationship between type A and AB thymomas is suggested by the similar high frequency (75–82%) of a *GTF2I* missense mutation in these thymomas, compared to the rarity of this mutation in the various type B thymomas (21–32%) {2044A}. Most alterations are shared with other thymoma types – namely, losses of genetic material on chromosomes 2, 4, 5, 6q23–25, 7p15.3, 8p, 13q14.3 (*RB*), 16q, and 18 {859,1434}. Mutations of *KIT* or *EGFR* have not been described {2047,2964}.

Prognosis and predictive factors
The overall survival is 80–100% at 5 and 10 years {402,1905,2488}. In the ITMIG database, the overall survival of R0 resected type AB thymoma at 10 years was 87% {2826}. Although type AB thymomas may present as stage II or stage III tumours, they can usually be cured by radical surgery {402,1360,2488}. Recurrence and metastasis are rare {1305,1967} but may occur {1129}, justifying long-term clinical monitoring. In the ITMIG database, the rate of recurrence is approximately 3% at both 5 and 10 years after R0 resection {2826}. Whether paraneoplastic myasthenia gravis has an impact on prognosis is controversial {369,1905,2107}.

Type B1 thymoma

M.A. den Bakker   F. Detterbeck   Y. Matsuno
A. Marx   N. Girard   K. Mukai
P. Ströbel   N.A. Jambhekar   A.G. Nicholson
S. Badve   A.M. Marchevsky W.I. Yang
V.L. Capelozzi   M. Marino
J.K.C. Chan   E.M. Marom

Definition

Type B1 thymoma is a neoplasm of thymic epithelial cells that closely resembles the normal thymus in terms of architecture and cytology. Accordingly, it is composed of dispersed epithelial cells that do not form clusters and are set in a dense background of immature T cells, mimicking the non-involuted thymic cortex. Areas of medullary differentiation are invariably present.

ICD-O code   8583/3

Synonyms

Lymphocyte-rich thymoma; lymphocytic thymoma; organoid thymoma; predominantly cortical thymoma (not recommended)

Epidemiology

Type B1 thymoma accounts for 17.5% (ranging from 5.9% to 52.8%) of thymomas {543,584,922,1578,1579,1580}. There is a slight female predominance {584}. Type B1 thymoma occurs most commonly in the fifth and sixth decades of life, with a mean age of 57 years and a wide age range (6–83 years) {358,584, 1469}. In the International Thymic Malignancy Interest Group (ITMIG) database, 17% of 3867 thymomas are coded as type B1 (with an average age of 53 years) {2826}.

Etiology

There are no established etiological factors. An origin from a putative thymic epithelial cell precursor with the potential for full bilineage corticomedullary differentiation has been proposed {2489}.

Clinical features

One third of patients are asymptomatic {586}. Others have variable autoimmune and local symptoms, such as chest pain, cough, and dyspnoea {586}. Myasthenia gravis occurs in 44% of patients (ranging from 7% to 70%) {584}. In the ITMIG database, 35% had myasthenia gravis {2826}. Pure red cell aplasia and hypogammaglobulinaemia (Good syndrome) – seen

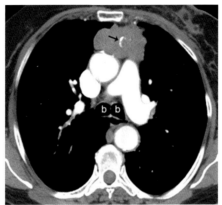

Fig. 3.15 Type B1 thymoma. Contrast-enhanced chest CT in a 78-year-old woman at the level of the main bronchi (b) demonstrates a lobular anterior mediastinal mass with curvilinear calcifications within it (arrow).

in 5% of cases each – and/or other autoimmune diseases can occur in isolation or together with myasthenia gravis.

The imaging features of type B1 thymoma have not been studied individually, and overlap with those seen in type A, AB, and B2 thymoma {2191}.

The imaging features of what have been called (in the published imaging series) low-risk thymomas (i.e. types A, AB, and B1) overlap with those of the so-called high-risk thymomas (i.e. types B2 and B3). Type B1 thymoma is almost always encapsulated, and extension to adjacent structures and pleural dissemination is very rare {402,1319,1521,1905,2150, 2151,2959}. About 50% of tumours are stage I, 37% stage II, 9% stage III, and < 5% stage IV.

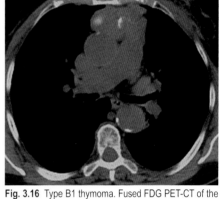

Fig. 3.16 Type B1 thymoma. Fused FDG PET-CT of the same patient as in the previous figure, at the same level, shows that the mass is focally FDG-avid, with a maximal standardized uptake value of 5.6.

Localization

Type B1 thymoma occurs in the anterior mediastinum. Ectopic localization is very rare.

Macroscopy

Type B1 thymoma is usually a nodular tumour with a well-defined capsule. The mean diameter ranges from 5.1 to 7.5 cm {369,2651}. The cut surface is soft, smooth, and tan-pink, with vague lobules delineated by fibrous septa. Necrosis or cystic change may be present {1738,1797,2651,2907}.

Cytology

Lymphocyte-rich smears may lead to the misdiagnosis of reactive lymph node, thymic hyperplasia, or T lymphoblastic

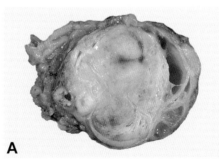
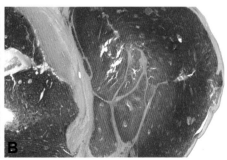

Fig. 3.17 Type B1 thymoma. A Macroscopic appearance of a type B1 thymoma with a nodular and focally cystic cut surface. B Low-power view showing an encapsulated tumour containing large angulated lobules separated by dense collagenous septa. Small pale-staining medullary islands are distributed in a dense lymphoid background.

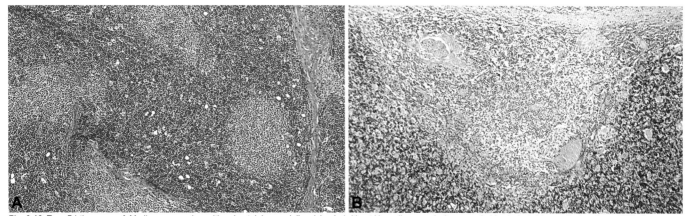

Fig. 3.18 Type B1 thymoma. **A** Medium-power view with pale-staining medullary islands (without Hassall corpuscles) surrounded by dark-staining cortical regions. **B** Medium-power detail of a light-staining medullary island containing Hassall corpuscles and abutting a fibrous septum.

lymphoma (T-LBL). The presence of inconspicuous epithelial cells can suggest the diagnosis {2795}.

Histopathology

Type B1 thymomas have thymus-like architecture, with a predominance of cortical areas. In some tumours, lobulation is virtually absent. In lobulated tumours, the lobules are often larger than those of the normal thymus, and are traversed by hypocellular, collagenous septa. The neoplastic epithelial cells, which are individually embedded within densely packed non-neoplastic immature lymphocytes, may be difficult to detect on low-power examination. A significant increase in epithelial cells beyond the density in the normal thymic cortex, or the presence of epithelial cell clusters (i.e. three or more contiguous epithelial cells), should suggest the possibility of type B2 thymoma. The epithelial cells have poorly defined, pale eosinophilic cytoplasm and oval to slightly irregular rounded nuclei with minor variation in size. The nuclei have pale chromatin, distinct nuclear membranes, and small variably conspicuous central

nucleoli. Any area with spindled epithelial cells suggests the alternative classification of type AB thymoma. Vaguely nodular, pale areas constituting foci of medullary differentiation (so-called medullary islands) are always present. They are less cellular, with no or few immature T cells, but have increased numbers of B cells and mature T cells, and may contain Hassall corpuscles and myoid cells. Perivascular spaces are often present, but are not a diagnostic requirement.

Two distinctive features of type B1 thymoma versus other thymomas are close resemblance to the normal, non-involuted thymic cortex, and the consistent presence of medullary islands.

Type B1 thymoma may be admixed with type B2 or B3 thymoma areas {2488}. The reporting of such cases is described in *Type A thymoma*.

Immunohistochemistry

The epithelial cells are diffusely positive for CK19 (and antibody AE1/AE3); focally positive for CK7, CK8, CK14, and CK18; and negative for CK20 {1361}. Almost all cases express p63 {424} and PAX8

{2832}. Lymphocytes are mostly immature T cells expressing a normal cortical marker profile: terminal deoxynucleotidyl transferase-positive, CD1a+, CD3+, CD4+, CD8+, and CD34−. Medullary islands are characterized by: 1) mainly mature T cells that are CD3+, terminal deoxynucleotidyl transferase-negative, CD1a−, and either CD4+ or CD8+; 2) a substantial B-cell population expressing CD20 and CD79a; and 3) epithelial cells that express CK19 diffusely and may be focally positive for CK10 and involucrin in association with Hassall corpuscles {1361} and (in about 50%) for the medullary marker AIRE (autoimmune regulator) {2489}.

Differential diagnosis

Type B1 thymoma is distinguished from hyperplastic thymus by larger lobules, a thicker fibrous capsule, the presence of fibrous septa, and the predominance of cortical areas over medullary islands, which often abut on fibrous septa, have fewer or no Hassall corpuscles, and have autoimmune regulator-positive epithelial cells {2489,2494}.

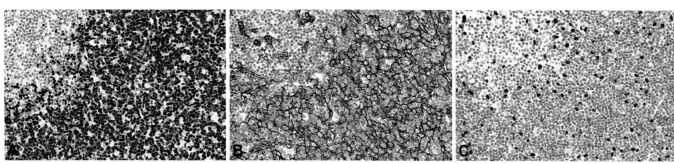

Fig. 3.19 Type B1 thymoma. Serial sections showing a medullary island (upper-left corner). **A** Medullary island largely devoid of terminal deoxynucleotidyl transferase-positive immature T cells, while there are abundant terminal deoxynucleotidyl transferase-positive T cells in the cortical areas. **B** Highlighting the delicate keratin-positive epithelial cell network in the medullary island and the cortical area. **C** Epithelial cells with p63-positive nuclei are individually interspersed among an abundance of p63-negative T cells in the medullary island and the cortical area. Reprinted from Marx A et al. {1595}.

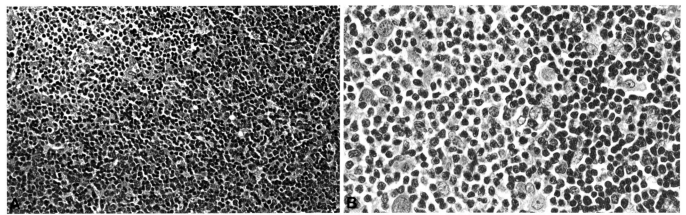

Fig. 3.20 Type B1 thymoma. **A** Medium power showing the organoid architecture of a B1 thymoma containing a light-staining medullary island (upper-left corner) and a dark-staining cortical area. Reprinted from Marx A et al. {1595}. **B** High-power detail of a B1 thymoma showing rare, unclustered epithelial cells with large, vesicular, clear nuclei and quite conspicuous nucleoli surrounded by abundant lymphocytes. Left field shows a medullary island.

Type B2 thymoma shows a higher content of epithelial cells and/or tumour cell clustering compared to type B1 thymoma, which may be confirmed by keratin immunohistochemistry. Medullary islands with or without Hassall corpuscles are obligatory in type B1, but rare in type B2 thymomas.

Rare type AB thymomas that show medullary islands in immature lymphocyte-rich (terminal deoxynucleotidyl transferase-positive) areas are distinguished from type B1 thymomas by at least focal occurrence of spindled tumour cells, a higher than normal content of keratin-positive tumour cells, and epithelial CD20 expression (in 50% of cases).

In T-LBL, corticomedullary architecture is effaced. Blasts infiltrate beyond the thymic epithelial networks into septa and mediastinal fat. Rearrangement of T-cell receptor genes is mostly monoclonal, while abnormal immunophenotypes of blasts are less common {2551}. Very rarely, type B1 thymomas fail to stain for individual keratins or even several other usually expressed epithelial markers. To avoid an erroneous diagnosis of T-LBL, identification of a preserved network of epithelial cells by a panel of epithelial markers including keratins and p63 is recommended {17}. Moreover, in type B1 thymoma, T cells lack atypia and show variable cytomorphology, whereas the neoplastic cells of T-LBL are monotonous and atypical, with frequent necrosis.

Genetic profile

Recurrent gene copy number alterations are uncommon in type B1 as compared to other type B thymomas {844,1434,2027,3011}. In one available study {1434} gene copy number alterations were less common in type B1 than other type B thymomas {844,2027,3011}. Losses of chromosomes 1p, 2q, 3q, 4, 5, 6q, 8, 13, and 18, and a gain of chromosome 9q have been identified using complementary DNA microarray {1434}. Recently, a missense mutation of the GTF2I gene has been reported in 32% of type B1 thymomas {2044A}.

Prognosis and predictive factors

Reported 10- and 20-year overall rates of survival range from 85% to 100% {402,952,1905,2154,2488}. About 90% of type B1 thymomas are completely resectable {1991,2488}, and recurrence is very rare (0–8%), particularly after R0 resection {1991,2488,2907}. In the ITMIG database, the overall survival rates of R0 resected type B1 thymoma at 5 and 10 years were 96% and 91%, respectively {2826}. The rates of recurrence after an R0 resection at 5 and 10 years were about 11% and 14%, respectively, overall (8% for stage I–II and 22% for stage III at 10 years). Whether resection status, stage, and tumour recurrence are significant prognostic factors in type B1 thymomas has not been explicitly addressed {369,543,583,586,1905,2129}.

Type B2 thymoma

A.M. Marchevsky
A. Marx
P. Ströbel
S. Badve
V.L. Capelozzi
J.K.C. Chan

M.A. den Bakker
F. Detterbeck
N. Girard
N.A. Jambhekar
M. Marino
E.M. Marom

Y. Matsuno
T.J. Molina
K. Mukai
A.G. Nicholson
W.I. Yang

Definition

Type B2 thymoma is a lymphocyte-rich tumour composed of polygonal neoplastic epithelial cells set in a background of numerous immature T cells. The epithelial cells usually occur in small clusters, and at a density that is consistently higher than that seen in type B1 thymoma or the normal thymus. Medullary differentiation may or may not be present.

ICD-O code   8584/3

Synonym

Cortical thymoma (not recommended)

Epidemiology

Type B2 thymomas account for 8.0–41.1% (averaging 26%) of the more than 2400 thymomas reported in multiple studies {543,584,922,1578,1579,1580}. They are usually diagnosed in adults in their fifth or sixth decade, with a mean age of 49 years {584} and a wide age range (4–83 years) {358,1469,2488}. There is no sex predominance {584,2141}. In the International Thymic Malignancy Interest Group (ITMIG) database, 28% of 3867 thymomas are coded as type B2 (with an average age of 52 years) {2826}.

Etiology

The etiology is unknown. An origin from a putative thymic epithelial cell precursor with the potential for variable bilineage corticomedullary differentiation has been proposed {2489}.

Clinical features

Some patients are asymptomatic. Others have local symptoms (e.g. chest pain, cough, dyspnoea, and superior vena cava syndrome) and/or variable autoimmune diseases. Myasthenia gravis is present in 54% (ranging from 24% to 71%). Pure red cell aplasia, hypogammaglobulinaemia (Good syndrome), and/or other autoimmune disorders occur in about 5% of cases {586,1594}.
The imaging features of type B2 thymoma overlap with those of type A,

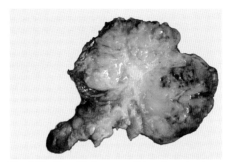

Fig. 3.21 Type B2 thymoma. Cut surface showing a grey-white, poorly circumscribed lesion with bosselated smooth borders and tumour nodules that are incompletely delineated by white fibrous septa.

AB, and B1 thymoma {2191}. Type B2 thymomas commonly show infiltration of the surrounding fat and adjacent structures, as well as pleural dissemination {402,1319,1521}.On average, 32% of tumours are in stage I, 29% in stage II, 28% in stage III, and 11% in stage IV. Distant metastasis (stage IVB) occurs in about 3% of cases.

Localization

Type B2 thymoma occurs in the anterior mediastinum. Ectopic localization is very rare.

Macroscopy

The tumours are encapsulated or show invasion of the mediastinal fat or adjacent organs. Their mean diameter ranges from 4 to 6.2 cm {369,2651}. The cut surface is grey-white and soft to firm, with lobules delineated by white fibrous septa. Necrosis, cystic changes, and/or haemorrhage may be present.

Cytology

Cytological diagnosis of thymoma is feasible, although reliable subclassification is generally not possible {45,422,2795}. Smears typically show isolated and/or clustered epithelial cells intermingled with numerous lymphocytes. Type B2 thymoma may be mistaken for reactive lymph node, thymic hyperplasia, or T lymphoblastic lymphoma if epithelial cells are sparse due to poor sampling {3005}.

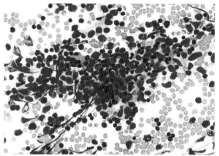

Fig. 3.22 Type B2 thymoma. Fine-needle aspirate showing single and clustered tumour cells intermingled with lymphocytes. The medium to large tumour cells show round or elongated nuclei and small nucleoli.

Histopathology

At low magnification in H&E-stained sections, type B2 thymomas appear blue due to the abundance of lymphocytes. They differ from lymphomas by the presence of a fibrous tumour capsule and a lobular architecture {1581,2377,2672}. The tumour lobules are irregular in size and shape, and are surrounded by delicate fibrous septa. Interspersed among the lymphoid cells are conspicuous singly arranged or poorly defined clusters of epithelial cells (≥ 3 cells). The epithelial cells show round or slightly oval nuclei with vesicular chromatin and small but prominent nucleoli. Rare cases show (usually focal) anaplasia.
Other typical features are the presence of perivascular spaces composed of a central venule surrounded by a clear space containing proteinaceous fluid or variable numbers of lymphocytes. Few cases show Hassall corpuscles. Medullary islands are uncommonly seen, and are usually inconspicuous. Particularly in patients with myasthenia gravis, lymphoid follicles may be seen in the fibrous septa and/or perivascular spaces. Treatment with corticosteroids may result in prominent histiocytic infiltrates, lymphocyte depletion, and necrosis.
Distinctive features of type B2 thymomas versus other thymomas are: 1) polygonal (non-spindle shaped) neoplastic thymic epithelial cells that usually occur in clusters and are more numerous than in the

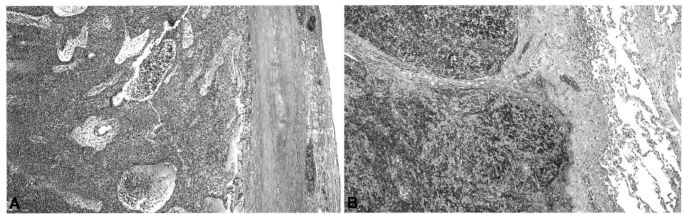

Fig. 3.23 Type B2 thymoma. **A** Tumour area that exhibits a thick fibrous capsule. **B** Pushing invasion front reaching into lung (Masaoka-Koga stage III).

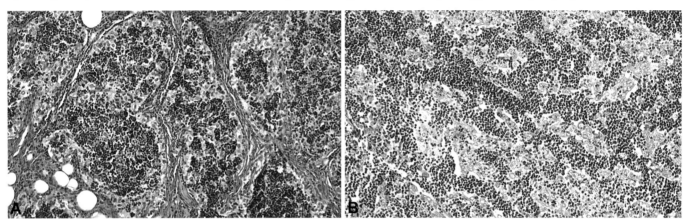

Fig. 3.24 Type B2 thymoma. **A** Fibrous septa within the tumour separate the lymphoepithelial elements into poorly formed lobules. This histopathological feature is helpful in distinguishing thymomas from malignant lymphomas. **B** Aggregates of epithelial cells admixed with lymphoid cells; the epithelial cells are larger than the lymphoid cells, and exhibit more prominent cytoplasm and hypochromatic nuclei with small nucleoli.

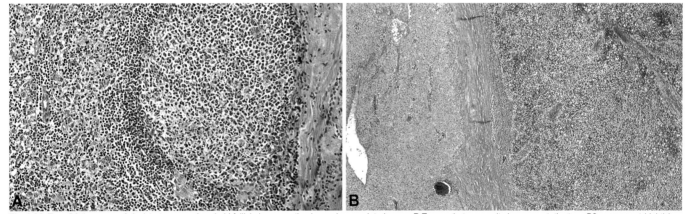

Fig. 3.25 Type B2 thymoma. **A** An intratumorous lymphoid follicle in a myasthenia gravis-associated case. **B** Tumour heterogeneity is apparent; the type B2 component (right) has a bluish appearance, while the type B3 component (left) is pink.

normal thymic cortex and B1 thymoma, and 2) a high content of intermingled immature T cells.

Heterogeneous areas with type B3 or B1 thymoma patterns are present in 42% and 4% of type B2 thymomas, respectively {2488}, and are reported as explained in *Type A thymoma*. Associated thymic carcinoma is rare {1358,2518}

(see *Combined thymic carcinomas*, p. 242).

Immunohistochemistry
The keratin-positive epithelial network is denser than that in B1 thymomas. Defective keratin expression is a rare pitfall {17} (see *Type B1 thymoma*, p. 196). Epithelial cells are admixed with highly

proliferative immature T cells (terminal deoxynucleotidyl transferase-positive, with a Ki-67 labelling index of about 90%) {1581,2377,2672}. Type B2 thymomas usually show strong expression of markers of cortical differentiation and variable expression of markers of medullary differentiation {2489}.

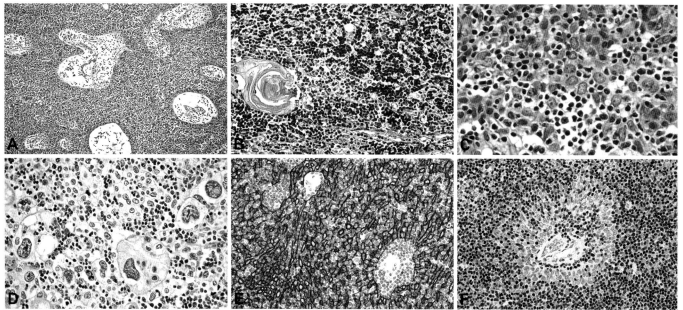

Fig. 3.26 Type B2 thymoma. **A** Perivascular spaces composed of a central venule surrounded by a clear space with variable numbers of lymphocytes. **B** A Hassall corpuscle in type B2 thymoma; epithelial cell abundance and clustering argue against type B1 thymoma. **C** Epithelial cells in a type B2 thymoma showing small but conspicuous nucleoli. **D** Anaplasia of tumour cells set in a background of abundant T cells, which are immature (i.e. immunoreactive for CD1a; not shown). **E** CK19 staining highlights perivascular spaces and an epithelial cell network that is denser than in type B1 thymoma and more open than in type B3 thymoma. **F** Terminal deoxynucleotidyl transferase staining reveals abundant immature T cells in the surroundings of a perivascular space; note the few terminal deoxynucleotidyl transferase-positive cells inside the perivascular space.

Differential diagnosis

Type B1 thymoma more closely resembles the normal thymus and shows fewer epithelial cells than type B2 thymoma. It lacks epithelial cell clusters and consistently shows medullary islands with or without Hassall corpuscles. Prominent perivascular spaces are more typical of type B2 than type B1 thymomas

Type B3 thymoma is a lymphocyte-poor tumour characterized by sheets of tumour cells sprinkled with immature T cells. In contrast with the blue colour seen on H&E staining in lymphocyte-rich type B2 thymoma, the solid epithelial growth pattern of type B3 thymoma imparts a pink colour.

T lymphoblastic lymphoma can mimic lymphocyte-rich thymomas (see *Type B1 thymoma*, p. 196). T lymphoblastic lymphoma can rarely arise in type B2 thymoma {684}.

The rare type B2 thymomas with anaplasia are distinguishable from thymic carcinomas by the maintenance of typical thymoma features (terminal deoxynucleotidyl transferase-positive T cells, perivascular spaces, lobular growth pattern, and absence of CD5/CD117 expression).

Genetic profile

Type B2 thymomas show more genetic alterations than type A thymomas, but fewer than B3 thymomas {844,1434,2027}. Recurrent losses of chromosomes 6q25.2–25.3 and 3p, and gain of 1q are found in both type B2 and B3 thymomas {844,1088,1434,2027,2046,3011}. No gain of *BCL2*, loss of *CDKN2A/B* {2045}, or mutations of *KIT* or *EGFR* has been observed in type B2 thymomas {2491}. Recently, a missense mutation of the *GTF2I*

gene has been reported in 22% of type B2 thymomas {2044A}.

Prognosis and predictive factors

Reported 10- and 20-year overall survival rates are 70–90% and 59–78%, respectively {402,952,1905,2154,2488}. Complete resection is achieved in 70–90% of cases {369,1905,1991,2488}. In the ITMIG database, the rates of recurrence after an R0 resection at 5 and 10 years were 14% and 32%, respectively, overall (13% for Masaoka-Koga stage I–II and 41% for stage III at 10 years). Advanced stage (III or IV) is a poor prognostic factor for tumour-related death {2488}. The prognostic significance of resection status, tumour size, and recurrence is unknown for type B2 and other types of thymomas, because studies have not stratified the thymic tumours by histological type {369,543,583,586,1905,2129}.

Type B3 thymoma

A. Marx
P. Ströbel
S. Badve
V.L. Capelozzi
J.K.C. Chan
M.A. den Bakker

F. Detterbeck
N. Girard
N.A. Jambhekar
A.M. Marchevsky
M. Marino
E.M. Marom

T.J. Molina
K. Mukai
A.G. Nicholson
W.D. Travis
W.I. Yang

Definition
Type B3 thymoma is an epithelium-predominant thymic epithelial tumour composed of mildly or moderately atypical polygonal tumour cells showing a sheet-like, solid growth pattern. In almost all cases, there are intermingled non-neoplastic immature T cells.

ICD-O code   8585/3

Synonyms
Atypical thymoma; epithelial thymoma; squamoid thymoma; well-differentiated thymic carcinoma (not recommended)

Epidemiology
Type B3 thymoma accounts for 16% of the more than 2400 thymomas reported in multiple studies {543, 584,922,1578,1579,1580}. The mean age at diagnosis is 55 years (ranging from 8 to 87 years) {584,1469}. A slight male predominance has been reported {584}. In the International Thymic Malignancy Interest Group (ITMIG) database, 21% of thymoma cases are coded as type B3 (with an average age of 52 years) {2826}.

Etiology
The etiology is unknown. An origin from a putative thymic epithelial cell precursor with minimal corticomedullary differentiation has been proposed {2489}.

Clinical features
Most patients have local symptoms, such as chest pain or superior vena cava syndrome. Myasthenia gravis has been reported in 50% of cases {369,584}. In the ITMIG database, 40% of patients had myasthenia gravis {2826}. Other autoimmune disorders are less common {586,1594}. Although there is overlap in the imaging features of type A through B3 thymoma, the few studies focusing on type B3 thymoma have shown it to be more likely to present with advanced-stage disease and higher FDG uptake than other types of thymoma {181,1585}. Type B3 thymomas commonly infiltrate the surrounding fat and adjacent

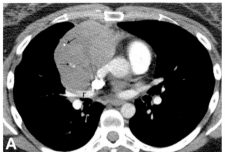
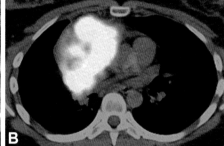

Fig. 3.27 Type B3 thymoma. **A** Axial contrast-enhanced chest CT in a 29-year-old woman at the level of the right superior pulmonary vein (r) shows a large heterogeneous anterior mediastinal mass with dense calcifications within it (arrows). **B** A fused image from FDG PET-CT of the same patient shows that the mass is markedly FDG-avid, with a maximal standardized uptake value of 15.5. Although there is overlap in the imaging features of the different histological types of thymoma, type B3 thymomas show much higher FDG uptake than thymomas of other types.

structures, and show pleural dissemination {402,1319,1521}. On average, 19% are stage I, 36% stage II, 27% stage III, and 18% stage IV. Distant metastasis (stage IVB) occurs in 3% (ranging from 0% to 15%).

Localization
Type B3 thymoma occurs in the anterior mediastinum. Ectopic localization is very rare.

Macroscopy
Type B3 thymomas are usually poorly circumscribed, with smooth extensions into the mediastinal fat or adjacent organs. The mean diameter ranges from 5.1 to 6.8 cm {369,2651}. The cut surface is firm and grey or yellow, with tumour nodules separated by fibrous bands.

Necrosis and haemorrhage may be present {2842}.

Cytology
Smears show sheets of tumour cells with some size variation, round nuclei, inconspicuous nucleoli, and rare admixed lymphocytes. Due to limited experience with type B3 thymoma, attempts at subtyping thymomas cytologically are currently not recommended {2795,3005}.

Histopathology
Typical findings include tumour lobules separated by fibrous septa, pushing borders at the invasion front, prominent perivascular spaces with epithelial palisading, and absence of intercellular bridges between tumour cells except in rare Hassall corpuscles or so-called squamous eddies. Tumour cells are

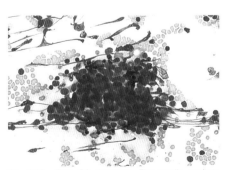

Fig. 3.28 Type B3 thymoma. Fine-needle aspirate showing sheets of relatively monotonous medium-sized tumour cells with round nuclei and inconspicuous small nucleoli; lymphocytes are virtually absent.

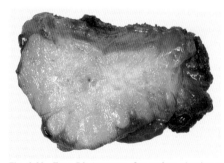

Fig. 3.29 Type B3 thymoma. Cut surface showing a grey-white, poorly circumscribed lesion with bosselated smooth borders and tumour nodules that are incompletely delineated by white fibrous septa.

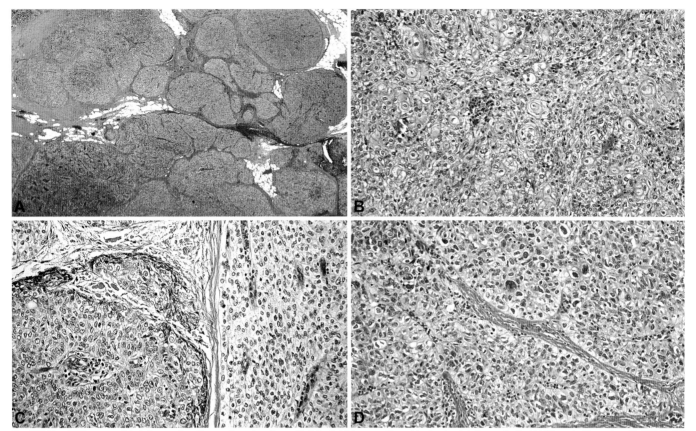

Fig. 3.30 Type B3 thymoma. **A** Lobular growth pattern and invasion of an epithelial cell-rich tumour with pushing borders into the mediastinal fat (Masaoka-Koga stage II). **B** Epithelial whorls resembling squamous eddies or abortive Hassall corpuscles; intercellular bridges can rarely be observed in such regions in type B3 thymoma. **C** A clear cell area (top and right) in an otherwise typical type B3 thymoma, with prominent perivascular space (the darker region in the lower-left part of the image). **D** Anaplasia in a type B3 thymoma; note the moderate cytological atypia throughout the image.

polygonal with eosinophilic or clear cytoplasm and slightly/moderately atypical, round to elongated, sometimes grooved or raisinoid nuclei. Nucleoli may be inconspicuous or prominent. Lymphoid follicles may occur in myasthenia gravis-associated tumours.

Distinctive features versus other thymoma types are: 1) predominance of polygonal epithelial cells that form solid sheets, resulting in a pink appearance on H&E stains at low magnification; and 2) paucity of admixed non-neoplastic immature T cells.

Thymomas that consist of type B3 and B2 components are common (2–16% of all thymomas), and may exceed the frequency of pure type B3 thymomas {402,543,2488}. Combined thymic carcinomas and type B3 thymomas are rare (0.2–1% of thymic epithelial tumours) {543,2488}. The reporting of such tumours is described in *Type A thymoma*.

Immunohistochemistry
The tumour cells usually react with pancytokeratin antibodies, and express CK19, CK5/6, CK7, CK8, and CK10, but not CK20. Other commonly positive markers are CD57, p63 {424,619,2912}, PAX8 {2832}, and (focally) epithelial membrane antigen {769}. TTF1, CD20, and thymic carcinoma markers are almost always negative (CD5 and CD117), or are focally expressed in rare cases (GLUT1 and MUC1) {1181,1314}. Terminal deoxynucleotidyl transferase (TdT)+ immature T cells occur in > 95% of cases. Type B3 thymomas show only occasional expression of markers of cortical differentiation and usually no expression of markers of medullary differentiation {2489}.

Type B3 thymoma variants
Focal spindle cell features can occur in an otherwise typical B3 thymoma. Whether a pure spindle cell variant of type B3 thymoma exists is currently unclear, and distinction from atypical type A thymoma will be difficult. The rare type B3 thymomas with anaplasia are distinguishable from thymic carcinomas by the maintenance of typical thymoma features (i.e. TdT+ T cells, perivascular spaces, a lobular growth pattern, the absence of CD5/CD117 expression, and usually the absence of desmoplasia).

Rare tumours with a type B3 thymoma morphology showing focal expression of CD5 and CD117 and/or lack of TdT+ T cells {975,1181,1595} should be labelled as type B3 thymomas, and not as thymic carcinomas {1793}.

Differential diagnosis
Unlike type B3 thymomas, type B2 thymomas are lymphocyte-rich. On H&E-stained sections, they appear blue rather than pink. However, since there is a morphological continuum between type B2 and B3 thymomas {2253,2525}, the distinction between type B2 and B3 may sometimes be arbitrary. Previously described distinguishing criteria (e.g. perivascular spaces and nuclear size) are not helpful for this distinction. Comparing diagnostic cases with images of epithelium-rich type B2 thymomas versus lymphocyte-rich type B3 thymomas may help with decision-making {1595}.

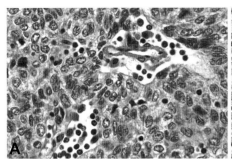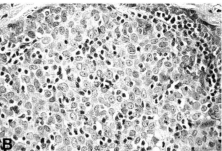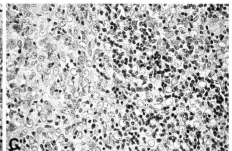

Fig. 3.31 Type B3 thymoma. **A** Details of slightly eosinophilic, mostly medium-sized, mildly to moderately atypical tumour cells showing round or oval nuclei of variable size, nuclear folds, and small inconspicuous nucleoli. The tumour cells form sheets that are sprinkled with few lymphocytes. Considerably more lymphocytes are present in the perivascular spaces. **B** Large cell features in a type B3 thymoma; the tumour cell nuclei and nucleoli are reminiscent of the large vesicular nuclei that are typical of type B2 thymoma. **C** Tumour heterogeneity at high power: type B3 thymoma (left) with sharp transition to a type B2 thymoma component (right).

Thymic squamous cell carcinoma (TSQCC) is distinguished from type B3 thymoma by the absence of a lobular growth, infiltrative rather than pushing-type invasion, prominent desmoplasia, a lack of perivascular spaces, more prominent nuclear atypia, and frequently the presence of intercellular bridges. TSQC-Cs commonly (in 80% of cases) express CD5 and CD117, while B3 thymomas do not {988,1314}, with rare exceptions {975,1181}. The cortical epithelial cell marker beta5t {2923} can be positive in B3 thymomas, but is typically negative in TSQCC. GLUT1 and MUC1, like CD5 and CD117, have also been reported to be more commonly positive in TSQCC than in type B3 thymomas {988,1181,1314}. However, since the literature on GLUT1 and MUC1 is still limited, further studies are needed to confirm their diagnostic value. With rare exceptions {1245}, TdT+ immature T cells are absent in TSQCC.

Genetic profile

Recurrent gene copy number alterations are more common in type B3 thymomas than in other thymomas {844,1434,2027,3011}. Recurrent losses of chromosomes 6q25.2–25.3 and 3p, and gains of 1q are found in both type B2 and B3 thymomas, while losses of 13q, 16q, and 17p, and gains of 4p and 17q have been found only in type B3 thymomas {844,2027,2046,3011}. Copy number gain of *BCL2* and loss of *CDKN2A/B* has been associated with a poor outcome {2045}. There are no mutations in the *EGFR/RAS* signalling pathway genes {844,1649} or *KIT* gene {841,844}. Recently, a missense mutation of the *GTF2I* gene has been reported in 21% of type B3 thymomas {2044A}.

Prognosis and predictive factors

Reported 10- and 20-year overall survival rates are 50–70% and 25–36%, respectively {402,952,1905,2488}. Recurrence occurs in up to 44% of cases, and in up to 20% of completely resected stage III cases {2488}. In the ITMIG database, the overall survival rates of R0 resected type B3 thymoma at 5 and 10 years were 89% and 81%, respectively. The rates of recurrence after an R0 resection at 5 and 10 years were about 23% and 29%, respectively, overall (11% for stage I–II and 28% for stage III at 10 years). Advanced stage (III or IV) is a poor prognostic factor for tumour-related death {2488}. The prognostic significance of resection status, tumour size, and recurrence is unknown for type B3 and other types of thymomas, because studies have not stratified the thymic tumours by histological type {369,543,583,586,1905, 2129}. Age and sex have no impact on prognosis {2488}. Myasthenia gravis was a favourable prognostic factor in recent studies, due to earlier tumour detection {369,543}.

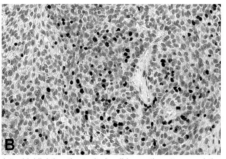

Fig. 3.32 Type B3 thymoma. **A** CK19 immunohistochemistry highlighting the typical solid growth pattern and the palisading of tumour cells around perivascular spaces. **B** Terminal deoxynucleotidyl transferase immunohistochemistry showing the paucity of immature T cells (so-called intraepithelial lymphocytes) interspersed among the tumour cells.

Micronodular thymoma with lymphoid stroma

H. Tateyama
A. Marx
P. Ströbel
F. Detterbeck
N. Girard
A.M. Marchevsky
E.M. Marom
K. Mukai

Definition
Micronodular thymoma with lymphoid stroma is a thymic epithelial tumour characterized by multiple small tumour islands composed of bland spindle or oval cells that are surrounded by an epithelial cell-free lymphoid stroma, which may contain lymphoid follicles.

ICD-O code   8580/1

Synonym
Micronodular thymoma with lymphoid B cell hyperplasia

Epidemiology
Micronodular thymoma with lymphoid stroma is a rare type of thymoma, accounting for about 1% of all cases. Patient ages range from 41 to 80 years (with a mean age of 64.5 years). There is a slight male predominance, with a male-to-female ratio of 1.5:1 {1967, 2492,2520,2602}. In the International Thymic Malignancy Interest Group (IT-MIG) retrospective database, micronodular thymoma with lymphoid stroma accounts for 1.4% of cases (with an average age of 71 years) {2826}.

Etiology
The etiology is unknown. The associated lymphoid stroma is thought to be recruited by chemokines that are abnormally expressed by the tumour cells {2492}. A putative thymic epithelial precursor is assumed to be the cell of origin.

Clinical features
Patients are usually asymptomatic and the tumour is an incidental radiographical finding. In very rare cases, myasthenia gravis has been reported {1967}.
There has been one case report describing the CT appearance of micronodular thymoma with lymphoid stroma, which overlaps with the imaging features of other types of thymoma {1261}.
Most micronodular thymoma with lymphoid stroma are localized; approximately 62% of the tumours are encapsulated (stage I) and 36% are minimally invasive (stage II) {1967,2492,2520,2602,2632}. An exceptional case showed wide invasion and multiple pleural implants {2520}. In the ITMIG database, 96% of micronodular thymomas with lymphoid stroma were stage I or II {2826}.

Localization
Micronodular thymoma with lymphoid stroma occurs in the anterior mediastinum. Ectopic localization is very rare.

Macroscopy
Micronodular thymoma with lymphoid stroma is usually well circumscribed and encapsulated. The cut surface is homogeneous and light tan, with occasional cystic spaces of variable size. Micronodular thymoma with lymphoid stroma is often soft and friable. Diameters range from 3 to 15 cm.

Histopathology
Micronodular thymoma with lymphoid stroma is characterized by multiple, discrete small solid nests or cords of tumour cells, separated by abundant lymphoid stroma, which usually contains lymphoid follicles with or without germinal centres and variable numbers of plasma cells.
The nodules are composed of bland, short spindle or oval cells with scant cytoplasm and oval to elongated uniform nuclei containing dispersed chromatin and indistinct nucleoli. Mitotic activity is lacking or minimal. A few interspersed lymphocytes may be observed within the nodules. Micro- and macrocystic changes are common. Rosette-like structures and glandular formation may be seen. However, Hassall corpuscles, perivascular spaces, and a lobular architecture are missing.
Areas corresponding to type A thymoma occur in up to 30% of micronodular thymomas with lymphoid stroma {2492,2602}. Associations with type AB {1967,2492} and B2 thymoma {2632} and thymic carcinoma {2520} are rare. The reporting of such tumours is described in *Type A thymoma*, p. 187.

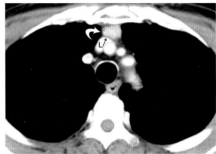

Fig. 3.33 Micronodular thymoma with lymphoid stroma in a 60-year-old man with a 1.8 cm stage I micronodular thymoma. Contrast-enhanced chest CT at the level of the left brachiocephalic vein (L) shows a smooth homogeneous anterior mediastinal mass (curved arrow) separated from the left brachiocephalic vein by fat (straight arrow).

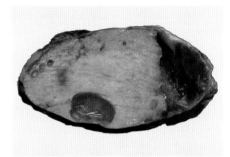

Fig. 3.34 Micronodular thymoma with lymphoid stroma. Macroscopy shows a homogeneous, light-tan cut surface with cyst formation.

Immunohistochemistry
The epithelial component in micronodular thymoma with lymphoid stroma shows positivity for pancytokeratin, CK5/6, and CK19, but typically lacks expression of CD20. The lymphoid stroma is devoid of keratin-positive epithelial cells, and contains mostly mature CD20+/CD79a+ B cells and CD3+/terminal deoxynucleotidyl transferase-negative T cells, but typically harbours a population of CD3+/CD1a+/CD99+/terminal deoxynucleotidyl transferase-positive immature T cells in the vicinity of the tumour nodules. In contrast, terminal deoxynucleotidyl transferase-positive cells are scarce within the epithelial nodules. Germinal centres in reactive follicles show CD20+/CD10+/Bcl2– B cells and CD23+ follicular dendritic cell networks.

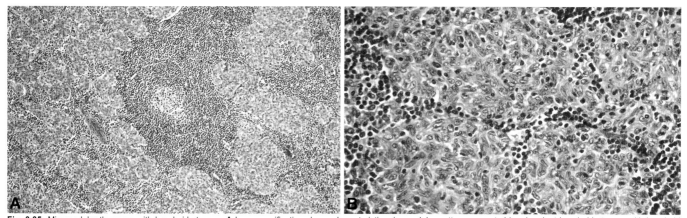

Fig. 3.35 Micronodular thymoma with lymphoid stroma. **A** Low magnification shows characteristic micronodular pattern separated by abundant lymphoid stroma, with lymphoid follicles having germinal centres. **B** Higher magnification shows small, solid nests composed of bland-looking spindle and oval cells.

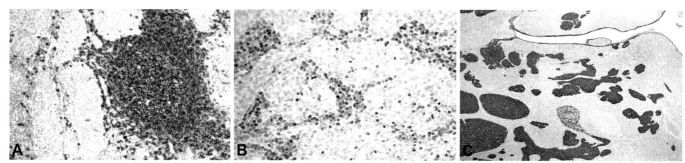

Fig. 3.36 Micronodular thymoma with lymphoid stroma. **A** A lymphoid follicle between epithelial micronodules shows positive immunostaining for CD20. **B** Immunostaining for terminal deoxynucleotidyl transferase shows a thin band of immature lymphocytes surrounding the tumour nodules, and a few scattered lymphocytes within the nodules. **C** Keratin staining shows epithelial nodules, but a lack of epithelial cells in the lymphoid stroma.

Many CD1a+/langerin-positive Langerhans cells are diffusely distributed within the tumour nodules, while fascin-positive mature dendritic cells are present mainly in the stroma {1103}. Plasma cells usually show a polyclonal pattern of immunostaining. However, monoclonal B and/ or plasma cells and even various low-grade so-called intratumorous lymphomas have been observed in rare cases of micronodular thymoma with lymphoid stroma {2492}.

Differential diagnosis
Thymic follicular hyperplasia, unlike micronodular thymoma with lymphoid stroma, is typically associated with myasthenia gravis and shows lymphoid follicles in the medulla and perivascular

spaces. Rarely, epithelial cells adjacent to lymphoid follicles become hyperplastic {220} to the extent that they resemble micronodular thymoma with lymphoid stroma. However, the lobular thymic architecture and Hassall corpuscles are maintained in thymic follicular hyperplasia.
Type AB thymoma is composed of spindle cells in variable lymphocyte-rich and lymphocyte-poor areas. Unlike in micronodular thymoma with lymphoid stroma, the lymphocyte-rich areas of type AB thymoma invariably contain abundant keratin-positive epithelial cells.
Micronodular thymic carcinoma with lymphoid hyperplasia shows a growth pattern and lymphoid stroma like those of micronodular thymoma with lymphoid stroma.

However, the tumour cells demonstrate high-grade cytological atypia, and immature T cells are absent {2837}.
Rare tumours show a micronodular thymoma-like growth pattern and stroma, but their nodules are composed of polygonal epithelial cells that resemble the tumour cells of type B2 thymoma {2602}. It is unclear whether these tumours represent an atypical variant of micronodular thymoma with lymphoid stroma or a micronodular variant of type B thymoma.

Prognosis and predictive factors
Micronodular thymoma with lymphoid stroma is usually diagnosed as stage I/ II disease. There have been no reports of recurrences, distant metastases, or tumour-related deaths.

Metaplastic thymoma

G. Chen
J.K.C. Chan
A.M. Marchevsky

E.M. Marom
A. Marx
K. Mukai
P. Ströbel

Definition
Metaplastic thymoma is a biphasic tumour of the thymus that consists of solid areas of epithelial cells in a background of bland-looking spindle cells, with sharp or gradual transitions between the two components.

ICD-O code   8580/3

Synonyms
Thymoma with pseudosarcomatous stroma; low-grade metaplastic carcinoma; biphasic thymoma; mixed polygonal and spindle cell type thymoma (not recommended)

Epidemiology
Metaplastic thymoma is an extremely rare type of thymoma. Only about 30 cases have been reported in the English-language literature. Metaplastic thymoma occurs in adult patients, with a median age of 50 years (ranging from 28 to 71 years). There is no sex predominance {402,1488,2526,2968,2969}.

Etiology
The etiology is unknown. Metaplastic thymomas appear to occasionally arise in the wall of thymic cysts {1753,2073}.

Clinical features
Most patients are asymptomatic, and are incidentally found to have an anterior mediastinal mass, but others present with cough, dyspnoea, or chest pain {1488}. The patients do not have myasthenia gravis or other paraneoplastic syndromes, with the exception of a single reported case {1202}.
The CT imaging features are similar to those of type A thymoma: a well-defined, smooth, homogeneous anterior mediastinal mass {1202,1488}. However, in one case report, the tumour was highly FDG-avid, with FDG uptake more similar to that found in more aggressive tumours such as thymic carcinoma {1102}.
Occasional tumours can show infiltration of adjacent tissues. Metastasis has not been reported. The stage distribution at

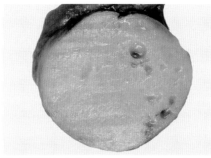

Fig. 3.37 Metaplastic thymoma. Macroscopy shows an encapsulated tumour with a homogeneous grey-white, firm cut surface and several small cysts.

presentation is as follows: 75% at stage I, 17% at stage II, and 8% at stage III {1488,1866,2526,2968,2969}.

Localization
Metaplastic thymoma occurs in the anterior mediastinum.

Macroscopy
The tumours are well circumscribed or encapsulated, but some may show invasive buds focally. The cut surfaces show homogeneous, solid, rubbery, grey-white to yellow tumour with a fascicular appearance. The reported maximum sizes range from 6 to 18 cm {1202,1488,2968}.

Histopathology
The tumours show a biphasic pattern, with a solid epithelial component merging gradually or abruptly with a spindle cell component. The two components are present in highly variable proportions from area to area and from case to case.

A lobular growth pattern and perivascular spaces, features commonly present in usual types of thymoma, are absent.
The epithelial cells form anastomosing islands or broad trabeculae, and may exhibit a squamoid or whorled quality. They are oval, polygonal, or plump spindly, with oval or grooved nuclei, granular chromatin, small nucleoli, and a moderate amount of eosinophilic cytoplasm. Some cells may exhibit enlarged pleomorphic nuclei with or without pseudoinclusions, but mitotic figures are usually absent. Commonly, some epithelial islands are traversed by twigs of eosinophilic hyaline material.
Between the solid epithelial islands, slender fibroblast-like spindle cells form short fascicles or storiform arrays. They are bland-looking, and their elongated nuclei have fine chromatin. Lymphocytes are usually sparse, and plasma cells can be present in occasional cases. Focal tumour necrosis has rarely been reported {1488}.
Distinctive features versus other types of thymomas are: 1) biphasic composition of epithelial cell islands and bland spindle cells, and 2) absence or paucity of lymphocytes throughout the tumour.
Rarely, areas of sarcomatoid carcinoma have been described in association with metaplastic thymoma, suggesting high-grade transformation {1519,1753}. The reporting of these so-called combined thymic carcinomas is described in *Type A thymoma*.

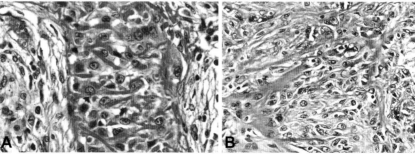

Fig. 3.38 Metaplastic thymoma. A Very often, some epithelial islands are traversed by thick twigs of hyaline material. B In some cases, significant nuclear pleomorphism can be observed in the epithelial cells; nuclear pseudoinclusions are also evident.

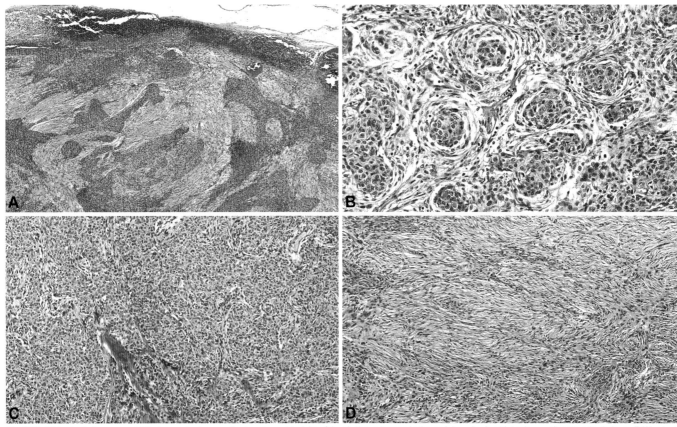

Fig. 3.39 Metaplastic thymoma. **A** The tumour is circumscribed, and a residual rim of thymic tissue is seen in the periphery (top); a biphasic growth pattern is obvious. **B** Whorls of epithelial cells scattered in a background of delicate spindly cells. **C** Epithelium-rich foci with few spindly cells. **D** Spindle cell-rich foci with few epithelial islands (at left).

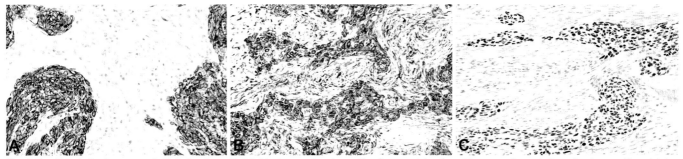

Fig. 3.40 Metaplastic thymoma. **A** Typically, the epithelial islands are strongly positive for pancytokeratin, while no or few spindle cells show positive staining. **B** Sometimes the spindle cells show extensive pancytokeratin immunoreactivity. **C** p63 staining is confined to the cells within the epithelial islands, and is not seen in the fibroblast-like spindle cells.

Immunohistochemistry

The epithelial islands are positive for keratins and p63, variably positive for epithelial membrane antigen, and negative for vimentin {1202}. The fibroblast-like spindle cells are negative or variably positive for keratins, negative for p63, focally positive for epithelial membrane antigen and actin, and positive for vimentin. The expression of keratins and epithelial membrane antigen, albeit only focal, in the fibroblast-like spindle cells supports their metaplastic nature. Both components are negative for CD5, CD20, CD34, and CD117. The Ki-67 index is low (< 5%) in both components. Immature terminal deoxynucleotidyl transferase-positive T cells are typically absent, but may be encountered in adjacent thymic remnants {1866}.

Differential diagnosis

Metaplastic thymoma is usually low-grade in contrast to sarcomatoid carcinoma, which is a highly aggressive malignant neoplasm, that invariably shows a high-grade spindle cell component with significant nuclear atypia, frequent mitotic figures, and (commonly) prominent coagulative necrosis. On immunohistochemistry, the Ki-67 proliferation rate is usually > 10% in sarcomatoid carcinoma {1753}.

Solitary fibrous tumour is a monophasic neoplasm with intercellular wiry collagen and a distinctive immunoprofile (CD34-positive, CD99-positive, Bcl2-positive, STAT6-positive, keratin-negative). Type A thymoma can show, in addition to spindle cells, a variety of histological patterns, including rosettes with or without central lumens, glandular or glomeruloid structures, papillary projections in cystic spaces, or meningioma-like whorls, mimicking a biphasic growth pattern. It is also often devoid of immature T cells. However, it is basically a monophasic tumour, lacks the anastomosing solid squamoid epithelial islands, and strongly expresses keratin and often CD20.

Genetic profile
Comparative genomic hybridization and microsatellite studies on a limited number of cases have shown no or few genetic alterations, suggesting a closer relationship to type A or type AB thymoma than to type B3 thymoma or thymic carcinoma {1488}. Tumour recurrence is apparently associated with the acquisition of multiple genetic aberrations. EBV is negative {1488}.

Prognosis and predictive factors
Among reported patients with follow-up information, the majority remained well after surgical excision at 1.5–20 years (median 10 years) {1488,1866,2526,2968,2969}. One patient developed local recurrence at 14 months, and died at 6 years {2969}. In two patients, there was progression to sarcomatoid thymic carcinoma at presentation, but the clinical course was uneventful after complete resection in one patient and unknown in the other {1519,1753}.

Other rare thymomas

G. Chen
L. Chalabreysse

Microscopic thymoma

Definition
The term microscopic thymoma is applied to the usually multifocal thymic epithelial proliferations of < 1 mm in diameter.

ICD-O code   8580/0

Synonym
Nodular hyperplasia of the thymic epithelium

Epidemiology
Microscopic thymoma was first described by Rosaï and Levine in 1976 {2193}. Since then, 13 additional cases

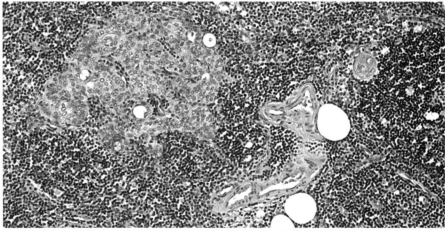

Fig. 3.42 Microscopic thymoma. A small, unencapsulated nodule of oval and spindle epithelial cells without interspersed lymphocytes at the corticomedullary junction of a non-atrophic thymus; no infiltrative growth.

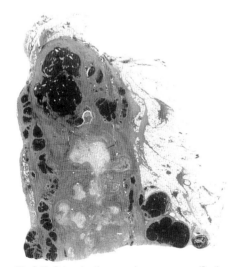

Fig. 3.41 Sclerosing thymoma. Low-power magnification showing extensive sclerosis, with only small remnants of the thymoma (blue nodules); many such thymomas may not be amenable to proper histological subtyping.

have been reported – in 8 females and 5 males with myasthenia gravis. The mean age is 39 years (ranging from 17 to 59 years) {368,492,2038,2096,2729}. The frequency of microscopic thymomas in thymectomy specimens of non-thymomatous myasthenia gravis patients ranges from 3.8 to 15% (with a mean of 4.7%), which overlaps with the frequency of identical-looking lesions in autopsy-derived control thymuses (4%) {2096}.

Etiology
The etiology is unknown. It is unclear whether myasthenia gravis is related to microscopic thymomas.

Clinical features
There are no local symptoms. Lesions are incidental findings in thymectomy specimens of patients with myasthenia gravis.
Microscopic thymoma is not detectable by imaging techniques.
Microscopic thymoma is either confined to the thymus parenchyma or can abut the perithymic adipose tissue. There is no infiltrative growth or metastasis. Staging according to the Masaoka staging system is not applied.

Localization
Microscopic thymoma occurs inside the thymus.

Histopathology
Lesions are usually composed of bland-looking plump spindle or polygonal cells forming well-circumscribed nodules that are embedded in the medulla or cortex,

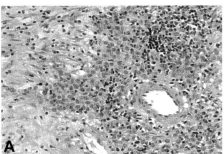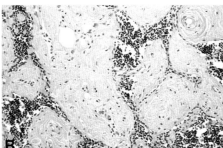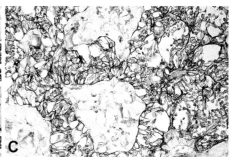

Fig. 3.43 Sclerosing thymoma. **A** Type B3-like thymoma remnants with few interspersed lymphocytes. **B** Tumour with abundant collagenous matrix that expands septa, obliterates perivascular spaces, and surrounds remnant lymphocyte-rich thymoma lobules. **C** CK19-expressing neoplastic epithelial cells surround obliterated perivascular spaces.

or that border the perithymic fat. Pleomorphism of epithelial cells is less common. Infiltrative growth is lacking. Interspersed immature T cells, lobulation, perivascular spaces, corticomedullary differentiation (including Hassall corpuscles), and a capsule are missing, leading some authors to advocate the term nodular hyperplasia of the thymic epithelium {419}. Multiple lesions prevail (present in 70% of cases). The accompanying thymus may show lymphofollicular hyperplasia or thymic atrophy. Expression of CK8/18 has been reported {2096}.

Microthymoma is defined as a conventional thymoma measuring < 1 cm {419}. Tumours with features of type AB, B1, and B2 thymoma have been reported {419,933,1745}.

Prognosis and predictive factors
Microscopic thymomas have no apparent impact on survival. Their prognostic relevance in terms of the remission of myasthenia gravis and their role as precursor lesions of conventional thymoma are unclear.

Sclerosing thymoma

Definition
Sclerosing thymoma is a very rare tumour exhibiting features of a conventional thymoma, but with exuberant collagen-rich stroma.

ICD-O code   8580/3

Synonym
Ancient thymoma

Epidemiology
Sclerosing thymoma accounts for < 1% of all thymomas. Patient ages range from 18 to 73 years, with incidence peaking

between 35 and 40 years. There is a slight male predominance {1731}.

Etiology
The etiology is unknown. Fibrogenic stimuli delivered by the neoplastic epithelium and/or regressive changes are thought to elicit stromal expansion {1356,1731}. Neoadjuvant chemotherapy rarely evokes similar changes {2842}.

Clinical features
Half of all patients with sclerosing thymoma are asymptomatic. Others have shortness of breath, chest pain, and/or myasthenia gravis {1731}.
Most tumours are in stage I or II.

Localization
Sclerosing thymoma occurs in the anterior mediastinum.

Macroscopy
The tumours form well-circumscribed masses with an average diameter of 8 cm (ranging from 2 to 18 cm). The cut surface is light tan and hard {1731}.

Histopathology
The tumour is dominated by a hyalinized, fibrosclerotic stroma that expands septa, perivascular spaces, and the tumour periphery. The embedded strands of neoplastic epithelial cells are often barely detectable on H&E staining, and may lack immature T cells. Thymoma subtyping is often impossible. Occasionally, areas of conventional thymoma (usually of type B2 and B3) occur, and should be reported explicitly {3002}. Dystrophic calcification, cholesterol granulomas, and small cysts are common {1270}.

Differential diagnosis
Neoplastic epithelial cells express keratins {1731}, while immature T cells, if

present, are terminal deoxynucleotidyl transferase-positive.
Sclerosing mediastinitis forms irregular solid masses composed of fibrosclerotic tissue with interspersed inflammatory infiltrates and at best minimal remnant thymic epithelial cells. The diagnosis requires exclusion of lymphomas; sarcomas (including desmoplastic small round cell tumours {1821}); germ cell tumours; metastases with desmoplastic stroma; fungal infections; and granulomatous, vasculitic, and IgG4-related disease.
The main sclerotic lymphomas are classical Hodgkin lymphoma and primary mediastinal large B-cell lymphoma (see *Lymphomas of the mediastinum*, p. 267). Solitary fibrous tumour is a spindle cell tumour with collagenous stroma. It has a CD34-positive, CD99-positive, Bcl2-positive, STAT6-positive immunophenotype, and lacks keratin-positive epithelial cells.

Prognosis and predictive factors
No tumour-related deaths have been reported.

Lipofibroadenoma

Definition
Lipofibroadenoma is a benign thymic tumour that resembles fibroadenoma of the breast.

ICD-O code   9010/0

Epidemiology
Only four lipofibroadenoma tumours have ever been reported, all in men aged 21–62 years {1357,1911,2104,2808}.

Etiology
No etiology is known. It is uncertain whether the epithelial or lipofibromatous components (or both) are neoplastic,

or whether the lesion is a hamartoma. Since the epithelial cells of two cases arose from an adjacent type B1 thymoma {1357,2808}, a putative thymic epithelial cell precursor is hypothesized to contribute to tumour development.

Clinical features
Three patients were asymptomatic. Another patient, with a lipofibroadenoma arising from a type B1 thymoma, had dyspnoea, dizziness, and pure red cell aplasia {1357}.
All cases were reported to be stage I.

Localization
Lipofibroadenoma occurs in the anterior mediastinum.

Macroscopy
The tumours are oval and well circumscribed, with maximal diameters of 3–10 cm. The cut surface is solid, grey, and firm.

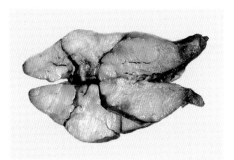

Fig. 3.44 Lipofibroadenoma of the thymus. Gross appearance of a lipofibroadenoma in continuity with a type B1 thymoma; the white areas represent the lipofibroadenomatous part of the composite neoplasm

Histopathology
The tumour resembles fibroadenoma of the breast. Fibrotic and hyaline stroma predominate over narrow strands of bland-looking epithelial cells, single or multiple fat cells, and few lymphocytes. Hassall corpuscles and calcifications can occur. Two cases arose adjacent to a type B1 thymoma {1357,2808}.

The epithelial cells are positive for AE1/AE3 and CK19. Lymphocytes express either CD3 or CD20, but not terminal deoxynucleotidyl transferase.

Differential diagnosis
Thymolipoma appears to be a related lesion, but is dominated by fat cells and lacks the dominant fibrous component of lipofibroadenoma.
Thymomas can show sclerosis, but are distinguished by broader islands or strands of polygonal tumour cells in a dense collagenous stroma without intermingled fat cells. Tumour cell palisades around perivascular spaces and lymphocytes may occur.

Prognosis and predictive factors
All patients were disease-free after complete resection, with a maximum of 8 years of follow-up.

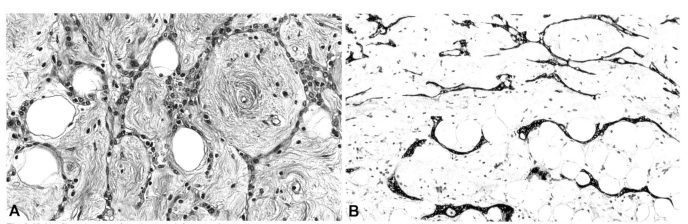

Fig. 3.45 Lipofibroadenoma of the thymus. **A** Strands of epithelium separated by fibrolipomatous stroma. **B** CK19 immunoreactivity of epithelial cells.

Thymic carcinomas
Squamous cell carcinoma

J.K.C. Chan
P. Ströbel
A. Marx
G. Chen
F. Detterbeck
N. Girard

A.M. Marchevsky
E.M. Marom
T.J. Molina
K. Mukai
W.D. Travis

Definition

Thymic squamous cell carcinoma (TSQCC) is a malignant neoplasm of the thymus with morphological features of squamous cell carcinoma as seen in other organs. Unlike thymomas, it generally lacks resemblance to the normal thymic cytoarchitecture, such as discrete lobulation, perivascular spaces, and admixed immature T lymphocytes.

ICD-O code   8070/3

Synonyms

Epidermoid keratinizing carcinoma; epidermoid non-keratinizing carcinoma; type C thymoma (not recommended)

Epidemiology

Thymic carcinomas account for approximately 22% of all thymic epithelial neoplasms {3022}, with squamous cell carcinoma being the most common type, accounting for approximately 70% of all cases {444,1899,2236,2839,2847,2847, 3022}. In the International Thymic Malignancy Interest Group (ITMIG) database, these figures are 17% and 79%, respectively {28}. TSQCC occurs in patients of various ages, but is most common in the sixth decade. In the ITMIG database, the average patient age is 56 years, and 56% of the patients are men {444,2838,2839}.

Etiology

The etiology is unknown. There is no

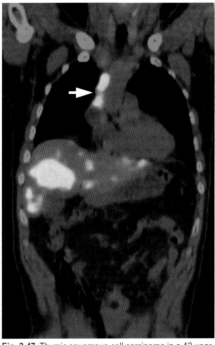

Fig. 3.47 Thymic squamous cell carcinoma in a 43-year-old man. Coronal fused PET-CT through the anterior mediastinal mass (arrow) shows that it is FDG-avid, with a maximal standardized uptake value of 6.9, and there are multiple FDG-avid liver metastases with a standardized uptake value of up to 10.9. Studies have shown that squamous cell carcinoma and other thymic carcinomas are more likely than thymomas to locally invade abutting mediastinal structures, to be heterogeneous and lobular, to contain calcifications, and to present with lymph node and distant metastases. They also have significantly higher FDG uptake than thymoma. FDG PET-CT is useful in the different forms of thymic carcinoma because it can identify distant metastatic disease sometimes overlooked by morphological imaging modalities.

known association with cigarette smoking or other environmental factors. A small proportion of cases appear to arise from the epithelial lining of unilocular or multilocular thymic cysts {1453,2835}. Rare cases are thought to arise from pre-existing thymomas, based on the observation of combined thymic epithelial tumours that harbour squamous cell carcinoma and conventional (usually type B3) thymoma components {1358,1750,2518} (see *Combined thymic carcinomas*, p. 242).

Clinical features

Signs and symptoms

The most frequent symptoms are related to mediastinal compression: chest pain, cough, and shortness of breath {1491,1888,2838,3022}. Less common symptoms include fever, superior vena cava syndrome, hoarseness, and haemoptysis {369,1888,2530,2838,2940}. One third of patients are asymptomatic, with the thymic tumour found incidentally {1888,2838,3022}, and < 5% of patients have associated myasthenia gravis {3022}, which is related to the presence of a coexisting thymoma component in at least some cases {2530}. Paraneoplastic polymyositis has also been rarely reported {1244}. In the ITMIG database, 12% of thymic carcinoma patients had a history of an extrathymic malignancy {28}.

Imaging

On imaging, TSQCCs present as an anterior mediastinal mass, and are more likely than thymoma to present with poorly defined, irregular lobular margins, or with necrotic or cystic changes that on CT manifest as low-attenuation regions and on MRI as greater tumour heterogeneity. Accompanying lymphadenopathy, pleural effusion, and distant metastases are more common than with thymoma {1086,2191}.

Tumour spread

Squamous cell carcinomas commonly show mediastinal and systemic

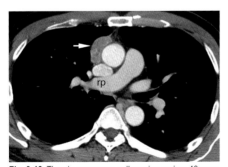

Fig. 3.46 Thymic squamous cell carcinoma in a 43-year-old man. Axial contrast-enhanced chest CT at the level of the right pulmonary artery (rp) shows a heterogeneous anterior mediastinal mass (arrow) with multiple low-attenuation regions within it.

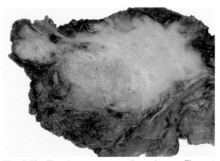

Fig. 3.48 Thymic squamous cell carcinoma. The cut surface of the thymus resection specimen shows a 9 cm infiltrative, solid, tan-whitish fleshy tumour. The tumour has invaded the left brachiocephalic vein (top) and the pericardium.

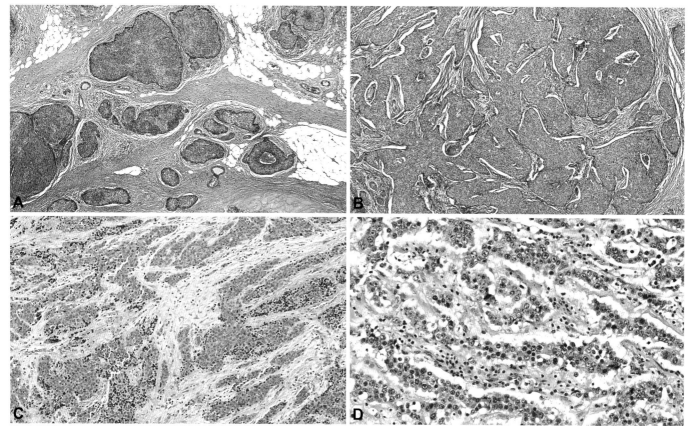

Fig. 3.49 Thymic squamous cell carcinoma. **A** Invasion in the form of smooth-contoured islands, resembling the growth pattern of invasive thymoma. **B** Growth predominantly in the form of anastomosing smooth-contoured islands. **C** Tumour invasion in the form of irregular jagged islands. **D** Tumour forming cords; coupled with the presence of some lymphocytes in the stroma, this may mimic seminoma.

involvement {2838}. The most frequently invaded mediastinal structures are the pericardium (40%), lung (40%), pleura (30%), and innominate veins and superior vena cava (20%) {2838,3022}. Mediastinal, cervical, and axillary lymph node metastases are common. Systemic metastases occur most frequently in the bone, liver, lung, adrenal glands, and brain {2784,2838}.

Staging
Tumour stage at diagnosis is I/II in < 15% of cases, stage III in 30–50%, stage IVA in 15–30%, and stage IVB in 30–50% {543,1318,1491,2838,2940,3022}. In the ITMIG database, the corresponding figures are 22%, 46%, 13%, and 19%, respectively {28} (see *Type A thymoma*, p. 187).

Localization
TSQCC occurs in the anterior mediastinum.

Macroscopy
TSQCCs are frankly invasive tumours, lacking the encapsulation or internal fibrous septation characteristic of

thymomas. The cut surfaces show firm to hard, tan-coloured tumour, with frequent foci of necrosis and haemorrhage. The mean maximum dimension is 7.2 cm (ranging from 2 to 17 cm) {3022}.

Cytology
Cytological smears of thymic carcinomas, unlike those of thymomas, show overt malignant features. Clustered and single large cells show enlarged nuclei, coarse chromatin, discrete macronucleoli, and a moderate amount of cytoplasm. Definitive classification is difficult, if not impossible, based on cytological features alone. The diagnosis should only be made with clinical and radiographical correlation. Immunohistochemistry performed on cell smears or cell block preparations may help {2794}.

Histopathology
TSQCCs consist of infiltrative sheets, islands, and cords of large polygonal cells, accompanied by broad zones of desmoplastic to sclerohyaline stroma that is variably infiltrated by chronic inflammatory cells. Unlike in squamous cell car-

cinoma of non-thymic origin, the tumour islands tend to be smooth-contoured, but the tumour can show predominantly jagged invasion in some cases. The tumour islands are frequently traversed by delicate blood vessels, which may mimic perivascular spaces when there is accompanying stromal oedema or retraction artefact. However, unlike in the perivascular spaces seen in thymomas, there is usually no optically empty space between the blood vessel and adjacent tumour cells (although fibrous tissue is present), there is usually no palisading of tumour cells around the space, and

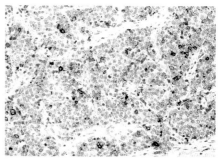

Fig. 3.50 Thymic squamous cell carcinoma. Chromogranin-positive tumour cells can be quite abundant.

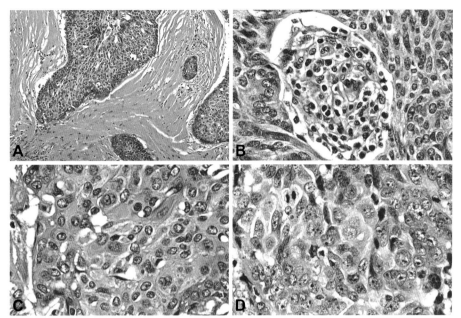

Fig. 3.51 Thymic squamous cell carcinoma. **A** Presence of prominent sclerohyaline stroma. **B** Shrinkage of the perivascular fibrous stroma results in a resemblance to perivascular spaces; in the stroma, there are some plasma cells in addition to lymphocytes, and there is no epithelial cell palisading around the space. **C** More obvious squamous differentiation (i.e. a greater amount of eosinophilic cytoplasm and the presence of intercellular bridges). **D** A poorly differentiated example, barely recognizable as squamous.

plasma cells are frequently present in addition to lymphocytes.

The polygonal tumour cells have large vesicular or hyperchromatic nuclei and distinct nucleoli. The cytoplasm is eosinophilic, and vague to obvious intercellular bridges can be identified in areas. Keratinization is present in some cases, and the keratinizing whorls may resemble Hassall corpuscles. The mitotic count varies from case to case. Foci of coagulative necrosis are common.

TSQCCs can show a range of differentiation from well to moderate to poor, based on the presence or absence of keratinization, the degree of nuclear pleomorphism, and the extent of squamous cell maturation. The relevance of grading is controversial: some studies have suggested that histological grading of thymic carcinomas has prognostic significance {1888,2530}, while more recent studies have shown no prognostic significance {2630,2940,3022}. Interpretation of these data is difficult, since there is currently no generally accepted tumour grading system.

Immunohistochemistry

TSQCCs are immunoreactive for keratins, and most are positive for p63 (83% of cases) and PAX8 (about 75% of cases) {95,619,1966,2832,2838}.

CD5, CD117, GLUT1, and MUC1 are frequently expressed in thymic carcinomas, but are much less common in thymomas, and therefore may potentially be of value in the differential diagnosis of difficult cases. Overall, these markers are expressed in approximately 70% of all thymic carcinomas, and in approximately 80% of TSQCCs (see Table 3.06).

However, since the literature on GLUT1 and MUC1 is still limited, further studies are needed to confirm their diagnostic value.

Proteasome subunit beta5t is not expressed in thymic carcinoma, in contrast to its almost universal expression in type B thymoma {975,2923}. FOXN1 and CD205 (thymic epithelial markers important for thymic organogenesis) are expressed in almost all cases of thymoma, and are positive in 68–76% and 10–59% of all thymic carcinomas, respectively {1871,2838}. Since these markers are uncommonly expressed in carcinomas of non-thymic origin, they are of value for confirming the thymic origin of a carcinoma {1871}.

In thymic carcinomas, focal expression of neuroendocrine markers is common (occuring in 64% of cases), but is rare in thymomas {1012,1416}.

Unlike in thymoma, the infiltrating lymphocytes include mature T cells and B cells. Terminal deoxynucleotidyl transferase-positive immature T lymphocytes are absent (with very rare exceptions).

Differential diagnosis

Pulmonary squamous cell carcinoma invading or metastasizing to the mediastinum can be difficult to distinguish from TSQCC, because the histological features are often identical. Clinical and radiological assessment are crucial for this distinction. Positive immunostaining for CD5, CD117, FOXN1, and/or CD205 can be of help, because these markers are uncommonly expressed in non-thymic squamous cell carcinomas. On the other hand, GLUT1 and MUC1 are not helpful for this purpose. Distinction from type B3 thymoma can be difficult (see p. 202). Other types of thymic carcinoma can show focal squamous differentiation or keratinization mimicking squamous cell carcinoma, such as

Table 3.06 Immunophenotypic profile of thymic carcinomas and thymomas {95,184,616,975,1183,1314,1330,1793, 1871,1965,2600,2630,2838}

	Proportion of cases showing positive staining			
	CD5	CD117	GLUT1	MUC1
Thymic carcinoma	113/181 (62%)	124/160 (78%)	24/29 (83%)	20/29 (69%)
Squamous cell carcinoma	90/121 (74%)	99/118 (84%)	16/18 (89%)	7/8 (88%)
Other types of thymic carcinoma	11/34 (32%)	6/17 (35%)	–	9/9 (100%)
Thymoma	7/246 (3%)	5/164 (3%)	8/17 (47% of B3 thymomas)	0/38 (0%)

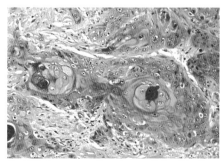

Fig. 3.52 Squamous cell carcinoma with keratinization.

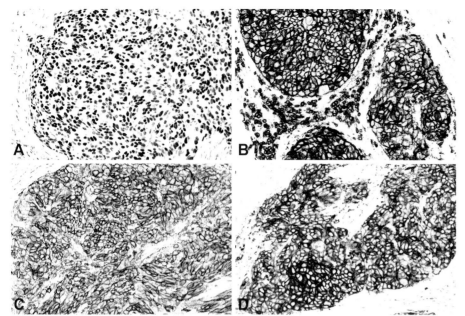

Fig. 3.53 Thymic squamous cell carcinoma. **A** Positive staining for p63 in the nuclei. **B** The tumour cells show cell membrane staining for CD5; the T lymphocytes in the stroma are also positive for CD5. **C** The tumour cells show cell membrane staining for CD117. **D** Positive staining for GLUT1.

lymphoepithelioma-like carcinoma, basaloid carcinoma, NUT carcinoma, and sarcomatoid carcinoma. They are diagnosed based on the presence of features characteristic of the respective tumour types in areas of the tumour not exhibiting squamous differentiation. Atypical carcinoid or large cell neuroendocrine carcinoma can be in the differential diagnosis because TSQCC frequently shows endocrine tumour-like vasculature and focal expression of neuroendocrine

markers. However, true neuroendocrine tumours show an even more prominent delicate vasculature and extensive immunoreactivity for neuroendocrine markers in > 50% of tumour cells.

Genetic profile
Loss of chromosomes 16q, 6, 3p, and 17p, and gain of 1q, 17q, and 18 are frequently observed in TSQCCs by comparative genomic hybridization {844,1703,2491,3011}. Among these

aberrations, deletion of chromosome 6 and gain of 1q are shared with type B3 thymoma {1087}. The pattern of chromosome gains and losses in TSQCC has been found to be different from that of pulmonary squamous cell carcinoma {844}. *KIT* mutation has been reported in up to 11% of thymic carcinomas {844,1964, 2047,2296,2487,2630,2691,2964}, and some dramatic responses to tyrosine kinase inhibitors have been recorded for *KIT* mutation-positive cases {2209,2490}. *TP53* mutation is found in about 20% of cases {844,999,2601,2825,2859}. Copy number gain of *BCL2* and loss of *p16* (*CDKN2A*) are common {999,1352,2045,2846}. *EGFR*, *KRAS*, *NRAS*, *BRAF*, *PIK3CA*, *APC*, *RET*, or *PTEN* gene mutations are rare or absent {844,1649,2487,2534,2846,2859, 2860,2924,2964}. *HER2* gene amplification is also rare, being found in 0–4% of cases {2846}. A recent study based on next-generation sequencing revealed a missense mutation of the *GTF2I* gene in < 10% of TSQCC, as compared with 21–82% in various thymoma types. In addition, rare recurrent mutations of the *TP53*, *CYLD*, *BAP1*, *CDKN2A*, and *PBRM1* genes were detected {2044A}.

Prognosis and predictive factors
The 5-year overall survival is 57.6–65.7% {51,241,369,402,543}. The prognosis is significantly associated with completeness of resection (hazard ratio = 3.692), tumour size, and lymph node status

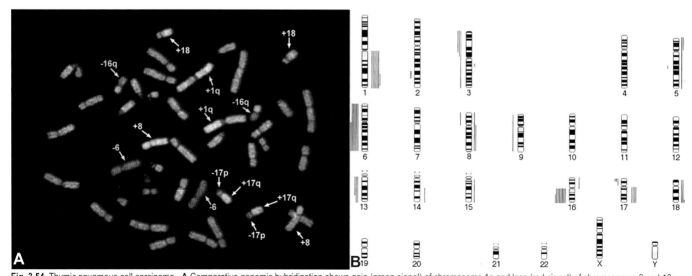

Fig. 3.54 Thymic squamous cell carcinoma. **A** Comparative genomic hybridization shows gain (green signal) of chromosome 1q and loss (red signal) of chromosomes 6 and 16q – the typical genetic alterations of this tumour type (highlighted by the yellow arrows). This case also showed loss of chromosome 17p and gain of chromosomes 8 and 17q (highlighted by the white arrows). **B** A chromosomal ideogram showing gains (bars on the right) and losses (bars on the left) of chromosomal material in 12 cases of thymic squamous cell carcinoma investigated by comparative genomic hybridization. The most frequent recurrent genetic imbalances in thymic squamous cell carcinoma are losses of chromosome 16q (67%), gains of chromosome 1q (60%), and losses of chromosome 6 (50%).

{2838,3022}. Most large series (including analysis of the SEER and ITMIG database) have found a significant association between tumour stage and survival {28,444,2847}. In the ITMIG database of >1000 patients with thymic carcinoma, multivariate analysis revealed that besides stage, resection status (R0) and the use of chemo- and radiotherapy were independent prognostic factors, whereas histological subtype and sex were not. These prognostic factors also appear to be relevant in an R0 cohort of patients.

Basaloid carcinoma

M. Papotti
P. Ströbel
A. Marx
J.K.C. Chan
F. Detterbeck

N. Girard
A.M. Marchevsky
E.M. Marom
K. Mukai
W.D. Travis

Definition

Basaloid carcinoma is a thymic carcinoma characterized by solid and cystic papillary nests of medium- to small-sized cells with a high nuclear-to-cytoplasmic ratio and peripheral palisading.

ICD-O code   8123/3

Epidemiology

Basaloid carcinoma accounts for < 5% of all thymic carcinomas {2530}. Only 35 cases are on record in the English-language literature {267,2254,2506, 2554,2697,2835,2921}. The tumour occurs in adults, with a median age of 60 years (ranging from 34 to 77 years) and a male-to-female ratio of 2.5:1. In the International Thymic Malignancy Interest Group (ITMIG) database, only 19 of the 6097 patients with thymic epithelial neoplasm have basaloid carcinoma; the average patient age is 58 years, and 63% of the patients are male {28}.

Etiology

Multilocular thymic cysts were observed in 17 (49%) of the 35 reported cases {267,2254,2506,2554,2697,2835,2921}, and may represent a precursor lesion {1066,2254}.

Clinical features

About 60% of cases are incidentally discovered to have a mediastinal tumour on chest radiographs {267}. The remaining cases present with non-specific symptoms related to mediastinal compression. Unlike in thymic squamous cell carcinoma, dyspnoea is more common than chest pain {267,2254,2506}. CT or MRI typically shows a multicystic anterior mediastinal mass with solid enhancing components {2506,2598}.

The tumour spread pattern is similar to that of thymic squamous cell carcinoma {267,2254,2506}. In the ITMIG database, 35% of basaloid carcinoma cases were in stage I/II, 35% in stage III, and 30% in stage IV {28}.

Localization

Basaloid carcinoma occurs in the anterior mediastinum.

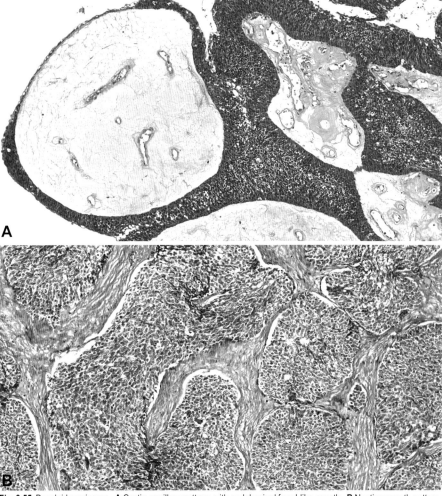

Fig. 3.55 Basaloid carcinoma. A Cystic-papillary pattern, with endoluminal frond-like growth. B Nesting growth pattern.

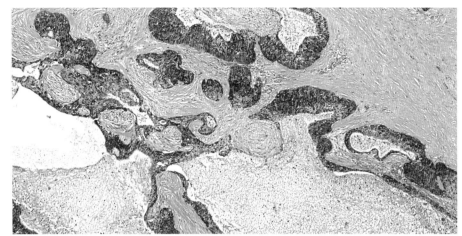
Fig. 3.56 Basaloid carcinoma. Tumour nests with cystic change.

Macroscopy

Basaloid carcinoma is generally a well-circumscribed greyish tumour with solid and cystic areas {267,2254,2506}. Mean tumour size is 8 cm (ranging from 2.8 to 20 cm).

Cytology

The literature on the cytopathological features of basaloid carcinoma is limited {2077}. Smears show a necrotic background with single and cohesive sheets of small monomorphic cells, and a high nuclear-to-cytoplasmic ratio. The cells have round nuclei, granular chromatin, and prominent nucleoli {2077}.

Histopathology

Basaloid carcinoma usually shows an admixture of cystic-papillary and nesting growth patterns {267}. The cystic-papillary pattern is characterized by cystic spaces lined by multiple layers of tumour cells, which occasionally generate papillary protrusions. The nesting pattern is similar to that of basaloid carcinomas of other locations, consisting of variably sized, compact nests of monotonous small or medium-sized tumour cells with peripheral palisading,

accompanied by variable amounts of sclerotic or desmoplastic stroma {2835}. The tumour cells are rounded or spindly, with indistinct cell borders, a high nuclear-to-cytoplasmic ratio, hyperchromatic nuclei, and distinct nucleoli. The mitotic count may exceed 30 mitoses per 2 mm² {267,2077}. Foci of comedo-type necrosis are common. Focal abrupt squamous differentiation is present in up to 40% of cases {267}. Small glands and deposits of amorphous basement membrane-like material may be present within the tumour nests. Rarely, there can be transformation to sarcomatoid carcinoma {267}. Cystic changes in basaloid carcinoma can result from pre-existing multilocular thymic cysts or cystic degeneration of the tumour. The cysts are lined by benign-looking squamous cells, sometimes in continuity with malignant basaloid cell nests (in the case of pre-existing multilocular thymic cysts), or all lined by neoplastic basaloid cells (in the case of cystic degeneration of the tumour).

Immunohistochemistry

Most basaloid carcinomas express p63/p40 and CD117, while CD5 is expressed in <50% of cases {267}. Single studied

cases expressed CK5/6 {2835}. TTF-1, chromogranin and synaptophysin are negative {267}.

Differential diagnosis

The main differential diagnoses are large cell neuroendocrine carcinoma (LCNEC), small cell carcinoma (SCC), adenoid cystic carcinoma-like tumour, NUT carcinoma, and poorly differentiated squamous cell carcinoma {267,600,2835}. Palisading is a feature of thymic basaloid carcinoma, mimicking LCNEC. However, LCNEC typically express multiple neuroendocrine markers in > 50% of tumour cells and are usually negative for p63/p40. Some basaloid carcinomas have small tumour cells that can resemble those of SCC, particularly if crush artefact is present. However, SCC usually do not show palisading, are often positive for neuroendocrine markers, and may express TTF1. In contrast to basaloid carcinoma, adenoid cystic carcinoma-like tumours usually show abundant pseudocystic spaces and are CD117 negative {600}. NUT carcinoma can resemble basaloid carcinomas in terms of small cell morphology and sharp transitions to focal squamous cell differentiation, but consistently show nuclear NUT immunoreactivity {925}. Distinction from poorly differentiated squamous cell carcinoma may be challenging if tumour cells are relatively small and basophilic; lack of palisading would favour the diagnosis of squamous cell carcinoma.

Genetic profile

The genetic data are limited to a single case demonstrating comparative genomic hybridization alterations similar to those of squamous cell carcinoma, including chromosomal gains in 1q and losses in 6 and 13 {3011}.

Prognosis and predictive factors

Fatal outcome due to pleural, liver, and lung metastases occurs in approximately 50% of cases {267,2530}. Combined surgical resection, chemotherapy, and radiotherapy was reported to effect a good response in one case {2554}. Predictive factors have not been investigated in this tumour type. In the ITMIG database, the survival and recurrence rates are similar to those of other types of thymic carcinoma (see *Squamous cell carcinoma*, p. 212).

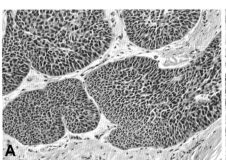 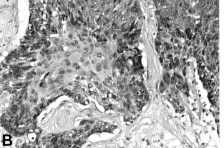

Fig. 3.57 Basaloid carcinoma. **A** Tumour nests composed of basaloid cells, with a high nuclear-to-cytoplasmic ratio and peripheral nuclear palisading. **B** Focal squamous differentiation.

Mucoepidermoid carcinoma

Y. Matsuno
J.K.C. Chan
F. Detterbeck
E.M. Marom
M. Wick

Definition
Mucoepidermoid carcinoma is a rare type of primary thymic carcinoma characterized by a combination of squamous cells, mucus-producing cells, and intermediate-type cells. It closely resembles mucoepidermoid carcinoma of other organs.

ICD-O code   8430/3

Epidemiology
In the literature, the reported ages of patients with mucoepidermoid carcinoma range from 8 to 84 years (with an average age of 49 years) {1872}. Men and women are affected almost equally. In the International Thymic Malignancy Interest Group (ITMIG) database, only 9 of the 6097 thymic epithelial tumours are mucoepidermoid carcinoma; the mean patient age is 64 years, and 66% of the patients are male {28}.

Etiology
Some cases of mucoepidermoid carcinoma appear to arise from associated multilocular thymic cysts {1719}. The rare association with thymoma supports the hypothesis of an origin from a putative thymic epithelial precursor {2913}.

Clinical features
Patients may present with dyspnoea or chest discomfort, although many are asymptomatic. Association with myasthenia gravis has not been reported.
The imaging features are similar to those of thymic squamous cell carcinoma {1862,2453,2949}.
Local invasion to the lung and/or pericardium is present in about half of all cases, even in cases with low-grade histology. Distant metastasis can also occur in advanced cases.
In the ITMIG database, 56% of mucoepidermoid carcinoma cases were stage I or II, and 44% were stage IV {28}.

Localization
Mucoepidermoid carcinoma occurs in the anterior mediastinum.

Macroscopy
Tumour size in reported cases ranges from 4 to 11 cm. The tumours are well demarcated in most cases, but infiltration to the pericardium is not uncommon. The cut surface demonstrates a combination of solid areas and cystic areas containing mucoid substance. Cases consisting solely of multilocular cysts have also been reported.

Cytology
Aspiration cytology smears are often cellular with a mucoid background. Epithelial cells are loosely cohesive, with a moderate amount of cytoplasm and round nuclei with small nucleoli. A small number of signet ring-like cells may be present {1207}.

Histopathology
The tumour shows features similar to those of mucoepidermoid carcinoma of the salivary glands. There are variable combinations of squamous (epidermoid) cells forming sheets or solid islands; mucus-secreting (goblet) cells (highlighted by mucicarmine or periodic acid–Schiff stain) forming nests, lining cystic spaces, or occurring as single cells; and intermediate cells forming nests or lobules, or intermingled with squamous or mucus-secreting cells. The majority of cases are histologically low-grade, showing mild cellular atypia such as small nucleoli and low mitotic activity {1719,1872}. Some cases show high-grade histology, with moderate atypia and high mitotic activity (> 7 mitoses per 2 mm^2) {1872}.
The tumour cells are positive for pancytokeratins and epithelial membrane antigen. There is variable staining for CK7 and CK20, but CK7 is less frequently positive (in only 1 of 5 cases in one study) {1872} than in mucoepidermoid carcinoma of the salivary glands. CK5/6 and p63 are often positive {2913}. MUC2 may be focally positive in goblet cells and intermediate cells {1872}. CD5 and CD117 (KIT) are negative in most reported cases. Cases with high-grade histology can be confused with

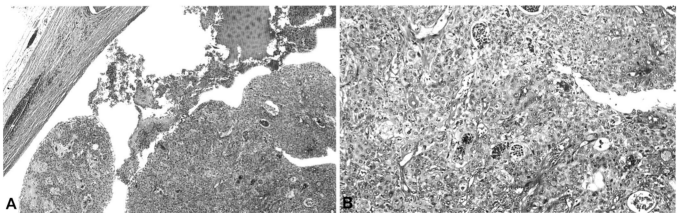

Fig. 3.58 Mucoepidermoid carcinoma. **A** Tumour associated with (occurring in) multilocular thymic cysts. **B** Solid islands of epidermoid cells punctuated by microcysts and admixed with mucin-containing cells.

adenosquamous carcinoma or mucinous adenocarcinoma.

Genetic profile

Translocation of *MAML2* (a member of the mastermind-like gene family), which is a characteristic feature of salivary gland mucoepidermoid carcinoma, has been detected by FISH analysis in 2 of 2 cases {2174}.

Prognosis and predictive factors

The prognosis depends on histological grade and stage. Survival is favourable in low-grade and low-stage (I or II) cases (3 of 3 patients with follow-up periods of > 2 years survived without recurrence after complete resection), whereas patients with tumours showing high-grade histology or advanced-stage disease have a much poorer prognosis {1872}.

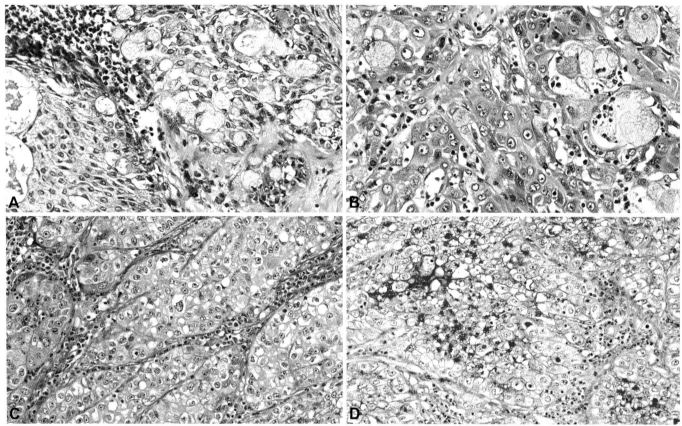

Fig. 3.59 Mucoepidermoid carcinoma. **A** Tumour composed of epidermoid and mucinous cells with low-grade cytology. **B** Nests of epidermoid cells with interspersed mucinous cells; this example is of higher grade, with distinct nucleoli. **C** The tumour, which contains solid islands of polygonal cells, is difficult to recognize as mucoepidermoid carcinoma. **D** Staining with mucicarmine reveals red-staining mucin in many tumour cells, indicating the presence of a morphologically inconspicuous mucinous cell component (same case as depicted in C).

Lymphoepithelioma-like carcinoma

J.K.C. Chan   E.M. Marom
L. Chalabreysse K. Mukai
F. Detterbeck   H. Tateyama

Definition
Lymphoepithelioma-like carcinoma is a primary thymic undifferentiated or poorly differentiated squamous cell carcinoma accompanied by a prominent lymphoplasmacytic infiltrate, and morphologically similar to nasopharyngeal carcinoma.

ICD-O code   8082/3

Synonyms
Lymphoepithelial carcinoma; lymphoepithelial-like carcinoma

Epidemiology
Thymic lymphoepithelioma-like carcinomas are very rare, accounting for 6–32% of all thymic carcinomas {366,402,452,2530,2838}. Patients range in age from 4 to 76 years, with a median age of 41 years and bimodal peaks at 14 years and 48 years. The male-to-female ratio is approximately 2:1 {960,1040, 1065,1069,1359,1854,1966,2467,2530, 2873,2914}. In the International Thymic Malignancy Interest Group (ITMIG) database, only 36 of the 6097 patients with thymic epithelial neoplasms have lymphoepithelioma-like carcinoma; the average patient age is 49 years {28}.

Etiology
The etiology is unknown. A proportion of cases are associated with EBV {2914}. Exceptionally, there is a concomitant component of thymoma, suggesting the possibility of transformation of

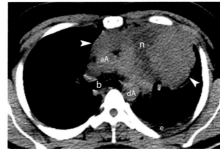

Fig. 3.61 Lymphoepithelioma-like carcinoma in a 21-year-old man. Axial unenhanced chest CT at the level of the main bronchi (b) demonstrates a large lobulated heterogeneous anterior mediastinal mass (between the arrowheads) with areas of necrosis (n) corresponding to the low-attenuation regions shown (n), displacing the mediastinum posteriorly, and associated with a left pleural effusion (e). The presence of a pleural effusion is more suggestive of a thymic carcinoma than of thymoma. aA, ascending aorta; dA, descending aorta.

lymphoepithelioma-like carcinoma from thymoma {2838}.

Clinical features
Although some patients are asymptomatic, most present with symptoms related to the mediastinal mass, such as dull chest pain, cough, and dyspnoea {960,2873}. Superior vena cava syndrome can occur in patients with more advanced disease {960,1040,1069,2873}. There is no association with myasthenia gravis, pure red cell aplasia, or hypogammaglobulinaemia. Rare cases are complicated by hypertrophic osteoarthropathy, polymyositis, or nephrotic syndrome {597,1040, 1040,1069,1247,1329,1854}.
Lymphoepithelioma-like carcinoma tends to be large at presentation and locally aggressive. At CT, low-attenuation regions within the tumour correspond to necrosis {1329}.
The tumour shows local spread into surrounding tissues, with frequent invasion of the pleura, lung, diaphragm, and pericardium {2944}. Lymph node, lung, liver, and bone are frequent sites for metastasis. In the ITMIG database, 25% of lymphoepithelioma-like carcinoma cases are in stage I/II, 43% in stage III, and 32% in stage IV.

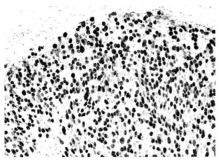

Fig. 3.60 Lymphoepithelioma-like carcinoma. The tumour cells show positive nuclear labelling for EBV-encoded small RNA on in situ hybridization.

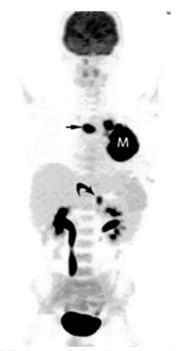

Fig. 3.62 Lymphoepithelioma-like carcinoma (same case shown in Fig. 3.61). A maximum-intensity projection image from FDG PET-CT shows that the avid FDG uptake is patchy – mostly located in the left hemithorax (M), with smaller FDG-avid foci scattered in the mediastinum bilaterally (straight arrow). This patchy distribution of FDG uptake in the primary tumour is due to the fact that there is no FDG uptake in the necrotic portions of the tumour. Paravertebral distant metastasis is seen adjacent to the T12 vertebral body (curved arrow). These features of low-attenuation regions and markedly FDG-avid tumour are typical of more aggressive thymic cancers, such as lymphoepithelioma-like thymic carcinoma.

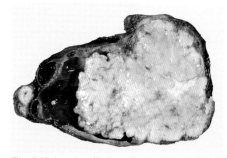

Fig. 3.63 Lymphoepithelioma-like carcinoma. A solid tumour with irregular borders and a yellow necrotic area; the tumour is growing into a multiloculated cyst on the left side.

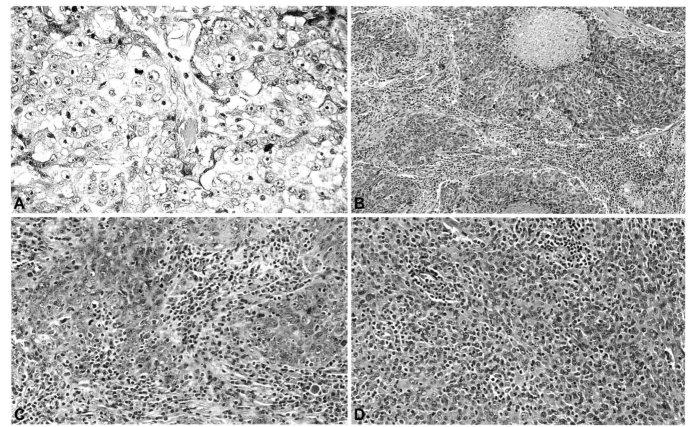

Fig. 3.64 Lymphoepithelioma-like carcinoma. **A** Lymphoepithelioma-like carcinoma without prominent lymphoid stroma, but showing a syncytial appearance of the large tumour cells, with large vesicular nuclei and conspicuous nucleoli; in situ hybridization for EBV-encoded small RNA is positive (not shown). **B** Irregular islands of carcinoma with coagulative necrosis; the stroma is heavily infiltrated by lymphocytes and plasma cells. **C** Islands of carcinoma with admixed lymphocytes and plasma cells. **D** The intimate intermingling of carcinoma cells (the cells with larger nuclei) with lymphocytes and plasma cells may make it difficult to recognize the epithelial nature of the tumour.

Localization

Lymphoepithelioma-like carcinoma occurs in the anterior mediastinum.

Macroscopy

The tumours typically show invasive borders. The cut surfaces are solid and yellow-white, with areas of necrosis.

Histopathology

The tumour consists of anastomosing sheets, nests, and cords of carcinoma cells accompanied by abundant lymphocytes and plasma cells. The carcinoma cells have indistinct cell borders, large vesicular nuclei, and one or more distinct nucleoli. The nuclei are unevenly crowded, and may appear overlapping. In general, there is no striking nuclear size variation or anaplasia.

In some cases, focal squamous differentiation can be present – the carcinoma cells are polygonal, with a greater amount of eosinophilic cytoplasm and vague intercellular bridges. Cells within the tumour islands can appear spindly. Mitotic activity is variable, but often pronounced. Coagulative necrosis is common. Many lymphocytes and plasma cells are present, both in the fibrous stroma and intimately admixed with the carcinoma cells. Germinal centres, eosinophils, and granuloma may be present.

The occasional cases of undifferentiated carcinoma with the features described above (syncytial-appearing large tumour cells with vesicular nuclei and distinct nucleoli) but lacking a significant lymphoplasmacytic infiltrate are also classified as lymphoepithelioma-like carcinoma if the tumour is shown to be EBV-positive.

Immunohistochemistry

Tumour cells are positive for pancytokeratins, and frequently for p63. CK7 and CK20 are negative. There is variable immunoreactivity for CD5, and frequent immunoreactivity for CD117 {616,1965}. The admixed lymphocytes include CD3+/ terminal deoxynucleotidyl transferase-negative mature T cells (the majority) and B cells. The plasma cells show polytypic staining for immunoglobulin.

Differential diagnosis

Thymic undifferentiated carcinoma is usually characterized by large anaplastic or pleomorphic tumour cells, with significant nuclear size variation. The tumour cells lack the syncytial quality and prominent lymphoplasmacytic infiltrate characteristic of lymphoepithelioma-like carcinoma, and EBV is negative.

The occasional cases of squamous cell carcinoma accompanied by a prominent lymphoplasmacytic infiltrate can be difficult to distinguish from lymphoepithelioma-like carcinoma. Overt squamous differentiation is lacking in lymphoepithelioma-like carcinoma, except in minor foci. EBV positivity favours a diagnosis of lymphoepithelioma-like carcinoma, although EBV negativity does not help in the differential diagnosis.

Micronodular thymic carcinoma with lymphoid hyperplasia {2837} shows a nodular rather than diffuse growth pattern of epithelial cells, and lacks syncytial growth. The lymphocytes lie adjacent to the epithelial componenent and are not intimately admixed with the tumour cells.

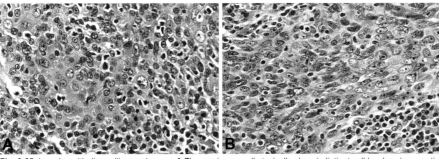

Fig. 3.65 Lymphoepithelioma-like carcinoma. **A** The carcinoma cells typically show indistinct cell borders (a syncytial appearance), vesicular nuclei, and conspicuous nucleoli. The nuclei often appear crowded. Lymphocytes and plasma cells are present within the tumour islands and in the stroma. Focal squamous differentiation is evident in the left field. **B** Some tumour islands predominantly contain spindly cells, but the nuclear morphology is no different from that of tumour islands with typical appearance.

An association with EBV has not been reported.

Metastatic lymphoepithelioma-like carcinoma from other sites (such as the lung) can be diagnosed with confidence only in conjunction with clinical and imaging findings.

Non-epithelial malignancies, such as large cell lymphoma, Hodgkin lymphoma, malignant melanoma, and malignant germ cell tumour can be readily excluded by immunohistochemistry.

Genetic profile

Approximately half of all cases of thymic lymphoepithelioma-like carcinoma are associated with EBV. EBV is almost always positive in children and young adults, but is uncommonly positive in adults aged > 30 years. Unlike in pulmonary and salivary gland lymphoepithelioma-like carcinomas, this association with EBV is not related to geographical or ethnic factors {405,1040,1065,1854,1966, 2467,2873}. The most reliable way to demonstrate EBV is in situ hybridization for EBV-encoded small RNA. Immunostaining for EBV LMP1 lacks sensitivity, and PCR may give false-positive results from bystander EBV-positive lymphocytes.

Prognosis and predictive factors

Thymic lymphoepithelioma-like carcinoma is a highly malignant neoplasm with a poor prognosis {366,2838}. The estimated average survival is only 16 months in 88% of patients {1065}. EBV status has no impact on prognosis. According to the ITMIG database, the survival and recurrence rates are similar to those of other types of thymic carcinoma (see *Squamous cell carcinoma*, p. 212).

Clear cell carcinoma

M. Marino
J.K.C. Chan
F. Detterbeck
E.M. Marom
K. Mukai
M. Wick

Definition

Clear cell carcinoma is a type of thymic carcinoma composed predominantly or exclusively of cells with optically clear cytoplasm.

ICD-O code   8310/3

Synonym

Carcinoma of the thymus with clear cell features {973}

Epidemiology

Thymic clear cell carcinoma is rare {1458,2417,2530}, with only 23 reported cases {394,1039,2650,2687,2900}. The tumours occur in the anterior mediastinal thymus, and one case was reported in an ectopic thymus in the posterior mediastinum {1900}. Patient ages range from 33 to 84 years, and there is a male predominance – with a male-to-female ratio of 1.6:1 {973,2163}. Because clear cells can occur in otherwise typical thymic squamous cell carcinoma, the clear cell phenotype could indicate either a distinct thymic carcinoma entity or a secondary change superimposed on other types of thymic carcinoma {2518}. However, the characteristic histological and clinical features and aggressive biological behaviour suggest that clear cell carcinoma is a distinctive type of thymic carcinoma {973,2874}. In the International Thymic Malignancy Interest Group (ITMIG) database, only 8 of the 6097 thymic epithelial neoplasms are clear cell carcinoma, with an average patient age of 55 years {28}.

Etiology

No established etiological factors have been reported. No EBV was detected in the single case investigated {766}. One case of combined thymoma and thymic carcinoma has been reported, with clear cell carcinoma arising in the necrotic areas of a thymoma {1358}. An associated thymic cyst was reported in a single case, in which there was transition of the clear cell carcinoma with benign cyst lining {366}.

Clinical features

Patients can be asymptomatic or present with symptoms such as dyspnoea, thoracic pain, and superior vena cava syndrome. No association with autoimmune phenomena or myasthenia gravis has been reported.

The imaging features of clear cell carcinoma are similar to those of squamous cell carcinoma, with a tendency for metastatic disease at presentation, including mediastinal lymphadenopathy {1387,1800}. The tumour often shows invasion of the surrounding structures. Metastasis is also common, such as to the mediastinal lymph nodes, lung, bone, skeletal muscle, brain, and spinal cord {973,2417}. In the ITMIG database, 17% of clear cell carcinoma cases are in stage I/II, 50% in stage III, and 33% in stage IV.

Most patients have stage II to III disease at presentation {973,2417}.

Localization

Thymic clear cell carcinoma occurs in the anterior mediastinum and ectopic thymus.

Macroscopy

The tumours can be totally encapsulated, partially encapsulated, or frankly invasive, with infiltration of the surrounding adipose tissue and large vessels. Cut surfaces are solid or partially cystic, and light brown to tan-coloured, with areas of haemorrhage and necrosis {366}. Tumour size ranges from 3 to 12 cm.

Cytology

Cytological preparations show clusters of tumour cells, most with vacuolated cytoplasm suggestive of signet ring cells. Focal glandular arrangement can also be present {1387}.

Histopathology

The tumour shows infiltrative growth, even in macroscopically well-demarcated tumours. It shows a lobulated architecture, with sheets, large islands, and trabeculae of tumour separated by a dense fibrous stroma. Rarely, small tumour nests are present in a loose fibrous stroma. Focal squamous differentiation can occasionally be found. The tumour cells are polygonal and show mild to moderate pleomorphism. The nuclei are round to oval, with finely dispersed chromatin and small nucleoli. The abundant clear cytoplasm, which contains glycogen, is lucent to granular, sometimes slightly eosinophilic. The mitotic count is usually < 10 mitoses

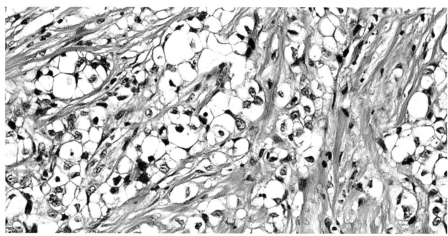

Fig. 3.66 Clear cell carcinoma. Islands and trabeculae of polygonal tumour cells infiltrate a fibrous stroma. The tumour cells show abundant, optically clear cytoplasm; a well-defined cell membrane; and moderately pleomorphic nuclei.

per 2 mm² {366,973}. Usually the tumour cells show diastase-sensitive cytoplasmic periodic acid–Schiff positivity {2468}. The tumours are often positive for epithelial membrane antigen and keratins (CK18 and high-molecular-weight keratins), but negative for vimentin, TTF1, carcinoembryonic antigen, S100, placental alkaline phosphatase, and leukocyte common antigen {973,1359,1800,1900}. CD5 is positive in a proportion of cases {616,1358}. CD117 was negative in the two investigated cases {110,1387}. No immature terminal deoxynucleotidyl transferase-positive T lymphocytes are present.

Metastases from renal, pulmonary, thyroid, and parathyroid carcinoma with clear cells must be excluded in the diagnosis of primary thymic clear cell carcinoma. The mediastinal non-epithelial clear cell neoplasms that must be excluded include seminoma, mediastinal large B-cell

lymphoma, PEComa, clear cell paraganglioma, clear cell melanoma, clear cell sarcoma, and glycogen-rich alveolar rhabdomyosarcoma {973,2870}. In type B3 thymoma, focal clear cell features are not uncommon, and the diagnosis rests on identification of areas with typical features of thymoma, and (usually) the presence of terminal deoxynucleotidyl transferase-positive T lymphocytes.

Prognosis and predictive factors

Clear cell carcinoma is an aggressive neoplasm, despite its relatively bland cytological appearance. Local recurrence and intra- and extrathoracic metastases are common, and patients often die of local or metastatic disease. The reported median survival {973} is only 13 months. In the ITMIG database, the survival and recurrence rates are similar to those of other types of thymic carcinoma (see *Squamous cell carcinoma*, p. 212).

Sarcomatoid carcinoma

K. Mukai   E.M. Marom
J.K.C. Chan   M. Wick
F. Detterbeck

Definition

Sarcomatoid carcinoma is a type of thymic carcinoma that consists partly or completely of spindle cells. Tumours with sarcomatous heterologous elements are called carcinosarcoma.

ICD-O code   8033/3

Synonyms

Spindle cell or metaplastic carcinoma

Epidemiology

Sarcomatoid carcinoma accounts for 5–10% of all thymic carcinomas {374,2530,2838}. It is a tumour of late adulthood, mostly the fourth to eighth decades. In the International Thymic Malignancy Interest Group (ITMIG) database, only 12 of the 6097 patients with thymic epithelial neoplasm have sarcomatoid carcinoma, with an average patient age of 47 years {28}.

Etiology

The etiology is unknown. It has been hypothesized that sarcomatoid carcinoma can develop through malignant transformation of type A thymoma or metaplastic thymoma, or progression of other thymic carcinomas {374,1753, 2516,2521,2530,2838}.

Clinical features

As with other high-grade mediastinal carcinomas, the most common symptoms include chest pain, cough, shortness of breath, and superior vena cava syndrome {374}.

The imaging features are similar to those of squamous cell carcinoma. The tumours tend to be large and lobular, with areas of low attenuation on CT correlating to tissue necrosis {1519,1857}.

The tumours often show invasion of the adjacent pleura, lung, and pericardium, and encroachment on the major vessels in the mediastinum. Metastases to regional lymph nodes and lung are common. In the ITMIG database 17% of sarcomatoid carcinoma cases are in stage I/II, 33% in stage III, and 50% in stage IV.

Localization

Sarcomatoid carcinoma occurs in the anterior mediastinum.

Macroscopy

The tumours are often large with infiltrative borders, although they can also (rarely) be encapsulated. The cut surfaces show fleshy white or grey tumour, often with areas of haemorrhage, necrosis, and cystic degeneration {374}.

Histopathology

Most spindle cell carcinomas consist of a mixture of conventional type A thymoma and areas of cytologically malignant spindle cells {2521}. However, tumours consisting entirely of malignant spindle cells are also reported. The transition between two components may be gradual or abrupt. The malignant areas frequently retain some architectural features of type A thymoma, such as lobular configuration, fascicular growth, and a pericytomatous vascular pattern. The nuclei of the malignant cells show coarse chromatin and prominent nucleoli. Mitoses are easily found {2521,2838}. Some cases may show small areas of lymphoepithelioma-like carcinoma or prominent squamous differentiation {2521}. Rare cases of spindle cell (sarcomatoid) carcinoma arising from metaplastic thymoma have also been reported {1519}.

Sarcomatoid transformation of thymic carcinoma is similar to pleomorphic carcinoma of the lung. This tumour contains both malignant epithelial (carcinomatous) and spindle cell (sarcomatous/sarcomatoid) components, sometimes with transition between the two. The carcinomatous component may consist of squamous cell carcinoma, adenocarcinoma, adenosquamous carcinoma, or undifferentiated carcinoma with significant nuclear pleomorphism {374,2516,2530}. However, it may be so subtle in some cases that the epithelial nature can only be demonstrated by immunohistochemistry or electron microscopy. The sarcomatoid component consists of fascicles and storiform arrays of spindle cells with pleomorphic nuclei, coarse chromatin, distinct nucleoli, and frequent mitotic figures.

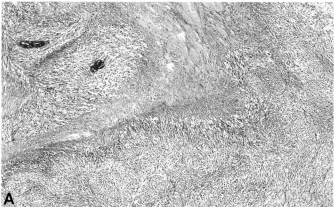
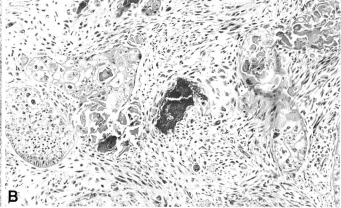

Fig. 3.67 Sarcomatoid carcinoma. **A** Spindle cells predominate, and there are areas of geographical necrosis. **B** A biphasic area composed of a squamous cell component that gradually merges into a spindle cell (sarcomatoid) component.

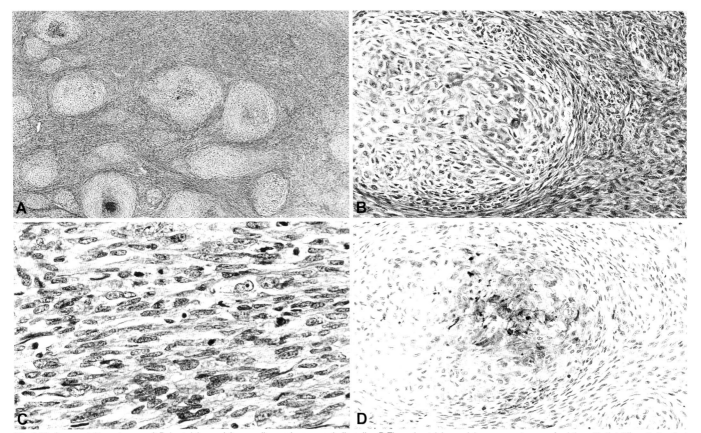

Fig. 3.68 Sarcomatoid carcinoma. **A** Pale-staining nodules are disposed among spindle cells. **B** The pale-staining nodules represent areas of subtle epithelial differentiation (but are cytokeratin-negative); this field shows a resemblance to metaplastic thymoma. **C** The sarcomatoid component contains closely packed spindle cells with moderate nuclear atypia and frequent mitoses. **D** Immunostaining for epithelial membrane antigen highlights nodular structures.

In addition to carcinomatous and spindle cell components, some sarcomatoid carcinomas contain heterologous mesenchymal elements, such as rhabdomyosarcoma, chondrosarcoma, or osteosarcoma {657,1901,2516}, with a rhabdomyosarcomatous component being most common. Such tumours were formerly designated as carcinosarcomas.

Immunohistochemistry
In spindle cell carcinoma, the type A thymoma component shows an immunohistochemical profile similar to that of the conventional counterpart. The neoplastic cells of spindle cell carcinoma are positive for low-molecular-weight keratins {2521}, and rare cases may show weak CD5 staining {1494}.
In sarcomatoid carcinoma, the epithelial component is variably positive for epithelial markers such as keratins and epithelial membrane antigen. CD5 may or may not be positive {366,1494,1519}. If a tumour consists of a spindle cell component only, the epithelial nature of the tumour must be confirmed by positive staining of epithelial markers (keratins or

epithelial membrane antigen) or electron microscopy. The spindle cells of the sarcomatous component may be diffusely positive, focally positive, or negative for keratin. Heterologous sarcomatous elements show appropriate markers for their differentiation.

Differential diagnosis
Distinguishing between atypical type A thymoma and spindle cell carcinoma can be very difficult, since the distinction criteria for this rare differential diagnosis are not well established. If CD5 or other markers of thymic carcinoma are positive, that supports the diagnosis of carcinoma. The mitotic count, presence of necrosis, or invasion to adjacent organs may not be useful for the differential diagnosis.
Thymic neuroendocrine tumours may be composed of spindle cells. However, the spindle cells usually form vague nesting pattern and are accompanied by prominent fibrovascular septa. Immunohistochemical studies demonstrating extensive staining for synaptophysin and/or chromogranin support the

neuroendocrine nature of the tumour {1726}.
Metaplastic thymoma may mimic sarcomatoid carcinoma. Although the cells within the epithelial islands often show nuclear pleomorphism, the spindle cells are bland-looking, with little or no mitotic activity.
Undifferentiated carcinoma predominantly consists of large polygonal cells with significant nuclear pleomorphism, and there should not be a significant spindle cell component.
Bland and non-proliferative myoid cells can occur in thymomas and thymic carcinomas, and must be distinguished from a heterologous rhabdomyosarcomatous component in sarcomatoid carcinoma.
Metastatic sarcomatoid carcinoma from other organs must always be excluded. Immunohistochemistry may help, if organ-specific markers (such as TTF1 for lung) can be demonstrated. Meticulous imaging and clinicopathological correlation is indispensable. Other biphasic tumours, such as mesothelioma and synovial sarcoma, can be diagnosed accurately by immunohistochemical staining

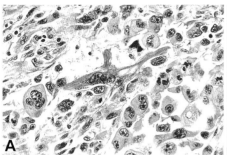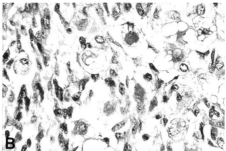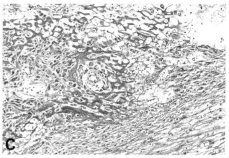

Fig. 3.69 Carcinosarcoma. **A** An elongated rhabdomyoblast with cross-striations is seen among polygonal carcinoma cells with pleomorphic nuclei. **B** Skeletal muscle differentiation characterized by rounded rhabdomyoblasts with vacuolated cytoplasm that are interspersed among spindle cells. **C** Malignant osteoid formation.

for specific markers and/or molecular studies.

Genetic profile
The information is limited. One case of sarcomatoid carcinoma showed a complex chromosomal abnormality including der(16)t(1:16)(q12;q12.1), a pattern identical to that of a case of thymic squamous cell carcinoma {657}.

Prognosis and predictive factors
This tumour type is highly aggressive; most patients die within 3 years of diagnosis. In the ITMIG database, the survival and recurrence rates are similar to those of other types of thymic carcinoma (see *Squamous cell carcinoma*, p. 212).

Adenocarcinomas

K. Mukai
J.K.C. Chan
F. Detterbeck
E.M. Marom

A. Marx
Y. Matsuno
W.D. Travis

Definition
Adenocarcinomas are a heterogeneous group of malignant thymic epithelial tumours showing glandular differentiation and/or mucin production.

ICD-O codes
Papillary adenocarcinoma	8260/3
Thymic carcinoma with adenoid cystic carcinoma-like features	8200/3
Mucinous adenocarcinoma	8480/3
Adenocarcinoma, NOS	8140/3

Synonyms
Colloid carcinoma;
tubular adenocarcinoma;
tubulopapillary adenocarcinoma

Epidemiology
Primary thymic adenocarcinomas are very rare, with most reports including only a single or a few cases. A published review of 26 cases of thymic adenocarcinoma reported that 10 cases had been identified as papillary adenocarcinoma; 9 cases as mucinous adenocarcinoma; 2 cases as papillotubular adenocarcinoma; 3 cases as conventional adenocarcinoma; and 2 cases as adenocarcinoma, not otherwise specified (NOS)

{1550}. The patients had a median age of 52.6 years (ranging from 15 to 82 years), and the male-to-female ratio was 2:1 {1550}.
Fewer than 10 cases of thymic carcinoma with adenoid cystic carcinoma-like features have been reported {600,1205}. In the International Thymic Malignancy Interest Group (ITMIG) database, only 29 of the 6097 patients with thymic epithelial neoplasm have thymic adenocarcinoma, with an average patient age of 56 years {28}.

Etiology
The etiology is unknown. Papillary adenocarcinomas often arise in type A or AB thymomas. Mucinous adenocarcinoma and adenocarcinoma, NOS may arise in multilocular thymic cysts {1550,2109}.

Clinical features
Patients either present with symptoms related to the thymic mass lesion (such as chest pain, cough, and dyspnoea) or are asymptomatic {1550}. Paraneoplastic syndromes such as myasthenia gravis and pure red cell aplasia have not been described.
The imaging features of adenocarcinoma are similar to those of squamous

cell carcinoma {438,2558}. However, because the main differential when biopsied is of metastatic disease, whole-body FDG PET-CT could be helpful, because these tumours are typically FDG-avid.
The tumours often show invasion of surrounding structures. Lymph node and distant metastases are not uncommon. In the ITMIG database, 39% of thymic

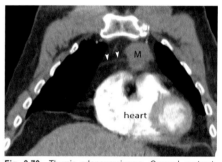

Fig. 3.70 Thymic adenocarcinoma. Coronal contrast-enhanced chest CT through the heart of a 68-year-old man with adenocarcinoma of the thymus. There is a homogeneous lobulated mass (M) involving the mediastinal fat and pericardium (arrowheads), confirmed at surgery. It showed substantial FDG avidity at PET-CT (not shown). The different forms of thymic carcinoma, including adenocarcinoma of the thymus, are more likely than thymoma to present with invasion into local structures such as the pericardium and major vessels, identified at imaging.

adenocarcinoma cases were in stage I/II, 35% in stage III, and 26% in stage IV.

Localization
Thymic adenocarcinomas occur in the anterior mediastinum.

Macroscopy
Most tumours are large and frankly invasive when discovered {6775,1550, 2516,2838}. They are solid, with or without cystic areas.

Histopathology
Papillary adenocarcinoma
This tumour shows an architectural resemblance to papillary thyroid carcinoma or malignant mesothelioma {775,1609}. It consists of tubulopapillary structures lined by cuboidal to polygonal cells with mildly atypical round to oval nuclei, small distinct nucleoli, and eosinophilic or clear cytoplasm. The papillary structures are variably supported by fibrovascular cores, and complex glomeruloid structures can also be formed. Psammoma bodies may be numerous. Coagulative necrosis can be present, and sometimes massive. This tumour is often associated with type A or AB thymoma with zones of transition, and is therefore assumed to represent malignant transformation of thymoma. Another associated lesion is multilocular thymic cyst. Cases with high-grade morphology and papillary features {438,1609} are more appropriately categorized as adenocarcinoma, NOS.

Thymic carcinoma with adenoid cystic carcinoma-like features
The histological features are very similar (but not identical) to those of salivary gland adenoid cystic carcinoma {600,1205}. They consist of nests of basaloid cells with variable numbers of pseudocysts filled with homogeneous

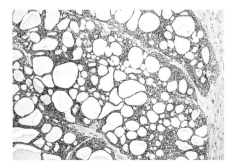

Fig. 3.71 Adenoid cystic carcinoma-like tumour showing a striking cribriform pattern, strongly resembling adenoid cystic carcinoma of the salivary glands.

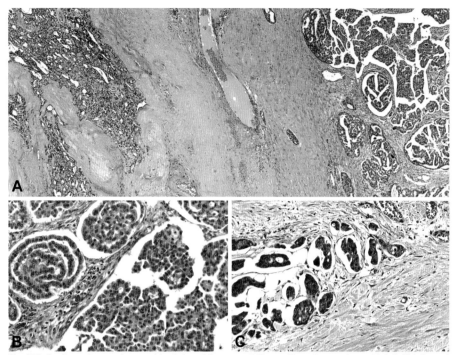

Fig. 3.72 Papillary adenocarcinoma arising in type A thymoma. **A** The papillary adenocarcinoma (right field) is located immediately adjacent to the type A thymoma (left field). **B** The papillary adenocarcinoma component, showing papillary tufts and glomeruloid structures lined by cells with mild nuclear atypia. **C** In papillary adenocarcinoma, a micropapillary growth can be present.

or granular basophilic basement membrane material. When pseudocysts predominate, cribriform structures are formed. True glands are rare among the basaloid cells. Nuclear atypia is slight to moderate. Tumour necrosis or perineural invasion is not a prominent feature.

Mucinous adenocarcinoma
These tumours resemble mucinous adenocarcinoma of the gastrointestinal tract, pancreas, breast, lung, or ovary {438,1550,2109,2558}. The carcinoma cells contain abundant mucin in the cytoplasm, and often assume goblet cell or signet ring cell morphology. The presence of abundant extracellular mucin results in dilated glands or mucin pools in which neoplastic cells (in the form of glands, strips, or single cells) float. This type of tumour is often associated with thymic cysts, and the presence of transition from benign cyst-lining epithelium to adenocarcinoma supports a primary thymic origin rather than metastatic mucinous adenocarcinoma.

Adenocarcinoma, not otherwise specified
Adenocarcinomas not conforming to any of the above three subtypes are tentatively grouped under adenocarcinoma, NOS, including high-grade adenocarcinoma with papillary features, tubular adenocarcinoma, and papillotubular adenocarcinoma. Histologically, the tumours show variable combinations of simple tubules, complex tubules and tubulopapillary structures that are lined by columnar cells {2288,2618}. Nuclear pleomorphism is significant. Debris is commonly found in the lumens, and coagulative necrosis is common.

Immunohistochemistry
Papillary adenocarcinoma of the thymus is positive for epithelial markers, including keratins, epithelial membrane antigen, and BerEP4. Focal positivity for CD5 may be present. Organ-specific markers of thyroid, lung, and mesothelium are negative {775}.

Thymic carcinoma with adenoid cystic carcinoma-like features shows extensive staining for keratin (34βE12) and p63. Unlike adenoid cystic carcinoma of the salivary glands, this tumour does not express myoepithelial markers such as smooth muscle actin or S100 protein. The pseudocysts contain basement membrane material positive for collagen IV, laminin, and stromal mucin. In some cases, scattered CD5-positive cells are present, but CD117 is negative. The Ki-67

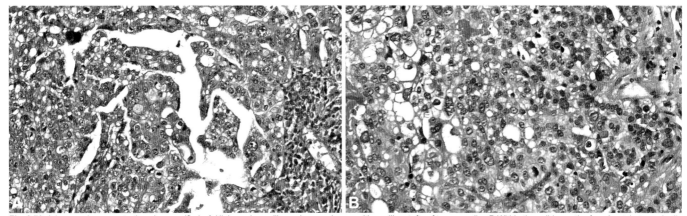

Fig. 3.73 Adenocarcinoma, not otherwise specified. **A** High-grade papillary adenocarcinoma with papillary tufts of tumour cells. **B** Within the solid growth of moderately to markedly pleomorphic cells, some abortive glandular spaces are present.

labelling index is < 10% {600,1205}. Mucinous adenocarcinomas and adenocarcinomas, NOS are positive for pancytokeratins, and sometimes also CD5. A proportion of them represent intestinal-type adenocarcinoma, as evidenced by a CK20-positive, CDX2-positive, MUC2-positive, and villin-positive immunophenotype {438,1550,2288}. Carbohydrate antigens, such as carcinoembryonic antigen or CA19-9, may be positive {6,1550}. Other cases express CK7 without enteric markers {2109,2558}. It remains to be determined whether categorization of these adenocarcinomas into intestinal-type and non-intestinal-type adenocarcinomas is of biological or prognostic importance.

Differential diagnosis
The most important differential diagnosis is metastatic adenocarcinoma from other organs. CD5 or CD117 has been used to confirm thymic origin, but negative results do not totally exclude this possibility, and positive results are not entirely specific. Organ-specific markers such as TTF1, GCDFP15, and thyroglobulin may be helpful to confirm the extrathymic origin of adenocarcinoma. Since adenocarcinoma of the thymus is often associated with or develops from thymic cyst, the presence of carcinoma in situ in the cyst epithelium supports a thymic origin. Association with conventional thymoma also favours a thymic primary.

Rare cases of thymoma with prominent glandular differentiation or signet ring cell-like features may also enter the differential diagnosis, especially in needle biopsy specimens. These tumours do not show significant cytological atypia or increased mitoses {2840,2843}.

Genetic profile
One case of adenocarcinoma with enteric differentiation showed a complex pattern of chromosomal imbalances including homozygous deletion at the HLA locus of chromosomal region 6p21.32 {1550}.

One case of adenoid cystic carcinoma-like tumours showed an isolated gain of whole chromosome 8 {600}.

Prognosis and predictive factors
Thymic adenocarcinomas have varying malignant potentials. Papillary adenocarcinoma is generally a low-grade carcinoma; recurrence or metastasis occurred in about half of the reported cases {775}. Most carcinomas with adenoid cystic-like features follow an indolent course, but distant metastasis has been reported {600,1205}.

Mucinous adenocarcinoma and adenocarcinoma, NOS are high-grade carcinomas, with most patients developing recurrence or dying of tumour {1550}. The prognosis is probably dependent on histological grade and clinical stage. In the ITMIG database, the survival and recurrence rates are similar to those of other types of thymic carcinoma (see *Squamous cell carcinoma*, p. 212).

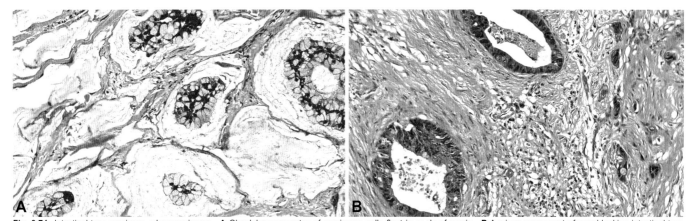

Fig. 3.74 Intestinal-type mucinous adenocarcinoma. **A** Glandular aggregates of carcinoma cells float in pools of mucin. **B** A minor component of usual-looking intestinal-type adenocarcinoma is often present.

NUT carcinoma

C.A. French
M.A. den Bakker

Definition

NUT carcinoma is a poorly differentiated carcinoma genetically defined by the presence of *NUT* gene rearrangement.

ICD-O code   8023/3

Synonyms

NUT midline carcinoma; t(15;19) carcinoma; thymic carcinoma with t(15;19); carcinoma with t(15;19) translocation; aggressive t(15;19)-positive carcinoma; midline lethal carcinoma; midline carcinoma of children and young adults with *NUT* rearrangement; *BET*-rearranged carcinoma

Epidemiology

Fewer than 100 cases of NUT carcinoma have been reported. NUT carcinoma affects males and females equally. Although it was originally thought to be a disease of children and younger adults (with a reported median age of 16

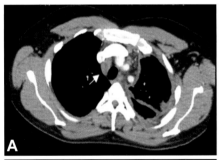

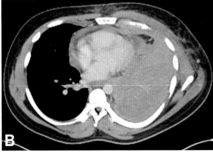

Fig. 3.75 NUT carcinoma. **A** Contrast-enhanced chest CT of early-stage mediastinal NUT carcinoma reveals a mediastinal mass (arrow) in a 30-year-old man. **B** The same patient's CT 2 months later demonstrated extension of the heterogeneously enhancing mass filling the hemithorax and invading the chest wall musculature and subcutaneous tissue.

years) {154,758}, NUT carcinoma can affect people of any age (with patient ages ranging from birth to 78 years) {154,756,2353,2463}. Thoracic/mediastinal NUT carcinoma accounts for 57% of all cases, but due to the involvement of both the lung and mediastinum in most cases at presentation, it is not possible to determine the fraction of these cases that originated within the mediastinum/ thymus {154}. In limited series, NUT carcinoma has been reported to account for approximately 3–4% of mediastinal/ thymic carcinomas {689,2048}.

Clinical features

Mediastinal NUT carcinoma usually presents at an advanced stage, with pleuritic chest pain, non-productive cough, weight loss, and shortness of breath {1428,1824,2616}.

Chest radiographs of mediastinal NUT carcinoma usually demonstrate a widened mediastinum with partial or complete opacification of the hemithorax due to pulmonary extension of tumour, making the distinction of a mass from effusion difficult or impossible. Extremely rapid disease progression is reported, with complete opacification of the thorax occurring within 2–8 weeks from initial presentation {2068}. On CT, NUT carcinoma appears as a hypoattenuating, heterogeneously enhancing, often extensively necrotic mass with poorly defined infiltrative borders {1824,2068,2464}. Invasion of adjacent structures, necrosis, and calcifications are frequent {1824,2068,2616}. MRI shows a hypointense T1-weighted and hyperintense T2-weighted lesion {2068}. High FDG uptake by NUT carcinoma is characteristic, thus PET-CT is the modality of choice to determine systemic disease burden {1852,2197,2315}, and is also helpful in monitoring response to treatment.

NUT carcinoma commonly spreads by local invasion and by lymphatic and haematogenous metastasis {154,758}. There is often invasion of the pleura. Distant metastases are common; bone metastases are observed early, and

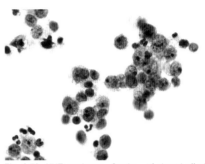

Fig. 3.76 NUT carcinoma. Cytology of pleural effusion reveals loosely cohesive, monomorphic, poorly differentiated epithelioid cells with prominent nucleoli and single cell necrosis (Papanicolaou stain).

multiorgan dissemination (such as to the ovaries, liver, and brain) is seen later in the course of disease {130,680,2068, 2097,2353,2590,2759}.

Localization

Thymic NUT carcinoma occurs in the anterior mediastinum.

Cytology

Aspirates yield cellular smears mainly composed of discohesive clusters and solitary cells of distinctly monomorphic, intermediate size, with irregular nuclear contours, variable granular to coarse chromatin, and discrete nucleoli. The cytoplasm varies from pale to dense eosinophilic (H&E stain); it may be vacuolated, but does not contain mucin. Larger sheets may be present. Mitotic figures, necrotic debris, and crush artefacts are common {175,3028}. The cytological characteristics are similar to those of other undifferentiated carcinomas, and are not specific for NUT carcinoma.

Histopathology

NUT carcinoma typically shows sheets and nests of small to intermediate-sized undifferentiated cells with a monomorphic appearance. The cells have evenly sized nuclei with irregular outlines and slightly coarse chromatin and small nucleoli. Occasional larger cells may be present. The cytoplasm varies from pale eosinophilic to basophilic, and may have a granular appearance. There is brisk mitotic activity, and necrosis is often present. NUT carcinomas commonly and characteristically demonstrate abrupt foci of keratinization {2462}. A brisk acute inflammatory infiltrate is commonly admixed with the tumour cells, although in some cases only minor chronic inflammation is seen. Glandular {1428} and mesenchymal {572} differentiation are distinctly uncommon. The histological features alone are those of undifferentiated carcinoma, poorly differentiated squamous carcinoma, or undifferentiated small round blue cell malignancy, and are not specific.

Immunohistochemistry

NUT carcinoma is consistently positive for nuclear protein in testis (NUT, aka NUTM1) protein on immunohistochemistry {925}. With the exception of weak focal nuclear staining in germinomas and embryonal carcinomas, staining with this antibody is limited to NUT carcinoma, and is thus a valuable screening tool. Pancytokeratin is positive in the majority of cases, although rare cases are negative {689,3028}. Variable results are obtained with other epithelial markers, such as epithelial membrane antigen, BerEP4, and carcinoembryonic antigen. Most cases show nuclear staining for p63/p40, indicating squamous differentiation.

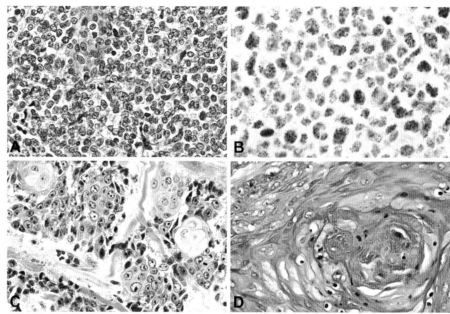

Fig. 3.78 NUT carcinoma. A Sheets of monomorphic, round to ovoid cells with scant cytoplasm can be so poorly differentiated that they may be confused with other small round blue cell neoplasms. B Diffuse nuclear immunohistochemical staining with nuclear protein in testis (NUT) antibody is diagnostic of NUT carcinoma. The speckled pattern of staining seen here is characteristic. C Focal squamous differentiation is characteristic, but not seen in all cases; also apparent are clear spaces between cells, which are also frequently seen in NUT carcinoma. D Rare cases resemble well-differentiated squamous cell carcinoma.

Occasional NUT carcinomas can stain for chromogranin, synaptophysin, or even TTF-1 {2590}. NUT carcinomas often stain for the haematopoietic stem cell marker CD34, which may lead to a misdiagnosis of acute leukaemia {758}. Germ cell, lymphoid, and myeloid markers are negative.

Differential diagnosis

The differential diagnosis includes any poorly differentiated malignant neoplasm {757}. NUT carcinoma is most commonly mistaken for thymic squamous cell carcinoma or undifferentiated carcinoma, but can also mimic small cell carcinoma, Ewing sarcoma, and acute leukaemia

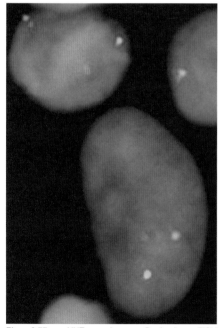

Fig. 3.77 NUT carcinoma. Dual-colour FISH demonstrates break-apart of red and green probes flanking the *NUT* breakpoint. Adapted from {755B, 756,760}.

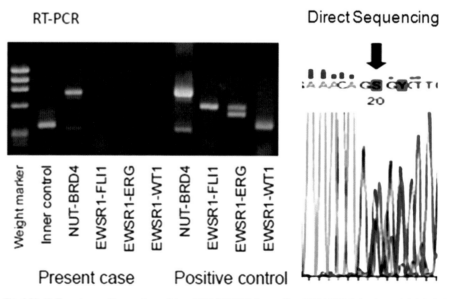

Fig. 3.79 NUT carcinoma. Reverse transcriptase PCR (RT-PCR) to amplify a BRD4-NUT fusion transcript. Adapted from French CA {756}.

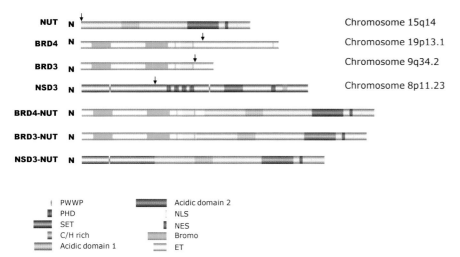

NUT	Chromosome 15q14
BRD4	Chromosome 19p13.1
BRD3	Chromosome 9q34.2
NSD3	Chromosome 8p11.23
BRD4-NUT	
BRD3-NUT	
NSD3-NUT	

PWWP
PHD
SET
C/H rich
Acidic domain 1
Acidic domain 2
NLS
NES
Bromo
ET

Fig. 3.80 A schematic of the known fusions present in NUT carcinoma: *BRD3-NUT*, *BRD4-NUT*, and *NSD3-NUT*. AD, acidic domain; ET, extraterminal; NES, nuclear export signal; NLS, nuclear localization signal. Adapted from French CA {756}.

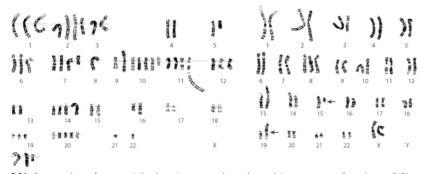

Fig. 3.81 A comparison of representative karyotypes seen in garden-variety squamous cell carcinoma (left) versus NUT carcinoma (right) reveals that NUT carcinoma is simpler. The red arrows point to derivative (der) 15 and 19 chromosomes. The *BRD4-NUT* fusion resides on the der 19. Adapted from French CA {756}.

{2048,2463}. In general, it is recommended that testing for NUT expression by immunohistochemistry be performed in all poorly differentiated carcinomas that lack glandular differentiation. A high-level suspicion on recognition of the monomorphic appearance of the tumour cells and abrupt keratinization, in combination with the clinical history of a rapidly growing mass with rapid dissemination, may point to the diagnosis.

Genetic profile

NUT carcinoma is characterized by chromosomal translocation and fusion of the *NUT* gene to *BRD4* – t(15;19) (q14;p13.1) (in 70% of cases), *BRD3* (15q14;9q34.2) (in 6% of cases), *NSD3* (8p11.23), or other unidentified gene(s) {154,758,759,759A,760}. Molecular demonstration of *NUT* rearrangement, such as by cytogenetic analysis, FISH, or reverse transcriptase PCR, is diagnostic of

NUT carcinoma. A unique characteristic is that unlike typical squamous carcinomas, its cytogenetics are often simple, with the chromosomal translocation sometimes being the only abnormality.

Prognosis and predictive factors

The prognosis and predicative factors of 54 NUT carcinomas with long-term follow-up were summarized by Bauer and colleagues {154}. NUT carcinoma is an extremely aggressive cancer, with a median survival of 6.7 months. Complete resection and initial treatment with radiotherapy are independently significantly associated with prolonged survival (both progression-free and overall survival). Survival is not significantly correlated with age, translocation type, sex, or tumour location, but progression-free survival is significantly shorter with mediastinal tumours. A significantly lower overall survival rate is associated with the presence of metastases. No specific chemotherapeutic regimen has demonstrated efficacy in treating NUT carcinoma, but two trials investigating the treatment of NUT carcinoma with small-molecule BET inhibitors that target BRD4 (a member of the BET family of proteins) are ongoing (ClinicalTrials.gov identifiers: NCT01587703 and NCT01987362).

Undifferentiated carcinoma

V. Thomas de Montpréville
J.K.C. Chan
F. Detterbeck
A. Marx

Definition

Undifferentiated carcinoma is a primary carcinoma of the thymus showing no morphological or immunohistochemical differentiation other than epithelial differentiation. This is a diagnosis of exclusion; poorly differentiated carcinomas that conform to defined types of thymic carcinoma (such as NUT carcinoma, lymphoepithelioma-like carcinoma, sarcomatoid carcinoma, and small cell carcinoma) are not included in this category.

ICD-O code   8020/3

Synonym

Anaplastic carcinoma

Epidemiology

Thymic undifferentiated carcinomas are very rare {2530}, with the largest reported series including only 7 cases {2530}. The patients are adults, with a median age of 54 years (ranging from 38 to 72 years). There is no sex predominance {366,1873,2630,2836}. In the International Thymic Malignancy Interest Group (ITMIG) database, only 16 of the 6097 patients with a thymic epithelial neoplasm have undifferentiated carcinoma; the average patient age is 46 years {28}.

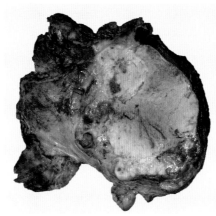

Fig. 3.82 Undifferentiated thymic carcinoma. A large, solid, fleshy tumour with prominent necrosis.

Etiology

The coexistence of undifferentiated carcinoma with thymoma in rare cases suggests that undifferentiated carcinoma may arise from a pre-existing more differentiated tumour {2630}.

Clinical features

Symptoms are related to local tumour growth, such as chest pain, cough, and dyspnoea {2836}. Some cases are asymptomatic.

The tumours show local spread into surrounding tissues and organs. Distant metastasis is frequent. In the ITMIG database, 0% of cases are in I/II, 38% are in stage III, and 62% are in stage IV.

Localization

Thymic undifferentiated carcinoma occurs in the anterior mediastinum.

Macroscopy

The tumours show infiltrative growth, and are often large (about 10 cm) {2836}.

Histopathology

Large polygonal tumour cells form infiltrative islands and sheets, usually with areas of coagulative necrosis. They typically show pronounced cellular pleomorphism, often with bizarre giant cells and atypical mitoses {2530,2630,2836}. Squamous, glandular, or sarcomatoid features should be absent. Rarely, there can be admixed bland-looking myoid cells (undifferentiated carcinoma with rhabdomyomatous differentiation).

A variant is characterized by a prominent inflammatory reaction mimicking the late stage of hyaline-vascular Castleman disease {1873}. Some tumour nests are located in the centres of the abnormal follicles. The tumour cells are positive for pancytokeratins {366,2630,2836}. Unlike

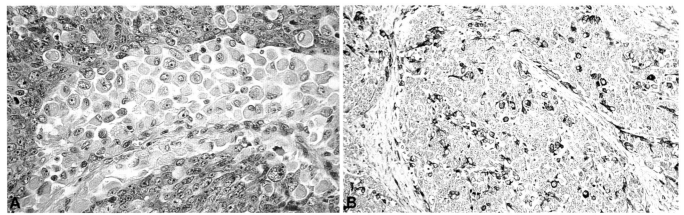

Fig. 3.83 Undifferentiated carcinoma with rhabdomyomatous differentiation. **A** Solid growth of large polygonal tumour cells with slightly basophilic cytoplasm and no evidence of differentiation; the admixed bland-looking and mitotically inactive myoid cells with round inconspicuous nuclei and eosinophilic cytoplasm should not be mistaken for a rhabdomyosarcomatous component (sarcomatoid carcinoma). **B** Immunostaining for desmin clearly highlights the myoid cells.

in poorly differentiated thymic squamous cell carcinoma, there is no expression of CK5/6, p63, or CD5 {2630}. Expression of CD117 and PAX8 is reported in 60% and 40% of cases, respectively {1793,2630,2836}. Malignant germ cell tumour markers (such as OCT3/4 and SALL4) and neuroendocrine markers are negative.

The main differential diagnoses are other thymic carcinomas (such as poorly differentiated squamous cell carcinoma, sarcomatoid carcinoma, and NUT carcinoma), poorly differentiated neuroendocrine carcinomas (small cell carcinoma and large cell neuroendocrine carcinoma), malignant germ cell tumours (such as embryonal carcinoma), other malignancies (such as melanoma and large cell lymphoma), invasion from a large cell or pleomorphic carcinoma of

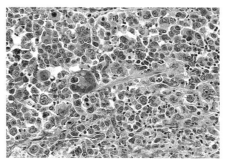

Fig. 3.84 Undifferentiated thymic carcinoma. The tumour contains large polygonal cells with prominent nuclear pleomorphism and mitotic activity. There is no squamous or glandular differentiation.

the lung, and metastatic undifferentiated carcinoma.

Genetic profile

There is no information on the genetic profile. Immunohistochemical and/or molecular studies for *NUT* gene translocation are helpful for the exclusion of NUT carcinoma, which is also morphologically undifferentiated {689}.

Prognosis and predictive factors

Undifferentiated carcinoma is a high-grade thymic carcinoma with a poor prognosis {2530}. Of 11 patients with follow-up information, 7 died at a median of 12 months, 1 developed recurrence at 4 years, and 3 were alive at 4 months to 22 years {366,1873,2630,2836}.

The presence of Castleman disease-like reaction is associated with a more protracted course {1873}. In the ITMIG database, the survival and recurrence rates are similar to those of other types of thymic carcinoma (see *Squamous cell carcinoma*, p. 212).

Other rare thymic carcinomas

D. Nonaka
H. Tateyama

ICD-O codes

Adenosquamous carcinoma	8560/3
Hepatoid carcinoma	8576/3
Thymic carcinoma, NOS	8586/3

There are rare reports of adenosquamous carcinoma {1359,2163,2687}, hepatoid carcinoma {749}, and rhabdoid carcinoma {2658} occurring as a primary tumour in the thymus. These tumours show features identical to those of their counterparts in other organs. One case reported as rhabdomyomatous carcinoma was actually a poorly differentiated adenosquamous carcinoma with a rhabdomyomatous component {555}; the interspersed skeletal muscle cells are bland-looking.

Micronodular thymic carcinoma with lymphoid hyperplasia {2837} is a rare form of thymic carcinoma resembling micronodular thymoma. It is characterized by multiple small nodules of cells with squamous differentiation, separated by an abundant lymphoid stroma. It shares some morphological features with undifferentiated large cell carcinoma associated with Castleman disease-like reaction {1873,2602}.

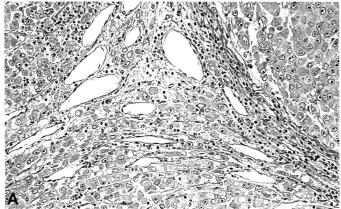
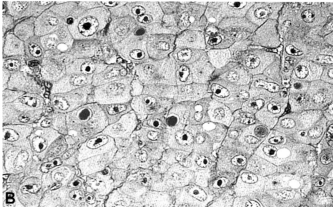

Fig. 3.85 Hepatoid thymic carcinoma. **A** Tumour nodules composed of large polygonal tumour cells resembling hepatocytes; there are no hepatic sinuses, portal structures, or tumour stroma. **B** Large polygonal cells with abundant eosinophilic cytoplasm; periodic acid–Schiff-positive globules (immunoreactive for alpha-1 antitrypsin, not shown) are present inside and between the tumour cells.

Thymic neuroendocrine tumours
Typical and atypical carcinoid

P. Ströbel
A. Marx
J.K.C. Chan
E.M. Marom

Y. Matsuno
A.G. Nicholson
W.D. Travis

Typical carcinoid

Definition

Typical carcinoid is a low-grade neuroendocrine epithelial neoplasm of thymic origin, with < 2 mitoses per 2 mm^2 and lacking necrosis.

ICD-O code   8240/3

Synonyms

Carcinoid tumour; well-differentiated neuroendocrine carcinoma (not recommended)

Epidemiology

Thymic neuroendocrine tumours are rare, accounting for only 2–5% of all thymic neoplasms {803,883,1727,2423}. Considering the paucity of data on clinicopathological correlations in thymic neuroendocrine tumours compared with the much better studied pulmonary neuroendocrine tumours, the approach taken in previous editions of the WHO classification (i.e. using the same nomenclature and criteria as for lung tumours) has been maintained in this edition. Thus, thymic neuroendocrine tumours are categorized into two major groups: 1) the low-grade typical carcinoids and intermediate-grade atypical carcinoids, which always show characteristic morphological and immunohistochemical neuroendocrine

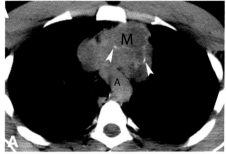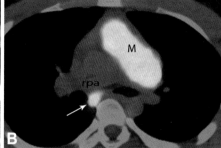

Fig. 3.86 Newly diagnosed atypical carcinoid in a 22-year-old man. **A** Unenhanced chest CT at the level of the transverse aorta (A) shows a lobular heterogeneous anterior mediastinal mass with areas of low attenuation corresponding to necrosis (M) and fine calcifications (arrowheads). **B** An axial fused image from FDG PET-CT at the level of the right pulmonary artery (rpa) shows that the primary mass (M) is markedly FDG-avid (with a maximum standardized uptake value of 25.7), and is associated with a mildly enlarged subcarinal FDG-avid lymph node consistent with a metastasis (arrow). This tumour shows aggressive imaging features commonly found in patients with neuroendocrine tumours, such as low-attenuation regions corresponding to areas of necrosis, calcifications, and avid FDG uptake. Imaging with FDG PET-CT is useful in patients with neuroendocrine tumours and other forms of thymic cancer because it highlights lymph nodes and distant metastases, which can be overlooked with morphological imaging early in the disease, when small.

features; and 2) the high-grade large cell neuroendocrine carcinomas (LCNECs) and small cell carcinomas, which may lack some neuroendocrine features. Unlike LCNEC, and small cell carcinoma of the lung, there is no established role of smoking in the development of thymic neuroendocrine tumours. Most of the tumours belong to the intermediate atypical carcinoid subgroup. Only typical carcinoid and atypical carcinoid (not LCNEC or small cell carcinoma) have been reported in the setting of multiple endocrine neoplasia type 1 (MEN1). The median

age at presentation is similar for all subgroups. Typical carcinoid and atypical carcinoid show a strong male predominance, which is less obvious in LCNEC and not seen in small cell carcinoma. For typical carcinoid, the average age at presentation is 49 years {2423}. MEN1-associated thymic neuroendocrine tumours have all been carcinoid tumours, and have occurred almost exclusively in male adults, with a mean patient age of 44 years (ranging from 31 to 66 years) {2612}. All thymic neuroendocrine tumours share a propensity for recurrence, lymph node or distant metastasis, and tumour-associated death {768,2423,2871}, and the risk increases from the low-grade to the high-grade group.

Etiology

About 25% of patients with thymic carcinoid tumours have a family history of MEN1 {2610}. Conversely, 8% of patients with MEN1 are found to have thymic carcinoid tumours {833}. Among patients with MEN1, smoking has been reported to be a risk factor in males {717,833,884}, but not females {2258}.

Table 3.07 Classification of thymic neuroendocrine tumours

Low-grade	Intermediate-grade	High-grade	
Typical carcinoid	Atypical carcinoid	Large cell neuroendocrine carcinoma (LCNEC)	Small cell carcinoma
• No necrosis • < 2 mitoses per 2 mm^2 (mean: 1 per 2 mm^2)	• Necrosis present and/or • 2–10 mitoses per 2 mm^2 (mean: 6.5 per 2 mm^2)	• Non-small cell cytology • Neuroendocrine markers • > 10 mitoses per 2 mm^2 (mean: 45 per 2 mm^2) • Frequent necrosis	• Small cell cytology • > 10 mitoses per 2 mm^2 (mean: 110 per 2 mm^2)
	Morphological variants • Spindle cell type • Pigmented type • With amyloid • Oncocytic/oxyphilic type • Mucinous type • Angiomatoid type • Combinations of the above variants	Combined large cell neuroendocrine carcinoma (with adenocarcinoma, squamous cell carcinoma, or spindle/giant cell carcinoma)	Combined small cell carcinoma (with LCNEC, adenocarcinoma, squamous cell carcinoma, or spindle/giant cell carcinoma)

Clinical features

About 50% of typical carcinoids present with local symptoms (chest pain, cough, dyspnoea, or superior vena cava syndrome) {883,1727,2423}. Paraneoplastic manifestations include Cushing syndrome (with or without cutaneous hyperpigmentation {799}), which occurs in 17–30% of adult and > 50% of childhood carcinoid tumours {554,2423,2523}. Another paraneoplastic manifestation is hypercalcaemia/hypophosphataemia, which results either from tumour production of parathyroid hormone-related protein {2980} or from primary hyperparathyroidism in MEN1 {2613}. Acromegaly {1133} and inappropriate production of antidiuretic hormone or atrial natriuretic peptide {1895} are uncommon, and carcinoid tumour syndrome is exceedingly rare (< 1%) {2423}. About 3% of patients develop synchronous malignancies {2423}.

On CT, neuroendocrine tumours are usually lobulated and heterogeneous (with low-attenuation regions within them), and enhance moderately to strongly with intravenous contrast injection {181,1168,1463}.

Approximately 50% of patients develop regional lymph node or distal metastasis. Bone and lung are frequently involved. Other (rare) sites include the liver, pancreas, and adrenal glands {2423}.

Localization

Typical carcinoids occur in the anterior mediastinum.

Macroscopy

Most tumours are unencapsulated and either circumscribed or grossly invasive. Their mean size is 8–10 cm (ranging from 2 to 20 cm) {549,1727,2423}. Cases associated with Cushing syndrome tend to be smaller (3–5 cm), due to earlier detection. Cut section is grey-white and firm, and can have a gritty consistency, often lacking the characteristic lobulated growth pattern of thymomas. Oncocytic variants may show a tan or brown cut surface. Calcifications are more common (present in 30% of cases) than in extrathymic neuroendocrine tumours {1727}.

Cytology

In fine-needle aspirates, tumour cells form loose clusters or small strands with indistinct cell borders. The cells are uniformly small, round to oval with scant

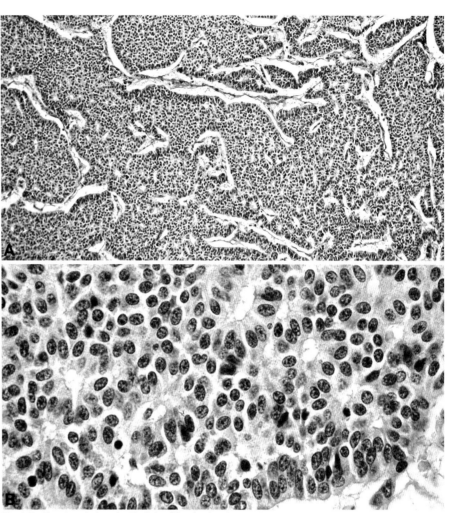

Fig. 3.87 Thymic typical carcinoid. **A** A solid and trabecular growth pattern; note the delicate vasculature between tumour masses; necrosis is absent. **B** High-power magnification showing rosettes, bland cytology, and no mitoses.

cytoplasm, and sometimes interspersed with larger cells with abundant granular cytoplasm {2800}. In pleural fluid, tumour cells form large spherical clusters, along with smaller groups of cuboidal cells {310}.

Histopathology

By definition, the tumours are devoid of necrotic areas and exhibit a low mitotic rate (< 2 mitoses per 2 mm^2) {2683} (see Lung *Carcinoid tumour*, p. 73) for mitosis-counting criteria). The tumour cells are uniform and polygonal, with relatively small, round nuclei; finely granular chromatin; and pale eosinophilic cytoplasm. Most tumours (> 50%) show trabecular and rosetting growth patterns, but several other patterns, such as festoons, solid nests, glandular structures, and nuclear palisading are also common. A delicate neuroendocrine tumour-type vasculature between the nests and trabeculae

is characteristic. Lymphovascular invasion is frequent. In addition to the various growth patterns, there are several recognized variants that can occur in either the typical or atypical carcinoid category. These carcinoid tumour variants include spindle cell {1457,1726,2872}, pigmented {1015,1285,1385}, with amyloid {1457}, oncocytic {1728,2925}, mucinous {1892,2517}, and angiomatoid {1725}.

Carcinoid tumours are immunoreactive for keratins (AE1/AE3, CAM5.2), often showing a dot-like staining pattern. Neuroendocrine markers such as synaptophysin, chromogranin, and NCAM/CD56 are usually strongly expressed. Most carcinoid tumours express at least two of these markers in > 50% of tumour cells {1012,1727,2423,2735}. One or more hormones (such as adrenocorticotropic hormone, human chorionic gonadotropin, somatostatin, calcitonin, and others) {990,2735,2871} can be detected in most

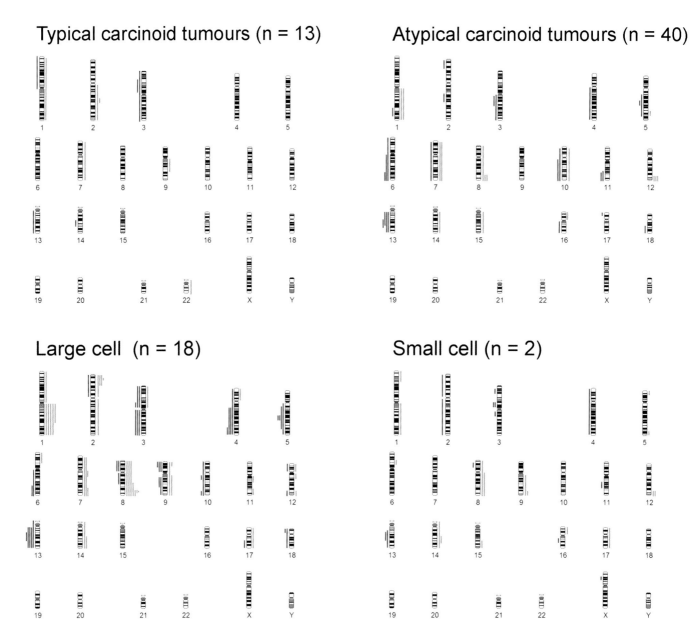

Fig. 3.88 The genomic profile of thymic neuroendocrine tumours (comparative genomic hybridization). There is an incremental increase in genomic alterations from typical carcinoids (average 0.8 alterations per case) to atypical carcinoids (average 1.1 alterations per case) to large cell neuroendocrine carcinomas (average 4.7 alterations per case) to small cell carcinomas (average 15.5 alterations per case). The chromosomal gains (green bars) and losses (red bars) are largely overlapping.

thymic neuroendocrine tumours, in a usually very low number of tumour cells. There is no close correlation between immunohistochemical hormone expression and clinical symptoms {32,990}. TTF1 is absent in most thymic carcinoid tumours {1906}.

Differential diagnosis
The major differential diagnoses include thymomas with spindle cell morphology (especially type A thymomas) and

paraganglioma. The carcinoid tumour variant with amyloid is indistinguishable from medullary thyroid carcinoma (extrathyroidal medullary carcinoma). The mucinous carcinoid tumour variant can resemble metastatic mucinous carcinoma, such as from the gastrointestinal tract or breast. The angiomatoid variant resembles haemangioma, with large blood-filled cystic spaces, but these spaces are lined by polygonal tumour cells and not endothelium {1725}. Carcinoid tumours

can be admixed with thymoma or different subtypes of thymic carcinoma {1359,2328,2519}, and have been reported as components of mature cystic teratomas of the thymus with somatic-type malignancy {1395,2220,2293,2333}.

Genetic profile
Typical thymic carcinoid tumours show the lowest number of genetic alterations among thymic neuroendocrine tumours. Up to 40% of cases do not show

alterations detectable by conventional comparative genomic hybridization {1968,2153,2495}. Recurrent aberrations include gains on chromosomes 1, 2q24, 7, 8p, 8q, 9q13, 11q23qter, and 22, and losses of 1p, 3p11, 6q, 10q, and 13q {1968,2153}. The gene locus of the *MEN1* gene on 11q13 is consistently unaltered {833,1968,2611,2613}. The pattern of chromosomal aberrations in thymic carcinoid tumours is significantly different from that of pulmonary carcinoid tumours {2495}.

Prognosis and predictive factors

There are few published data on the prognosis of thymic carcinoid tumours. The available data suggest that the prognosis of typical carcinoids is slightly better than that of atypical carcinoids {2495}. Published 5-year survival rates are in the range of 50–70% {1727,2423,2495}, with a median survival of 126 months {2495}.

Atypical carcinoid

Definition

Atypical carcinoid is an intermediate-grade neuroendocrine epithelial neoplasm of thymic origin, exhibiting 2–10 mitoses per 2 mm^2 and/or foci of necrosis.

ICD-O code   8249/3

Synonym

Moderately differentiated neuroendocrine carcinoma (not recommended)

Epidemiology

In the thymus, atypical carcinoids are far more common than typical carcinoids {32,883,1727,2495}. They are mainly tumours of adults, with a mean patient age of 48–55 years in both males and females (ranging from 18 to 82 years) {883,1727,2423,2735}, but they have also been rarely observed in children ranging in age from 8 to 16 years {799,1476}. There is a male predominance, with the male-to-female ratio ranging from 2:1 to 7:1 {652,883,1727,2423}.

Etiology

See *Typical carcinoid*, p. 234.

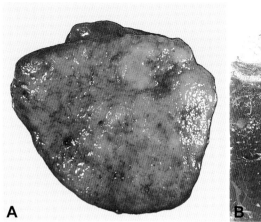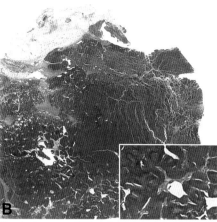

Fig. 3.89 Thymic atypical carcinoid. A macroscopic image (**A**) and a low-power H&E section (**B**) of a thymic atypical carcinoid. The H&E section shows vague circumscription and infiltrative growth of the tumour. The inset figure highlights multiple microscopic foci of necrosis.

Clinical features

Half of all patients with atypical carcinoids already have mediastinal, cervical, or supraclavicular lymph node metastases at presentation {883,1727,2735}. Invasion into adjacent organs (40–50%) or pleural or pericardial cavity (10%) is common {883,2735}. Sites of distant metastasis include the lung, brain, lumbar spine, bone, liver, kidney, adrenals, skin, and soft tissues {32,883,883,1727,2423}.

Localization

Atypical carcinoids occur in the anterior mediastinum.

Macroscopy

See *Typical carcinoid*, p. 234.

Cytology

Atypical carcinoids cannot be distinguished from typical carcinoids based on cytological features.

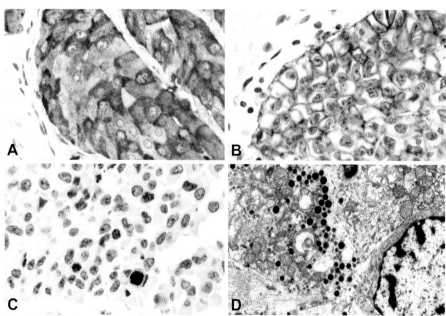

Fig. 3.90 Thymic atypical carcinoid. **A** Chromogranin staining. **B** Strong membranous staining of CD56. **C** Low Ki-67 index. **D** Transmission electron microscopy shows distinct electron-dense neurosecretory granules of variable sizes in the cytoplasm of a tumour cell.

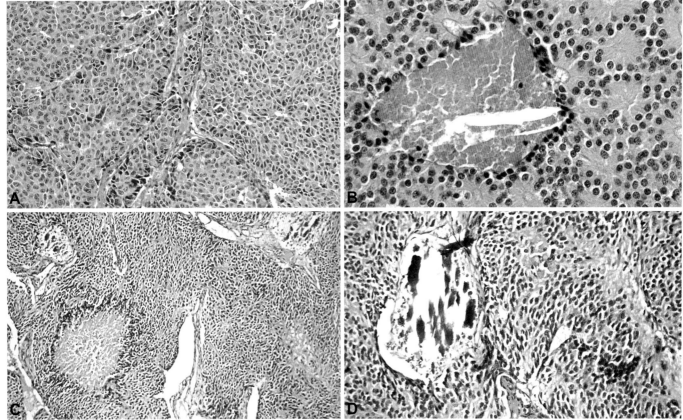

Fig. 3.91 Thymic atypical carcinoid. **A** Solid growth pattern. **B** Striking rosette formation and a punctate area of necrosis (comedo-type necrosis). **C, D** More diffuse growth, with foci of necrosis and calcifications.

Histopathology

All architectural features of typical carcinoids can occur. Even a small punctate area of necrosis in an otherwise typical carcinoid justifies a diagnosis of atypical carcinoid. Compared to typical carcinoids, atypical carcinoids more frequently show some degree of nuclear pleomorphism, including rare anaplastic cells {883}, a focal diffuse (so-called lymphoma-like) growth pattern {883,1727,2735}, or extensive desmoplastic stroma with single-cell filing of tumour cells {2868}. Calcifications are also frequent {1727}.

The immunohistochemical features of atypical carcinoids are identical to those of typical carcinoids.

Genetic profile

The genetic alterations overlap with those of thymic typical carcinoid, but the average number of alterations per tumour is slightly higher. Recurrent chromosomal gains include 1q, 5p, 5q, 7p, 7q, 8q, 12q24, 17q, and 20q. Chromosomal losses include 3p, 3q, 4q, 5q, 6q, 10q, 11q, and 13q {2153,2495}. The pattern of chromosomal aberrations in thymic carcinoid tumours is significantly different from that of pulmonary carcinoid tumours {2495}.

Prognosis and predictive factors

In published series, the overall survival rates of atypical carcinoids vary from 20–70% {1727,2423,2495} to up to 80% {503,883}, with a median survival of 52 months {2495}. Late recurrences up to 9 years after resection have been reported {2692}.

Large cell neuroendocrine carcinoma

A.G. Nicholson
J.K.C. Chan
E.M. Marom
A. Marx

Y. Matsuno
P. Ströbel
W.D. Travis

Definition

Large cell neuroendocrine carcinoma (LCNEC) is a high-grade thymic tumour composed of large cells with neuroendocrine morphology and either neurosecretory granules on electron microscopy or positive neuroendocrine immunohistochemical markers. Necrosis is usually extensive, and the mitotic rate is high.
Combined LCNEC has an additional component of other thymic epithelial tumours (including thymoma and thymic carcinoma).

ICD-O codes

Large cell neuroendocrine
   carcinoma   8013/3
Combined large cell
   neuroendocrine carcinoma   8013/3

Synonym

Poorly differentiated (high-grade) neuroendocrine carcinoma
(not recommended)

Epidemiology

LCNECs account for 14–26% of all thymic neuroendocrine neoplasms {32,2495,2644}, with an estimated incidence of 1 case per 20 million individuals {803}. Males are affected twice as often as females, and the median patient age

is 51 years (ranging from 16 to 79 years) {32,331,414,1887,2495}.

Etiology

The etiology is unknown. LCNEC does not occur as a component of multiple endocrine neoplasia type 1 {717,833,884,2258,2644}.

Clinical features

Half of all patients with LCNEC are asymptomatic {32,2383}. Most symptomatic patients present with chest pain, dyspnoea {644}, or superior vena cava syndrome. Cushing syndrome appears to be exceptional {2644}, but has been reported in single cases {2247}.
About 75% of tumours are in an advanced stage, with invasion of neighbouring organs or distant metastases (e.g. to the spine and liver) {331,366,414,1641,2495}.

Localization

LCNEC occurs in the anterior mediastinum.

Macroscopy

The macroscopy is the same as in other thymic neuroendocrine tumours.

Histopathology

LCNEC is a high-grade tumour with non-small cell morphology and a mitotic rate

that by definition exceeds 10 mitoses per 2 mm², but is often much higher. Necrosis is almost always present, and often extensive. Large tumour cell size (including frankly anaplastic giant cells) is more common than in atypical carcinoids {414,883,1727}. However, the morphology of some tumours is identical to that of atypical thymic carcinoid tumours, but with too many mitoses. Architectural features common to neuroendocrine tumours (e.g. nesting, trabeculae, and rosettes) are often less well developed than in atypical carcinoids.
LCNECs are usually strongly positive for neuron-specific enolase, chromogranin, synaptophysin, and CD56 {414,414,2644}, and express keratins such as CAM5.2 or AE1/AE3, sometimes with a cytoplasmic dot-like pattern {414}. Single cases have been reported to express CD117. CD5 is negative {414,644}. The higher mitotic rate is the essential feature distinguishing LCNEC from atypical carcinoid. LCNEC must be differentiated from metastatic LCNEC (e.g. of the lung), and positive TTF1 immunostaining favours a lung primary, although TTF1 can be expressed in extrapulmonary tumours. Careful clinical and radiological correlation is currently the primary way to distinguish pulmonary from thymic LCNEC. True LCNEC (with strong and

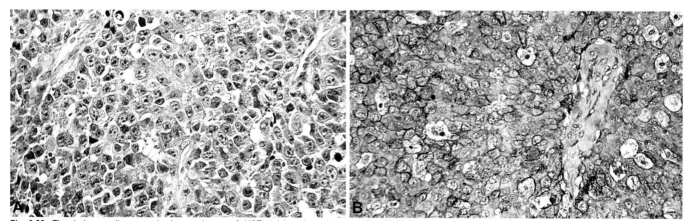

Fig. 3.92 Thymic large cell neuroendocrine carcinoma. A H&E staining shows tumour cells with high-grade morphology, prominent nucleoli, and multiple apoptotic bodies. B Immunohistochemistry shows strong diffuse membranous staining for CD56.

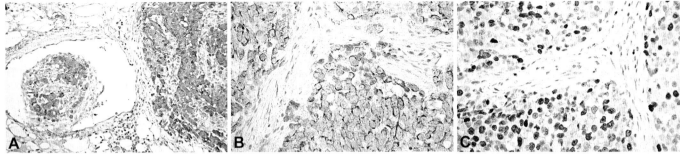

Fig. 3.93 Thymic large cell neuroendocrine carcinoma. **A** Strong chromogranin staining with a tumour plug in an adjacent blood vessel. **B** Synaptophysin staining. **C** High Ki-67 index.

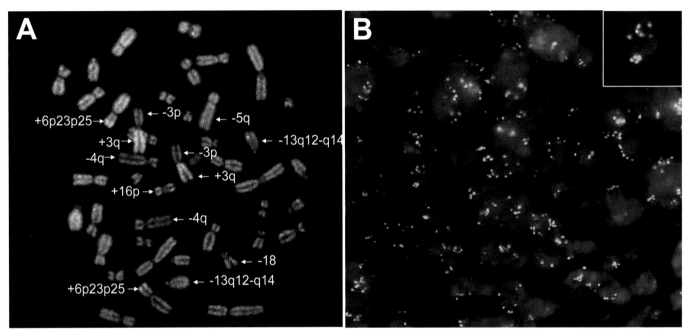

Fig. 3.94 Thymic large cell neuroendocrine carcinoma. **A** Comparative genomic hybridization of metaphase chromosomes shows multiple chromosomal gains (green) and losses (red). **B** FISH shows *MYC* gene amplification (green signals). Reprinted from Ströbel P et al. {2495}.

diffuse expression of usually more than one endocrine marker in > 50% of tumour cells) must be distinguished from non-neuroendocrine thymic carcinomas, which commonly show focal and/or weak expression of neuroendocrine markers {1012,1416}.

Genetic profile

The genetic alterations in LCNEC – e.g. gains on chromosomes 1q, 6p, 7, 8q (*MYC*), 12q, and 14, and losses on chromosomes 3, 4q, and 13q – overlap with those in thymic carcinoid tumours, but occur at a higher frequency. Alterations found only in LCNEC include gains at 2p, 9p, and 17q, and losses at chromosome 4p, 8p, 9p, and 18p {2495}. The pattern of chromosomal aberrations found in thymic LCNEC is not different from that found in their pulmonary counterparts {2495}.

Prognosis and predictive factors

Reported 5-year overall survival ranges from 30 to 66% {331,366,1641, 2495,2644}.

Small cell carcinoma

W.D. Travis
P. Ströbel
A. Marx
J.K.C. Chan

E.M. Marom
Y. Matsuno
A.G. Nicholson

Definition

Small cell carcinoma is a high-grade thymic tumour that consists of small cells with scant cytoplasm, poorly defined cell borders, finely granular nuclear chromatin, and absent or inconspicuous nucleoli. The cells are round, oval, or spindled, and nuclear moulding is prominent. Necrosis is typically extensive and the mitotic count is high.

Combined small cell carcinoma has an additional component of other thymic epithelial tumours (including thymoma and thymic carcinoma).

ICD-O codes

Small cell carcinoma   8041/3
Combined small cell carcinoma 8045/3

Synonyms

Oat cell carcinoma; poorly differentiated (high-grade) neuroendocrine carcinoma (obsolete)

Epidemiology

Small cell carcinomas account for approximately 10% of all thymic neuroendocrine neoplasms {367,783,1727,2495,2644}, with an estimated incidence of one case per 50 million individuals {803}. Males and females are equally affected, and the median patient age is 58 years (ranging from 37 to 63 years) {984,1359,2495,2687,2873}.

Etiology

The etiology of small cell carcinoma is unknown. Small cell carcinomas do not occur in multiple endocrine neoplasia type 1 {717,833,884,2258,2644}. There are no data on the etiological role of smoking.

Clinical features

Symptoms include weight loss, sweating, chest pain, cough, and superior vena cava syndrome {1359,2644,2873}. Exceptional patients may present with Cushing syndrome due to ectopic adrenocorticotropic hormone production {984}. Most tumours show invasion of neighbouring structures such as the lung, pericardium, pulmonary artery, phrenic

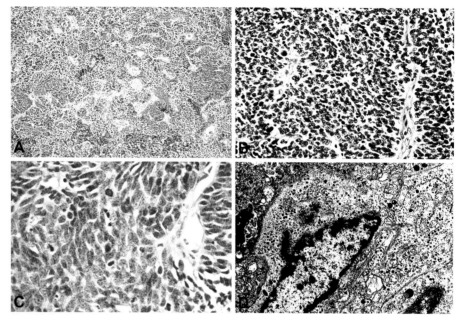

Fig. 3.95 Thymic small cell carcinoma. A Small cell carcinoma showing focal crush artefacts at low-power magnification. B Primary small cell carcinoma of the thymus. C Cytological details at high-power magnification: cellular crowding, elongated nuclei with salt-and-pepper chromatin structure, no recognizable nucleoli, scant cytoplasm, and high mitotic activity. D Dense core granules are numerous in the cytoplasm of the tumour cells.

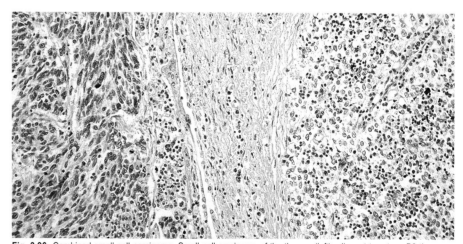

Fig. 3.96 Combined small cell carcinoma. Small cell carcinoma of the thymus (left) adjacent to a type B3 thymoma (right). Such tumours should be classified as combined small cell carcinomas.

nerve, or aortic arch {984,1359,2873}, or distant metastases to the lung, bone, brain, liver, and abdominal lymph nodes {1359,2495,2644,2687,2873}.

Localization

Small cell carcinomas occur in the anterior mediastinum.

Macroscopy

The macroscopy of small cell carcinoma is similar to that of other thymic neuroendocrine tumours, but necrosis and haemorrhage can be extensive. The tumours may be large, measuring 10–15 cm in diameter {1359,2873}.

Cytology

The tumour cells show a high nuclear-to-cytoplasmic ratio, scant cytoplasm, nuclear moulding, and finely granular nuclear chromatin. The nucleoli are inconspicuous or absent. Crush artefacts, nuclear breakdown, and apoptotic bodies are common.

Histopathology

The histology of thymic small cell carcinoma is identical to that of small cell carcinomas in other organs. Tumour cells are small (usually less than 3 times the size of a small resting lymphocyte). Nuclei can be round, oval, or spindle-shaped; the chromatin is finely granular; and nucleoli are inconspicuous. Apoptotic bodies are often numerous. Neuroendocrine differentation can be demonstrated in some cases by electron microscopy {2644,2687}.

The combination with thymoma, squamous cell carcinoma or adenosquamous cell carcinoma has been reported. Most cases stain for keratins, with rare exceptions {984,1359,2687}, and most tumours stain with neuroendocrine markers such as chromogranin, synaptophysin, or CD56 {984,1359,2644,2687}, although expression of neuroendocrine markers is not required for the diagnosis. Adrenocorticotropic hormone may be expressed.

The main differential diagnosis is metastasis from pulmonary small cell carcinoma, which requires careful correlation with clinical findings and imaging. TTF1 staining in thymic small cell carcinoma has not been analysed. The diagnosis of small cell carcinoma with negative keratin should be made with great caution after exclusion of lymphoma (CD45, terminal deoxynucleotidyl transferase, and CD3), and primitive neuroectodermal tumour (e.g. CD99).

Genetic profile

There are only two published cases with genetic data available {2495}. Both cases were highly aberrant, with multiple chromosomal gains and losses that were mostly overlapping with the more stable thymic carcinoid tumours and large cell neuroendocrine carcinomas.

Prognosis and predictive factors

Prognosis is poor, with a 5-year survival rate of 0% {1729}. Median survival is 13.75 months (ranging from 13 to 26 months) {1359,2495,2644,2873}.

Combined thymic carcinomas

K. Mukai
M. Marino
P. Ströbel
W.D. Travis

Definition

Combined thymic carcinomas are tumours that are composed of at least one type of thymic carcinoma and another thymic epithelial tumour, which may be any type of thymoma or thymic carcinoma. Tumours with a small cell or large cell neuroendocrine carcinoma component are by definition excluded from this category, and are diagnosed as combined small cell carcinomas and combined large cell neuroendocrine carcinomas respectively.

ICD-O codes

Code the most aggressive component.

Synonyms

Composite thymoma-thymic carcinoma; combined thymic epithelial tumours

Clinical features

The clinical manifestations, imaging findings, tumour spread, and staging of combined carcinomas are the same as those of thymic epithelial tumours of a single histological type {1898,2518,2838,2839}.

Localization

Almost all cases of combined thymic carcinomas were observed in the anterior mediastinum.

Macroscopy

The macroscopic features of these tumours are the same as those of non-combined thymic carcinomas {2518,2838}.

Histopathology

The different components of a combined thymic carcinoma should be apparent on

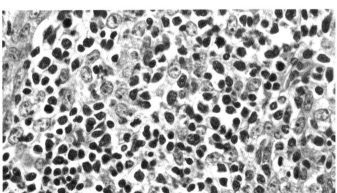
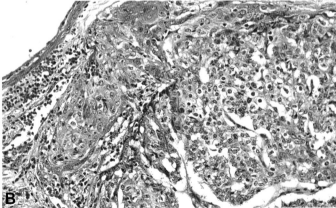

Fig. 3.97 Combined squamous cell carcinoma and type B2 thymoma. **A** The B2 thymoma component shown in this figure is rich in lymphocytes. **B** In the squamous cell carcinoma component, the cells show moderate nuclear pleomorphism, and squamous differentiation is evident in the upper field.

H&E staining. Heterogeneous differentiation that is apparent only by immunohistochemistry or electron microscopy is not sufficient to call a tumour combined thymic carcinoma. The carcinoma component may be any type of thymic carcinoma or carcinoid tumour, but excluding small cell carcinoma and large cell neuroendocrine carcinoma {1769}. The thymoma component may be any type of thymoma.

The most common combinations are thymic squamous cell carcinoma and type B3 thymoma {2518,2838}; and papillary adenocarcinoma or sarcomatoid carcinoma associated with type A thymoma {1610,2838}. The components may show gradual transition or be sharply separated from each other. Two thymic carcinoma components in a combined thymic carcinoma are rare.

Reporting the diagnosis of thymic carcinomas with more than one histological pattern

Tumours that consist of a thymic carcinoma or carcinoid tumour component of whatever size/percentage next to a thymoma should be labelled as thymic carcinoma or carcinoid tumour (specifying the percentage and histological type), followed by a listing of the accompanying thymoma component(s) and their relative percentage, starting with the predominant thymoma component; minor components should be reported in 10% increments {1595}. If a tumour consists of two or more different carcinomas, or a combination of a carcinoma and a carcinoid tumour, the diagnosis should list all

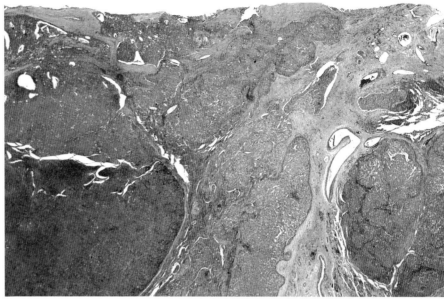

Fig. 3.98 Combined squamous cell carcinoma and type B2 thymoma. The blue areas in the left field represent type B2 thymoma, and the pink areas represent supervening squamous cell carcinoma.

subtypes, starting with the predominant component; minor components should be reported in 10% increments, e.g. "Combined thymic carcinoma composed of squamous cell carcinoma and lymphoepithelioma-like carcinoma, with proportions of 70% and 30%, respectively".

Immunohistochemistry

The immunohistochemical findings are similar to those in corresponding non-combined tumours. CD5, CD117, GLUT1, or MUC1 may be used to delineate thymic squamous cell carcinoma from type B3 thymoma, as described in *Type B3 thymoma*.

Genetic profile

The components of combined thymic carcinomas are expected to show changes similar to their single counterparts, but no systematic study has been done. Genetic overlaps between different components (e.g. between thymic squamous cell carcinoma and type B3 thymoma) have supported clonal relationships {2491}.

Prognosis and predictive factors

The prognosis of this type of tumour depends on the most aggressive component {2518}.

Germ cell tumours of the mediastinum
Seminoma

A.L. Moreira
J.K.C. Chan
L.H.J. Looijenga
A. Marx
P. Ströbel
T.M. Ulbright
M. Wick

Definition

Seminoma is a malignant neoplasm composed of cells resembling primordial germ cells. Mediastinal seminomas are morphologically indistinguishable from their gonadal counterparts.

ICD-O code   9061/3

Synonym

Germinoma; in women: dysgerminoma

Epidemiology

Both clinically and biologically, germ cell tumours of the mediastinum are separated into pre- and postpubertal entities {1912}. While prepubertal germ cell tumours consist only of teratomas and yolk sac tumours (either pure or mixed tumours), postpubertal germ cell tumours can be almost any of the histological types of germ cell tumours seen in the gonads, with the exception of spermatocytic seminoma. For therapeutic purposes, germ cell tumours are grouped into seminomas and non-seminomatous germ cell tumours (NSGCTs), which include embryonal carcinoma, yolk sac tumour, choriocarcinoma, mixed germ cell tumours (which may or may not include a seminomatous component), and teratoma. The distribution of the histological types of mediastinal germ cell tumours varies from study to study. Seminoma is the most common in some studies {882,1291}, and mature teratoma (followed by seminoma) is the most common in others {2192,2566}. This variability in the reported frequency may be the result of different patterns of referral between institutions {2144}.

The reported frequency of postpubertal pure primary mediastinal seminomas in males is 32% (ranging from 9% to 39%) {223,634,1722,1737,2567}.

Almost all reported mediastinal seminomas have occurred in men {634,1722, 1737,2567}, with rare case reports of dysgerminoma (the histological counterpart of seminoma) occurring in women {634,2567}. For postpubertal mediastinal germ cell tumours, the peak age distribution for seminoma is between 33 and 39 years (ranging from 18 to 65 years) {223,882,965,1291,2192,2566}.

Etiology

The etiology of mediastinal germ cell tumours, including seminoma, is unknown. Although mediastinal germ cell tumours in general tend to be particularly common in patients with Klinefelter syndrome (XXY) {511,1440,2295,2425,2477,2704}, this is not true of seminoma {969}. Interestingly, individuals with Klinefelter syndrome are not at increased risk for testicular germ cell tumours (either seminoma or others). This has been explained by the lack of a proper microenvironment for the survival of XXY germ cells in the testis {2327,2877,2878}. There is one report of a mediastinal seminoma in a patient with Down syndrome {1099}.

It has been hypothesized that extragonadal germ cell tumours in general are a consequence of aberrant midline migration of primordial germ cells {2881}. In postpubertal males, the mediastinum is the most frequent site of extragonadal germ cell tumours. There are some data to suggest that the thymus produces KIT ligands {573,1913} that favour the survival and proliferation of such mismigrated primordial germ cells, which ultimately could develop into germ cell tumours.

Clinical features

Signs and symptoms

The clinical symptoms are non-specific. Presenting symptoms are related to the size of the tumour, and include chest pain, dyspnoea, respiratory distress, cough, hoarseness, and superior vena cava syndrome {1341,1737,2566}. The size of the tumour may be relatively large, due to slow growth with few clinical symptoms overall.

Some patients are asymptomatic, with the tumour detected by unrelated imaging studies or thoracotomy {1737}. Mild serum elevation of the β-subunit of human chorionic gonadotropin (βhCG) (≤ 100 IU/L in adults and ≤ 25 IU/L in children; normal range, ≤ 5 IU/L) can be found in up to a third of patients with pure seminoma {221,855}.

α-Fetoprotein (AFP) levels are never elevated in pure seminoma. Lactate dehydrogenase is elevated in both pure seminoma and NSGCTs, although it is not a specific tumour marker. High lactate dehydrogenase levels are an independent unfavourable prognostic factor for germ cell tumours. In adults, serum tumour marker (including lactate dehydrogenase) levels at diagnosis are important

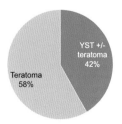

Mediastinal Germ Cell Tumors in Prepubertal Patients (N=48)

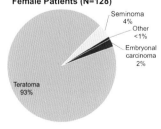

Mediastinal Germ Cell Tumors in Postpubertal Female Patients (N=128)

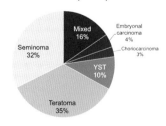

Mediastinal Germ Cell Tumors in Postpubertal Male Patients (N=519)

Fig. 3.99 Distribution of primary mediastinal germ cell tumour subtypes according to age and sex. YST, yolk sac tumour. Reprinted from Williamson WR, Ulbright TM {1581}.

criteria for risk stratification according to the International Germ Cell Cancer Collaborative Group (IGCCCG) system {1089}. However, unlike for NSGCT, the use of serum markers to guide or monitor treatment for seminoma is not recommended {838}.

A diagnosis of primary mediastinal germ cell tumour requires the absence of a testicular or ovarian tumour on physical examination, CT, high-resolution ultrasonography, or MRI {222}. A bilateral testicular biopsy is not mandatory, since mediastinal germ cell tumours are usually not associated with intratubular germ cell neoplasia {927}. Although it is prudent to rule out metastatic disease from a primary gonadal seminoma, mediastinal metastases are rare in gonadal seminomas, particularly in the absence of retroperitoneal lymph node metastasis {1237}.

The frequency of other neoplasms is not increased in patients with seminoma or other mediastinal germ cell tumours {223,963}. The risk for the development of metachronous testicular cancer is low {223,962}.

Imaging

Pure seminomas form uncalcified, homogeneous masses that are indistinguishable from lymphoma {2498}, whereas NSGCTs are usually heterogeneous masses, exhibiting central attenuation and a frond-like periphery {2498}. Multilocular cystic lesions can accompany any mediastinal germ cell tumour (particularly seminoma), but can also be seen in thymomas, thymic carcinomas, Hodgkin or non-Hodgkin lymphomas, and metastasis to the mediastinum. These lesions are also included in the radiographical differential diagnosis of germ cell tumour.

Tumour spread and staging

At the time of diagnosis, most mediastinal seminomas are localized, circumscribed masses without macroscopic or microscopic evidence of invasion into neighbouring structures such as the pleura, pericardium, and great vessels {1737}. Metastasis occurs in approximately 40% of cases {221,223}. The preferential sites of distant spread are the lymph nodes, lung, chest wall, brain, pleura, liver, adrenal glands, and bone {1714,1722}. Lymph node metastases most commonly occur in the neck and abdomen (in 25% and 8% of

cases, respectively, in one series) {221}. Metastasis to viscera other than the lung is a major adverse prognostic factor in seminomas {965} and other malignant NSGCTs {223,965}. Germ cell tumour staging is controversial. Some authors use a modified TNM classification of soft tissue tumours {2853}. A specific staging for mediastinal germ cell tumours based on the degree of local invasiveness and metastasis has also been proposed {1722,2841}, but is not widely used {2278}.

Table 3.08 Comparison of the general features of mediastinal germ cell tumours and seminomas

Feature	Mediastinal germ cell tumour	Seminoma
Incidence	Rare • 3–4% of all germ cell tumours • Up to 16% of all mediastinal tumours in adults and 19–25% in children {1291,1722, 2080,2566}	Rare • 10–20% of all mediastinal germ cell tumours {882,1291,2192,2566}
Age distribution	All age groups (range: 0–79 years)[a] {1722,2302,2566} • Prepubertal (< 8 years): teratoma and yolk sac tumour {2302,2567} • Postpubertal: 25–29 years (range: 14–51 years); all histological types {223,882,965}	Postpubertal: 33–39 years (range: 14–65 years) {223,882,965,1291,2192,2566}
Classification	Pure and mixed forms[b]	Pure and mixed forms[b]
Etiology	Unknown Klinefelter syndrome is a risk factor for non-seminomatous germ cell tumour {968,970}	Unknown No associated risk with Klinefelter syndrome {969}
Clinical associations	Non-seminomatous germ cell tumours are associated with haematological malignancies No increased risk of gonadal germ cell tumour	No association with haematological malignancies No increased risk of gonadal germ cell tumour
Genetics	Isochromosome 12p	Isochromosome 12p

[a] Children and adolescents (< 18 years) account for 16–25% of all cases, which are divided into prepubertal and postpubertal mediastinal germ cell tumour; in prepubertal germ cell tumour, yolk sac tumour has a female predominance; in postpubertal germ cell tumour, malignant tumour (seminoma and non-teratoma germ cell tumour) has a male predominance. Teratoma affects males and females equally, independent of age;
[b] All histological types of germ cell tumour that can be seen in the gonad can occur in the mediastinum except spermatocytic seminoma. For therapeutic purposes, the tumours are diagnosed as seminomas and non-seminomatous germ cell tumours, which include embryonal carcinoma, yolk sac tumour, choriocarcinoma, mixed germ cell tumours (which may or may not include a seminomatous component), and teratoma.

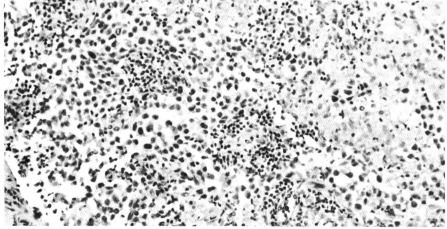

Fig. 3.100 Seminoma. Large monotonous tumour cells associated with a dense lymphoid infiltrate and granulomatous inflammation.

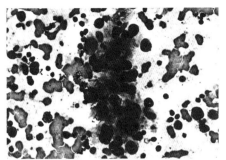

Fig. 3.101 Seminoma. Note the large cells dispersed or arranged in small clusters. The tumour cells are often devoid of cytoplasm. The nuclei are large, with prominent nucleoli. Note the presence of lymphocytes in the background, in close association with tumour cells (modified Giemsa stain).

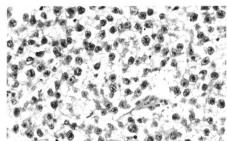
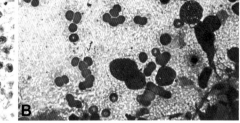

Fig. 3.103 Seminoma. **A** The tumour cells have round vesicular nuclei with prominent eosinophilic macronucleoli, abundant pale cytoplasm, and well-defined cell membranes. A few lymphocytes with small dark nuclei are scattered among the seminoma cells. **B** Characteristic tigroid background seen in smears stained with modified Giemsa.

Localization

Seminomas occur in the anterior mediastinum.

Macroscopy

Mediastinal seminomas are morphologically identical to their gonadal counterparts. Macroscopically, they are mostly well-circumscribed, fleshy tumours with a homogeneous, slightly lobulated to multinodular, tan-grey or pale cut surface. Punctate focal haemorrhage and yellowish foci of necrosis may be observed. The median tumour size is 4.6 cm (ranging from 1 to 20 cm) {221,1737}.

Cytology

In the era of neoadjuvant therapy for germ cell tumour before surgical excision, small biopsy and cytology specimens are the main materials available for diagnosis. Seminoma has a characteristic cytological appearance: small clusters or dispersed monotonous large cells with central nuclei and large, prominent nucleoli. Due to the fragility of the glycogen-rich cytoplasm, most of the nuclei are stripped of cytoplasm. A classical tigroid background is present in hypercellular smears corresponding to dispersed glycogen particles, but can be difficult to identify in paucicellular smears. Dispersed polymorphous populations of lymphocytes and small clusters of epithelioid macrophages (granuloma) are often seen {326,393,923}.

If the cytological features are diagnostic of seminoma, but the patient has high AFP or βhCG levels, a diagnosis of mixed germ cell tumour should be considered. Mildly elevated βhCG levels (see above) are still compatible with a fine-needle aspiration biopsy-based diagnosis of pure seminoma {221,855,2302}.

Histopathology

Mediastinal seminomas are composed of round to polygonal, fairly uniform tumour cells with round to oval, central, slightly squared, non-overlapping nuclei and one or more large central nucleoli. The tumour cells commonly have abundant, glycogen-rich, clear to lightly eosinophilic cytoplasm and distinct cell membranes. Rarely, the tumour cells may show dense eosinophilic cytoplasm or a greater degree of cellular pleomorphism. The tumour cells grow in confluent multinodular clusters, sheets, cords, strands, or irregular lobules. The tumour is traversed by delicate fibrous septa, where there is frequently an infiltrate of small mature lymphocytes, plasma cells, and occasional eosinophils, sometimes with germinal centre formation. The lymphoid infiltrate can also be intermingled with the tumour cells. A granulomatous reaction ranging from poorly defined clusters of epithelioid histiocytes to well-defined epithelioid granulomas with Langhans giant cells may be present. The brisk inflammatory or granulomatous reaction and scar formation can be very extensive, and may obscure the underlying seminoma {1718,1737,2844}. The tumour can also be interspersed by epithelium-lined thymic cysts.

In some cases, syncytiotrophoblastic cells (the source of elevated βhCG) are scattered throughout the tumour, often in close proximity to capillaries and/or focal punctate haemorrhage. These

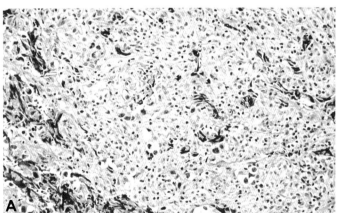
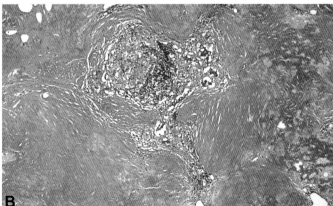

Fig. 3.102 Seminoma. **A** Seminoma can be obscured by inflammatory or granulomatous reaction and scar formation. **B** Massive fibrosclerotic change with only small tumour remnants.

Table 3.09 Immunohistochemical profiles of various types of germ cell tumours

Germ cell tumour type	Cytokeratin	OCT4 (OCT3/4)	SALL4	CD117	CD30	α-Fetoprotein	β-Subunit of human chorionic gonadotropin	Glypican 3
Seminoma	– [a]	+	+	+	–	–	– [b]	–
Embryonal carcinoma	+	+	+	–/+	+	+/–	– [b]	–
Yolk sac tumour	+	–	+	+/–	–	+	–	+
Choriocarcinoma	+	–	+ (mononuclear trophoblast)	–	–	–	+	+ (syncytiotrophoblast)
Teratoma	+ (epithelial component)	–	–/+ (focal staining in enteric glands, primitive neuroepithelium, and blastema-like stroma of immature teratoma)	–/+	–	–/+ [c]	–	+/–

[a] Can show positive staining in a dot-like pattern;
[b] Positive in scattered syncytiotrophoblasts;
[c] AFP can be positive in fetal gut, liver, or neuroepithelium in immature teratoma.
Note: A few new markers are emerging, such as SOX2 (positive in embryonal carcinoma, negative in seminoma);
SOX17 (positive in seminoma, negative in embryonal carcinoma) {542},
and LIN28 (positive in most germ cell tumours, except teratoma {839}.

multinucleated giant cells have abundant basophilic cytoplasm and occasional intracytoplasmic lacunae. However, there are no cytotrophoblast cells or confluent nodules as seen in choriocarcinoma. Seminoma can occur as a component in mixed germ cell tumours. Spermatocytic seminomas have not been described in the mediastinum, most likely because spermatocytic seminomas are derived from a more mature germ cell that can only be found in the testis {1506}.

Immunohistochemistry and differential diagnosis

The immunohistochemical profiles of germ cell tumours very closely reflect the differentiation and maturation markers of normal embryonic stem cells, including germ cells {1507,1912}.
Accordingly, seminomas are positive for OCT4 (OCT3/4) and SALL4 {376,1507,2514}. CD117 positivity in a cell membrane or paranuclear Golgi pattern is seen in approximately 70% of cases {2093,2514}. D2-40 is also commonly positive. PLAP is rarely used as a seminoma or germ cell tumour marker nowadays, because of its lack of specificity and the frequent presence of background staining. Immunostaining for βhCG often highlights scattered syncytiotrophoblastic cells. AFP is negative {1722,1737,2527}.
Up to 70% of seminomas show staining for keratins (such as AE1/AE3), but the staining is often focal and weak, usually

with a paranuclear distribution. The scattered syncytiotrophoblastic cells are also strongly positive for keratins. Other germ cell tumours (i.e. embryonal carcinoma, yolk sac tumour, and choriocarcinoma) and metastatic carcinoma to the mediastinum show diffuse strong staining for keratin. Other differential diagnoses include metastatic melanoma, primary mediastinal large B-cell lymphoma, thymoma, thymic carcinoma, and particularly clear cell carcinoma (primary or metastatic).

Genetic profile

The genetic changes described in mediastinal seminomas are the same as those reported in testicular seminomas, with 69% demonstrating the isochromosome i(12p), and approximately 87% showing the 12p amplification {2514} characteristic of postpubertal malignant germ cell tumours at all sites. Mediastinal seminomas are most commonly aneuploid, with a minority having near-tetraploid DNA content. A single study reported partially non-coding *KIT* mutations (in 4 out of 8 cases) in mediastinal seminoma {2093}.

Prognosis and predictive factors

In the era of cisplatin-based chemotherapy for malignant germ cell tumours, the most important prognostic factors in extragonadal germ cell tumours are localization of the primary tumour and histology {1239,2567}.

Mediastinal localization of a germ cell tumour is associated with a worse prognosis in general than localization at other extragonadal and gonadal sites {133,965, 1089,1341,1448,1569,2302}.
However, recent cisplatin-based neoadjuvant strategies have provided dramatically improved outcomes in both children {2302} and adults {222,223,733}. Initial AFP levels > 10 000 ng/mL (normal range is variable, but is usually < 50 ng/mL) indicate a worse prognosis in children {133}. Elevated βhCG is usually an independent adverse prognostic factor for survival in adults {223}.
Seminomas show a favourable response to radiotherapy and cisplatin-based chemotherapies, and have an excellent prognosis, with a 5-year survival rate of 90% (which is not different from that of seminomas from other locations) {222,223,965,1448,2567}. If residual lesions persist after completion of chemotherapy, investigation by PET is helpful in distinguishing viable from necrotic tumour {557}. Unlike in NSGCT, surgical resection of residual mass is usually not indicated. Adverse prognostic parameters in seminomas are liver metastasis and metastases to multiple other sites {965,1089}.
For mixed germ cell tumour with or without a seminomatous component, the favourable prognostic indicators following preoperative cisplatin-based chemotherapies are completeness of resection {961,962,2302}, < 10% viable cells {733},

Table 3.10 Therapy for various types of germ cell tumours[a]

Histological diagnosis	Therapeutic option
Seminoma	Chemotherapy
Yolk sac tumour	Chemotherapy, followed by resection of remaining tumour mass
Embryonal carcinoma	Chemotherapy, followed by resection of remaining tumour mass
Choriocarcinoma	Chemotherapy, followed by resection of remaining tumour mass
Mixed germ cell tumour	Chemotherapy, followed by resection of remaining tumour mass
Teratoma, mature	Surgical resection
Teratoma, immature	Surgical resection

[a] Histological classification of germ cell tumours has therapeutic implications; in the era of neoadjuvant therapy for germ cell tumours, the diagnosis is usually based on fine-needle aspiration biopsies, serum tumour marker (α-fetoprotein and the β-subunit of human chorionic gonadotropin) levels, and imaging studies.

and low-risk features according to the International Germ Cell Cancer Collaborative Group (IGCCCG) staging system {1089}. Decreased survival is associated with failure to respond to cisplatin and higher rates of relapse {965}. Unsatisfactory decline of AFP and/or βhCG levels during the early phase of chemotherapy appears to herald a worse outcome {1619}. Treatment failure is among the worst prognostic factors; it is more common in mediastinal than other germ cell tumours, and is significantly associated with non-seminomatous histology and metastasis to the liver, lung, and brain {965}.

Embryonal carcinoma

J.K.C. Chan
L.H.J. Looijenga
A. Marx
A.L. Moreira
T.M. Ulbright
M. Wick

Definition
Embryonal carcinoma is a germ cell tumour composed of large primitive cells of epithelial appearance, resembling cells of the embryonic germ disc.

ICD-O code   9070/3

Synonym
Malignant teratoma undifferentiated (obsolete)

Epidemiology
Pure embryonal carcinoma accounts for up to 2% of all mediastinal germ cell tumours {1291,1722}, and for 4% of all postpubertal non-seminomatous germ cell tumours (NSGCTs) {1239,1581, 1722,2567}. It is predominantly a tumour of young males (with a male-to-female ratio > 10:1) {1291,2567}. The mean age of adult patients is 27 years (ranging from 18 to 67 years) {1290,2567}. Embryonal carcinoma in childhood is very rare but peaks between the ages of 1 and 4 years (usually occurring as part of a mixed germ cell tumour), and again after the age of 14 years {2301,2302}.

Etiology
The etiology is unknown. Like other mediastinal NSGCTs, embryonal carcinoma is associated with Klinefelter syndrome {183,1568,1636,1834,2787}. The rare occurrence of familial cases suggests a possible role of genetic predisposition {39,1587}. In terms of histogenesis, the primordial germ cell is thought to be the cell of origin {1913,2395}.

Clinical features
Patients present with thoracic or shoulder pain (60%), respiratory distress (40%), hoarseness, cough, fever, or superior vena cava syndrome {2567}. Virtually all patients have increased serum α-fetoprotein levels, and some have elevated levels of the β-subunit of human chorionic gonadotropin (βhCG) {2567}. Imaging findings are not different from those reported for other NSGCTs {2192}. Local tumour spread is common, and can lead to compression and infiltration of the lung. There is a high rate (about 50%) of haematogenous metastasis (to the lung, liver, brain, and bones), while lymphogenous metastasis is much rarer {223,2567}. A quarter of all patients already have pulmonary metastasis at presentation.

Localization
Embryonal carcinomas occur in the anterior mediastinum.

Macroscopy
Embryonal carcinomas are large tumours with invasion of the surrounding organs and structures. The cut surface often reveals soft, fleshy, grey-white or pink-tan tumour with large areas of necrosis and haemorrhage. When embryonal carcinoma occurs as a component of mixed germ cell tumour, interspersed cystic spaces are common.

Cytology
Smears of embryonal carcinoma are often cellular and composed of a high-grade epithelial neoplasm resembling a poorly differentiated carcinoma. The malignant cells are arranged in three-dimensional clusters or flat sheets, and can form papillary structures and acini. The nuclei are large and pleomorphic, with coarse chromatin and prominent nucleoli. Without immunohistochemical stains, it is almost impossible to distinguish embryonal carcinoma from a poorly differentiated carcinoma. Cytological diagnosis should always be correlated with clinical and radiographical studies {37,480,923}.

Histopathology
Embryonal carcinomas grow in the form of solid sheets, tubules, and papillary structures. They consist of large polygonal or columnar cells, often with indistinct cell borders. The nuclei are large, round or oval, and often vesicular, but can be hyperchromatic or have light chromatin. They are often crowded and sometimes overlapping. Large single or multiple eosinophilic nucleoli are common. The cytoplasm is amphophilic, but can be basophilic, eosinophilic, pale, or clear. Mitoses are numerous and often atypical. There are often many apoptotic bodies, and coagulative necrosis is common. The stroma is usually scant in viable tumour areas, but fibrotic adjacent to areas with regressive changes. Granulomas are uncommon. In about a third of cases, there are scattered single or small groups of syncytiotrophoblasts.

When embryonal carcinoma occurs as a component of mixed germ cell tumour, other germ cell tumour components

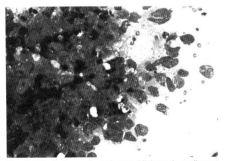

Fig. 3.104 Embryonal carcinoma. High-grade malignant tumour with large, pleomorphic tumour cells with coarse chromatin and prominent nucleoli (modified Giemsa stain).

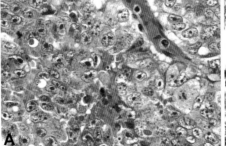
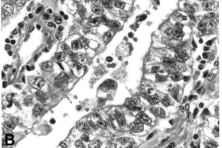

Fig. 3.105 Mediastinal embryonal carcinoma. A Large tumour cells with indistinct cell borders, crowded nuclei, vesicular chromatin, and large eosinophilic nucleoli; the cytoplasm ranges from amphophilic to pale. B Columnar tumour cells with disarrayed nuclei, a mildly hyperchromatic chromatin pattern, and large nucleoli; the cytoplasm is pale to clear.

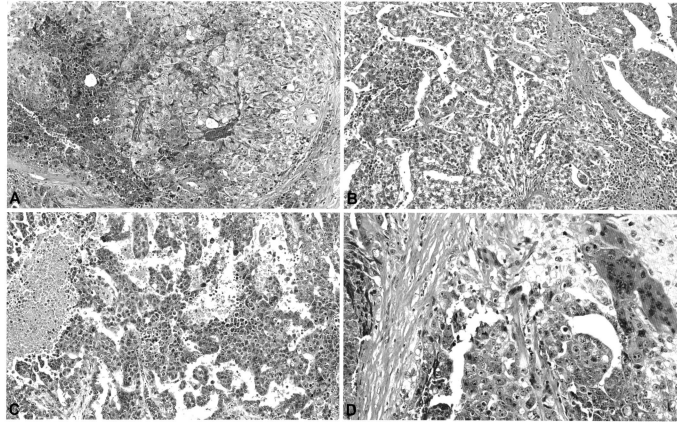

Fig. 3.106 Mediastinal embryonal carcinoma. **A** Solid growth pattern. **B** Complex glandular pattern. **C** Papillary pattern. **D** In the right upper field, several multinucleated syncytiotrophoblastic cells are seen, in the absence of accompanying cytotrophoblasts.

include teratoma (56%), choriocarcinoma (22%), or seminoma (22%) {1290,2566}. Association with yolk sac tumour is rare in adults {2567}, but more common in adolescents {1736}. Embryonal carcinomas uniformly stain for low-molecular weight keratins, while epithelial membrane antigen, carcinoembryonic antigen, and vimentin are usually negative. CD30 is expressed in 85–100% of cases {1412,1962}. SOX2 expression distinguishes embryonal carcinoma from seminoma {542}. The embryonic stem cell transcription factors OCT4 (OCT3/4), SALL4, and NANOG are uniformly positive {1064,1169,1487}.

Immunostaining for α-fetoprotein {18, 1736} occurs in scattered tumour cells or small foci in about 30% of cases. The scattered syncytiotrophoblastic cells, when present, are positive for βhCG.

Differential diagnosis
When syncytial-appearing areas are extensive, embryonal carcinoma can mimic choriocarcinoma {1736}. However, a biphasic plexiform pattern produced by a mixture of syncytiotrophoblasts and cytotrophoblasts is lacking, and pure embryonal carcinomas lack the extensive βhCG immunoreactivity of choriocarcinoma {1736}.

Yolk sac tumour can be distinguished from embryonal carcinoma by its more varied growth pattern (most commonly microcystic and reticular); smaller cell size; presence of Schiller-Duval bodies; and characteristic immunoprofile of CD30 negativity, OCT4 negativity, SALL4 positivity, and glypican 3 positivity.
Embryonal carcinoma can be distinguished from seminoma by its greater degree of nuclear pleomorphism, at least focal definite epithelial characteristics (such as gland formation), and uniform strong staining for keratin, frequent CD30 and SOX2 expression, and infrequent CD117 expression {2527}.

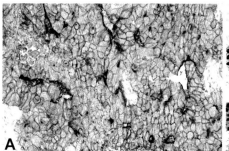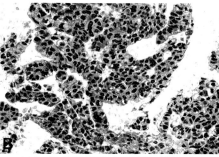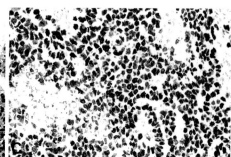

Fig. 3.107 Mediastinal embryonal carcinoma. **A** Cell membrane staining for CD30. **B** Nuclear OCT4 staining. **C** Nuclear staining for SALL4.

Mediastinal metastasis from large cell carcinoma of the lung may mimic embryonal carcinoma {1736}. The young age of most patients with embryonal carcinoma, CD30 expression, OCT4 expression, and the presence of tumour markers in the serum (such as α-fetoprotein and βhCG) are distinguishing features. Metastasis to the mediastinum from a testicular embryonal carcinoma or mixed germ cell tumour {1155,1237} must be excluded.

Genetic profile
The genetic changes are the same as those reported in their testicular counterparts – isochromosome 12p characteristic of postpubertal malignant germ cell tumours at all sites. A cell line established from a mediastinal embryonal carcinoma showed regional amplification of *SOX2* {658}.

Prognosis and predictive factors
The long-term survival rate of about 50% in adult patients with mediastinal embryonal carcinoma after cisplatin-based chemotherapy {2567} is very similar to the rates published for large series of adult NSGCTs. For children with embryonal carcinoma, the 5-year survival rates are significantly better (> 80%) {2302}.

Yolk sac tumour

A. Marx
A.L. Moreira
J.K.C. Chan
L.H.J. Looijenga
P. Ströbel
T.M. Ulbright
M. Wick

Definition
Yolk sac tumour is a malignant tumour characterized by numerous patterns that recapitulate the yolk sac, allantois, and extra-embryonic mesenchyme.

ICD-O code   9071/3

Synonym
Endodermal sinus tumour
(not recommended)

Epidemiology
In patients aged < 15 years, yolk sac tumour is the second most common mediastinal germ cell tumour (after teratomas), and the most common malignant germ cell tumour, with an incidence rate of about 0.25 cases per 100 000 children. After puberty, yolk sac tumour occurs almost exclusively in males (with rare exceptions) {1226,2935}, and shows an increasing incidence that peaks in the third decade and then decreases thereafter {2230}. Patient ages range from 15 to 59 years, and the incidence rate is 0.3 cases per million individuals per year {2230}. Pure yolk sac tumour in adolescents and adults is the fourth most common germ cell tumour (after teratoma, seminomas, and mixed germ cell tumours), accounting for 10% of all cases {1240,1722,2278}.

Etiology
The etiology is unknown. For unclear reasons, Klinefelter syndrome is a risk factor after puberty but not before {2787}. The

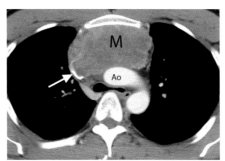

Fig. 3.108 Yolk sac tumour. Contrast-enhanced chest CT of a 40-year-old man at the level of the main bronchi shows a lobulated, poorly marginated, heterogeneous anterior mediastinal mass (M) invading the superior vena cava (arrow). The mass displaces the aorta (Ao) and airways posteriorly. Superior vena caval involvement by yolk sac tumour was confirmed at surgery.

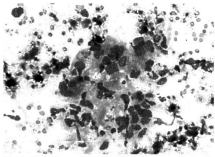

Fig. 3.109 Yolk sac tumour. A high-grade neoplasm with large irregular nuclei. Note the presence of metachromatic material around tumour cells (hyaline balls, modified Giemsa stain) and the necrotic background. Schiller-Duval bodies cannot be seen in cytology preparation.

mismigration of a primordial germ cell has been postulated for the histogenesis {1913,2395}. Associated thymic cysts are probably a secondary phenomenon {1721}.

Clinical features
Patients with mediastinal yolk sac tumour often present with chest pain, dyspnoea, chills, fever, and superior vena cava syndrome {1736,2566,2567}. α-fetoprotein (AFP) levels are almost always elevated. No specific imaging findings have been published. FDG PET may be instrumental for the detection of even tiny tumour recurrences {2561}.
Mediastinal yolk sac tumour almost always shows extension into the surrounding fat and adjacent structures, including the lung, while pleural dissemination is rare {1736,2935}. Before puberty, pure

and mixed mediastinal yolk sac tumours have a 30% risk for distant metastasis {2303}; mainly to the lung, lymph nodes, liver, bone, and brain {856,857,2302}. After puberty, 50% of mediastinal yolk sac tumours show metastases in the lung

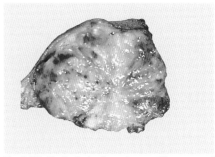

Fig. 3.110 Mediastinal yolk sac tumour. Macroscopy of pure mediastinal yolk sac tumour, showing a grey-white and gelatinous cut surface; there is no haemorrhage and no necrosis.

or intrathoracic lymph nodes, while extrathoracic metastases occur in < 10% of cases {1722,1736}. Bone metastasis, although rare overall, is typical of mediastinal germ cell tumours, particularly yolk sac tumours {814}.

There is no validated staging system for mediastinal germ cell tumours. Some paediatric studies adopted the TNM system for sarcomas {2302}, while others used the four-tiered system for extragonadal germ cell tumours that combines resection and metastatic status {513}. The system proposed by Moran {1722}

has been used in studies with adults {1736,2278}.

Localization

Yolk sac tumours occur in the anterior mediastinum.

Macroscopy

Macroscopically, pure yolk sac tumours are solid and soft. The cut surface is typically pale grey or grey-white, with a gelatinous or mucoid quality. After neoadjuvant treatment protocols, mediastinal germ cells tumours typically show

haemorrhage and necrosis. Cyst formation may be treatment-related, or may suggest a mixed germ cell tumour with yolk sac tumour component.

Cytology

Smears of yolk sac tumour show aggregates of medium to large cells with variable nuclei, prominent nucleoli, moderate to occasionally abundant cytoplasm, and a variable background of debris and mucoid or metachromatic material (modified Giemsa stain). Lymphoid cells and granulomas are typically not present. Cytological diagnosis should always be correlated with clinical and radiographical studies {37,480,923}.

Histopathology

There is a wide spectrum of histological patterns in yolk sac tumours: microcystic (reticular), macrocystic, glandular-alveolar, endodermal sinus (pseudopapillary), myxomatous, hepatoid, enteric, polyvesicular, vitelline, solid, and spindle; and a given tumour usually shows more than one pattern {1206,1633,1736,2615}. The different patterns have no apparent prognostic or biological significance.

The reticular or microcystic variant is the most common pattern, characterized by a loose network of cystic spaces and channels lined by flat or cuboidal cells with scant cytoplasm. The myxomatous pattern is characterized by a stroma rich in glycosaminoglycans, in which the epithelial cells are suspended. The endodermal sinus pattern typically shows pseudopapillary structures and Schiller-Duval bodies – i.e. glomeruloid structures with a central blood vessel covered by an inner rim of tumour cells, surrounded by a capsule lined by an outer (parietal) rim of tumour cells. The polyvesicular-vitelline pattern is defined by cysts that are lined by cuboidal to flat tumour cells surrounded by a dense fibrous stroma. The solid pattern is usually seen only focally, and may resemble embryonal carcinoma or seminoma; however, the cells of yolk sac tumour are usually smaller and less pleomorphic than those of embryonal carcinoma, and more pleomorphic than is typical of seminoma. It typically retains the usual immunohistochemical profile although with lesser positivity for AFP {1206}. Yolk sac tumour with a hepatoid pattern {1720,2715} has cells with abundant eosinophilic cytoplasm resembling fetal or adult liver {2082}. The enteric

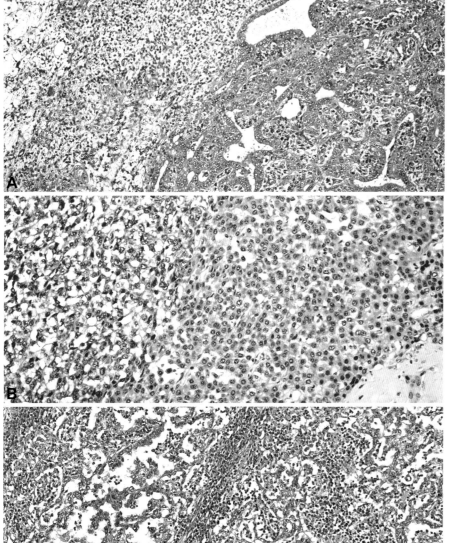

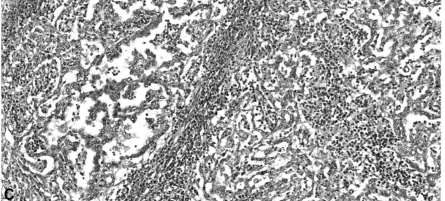

Fig. 3.111 Yolk sac tumour. **A** Enteric and microcystic growth pattern. **B** Hepatoid growth pattern. **C** Glandular pattern and prominent lymphocyte-rich stroma.

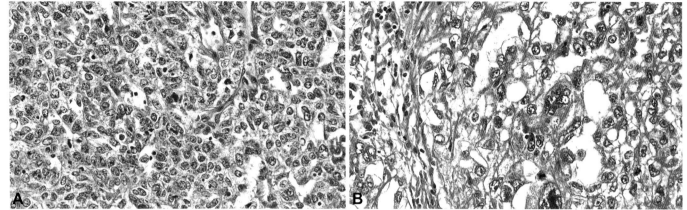

Fig. 3.112 Yolk sac tumour. **A** Solid growth pattern. **B** Focal anaplasia.

and endometroid patterns show glandular features resembling the fetal human gut and secretory endometrial glands, respectively {463,470}. If these patterns are seen within an immature teratoma, immunohistochemistry may be necessary to determine whether they represent immature fetal tissue or yolk sac tumour {1863}.

The occurrence of admixed syncytiotrophoblasts in otherwise typical yolk sac tumour is of unknown prognostic significance, and does not warrant a diagnosis of mixed germ cell tumour {1633}.

Sarcoma development in yolk sac tumour represents somatic-type malignancy, and is very rare in pure mediastinal yolk sac tumour {1556}, but more common in mixed germ cell tumour {2144,2712} (see *Germ cell tumours with somatic-type solid malignancy*, p. 263).

Associated haematological malignancies (mainly acute leukaemias and myelodysplastic syndromes) are particularly common in mixed germ cell tumours with a yolk sac tumour component (58%) and pure yolk sac tumours (25%) {964,1633}, and are clonally related to the underlying germ cell tumour {621,964,1381,1837}.

Immunohistochemistry

Yolk sac tumours are consistently immunoreactive for cytokeratins (AE1/AE3), glypican 3 {3035}, and the more recently described stem cell markers SALL4 {321,1487,2801} and LIN28 {323,2855}, while they are negative for OCT4, NANOG {126,1507}, SOX2 {1487,1505,1869,2271}, and D2-40 {126,1064,1415}. Single syncytiotrophoblastic cells that occur in a minority of yolk sac tumours express the β-subunit of human chorionic gonadotropin {1633}. AFP and PLAP may be expressed in up to 70% of yolk sac tumours, KIT/CD117 (mostly faintly) in up to 40% {1064}, and CD30 in up to 25% {322,323,1206,1487,2527,2801}, while epithelial membrane antigen is rarely detectable (in < 25% of cases), and even then in a minority of tumour cells only {1064,2801}. For details, see *Seminoma*, p. 244.

Differential diagnosis

Mediastinal seminoma can resemble solid variant of yolk sac tumour and reacts with antipancytokeratin antibody CAM5.2 in up to 80% of cases; however, generally in a dot-like, paranuclear pattern {1737}.

Unlike yolk sac tumour, seminoma is typically OCT4-positive, KIT-positive, D2-40-positive, and glypican 3-negative on immunohistochemistry.

Embryonal carcinoma is commonly composed of larger and more atypical tumour cells, shows less varied growth patterns, lacks microcystic and reticular areas and Schiller-Duval bodies, and exhibits a characteristic immunoprofile: CD30 positivity, OCT4 positivity, SOX2 positivity, and glypican 3 negativity.

Choriocarcinoma may resemble yolk sac tumour due to complex biphasic growth patterns produced by intermingled syncytiotrophoblasts and cytotrophoblasts, and due to focal immunoreactivity for SALL4 {322} and LIN28 {839}. However, pure yolk sac tumour lacks the β-subunit of human chorionic gonadotropin immunoreactivity {1736}.

Immature teratoma with primitive endodermal (including hepatic), neuroectodermal, and spindle cell mesenchymal components may mimic the varied growth patterns of yolk sac tumour, and may focally express glypican 3, AFP, SALL4, LIN28, HepPar-1, and CDX2 {320,1633,1863}. However, unlike yolk sac tumour, immature teratoma typically

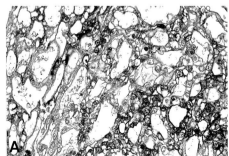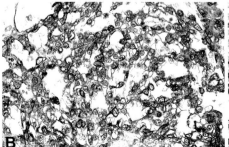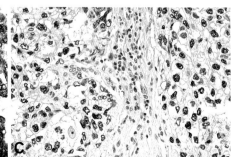

Fig. 3.113 Yolk sac tumour. **A** Expression of α-fetoprotein. **B** Expression of glypican 3. **C** Expression of SALL4.

has a component of embryonic-appearing neuroepithelium that may be CD56-positive and/or OCT4-positive {8}, and other components that are immunoreactive for epithelial membrane antigen.

Thymic carcinoma and mediastinal yolk sac tumour can share a solid growth pattern, expression of keratins and CD117, and lack of AFP expression {988,1064,1206,1965}. However, thymic carcinoma is often CD5-positive {1011}, while negative for glypican 3 {1487}, SALL4 {1113}, and LIN28 {323}.

Metastatic carcinoma to the mediastinum, including pulmonary, intestinal, hepat cellular, and hepatoid carcinomas can resemble glandular, solid, or hepatoid variants of yolk sac tumour, with which they can share expression of glypican 3, AFP, CDX2, and HepPar-1 in addition to cytokeratins {126}. Metastatic carcinomas are typically negative for SALL4 and LIN28 {126,1863}; however, exceptions occur {322,323}. Metastasis from a gonadal or retroperitoneal pure yolk sac tumour or mixed germ cell tumour to the mediastinum must be excluded {1237}.

Genetic profile

Mediastinal yolk sac tumours show the same genetic alterations as yolk sac tumours elsewhere. Yolk sac tumours in children aged < 8 years exhibit losses at 1p, 4q, and 6q, and gains at 1q, 3, 20q, and 20, but neither i(12p) nor sex chromosome alterations. In contrast, yolk sac tumours occurring after the age of 8 years show i(12p) in 60% of cases, gains of chromosomes 21 and X in 20% of cases each, and loss of chromosome 13 in 30% of cases {2303}.

Age-related genetic alterations are accompanied by distinct imprinting patterns {1912,2304} and gene expression profiles {1963}.

Prognosis and predictive factors

The 5-year event-free and overall survival rates of children aged < 15 years with malignant non-seminomatous germ cell tumours are 83% and 87%, respectively, with no difference between yolk sac tumour and mixed germ cell tumour {2302}. The most important favourable prognostic factor is complete resection. Following incomplete resection, the 5-year survival rate drops to 42% {2302}. Brain metastasis is a poor prognostic sign {856,857}.

After the age of 15 years, the 5-year overall survival in mediastinal non-seminomatous germ cell tumour is 45–54% {707,965,2178,2278}. Lack of metastasis {1722,1736,2178,2278}, complete resection, postoperative normalization of tumour markers {1201, 2278}, low preoperative levels of the β-subunit of human chorionic gonadotropin {2178}, pure yolk sac tumour histology {2178}, and complete tumour necrosis after chemotherapy {1240} are favourable prognostic factors. Somatic-type malignancy and clonally related haematological malignancies portend a poor prognosis, due to therapeutic refractoriness {621,964,1381,1837}.

Choriocarcinoma

P. Ströbel
J.K.C. Chan
L.H.J. Looijenga
A. Marx

A.L. Moreira
T.M. Ulbright
M. Wick

Definition
Choriocarcinoma is a highly malignant trophoblastic neoplasm composed of syncytiotrophoblast, cytotrophoblast, and variably intermediate trophoblast. Mediastinal choriocarcinomas are morphologically indistinguishable from their gonadal or uterine counterparts.

ICD-O code   9100/3

Synonyms
Chorioblastoma; chorioepithelioma; chorionic carcinoma (obsolete)

Epidemiology
Almost all reported cases of choriocarcinoma have occurred in adult male patients (with an age range of 17–63 years) {317,634,802,1217,1723,2389, 2567}. Only 3% of mediastinal germ cell tumours are pure choriocarcinomas {1239,1291,1722,1736}; however, estimates are biased by the referral patterns of the reporting institutions. The crude estimated incidence of choriocarcinomas is 1 case per 12 million individuals {2567}.

Etiology
Choriocarcinoma, either pure or as part of a mixed germ cell tumour, tends to be particularly common in patients with Klinefelter syndrome {511,1440,2295,2425,2477,2704}. It has been hypothesized that extragonadal germ cell tumours in general are a consequence of aberrant midline migration of primordial germ cells {2881}.

Clinical features
The tumours are rapidly growing {3001}, and early bronchial invasion is typical. Reported symptoms at presentation include shortness of breath, chest pain, cough, superior vena cava syndrome, syncopal episodes, persistent headache, and cardiac tamponade {531,1217,1440,1723}. Some patients present with gynaecomastia {317} due to human chorionic gonadotropin production {317,634,802,1722,2389}. Since the polypeptide alpha chain of human cho-

rionic gonadotropin is similar to thyroid-stimulating hormone, patients may also develop thyrotoxicosis {1440,1754,2295}. The tumours often appear as well-circumscribed anterior mediastinal masses on chest radiograms {1723,2567} and CT {802}, often with protrusion into one lung field or lung collapse {2567}. The tumours often show evidence of necrosis {802}. Primary choriocarcinomas have also been observed in the posterior mediastinum {1723}.
Mediastinal choriocarcinomas are highly aggressive neoplasms, with early haematogenous dissemination {1722}. Common metastatic sites are the lungs, liver, kidney, and spleen {1723}. Others include the brain, choroids, heart, adrenals, and bone {1291,1346,1723,2389}.
There is currently no established staging system for mediastinal germ cell tumours. Most cases of choriocarcinoma present with infiltration of neighbouring organs such as the great vessels, lung, and chest wall, and/or with intra- and extrathoracic metastases {802,1722,1736}.

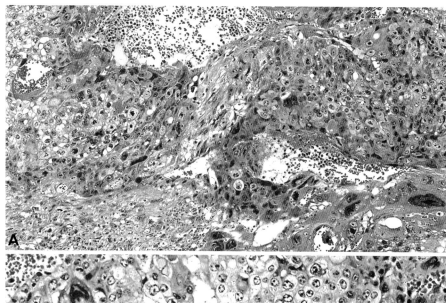
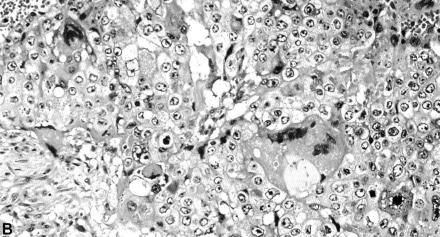

Fig. 3.114 Choriocarcinoma. A A low-power view showing a highly polymorphic malignant tumour forming lacunae filled with blood. B High-power magnification shows multinucleated syncytiotrophoblast cells capping mononucleated cytotrophoblast cells.

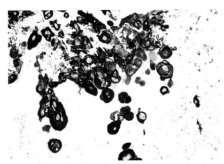

Fig. 3.115 Choriocarcinoma immunohistochemistry. Strong, diffuse expression of the β-subunit of human chorionic gonadotropin.

Localization
Choriocarcinomas occur in the anterior and posterior mediastinum.

Macroscopy
Most tumours are large (with an average size of 10 cm), soft, friable, and extensively haemorrhagic. Most also contain foci of necrosis {1217,1723}.

Cytology
The cytology is characterized by syncytiotrophoblasts and mononucleated cytotrophoblasts. In H&E stain, syncytiotrophoblasts are very large cells with eosinophilic cytoplasm, one to several nuclei, and distinct nucleoli. Mononucleated cytotrophoblasts are medium-sized cells with vacuolated, basophilic cytoplasm and eccentric nuclei {393,480}.

Histopathology
Mediastinal choriocarcinoma can occur in a pure form or as part of a mixed germ cell tumour. The histology is not different from that of its gonadal counterpart. Syncytiotrophoblasts and cytotrophoblasts are typically intermingled in a bilaminar plexiform pattern or in disordered sheets. Occasionally, scattered clusters of syncytiotrophoblasts cap cytotrophoblast nodules. Syncytiotrophoblasts are large multinucleated cells with numerous, pleomorphic, dark-staining nuclei, variably distinct nucleoli, and abundant densely eosinophilic or amphophilic cytoplasm, which may contain cytoplasmic lacunae. Cytotrophoblasts are more uniform, polygonal cells with round nuclei, prominent nucleoli, and clear or eosinophilic cytoplasm. Atypical mitosis and cellular atypia are common. There can be sheets of nondescript mononuclear cells that resemble intermediate trophoblasts. Choriocarcinomas are typically intimately associated with dilated vascular sinusoids. Partial or complete replacement of the walls of blood vessels is common. There are often vast areas of haemorrhage and necrosis {802,1217,1723}.

Choriocarcinomas express keratins, and are negative for OCT4, PLAP, α-fetoprotein, carcinoembryonic antigen, CD30, and vimentin. The syncytiotrophoblastic cells express human chorionic gonadotropin {802,1217,2527}, glypican 3 {3036}, and inhibin alpha, while the mononuclear trophoblastic cells are often positive for SALL4.

Clinical information is needed to rule out metastatic gonadal choriocarcinoma, although mediastinal metastasis of gonadal germ cell tumours seems to be exceptional {1155,1239}. Mediastinal metastasis from a poorly differentiated carcinoma with choriocarcinoma-like features is another differential diagnosis. Single cases of placental site trophoblastic tumour, another trophoblastic tumour, have been reported in the mediastinum {2852}.

Genetic profile
Mediastinal choriocarcinomas have been described to harbour an isochromosome i(12p) characteristic of postpubertal malignant germ cell tumours {364}.

Prognosis and predictive factors
In most reported cases, the patients died of disseminated disease shortly after diagnosis (with an average survival time of 1–2 months) {317,802,1723,1736,2389}. However, treatment with cisplatin-based chemotherapy may improve the outcome {223,531,1406,1440,2567}.

Mature and immature teratoma

A.L. Moreira   P. Ströbel
J.K.C. Chan   T.M. Ulbright
L.H.J. Looijenga M. Wick

Definition

Teratoma is a germ cell tumour composed of somatic tissues derived from two or three of the germ layers (ectoderm, endoderm, and mesoderm). Teratomas can be further classified as mature teratomas, which are composed exclusively of mature, adult-type tissues; and immature teratomas, which contain immature, embryonic, or fetal tissues either exclusively or in addition to mature tissues.

ICD-O codes

Teratoma, mature   9080/0
Teratoma, immature   9080/1

Epidemiology

Teratomas are rare neoplasms, accounting for < 10% of all mediastinal masses. They occur in both pre- and postpubertal males and females, with no sex predominance {1459,1459,2301}. In prepubertal patients, pure teratomas account for 58% of all mediastinal germ cell tumours, and can occur even in fetuses as young as 18 weeks of gestation {829,1656,2404}. In postpubertal patients, they account for 93% of germ cell tumours in females and 35% in males {564,634,928,1581,1722,1833,2498,2820}. Similar to other non-seminomatous germ cell tumours, mature and immature teratomas (often associated with another histological type of germ cell tumour) can occur in patients with classical (i.e. 47,XXY karyotype) Klinefelter syndrome and, very rarely, mosaic Klinefelter syndrome {578,2502,2787}. Immature teratomas are much rarer than mature teratomas {1327,1722}. Unlike mature teratomas, immature teratomas occur more frequently in men than in women.

Etiology

The etiology is unknown, but may differ between pre- and postpubertal teratomas. Postpubertal teratomas are thought to derive from a primordial germ cell, but at least some prepubertal teratomas are thought to derive from an embryonic stem cell {2304}.

Clinical features

Signs and symptoms

Mature teratomas are asymptomatic in 50% of children and 66% of adults, with the tumour being detected by unrelated imaging studies or during unrelated thoracotomy {1737}. The tumour may be relatively large, due to slow growth with few clinical symptoms {527,1459,1696,2567}. Symptomatic cases can be associated with chest, back, or shoulder pain; dyspnoea; cough; and fever due to chronic pneumonia {527,2302,2727}. Respiratory compromise is more common in neonates and children than in adults, usually due to the size of the space-occupying lesion {2330}. Rare symptoms include superior vena cava syndrome, Horner syndrome, and pneumothorax, which are more common in adults {855,2302}. An unusual presentation is coughing up hair (trichoptysis) or other materials due to the formation of a tumour–bronchial fistula, possibly resulting from proteolytic enzymes produced by exocrine pancreatic tissue present in the tumour {910,1489}. Tumour rupture is rare, but appears to be more common in mediastinal teratomas than in teratomas of other sites {29,532,1005,1489}. Rupture of a teratoma can result in pleural effusions, empyema, or cardiac tamponade. The presence of endocrine pancreatic component can cause hyperinsulinism and hypoglycaemia {685,1028}. The usual serum tumour markers (α-fetoprotein and the β-subunit of human chorionic gonadotropin) are not elevated.

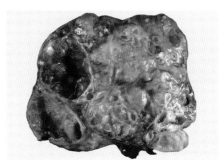

Fig. 3.116 Mature teratoma. A circumscribed multilocular cystic tumour.

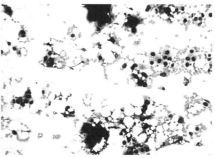

Fig. 3.117 Mature teratoma. Smears show bland epithelial cells in a cystic background. Note the presence of metachromatic material (cartilaginous material, modified Giemsa stain). These features mimic normal structures. The cytological diagnosis of teratoma can only be reached with clinical and radiographical correlation.

Teratomas more commonly arise in the anterior mediastinum, but have also been reported in the posterior mediastinum {1063,1130,2567}, in an intrapericardial location {212,471,1648}, and within the myocardium {2302}. Hydrops fetalis is a complication of congenital intra- and extrapericardial mediastinal teratoma {829,2011}. Teratomas can extend deeply into one or both thoracic cavities and elicit atelectasis {2727}.

Imaging

A mature teratoma can be mistaken for a large pleural effusion on routine chest radiographs. CT is the modality of choice for tumour diagnosis {442}. Mature teratomas are well-demarcated tumours, and show multilocular cystic structures in almost 90% of cases {1696,2004,2498}. Attenuation is heterogeneous, with varying combinations of soft tissue, fluid, fat, and calcium {1696}. Calcifications occur in 26% {1459} to 53% {1696} of cases. A shell-like tumour wall calcification or identifiable bone and teeth each occur in up to 8% of cases {1459,1696}.
Immature teratomas appear more often as solid masses {2498}. There are no detailed reports on imaging studies for pure immature teratoma.

Tumour spread

Pure teratomas are localized tumours, and there have been no reports of tumour spread. However, in mixed germ

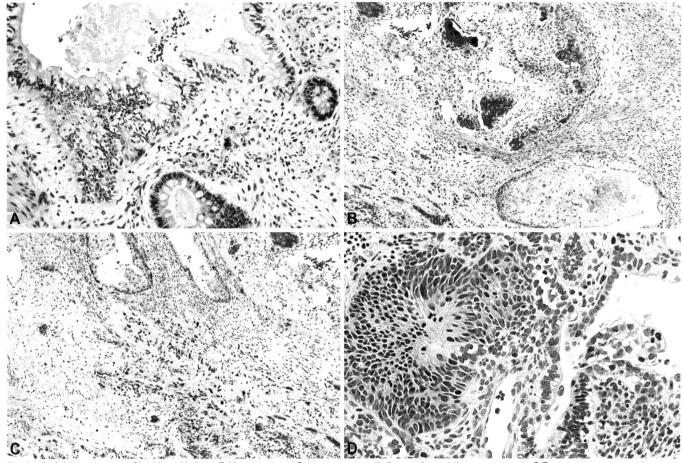

Fig. 3.118 A Mature teratoma. Glandular epithelium. **B** Mature teratoma. Bone, squamous epithelium, and neural tissue are present. **C** Teratomatous component in a post-chemotherapy resection specimen. Neurogenic tissue shows reactive atypia, not to be confused with somatic transformation or immature component. **D** Immature teratoma. Primitive neuroepithelium forming rosettes and immature glands.

cell tumour post-chemotherapy resection specimens, teratomatous components (either mature or immature) are often seen in metastatic sites.

Localization
Teratomas occur in the anterior and posterior mediastinum.

Macroscopy
Mature mediastinal teratomas are usually encapsulated masses, with a mean diameter of 10 cm (ranging from 3 to 25 cm) {2144,2820}, but there can also be adhesions to the surrounding lung or great vessels {2144,2727}. The cut surface is variegated, showing unilocular or multilocular cysts varying in size from millimetres to several centimetres. The cysts can contain clear fluid, mucoid material, sebaceous and keratinaceous debris, hair, fat, cartilage, and (rarely) teeth or bone {2498}.
Immature teratomas have a similar size distribution as mature teratomas {1327}.

They have a soft to fleshy consistency or are extensively fibrous or cartilaginous. Unlike in mature teratomas, haemorrhage and necrosis are common {2144}.

Cytology
Cytological diagnosis of mature teratoma is difficult {7}. The aspirates may be paucicellular with a few anucleated squamous cells and macrophages in a proteinaceous (cystic) background. The presence of ciliated bronchial epithelium, smooth muscle, and cartilage – common components of a mature teratoma – can be mistaken for contamination by bronchopulmonary tissue. A mucoid background with bland-looking signet ring cells can be seen, but the diagnosis can only be made if other cellular types are also present. Other epithelial cells, such as pancreatic acini and intestinal-type mucosa, may suggest the possibility of a teratomatous lesion {7,2504}.
The cytological smears of immature teratomas may be cellular and show a

cytological pattern of small blue cell tumour. Tumour cells may be isolated or grouped in small aggregates forming branching sheets. The cells have small, round, hyperchromatic nuclei with inconspicuous nucleoli and a high nuclear-to-cytoplasmic ratio. Rosettes with neuropils are rarely seen, as are rhabdomyoblasts, immature cartilage, and blastema-like stromal cells {7,2115}.
The diagnosis of teratoma in cytological specimens or small biopsies should be made only after careful correlation with imaging and serological studies that can exclude mixed germ cell tumour.

Histopathology

Mature teratoma
Mature tissues representing two or three of the germ layers are seen throughout the tumour in a haphazard distribution. Skin and cutaneous appendages are commonly found forming cyst linings. Despite the high frequency of skin and

adnexa, monodermal teratomas (dermoid cysts) are very rare in the mediastinum {2343,2934}. Other commonly found tissues are bronchial mucosa and glands, gastrointestinal mucosa, nerves and mature brain tissue, smooth muscle, and adipose tissue. These elements are seen in approximately 80% of tumours. Skeletal muscle, bone, and cartilage are less common, and are often seen in the solid component of the tumour. Pancreatic tissues, including both exocrine and endocrine glands, are found in up to 60% of cases, but are rare or absent in teratomas of other sites {641,822}. Salivary glands, prostate, liver, and melanocytes are less common.

Extensive granulomatous inflammation may be seen in association with ruptured cysts {2144}. Remnant thymic tissue is found outside the capsule in 75% of mature teratomas.

Immature teratoma

These tumours consist of embryonic tissues derived from the various germ layers, such as immature glands lined by tall columnar cells, fetal lung, mesenchymal and primitive cartilage, bone, rhabdomyoblasts, blastema-like stromal cells. The most common immature component is neuroectodermal tissue, with neuroepithelial cells forming tubules and rosettes {2144,2820}. The proportion of immature teratomas in combination with mature tissue varies from 20% to 40% {111,141,1327,1722,2820}. There are insufficient data to support a grading system for immature teratomas of the mediastinum, and some studies show no prognostic significance of grading in children {855,1583,2302}.

Teratomatous component of mixed germ cell tumour

In mixed germ cell tumour, the term used to describe differentiated somatic tissues is teratomatous component. In resected post-chemotherapy residual masses, as well as in metastatic diseases, the teratomatous component often appears immature or atypical {2144}.

Immunohistochemistry

Immunohistochemistry is generally not required for diagnosis of teratoma, but may help in characterizing immature components, such as rhabdomyoblasts (using desmin and myogenin), neural components (using S100 and synaptophysin), and immature cartilage (using S100 and glial fibrillary acidic protein) {1878}. Pure teratomas are negative for the β-subunit of human chorionic gonadotropin and CD30. α-fetoprotein is usually negative, although liver cells and immature neuroepithelium may express α-fetoprotein.

Differential diagnosis

The main differential diagnoses are other cystic lesions of the mediastinum. The diagnostic challenge is often encountered in cytological specimens or small biopsies, since the finding of mature elements could represent normal tissue contaminant, and not a true representation of the lesion. The findings of immature elements in small biopsy could suggest the diagnosis of small blue cell tumour and sarcoma. To avoid these pitfalls, careful correlation with clinical and radiographical studies is imperative. In resection specimens, the main differential diagnosis is mixed germ cell tumour with a teratomatous component. Immature teratoma may be difficult to distinguish from teratoma with somatic-type malignancy, but the latter usually forms a defined nodule within the tumour mass, and shows frank cytological atypia and invasiveness that are absent in pure immature teratomas. The teratomatous component of a post-chemotherapy resected specimen can show significant cellular atypia, and should not be confused with a somatic-type malignancy {2144}.

Genetic profile

Unlike malignant germ cell tumours, the pure mature and immature teratomas analysed and reported to date have not shown recurrent genetic gains or losses. Rare cases of immature teratomas in adults showed t(6;11) associated with a high risk of haematogenous metastasis and subsequent death {2402,2403,2747}.

Prognosis and predictive factors

Mediastinal mature teratomas have an excellent prognosis after complete resection in all age groups {882,1448, 1583,2302,2567}. In infants, tumours may be quite large, and associated with developmental abnormalities due to compression of adjacent structures during development.

The prognosis of pure immature teratoma is still debated, due to limited experience {2820}. In children, pure immature teratoma has an excellent prognosis, with no risk of recurrence or metastasis {1327,1583,2302}. In adults, most studies also show a good prognosis, with no recurrences after complete excision {1722,2278}.

Mixed germ cell tumours

J.K.C. Chan
L.H.J. Looijenga
A. Marx
A.L. Moreira
P. Ströbel
T.M. Ulbright
M. Wick

Definition
Mixed germ cell tumours are neoplasms composed of two or more types of germ cell tumours. The diagnosis should be supplemented by a listing of the germ cell tumour components and their approximate proportions.

ICD-O code   9085/3

Synonyms
Malignant teratoma intermediate; teratocarcinoma (obsolete)

Epidemiology
In adults, mixed germ cell tumours account for 16% of all mediastinal germ cell tumours {564,634,1246,1291,2820}, second only to teratomas and seminomas {634,1246,1581,1722,2820}. Virtually all patients are male {1246,1722}. In children, mixed germ cell tumours account for about 20% of all mediastinal germ cell tumours. Among children aged < 8 years, some (but not all) studies have reported a female predominance {203,1246,2303}, while all patients aged > 8 years are male {2303}.
The components of mixed germ cell tumours are different in pre- and postpubertal tumours. In children, most tumours are a combination of yolk sac tumour and teratoma (mature or immature). Other types are virtually non-existent during the first 4 years of life {2302}.
In adults, the two most common components are teratoma (in a mean of 65% of cases, ranging from 50% to 73%) and embryonal carcinoma (in a mean of 66% of cases, ranging from 22% to 100%) {275,536,634,1246,2567}. Less common components are yolk sac tumour (in a mean of 48% of cases, ranging from 0% to 83%), seminoma (in a mean of 38% of cases, ranging from 22% to 50%), and choriocarcinoma (in a mean of 28% of cases, ranging from 10% to 67%) {634,1246,1291,1722,2567}. The teratoma component is more often immature than mature {16,1291}. Adult (but not childhood) mediastinal mixed germ cell tumours are frequently associated with somatic malignancies.

Etiology
Mixed germ cell tumours can be associated with Klinefelter syndrome {183,969,970,1371,2303}.

Clinical features
Only about 10% of mixed germ cell tumours are asymptomatic at diagnosis {2567}. Most patients present with symptoms similar to those of other mediastinal germ cell tumours: chest pain, cough, dyspnoea, hoarseness, superior vena cava syndrome, and cardiac tamponade {2311,2567}. Precocious puberty and gynaecomastia are uncommon {1371}. In rare cases, endocrinological symptoms induced by production of the β-subunit of human chorionic gonadotropin (βhCG) may precede tumour diagnosis by years {2314}. A minority of patients present with symptoms attributable to metastases {872,927,2567}.
Most cases (about 90%) show elevated serum tumour marker levels {1246}. Raised α-fetoprotein (AFP) (in about 80% of cases) is strongly correlated with the presence of a yolk sac tumour component, although teratomatous hepatoid cells and teratomatous neuroepithelium can also produce small amounts of AFP. Increased βhCG levels (in about 30% of cases) occur in mixed germ cell tumours with a choriocarcinoma component or with syncytiotrophoblasts {2904}.
Imaging studies typically show a large, inhomogeneous mass with necrosis, haemorrhage, and infiltration of adjacent structures. The presence of cystic spaces or adipose tissue suggests the presence of a teratomatous component {927,2498}.
Most mixed germ cell tumours exhibit extensive infiltration into mediastinal structures and adjacent organs. The reported rates of metastasis at the time of diagnosis vary widely, from 20–36% {634,2302,2567} up to > 80% {1239, 2904}. Common sites of metastasis include the lung, pleura, lymph node, liver, bone, and brain {187,1246,2303,2567}.

Localization
Mixed germ cell tumours occur in the anterior mediastinum.

Macroscopy
The tumours are often frankly infiltrative, and show a heterogeneous cut surface, with solid fleshy tumour interspersed with areas of haemorrhage and necrosis. The presence of cystic spaces usually indicates the presence of a teratomatous component. Tumours range from 3 to 20 cm, with a mean size of 10 cm {1097}.

Cytology
Cytological diagnosis of mixed germ cell tumour is difficult, since only one element may be present in a preparation. The cytomorphological features of the germ cell tumour components are similar to those described for pure germ cell tumours (see *Seminoma*, *Embryonal carcinoma*, and *Yolk sac tumour*, pp. 244–254). Cytological diagnosis should always be correlated with clinical, serological, and radiographical studies.

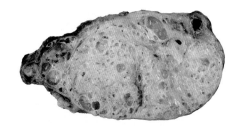

Fig. 3.119 Mixed germ cell tumour. Macroscopy of a mixed germ cell tumour of the anterior mediastinum resected after four cycles of BEP chemotherapy in a 27-year-old man; α-fetoprotein levels had decreased from 1100 to 40.8 ng/mL. Pathological examination showed foci of yolk sac tumour associated with teratomatous component.

Histopathology

Various types of germ cell tumours can occur in any combination, and their morphologies are identical to those of pure germ cell tumours. The individual germ cell tumour components can be discrete or (more commonly) intricately intermingled. The reported frequencies of the various germ cell tumour types vary widely in the literature (see above).

In children, unlike in adults, the teratoma components are more often mature than immature {203,2248,2303}. The diagnostic label polyembryoma is often used when there are prominent embryoid bodies in postpubertal tumours (so named because of their resemblance to early embryo). These are characterized by a central embryonic disc formed by pseudostratified columnar cells, with an amniotic cavity lined by flat to cuboidal cells on one side of the disc and a yolk sac on the other side, surrounded by loose mesenchyme. Polyembryoma is essentially a mixed germ cell tumour with at least embryonal carcinoma and yolk sac tumour components {183,2433}.

Histology of metastasis

The histology of metastases usually reflects the histology of the primary germ cell tumour or one of its components {16}, but other germ cell tumour histologies and somatic-type malignancies may also occur, particularly after chemotherapy {63,1566,1601,2711}.

Post-chemotherapy histology, including growing teratoma syndrome

After chemotherapy, residual viable non-teratomatous tumour is found in up to 50% of cases, even after normalization of serum tumour markers {2714}. In the remaining cases, necrosis, teratoma structures, inflammatory infiltrates (including xanthogranulomatous reaction), and fibrosis can be encountered. Chemotherapy may unmask a previously overlooked somatic-type tumour or teratomatous component. Metastases do not necessarily reflect the histology of remnant viable tumour in the primary location {63,1601}.

During or following chemotherapy, patients with germ cell tumour can show {2904}: 1) normalization of tumour markers and resolution of the tumour mass (10%), 2) persistent elevation of tumour markers and tumour mass due to resistance to chemotherapy (10%), or 3)

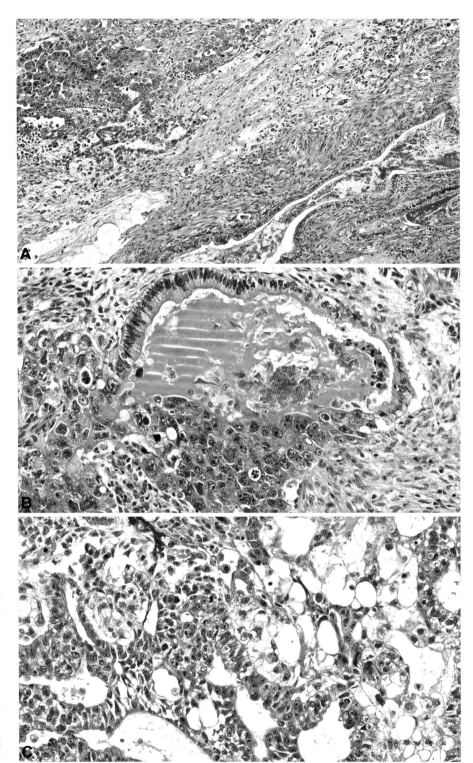

Fig. 3.120 Mediastinal mixed germ cell tumour. **A** The upper field shows embryonal carcinoma with a solid to glandular growth pattern; the lower field shows teratoma composed of glands lined by more bland-looking cells. **B** The embryonal carcinoma component (lower field) merges intricately with the teratomatous component (upper field), giving the impression of maturation of the former to the latter. **C** The embryonal carcinoma component (left field) merges into the yolk sac tumour component (right field), which shows a microcystic growth pattern and smaller cells with less conspicuous nucleoli.

normalization of tumour markers with residual tumour mass (80%). In the last group, 10–20% of patients exhibit tumour enlargement, which can be attributable to chemotherapy-resistant germ cell tumour components that do not secrete

AFP or βhCG, development of somatic-type malignancy, or growing teratoma syndrome. Growing teratoma syndrome is a rare complication of mixed germ cell tumours {21}, and defined by an increase in tumour size during or after chemotherapy, normalization of serum tumour markers, and the presence of mature teratoma only on histological analysis of the resected tumour specimen {1501}. The growing mediastinal mass can be asymptomatic or can produce symptoms such as fever, dyspnoea, or cardiopulmonary deterioration, sometimes necessitating urgent surgical intervention {21,1238,1601}. Lymphatic spread can involve mediastinal and supraclavicular lymph nodes {63}. Late complications are local or metastatic development of malignant non-seminomatous germ cell tumours (NSGCTs) and development of somatic-type sarcoma, carcinoma, or leukaemia {63,1601}.

Immunohistochemistry
The immunohistochemical profiles of the individual germ cell tumour components are identical to those of their pure counterparts.

Differential diagnosis
Embryonal carcinomas or seminomas containing scattered syncytiotrophoblastic cells do not qualify as mixed germ cell tumours, but are classified as the respective germ cell tumours. Unlike choriocarcinomas, they lack a cytotrophoblastic component that blends intricately with syncytiotrophoblasts to form a bilaminar pattern.

Genetic profile
In adults and children aged > 8 years, i(12p) and sex chromosomal abnormalities (often associated with Klinefelter syndrome) are the most common recurrent abnormalities of mediastinal mixed germ cell tumours {297,2303}. Additional recurrent changes include gain of chromosome 21 and loss of chromosome 13. These abnormalities are also encountered in the mature teratoma component and/or somatic-type malignant components of mixed germ cell tumours, while pure teratomas are typically devoid of genetic imbalances {1761,2303}.
In children aged < 8 years, i(12p) does not occur {2303}, and gain of the X chromosome and trisomy 21 {297,2303} are rare findings. Instead, gain of 1q, 3, and

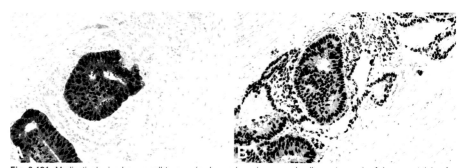

Fig. 3.121 Mediastinal mixed germ cell tumour (embryonal carcinoma and yolk sac tumour). **A** Immunostaining for OCT4 selectively highlights the embryonal carcinoma component. **B** Immunostaining for SALL4 highlights the yolk sac tumour component (which is OCT4-negative), in addition to embryonal carcinoma component.

20q, and loss of 1p, 4q, and 6q are common {297,2303} in yolk sac tumour; teratomatous elements show no chromosomal abnormalities.

Prognosis and predictive factors
In adults, mixed germ cell tumours exhibit a long-term survival rate of 40–50% {41,1492,1724}, and there appears to be no significant difference between mixed and pure NSGCTs {2567}. High tumour stage (particularly metastasis to the brain, liver, lung, and bone) and elevated βhCG levels are major risk factors for poor outcome with mixed germ cell tumours, as for NSGCTs {223,965}. Modern cisplatin-based chemotherapies and resection are the treatments of choice {41,223,274,1838,2906}.
In children, the prognosis of mixed germ cell tumour (teratoma and yolk sac tumour) is not different from that of pure yolk sac tumour {2302}; 5-year overall survival rates of > 80% can be achieved with modern therapies {2302}. Local stage, distant metastasis, and AFP levels were not shown to be of prognostic significance in a paediatric series of NSGCTs that included 24% mixed germ cell tumours {2302}. In young children, mixed germ cell tumours that consist of teratomas with only minor foci of yolk sac tumour have a good prognosis after complete resection and chemotherapy {1583}.
Small series suggest that an extensive seminoma component has a beneficial impact on survival {1714,1724}, while a choriocarcinoma component portends an aggressive clinical course {564,2820}.

Post-chemotherapy prognostic factors
Post-chemotherapy findings are the most important prognostic factors in the era of multimodality treatment. Primary

complete response (i.e. normalization of tumour marker levels and disappearance of the mediastinal mass after chemotherapy) occurs in 10% of patients with NSGCTs, and is associated with a long-term survival rate of 80% {732}. About 20% of patients relapse, usually within 2 years after chemotherapy, and may be amenable to salvage therapy {2904}.
Among patients who show normalization of tumour markers and a residual tumour mass (80% of patients) {732,733,2278,2904,2906}, completeness of resection is the most important prognostic factor in both adults {2278} and children {10,2302}. The salvage rates after incomplete resection are < 10% in adults and < 50% in children.
Post-chemotherapy histology has a bearing on prognosis {791,2144}: a complete lack of viable tumour cells is associated with a 90% disease-free survival rate, and the rate drops to 60% if viable teratoma (including growing teratoma syndrome) is present. The presence of viable non-teratomatous germ cell tumour or somatic-type malignancy is associated with a 30% and < 10% survival rate, respectively.
Patients with persistently elevated tumour markers have a worse prognosis than those with normalization of tumour markers, even though viable tumour is detectable in only half of the resection specimens from both groups {1239}. Relapses after chemotherapy and surgery, and primary resistance to chemotherapy are poor prognostic factors, due to low salvage rates {223}.

Germer cell tumours with somatic-type solid malignancy

P. Ströbel
J.K.C. Chan
L.H.J. Looijenga
A. Marx

A.L. Moreira
T.M. Ulbright
M. Wick

Definition

A germ cell tumour with somatic-type solid malignancy is a mediastinal germ cell tumour accompanied by a non-germ cell (i.e. somatic-type) malignant component of sarcoma or carcinoma.

Germ cell tumours with associated haematological malignancy (see p. 265) are a unique mediastinal variant of germ cell tumours with somatic-type malignancy.

ICD-O code   9084/3

Synonyms

Germ cell tumour with malignant transformation; germ cell tumour with non-germ cell malignancy

Epidemiology

Overall, germ cell tumours with somatic-type malignancy are rare, accounting for only about 2% of all male germ cell tumours {30}. However, about 25–30% of these cases occur in the mediastinum {2712}, and somatic-type malignancy seems to arise more frequently in mediastinal tumours than in gonadal or retroperitoneal primary tumours. Germ cell tumours with somatic-type malignancy can occur in patients with Klinefelter syndrome {2927}. Many of the germ cell tumours are of mixed type or teratomas {872,1566,1908,2711}, but somatic-type malignancy has also been observed in pure yolk sac tumours {2713} and seminomas {1055,2712}. With few exceptions {318,512,1291}, these tumours occur in adult males, with the incidence rate peaking between the ages of 20 and 40 years {491,1246,1291,1566,1722}. Somatic-type solid malignancy may arise in the primary germ cell tumour or only in the metastases {96,318,1761,1749}. It is more common after chemotherapy and in late tumour relapses.

Etiology

The etiology of somatic-type malignancy is unknown. It is not believed to be a direct consequence of cisplatin-based chemotherapy of the mediastinal germ cell tumour {1837}. There is evidence that cells from malignant germ cell tumours show remarkable plasticity and pluripotency (or even totipotency), which could explain the emergence of cells with somatic tissue-type differentiation {839,1025}. The malignant cells may retain some of the functional properties of their presumptive normal counterparts: the yolk sac is the common embryological origin of both primordial germ cells and haematopoietic progenitors, which could explain the preferential association of yolk sac tumours with haematological malignancies {1837}. However, the association between yolk sac tumour and haematological malignancy exists only in the mediastinum, and is not seen with gonadal yolk sac tumours. The available data support the conclusion that the germ cell tumour and the somatic-type malignancy component are clonally related {964,1381,1761,1837,2293}.

Clinical features

Germ cell tumours with somatic-type solid malignancy show the same local symptoms as other mediastinal germ cell tumours, but they are more frequently symptomatic (in about 90% of cases) than pure teratomas (in about 50% of cases). Symptoms due to metastatic disease may accompany or follow local symptoms {1761}. Most but not all cases show elevated α-fetoprotein and/or β-subunit of human chorionic gonadotropin levels in the serum. Other tumour markers (e.g. carcinoembryonic antigen or neuron-specific enolase) may be elevated depending on the malignant components present. Germ cell tumours with somatic-type solid malignancy have been described to be associated with fatal haemophagocytic syndrome {398,1067,2242}.

Imaging studies typically reveal a solid mass (representing the sarcoma or carcinoma component) associated with either a cystic teratomatous structure or a lesion showing heterogeneous attenuation, predominantly areas of enhancing soft tissue elements, calcifications, and massive necrosis {96,1961,2238,2498, 2562}.

Tumours infiltrate into the mediastinal structures and the lung {1566}. Metastases have been reported in the majority of cases {1566,1894}, and involve lung {491,1761}, regional lymph nodes {49,1239}, bone {1908,2927}, brain {2712,2927}, liver {49,2712}, and spleen {1761,2712}. Metastases can be composed of the somatic-type tumour {491,1566}, the germ cell tumour, or one of its components {1566}, or both {1566,2711}.

Localization

Germ cell tumours with somatic-type malignancy occur in the anterior mediastinum.

Macroscopy

The tumours range in size from 6 to 30 cm {1566,1722}. They usually exhibit a partially cystic and often variegated cut surface, with focally necrotic areas. The somatic-type malignancy component is firm and grey (carcinoma or sarcoma) or haemorrhagic (e.g. angiosarcoma), and often adherent to adjacent mediastinal structures {2712}.

Histopathology

Mature {318,512,1291,1749} and immature {634,1500,1894,2927} teratomas,

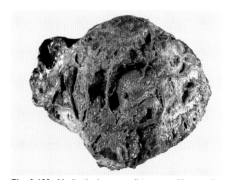

Fig. 3.122 Mediastinal germ cell tumour with somatic-type malignancy. This post-chemotherapy resection specimen is mostly necrotic, with focal areas of viable mature teratoma and yolk sac tumour. Histology revealed somatic-type malignancy (sarcoma).

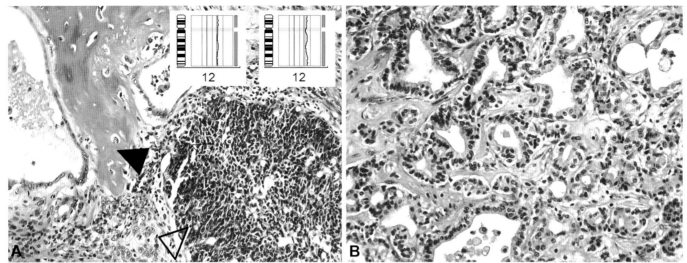

Fig. 3.123 Germ cell tumour with somatic-type solid malignancy. **A** Mediastinal mature teratoma with epithelial cysts and bone (black arrowhead) and neuroendocrine carcinoma (open arrowhead); both components show a gain of chromosome 12 (inset). **B** Enteric-type adenocarcinoma in mediastinal mature teratoma.

seminomas, yolk sac tumours, and mixed germ cell tumours can be associated with various sarcomas (in 63% of cases) {512,2711,2712}, carcinomas (in 37%) {1749}, or combinations of both {1255,1291,1664,2246,2712}. The somatic malignancy can be intimately intermingled with the germ cell tumour component, or can form an expansile nodular proliferation of atypical cells, often with increased mitotic rate and necrosis. Embryonal rhabdomyosarcoma {491,512,1566,2712} is the most common somatic-type malignancy. Angiosarcoma {488,1566,2711}, leiomyosarcoma {2712}, and neuroblastoma {482,1894} are also common, but any type of sarcoma (including chondrosarcoma, osteosarcoma, malignant peripheral nerve sheath tumour, primitive neuroectodermal tumour {2144}, glioblastoma, and liposarcoma {1724}) may occur. The epithelial malignancies associated with germ cell tumour are mostly colonic type adenocarcinomas {387,1255,1664,1749,1961, 2261}, but also include adenosquamous and squamous cell carcinomas {2144,2712}, while carcinoid tumours are rare {1395,2220,2293,2333}.

Immunohistochemistry
The somatic-type malignancy components stain like their counterparts elsewhere in the body, and generally do not express germ cell tumour markers such as PLAP, α-fetoprotein, or the β-subunit of human chorionic gonadotropin. However, rhabdomyoblasts, embryonal rhabdomyosarcomas, and leiomyosarcomas can express PLAP {864}, and hepatoid carcinomas can be α-fetoprotein-positive.

Differential diagnosis
Germ cell tumour with somatic-type malignancy may be difficult to distinguish from immature teratoma. Frank atypia and infiltrative growth favour somatic-type malignancy. Chemotherapy-induced atypia is usually diffusely distributed throughout the tumour, while somatic-type malignancy is a focal process, often forming a recognizable mass and invading adjacent structures {2498}. Scattered rhabdomyoblasts are a common feature of mature and immature teratomas, and do not justify a diagnosis of rhabdomyosarcoma unless they show nodular tumour formation and/or infiltration of adjacent structures. Rhabdomyoblasts can rarely occur in thymic carcinomas, but the thymic carcinoma is morphologically different from germ cell tumour and commonly expresses CD5, and the rhabdomyoblasts do not show atypia or proliferative activity.

Genetic profile
An isochromosome i(12p) genotype shared by the somatic-type neoplasia and the associated germ cell tumour component is typical {445,964, 1381,1761,2293,2998}. In one case of teratoma-associated rhabdomyosarcoma, an add(2)q35–37 genetic abnormality characteristic of rhabdomyosarcoma was detected in the sarcoma, but not the germ cell component {1761}, suggesting that tissue-specific secondary chromosomal aberrations may be necessary for the development of somatic-type malignancy in germ cell tumour.

Prognosis and predictive factors
The presence of somatic-type malignancy in germ cell tumour confers a dismal prognosis {634,872,1239,1246,1761}. There is no response to chemotherapies used for the treatment of germ cell tumours, and treatment should be tailored according to the transformed histology {614,1761}. Only a minority of patients survive after chemotherapy and complete surgical removal of the mediastinal tumour {1761,2712}. Advanced local infiltration, metastatic disease, and incomplete resection are adverse prognostic factors {1239,1566,2712}, while the type of somatic malignancy in the primary biopsy seems to have no major impact on survival {1761}. The persistence of viable tumour after chemotherapy heralds an unfavourable outcome {791,1239,2904}. The median survival is approximately 9 months {634,872,1239,1246, 1761}.

Germn cell tumours with associated haematological malignancy

A. Orazi   A.L. Moreira
J.K.C. Chan   T.M. Ulbright
L.H.J. Looijenga

Definition

Germ cell tumours with associated haematological malignancy are germ cell tumours accompanied by haematological malignancies that are clonally related to the underlying germ cell tumours. This association is a variant of somatic-type malignancy that is unique to mediastinal germ cell tumours. The haematological malignancies can involve the mediastinum, or can present as infiltration of bone marrow or lymphatic organs, leukaemia, or myeloid sarcoma. Haematopoietic malignancies that arise due to chemotherapy are not included in this category.

ICD-O code   9086/3

Epidemiology

Haematological malignancies develop in 2–6% of malignant non-seminomatous mediastinal germ cell tumours {962,1823} (i.e. in 0.5–1.5% of all mediastinal germ cell tumours), but virtually never occur in germ cell tumours of other sites {1582}. Patients are typically adolescents or young adults (patient age ranges from 9 to 48 years), and virtually all patients are male {363,570,1837}. About 10–20% of cases have been associated with Klinefelter syndrome {160,595,1837}.

Etiology

It is hypothesized that a totipotent or pluripotent primordial germ cell gives rise to a leukaemic clone. Alternatively, the presence of foci of extramedullary haematopoiesis within the yolk sac tumour component (which has been documented in some cases of mediastinal germ cell tumours) suggests the alternative possibility that these haematological malignancies may develop from more committed, somatic-type haematopoietic cells {1916}.

An association between mediastinal germ cell tumours and haematological malignancies has been recognized since the 1970s {3020}. Origin from a germ cell tumour-derived pluripotent cell and independence from previous radiochemotherapy have been hypothesized since the 1980s {1835,1836}. Genetic studies have demonstrated chromosomal aberrations shared between germ cell tumours and associated haematological malignancies {363,1381}, providing evidence for a clonal relationship. Extramedullary haematopoiesis in a subgroup of mediastinal germ cell tumours {1916} suggests that committed haematopoietic precursors could be an alternative origin. The predilection of the syndrome for mediastinal germ cell tumours remains unexplained. It has been speculated that the expression of haematopoietic growth and differentiation factors in some mediastinal germ cell tumours could drive the differentiation of primordial germ cells into haematopoietic progeny. The profile of differentiation factors expressed may also underlie the preferred commitment of transformed precursors to the megakaryocytic and monocytic lineage {1823,1916}. Concomitant mediastinal and extramediastinal leukaemias show a comparable immunophenotype and genotype, suggesting the spread of haematopoietic tumour cells from germ cell tumours to blood, bone marrow, and extramedullary sites {363,1381,1761}.

Clinical features

The most common clinical features at diagnosis of this haematological disorder include pancytopenia, hepatosplenomegaly, and thrombocytopenia – each occuring in 20–35% of cases. Bleeding complications and infections arise due to cytopenias in myelodysplastic syndromes, and acute leukaemias are also common events. Thromboembolic complications (due to thrombocytosis and megakaryocytic hyperplasia) {1837} and mediastinal mass formation (due to myeloid sarcoma) are rare {2246}. Other clinical signs are leukaemic skin lesions, flushing {964}, and the development of haemophagocytic syndromes {2719}. Haematological complications can accompany, follow {223,2719,2785}, or precede local symptoms. Leukaemias most commonly become apparent within the first year after diagnosis of germ cell tumours (at a median of 6 months after, with a range of 0–122 months) {570,964,1761,1837,1916}. There is no increased overall risk for other secondary tumours in patients with mediastinal germ cell tumours {221,223}.

Localization

Germ cell tumours with associated haematological malignancy occur in the anterior mediastinum.

Macroscopy

The gross findings are identical to those of non-seminomatous malignant germ cell tumours.

Histopathology

The germ cell tumours underlying the haematological malignancies are typically

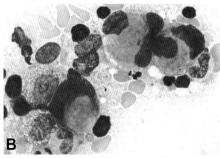

Fig. 3.124 Mediastinal germ cell tumour with associated haematological malignancy. **A** Bone marrow biopsy showing high-grade myelodysplastic syndrome (refractory anaemia with excess blasts); note the increased number of blasts and the presence of severe dysmegakaryopoiesis. **B** A bone marrow touch preparation of the same biopsy, showing high-grade myelodysplastic syndrome (refractory anaemia with excess blasts); note the presence of severe dysmegakaryopoiesis.

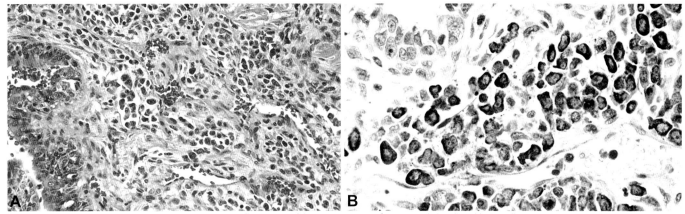

Fig. 3.125 Mediastinal germ cell tumour with haematopoietic differentiation. **A** Note the presence of haematopoietic cells within the yolk sac tumour blood vessels. **B** Intravascular proliferation of immature myeloid precursors showing myeloperoxidase immunoreactivity

non-seminomatous malignant germ cell tumours – most often yolk sac tumours or mixed germ cell neoplasias with a yolk sac component, although immature teratomas and mixed germ cell tumours with somatic-type sarcomas have also been observed {93,363,964,1380,1761,1837}. The categories of reported haematological malignancies are: acute leukaemias {223,1408}, disseminated histiocytic sarcoma (malignant histiocytosis) {93,160,570,1380,1837}, and (rarely) localized histiocytic proliferations {3033}, myelodysplastic syndromes {445,1823,2428,2785}, myeloproliferative diseases {363,1381,1837}, and mastocytosis {396}. Among the acute leukaemias, acute megakaryoblastic leukaemia and acute myeloid leukaemia with monocytic differentiation {891,1381,2760,2998} are the most common, accounting for about half of all cases {223,1837,1916}. Acute myeloid leukaemia, differentiated {2785}; erythroleukaemia {1823,2262}; acute undifferentiated leukaemia {1837}; and acute lymphoblastic leukaemia {1408,1837} have also been described. Myelodysplastic syndromes include refractory anaemia with excess blasts {2428} and cases with megakaryocytic hyperplasia {1835}. Myelodysplasia can precede acute myeloid leukaemias {2785}. Essential thrombocythaemia and primary myelofibrosis are the types of myeloproliferative neoplasms encountered in association with mediastinal germ cell tumours {797,1837}. Leukaemias may diffusely or focally infiltrate the underlying germ cell tumour {1916}, or can form tumorous lesions (myeloid sarcoma) in the

mediastinum {2246}. Extramediastinal manifestations (e.g. organomegaly and leukaemia) can occur in the presence or absence of detectable haematopoietic malignancy in the mediastinal germ cell tumour {1916}.

Immunohistochemistry
Interpretation of cytochemical findings in blood or bone marrow smears, and of immunophenotypic profiles follows the criteria of the *WHO classification of tumours of haematopoietic and lymphoid tissues* {2548}. CD34 and terminal deoxynucleotidyl transferase can be used to identify the presence of blasts. Useful immunohistochemical stains for myeloid-associated antigens include myeloperoxidase, CD33, CD117, CD68, CD14, CD163, lysozyme, CD61 (or CD42b), and CD71 (or glycophorin). Additionally, CD10, CD19, CD79a, CD7, and CD3 may be useful for excluding the possibility of acute lymphoblastic leukaemia. If blastic plasmacytoid dendritic cell tumour is under consideration, then CD123, CD4, and CD56 must be added.

Differential diagnosis
Clonally related haematological malignancies must be distinguished from secondary myelodysplastic syndromes and acute myeloid leukaemias that are related to salvage chemotherapy regimens (including etoposide treatment) in patients with mediastinal germ cell tumour {1316,2246}. In one large series, secondary myelodysplastic syndromes and acute myeloid leukaemias occurred in 0.7% and 1.3% of cases, respectively

{1316}. Chemotherapy-related acute myeloid leukaemias do not show i(12p), and usually manifest later (25–60 months after chemotherapy) than germ cell-related acute myeloid leukaemias (which have a median time to onset after chemotherapy of 6 months, ranging from 0 to 122 months) {964,1837}.

Genetic profile
Isochromosome i(12p) is the most specific and most common chromosomal marker shared by germ cell tumours and the associated haematological malignancies {363,445,1761,1837,2998}. The haematological malignancies can also harbour other genetic alterations more typically seen in various haematological malignancies – such as del(5q) and trisomy 8 – suggesting that aberrations not specific to germ cell tumour determine the phenotype of the associated haematological malignancy {1761}.

Prognosis and predictive factors
The occurrence of a clonally related acute leukaemia in a patient with mediastinal germ cell tumour is among the most adverse prognostic factors. In a published series, none of the reported patients survived for > 2 years after the onset of leukaemia; the median survival was 6 months {964}. These leukaemias appear to be refractory to current treatment protocols, including aggressive induction chemotherapy and allogeneic bone marrow transplantation {1067,3020}. However, the clinical course in patients with myeloproliferative neoplasms may be more protracted {797}.

Lymphomas of the mediastinum
Primary mediastinal large B-cell lymphoma

W. Klapper   R. Gascoyne
E.S. Jaffe   P. Möller
P. Gaulard   S. Nakamura
N.L. Harris   A. Rosenwald

Definition

Primary mediastinal (thymic) large B-cell lymphoma is an aggressive large B-cell lymphoma arising in the mediastinum, of putative thymic B-cell origin, and with distinctive clinical, immunophenotypic, genotypic, and molecular features.

ICD-O code   9679/3

Synonyms

Not recommended: primary mediastinal clear cell lymphoma of B-cell type {1706}; mediastinal diffuse large cell lymphoma with sclerosis {1653}

Epidemiology

Primary mediastinal large B-cell lymphoma (PMBL) accounts for about 2–3% of all non-Hodgkin lymphomas, and occurs predominantly in young adults (during the third and fourth decade), with a female predominance {346,956,1421,2627,3029}.

Etiology

No evidence of extrinsic risk factors for the development of PMBL has been identified. It is unrelated to EBV or other known viruses {346}. Exome sequencing of a family with three PMBL patients identified *MLL* as a candidate predisposition gene {2239}.

Clinical features

Patients present with a localized anterior-superior mediastinal mass. Symptoms, which are related to the mediastinal mass, include superior vena cava syndrome (most frequently), airway obstruction, and pleural and/or pericardial effusion. B symptoms may be present.
On imaging, the mass is often bulky, and invades adjacent structures such as the lung, pleura, or pericardium. Local spread to supraclavicular and cervical lymph nodes can occur. A characteristic feature of PMBL is its regular contour and the absence of (or presence of only minimal) cervical and abdominal lymphadenopathy on imaging {2599}.

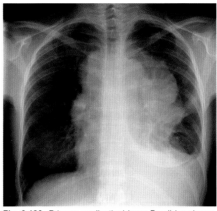

Fig. 3.126 Primary mediastinal large B-cell lymphoma. A chest radiograph showing a large mediastinal mass.

About 80% of cases are stage I–II at the time of diagnosis, with a mediastinal tumour > 10 cm (i.e. a bulky mass) in 60–70% of patients. Infiltration of the lung, chest wall, pleura, and pericardium is frequent. Pleural or pericardial effusions are present in one third of cases {3029}. Leukaemia is never observed, and bone marrow involvement is infrequent. At progression, dissemination to distant extranodal sites such as the kidney, adrenal glands, liver, and central nervous system is relatively common, but disseminated lymph node or bone marrow involvement is rare.
Staging is performed according to the Ann Arbor scheme for lymphomas {483}. Stage is established using both standard radiological procedures and PET. Stage is combined with other clinical factors to evaluate prognostic risk using the International Prognostic Index {3027}.

Localization

Virtually all patients with PMBL present with a tumour in the thymic area (anterior-superior mediastinum), which is thought to be the origin of the neoplasm {19}.

Macroscopy

PMBL presents as a solid mass lesion, tan to light brown, and sometimes with central necrosis.

Cytology

Fine-needle aspiration biopsy can be used successfully in most cases to differentiate between lymphoma and other malignant tumours, but definitive diagnosis and subclassification of lymphoma is not advised based on fine-needle aspiration biopsy alone.

Histopathology

Histomorphology
The growth pattern is diffuse and the large cells usually form clusters or sheets. The centre of the lesion contains predominantly neoplastic cells. However, at the periphery of the mass, a variable number of reactive cells such as lymphocytes, macrophages, and granulocytes may be present. A frequent but not consistent feature is a distinctive fibrosis made up of irregular collagen bands compartmentalizing cellular areas of varying size {1706,2009,2993}. This stromal component is frequently absent if lymph nodes are involved. In cases with locoregional lymph node involvement, the invasion

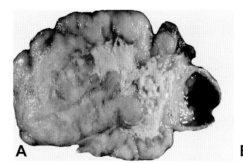 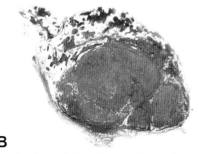

Fig. 3.127 Primary mediastinal large B-cell lymphoma. **A** Gross view shows a fleshy tan tumour with areas of necrosis. **B** Low-power magnification shows intrathymic tumoural growth of the primary mediastinal large B-cell lymphoma.

pattern is carcinoma-like, starting from marginal sinuses, with gradual replacement of the normal lymphoid tissue.

PMBL has a wide range of cytomorphology. The cells range from medium-sized to large (2–5 times the size of a small lymphocyte); have abundant, frequently clear cytoplasm; and have irregularly round or ovoid (occasionally multilobated) nuclei, usually with small nucleoli {2009}. Some cases may contain cells with pleomorphic nuclei and abundant amphophilic cytoplasm, and may resemble Hodgkin lymphoma or non-lymphoid tumours {2009,2667}. Rarely, there are so-called grey zone borderline lesions combining features of PMBL and classical Hodgkin lymphoma. Examples of composite PMBL and nodular sclerosis classical Hodgkin lymphoma have been described, and PMBL may occur either before or at relapse of nodular sclerosis classical Hodgkin lymphoma {2667}.

Immunohistochemistry
PMBL expresses B-cell lineage antigens such as CD19, CD20, CD22, and CD79a, but characteristically lacks immunoglobulin expression, despite a functional immunoglobulin gene rearrangement and expression of the transcription factors PAX5, BOB.1, OCT2, and PU.1 {1198,1498,2057}. CD30 is present in > 80% of cases, but unlike in classical Hodgkin lymphoma, the expression is usually weak and heterogeneous {994,2057}. CD15 expression has not been extensively studied. Tumour cells are frequently positive for IRF4/MUM1 (75%) and CD23 (70%), and have variable expression of Bcl2 and Bcl6. CD10 expression is uncommon {307,546,2057}. Tumour cells are also positive for MAL antigen, CD54, CD95, TRAF1, p63, and nuclear REL {489,490,2057,3008}. PMBLs often lack HLA class I and/or class II molecules {1706,1707}. PMBL is CD11c-positive in about 40% of cases {2165}. TNFAIP2 was recently identified to be aberrantly expressed in PMBL, a feature in common with classical Hodgkin lymphoma but rarely found in diffuse large B-cell lymphoma (DLBCL), not otherwise specified {1321}.

Differential diagnosis
The diagnosis of PMBL requires a combination of pathological and clinical data. Absence of widespread extrathoracic lymph node or bone marrow involvement is required to exclude DLBCL with mediastinal involvement, since no histopathological, immunohistochemical, or genetic features readily differentiate between these diseases. DLBCL involving the mediastinum often shows involvement of mediastinal lymph nodes rather than the thymic area, and more abundant extramediastinal involvement than PMBL. Classical Hodgkin lymphoma has a prominent inflammatory background, which is generally absent in PMBL. CD45 is negative in classical Hodgkin lymphoma, but often difficult to evaluate by immunohistochemistry. Lymphomas sharing histopathological features of both classical Hodgkin lymphoma and PMBL have been described, and are categorized as B-cell lymphoma, unclassifiable, with features intermediate between DLBCL and classical Hodgkin lymphoma

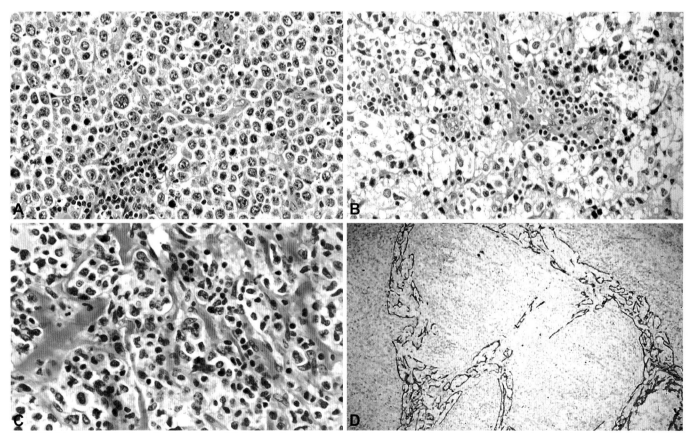

Fig. 3.128 Primary mediastinal large B-cell lymphoma. **A** In this case, there are intermingled Hodgkin/Reed-Sternberg-like cells in a background of more typical monomorphous tumour cells. **B** This case is composed predominantly of large cells with abundant clear cytoplasm, resembling the lacunar cells of nodular sclerosis classical Hodgkin lymphoma. **C** There is delicate sclerosis creating an alveolar-like pattern. **D** The tumour has infiltrated thymic tissue, as indicated by staining for cytokeratin.

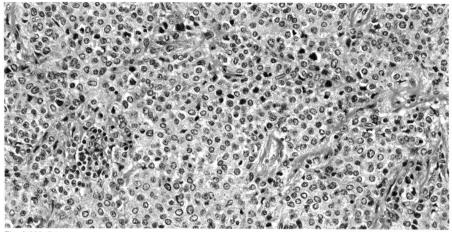

Fig. 3.129 Primary mediastinal large B-cell lymphoma. The histopathology of a typical primary mediastinal large B-cell lymphoma shows diffuse sheets of large blastic cells with clear or pale eosinophilic cytoplasm.

(sometimes referred to as mediastinal grey zone lymphoma).

Genetic profile

Immunoglobulin genes are rearranged, and may be class-switched, with a high load of somatic hypermutation without ongoing mutations {1447}. Rearrangements of *BCL2*, *BCL6*, and *MYC* genes are absent or rare {2689}. Breaks in the HLA class II transactivator *CIITA* at 16p13.13 have been reported in 38% of PMBL, associated with downregulation of HLA class II molecules and overexpression of ligands of the receptor molecule PD1 (PDL1 and PDL2) {2460}. The genomic profile typically contains gains

such as amplified regions in chromosomes 9p24.1, including the *JAK2/PDL2* locus (up to 75%); 2p16.1, including the *REL/BCL11A* locus (51%); Xp11.4–21 (33%); and Xq24–26 (33%). This profile is relatively unique among DLBCLs, but similar to that of classical Hodgkin lymphoma {180,1162,2854}. Copy number gains and high-level amplification (29%), as well as rearrangements (20%) of PDL1 and PDL2 occur almost exclusively in PMBL {2707}. Further gains map to 12q31 (30%), 7q22 (32%), and 9q34 (32%) {180}. Candidate genes include *REL* and *BCL11A*, which are amplified in a proportion of PMBL leading to a frequent (albeit inconsistent) nuclear accumulation

of their proteins {2177,2850,2851}, and *JAK2* {1162,1651}. PMBL has a unique transcriptional signature that is distinct from those of other forms of DLBCL, but shares similarities with that of classical Hodgkin Lymphoma {2200,2286}. PMBL has constitutively activated NF-κB {721}, possibly due to deleterious mutations in the *TNFAIP3* gene, which is found in 36% of PMBL and encodes A20 (a zinc finger protein and negative regulator of NF-κB) {2300} and JAK-STAT signalling pathways (also found in classical Hodgkin lymphoma) {2696,2851}. Mutations of *BCL6* are detected in about 54% of PMBLs {1561}. Mutations affecting the *STAT6* DNA-binding domain occur in 36% of PMBLs, and are not found in DLBCL {2164}. Recurrent mutations in *PTPN1*, a negative regulator of JAK-STAT signalling, are found in 22% of PMBLs {920}. There are no *BRAF* or *KRAS* hotspot mutations in PMBL {1788}.

Prognosis and predictive factors

Variations in the cytomorphology of PMBL have not been associated with prognosis {2009}. Extension into adjacent thoracic viscera or pleura, pericardial effusion, and poor performance status are associated with inferior outcome {346,1421,1422,2286}. In adults, the prognosis of PMBL seems to be at least as good as that of DLBCL, not otherwise specified, with a plateau in the survival curve {2152,3029}. Recently adopted immunochemotherapy protocols have shown a high cure rate in adults as well as in children {639,2899}, without requiring adjuvant radiotherapy.

Fig. 3.130 Primary mediastinal large B-cell lymphoma. **A** Immunohistochemistry for CD20 shows strong staining of all cells. **B** The cells are positive for CD23. **C** There is variable staining for CD30. **D** Immunohistochemistry for CD11c shows that a subset of the cells are positive.

Extranodal marginal zone lymphoma of mucosa-associated lymphoid tissue (MALT lymphoma)

H. Inagaki
J.K.C. Chan
E.S. Jaffe
N.L. Harris
P. Möller
S. Nakamura

Definition
Thymic extranodal marginal zone lymphoma of mucosa-associated lymphoid tissue (MALT lymphoma) consists of heterogeneous populations of small B cells, which include centrocyte-like, monocytoid, plasmacytoid, and plasma cells that surround reactive lymphoid follicles and infiltrate the thymic epithelium to form lymphoepithelial lesions.

ICD-O code   9699/3

Synonyms
Primary thymic extranodal marginal zone lymphoma; thymic extranodal marginal zone B-cell lymphoma of MALT

Epidemiology
Thymic MALT lymphoma is rare {1078, 1094,1515,1996,2557}. Most patients are in their sixth or seventh decade, with patient ages ranging from 14 to 75 years. Male patients tend to be about 10 years older than female patients on average. There is a female predominance (with a female-to-male ratio of 3:1) and approximately 80% of reported cases have occurred in Asian patients.

Etiology
Thymic MALT lymphoma is strongly associated with autoimmune disease (> 60% of cases), especially Sjögren syndrome {1078}. An association of thymic MALT

lymphoma with micronodular thymoma has also been reported {2492}. There is no association with EBV {1078}. There is currently no evidence for a histogenetic link with primary mediastinal (thymic) large B-cell lymphoma.

Clinical features
Patients are usually asymptomatic, with the mediastinal tumour discovered incidentally on chest radiograph. A minority of patients present with chest pain, shortness of breath, haemoptysis, or back pain. In cases associated with autoimmune disease (most commonly Sjögren syndrome), the time interval between the onset of autoimmune disease and the discovery of the thymic tumour ranges from 2 to 25 years {1078}. Monoclonal gammopathy (frequently IgA and occasionally IgG or IgM) is common {1515}.
The bulk of the disease is in the anterior mediastinum, but the regional lymph nodes are sometimes involved. Concurrent MALT lymphoma at other sites (e.g. the salivary gland or lung) occurs in about 20% of cases.
Most tumours are of low stage (I or II) at presentation {1078}.

Localization
By definition, the tumour involves the thymus. Regional lymph nodes may also be involved.

Macroscopy
Grossly, the tumour is often encapsulated and consists of solid greyish-white fleshy tissue, commonly interspersed with multiple, variable-sized cysts. The tumours range from 1.5 to 17.5 cm in greatest dimension. Invasion into the adjacent pericardium and pleura is sometimes found.

Histopathology
The normal thymic lobular architecture is effaced by a dense lymphoid infiltrate, but residual Hassall corpuscles can still be identified. There are commonly many interspersed epithelium-lined cystic spaces. Reactive lymphoid follicles are scattered within the lymphoid infiltrate,

surrounded by small lymphocytes, centrocyte-like cells, plasmacytoid lymphocytes, and scattered centroblast-like cells. The centrocyte-like cells have small to medium-sized irregular nuclei, indistinct nucleoli, and a moderate amount of pale cytoplasm. They show extensive invasion of the thymic epithelium, forming lymphoepithelial lesions. The lymphoid cells within and immediately around the epithelial structures usually possess an even greater amount of clear cytoplasm, reminiscent of monocytoid B cells. There are often interspersed aggregates of plasma cells, which show immunoglobulin light chain restriction on immunohistochemical staining. This finding is very useful in establishing a diagnosis, especially for early lesions, in which neoplastic cells are found only focally in the lymphoid proliferation. In some cases, the immunoglobulin product may form crystals, which then accumulate in benign histiocytes, producing the picture of crystal-forming histiocytosis. Transformation to diffuse large B-cell lymphoma has only rarely been reported {1515}.
The tumour cells express B cell-specific markers, such as CD20 and CD79a. They are negative for CD3, CD5, CD10, CD23, CD43, and cyclin D1, but positive for the marginal zone cell marker IRTA1 {696}. They commonly express Bcl2, and > 70% of the cases express IgA.

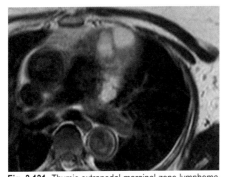

Fig. 3.131 Thymic extranodal marginal zone lymphoma of mucosa-associated lymphoid tissue. Chest MRI (T2-weighted image) shows an anterior mediastinal mass (at the upper middle of the figure) with solid and cystic components.

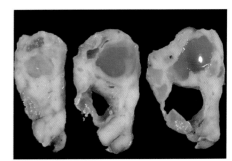

Fig. 3.132 Thymic extranodal marginal zone lymphoma of mucosa-associated lymphoid tissue. The cut surface of the tumour (the same case as in the previous figure), shows fleshly, tan-coloured tumour tissue (approximately 4 cm in the major axis) interspersed with multiple cystic spaces containing greenish fluid.

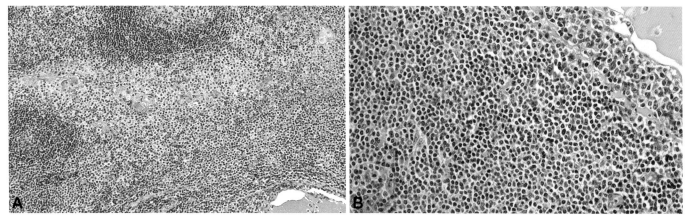

Fig. 3.133 Thymic extranodal marginal zone lymphoma of mucosa-associated lymphoid tissue. **A** Lymphoid follicles with intact mantle zone are surrounded by a diffuse small lymphoid infiltrate; the middle field shows thymic epithelium (including Hassall corpuscles), heavily infiltrated by lymphoma cells with pale cytoplasm; in the lower-right corner, there is an epithelium-lined cyst containing eosinophilic proteinaceous fluid. **B** The epithelium lining the cyst is invaded by neoplastic B cells forming a lymphoepithelial lesion.

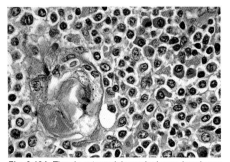

Fig. 3.134 Thymic extranodal marginal zone lymphoma of mucosa-associated lymphoid tissue. A Hassall corpuscle surrounded by neoplastic B cells and plasma cells.

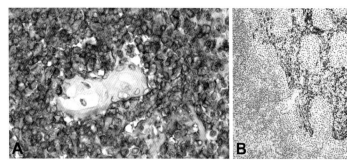

Fig. 3.135 Thymic extranodal marginal zone lymphoma of mucosa-associated lymphoid tissue. **A** Dense infiltrate of CD20+ neoplastic B cells around a Hassall corpuscle. **B** Keratin staining showing lymphoepithelial lesions.

Differential diagnosis

The main differential diagnoses are multilocular thymic cyst, lymphoepithelial sialadenitis-like thymic hyperplasia, and thymic follicular hyperplasia (which is most frequently associated with myasthenia gravis) {1996}. In these reactive processes, the thymic lobular architecture is fairly well preserved, there is no band-like or sheet-like proliferation of centrocyte-like cells or monocytoid cells, CD20+ cells do not occur in dense sheets, and the plasma cells show polytypic staining for immunoglobulin. Other differential diagnoses include Castleman disease, IgG4-related sclerosing disease, thymoma, seminoma, Hodgkin lymphoma, and diffuse large B-cell lymphoma.

Genetic profile

This lymphoma is derived from postgerminal centre marginal zone B cells. Immunoglobulin genes are clonally rearranged {1078,2557}. A biased use of the *VH* genes is reported, suggesting that thymic MALT lymphomas may originate from specific subsets of B cells {2976}. Only one case has been studied by cytogenetics, with the finding of 46,X,dup(X)(p11p22) {950}. Thymic MALT lymphoma shows a high frequency of trisomy 3, a low incidence of trisomy 18, and an absence of translocations involving the *MALT1* or *IGH* genes {854,1317}. Deletion of the *A20* gene (an NF-κB inhibitor) has been reported in one case {854}. There is no known genetic susceptibility.

Prognosis and predictive factors

Thymic MALT lymphoma is associated with an excellent outcome. Only one tumour-related death has been reported {1078}. High tumour stage at presentation or concurrent involvement of other MALT sites is not necessarily associated with a poor prognosis. Most patients have undergone surgical resection both for diagnosis and treatment of low-stage disease. Chemotherapy and radiotherapy have also resulted in complete remission in some cases.

Other mature B-cell lymphomas

A. Rosenwald
R. Gascoyne
N.L. Harris

E.S. Jaffe
P. Gaulard

Hodgkin lymphoma; primary mediastinal large B-cell lymphoma; B-cell lymphoma, unclassifiable, with features intermediate between diffuse large B-cell and classical Hodgkin lymphoma; and extranodal marginal zone lymphoma of mucosa-associated lymphoid tissue are the main mature B-cell lymphomas, but there are also several others. These other mature B-cell lymphomas involve mediastinal lymph nodes or soft tissue, and generally reflect the spectrum of other systemic nodal and extranodal B-cell lymphomas. However, due to the mediastinum's inaccessibility as a biopsy site, the primary diagnosis is rarely made on mediastinal biopsies. The mature B-cell lymphomas that arise in or (more frequently) involve the mediastinum include follicular lymphoma, small lymphocytic lymphoma, nodal marginal zone lymphoma, mantle cell lymphoma, diffuse large B-cell lymphoma, and Burkitt lymphoma. The epidemiology, etiology, clinical features, cytology, macroscopy, localization, histopathology, genetic profile, prognosis, and predictive factors of these lymphomas are detailed in the *WHO classification of tumours of haematopoietic and lymphoid tissues* {2548}

T lymphoblastic leukaemia / lymphoma

T.J. Molina
N.L. Harris
E.S. Jaffe
W. Klapper

Definition
T lymphoblastic leukaemia/lymphoma is a neoplasm of lymphoblasts committed to the T-cell lineage, typically composed of small- to medium-sized blast cells with scant cytoplasm, moderately condensed to dispersed chromatin, and indistinct nucleoli. The neoplasm variably involves the thymus, lymph nodes, bone marrow, and peripheral blood. T lymphoblastic lymphoma (T-LBL), by convention, is the term used when the process is confined to a mass lesion with no or minimal evidence of peripheral blood and bone marrow involvement. T acute lymphoblastic leukaemia (T-ALL) is the appropriate term when there is extensive peripheral blood and bone marrow involvement. If a patient presents with a mass lesion and lymphoblasts in the bone marrow, the distinction between T-ALL and T-LBL is arbitrary. For many treatment protocols, the presence of > 25% bone marrow blasts is used to define leukaemia.

ICD-O code   9837/3

Synonym
Precursor T-ALL/precursor T-LBL

Epidemiology
T lymphoblastic neoplasms occur most commonly in late childhood, adolescence, and young adulthood. There is a male predominance, and 15% of childhood and 25% of adult acute lymphoblastic leukaemias are of T-cell type {242}. Cases presenting without bone marrow and peripheral blood involvement (i.e. lymphoblastic lymphomas) account for 85% of all lymphoblastic lymphomas, for 25–30% of childhood non-Hodgkin lymphomas, and for only 2% of adult non-Hodgkin lymphomas worldwide {2627}. Some studies have reported that there is an increased prevalence of T lymphoblastic neoplasia in developing countries, while B-cell lymphoblastic neoplasms are more common in industrialized countries {2659}.

Etiology
The etiology is unknown. No association with viruses or immune status has been demonstrated. Patients with ataxia telangiectasia are at increased risk for development of T-ALL, but the *ATM* gene has not been implicated in sporadic T lymphoblastic neoplasia {2575}. In early childhood T-ALL, the neoplastic clone can be detected at birth by clone-specific T-cell receptor gene rearrangement, suggesting that the transforming event occurs in utero {703}.

Clinical features
Patients typically present acutely with symptoms related to a large mediastinal

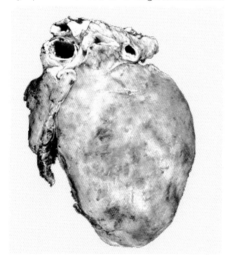

Fig. 3.136 T lymphoblastic lymphoma. A solid tumour mass with infiltration of mediastinal fat and involvement of the great vessels.

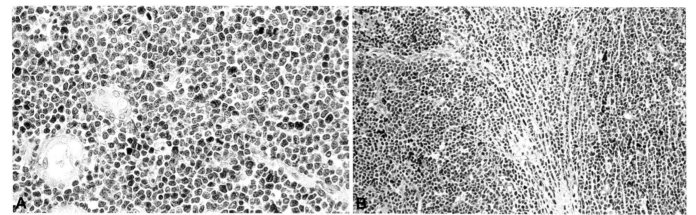

Fig. 3.137 T lymphoblastic lymphoma. A Diffuse destructive tumour growth effacing corticomedullary compartments; note the residual Hassall corpuscles; this pattern must not be confused with type B thymoma. B Diffuse tumour growth and a streaming pattern in interlobular septa.

mass, often with pleural or pericardial effusions. Airway compromise is common, and the presentation is often as a medical emergency.

Localization
The tumour typically involves the mediastinum (specifically the thymus), and often the mediastinal lymph nodes. The supradiaphragmatic lymph nodes may also be involved, and tumour cells are often shed into the pleural fluid. The bone marrow and peripheral blood are involved at some point during the clinical course in the majority of cases. Central nervous system involvement is also common.

Cytology
On smears, lymphoblasts vary from small cells with scant cytoplasm, condensed nuclear chromatin, and indistinct nucleoli to larger cells with a moderate amount of cytoplasm, dispersed chromatin, and multiple nucleoli. Azurophilic granules may be present. Fine-needle aspiration biopsy and/or core biopsies, even with flow cytometry, may not be reliable for distinguishing T-LBL from thymoma, since the immunophenotype of the blast cells may be indistinguishable from that of cortical thymocytes.

Histopathology
The thymus and mediastinal soft tissue, as well as adjacent lymph nodes, are involved. The epithelial meshwork is destroyed, septa are effaced, and the tumour cells spread through the capsule into adjacent mediastinal tissue. In tissue sections, the cells are small to medium-sized, with scant cytoplasm and round, oval, or convoluted nuclei with fine

chromatin and indistinct or small nucleoli. Occasional cases have larger cells with prominent nucleoli. In lymph nodes, the pattern is infiltrative rather than destructive, often with partial preservation of the subcapsular sinus and germinal centres. Mitotic figures are typically numerous. A starry-sky pattern may be present, but is usually less prominent than in Burkitt lymphoma. Pleural or pericardial fluid may be the initial diagnostic specimen. Cases with increased tissue eosinophils should be assessed for translocation involving the *FGFR1* gene on chromosome 8p11, which is associated with both myeloid and lymphoid differentiation and a poor prognosis {1084}.

Immunophenotype
T-ALL and T-LBL share common immunophenotypic features. Flow cytometry in addition to immunohistochemistry is often helpful for optimal classification of the precursor cell neoplasia. The lymphoblasts are usually positive for terminal deoxynucleotidyl transferase (TdT). In addition to TdT, the most specific markers to indicate the precursor nature of T lymphoblasts are CD34 and CD1a. CD99 is also a marker of immaturity, but is also expressed in peripheral T-cell lymphomas, small round cell tumours, and small cell carcinoma, and might be misleading – especially if the tumour is TdT-negative.
Only CD3 expression is considered truly T-cell lineage-specific. Cells variably express CD2, CD7, CD5, CD1a, CD4, and/ or CD8 and CD10. The constellation of antigens resembles stages of thymic T-cell differentiation, ranging from early or pro-T and pre-T (cytoplasmic CD3+,

CD1a–, CD4–, and CD8–), to cortical thymocyte (CD1a+, surface CD3+, CD4+, and CD8+), to late thymocyte (CD1a–, surface CD3+, CD4+, or CD8+). There is some correlation with presentation and differentiation stage (cases with bone marrow and blood presentation may show earlier differentiation stage than cases with thymic presentation {189,888}), but there is overlap {2108}.
Among cases that express T-cell receptor proteins, the majority express the alpha/beta type, and a minority express the gamma/delta type (which appear to have a more immature phenotype) {308,2551}. Rare cases of lymphoblastic lymphoma presenting in the mediastinum have the immunophenotype of immature NK cells (cytoplasmic CD3+ and CD56+) {379,1310,2354}. Thus, the minimal histopathological criteria for classification as T-LBL are expression of CD3 in a TdT-positive lymphoma when B-cell CD19 and myeloid differentiation (i.e. myeloperoxidase or monocytic markers) is not detectable. About 12% of T-LBLs express CD79a, and a subset of T-LBLs express CD13 and/or CD33; these features are not considered evidence of a mixed phenotype. If either CD19 or CD22, and PAX5 or myeloperoxidase are expressed in a CD3-positive precursor cell neoplasm, the criteria of a mixed phenotype acute leukaemia/lymphoma are fulfilled {1936}.
A small subset of TdT-negative T-LBL/T-ALL has been reported, and is considered to be of high risk {3026} and closely related to high-risk early thymic progenitor T-ALLs {499} that coexpress (in addition to CD3) early myeloid markers (i.e. CD13, CD33, and HLA-DR) and

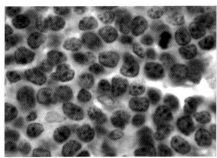

Fig. 3.138 Mediastinal T lymphoblastic lymphoma. The tumour cells have dispersed chromatin, small nucleoli, and scant cytoplasm, such that the nuclei appear to overlap.

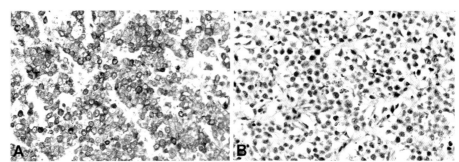

Fig. 3.139 T lymphoblastic lymphoma. **A** Immunohistochemistry for CD3 shows only cytoplasmic staining. **B** Immunohistochemistry shows nuclear terminal deoxynucleotidyl transferase staining.

early stem cell markers (i.e. CD117 and CD34).

Differential diagnosis

On biopsy specimens, the differential diagnosis often includes thymoma with a prominent immature T-cell population (type B1 or B2 thymoma). The immunophenotype of T-LBL can be identical to that of the normal cortical thymocytes in thymoma. The infiltrative growth of the lymphoblasts in T-LBL, with replacement of the thymic epithelium and invasion of mediastinal fat, is an important distinguishing feature. Demonstration of clonality by molecular genetic analysis or identification of a molecular abnormality (such as *NOTCH1* mutation) or cytogenetic abnormality can be helpful in confirming the diagnosis of lymphoma.

In patients with a mediastinal mass and lymphocytosis, a diagnosis of peripheral T-cell lymphocytosis associated with thymoma should be considered {144,541,1713}. In such cases, the circulating T cells are polyclonal.

Genetic profile

Molecular and cytogenetic studies suggest that T-ALL and T-LBL share many characteristics, although there are some subtle differences in their biological profile {151,292}.

The T-cell receptor genes are clonally rearranged in most (but not all) cases, and T-cell receptor immunogenetic analysis identifies different subsets of lymphoblastic lymphoma, based on maturational stages of T-cell development, which correlate with some clinical features, mainly age at presentation {129}.

Mutations in *NOTCH1* (48–60%), or in *NOTCH1* and/or *FBXW7* (55–64%) are most frequent {228,308}; loss of heterozygosity of chromosome 6q occurs in 12% of cases {228,293} in paediatric lymphoblastic lymphoma protocols. Other genetic aberrations have been described in T-LBL, but due to the low number of analysed cases, the frequency and clinical relevance of these aberrations remain uncertain. These lesions include loss of heterozygosity of 9p21 (*CDKN2A/B*), 11q

(*ATM*), and 17p {1347}; cytogenetic aberrations in the *CDKN2A* locus {2725}; t(9;17)(q34;q23) {1200,1503,2325}; translocations involving the *TCRA/TCRD* locus on 14q11 {1503}; and fusion transcripts *PICALM-MLLT10* (*CALM-AF10*) and *NUP214-ABL1* {129}. All of these lesions except t(9;17)(q34;q23) have been detected in T-ALL.

Prognosis and predictive factors

With aggressive therapy, the prognosis is similar to that of B-cell lymphoblastic neoplasms, and does not appear to correlate with immunophenotype or genetic abnormalities {861}. Mutations of *NOTCH1/FXBW7* are associated with a favourable prognosis, while loss of heterozygosity at 6q and absence of T-cell receptor gamma gene biallelic deletion predict a potentially worse prognosis {228,293,308}.

Anaplastic large cell lymphoma and other rare mature T- and NK-cell lymphomas

L. Lamant
P. Gaulard
J.K.C. Chan
E.S. Jaffe

S. Nakamura
T.J. Molina
L. de Leval

Definition

Peripheral NK- and T-cell lymphoma is a term that collectively designates all lymphoid neoplasms derived from mature (post-thymic) NK and T cells. Anaplastic large cell lymphoma (ALCL) is emphasized in this section, because of its peculiar features and the likelihood of it being confused with non-haematological malignancies.

ALK-positive ALCL is a mature T-cell lymphoma associated with translocation of *ALK* with a variety of other genes, most commonly *NPM1*. A characteristic feature is strong expression of CD30 and the presence of hallmark cells.

ICD-O codes

ALK-positive anaplastic large
   cell lymphoma   9714/3
ALK-negative anaplastic large
   cell lymphoma   9702/3

Synonym

Ki1 lymphoma (obsolete)

Epidemiology

ALCL accounts for 3% of adult non-Hodgkin lymphomas {2461}, and for 15–20% of childhood mature non-Hodgkin lymphomas. It is the most prevalent mature T/NK-cell lymphoma in children {626,1018}. ALK-positive ALCL accounts for more than 90% of all ALCLs in children {269}, but for only 50% of adult cases {2386}.

Clinical features

Patients may present with cough, dyspnoea, or chest pain related to a mediastinal mass. Extranodal involvement (skin, bone, soft tissue, lung, or liver) is more common in ALK-positive than ALK-negative ALCL. Most patients present with advanced-stage (III or IV) disease. Staging is performed according to the Ann Arbor staging classification.

Localization

The thymus and mediastinum are not primary sites of predilection, but mediastinal involvement is not uncommon, and most commonly occurs in the context of advanced-stage disease.

Histopathology

ALCL is characterized by a tendency for a cohesive growth pattern and sometimes an intrasinusoidal growth in lymph nodes. All cases contain a variable proportion of characteristic cells (hallmark cells) with abundant cytoplasm, a kidney-shaped nucleus, and a prominent Golgi region {2548}. In ALK-positive cases, several morphological patterns are recognized (common, small cell, lymphohistiocytic, and Hodgkin-like), and can coexist in a single lesion (composite pattern). ALK-negative ALCL is currently included as a provisional entity in the *WHO classification of tumours of haematopoietic and lymphoid tissues*; it is defined as a tumour morphologically indistinguishable from ALK-positive ALCL {2548}, but lacking the ALK protein.

In ALCL, the tumour cells are strongly positive for CD30 in a membranous and Golgi pattern, and virtually all cases co-express epithelial membrane antigen. The loss of several pan-T-cell antigens is frequently observed, while expression of cytotoxic molecules is common {1392,2285}. In ALK-positive ALCL, the tumour cells express the ALK fusion protein, for which the subcellular distribution depends on the *ALK* partner gene

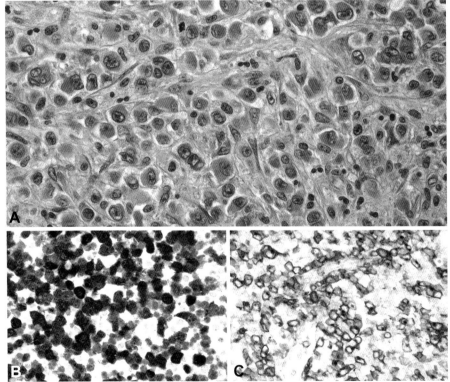

Fig. 3.140 ALK-positive anaplastic large cell lymphoma. **A** Predominant population of large cells, including so-called hallmark cells with kidney-shaped nuclei. **B** In a case associated with the t(2;5) translocation, ALK staining is cytoplasmic, nuclear, and nucleolar (expression of the nucleophosmin-ALK fusion protein). **C** Strong expression of CD30 highlights the perivascular accentuation of tumour cells, frequently observed in anaplastic large cell lymphoma.

involved in the chromosomal translocation {2548}.

Differential diagnosis
ALCL may mimic carcinoma or melanoma due to its growth pattern, and cases
with nodular fibrosis and capsular thickening may resemble mediastinal large
B-cell lymphoma or classical Hodgkin
lymphoma. However, these diagnoses
can be ruled out by immunophenotyping
for keratin, S100, pan-B-cell and pan-T-
cell antigens, CD15, epithelial membrane
antigen, and ALK.
For ALK-negative ALCL, the most difficult differential diagnosis is peripheral
NK- and T-cell lymphoma, not otherwise
specified with CD30 expression, because
there are no unique defining immunophenotypic or genetic features {210,2548}.

Genetic profile
A monoclonal rearrangement of the T-
cell receptor genes is observed in 90%
of cases. ALK-positive ALCLs are associated with a chromosomal translocation
involving the *ALK* gene. The majority are
associated with t(2;5)(p23;q35) juxtapos-
ing *ALK* to the *NPM1* gene, but *ALK* can
also be fused with many other partner
genes {1351,1758}. A recurrent t(6;7)
(p25;q32) translocation has been identified in a small subset of ALK-negative
ALCL {710}.

Prognosis and predictive factors
The prognosis is generally favourable
with systemic chemotherapy. However,
along with other clinical and biological
factors, mediastinal involvement is associated with a poor outcome in childhood
series {269,626,1424,2321,2880}. No
study has addressed the prognostic significance of mediastinal involvement (observed in 30% of adult cases) {2386}. In
adults, the positive prognostic impact of
ALK expression is partially dependent on
age {2386}. Younger patients with ALCL
with and without ALK expression have
similar outcomes.

Hodgkin lymphoma

S. Nakamura
E.S. Jaffe
N.L. Harris
A. Rosenwald

Definition

Hodgkin lymphoma is a monoclonal B-cell lymphoid neoplasm diagnosed by the identification of Reed-Sternberg (RS) cells or variants in the appropriate cellular environment. The two major types are classical Hodgkin lymphoma and nodular lymphocyte-predominant Hodgkin lymphoma {648,1564}. A subtype of classical Hodgkin lymphoma – nodular sclerosis classical Hodgkin lymphoma (NSCHL) – is the most common subtype worldwide, especially in industrialized countries. It frequently presents in the mediastinum, sometimes with involvement of the thymus. Other subtypes are exceedingly rare in mediastinal biopsies, and are described in the *WHO classification of tumours of haematopoietic and lymphoid tissues* {2548}.

ICD-O code   9650/3

Synonym

Hodgkin disease

Epidemiology

Lymphomas account for approximately 15% of all mediastinal masses {2363}, and 10% of them are primary {645}. NSCHL accounts for 50–70% of primary mediastinal lymphomas, and is most prevalent between the ages of 15 and 34 years. The disease is more common in industrialized countries, is associated with higher socioeconomic status, and has continued to slightly increase in incidence over the past few decades {462}. Females are more often affected than males. The disease is less common in Blacks and Asians.

Etiology

The pathogenesis of mediastinal NSCHL remains to be elucidated. This lymphoma is rarely associated with EBV, and possibly originates from thymic B cells {1702,2200,2286,2667}. Genetic predisposition may play a role, and familial cases have been reported {863}. HLA-DR2 and HLA-DR5 are overrepresented in EBV-negative Hodgkin lymphoma {1046}.

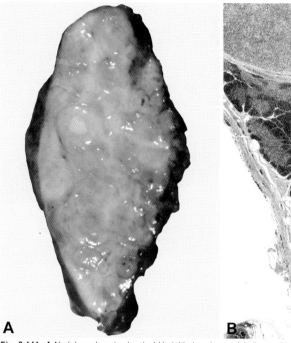

Fig. 3.141 A Nodular sclerosis classical Hodgkin lymphoma. A bulky mediastinal mass that was surgically resected. The cut surface shows lobulated, firm, yellowish nodules divided by fibrous bands. **B** Nodular sclerosis classical Hodgkin lymphoma involving the thymus. The tumour is sharply demarcated from the residual thymus, but infiltrates into the adjacent thymic medulla.

Clinical features

Symptoms directly attributable to a large anterior mediastinal mass may include chest discomfort, dyspnoea, and cough. NSCHL tends to simultaneously involve the lower cervical, supraclavicular and mediastinal lymph nodes.

Hodgkin lymphoma typically spreads to contiguous lymph node regions, rather than showing discontinuous dissemination. Mediastinal Hodgkin lymphoma may directly invade adjacent lung and pericardium. Large mediastinal masses may show direct extension through the chest wall.

Classical Hodgkin lymphoma is staged according to the Ann Arbor staging classification with the Cotswolds modification {1486}.

Localization

Mediastinal Hodgkin lymphoma commonly arises from the thymus, the mediastinal lymph nodes, or both.

Macroscopy

NSCHL sometimes forms a very large mass and shows multiple, firm, white or yellowish nodules, with or without visible fibrous bands, on the cut surface. The tumour is sharply demarcated from residual thymic remnants or frankly infiltrative. Thymic involvement may be accompanied by cyst formation.

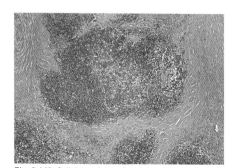

Fig. 3.142 Cellular nodules of nodular sclerosis classical Hodgkin lymphoma are completely separated by concentric fibrous bands of mature collagen.

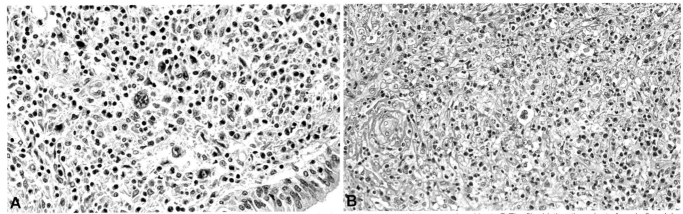

Fig. 3.143 A Mediastinal nodular sclerosis classical Hodgkin lymphoma involving the lung; adjacent bronchial mucosa is evident. **B** The fibrohistiocytic variant of grade 2 nodular sclerosis classical Hodgkin lymphoma is characterized by a marked infiltrate of histiocytes and inflammatory cells, which may obscure the Hodgkin/Reed-Sternberg cells.

Cytology

The cytology of Hodgkin lymphoma of the mediastinum is the same as that observed in other sites.

Histopathology

The diagnosis is based on the presence of RS cells and variants in a rich inflammatory background {648,955,2548}. Classical RS cells are large, with abundant eosinophilic or amphophilic cytoplasm, and contain double or multiple nuclei with large, eosinophilic nucleoli and perinucleolar clearing. Mononuclear variants are called Hodgkin cells. Classical RS cells generally make up only a minority of the neoplastic population, and mononuclear cells predominate. Degenerated RS cells with condensed cytoplasm and pyknotic nuclei are called mummified cells. The lacunar variant of the RS cell is common in NSCHL. Lacunar cells are characterized by relatively small, hyperlobated nuclei, small nucleoli, and abundant pale cytoplasm that is retracted in formalin-fixed tissues. Paradoxically, classical RS cells may be difficult to identify in NSCHL. The cellular constituents and the degree of collagen

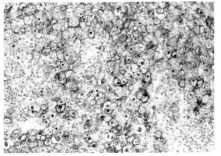

Fig. 3.144 Nodular sclerosis classical Hodgkin lymphoma. Strong expression of CD30 in Hodgkin/Reed-Sternberg cells.

formation vary widely, even within the same specimen. The criteria of both lacunar cells and collagen bands are highly reproducible for the definite diagnosis of NSCHL. Cases demonstrating typical lacunar cells with minimal or absent fibrosis are designated as the cellular phase of NSCHL. Lacunar cells may occur in clusters in the syncytial variant. The fibrohistiocytic variant is characterized by increased histiocytes and fibroblasts, without heavy collagen deposition. The inflammatory background of NSCHL consists of lymphocytes, plasma cells, and granulocytes. Eosinophilic abscesses and geographical necrosis are common. Two grades of NSCHL have been proposed, based on nuclear pleomorphism, lymphocyte depletion, or increased eosinophils {1542}, but grading is considered optional {2756}.

To establish the primary diagnosis of classical Hodgkin lymphoma in small biopsies, either classical multinucleated RS cells or lacunar cells showing the typical immunophenotype should be identified, and this may require examination of multiple levels of the biopsy.

Immunohistochemistry
The most reliable markers for classical Hodgkin lymphoma are CD30 and CD15. CD30 is expressed on RS cells and variants in 85–96% of cases, in a membranous pattern with accentuation in the Golgi area of the cytoplasm {2548}. CD15 is found in 75–85% of cases, although staining may be restricted to a minority of the neoplastic cells. In < 20–40% of cases, CD20 is detectable, usually on a minority of the neoplastic cells, with varied intensity. PAX5 and fascin are also useful markers for classical

Hodgkin lymphoma. PAX5 is expressed more weakly in RS cells than in normal B cells. IRF4/MUM1 is positive, but Bcl6 is usually negative. Aberrant expression of T-cell antigens may be seen, usually in cases of higher grade {2771}. Association with EBV, demonstrated by EBV-encoded small RNA, is infrequent (10–25%) in NSCHL. The reactive background contains variable numbers of B and T lymphocytes, with the latter forming rosettes around individual tumour cells.

Differential diagnosis
The differentiation of classical Hodgkin lymphoma from diffuse large B-cell lymphoma is easily made by morphology and immunohistochemistry in most cases. Primary mediastinal (thymic) large B-cell lymphoma is a distinct form of diffuse large B-cell lymphoma. Some cases show overlapping features between primary mediastinal large B-cell lymphoma and classical Hodgkin lymphoma. These cases are referred to as B-cell lymphoma, unclassifiable, with

Table 3.11 Genetic features that provide evidence for the B-cell origin of classical Hodgkin lymphoma

Clonal Ig heavy and light chain gene rearrangement in Hodgkin/Reed-Sternberg (HRS) cells
Somatic mutations in *V* genes of HRS cells
Aberrant somatic mutation of several proto-oncogenes in HRS cells
Class switch recombination in classical Hodgkin lymphoma cell lines
Clonally related composite lymphomas of classical Hodgkin lymphoma and B-cell non-Hodgkin lymphoma
Ig loci-associated chromosomal translocations in HRS cells of about 20% of classical Hodgkin lymphoma

Table 3.12 Somatic genetic aberrations in Hodgkin/Reed-Sternberg cells (only genes in which mutations were found are listed); data summarized in {1362}

Gene	Approximate frequency	Pathway/function
Main tumour suppressor gene mutations		
NFKBIA	15%	NF-κB
NFKBIE	15%	NF-κB
TNFAIP3	40% (70% in EBV-negative cases)	NF-κB
SOCS1	40%	JAK-STAT
TP53	8%	DNA damage response, apoptosis, and cell-cycle regulation
CD95 (FAS)	6%	Extrinsic apoptosis
Gains and amplifications of proto-oncogenes		
REL	50%	NF-κB
MAP3K14	25%	NF-κB
JAK2/JMJD2C/PDL1/PDL2	35%	JAK-STAT, histone modification, immune evasion
MDM2	60%	Apoptosis regulation
BCL3	15%	NF-κB
Chromosomal translocations		
CIITA	15%	HLA class II expression
BCL6	1%	Regulation of germinal centre
JAK2	3%	JAK-STAT
BCL3	10%	NF-κB
Ig loci[a]	20%	

[a] Translocations with various partners (e.g. BCL1, BCL2, BCL3, BCL6, and MYC), mostly still unknown.

features intermediate between diffuse large B-cell lymphoma and classical Hodgkin lymphoma, also known as grey zone lymphoma {650,1564,2667} (see *B-cell lymphoma, unclassifiable, with features intermediate between diffuse large B-cell lymphoma and classical Hodgkin lymphoma*, p. 280). Synchronous or metachronous cases of both neoplasms are excluded from this category. Only rare cases of anaplastic large cell lymphoma (ALK-positive) have histology resembling NSCHL {2761}.

Genetic profile

Immunoglobulin gene rearrangement studies of isolated single cells have verified the clonal nature of Hodgkin/Reed-Sternberg cells in almost all cases {1362,1363}. The high load of somatic mutations in the rearranged immunoglobulin genes supports a germinal centre derivation, specifically preapoptotic germinal centre B cells. Therefore, escape from apoptosis is assumed to represent the major oncogenic event in classical Hodgkin lymphoma lymphomatogenesis.

Hodgkin/Reed-Sternberg cells have a much higher number of chromosomal aberrations, including multiple numerical as well as structural abnormalities, than most other lymphomas. However, it is still unclear whether this is mostly a side-effect of some type of genetic instability, or whether the expression of specific oncogenes or tumour suppressor genes is recurrently affected by these lesions. Several recurrent genetic lesions have been identified in classical Hodgkin lymphoma. The most frequently found lesions affect members of the NF-κB or JAK-STAT signalling pathways.

By gene expression profiling, classical Hodgkin lymphoma and primary mediastinal large B-cell lymphoma are closely related {2200,2286,2667}.

Interactions between Hodgkin/Reed-Sternberg cells and background inflammatory cells play a role in the prognosis of classical Hodgkin lymphoma. The cytokine milieu plays a role in creating this microenvironment {898,1362,2457}.

Prognosis and predictive factors

Patients are usually treated with chemotherapy (with or without radiotherapy) adapted to clinical stage, which has greatly improved prognosis with recent protocols {1029}. Stage is the single most important prognostic factor. In situ evaluations of biological markers related to the tumour microenvironment have been shown to be prognostically relevant, but are not applied in routine clinical practice {2457,2459,2588}. The use of PET to evaluate response to chemotherapy is very helpful for clinical management {486}.

B-cell lymphoma, unclassifiable, with features intermediate between diffuse large B-cell and classical Hodgkin lymphoma

E.S. Jaffe
R. Gascoyne
S. Nakamura
S.A. Pileri
A. Rosenwald

Definition
B-cell lymphoma, unclassifiable, with features intermediate between diffuse large B-cell and classical Hodgkin lymphoma is a B-cell lineage lymphoma with clinical, morphological, and/or immunophenotypic features that overlap between classical Hodgkin lymphoma (especially nodular sclerosis classical Hodgkin lymphoma, NSCHL), and diffuse large B-cell lymphoma (especially primary mediastinal large B-cell lymphoma PMBL). Most cases present with a mediastinal mass. In the mediastinum, the term mediastinal grey zone lymphoma (MGZL) is also used.

ICD-O code   9596/3

Synonyms
Mediastinal grey zone lymphoma; Hodgkin-like anaplastic large cell lymphoma (obsolete)

Epidemiology
The epidemiology of MGZL is similar to that of NSCHL, with the exception that MGZL is more common in males than in females {1161,2667}. It usually presents in patients aged between 20 and 40 years. Cases occurring outside the mediastinum are seen in older patients {650}. Most cases have been reported

from Western countries. Like NSCHL, the disease is less common in Blacks and Asians.

Etiology
The etiology is unknown. Like NSCHL, MGZL is infrequently positive for EBV {1161,2667}.

Clinical features
Most patients present with a large mediastinal mass that may be associated with superior vena cava syndrome. The mass may cause tracheal compression and respiratory distress {1161,2667}.

Localization
The most common presentation is with a large anterior mediastinal mass, with or without involvement of the supraclavicular lymph nodes. Other peripheral lymph node groups are less commonly involved. There may be spread to the lung

by direct extension, as well as spread to the liver, spleen, and (less commonly) bone marrow. Non-lymphoid organs are rarely involved, unlike in PMBL {638}.

Macroscopy
The tumour has a tan, fish-flesh appearance, often with extensive areas of necrosis. Areas of fibrosis may also be present.

Cytology
Cytological features are not reliable for distinguishing this tumour from other mediastinal lymphomas.

Histopathology
The tumour is composed of a confluent, sheet-like growth of pleomorphic tumour cells in a diffusely fibrotic stroma. Focal fibrous bands may be seen in some cases. The cells are larger and more pleomorphic than in the typical case of

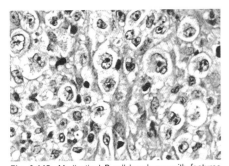

Fig. 3.145 Mediastinal B-cell lymphoma with features intermediate between diffuse large B-cell lymphoma and classical Hodgkin lymphoma, showing a sheet-like growth of large cells, with fibrillary fibrosis. Some cells resemble lacunar cells and mononuclear Hodgkin cells.

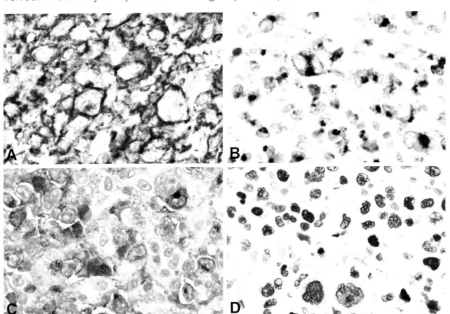

Fig. 3.146 B-cell lymphoma with features intermediate between diffuse large B-cell lymphoma and classical Hodgkin lymphoma. A The CD20 stain is strongly positive in all tumour cells. B CD15 is positive in the tumour cells, including cells both with and without Hodgkin/Reed-Sternberg-like features. C CD30 is positive, with some cells showing strong Golgi staining. D Staining for OCT2 is strongly positive in all tumour cells, including those with Hodgkin/Reed-Sternberg-like features.

PMBL, although some centroblast-like cells may be present. Pleomorphic cells resembling lacunar cells and Hodgkin cells are readily seen. A characteristic feature is the broad spectrum of cytological appearances, with different areas of the tumour showing variations in cytological appearance. The background inflammatory infiltrate is less evident than in NSCHL, although scattered eosinophils, lymphocytes, and histiocytes may be present. Necrosis is usually evident {1161,2667}.

In immunohistochemical stains, the B-cell programme is often preserved, with expression of both CD20 and CD79a. Both CD30 and IRF4/MUM1 are usually positive, but CD15 is less commonly expressed. Surface and cytoplasmic immunoglobulins are absent. The transcription factors PAX5, OCT2, and BOB.1 are usually positive. Bcl6 is variable, and CD10 and ALK are negative. The background lymphocytes are predominantly CD3+/CD4+, as seen in classical Hodgkin lymphoma. MAL, a marker associated with PMBL, is expressed in at least a subset of the cases. Nuclear cREL/p65 protein has been identified in those cases tested {1161,2667}.

Genetic profile
Clonal immunoglobulin gene rearrangement is often positive. The tumour cells show many of the genetic aberrations reported in PMBL and NSCHL {2458}. In particular, gains at 2p16.1 (the *REL* locus) and alterations at 9p24.1 involving the *JAK2/PDL2* locus are common {650}. Genetic and epigenetic profiling show differences with both classical Hodgkin lymphoma and PMBL {649,2758}.

Prognosis and predictive factors
These lymphomas generally have a more aggressive clinical course and worse outcome than either classical Hodgkin lymphoma or PMBL. There is no consensus on the optimal treatment, although there is evidence that combined-modality treatment is required, with both chemotherapy and radiation therapy used for patients with a residual PET-positive mass at the completion of the chemotherapy regimen {638,2887A}.

Histiocytic and dendritic cell neoplasms of the mediastinum

J.K.C. Chan
E.S. Jaffe
S.A. Pileri

Langerhans cell lesions

Definition

Langerhans cell histiocytosis is a neoplastic proliferation of Langerhans cells that show immunoreactivity for CD1a, S100 protein, and langerin, as well as the ultrastructural presence of Birbeck granules. Langerhans cell sarcoma differs from Langerhans cell histiocytosis in that it has overtly malignant cytological features. It can present de novo or can (exceptionally) progress from antecedent Langerhans cell histiocytosis.

ICD-O codes

Thymic Langerhans cell
  histiocytosis   9751/1
Langerhans cell sarcoma   9756/3

Synonyms

Eosinophilic granuloma; histiocytosis X (not recommended)

Epidemiology

Involvement of the thymus or mediastinal lymph node by Langerhans cell histiocytosis is rare {1471}, usually occuring in the setting of disseminated disease {248,1167,2299}. Langerhans cell sarcoma is even rarer, but a case was reported to have arisen from a mediastinal germ cell tumour, with involvement of the thymus, mediastinal lymph nodes, and other sites {2054}.

Clinical features

Rare cases of Langerhans cell histiocytosis presenting with thymic involvement have been reported {260,836, 1431,1880,1880,2796}. In children, the thymus is often markedly enlarged due to extensive involvement; there can be invasion of the surrounding mediastinal structures. In adults, the thymic involvement is usually subtle, and is discovered incidentally in thymi removed primarily for another indication; thus, the reported association with myasthenia gravis is probably fortuitous {260,836,1880,2796}.

Histopathology

The key histological feature of Langerhans cell histiocytosis is a diffuse infiltrate of non-cohesive Langerhans cells with grooved or markedly contorted nuclei, thin nuclear membranes, fine chromatin, and eosinophilic cytoplasm. There are commonly admixed multinucleated giant cells and eosinophils. Necrosis can be present. The Langerhans cells typically express S100 protein, CD1a, and langerin (CD207). The ultrastructural hallmark is presence of Birbeck granules.

The thymus can be involved diffusely or focally. The involved areas show destruction of the normal thymic parenchyma, damage to Hassall corpuscles, interlobular connective tissue infiltration, and scattered calcospherites {2299,2393}. Localized thymic involvement in adults often

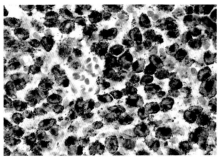

Fig. 3.148 Langerhans cell histiocytosis. Immunostaining for langerin (CD207) shows granular staining in the tumour cells.

takes the form of scattered small nodular aggregates of Langerhans cells. This can be accompanied by reactive lymphoid hyperplasia or multilocular thymic cyst {2796}.

An important differential diagnosis is histioeosinophilic granuloma of the mediastinum, a reactive lesion resulting from iatrogenic pneumomediastinum, akin to reactive eosinophilic pleuritis {931,1662}. Although both histioeosinophilic granuloma and Langerhans cell histiocytosis feature histiocytes and eosinophils, the histiocytes in the former are confined to the capsule or septa of the thymus with sparing of the parenchyma, the nuclei are uncommonly grooved, and S100 protein immunostain is negative.

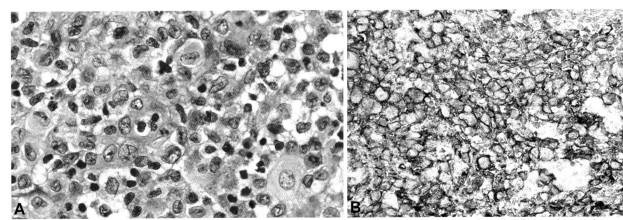

Fig. 3.147 Langerhans cell histiocytosis presenting as a thymic mass. **A** There is a diffuse infiltrate of cells with grooved nuclei, delicate nuclear membrane, and eosinophilic cytoplasm; note the presence of some admixed eosinophils. **B** Immunostaining shows CD1a expression in the tumour cells; macrophages are spared.

Genetic profile

BRAF V600E and V600D mutations are found in about half of all cases of Langerhans cell histiocytosis {954,1204}.

Prognosis and predictive factors

In children with thymic/mediastinal node involvement in the setting of multi-system disease, the 5 year overall survival is 87% {631A}. In children or adults with thymic involvement alone, outcome appears excellent with or without treatment, but available data are limited {631A}.

Histiocytic sarcoma

Definition

Histiocytic sarcoma is a malignant proliferation of cells with morphological and immunophenotypic features of mature tissue histiocytes. Neoplastic proliferations associated with acute monocytic leukaemia are excluded, but may show overlapping features due to closely related cell lineage.

ICD-O code   9755/3

Synonym

True histiocytic lymphoma (obsolete)

Epidemiology

Histiocytic sarcoma is a rare neoplasm. It affects a wide age range, from infants to the elderly; however, most cases occur in adults (with a median age of approximately 50 years). A male predominance has been found in some studies, but not in others {2058}. Only a single case has been reported to show predominant involvement of the mediastinum {1196}.

One reported case of primary central nervous system histiocytic sarcoma relapsed in the mediastinum after 3.5 years {324}.

Etiology

The etiology is unknown. A subset of cases occur in patients with mediastinal non-seminomatous germ cell tumour, most commonly malignant teratoma, and often with a yolk sac tumour component {2507}. The histiocytic sarcomas that arise in this setting often show systemic involvement. Since teratocarcinoma cells may differentiate along haematopoietic lines in vitro, these histiocytic neoplasms probably arise from pluripotent germ cells. Some cases appear to arise by transdifferentiation from either B-cell or T-cell neoplasms {709}.

Clinical features

Patients may present with a solitary mass, but systemic symptoms are relatively common. The mediastinum is an extremely uncommon site of presentation, with most cases arising in other extranodal sites, including the skin, bone, soft tissue, intestine, lymph nodes, and spleen {1033,2058}.

Macroscopy

The tumour may have a very heterogeneous appearance, especially when associated with a germ cell neoplasm.

Histopathology

Histiocytic sarcomas are composed of a diffuse proliferation of large, non-cohesive cells with abundant cytoplasm. The proliferating cells may be monomorphic or (more commonly) pleomorphic. The individual neoplastic cells are usually large and round to oval in shape; however, focal areas may show sarcomatoid features with a spindle cell component {1033,2058}.

The cytoplasm is usually abundant and eosinophilic, often with some fine vacuoles. Haemophagocytosis may occasionally be seen in the neoplastic cells. The nuclei are generally large, round to oval or irregularly folded, and often eccentrically placed; large multinucleated forms are commonly seen. Chromatin is usually dispersed, with a vesicular appearance. A variable number of reactive cells may be seen, including small lymphocytes, plasma cells, benign histiocytes, neutrophils, and eosinophils.

Immunohistochemistry and differential diagnosis

Immunostaining is essential for distinction from other large cell neoplasms, such as diffuse large B-cell lymphoma, anaplastic large cell lymphoma, melanoma, and carcinoma.

By definition, there is expression of one or more histiocytic markers, including CD163, CD68 (such as clones KP1 and PG-M1), and lysozyme, with typical absence of Langerhans cell markers (CD1a and langerin), follicular dendritic cell markers (CD21 and CD35), and myeloid cell markers (myeloperoxidase) {1033,2058,2790}. However, CD33 and CD13, often used as myeloid markers, may be positive in histiocytic sarcoma {1495}. CD4 and CD14 are both often positive, as are the transcription factors CEBPA or CEBPB, PU.1, and BOB.1 {709}. In addition, CD45 and HLA-DR are usually positive. Rarely, weak expression of CD15 occurs. There may be expression of S100 protein, but it is usually weak

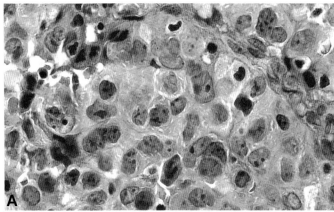
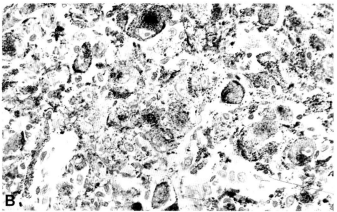

Fig. 3.149 Histiocytic sarcoma. **A** The neoplastic cells are large, and have abundant eosinophilic cytoplasm; this case was associated with a mediastinal germ cell neoplasm. **B** The tumour cells show granular immunostaining for CD68 (PG-M1).

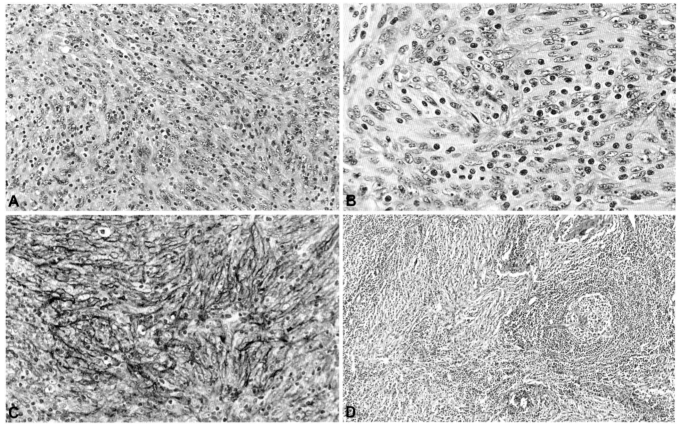

Fig. 3.150 Follicular dendritic cell sarcoma of the thymus. **A** A fascicular to storiform growth pattern; irregular clustering of nuclei and sprinkling of small lymphocytes are evident. **B** The tumour contains spindle cells with indistinct cell borders, elongated pale nuclei, and small distinct nucleoli; the nuclei appear irregularly clustered, and there are many admixed lymphocytes. **C** Immunostaining for CD21 highlights the tumour cells, which are elongated and form a meshwork. **D** On the right is a component of coexisting hyaline-vascular Castleman disease.

or focal, in contrast to the stronger reactivity in Langerhans cells and interdigitating dendritic cells {2790}. The Ki-67 index is variable.

Genetic profile
Histiocytic sarcomas usually lack clonal immunoglobulin or T-cell receptor gene rearrangements, but some cases have been reported to show antigen receptor gene rearrangements, most likely representing examples of transdifferentiation from lymphomas {408,709}.
The rare cases arising in mediastinal germ cell tumour show isochromosome 12p, identical to the genetic change in the germ cell tumour.

Prognosis and predictive factors
Histiocytic sarcoma is usually an aggressive neoplasm, with a poor response to therapy, although some exceptions have been reported. Most patients (60–80%) die of progressive disease, reflecting the high clinical stage at presentation (stage III or IV) in the majority (70%) of patients. Patients with clinically localized disease

and small primary tumours have a more favourable long-term prognosis {1033}.

Follicular dendritic cell sarcoma

Definition
Follicular dendritic cell sarcoma is a neoplastic proliferation of spindled to ovoid cells showing morphological and phenotypic features of follicular dendritic cells.

ICD-O code   9758/3

Synonyms
Follicular dendritic cell tumour; dendritic reticulum cell tumour (not recommended)

Epidemiology
Follicular dendritic cell sarcoma is an uncommon tumour that can involve the lymph nodes or extranodal sites. The patients are usually adults, with a mean age of 50 years. There is no sex predominance {2289}. Approximately 12% of reported cases show involvement of the thymus or mediastinal lymph

nodes {65,377,580,704,1147,1350,2029, 2058,2289,2503}. Most patients present with localized disease; distant metastasis at presentation is uncommon.

Etiology
Some cases appear to arise in the setting of hyaline-vascular Castleman disease, sometimes with a recognizable intermediary phase of follicular dendritic cell proliferation outside the follicles {372,377,1477}. Components of hyaline-vascular Castleman disease and follicular dendritic cell sarcoma may be identified in the same tumour mass {580}.

Clinical features
Patients are asymptomatic or present with symptoms related to the mediastinal mass, such as cough, haemoptysis, or chest discomfort. Paraneoplastic pemphigus or paraneoplastic myasthenia gravis occurs in a small proportion of patients {958,2289}.

Localization
Follicular dendritic cell sarcoma occurs in the anterior and posterior mediastinum.

Macroscopy
Follicular dendritic cell sarcoma of the mediastinum is often large. It is well circumscribed or invasive. The cut surfaces are solid and light tan-coloured.

Histopathology
The histological spectrum is broad; the growth pattern can be storiform, whorled, fascicular, nodular, diffuse, or even trabecular. The individual tumour cells are spindle-shaped or ovoid, with indistinct cell borders and lightly eosinophilic cytoplasm. The nuclei are elongated or oval with thin nuclear membranes, vesicular chromatin, and small distinct nucleoli. Nuclear pseudoinclusions are common. There is often an irregular clustering of the nuclei, and occasional multinucleated tumour giant cells can be present. In most cases, nuclear pleomorphism is mild, but some cases show significant nuclear pleomorphism, mitotic activity, and coagulative necrosis. Uncommon morphological features include epithelioid tumour cells with hyaline cytoplasm, clear cells, oncocytic cells, myxoid stroma, fluid-filled cystic spaces, blood-filled cystic spaces, prominent fibrovascular septa, and jigsaw puzzle-like lobulation. Typically, dispersed among the tumour cells are small to moderate numbers of lymphocytes, which can show clustering around blood vessels. Ultrastructurally, the tumour cells typically show numerous long slender cytoplasmic processes, often connected by scattered mature desmosomes. Birbeck granules are absent, and there are few lysosomes.

Immunohistochemistry
The diagnosis of follicular dendritic cell sarcoma requires confirmation by immunohistochemical studies. The tumour should show positive staining for one or more follicular dendritic cell markers, such as CD21, CD35, and CD23. Clusterin, D2-40, and CXCL13 are frequently positive, but are not entirely specific {2775,2996}. Activated follicular dendritic cells in both hyaline-vascular Castleman disease and follicular dendritic cell sarcomas express epidermal growth factor receptor more strongly than resting dendritic cells {2774}. CD68 and S100 may be variably and weakly expressed, while

CD1a and CD30 are negative {2058}. Keratin is negative, but epithelial membrane antigen is expressed in 40–88% of cases, which may lead to confusion with other entities such as thymoma and meningioma {377,2058}.

The intermingled lymphocytes usually represent a mixture of mature T cells and B cells, although one type may predominate. In rare cases, there are abundant immature (terminal deoxynucleotidyl transferase-positive) T cells, and this feature is apparently associated with the development of autoimmune phenomena, such as paraneoplastic pemphigus and myasthenia gravis {958,1264}.

Differential diagnosis
Type A thymoma can be distinguished from follicular dendritic cell sarcoma by the lobulated growth pattern, focal gland formation, paucity of lymphocytes, keratin immunoreactivity, and lack of expression of follicular dendritic cell-associated markers.

Type B thymoma may mimic follicular dendritic cell sarcoma due to the admixture of syncytial-appearing plump tumour cells with lymphocytes. Distinguishing features are a lobulated growth pattern (although rare cases of follicular dendritic cell sarcoma can exhibit jigsaw puzzle-like lobulation), the presence of perivascular spaces, keratin immunoreactivity, and an abundance of immature terminal deoxynucleotidyl transferase-positive T cells {437}.

Other differential diagnoses include interdigitating dendritic cell sarcoma, meningioma, carcinoma (including lymphoepithelioma-like carcinoma), melanoma, and various sarcomas. In general, the distinction can be readily achieved by immunohistochemistry.

Genetic profile
The limited cytogenetic data show complex cytogenetic abnormalities {2033}. In one study, 3 of 8 cases of follicular dendritic cell sarcoma showed clonal rearrangements of the immunoglobulin genes {408}; but whether this indicates transdifferentiation from a pre-existing B-cell neoplasm is unclear.

Prognosis and predictive factors
Follicular dendritic cell sarcoma is of intermediate-grade malignancy, with local recurrence and distant metastasis rates of 28% and 27%, respectively {2289}. The 2-year survival rates for early, locally advanced, and distant metastatic disease are 82%, 80%, and 42%, respectively {2289}. Large tumour size ($\geq$ 6 cm), coagulative necrosis, high mitotic count ($\geq$ 5 mitoses per 2 mm^2), and significant cytological atypia are associated with a worse prognosis {2289}. Some patients may die from refractory paraneoplastic pemphigus.

Interdigitating dendritic cell sarcoma

Definition
Interdigitating dendritic cell sarcoma is a neoplastic proliferation of spindled to ovoid cells with phenotypic features of interdigitating dendritic cells. Immunohistochemistry is pivotal for its distinction from follicular dendritic cell sarcoma, which has almost identical morphological features.

ICD-O code   9757/3

Synonym
Interdigitating dendritic cell tumour

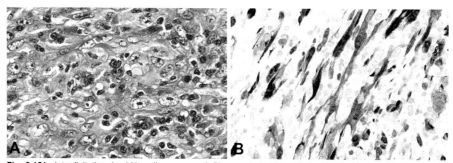

Fig. 3.151 Interdigitating dendritic cell sarcoma. **A** Plump spindled to oval, moderately pleomorphic tumour cells are admixed with lymphocytes and plasma cells; the tumour cells have indistinct cell borders, eosinophilic cytoplasm, vesicular nuclei, and large nucleoli. **B** The tumour cells show immunoreactivity for S100 protein; the presence of multiple dendritic cell processes is evident in at least some tumour cells.

Epidemiology

Interdigitating dendritic cell sarcomas are very rare (with only about 100 cases reported in the literature), and mediastinal involvement is even rarer {2289}. The few reported cases involved the mediastinal lymph nodes as a component of disseminated disease {711,1667,2110,2213,2743}.

Histopathology

The tumour shows a fascicular, storiform, whorled, or diffuse growth pattern, consisting of spindle-shaped or plump cells with indistinct cell borders and abundant eosinophilic cytoplasm. The nuclei often exhibit finely dispersed chromatin and distinct nucleoli. Cytological atypia is variable. Foci of necrosis may be seen. A variable number of T lymphocytes are scattered throughout. The diagnosis requires confirmation by immunohistochemistry, with or without ultrastructural studies (complex interdigitating cell processes lacking well-formed macula adherens-type desmosomes and lacking Birbeck granules).

The neoplastic cells strongly express S100 protein, and often show variable weak staining for CD68, lysozyme, CD4, CD11c, CD14, and CD45. They should be negative for CD1a, langerin (CD207), follicular dendritic cell markers, myeloperoxidase, T-cell lineage-specific markers, and B-cell lineage-specific markers. Melanocytic markers such as HMB45, melan A, microphthalmia transcription factor, and SOX10 are negative.

The most important differential diagnosis is malignant melanoma (primary or metastatic), which is far more common than interdigitating dendritic cell sarcoma. Unlike in interdigitating dendritic cell sarcoma, S100 staining usually reveals only bipolar tapering cell bodies, but not multiple cell processes arising from each cell. Other differential diagnoses include various types of dendritic cell tumour, S100-positive mesenchymal tumours (such as malignant peripheral nerve sheath tumour), and myoepithelial neoplasms.

Genetic profile

To date, only 4 cases have been studied using molecular techniques. Alterations of chromosome 12 were observed in 2 of these {1883}.

Prognosis and predictive factors

In two series, the median survival ranged from 30 to 35 months {2031,2289}. Overall, cases with localized disease have a more favourable outcome, although local relapses can occur. Patients with widespread or metastasizing tumour have an average survival of 9 months.

Fibroblastic reticular cell tumour

Definition

Fibroblastic reticular cell tumour is a neoplasm with morphological and immunophenotypic features of fibroblastic reticular cells. Fibroblastic reticular (reticulum) cells are stromal support cells located in the paracortical and medullary regions of lymph nodes, the periphery of the white pulp in the spleen, and the extrafollicular areas of the tonsil {608,750,885,1586}. These cells have multiple long delicate cell processes and express vimentin. They may also variably express keratin, actin, and desmin.

ICD-O code   9759/3

Synonyms

Fibroblastic dendritic cell tumour; cytokeratin-positive interstitial reticulum cell (CIRC) tumour

Epidemiology

Fibroblastic reticular cell tumour is very rare; a review of dendritic cell tumours identified only 19 cases in the English-language literature, with 8 of the cases showing involvement of the mediastinum or mediastinal lymph nodes (either alone or in combination with other sites) {373,885,2289}. The tumour occurs over a wide age range of 13–80 years, with a median patient age of 61 years. There is a slight male predominance.

Clinical features

Fibroblastic reticular cell tumour usually involves the lymph nodes (most commonly the cervical and mediastinal lymph nodes), but can also involve various extranodal sites {65,373,887,1586,2289,2309}. Patients usually present with symptoms related to the mass lesion, although some are asymptomatic.

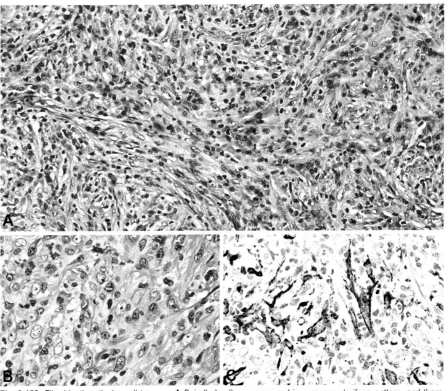

Fig. 3.152 Fibroblastic reticular cell tumour. A Spindled cells are arranged in a coarse storiform pattern, and there are admixed lymphocytes and plasma cells. B The atypical plump spindle-shaped cells have indistinct cell borders, eosinophilic cytoplasm, vesicular nuclei, and distinct nucleoli; admixed lymphocytes, plasma cells, and eosinophils are present. C The tumour cells show a dendritic pattern of immunostaining for smooth muscle actin.

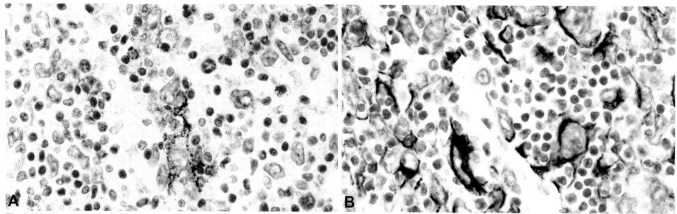

Fig. 3.153 Hybrid follicular dendritic cell sarcoma and fibroblastic reticular cell tumour. **A** Some tumour cells show positive immunostaining for CD35. **B** Many tumour cells show positive immunostaining for desmin; the dendritic cell processes of the tumour cells are evident.

Histopathology

The tumour is histologically similar to follicular dendritic cell sarcoma or interdigitating dendritic cell sarcoma. Spindle-shaped tumour cells with indistinct cell borders show a whorled, fascicular, or storiform growth pattern. The nuclei are often vesicular, with distinct nucleoli. In some cases, pleomorphic or bizarre nuclei are present. There are often interspersed delicate collagen fibres. Coagulative necrosis can be present. There are usually lymphocytes and plasma cells admixed with the tumour cells. Ultrastructurally, the spindle cells show delicate cytoplasmic processes and features reminiscent of myofibroblasts (i.e. filaments with occasional fusiform densities, well-developed desmosomal attachments, rough endoplasmic reticulum, and basal lamina-like material).

The tumour cells are positive for vimentin, and show variable immunoreactivity for keratins, smooth muscle actin, and desmin, in a dendritic pattern. There can also be immunoreactivity for CD68. The tumour should not express markers of follicular or interdigitating dendritic cells. However, fibroblastic reticular cells and follicular dendritic cells probably share a common mesenchymal origin.

For keratin-positive cases, the main differential diagnoses are undifferentiated carcinoma (thymic or metastatic), sarcomatoid carcinoma (thymic or metastatic), and atypical type A thymoma. For keratin-negative cases, the main differential diagnoses are various types of dendritic cell tumours; and for those with expression of myoid markers, smooth muscle tumours, myofibroblastic tumours, and angiomatoid fibrous histiocytoma must also be considered.

Prognosis and predictive factors

Local recurrence and distant metastasis are common, occurring in 36% and 45% of patients, respectively, at a median of 7 months. Common sites of metastasis are the lymph nodes, lung, and liver {2289}.

Other dendritic cell tumours

Definition

There are rare types of dendritic cell tumour other than the better-delineated entities covered in the previous sections. These include indeterminate dendritic cell tumour, dendritic cell tumours with hybrid features, and dendritic cell tumours that defy classification (which can be designated as dendritic cell tumour, not otherwise specified).

ICD-O code

Indeterminate dendritic
   cell tumour   9757/3

Indeterminate dendritic cell tumour

Indeterminate dendritic cell tumour (also called indeterminate cell histiocytosis or indeterminate cell tumour) is a neoplastic proliferation of spindle-shaped or oval cells with immunophenotypic features similar to those of normal indeterminate cells {404,417,2147,2198}. It is morphologically similar to Langerhans cell histiocytosis or Langerhans cell sarcoma, except that there are usually few admixed eosinophils. Immunophenotypically, it is similar to Langerhans cell lesions in that it is positive for S100 and CD1a, but it differs in being langerin (CD207)-negative. Ultrastructurally, the cells typically show complex interdigitating processes, but no Birbeck granules. Indeterminate dendritic cell tumour is very rare, with skin involvement being the most common manifestation. To date, this tumour has not been reported to occur as a primary neoplasm in the thymus or mediastinum.

Hybrid dendritic cell tumour

Rare hybrid tumours exhibit morphological, immunohistochemical, or ultrastructural features of more than one distinctive type of dendritic cell neoplasm, such as follicular dendritic cell sarcoma and fibroblastic reticular cell tumour {603,1160,3019}. One case occurring in the mediastinum has been reported; the immunophenotypic features of the tumour were consistent with those of interdigitating dendritic cell sarcoma, but the ultrastructural features were more consistent with those of follicular dendritic cell sarcoma {603}.

Myeloid sarcoma and extramedullary acute myeloid leukaemia

A. Orazi

Definition
Myeloid sarcoma is a mass-forming neoplastic proliferation of myeloblasts with or without maturation, occurring in an extramedullary site. It may occur de novo or simultaneously with acute myeloid leukaemia, myeloproliferative neoplasms, myelodysplastic/myeloproliferative neoplasms, or myelodysplastic syndromes. It may also be the first manifestation of leukaemic relapse in a previously treated patient {2055}. Interstitial infiltration of myeloid blasts without a nodular mass is termed extramedullary acute myeloid leukaemia.

ICD-O code
9930/3

Synonyms
Extramedullary myeloid tumour; granulocytic sarcoma; chloroma

Clinical features
Mediastinal myeloid sarcoma has been reported in association with superior vena cava syndrome {2116,2125}. Most mediastinal cases occur simultaneously with acute myeloid leukaemia or are followed shortly by acute myeloid leukaemia. All patients who presented with primary mediastinal myeloid sarcoma without concurrent acute myeloid leukaemia eventually relapsed with frank leukaemia {450}.

Localization
Most documented cases arose in the anterior mediastinum.

Histopathology
The most common type of myeloid sarcoma occurring in the mediastinum is granulocytic sarcoma {2931}, a tumour composed of myeloblasts and promyelocytes. The degree of maturation varies in different cases. The blastic subtype is entirely composed of myeloblasts; in the more differentiated subtypes, promyelocytes are also present {1122,2809}. Rare cases composed of monoblasts (called monoblastic sarcoma), can also occur in this location. Cases associated with acute transformation of an underlying myeloproliferative neoplasm may show areas containing a preponderance of mature myeloid cells (e.g. granulocytes)

or foci of trilineage extramedullary haematopoiesis in association with the blastic proliferation.

Cytochemistry and immunophenotype
Cytochemical stains to detect myeloid differentiation in acute myeloid leukaemia can be applied to imprints of biopsy material. Flow cytometry may demonstrate myeloid antigen expression. Myeloid-associated markers that can be helpful in confirming the diagnosis include lysozyme, myeloperoxidase, CD33, CD43, CD117, CD68, and CD61. The lack of expression of lymphoid-associated antigens helps in the differential diagnosis with large cell lymphomas and lymphoblastic lymphoma. The histochemical stain for chloroacetate esterase may be helpful in identifying promyelocytes and better-differentiated myeloid elements present in better-differentiated subtypes of myeloid sarcoma.

Differential diagnosis
The major differential diagnoses are with non-Hodgkin lymphomas, lymphoblastic lymphoma, and diffuse large cell lymphoma; in children, the differential diagnosis also includes various metastatic small round cell tumours. Cases of myeloid sarcoma with prominent sclerosis may closely mimic primary mediastinal (thymic) large B-cell lymphoma. In patients with mediastinal germ cell tumours, the possibility of a local origin of the myeloid sarcoma from immature haematopoietic precursor

cells occurring within the germ cell tumour should also be considered {1916} (see also *Germ cell tumours with associated haematological malignancy*, p. 265).

Genetic profile
A significant proportion of mediastinal myeloid sarcomas have complex cytogenetic abnormalities {2116}. Most of those occurring in acute myeloid leukaemia can also be seen {2055}. The presence of genetic abnormalities in myeloid sarcoma can be detected by conventional cytogenetics or FISH, as well as by PCR-based techniques. Mutational analysis may be indicated in cases with normal karyotype, following the usual guidelines used to treat patients with acute myeloid leukaemia.

Prognosis and predictive factors
Mediastinal myeloid sarcoma is an aggressive disease. Patients who presented with a primary mediastinal myeloid sarcoma and were treated with local irradiation only (before developing acute myeloid leukaemia) eventually all relapsed with frank leukaemia and died soon after {450}. In contrast, patients who were considered to have acute myeloid leukaemia and given upfront systemic chemotherapy had better outcomes, their prognosis being that of the underlying leukaemia {450,1122}. Allogeneic bone marrow transplantation is the only available potentially curative treatment {1435}.

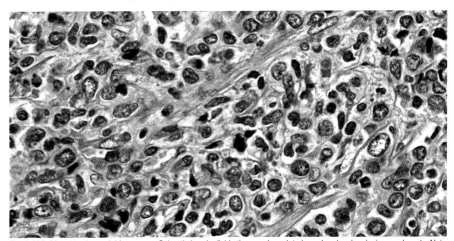

Fig. 3.154 Monoblastic myeloid sarcoma. Sclerotic bands divide the neoplasm into irregular alveolar clusters and cords. Note the kidney-shaped immature nuclei with vesicular or granular chromatin, multiple small nucleoli, and abundant pale cytoplasm.

Soft tissue tumours of the mediastinum

Thymolipoma

R.J. Rieker

Definition
Thymolipoma is an encapsulted tumour that consists of mature adipose tissue with interspersed non-neoplastic thymic tissue.

ICD-O code 8850/0

Synonym
Thymolipomatous hamartoma (not recommended)

Epidemiology
Thymolipomas are rare tumours of the anterior mediastinum, accounting for 2–9% of all thymic neoplasms. The tumours occur at any age, with no sex predominance {1716,2155}.

Etiology
It is still a matter of speculation whether thymolipoma is a benign tumour of specialized thymic stroma (fat) arising in relationship to the thymic epithelium, an aberrant development of the third pharyngeal pouch, or a fatty regression of a hyperplastic thymus or thymoma {976,1047,2155}.

Clinical features
Most thymolipomas are detected incidentally, others due to local symptoms (e.g. cough, dyspnoea, chest pain, hoarseness, and cyanosis) or paraneoplastic syndromes. Myasthenia gravis is the most common symptom {1969,2190}, while aplastic anaemia, Graves disease, and hypogammaglobulinaemia are rare {528,1943}.

On radiographs, thymolipoma may resemble cardiomegaly or lymphoma {1699}. However, CT and MRI are usually diagnostic, showing predominant areas of mature fat (high signal intensity on T1-weighted images and low signal intensity on fat-saturated sequences) with interspersed islands of soft tissue {694,1607}.

Localization
Thymolipomas occur in the anterior mediastinum.

Macroscopy
Thymolipomas are encapsulated tumours. They range in size from 3 cm to > 30 cm {2155}. The tumours are fairly well circumscribed, soft, and yellow on the cut surface. Scattered streaks or solid areas representing entraped thymic tissue may be evident on gross inspection.

Histopathology
Histologically, the tumours consist of mature adipose tissue with strands or even large areas of thymic tissue that is mostly atrophic, but may contain lymph follicles and Hassall corpuscles. Atypia and mitotic activity are missing. Thymolipomas may rarely contain thymomas or carcinoid tumours {80,913,2455}. Immunohistochemistry is usually not necessary.

Lipoma of the mediastinum is distinguished by its lack of thymic epithelial components. Liposarcoma is characterized by a higher degree of atypia (see *Liposarcoma*, p. 290).

Genetic profile
In one case, a translocation involving the *HMGA2* gene on chromosome 12q15 was found {1047}.

Prognosis and predictive factors
Complete resection is curative. No metastases, recurrences, or tumour-related deaths have been reported.

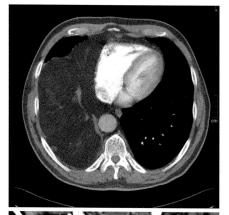
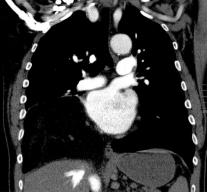

Fig. 3.156 Mediastinal lipoma. CT showing a well-circumscribed tumour.

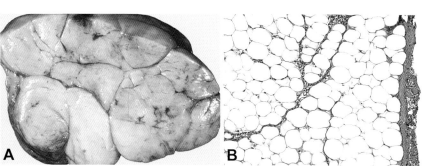

Fig. 3.155 Thymolipoma. **A** A thinly encapsulated thymolipoma in a 6-year-old boy; the cut surface is yellow, bulging, and lobulated, resembling lipoma. Reprinted from Shimosato Y, Mukai K {2376}. **B** Adipocytic cells with thin septa containing thymic tissue.

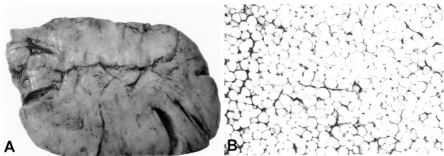

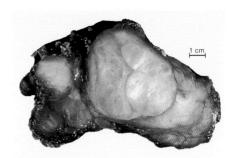

Fig. 3.157 Mediastinal lipoma. **A** Macroscopy of a well-encapsulated tumour. **B** Mature adipocytes with small eccentric nuclei.

Fig. 3.159 Mediastinal liposarcoma. Macroscopy of a recurrent tumour (2 years after first treatment): a well-circumscribed and partially encapsulated tumour from the anterior mediastinum.

Lipoma

R.J. Rieker

Definition

Lipomas are very rare tumours in the mediastinum, but they are common benign tumours among mesenchymal tumours. Other benign lipomatous tumours include lipoblastoma/lipoblastomatosis {632}, hibernomas {31}, and angiolipomas {1289}. Histologically, mediastinal lipomas are identical to their cutaneous and soft tissue counterparts. In doubtful cases and cases with mild cytological atypia, MDM2 and CDK4 immunostaining and FISH analysis are useful to exclude atypical lipomatous tumour/well-differentiated liposarcoma {204,2405}.

ICD-O code   8850/0

Liposarcoma

J-M. Coindre

Definition

Liposarcoma is a malignant mesenchymal tumour with adipocytic differentiation.

ICD-O codes

Well-differentiated liposarcoma   8850/3
Dedifferentiated liposarcoma   8858/3
Myxoid liposarcoma   8852/3
Pleomorphic liposarcoma   8854/3

Synonyms

Well-differentiated liposarcoma/adipocytic liposarcoma; myxoid liposarcoma/round cell liposarcoma

Epidemiology

Liposarcoma is the most common sarcoma of the mediastinum. It usually occurs in adults aged > 40 years, and is rare in children {224,926,1288}.

Clinical features

The presenting symptoms are most commonly dyspnoea and cough. Imaging usually shows a large tumour with a mature lipomatous component.

Localization

Liposarcoma occurs in all mediastinal compartments, particularly in the anterior and posterior mediastinum {224,926,1288}. Some cases may occur in the thymus.

Macroscopy

Mediastinal liposarcoma is usually a large, well-circumscribed, multinodular mass, with a mixture of lipomatous and myxoid areas.

Histopathology

The histopathological findings are identical to those of liposarcomas elsewhere (particularly the retroperitoneum) {926}. Well-differentiated and dedifferentiated liposarcomas are the most common subtypes in the mediastinum {224,926}.

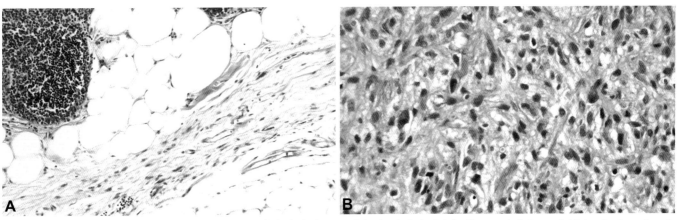

Fig. 3.158 **A** Well-differentiated liposarcoma. Lipomatous tumour developing in the thymus and showing atypical cells in the fibrous septa that separate lobules of mature adipocytic cells. **B** Dedifferentiated liposarcoma. Poorly differentiated spindle and pleomorphic cell sarcoma developed in the anterior mediastinum.

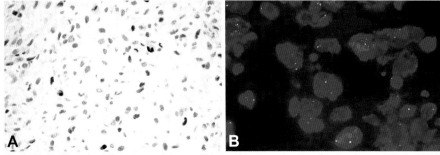

Fig. 3.160 Dedifferentiated liposarcoma. **A** Immunohistochemistry showed a strong focal nuclear positivity for MDM2. **B** FISH analysis demonstrated *MDM2* amplification, leading to the diagnosis of dedifferentiated liposarcoma. Red: *MDM2* probe (numerous signals in dots). Green: *CEP12* with one or two signals per cell.

Well-differentiated liposarcoma with lipoma-like, sclerosing, and inflammatory subtypes should be distinguished from lipoma by *MDM2* status analysis (immunohistochemistry and FISH analysis) when needed. Dedifferentiated liposarcomas show a poorly differentiated sarcomatous component (i.e. undifferentiated pleomorphic sarcoma, myxofibrosarcoma, fibrosarcoma, or inflammatory malignant fibrous histiocytoma-like areas), with a possible heterologous component (such as a rhabdomyosarcoma, leiomyosarcoma, or osteochondrosarcoma component) associated with a well-differentiated liposarcomatous component. Small samples often show the poorly differentiated component only, but the differential diagnosis of dedifferentiated liposarcoma should be raised in this location. Immunohistochemistry usually shows an overexpression of *MDM2* and *CDK4*, but the gold standard for the diagnosis is FISH analysis showing *MDM2* amplification. Pleomorphic liposarcoma and (rarely) myxoid liposarcoma have also been reported in this location

Genetic profile
Well-differentiated and dedifferentiated liposarcomas are characterized by a 12q13–21 amplicon with a constant *MDM2* amplification demonstrated by FISH and comparative genomic hybridization analyses. Myxoid liposarcoma is characterized by a recurrent translocation involving *DDIT3*, which can be shown by FISH analysis. Pleomorphic liposarcoma shows a complex genomic profile with no specificity

Prognosis and predictive factors
Overall prognosis is poor, and 44% of patients die from the disease {224}. As with retroperitoneal liposarcomas, local recurrences are common, related to the difficulties in achieving total resection in the mediastinum. Distant metastases are also observed, particularly with the pleomorphic and myxoid subtypes {224}.

Solitary fibrous tumour

C.D.M. Fletcher

Definition
Solitary fibrous tumour in the mediastinum is a rare fibroblastic neoplasm that often shows a prominent branching vascular pattern and exhibits varied biological behaviour.

ICD-O codes
Solitary fibrous tumour   8815/1
    Malignant   8815/3

Synonyms
Obsolete: localized fibrous tumour; sub-mesothelial fibroma

Epidemiology
Mediastinal/thymic solitary fibrous tumour is rare, but typically occurs in adults of either sex.

Clinical features
The clinical features are essentially the same as those of pleural solitary fibrous tumour {735A,2897}.

Localization
The anterior mediastinum is the most common location for solitary fibrous tumours. Occasionally, cases also involve the thymus {2897}.

Macroscopy
Mediastinal solitary fibrous tumour is usually a large, well-circumscribed, fibrous mass, which may rarely be pedunculated.

Histopathology
The histological and immunohistochemical features of mediastinal/thymic solitary fibrous tumours are essentially indistinguishable from those of the pleural lesions {735A,2897}. STAT6 is the most specific marker for solitary fibrous tumour {624}. The differential diagnosis is the same as for pleural solitary fibrous tumour, but in the mediastinum also includes thymomas with spindle cell morphology, particularly type A thymomas.

Genetic profile
See *Solitary fibrous tumour* in {735A}.

Prognosis and predictive factors
A mitotic rate of > 4 mitoses per 2 mm^2 is the best predictor of malignant behaviour in solitary fibrous tumour {623}. It has been suggested that the prognosis of mediastinal solitary fibrous tumour is worse than that of pleural solitary fibrous tumour, but this may reflect tumour size as well as problems regarding resectability.

Synovial sarcoma

J-M. Coindre

Definition
Synovial sarcoma in the mediastinum is a rare mesenchymal tumour that displays a variable degree of epithelial differentiation and has a specific chromosomal translocation – t(X;18), which leads to the formation of an *SS18-SSX* fusion gene.

ICD-O codes
Synovial sarcoma, NOS   9040/3
Synovial sarcoma, spindle cell   9041/3
Synovial sarcoma, epithelioid cell   9042/3
Synovial sarcoma, biphasic   9043/3

Synonyms
Not recommended: tenosynovial sarcoma; synoviosarcoma; synovioblastic sarcoma

Epidemiology
Mediastinal synovial sarcoma is rare, accounting for about 10% of intrathoracic

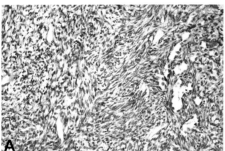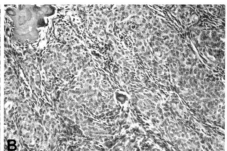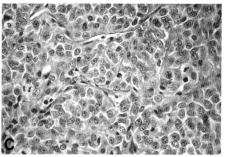

Fig. 3.161 Synovial sarcoma. **A** Monophasic spindle cell synovial sarcoma focally with gaping vessels resembling solitary fibrous tumour. **B** Spindle cell component of calcifying synovial sarcoma (30% of all synovial sarcoma cases), showing an unusual biphasic type: solid epithelial cords and few spindle cells. **C** High-power view of the solid epithelial component; if this were the only component, the tumour would be called monophasic epithelial synovial sarcoma.

synovial sarcomas {957}. The median patient age is 35 years {2524}.

Clinical features
The most common presenting symptoms are dyspnoea, chest pain, and cough.

Localization
Synovial sarcoma occurs in the anterior or posterior mediastinum {957,2524}.

Macroscopy
Mediastinal synovial sarcoma is well circumscribed or invades adjacent anatomical structures. The tumour size ranges from 5 to 20 cm {2524}.

Histopathology
The histological and immunohistochemical features are essentially indistinguishable from those of synovial sarcomas elsewhere {2532}, but with more frequent monophasic spindle cell and poorly differentiated subtypes {167,957,2524}. The differential diagnosis is principally the same as for lung and pleural synovial sarcoma; however, in the mediastinum,

type A thymoma also enters the differential diagnosis, and can be excluded by strong diffuse keratin expression and absence of t(X;18)(p11;q11) on FISH.

Genetic profile
Synovial sarcoma is characterized by the t(X;18)(p11;q11) translocation, which is specific {2532}.

Prognosis and predictive factors
Most reported cases followed an aggressive clinical course. About half of all patients died of the disease within 5 years {957}.

Vascular neoplasms

P. Ströbel

Definition
Vascular neoplasms are a variety of primary tumours of the mediastinum that display unequivocal features of vascular differentiation by

morphology, immunohistochemistry, and ultrastructure.

ICD-O codes
Lymphangioma	9170/0
Haemangioma	9120/0
Epithelioid haemangioendothelioma	9133/3
Angiosarcoma	9120/3

Epidemiology
With the exception of paediatric lymphangiomas {132,2544}, vascular tumours of the mediastinum are rare, accounting for only 1–4.5% of all tumours in this location {538,1646,1937, 2355,2879,2917}. In adults, most of these tumours occur in middle-aged patients, with no sex predominance {406,831,1213,1717,2528,2830}.

Clinical features
Symptomatic tumours, regardless of their histology, often manifest with retrosternal pain, dyspnoea, cough, or stridor {538,1717,1937,2528,2830,2879}. Haemangiomas tend to be multifocal, with

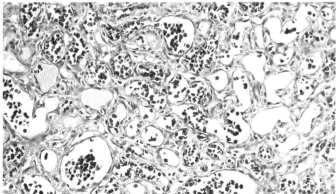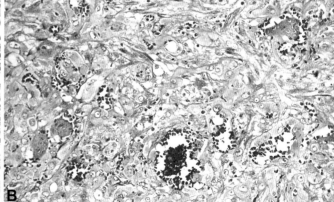

Fig. 3.162 Vascular neoplasms of the mediastinum. **A** Capillary haemangioma of the anterior mediastinum. The tumour forms distinct lobules separated by a loose stroma. **B** Epithelioid haemangioendothelioma. Cords of epithelioid tumour cells with abundant eosinophilic cytoplasm; occasional tumour cells show vacuolation; some primitive vascular channels contain blood; this case also shows interspersed osteoclastic giant cells.

involvement of the spleen, liver, and kidneys {2528}.

Infantile haemangioendothelioma can be associated with consumptive thrombocytopenia (Kasabach-Merritt syndrome) {1001}. Haemorrhagic pericarditis, pneumonia, swelling of the face and neck, and dizziness have also been described in some angiosarcomas {2830}.

On CT, lymphangiomas are usually cystic lesions with smooth margins and a density close to the signal of water or protein {1937}. Haemangioendotheliomas and angiosarcomas are usually mass lesions with indistinct borders, and may show calcifications and encroachment of neighbouring structures {2528,2830,2879}. Aggressive tumours infiltrate the thymus, pericardium, and carotid sheaths {2879}. Angiosarcoma metastases to the liver {596} and the extremities {406} have been described.

Localization
Vascular neoplasms can involve both the anterior and posterior mediastinum.

Macroscopy
Both benign and malignant lesions tend to be large (3–20 cm) {1717, 1937,2528,2830}. In malignant tumours, there are poorly defined margins, haemorrhage, and necrosis {2830}. Calcifications occur in haemangiomas and angiosarcomas {1717,2830}.

Histopathology
All vascular lesions resemble their respective counterparts elsewhere in the body. Lymphangiomas are composed of medium-sized or small lumina containing lymphatic fluid and a mixture of loose collagen tissue and adipose tissue {1937}. Haemangiomas can be of the capillary or the cavernous type, and can show infiltrative margins, regressive changes, and foci with increased mitotic activity {1717}. Epithelioid haemangioendotheliomas show glomeruloid nests of epithelioid cells containing intracytoplasmic lumina {2528,2879}. Occasional mitoses are present. Haemosiderin pigment can be abundant. Occasionally, tumours contain metaplastic bone or osteoclast-like giant cells {2528}. Angiosarcomas are characterized by dissecting vascular spaces lined by atypical endothelium with variable (but often high) numbers of mitoses {596}, depending on the degree of differentiation. Some cases with

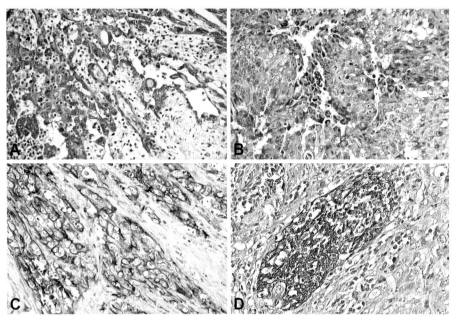

Fig. 3.163 Angiosarcoma. **A** The tumour forms anastomosing channels, and the lining cells show significant nuclear pleomorphism and atypia. **B** Angiosarcoma can show a solid growth, obscuring the vascular nature of this malignant tumour. **C** Typical immunostaining of tumour cell membranes for CD31. **D** Immunostaining of remnant thymic epithelial cell network for CK19.

epithelioid morphology have been described {406,2830}.

Markers of lymphatic or vascular endothelial cells (such as CD31, CD34, ERG, and lectin) are usually present. CD34 can be absent in haemangioendotheliomas {2528} and angiosarcomas. Keratins are negative {2528,2830}.

The major *differential diagnostic* challenge is to distinguish the different vascular tumours from each other. Type A thymoma may occasionally be very cystic, and may superficially resemble cavernous haemangioma. The differential diagnoses of angiosarcoma include haemangioendothelioma, haemangioma, and carcinoma. Pure angiosarcomas must be differentiated from angiosarcomas that arise as part of a mediastinal germ cell tumour with somatic-type malignancy and herald a poor prognosis {488,872,1556}. A lymphangioma associated with a thymic carcinoma has been reported {1068}.

Genetic profile
Epithelioid haemangioendothelioma has a t(1;3)(q36;q23–25) translocation that results in a fusion of *WWTR1* with *CAMTA1* in virtually all cases {2827}.

Prognosis and predictive factors
Despite sometimes worrisome histological features, mediastinal haemangiomas

are benign tumours {1717}. The prognosis of epithelioid haemangioendothelioma also seems favourable, with most patients alive after extended follow-up periods {2528}. Angiosarcomas are aggressive tumours, with survival times ranging from 2 to 36 months from the time of diagnosis in previous reports {596,743}, while a recent series suggested that the clinical course of mediastinal angiosarcomas may be more protracted than that of angiosarcomas in other organs {2830}.

Neurogenic tumours

C.D.M. Fletcher

Although soft tissue tumours as a group are rare in the mediastinum, peripheral nerve sheath tumours are among the most common. Such tumours arise much more often in the posterior than the anterior mediastinum, and origin in the thymus itself is truly exceptional. The most commonly encountered lesions are benign schwannoma and malignant peripheral nerve sheath tumour {1340,1575}. Cellular schwannoma, which may be mistaken for malignant peripheral nerve sheath tumour, has a predilection for the paravertebral region in both the mediastinum and the retroperitoneum {2861}. Melanotic schwannoma {2661}, neurofibroma, granular cell tumour, and paraganglioma may also occur in this location, as may ganglioneuroma and (less often) ganglioneuroblastoma/neuroblastoma (see the next section). Paraganglioma and peripheral nerve sheath tumours arising in the mediastinum have no special or distinct clinicopathological features compared to their more common somatic counterparts {736}.

Ganglioneuroma, ganglioneuroblastoma, and neuroblastoma

A. Marx

Definition
Ganglioneuroma is a benign neoplasm of mature ganglion cells within dominant Schwannian stroma. Ganglioneuroblastoma and neuroblastoma are malignant tumours composed of primitive or maturing neuroblasts, or neuroblasts and mature ganglion cells with variable Schwannian stroma.

ICD-O codes
Ganglioneuroma   9490/0
Ganglioneuroblastoma   9490/3
Neuroblastoma   9500/3

Epidemiology
The incidence of neuroblastoma and ganglioneuroblastoma is about 1 case per 100 000 individuals per year {801}, with no sex predominance. About 95% of

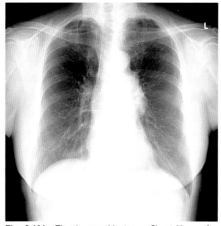

Fig. 3.164 Thymic neuroblastoma. Chest X-ray of a 65-year-old woman with an incidentally detected anterior mediastinal mass showing smooth borders projecting to the left hilum.

neuroblastomas and ganglioneuroblastomas occur in patients aged < 5 years, and many ganglioneuroma occur in patients aged ≥ 5 years {817}. The rare thymic cases occurred in elderly patients {81,88,1886,2013,2709}.

Etiology
The etiology is unknown. Rare familial neuroblastoma cases are related to mutations of ALK, PHOX2B, ATRX, and unknown genes. Neurofibromatosis and multiple endocrine neoplasia type 2B predispose individuals to ganglioneuroma {1947,2449}. Posterior mediastinal cases are neural crest derivatives. Thymic cases hypothetically arise from aberrantly localized ganglia or pluripotent thymic epithelial progenitors {81,2709}.

Clinical features
Symptoms due to compression of vital

organs are common, while hypertension, opsomyoclonus, and vasoactive intestinal peptide secretion are rare {1057}. Inadequate antidiuretic hormone secretion can occur in thymic neuroblastoma {88,2013}.

On imaging, neuroblastoma and ganglioneuroblastoma are heterogeneous masses, commonly with calcification, haemorrhage, and MIBG positivity on PET {1947}. Ganglioneuromas often appear circumscribed and homogeneous, and are negative on MIBG scans {817}.

Localization
About 20% of neuroblastomas and ganglioneuroblastomas, and 40–50% of ganglioneuromas arise in the mediastinum, mainly (in 95% of cases) in the posterior compartment {200,817,1947,2578}. Rarely, neuroblastomas {81,88,1886,2013,2709} and ganglioneuroblastomas {88} have been described in the thymus.

Macroscopy
The tumours are circumscribed or irregular, usually measuring up to 10 cm, but rarely > 25 cm. On cut surfaces, haemorrhage, cystic changes, and necrosis are common in neuroblastoma and ganglioneuroblastoma. Ganglioneuromas are more homogeneous, and grey-white to tan-yellow {1378}.

Cytology
Cytology shows small neuroblasts with finely dispersed chromatin, alone or with ganglion-like or hyperchromatic cells. They may occur singly or in clusters, often connected by fibrillary material.

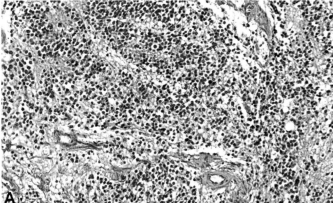
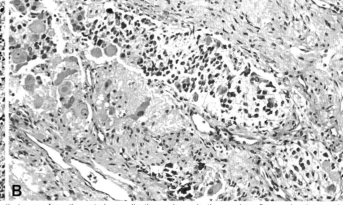

Fig. 3.165 A Thymic neuroblastoma. Histology of the solid region of the partially cystic tumour from the anterior mediastinum shown in the previous figure, showing poorly differentiated, Schwannian stroma-poor neuroblastoma with abundant neuropil. B Ganglioneuroblastoma, intermixed, Schwannian stroma-rich. From the posterior mediastinum of a child. Note the clusters of mature and maturing ganglion cells, the hyperchromatic small neuroblasts, the Schwannian spindle cell component, and the calcification.

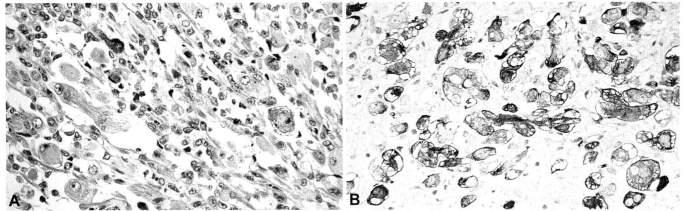

Fig. 3.166 Embryonal rhabdomyosarcoma of the mediastinum. **A** H&E staining showing numerous rhabdomyoblasts. **B** Desmin expression with occasional cells showing cross-striations.

Histopathology

The histopathological findings are identical to those of neuroblastic tumours occuring elsewhere {1378}. Thymic neuroblastoma consistently contains numerous maturing neuroblasts {2013}.

Genetic profile

Recurrent genetic aberrations in neuroblastoma and (less frequently) ganglioneuroblastoma include *MYCN* amplification, imbalanced 11q and 1p losses, and gains of 17q {1947}. Molecular data are lacking for thymic neuroblastoma/ganglioneuroblastoma.

Prognosis and predictive factors

Stage IV disease is less common (15%) in patients with mediastinal primaries {571} than in neuroblastoma patients overall (30%) {631}. Metastases involve the bone marrow, bone, lymph nodes, and liver (30–70%), but rarely the lung (3.6%) or the brain (< 1%). Pre- and postoperative staging and risk stratification systems apply to mediastinal cases {264,473}. The 5-year survival rate of neuroblastoma/ganglioneuroblastoma is 90% {801}. Favourable prognostic factors are younger age {2368}, hyperdiploidy, non-amplified *MYCN*, and the absence of aberrations of 11q and 1p {818,1947,2555}.

Other rare mesenchymal tumours

J.K.C. Chan

Other mediastinal/thymic mesenchymal tumours, in order of frequency of occurrence, include: undifferentiated pleomorphic sarcoma {407,991,1075}; leiomyomatous tumours (including leiomyomas {2336} and leiomyosarcomas {2766}); Ewing sarcoma {671,847,1313,2127,2316}; rhabdomyosarcoma of embryonal, alveolar, or pleomorphic type (which should be distinguished from rhabdomyosarcoma arising from germ cell tumours with somatic-type malignancy and from heterologous components in sarcomatoid carcinoma and dedifferentiated liposarcoma) {2529}; desmoid-type fibromatosis {1303}; inflammatory myofibroblastic tumour {500,907,1555}; desmoplastic small round cell tumour {1821}; and osteosarcoma {1010,1442}. Other very rare tumours have also been reported: calcifying fibrous tumour {1817}, myelolipoma {669,1256,2767}, elastofibrolipoma {552}, deep benign fibrous histiocytoma {848}, rhabdomyoma {1676,2392,3032}, ependymoma (including myxopapillary type) {607,687, 1547,1747,2886}, angiomatoid fibrous histiocytoma {89,401}, giant cell tumour of soft tissue {765,860}, PEComa {306}, low-grade fibromyxoid sarcoma {1344}, chondrosarcoma {2124}, clear cell sarcoma of soft tissue {2646}, malignant rhabdoid tumour {794,924,1599}, alveolar soft part sarcoma {740}, and chordoma {1606,2182,2438}.

Ectopic tumours of the thymus

J.K.C. Chan

Ectopic thyroid tumours

Definition
Ectopic thyroid tumour is a thyroid neoplasm that occurs in sites other than the cervical thyroid gland proper.

ICD-O codes
Follicular adenoma	8330/0
Follicular carcinoma	8330/3
Oncocytic (Hurthle cell) carcinoma	8290/3
Medullary thyroid carcinoma	8345/3

Epidemiology
Thyroid tumours occurring in the mediastinum are often of cervical thyroid gland origin that has extended into the mediastinum. Genuine ectopic thyroid tumours arising in the mediastinum without connection to the cervical thyroid gland are very rare.

Etiology
The etiology is unknown. Thyroid tissue that has aberrantly migrated to the mediastinum during embryological development is the cell of origin for ectopic thyroid tumours in the mediastinum.

Clinical features
Patients are either discovered to have a mediastinal tumour incidentally, or present with symptoms referable to a mediastinal mass.

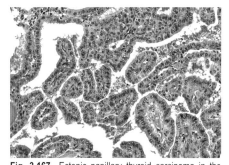

Fig. 3.167 Ectopic papillary thyroid carcinoma in the anterior mediastinum. The tumour is composed of papillae lined by cells with overlapping and pale-staining nuclei with frequent grooves.

Histopathology
Both benign and malignant thyroid tumours can occur in the mediastinum; their nomenclature and diagnostic criteria should follow the *WHO classification of tumours of endocrine organs* {567}. Follicular adenoma and papillary carcinoma are the most common ectopic thyroid tumours, but other tumour types have also been described, such as follicular carcinoma, oncocytic (Hurthle cell) carcinoma, poorly differentiated carcinoma, and medullary carcinoma {612, 1105,1218,1482,1684,1945,2052,2497, 2807,2866}.

Thyroid follicular cell tumours are immunoreactive for keratins, thyroglobulin, and TTF1, but not chromogranin. Medullary carcinoma is positive for keratin, chromogranin, and calcitonin, and variably positive for TTF1.

Ectopic papillary thyroid carcinoma may raise the differential diagnoses of primary thymic adenocarcinoma of papillary type and metastatic adenocarcinoma. Ectopic follicular adenoma or adenocarcinoma may raise the differential diagnoses of thymic germ cell tumour, ectopic parathyroid neoplasm, and thymic adenocarcinoma.

Prognosis and predictive factors
Information on the behaviour of these ectopic tumours is limited, but the outcome is probably similar to that of tumours of comparable stage occurring in the cervical thyroid gland {2866}.

Ectopic parathyroid tumours

Definition
Ectopic parathyroid tumour is a parathyroid cell neoplasm occurring in sites other than the usual locations (i.e. the parathyroid glands in the neck) {2497}.

ICD-O codes
Parathyroid adenomas	8140/0
Parathyroid carcinomas	8140/3

Epidemiology
Approximately 10–20% of all parathyroid neoplasms occur in the mediastinum, most commonly in the anterosuperior mediastinum in the vicinity of or within the thymus gland {461,485,1820,1879, 2798,2872}.

Etiology
The inferior parathyroid glands and the thymus share a common origin from the third branchial pouch {2872}, accounting for the occurrence of ectopic or supernumerary parathyroid glands in the anterosuperior mediastinum, which gives rise to ectopic parathyroid tumours {1405}.

Clinical features
Patients usually present with symptoms due to hyperparathyroidism (such as bone pain or renal stones), but some may be found to have hypercalcaemia incidentally {1732}. There is often radiological evidence of a mediastinal mass {566,1233,1732,1732,1776,2099}.

Localization
Ectopic parathyroid tumours occur in the anterior mediastinum and thymus.

Histopathology
The nomenclature and diagnostic criteria for parathyroid tumours should follow the *WHO classification of tumours of endocrine organs* {567}.

Parathyroid adenomas are circumscribed tumours that consist of sheets and trabeculae of polygonal cells traversed by a delicate vasculature. There is often a mixture of cells with clear, eosinophilic, amphophilic, or oxyphilic cytoplasm. The nuclei are usually uniform and round, but there can also be interspersed pleomorphic nuclei. Mitotic figures are absent or rare. Rare tumours can have abundant interspersed adipose cells (lipoadenomas) {1820,2901} or lymphocytes {697}.

Parathyroid carcinomas are generally similar to parathyroid adenomas, but often show capsular or vascular invasion,

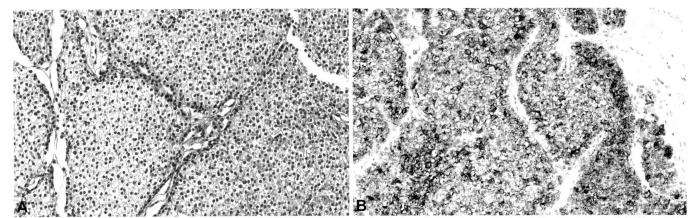

Fig. 3.168 Ectopic parathyroid adenoma in the anterior mediastinum. **A** Sheets of polygonal cells with clear cytoplasm, traversed by delicate fibrovascular septa. **B** Positive granular immunostaining for parathyroid hormone supports the parathyroid nature of the neoplasm.

sclerotic bands, mitotic figures, and coagulative necrosis. The nuclei can be uniform, or can show significant pleomorphism and macronucleoli.

Parathyroid tumours are immunoreactive for keratins, chromogranin, and parathyroid hormone {1242}. They are negative for thyroglobulin, TTF1, and PAX8 {1242}. Various neuroendocrine tumours (such as carcinoid tumour, atypical carcinoid, large cell neuroendocrine carcinoma, paraganglioma, and medullary thyroid carcinoma) are in the differential diagnosis. A definitive diagnosis can be made if parathyroid hormone is demonstrated by immunohistochemistry. Parathyroid

neoplasms with pleomorphic cells may be mistaken for thymic carcinoma.

Prognosis and predictive factors

Complete excision is curative for parathyroid adenoma {1062,2817}. Parathyroid carcinoma can recur or metastasize.

Other rare ectopic tumours

Extremely rarely, ectopic sebaceous glands and ectopic salivary gland tissues can occur in the thymus {1677,2902}. To date, ectopic sebaceous neoplasms have not been reported in the thymus or

mediastinum. The one reported case of mixed tumour of the thymus/mediastinum was probably derived from ectopic salivary gland tissue {708}. The occurrence of mucoepidermoid carcinoma in the thymus may suggest a possible origin from ectopic salivary gland tissue, but this seems unlikely, because the carcinomas often show transition with multilocular thymic cysts, suggesting an origin from thymic epithelium instead.

Rare examples of ectopic meningioma have been reported in the mediastinum, with a disproportionally high frequency of the tumours considered to be malignant {400,1697,1960,2938}.

Metastasis to the thymus or mediastinum

M.O. Kurrer
A. Marx
A.G. Nicholson
P. Ströbel

Definition

Metastasis to the thymus or mediastinum is a malignant tumour that originates outside of the mediastinum and spreads to the thymus or the mediastinum by lymphatic or haematogenous route. Direct extension by contiguous growth into the thymus is technically not a metastasis, but may require similar clinical considerations.

Etiology

Tumours can spread to the thymus or anterior mediastinum either from adjacent organs (i.e. the lung, thyroid, and breast {1195}) or from distant organs {1634,1665}, including the prostate {1478}. The presence of multiple thymic tumours does not exclude primary thymic tumours {1746,1868,1875}. Soft tissue tumours that metastasize to the thymus or mediastinum are indistinguishable from their primary mediastinal counterparts, but can differ in their clinical features.

Histopathology

Depending on the patient's sex and age, and the clinical context, a battery of immunohistochemical markers may be required to differentiate between a thymic primary tumour and a metastatic lesion. However, a definite distinction may not be possible in all instances. In squamous cell carcinomas, PAX8, CD5, CD117, CD70, FOXN1, and CD205 support a thymic origin {95,1013,1871}. Mediastinal adenocarcinomas are so rare that metastasis is much more likely than a mediastinal primary. Expression of TTF1, GATA3, hormone receptors, and WT1 favour metastatic disease, while CDX2 does not exclude a primary thymic adenocarcinoma with enteric differentiation. CD5 is expressed in a substantial number of primary and metastatic adenocarcinomas, and is thus not helpful. Specific markers for the distinction between neuroendocrine tumours of pulmonary and thymic origin have not been reported, but a PAX8-positive/TTF1-negative immunophenotype may suggest a thymic primary site, while a PAX8-negative/TTF1-positive

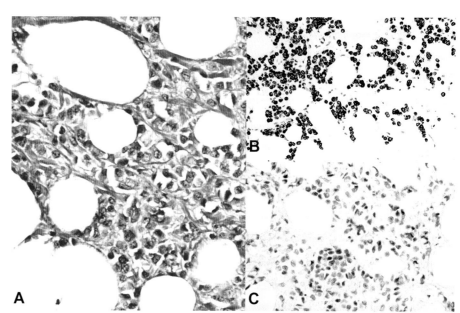

Fig. 3.169 **A** Metastasis of breast carcinoma involving mediastinal fat. **B** Tumour cells stain for cytokeratin 7. **C** Tumour cells stain for estrogen receptor.

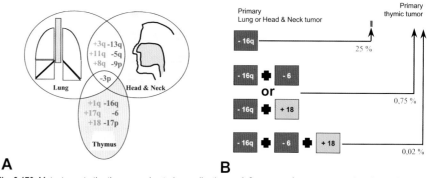

Fig. 3.170 Metastases to the thymus and anterior mediastinum. **A** Summary of recurrent genetic gains and losses (as determined by comparative genomic hybridization) discriminating between squamous cell carcinomas of the thymus, lung, and head and neck region. There is considerable overlap between the carcinomas arising in the lung and those arising in the head and neck. In contrast, the major genetic aberrations of thymic carcinomas are not shared with carcinomas of the lung or the head and neck. **B** The diagnostic value of comparative genomic hybridization-based genetic profiles for the distinction between squamous cell carcinomas of the thymus and mediastinal metastases of primary lung and head and neck tumours. The percentages indicate the probabilities for a primary lung or head and neck carcinoma in the presence of highly discriminating genetic alterations {216,1614,2448,3011}.

immunophenotype may be more suggestive of metastasis from a pulmonary primary {2845}.

Genetic profile

Distinct genetic aberrations that aid in the distinction between primary thymic and metastatic squamous cell carcinoma include gains of 1q and loss of 6q25.2–25.3 and 16p {3011}.

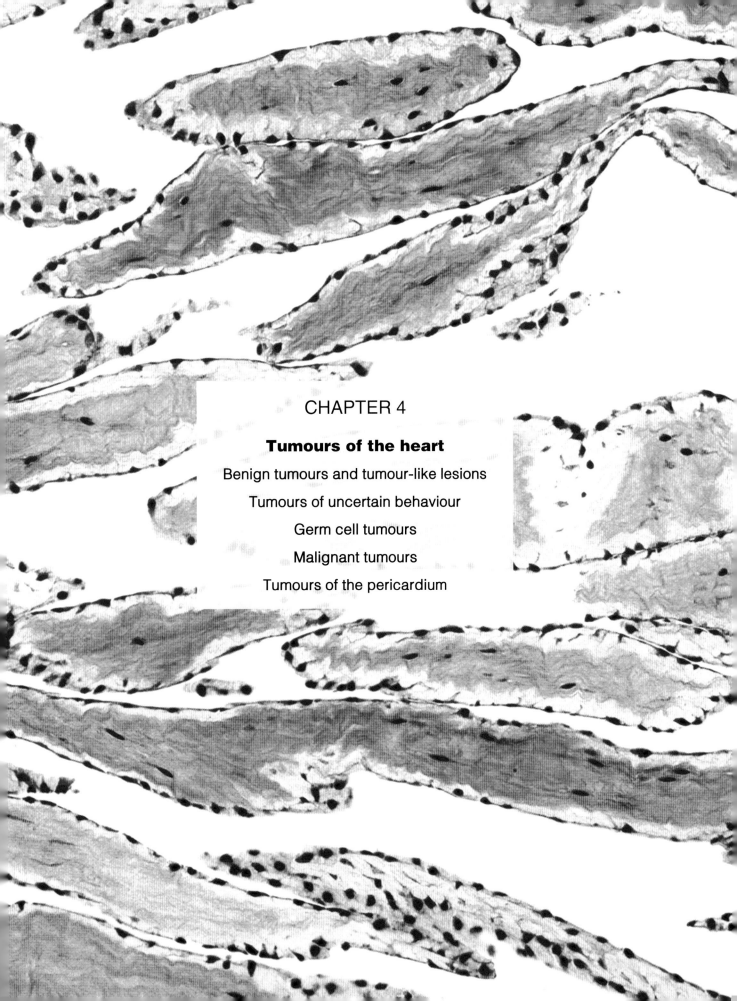

CHAPTER 4

Tumours of the heart

Benign tumours and tumour-like lesions

Tumours of uncertain behaviour

Germ cell tumours

Malignant tumours

Tumours of the pericardium

WHO classification of tumours of the heart[a,b]

Benign tumours and tumour-like lesions

Rhabdomyoma	8900/0
Histiocytoid cardiomyopathy	
Hamartoma of mature cardiac myocytes	
Adult cellular rhabdomyoma	8904/0
Cardiac myxoma	8840/0
Papillary fibroelastoma	
Haemangioma, NOS	9120/0
Capillary haemangioma	9131/0
Cavernous haemangioma	9121/0
Arteriovenous malformation	
Intramuscular haemangioma	9132/0
Cardiac fibroma	8810/0
Lipoma	8850/0
Cystic tumour of the atrioventricular node	8454/0
Granular cell tumour	9580/0
Schwannoma	9560/0

Tumours of uncertain behaviour

Inflammatory myofibroblastic tumour	8825/1
Paraganglioma	8680/1

Germ cell tumours

Teratoma, mature	9080/0
Teratoma, immature	9080/3
Yolk sac tumour	9071/3

Malignant tumours

Angiosarcoma	9120/3
Undifferentiated pleomorphic sarcoma	8830/3
Osteosarcoma	9180/3
Myxofibrosarcoma	8811/3
Leiomyosarcoma	8890/3
Rhabdomyosarcoma	8900/3
Synovial sarcoma	9040/3
Miscellaneous sarcomas	
Cardiac lymphomas	
Metastatic tumours	

Tumours of the pericardium

Solitary fibrous tumour	8815/1
Malignant	8815/3
Angiosarcoma	9120/3
Synovial sarcoma	9040/3
Malignant mesothelioma	9050/3
Germ cell tumours	
Teratoma, mature	9080/0
Teratoma, immature	9080/3
Yolk sac tumour	9071/3

[a] The morphology codes are from the International Classification of Diseases for Oncology (ICD-O) {763}. Behaviour is coded /0 for benign tumours; /1 for unspecified, borderline or uncertain behaviour; /2 for carcinoma in situ and grade III intraepithelial neoplasia; and /3 for malignant tumours. [b] The classification is modified from the previous WHO classification {2672}, taking into account changes in our understanding of these lesions.

Tumours of the heart
Introduction

V. Thomas de Montpréville
A.P. Burke
A.W. ElBardissi
A.A. Frazier
T. Strecker

Epidemiology

Primary cardiac tumours are rare, and their prevalence in the general population is not known. Most epidemiological data are obtained from autopsy or surgical pathological series, which are subject to multiple biases {2628}. The autopsy prevalence of primary cardiac tumours reported in the literature varies greatly {56}, but may be estimated to be between 1 in 2000 {2628} and 2 in 1000 {2005}. The proportion of heart surgeries that are performed for tumours was only about 0.45–0.85% in several large series {2456,2482,2997}, and 0.093% in a multicentre paediatric series {201}. In Japan, the incidence of operated cardiac tumours is estimated to be about 500 cases per year {56}. However, surgical data certainly underestimate tumours that do not require surgery (e.g. rhabdomyomas and metastases), as well as tumours possibly revealed by sudden death. Pathological data from referral centres overestimate the rarest types of tumours, and the tumours that present diagnostic difficulties in histology, such as malignant neoplasms {2005}.

The histological variety of primary cardiac tumours is great {56,283,1128,2628}. The prevalence of each histological type is highly age-related. Nearly 90% of primary heart tumours are benign, in both children and adults {283,2628}. Each histological type has preferential anatomical locations (endocardium-valve-myocardium-pericardium; atrium-ventricle; left-right heart) {662,663,1954}. Primary cardiac tumours can be classified into three clinicopathological groups: benign congenital tumours, benign acquired tumours, and malignant tumours {2631}.

Myxomas account for 70–80% of all primary cardiac tumours in most surgical series {238,663,2456,2482}. In Iceland, an incidence rate of 0.11 per 100 000 has been calculated using more than 25 years' worth of data from centralized national registries {2397}. The peak of incidence is between the fourth and sixth decade {2628}. There is a female predominance, with about 60–70% of myxomas occurring in women {143,238,663,2631}. Myxomas other than those associated with Carney complex are very rare in children {2210}. In Carney complex, there is no female predominance of myxomas, and the tumours are generally multiple and atypically located. Aside from myxomas, the other benign acquired tumours included in most large series are, in order of decreasing frequency, papillary fibroelastomas, lipomas, and haemangiomas {238,663,2456,2631}. Other tumours (i.e. tumours of neural tissue, inflammatory myofibroblastic tumour, adult-type rhabdomyoma, etc.) are exceptional, and are generally reported as single or few cases.

Congenital benign tumours occur in children and infants, and are increasingly diagnosed in utero {283}. Paediatric series show that rhabdomyomas are the most common of these tumours, and that other types include, in order of decreasing frequency, fibromas, teratomas, and congenital haemangiomas {201,1954,2631}. Histiocytoid cardiomyopathy and cystic tumour of the atrioventricular node are very rare diseases. The heart may also rarely be involved by other congenital conditions, such as myofibromatosis {551}. Fibromas {662,1021,2631} and teratomas {471,2628} are rarely diagnosed in adults.

The proportion of primary cardiac tumours that are malignant is estimated to be about 10% {1827,2628}, and even less in children {1954}. In recent series, this proportion ranged from less than 10% {238,663,1954,2456} to 15–20% {143,2631}, and even up to 30% {56,2005}. The highest prevalence rates are typically observed in tertiary referral centres for difficult cases. Primary malignant tumours are mainly sarcomas {1248,1828}. Only about 1% of primary malignant cardiac tumours are lymphomas {1144}. In children, teratomas may rarely be malignant {1954}.

Tumours that have metastasized to the heart are much more common than primary cardiac tumours {56,296}, but are rarely surgically excised. They are often asymptomatic, and unlike most primary tumours, they seldom require histological confirmation or surgical treatment. Cardiac metastases are found in about 7–9% of autopsies of patients with malignant tumours {56,296}. The pericardium is the most common site of metastases, especially from lung and breast carcinomas {296}. Cardiac metastases are also frequently melanomas, lymphomas, or sarcomas {2482,2631}. Endocardial metastases, in the right heart preferentially, result from endovascular extension of renal, hepatic, and uterine cancers {56,296}.

Etiology

Some cardiac tumours occur in the setting of genetic predispositions or are part of genetic syndromes. This may have implications for genetic counselling, as well as therapeutic implications for targeted therapies.

Cardiac rhabdomyomas are associated with tuberous sclerosis – an autosomal dominant disorder characterized by the development of hamartomas in multiple organs. The disease is caused by mutations of the tumour suppressor genes *TSC1* or *TSC2*, at chromosomes 9q34 and 16p13.3, respectively. These mutations result in the loss of expression of hamartin and tuberin, respectively. The role of these proteins in the mTOR pathway, which has been demonstrated in cardiac rhabdomyoma {1164}, may have therapeutic implications {1694}. Most cardiac rhabdomyomas in children are associated with tuberous sclerosis, especially when the rhabdomyomas are multiple. Rhabdomyomas are usually the revealing symptom. Cardiac rhabdomyomas are found in about half of all children with tuberous sclerosis, especially in the case of *TSC2* mutation {1165}.

Cardiac fibromas may be associated with Gorlin syndrome (also called basal cell naevus syndrome and nevoid basal cell carcinoma syndrome) – an autosomal dominant disorder characterized by developmental abnormalities and a predisposition to neoplasia {1388}. This syndrome mainly results from germline mutations in the *PTCH1* gene at chromosome 9q22.3. This gene encodes a tumour suppressor protein, which inhibits the Hedgehog signalling pathway. Mutations of this gene are present in cutaneous basal cell tumours associated with Gorlin syndrome, as well as in most sporadic cutaneous basal cell carcinomas, with therapeutic implications {2595}. Interestingly, mutations of this gene have also been found in sporadic cardiac fibromas unassociated with Gorlin syndrome {2291}.

Histiocytoid cardiomyopathy sometimes occurs in families {283}, but the exact genetic abnormalities are unknown. Mitochondrial DNA mutations have been described {727}. A recent whole-genome expression analysis suggests a down-regulation of the IL33-IL1RL1/p38-MAPK/S100A8-S100A9 axis, and provides several candidate genes on 1q21.3c and 2q12.1a for predisposing inherited mutations {2351}.

Cardiac myxomas may be part of Carney complex – an autosomal dominant syndrome. This syndrome includes cardiac, cutaneous, and breast myxomas; cutaneous and mucosal pigmented lesions; Sertoli cell testicular tumours; thyroid tumours; and endocrine abnormalities, especially Cushing syndrome {2210}. About 70% of patients with Carney complex have germline mutations in the *PRKAR1A* gene on chromosome 17q22–24, which may function as a tumour suppressor gene {2210}. A mutation on chromosome 2p16 is less common. However, genetic abnormalities of these loci have not been definitely found to date in sporadic cases (which account for more than 90% of cardiac myxomas).

It is possible that some cardiac tumours are in part a reactive process. Papillary fibroelastomas may be giant forms of Lambl excrescences, and have been reported after cardiac instrumentation and thoracic irradiation {1370}. Calcified amorphous tumours may be ancient thrombi. The accumulation of fat in the atrial septum may be considered a true lipoma {2005}, but a subset in elderly and obese patients may simply be lipomatous hypertrophy.

The genomic profile of most cardiac undifferentiated sarcomas is similar to that

Table 4.01 Clinicopathological features of the main primary cardiac tumours

	Demographics			Location		Multiple tumours	Syndromic associations	Clinical presentation
	Infants/ fetuses	Children	Adults	Cardiac wall layer	Cardiac location			
Benign acquired tumours								
Myxoma		+/–	+ +	Endocardium (E)	Left atrium (P)	Rare (Carney complex)	Carney complex (5–10%)	Haemodynamic obstruction, embolization, constitutional symptoms
Papillary fibroelastoma		+/–	+ +	Endocardium (E)	Left-sided valves (P)	Occasional		Embolization
Haemangioma	+	+	+	Any	Any			
Lipoma		+/–	+	Any	Any		Tuberous sclerosis (rare)	
Inflammatory myofibroblastic tumour	+/–	+	+/–	Endocardium (P)	Any			
Benign congenital tumours								
Rhabdomyoma	+ +	+		Myocardium (E)	Ventricles (near E)	Common	Tuberous sclerosis (> 90%)	Haemodynamic obstruction, arrhythmia, spontaneous regression
Fibroma	+	+	+/–	Myocardium (E)	Ventricles (near E)		Gorlin syndrome (< 10%)	Haemodynamic obstruction, arrhythmia
Teratoma	+	+	+/–	Pericardium (near E)	Ventricular septum (rare)			Hydrops fetalis, tamponade, haemodynamic obstruction
Haemangioma	+/–			Myocardium (P)	Right atrium (P)			Spontaneous regression
Histiocytoid cardiomyopathy	+/–			Subendocardium (P)	Ventricles (near E)	Common	Familial cases	Arrhythmia
Malignant tumours								
Angiosarcoma		+/–	+	Any	Right atrioventricular groove (P)			
Undifferentiated pleomorphic sarcoma/ myxofibrosarcoma		+/–	+	Any	Left-sided chambers (P)			Pericardial effusion, Constitutional symptoms, Infiltration on imaging, Positron emission tomography (PET) positivity
Other sarcoma	+/–	+/–	+/–	Any	Any			
Lymphoma		+/–	+/–	Any	Right atrium (P)			
E, exclusive; P, predominant.								

of pulmonary artery intimal sarcomas, with recurrent alterations in *MDM2*, *PDG-FRA*, and *CDKN2A* genes, which could allow for the development of new targeted therapies {1828}.

Clinical features

Signs and symptoms

The clinical symptoms of the various cardiac tumours are often non-specific and insidious, which can delay diagnosis and surgical management. The symptoms may relate to processes in the heart, such as valvular dysfunction, pericardial effusion with tamponade, intracardiac blood flow obstruction, arrhythmia, and congestive heart failure. Alternatively, peripheral embolization may lead to systemic deficits, dyspnoea, chest pain, syncope, haemolysis, and sudden death. Constitutional symptoms include fever, malaise, and weight loss. An increasing proportion of cardiac tumours induce no symptoms at all, and become evident only as incidental findings {23,2482}. The clinical manifestations depend on the tumour's size, anatomical location, growth, and invasiveness {24,899,2484}. Most benign cardiac tumours form well-circumscribed nodular masses that can be completely resected. Malignant primary or metastatic cardiac tumours are often not entirely resectable, due to their large dimension, anatomical location, and infiltrative growth. In such cases, tumour debulking may be the only feasible surgical strategy {810,1467,1990}. A series of cardiac sarcomas showed a median survival of 39 months for completely resected tumours, 18 months for tumours that could not be entirely resected, and 11 months for unresectable tumours {1096}. Benign symptomatic cardiac tumours often present as intracavitary lesions with signs of embolization or obstruction, or constitutional manifestations {347,2181,2452}. Left-sided cardiac tumours (especially atrial myxomas) may cause systemic embolism involving the coronary, cerebral, and peripheral arteries, resulting in myocardial infarction, stroke, and ischaemic viscera or extremities {356,2730}. Left-sided tumours, especially papillary fibroelastomas, may also interact with mitral or aortic valve function, resulting in regurgitation or stenosis. These valve dysfunctions manifest as heart failure with progressive dyspnoea, pulmonary oedema,

fatigue, dizziness, syncope, and arrhythmia {1322,2480}. Right-sided cardiac tumours may lead to pulmonary embolism, with subsequent infarction and/or pulmonary hypertension. Obstruction of the atrioventricular or pulmonary outflow tract results in heart failure with signs of peripheral oedema, ascites, dyspnoea, hepatomegaly, and arterial hyper- or hypotension {1260,2481}. Cardiac congenital tumours (especially rhabdomyomas {1165}, fibromas {2631}, and congenital haemangiomas {1541}) generally and spontaneously become non-growing lesions or undergo regression.

Malignant primary and metastatic cardiac tumours may occur in any anatomical part of the heart; in the cavities as well as in the myocardium, pericardium, and contiguous structures. Clinical symptoms may be absent, or these tumours may cause haemodynamic instability (often at a later stage), with systemic disorders like fever, malaise, fatigue, anorexia, and weight loss. Pericardial effusion is a common presentation of cardiac metastases. Further infiltrating growth and extension may result in life-threatening complications or sudden death {23,2483,3016}.

Endomyocardial biopsy under echocardiographical guidance is useful for diagnosis, and facilitates therapeutic planning of malignant cardiac neoplasms, particularly in the setting of unresectable masses that require histological characterization before chemotherapy is started {2628}.

Imaging

Imaging evaluation of a suspected cardiac mass is performed to assess its location, morphology, and tissue character, as well as the extent of local invasion and vascular involvement, the impact on valve structures and blood flow, and extracardiac findings {288,2549}. Radiological investigation may include chest radiography, echocardiography, electrocardiography-gated cardiac CT angiography, MRI, and even coronary angiography {193,903,1021,2442}. The spectrum of cardiac masses includes benign, malignant, and secondary tumours, but the radiological differential diagnosis acknowledges that metastatic disease, thrombi, and vegetations are far more common than primary cardiac tumours. Additional clues that help to refine differential diagnosis include patient age, the presence of extracardiac malignancy,

genetic predisposition, HIV positivity, and prior organ transplantation.

Transthoracic echocardiography is inexpensive, simple, and widely available. It is generally the initial imaging method. Transoesophageal echocardiography is especially useful for assessing masses within the atria or associated with the valves. Pregnancy sonography may detect fetal organ anomalies, including heart tumours, usually from 18 to 23 weeks of gestation.

CT angiography, optimized with intravenous contrast administration and electrocardiography-synchronized data acquisition, provides excellent visualization of the cardiac anatomy, valvular configuration, and coronary vessels. Visual information is provided on contiguous axial images, complemented by coronal and sagittal multiplanar reconstructions, as well as three-dimensional renderings. In addition to localization and lesion contour, other CT features of a cardiac mass include tissue attenuation (soft tissue, fat, calcium, and fluid) and heterogeneity, along with patterns of contrast enhancement. Cardiac MRI sequences enhance the soft tissue differentiation of a cardiac mass (especially an intramural lesion) from adjacent myocardium, and reveal characteristic patterns of contrast enhancement (absent, early, or delayed). MRI acquires data over several cardiac cycles, providing dynamic information pertaining to myocardial perfusion, cardiac wall motion, lesion mobility, and valvular function.

Radiological features that strongly suggest benignity include well-defined margins, intracavitary location, narrow mural attachment, mobility, left-sided location, and the absence of associated pulmonary or pericardial nodules. For example, a cardiac myxoma is usually a smoothly marginated, intracavitary, pedunculated mass in the left atrium arising from the atrial septum. Papillary fibroelastomas are subcentimetre, pedunculated valvular masses, often discovered incidentally on an aortic or mitral valve leaflet. Cardiac fibromas are generally well circumscribed, ventricular, and partly calcified. Rhabdomyomas tend to be intramural, ventricular, and multiple in number. Lipomas and lipomatous hypertrophy of the atrial septum are distinguished by their uniform fat content and location. Contrast-enhanced CT or MRI may help to distinguish between a bland thrombus (a non-enhancing lesion) and a cardiac neoplasm.

Imaging findings that are more suggestive of malignancy are right-sided location, poorly defined tumour margins, intramyocardial location, wide-based mural attachment (if intracavitary), heterogeneity, and – most importantly – invasion of regional structures (including valves, pericardium, pleura, regional vessels, and mediastinum). Multifocal intracardiac or pericardial lesions and/or pulmonary metastases further support a malignant character. On CT, cardiac angiosarcoma typically appears as a right atrial mass (in 90% of cases), with high-attenuation pericardial effusion (haemopericardium) and enhancing pericardial nodularity (reflecting tumour hypervascularity). The characteristic MRI features of angiosarcoma include focal high-intensity areas on T1-weighted images (corresponding to areas of haemorrhage) and strong post contrast enhancement. Primary cardiac osteosarcoma variably demonstrates calcification, and arises almost exclusively (in > 95% of cases) in the left atrium, whereas metastatic osteosarcoma is usually centred in the right atrium. Primary cardiac lymphoma is typically multifocal, intramural, and accompanied by pericardial effusion on CT and MRI.

Critical companion findings of cardiac neoplasia that may be revealed on imaging include superior vena caval obstruction, valvular dysfunction, valvular tumour entrapment, pericardial tumour infiltration, large and/or haemorrhagic pericardial effusion, cardiac tamponade, and pulmonary or systemic embolization. In addition to directing prompt clinical intervention, imaging is also a practical tool for planning the surgical treatment of a cardiac mass, revealing the relationship of a mass to its adjacent coronary arterial anatomy.

Benign tumours and tumour-like lesions

C. Basso

Rhabdomyoma

Definition

Rhabdomyoma is a benign tumour of the striated cardiac myocytes.

ICD-O code   8900/0

Synonym

Cardiac rhabdomyoma

Epidemiology

Rhabdomyoma is the most common heart neoplasm in infants and children, estimated to account for > 60% of all heart tumours {162,165,755,2628}. It is also by far the most common tumour diagnosed in utero {1022}. Up to 86% of cardiac rhabdomyomas have been reported in association with tuberous sclerosis {237,949,2339}, and up to 60% of children with tuberous sclerosis are diagnosed with a cardiac rhabdomyoma by echocardiography {2815}. However, because many affected infants have no cardiac symptoms, cardiac rhabdomyomas not associated with tuberous sclerosis may go unrecognized, and the true incidence remains unknown.

Etiology

The striated muscle characteristics of rhabdomyoma cells and the absence of proliferative activity support the concept that rhabdomyoma is a hamartoma rather than a neoplasm.

Clinical features

Signs and symptoms

The clinical features of rhabdomyomas depend on their localization,

number of masses, and dimensions {237, 729,2339,2628}. Children may be asymptomatic or only mildly symptomatic, presenting with a cardiac murmur at physical examination {162,165,755}. Usually, prenatal diagnosis occurs when arrhythmias, hydrops, delayed fetal growth, or family history for tuberous sclerosis have been detected on routine fetal screening {116,1022,2726}.

A large intramural or intracavitary mass may cause ventricular outflow obstruction, or atrioventricular or semilunar valve distortion. Congestive heart failure, respiratory distress, or even low cardiac output syndrome may occur in neonates or infants. In the most severe cases, the ventricular obstruction may even mimic a severe subvalvular aortic stenosis, hypoplastic left heart syndrome, or pulmonary stenosis {5,540,761}. Exceptionally, the tumoural masses may diffusely infiltrate the myocardium and cause severe contractile and diastolic dysfunction, even mimicking a restrictive cardiomyopathy {205,1953}.

All the common arrhythmias, both atrial and ventricular, have been described in association with cardiac rhabdomyomas. Direct compression of the conduction system may account for conduction disturbances such as left axial deviation, bundle branch block, and various degrees of atrioventricular block. ST segment and T wave abnormalities are common {205,237,2339}. When located in the atrioventricular junction, the tumour may act like an accessory pathway, with resultant pre-excitation on 12-lead electrocardiogram {1597}. Tumour regression is

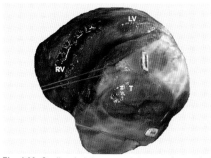

Fig. 4.02 Cardiac rhabdomyoma, intraoperative surgical view of the tumour during resection. LV, left ventricle; RV, right ventricle; T, tumour. Reprinted from Padalino MA et al. {1953}.

often associated with spontaneous resolution of the delta wave.

Imaging

Two-dimensional echocardiography remains the main diagnostic tool. Typically, rhabdomyomas are multiple, well-circumscribed nodular masses, which are highly echogenic, either intramural or pedunculated intracavitary, and localized everywhere in the myocardium {237,729}. Rhabdomyomas present with a homogeneous echogenicity due to the absence of fibrosis, necrosis, calcification, cystic areas, and haemorrhagic areas. This is an important feature to distinguish them from thrombi, myxomas, and others tumours. Pericardial effusion is rarely detected on echocardiography. The cardiac MRI signal characteristics of these well-defined homogeneous nodules are almost identical to those of the normal myocardium {193}.

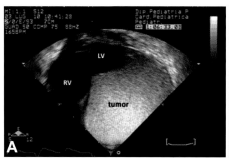
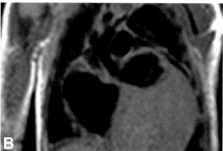
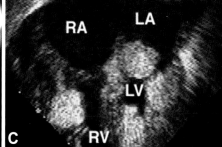

Fig. 4.01 A Two-dimensional echocardiographic detection of cardiac rhabdomyoma. Large intramural cardiac mass located at the posterior wall and apex of the left ventricle and involving the ventricular septum. **B** Cardiac MRI of a huge intramural left ventricular cardiac rhabdomyoma. Proton density T1-weighted fast spin echo in coronal plane, showing a large homogeneous, isointense mass involving the left ventricular wall. **C** Two-dimensional echocardiographic detection of cardiac rhabdomyoma. Multiple endocavitary masses involving the left and right ventricles. LA, left atrium; LV, left ventricle; RA, right atrium; RV, right ventricle. A and B reprinted from Padalino MA et al. {1953}.

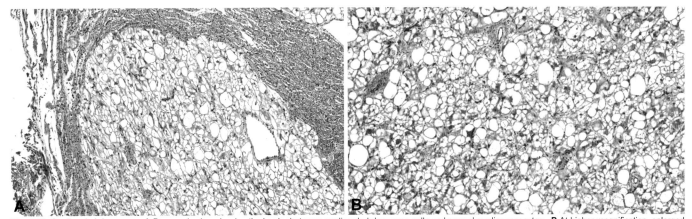

Fig. 4.03 Cardiac rhabdomyoma. **A** Panoramic view showing the border between cardiac rhabdomyoma cells and normal cardiac myocytes. **B** At higher magnification, enlarged swollen myocytes with clear cytoplasm and centrally located nucleus are visible; strands of cytoplasm are connected with the periphery of the cell (spider cells). B reprinted from Padalino MA et al. {1953}.

Localization

Rhabdomyomas may occur anywhere in the heart, most often in the ventricular myocardium. Although mostly intramural, they may sometimes protrude into the ventricular cavity, or they may occur as pedunculated or sessile masses.

Macroscopy

Rhabdomyomas are well-defined, unencapsulated, whitish or greyish nodular masses that range in size from millimetres to several centimetres. They are usually multiple, appearing as solitary masses in only 10% of cases.

Histopathology

Rhabdomyomas are well-demarcated nodules of enlarged vacuolated cells with clear cytoplasm due to abundant glycogen deposits. A characteristic feature is the so-called spider cell appearance, i.e. cells characterized by cytoplasmic radial extensions with contractile myofilaments from the central nucleus to the cell periphery {162,1952}. At transmission electron microscopy, rhabdomyoma cells look like myocytes, with abundant glycogen, rare mitochondria, and intercalated discs sparse all around the periphery of the cell instead of being localized at the cell poles.

On immunohistochemistry, the typical features of striated muscle cells are present (i.e. positive expression of myoglobin, desmin, actin, and vimentin). There is no evidence of cell proliferation by immunohistochemistry.

Cardiac fibroma is the other mural tumour occurring in infants and children, but has different histological features. Very rare cardiac sarcomas may occur in the ventricles of children, and are infiltrating tumours with histological features characteristic of sarcoma.

Genetic profile

Almost 50% of patients with rhabdomyoma present with a family history of tuberous sclerosis (an autosomal dominant disease with variable penetrance and expression).

To date, two genes have been found to be associated with tuberous sclerosis: *TSC1*, which encodes the protein hamartin (9q34); and *TSC2*, which encodes the protein tuberin (16p13.3) {2079,2755}. These two proteins are involved in the tumour suppression mechanism, but their precise role in cardiac tumour development remains unknown.

Prognosis and predictive factors

The natural history of rhabdomyomas is characterized by the possibility of spontaneous regression, either partial or complete. Complete resolution of > 80% of tumours may occur during early childhood {237}. Thus, surgery is reserved only for severely symptomatic patients; otherwise, clinical follow-up, associated with oral medication, is usually indicated {165,1121,1952,1954}. The most common reason for surgical referral is ventricular arrhythmia, which does not respond to drug therapy, and ventricular outflow obstruction. Although surgical resection should ideally be as radical as possible, the well-known possibility of spontaneous mass regression allows surgeons to safely perform a partial resection whenever a greater removal of tissue may jeopardize important cardiac structures.

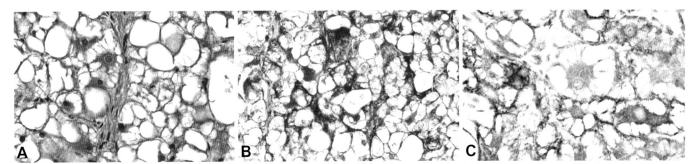

Fig. 4.04 Cardiac rhabdomyoma. **A** At higher magnification, enlarged swollen myocytes with clear cytoplasm and centrally located nucleus are visible; strands of cytoplasm are connected with the periphery of the cell (spider cells). **B** The enlarged cells are vacuolated due to abundant glycogen deposits in the cytoplasm. **C** At immunohistochemistry, cells are positive for striated muscle markers. B and C reprinted from Padalino MA et al. {1953}.

Histiocytoid cardiomyopathy

B.M. Shehata

Definition
Histiocytoid cardiomyopathy is a hamartomatous lesion of the sinoatrial node, atrioventricular node, and Purkinje fibres of the cardiac conduction system {2351}.

Synonyms
Infantile cardiomyopathy; oncocytic cardiomyopathy; infantile cardiomyopathy with histiocytoid changes; myocardial or conduction system hamartoma.
Obsolete: focal lipid cardiomyopathy; isolated cardiac lipidosis; foamy myocardial transformation; infantile xanthomatous cardiomyopathy; arachnocytosis of the myocardium {2352}

Epidemiology
Histiocytoid cardiomyopathy occurs predominately in the first 2 years of life; 20% of cases are diagnosed within the first month, and 60% within the first year. No case has been reported after 2.5 years of age.
The female to male ratio is 3:1. Histiocytoid cardiomyopathy appears to be most common in Caucasian infants, followed by African-American and Latin-American infants; it is rare in Asian infants {2352}.
About 100 cases have been reported in the literature, and over 120 cases are included in the histiocytoid cardiomyopathy registry. The prevalence of this disease may be higher than reported, since some cases are misdiagnosed as sudden infant death syndrome.

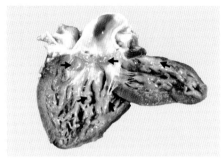

Fig. 4.06 Histiocytoid cardiomyopathy. Gross view of the heart, showing multiple histiocytoid nodules in the aortic valve leaflets, endocardium, and papillary muscles (arrows).

Etiology
Many theories have been proposed, including viral infection, toxic exposure, metabolic disorders, and mitochondrial myopathies.
The involvement of the sinoatrial and atrioventricular nodes, and the prevalence of histiocytoid cells along the Purkinje fibre distribution point to an origin from the cardiac conduction system. The primitive Purkinje cells of the developing heart show a striking resemblance to histiocytoid cells. Both types of cells show strong positivity for cholinesterase (present only in the conduction tissue) {2352}, and for neutral lipids with a Sudan black stain.

Clinical features
Histiocytoid cardiomyopathy is a distinct arrhythmogenic disorder, with 70% of cases presenting with arrhythmias and electrical disturbances {2168}, including paroxysmal atrial tachycardia, atrial fibrillation, ventricular fibrillation, ventricular tachycardia, premature atrial and ventricular contractions, Wolff-Parkinson-White syndrome, and right or left bundle branch block.
Approximately 20% of cases present as sudden death, and can be misclassified as sudden infant death syndrome. Other infants experience flu-like symptoms preceding or accompanying cardiac manifestations. Over 95% of patients show cardiomegaly.
Infants with histiocytoid cardiomyopathy show a spectrum of associated anomalies, including cardiac malformation (16%), extracardiac anomalies (17%), and combined cardiac and extracardiac anomalies (4%). Extracardiac oncocytic cells in exocrine and endocrine glands are reported in 7% of cases {2352}.

Localization
Histiocytoid cardiomyopathy nodules may occur in both ventricles, in the septum, and on the cardiac valves. Although they mainly occur beneath the endocardium following the distribution of the bundle branches of the conduction system, they can also occur in the inner myocardium, and (rarely) in subepicardial areas.

Macroscopy
Grossly, histiocytoid cardiomyopathy is characterized by single or multiple subendocardial yellow-tan nodules/plaques, ranging in size from 1 to 15 mm. The

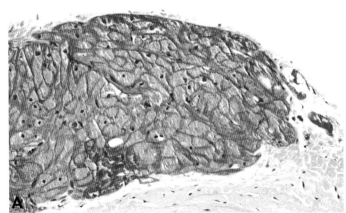
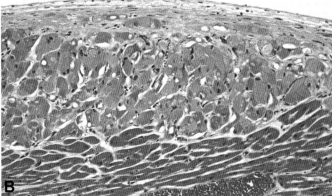

Fig. 4.05 Histiocytoid cardiomyopathy. **A** Microscopic view of the valve leaflet, with histiocytoid nodule. **B** Subendocardial histiocytoid nodule; note the poorly defined border with adjacent myocardial fibres.

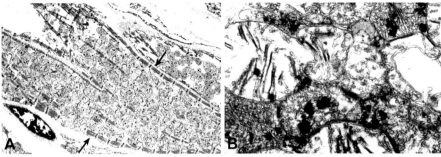

Fig. 4.07 Histiocytoid cardiomyopathy. **A** Electron microscopy showing histiocytoid cells packed with mitochondria; the diminished myofibrils are displaced to the periphery of the cell (arrows). **B** Higher magnification showing swollen mitochondria with disorganized cristae and dense membrane-bounded granules.

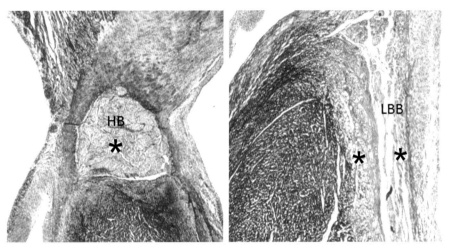

Fig. 4.08 Histiocytoid cardiomyopathy. A serial histological sections study of the specialized conducting tissue reveals foci of histiocytoid cells (asterisks) in the His bundle (HB) and left bundle branch (LBB) as well as adjacent myocardium. Reprinted from Rizzo S et al. {2168}.

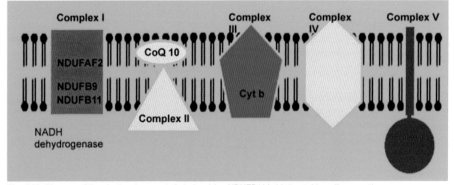

Fig. 4.09 Diagram of the electron transport chain involving NDUFB11 in histiocytoid cardiomyopathy.

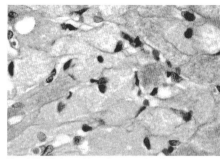

Fig. 4.10 Histiocytoid cardiomyopathy. Histiocytoid cells resembling foamy macrophages in the myocardium.

vimentin, or cytokeratin (CAM5.2), whereas S100 staining is variable. Cell proliferation markers such as Ki-67 (MIB1) are negative {835,2233}.

Ultrastructurally, the histiocytoid cardiomyopathy cells show poorly developed intercellular junctions. Their cytoplasm is characterized by a superabundance of swollen mitochondria containing dense membrane-bound granules with disorganized cristae. The diminished myofibrils are pushed to the periphery of the cell. Lipid droplets of variable size are also observed.

Mitochondrial cardiomyopathy shows no discrete nodules, all myocytes are affected, and the mitochondria are consistently abnormal (i.e. enlarged and variable in size and shape, with occasional glycogen particles). The cristae are increased in number and on cross-section are arranged in a concentric fashion surrounding occasional dense bodies. Chronic ischaemia may show subendocardial myocyte vacuolization.

Genetic profile

A familial tendency is reported in 5% of cases. However, the familial recurrence rate may actually be higher, due to the recurrent miscarriages in histiocytoid cardiomyopathy families.

A missense mutation in the *CYB* gene pointed towards a mitochondrial etiology {64}. A second mitochondrial mutation was found at A8344G in the mitochondrial DNA, within the *MT-TK* gene that encodes tRNA[Lys] {2734}. However, these mutations were not seen in histiocytoid cardiomyopathy registry cases {2351}.

Genomic expression profiling did not provide evidence for these putative causal genes for histiocytoid cardiomyopathy. Seven differentially expressed genes in histiocytoid cardiomyopathy that relate to interleukin signalling have been identified, but a causative role has not been

lesions may not be discernible as nodules, but multiple sections of the myocardium may show a mottled appearance, with irregular, poorly defined, yellowish-tan areas.

Histopathology

Histiocytoid cardiomyopathy lesions appear as multifocal, poorly defined islands of large polygonal cells with a granular eosinophilic cytoplasm, a small round to oval-shaped nucleus, and occasional nucleoli· The cytoplasmic appearance is due to extensive accumulation of mitochondria. These cells are distributed along the Purkinje fibres of the conduction system. The sinoatrial and atrioventricular nodes were involved in the majority of cases in which the conduction system was examined {2168,2352}.

Histiocytoid cardiomyopathy cells stain positive for desmin, myoglobin, myosin, and muscle-specific actin by immunohistochemistry. There is no expression of macrophage/histiocyte antigens (CD68, CD69, MAC387, LN3, and HAM56),

demonstrated {2351}. The female pre-dominance suggested an X-linked muta-tion, which was confirmed by a recent dis-covery of *NDUFB11* mutation in Xp11.23 in more than one case {206,2351A}.
In general, the findings suggest that his-tiocytoid cardiomyopathy is a genetically heterogeneous disease.

Prognosis and predictive factors
If left untreaed, this condition is usually fatal {2168}. However, the outcome has improved over the past two decades due to developments in surgical inter-vention, electrophysiological mapping, and ablation of the arrhythmogenic foci, with a survival rate of approximately 80%.

A few patients with extensive disease had cardiac transplant. Aggressive an-tiarrhythmic treatment may even allow the histiocytoid cardiomyopathy lesion to regress without the need for surgery {798,826,1229,1632}.

Hamartoma of mature cardiac myocytes

J.J. Maleszewski

Definition
Hamartoma of mature cardiac myocytes is a benign overgrowth of differentiated, mature striated cardiac myocytes.

Synonyms
Hamartoma of adult cardiac myocytes; cardiac hamartoma

Epidemiology
Hamartoma of mature cardiac myocytes is among the rarest primary cardiac tumours, with fewer than 25 cases reported in the literature. It has been reported in patients aged from 6 months to 76 years, although it tends to occur in younger patients, with a median age of 24 years {448,706}. Two thirds of cases occur in males.

Clinical features
Most are asymptomatic and found inci-dentally at the time of autopsy. In symp-tomatic cases, the clinical features are often related to arrhythmia (e.g. palpi-tations, syncope, chest pain, and sud-den death) {568}. Variable electrocar-diographical abnormalities have been reported {706}. Echocardiography, CT, and cardiac MRI visualize the size and location of these tumours {840}.

Localization
Hamartomas of mature cardiac myocytes usually arise in the ventricles, but atrial involvement has also been reported. They may arise as multiple or (more com-monly) solitary lesions {706}.

Macroscopy
Hamartoma of mature cardiac myocytes consists of firm, poorly defined areas of pale (fibrotic) tissue. The lesions are usually < 5 cm in greatest dimension, although tumours measuring up to 9 cm have been reported {706}. The poorly cir-cumscribed nature of these lesions can make complete surgical excision difficult {2113}.

Histopathology
The lesions are composed of enlarged, disorganized, striated cardiac myo-cytes with sarcoplasmic vacuolization and bizarre nuclei. The myocytes may be arranged in disorganized whorls or a herringbone pattern {286}. Tumour myocytes may merge with the normal myocardium or form a relatively abrupt transition. Variable amounts of interstitial fibrosis, adipose tissue, and nerves may be present. When significant collections

of blood vessels, smooth muscle, fat, and nerves have been identified, the term mesenchymal hamartoma has been em-ployed {252}.
The tumours express muscle markers such as desmin, troponin, actin, and myosin. Ki-67 studies have shown the le-sions to be non-proliferative {286}.
The differential diagnoses include car-diac rhabdomyoma (but so-called spider cells are not seen), cardiac fibroma (due to abundant interstitial collagen, com-bined with the pale and firm nature of the tumour), and hypertrophic cardiomyopa-thy (but such does not present as a dis-crete mass lesion). Genetic testing and family history may prove useful in distin-guishing between these entities.

Prognosis and predictive factors
Though histopathologically benign, these tumours can have fatal consequences, such as intractable arrhythmias or sud-den death {706}. Surgical excision (even when incomplete) has proven very effec-tive in cases where the tumours cause ar-rhythmia and/or haemodynamic obstruc-tion {568,2113}.

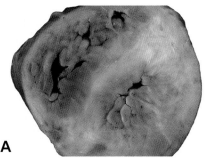 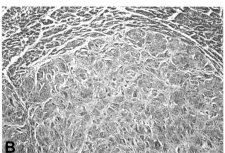 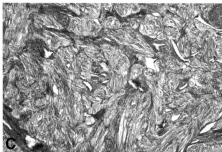

Fig. 4.11 Hamartoma of mature cardiac myocytes. **A** A poorly defined, vaguely circular area of apparent fibrosis can be seen in the anteroseptal region of this mid-ventricular, short-axis specimen. **B** Enlarged and disorganized myocytes can be seen in this photomicrograph, forming a distinct border with the adjacent normal myocardium. **C** A Masson trichrome stain highlights the degree of myocyte disorganization within the tumour, as well as the fibrosis interspersed throughout.

Adult cellular rhabdomyoma

A.P. Burke

Definition
Adult cellular rhabdomyoma is a benign neoplasm showing skeletal muscle differentiation, composed of round or spindle cells, and occurring in adult myocardium.

ICD-O code   8904/0

Synonym
Adult intracardiac rhabdomyoma

Epidemiology
Adult cellular rhabdomyomas are extremely rare, with few reported cases {285,2995}. Cardiac rhabdomyomas have been diagnosed in adults based on imaging findings, but without histological confirmation {651,2792}. Both men and women are affected.

Clinical features
The presenting symptoms include cardiac arrhythmias, but adult cellular rhabdomyoma can also be an incidental finding. Surgical excision has been successful in all cases, without reported recurrence.

Localization
The reported lesions occurred in the right atrium and in the right ventricle.

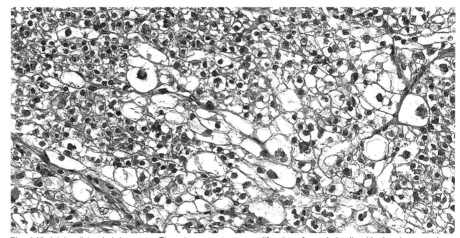

Fig. 4.12 Adult cellular rhabdomyoma. There is a monotonous proliferation of rounded cells with abundant cytoplasm and focal vacuolization.

Macroscopy
These tumours are soft, homogeneous masses that may be lobulated.

Histopathology
These tumours are composed of monomorphic, rounded or slightly spindled cells with abundant cytoplasm and focal cytoplasmic clearing. The histological appearance is similar to that of the adult type of extracardiac rhabdomyoma. Immunohistochemical stains for striated muscle are positive. There are few, if any, of the large vacuoles with cytoplasmic streaming (so-called spider cells) that are present in congenital rhabdomyoma. Unlike in congenital rhabdomyoma of the heart, which lacks proliferation, Ki-67 immunohistochemical staining shows a low proliferative rate.

Prognosis and predictive factors
There are no known recurrences.

Cardiac myxoma

D. Jain
J.J. Maleszewski

Definition
Cardiac myxoma is a benign neoplasm that consists of stellate, ovoid, or plump spindle cells within a vascular myxoid matrix.

ICD-O code   8840/0

Epidemiology
Cardiac myxoma is the most common true primary cardiac neoplasm.

It occurs in all age groups (having been described prenatally through the age of 97 years), but it manifests most commonly between the fourth and seventh decades of life {1364,1393,2161,2628}. Cardiac myxomas occur, on average, twice as commonly in women than in men {2970}, but this female predominance is not as striking in patients aged > 65 years {233}.

More than 90% of cardiac myxomas arise in an isolated fashion. The remaining cases arise in association with Carney complex (myxoma syndrome) – an autosomal dominant condition. Syndromic tumours generally occur in younger patients, with no sex predominance {879}.

Etiology
There has been controversy about the histogenesis of cardiac myxomas since they were first described. Initially they were thought to be reactive lesions or organizing thrombi; however, their locations within the heart, their genetics, and their overall histology are more characteristic of a neoplastic process. The origin of the myxoma cell (or lepidic cell) has also proven enigmatic. It was initially thought to originate from senescent endothelial cells in the region of the fossa ovalis (Prichard structures), but little evidence supported this notion {2733}. Recent molecular characterization studies have revealed protein expression profiles similar to those seen in endocardial-mesenchymal transformation of the endocardial cushion {1304,1930}. Whether these cells ultimately derive from developmental remnants or from re-expression by a terminally differentiated cardiac cell is

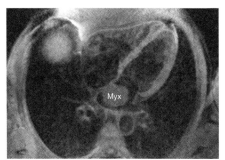

Fig. 4.13 Cardiac myxoma. Four-chamber, T1-weighted MRI at fat saturation shows a mass in the left atrium adherent to the atrial septum. The majority of the signal intensity is similar to that of myocardium. Myx, myxoma.

not yet clear. Immunohistochemical, ultrastructural, and in vitro studies, as well as the presence of glandular structures in a minority, seem to corroborate their neoplastic nature {2095,2145}.

Clinical features

Signs and symptoms
The clinical presentation of cardiac myxoma is diverse and (as is the case with most cardiac tumours) primarily dependent on tumour location, size, shape, mobility, and rate of growth. Patients with cardiac myxomas may be entirely asymptomatic (10–20%) or have symptoms of abrupt heart failure {1364}.

Cardiac symptoms
Cardiac myxomas can produce several cardiac symptoms, including syncope, dyspnoea, chest pain, and palpitations {2331}. Most cardiac symptoms are related to the tumours obstructing the normal flow of blood through the heart, either intermittently or throughout the cardiac cycle. Occasionally, atrial myxomas may obstruct the atrioventricular valve orifice, causing a diastolic tumour plop on auscultation. Some authors have noted an association between septal tumour location and heart failure, and between extraseptal location and neurological events {2547}.

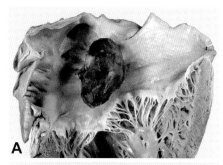

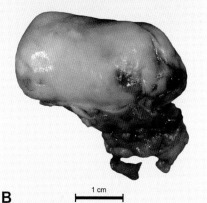

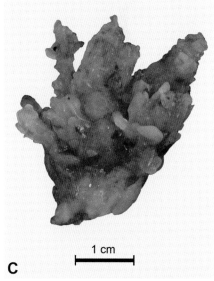

Fig. 4.14 Cardiac myxoma. **A** A cardiac myxoma arising from the left atrium, in the region of the fossa ovalis. Reprinted from Thiene G et al. {2628A}. **B** A pedunculated, solid-type myxoma with a smooth, undulating surface arising from a pedicle. **C** Villous-type myxoma with numerous, friable fronds; the cut surface of a myxoma exhibits a variegated appearance, with yellow, opalescent mucoid tissue and areas of focal haemorrhage.

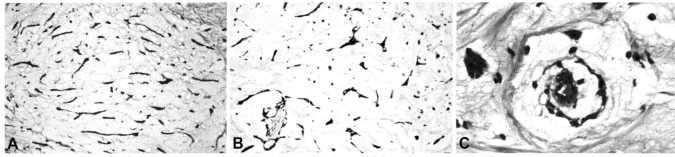

Fig. 4.15 Cardiac myxoma. **A** Myxoma cells existing as cords and nests in a myxoid background. **B** Reactivity of myxoma cell with antibodies directed against calretinin. **C** Myxoma cells forming rings around small intratumoural vessels (so-called vasoformative rings).

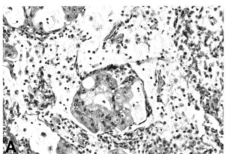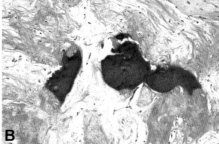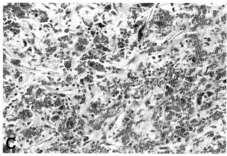

Fig. 4.16 Cardiac myxomas – unusual histological findings. **A** Gland formation. **B** Calcification. **C** Recent and chronic haemorrhage within the tumour.

Embolism

Villous tumours and those with abundant myxoid stroma are more likely to be associated with embolization. Tumour degeneration by over-expression of matrix metalloproteinases may hasten embolization {1931}. In addition to the tumour itself, embolization of surface thrombi is reported. Embolization to both the pulmonary and systemic circulation may occur, depending primarily on the site of the tumour and can result in pulmonary embolism, acute myocardial ischaemia or stroke {1324,2717}.

Table 4.02 Diagnosis of Carney complex requires the presence of two major criteria or one major and one supplemental criterion {2479}

Major criteria
Cardiac myxoma
Other myxoma (e.g. breast, cutaneous, or mucosal)
Spotty skin pigmentation or blue naevus
Cushing syndrome
Acromegaly
Large cell calcifying Sertoli cell tumour
Psammomatous melanotic schwannoma
Osteochondromyxoma
Supplemental criteria
Affected first-degree relative
Inactivating mutation of the *PRKAR1A* gene

Constitutional symptoms

Constitutional symptoms can include fever, weight loss, and arthralgias and are frequently associated with large or multiple tumours {673}. Clinical signs such as anaemia, leukocytosis, and elevated erythrocyte sedimentation rate may also be observed. Many of the phenomena are believed to be related to cytokine elaboration by the tumours themselves, including IL6, IL4, IL12p70, IFN gamma, and tumour necrosis factor {2413}. A wide range of paraneoplastic syndromes (including vasculitis/vasculopathy, pancreatitis, demyelinating neuropathy, and epistaxis) have been reported {2007,2273,2413}.

Carney complex

Less than 10% of cardiac myxomas arise in the setting of Carney complex, which includes previously described LAMB (lentigines, atrial myxomas, mucocutaneous myxomas, and blue naevi) and NAME (naevi, atrial myxoma, myxoidneurofibroma, and ephelides) syndromes. Carney complex is an autosomal dominant disorder characterized by the constellation of myxomas (cardiac or otherwise), endocrinopathy (Cushing syndrome and acromegaly), and spotty skin pigmentation. Clinical diagnosis is reliant on demonstration of a set of features that includes two major criteria or one major and one supplemental criterion {2479}.

Imaging

Transthoracic echocardiography is the diagnostic imaging modality of choice {276}. Echocardiographically, a cardiac myxoma usually appears as a mobile endocardial mass of irregular shape, most often arising in the left atrium in the region of the fossa ovalis. Areas of variable echogenicity and calcification may be seen. More advanced echocardiographical modalities, such as contrast and three-dimensional echocardiography, may help provide a more complete characterization of the tumour appearance, size, and location {1571,1907,2628,2649}.
If a definitive tumour stalk is not visible, cardiac MRI and CT may help to exclude the myocardial infiltration seen in malignant processes. Hypointensity in T1- and hyperintensity in T2-weighted images due to the gelatinous nature or high extracellular water content of myxomatous tissue are seen. Myxomas often show contrast enhancement due to their vascularity. Selective coronary angiography can visualize the blood supply of myxoma, sometimes with a tumour blush appearance.

Tumour spread

Myxomas can recur locally, a phenomenon that is usually explained by incomplete resection {1558,2121}. They can also spread to distant sites through embolization. After that, myxomas can infiltrate the arterial wall and produce histologically identical tumours at the embolization site. Intracranial aneurysm due to embolization is also a rare and morbid complication {2779}. Occasionally, myxoma cells may infiltrate the vascular wall, causing weakening and aneurysm {1139}.

Localization
Cardiac myxomas are intracavitary endocardial lesions, most often arising in the left atrium (80–90% of cases), in the region of the fossa ovalis {1558,2997}. The tumours have also been reported in all other cardiac chambers, and very rare examples of valvular myxomas have been described {712,2282,2979}. About half of the cardiac myxomas that arise in the setting of Carney complex occur outside of the left atrium, whereas < 20% occur outside of the left atrium in nonsyndromic circumstances {1558}. The tumours can also be multicentric, which is usually the case in the setting of Carney complex {2662}.

Macroscopy
The gross appearance of cardiac myxomas is quite variable. The tumours can be < 1 cm or > 15 cm in size {434,2060,2184,3015}. They may be either sessile and broad-based or pedunculated – arising from a stalk. Tumour stalks may occasionally be long, resulting in free mobility of the tumour within the chamber or through a valvular orifice. Two basic gross subtypes have been described: solid and villous. Tumours of the solid type may be globular or elongated, with a smooth, shiny, and sometimes undulant surface. Tumours of the villous type (as the name would imply) have irregular, often friable, papillary surfaces. Embolization may occur from the friable fronds themselves or from surface thrombi {1163}. The cut surface is variegated, usually owing to the myxoid tissue and areas of intratumoural haemorrhage, which is very common. The myxoid tissue has a mucoid appearance and can be pearly white, grey, or green-yellow. Areas of necrosis, cystic change, fibrosis, and calcification can also be seen {15,1987}. Rarely, cardiac myxomas show extensive calcifications with a stone-like appearance – the so-called lithomyxoma {150}.

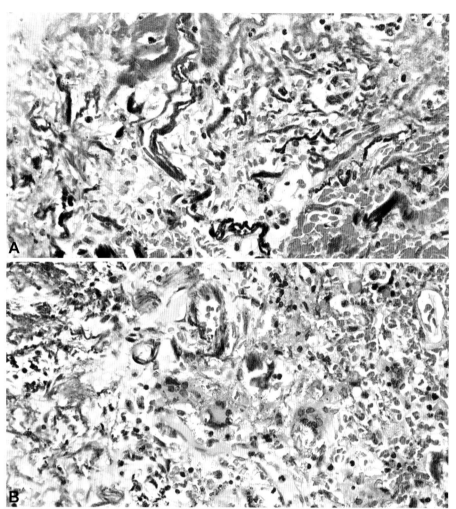

Fig. 4.17 Cardiac myxomas – unusual histological findings. **A** Gamna-Gandy bodies. **B** Macrophage giant cells.

Cytology
Cytological descriptions are scarce, with fewer than 15 cases reported in the literature {1112,1644}. The characteristic features are polyhedral or stellate tumour cells in a myxoid or mucinous background. Interspersed inflammatory cells, haemosiderin-laden macrophages, and Gamna-Gandy bodies may also be seen {1150}.

Histopathology
Cardiac myxomas exhibit considerable histological variability, sometimes even in different regions of the same tumour. The one defining characteristic is the presence of the so-called myxoma cell (or lepidic cell), a cytologically bland cell with eosinophilic cytoplasm and an oval or round nucleus. These stellate, ovoid, or plump spindle cells may occur singly or in groups. When in groups, the cells can form cords, nests, or rings. Rings frequently occur around capillaries or small vessels, and have been termed vasoformative rings.

The cells are typically within a myxoid matrix, rich in mucopolysaccharides with a variable amount of proteoglycan, collagen, and elastin {1128}. It shows strong reactivity with Alcian blue, is resistant to hyaluronidase, and shows patchy positivity with mucicarmine and periodic acid–Schiff stains. The background may also contain variable numbers of inflammatory cells and (rarely) multinucleated giant cells {290,986}.

Larger, thick-walled vessels are often present near the stalk or base of the lesion, while smaller vessels are present throughout {1930}. Haemorrhage, both recent and remote, is frequently encountered and is likely a product of the vascularity and trauma throughout the cardiac cycle. Remote haemorrhage can manifest as haemosiderin-laden macrophages and/or iron encrustation of the elastic fibres of the tumour

Table 4.03 The main differential diagnoses of endocardial-based masses

Mass	Location	Gross features	Histological features	Immunohistological features
Myxoma	Atrial, usually at the septum	Mucoid, variegated, smooth, or villous	Myxoma cells, myxoid matrix, haemorrhage	Calretinin-positive
Thrombus	Usually atrial	Homogeneous, rough surface, friable, may be heavily calcified (calcified amorphous tumour)	Fibrin-positive or -negative fibroblasts and granulation tissue	Calretinin-negative
Papillary fibroelastoma	Usually valvular	Many delicate fronds (when in solution)	Avascular fibroelastic fronds with bland, endothelial lining	CD34/CD31-positive lining cells, calretinin-negative
Sarcoma	Usually left atrial, not typically at the septum	Mucoid, usually with infiltration of normal structures	Myocardial infiltration, pleomorphism, necrosis, and mitoses	Smooth muscle actin-positive or -negative, calretinin-negative (dependent on histological type)
Haemangioma	Any cardiac chamber	Dark red to purple, not mucoid	Variably sized blood vessels	CD31/CD34-positive, calretinin-negative, actin-positive in pericytes
Rhabdomyoma	Any cardiac chamber	Well-defined, unencapsulated, whitish or greyish nodular masses	Enlarged vacuolated cells with clear cytoplasm due to abundant glycogen (spider cells)	Positive for myoglobin, desmin, actin, and vimentin
Metastatic carcinoma	Most commonly in the right atrium and right ventricle	Firm, well circumscribed, tan to yellow	Infiltrating malignant glands	Depends on primary site (kidney, uterus, liver, lung, etc.)

matrix (Gamna-Gandy bodies). Secondary degenerative changes such as fibrosis, cystic change, necrosis, thrombosis, calcification, and metaplastic bone formation can also be seen {150}.

Glandular elements are very rare – identified in < 3% of all myxomas {3014}. The glands are predominantly located at the base of the tumour, without local infiltration. Mucinous adenocarcinoma arising in glandular variant has also been reported {185}. Similarly, diffuse large B-cell lymphomas, some associated with EBV, have been described in the background of an otherwise classical cardiac myxoma {2542}.

Foci of extramedullary haematopoiesis may be seen in 7% of myxomas {1430}. Thymic rests and cellular thymoma-like elements have been observed {1675}. There have also been rare reports of gastric heterotopia, chondroid differentiation, and prominent oncocytic change {172,325,2098,2882}.

Immunohistochemistry
Myxoma cells exhibit reactivity with antibodies directed against calretinin in nearly all cases, while variable reactivity has been observed with antibodies directed against PGP9.5, neuron-specific enolase, S100 protein, synaptophysin, smooth muscle actin, and desmin {13}. The cells are non-reactive with epithelial and monocyte/macrophage markers. Endothelial markers (e.g. factor VIII, ulex europaeus agglutinin, CD31, CD34, thrombomodulin, and endothelin) are, as expected, positive in endothelium, with variable reactivity reported in myxoma cells {2255}.

Differential diagnosis
The primary differential diagnoses of cardiac myxoma include organizing thrombus, so-called calcified amorphous tumour (when calcification is present), papillary fibroelastoma (particularly when the myxoma is of the villous variety), and

other rare entities. When heterologous glands are identified, differentiation from metastatic adenocarcinoma is paramount, and can usually be achieved with clinical history, imaging, and ancillary studies.

Genetic profile
Study of syndromic myxomas has provided the most compelling genetic basis for myxoma formation. Genetic linkage analysis has implicated two independent loci in Carney complex: 17q23–24 and 2p16. Inactivating mutations in the *PRKAR1A* gene located at 17q23–24, coding for the cAMP-dependent protein kinase type I-alpha regulatory subunit, have been described in two thirds of Carney complex cases {2776}. The gene at locus 2p16 remains unknown; however, the presence of an activated oncogene at this locus is considered to be responsible for tumorigenesis in at least a subset of patients {1615,2963}. Although initially thought to play a role only in syndromic tumour formation {1533,1572}, *PRKAR1A* has also been implicated in a subset of patients without Carney complex {1560}. Cytogenetic data on myxoma are limited, but 15 previously analysed myxomas contained clonal numerical or non-clonal structural abnormalities. Cytogenetic analyses of 3 cases of Carney complex revealed similar chromosome patterns of non-syndromic cases {601,908}.

Prognosis and predictive factors
Non-syndromic and familial myxomas differ not only in their clinical features and etiology, but also in prognosis. The tumour recurrence rate is relatively low in non-syndromic patients (< 5%), but approaches 10–20% in Carney complex patients. Patients with Carney complex may also develop more than one tumour (in a synchronous or metachronous fashion), and are more likely to have atypical cardiac locations {207,2360}. The finding of any cardiac myxoma should lead to evaluation for Carney complex, a diagnosis that necessitates follow-up for the patient and their relatives {1558,1951}.

Papillary fibroelastoma

J.J. Maleszewski
A. Agaimy

Definition
Papillary fibroelastoma is a benign endocardial papillary growth that consists of endothelium overlying avascular fibroelastic fronds.

Synonyms
Fibroelastic papilloma; cardiac papilloma; giant Lambl excrescence

Epidemiology
Papillary fibroelastoma is the most common tumour or tumour-like lesion excised from the heart at many institutions {2584}. Due to increasing recognition through higher-resolution imaging techniques, they are now encountered more frequently than in the past {2628}. Papillary fibroelastoma is the most common primary cardiac valvular tumour-like lesion, accounting for 73% of the cases in one large series, and 89% of the cases in another {655,2234}. Patients are typically 60–70 years old, but lesions have been reported from the neonatal period up through 92 years of age, with no clear sex predominance {655,893,2584}.

Etiology
It is unclear whether papillary fibroelastomas are reactive growths, hamartomatous lesions, or neoplastic processes. There is no histological or molecular evidence that these lesions are true neoplams.
Associations have been described with rheumatic heart disease, hypertrophic cardiomyopathy, valvular heart disease, and congenital heart disease {2164,1370}. The fact that papillary fibroelastomas frequently arise on areas of damaged endothelium or haemodynamic trauma (e.g. in structural heart disease or at sites of prior surgery, instrumentation, or irradiation) seems to support the notion that they are reactive phenomena. Initially, some authors speculated that the association of papillary fibroelastoma with congenital heart defects was evidence of a hamartomatous nature {530}, but the abnormal haemodynamics/endothelial injury hypothesis may explain these examples as well.

Clinical features
The clinical presentation of papillary fibroelastomas varies greatly, from asymptomatic to symptoms of heart failure, syncope, embolic phenomena, or sudden death {148}. As is the case with most cardiac tumours, the clinical symptoms are dependent primarily on the size and location of the mass. Tumours arising from the aortic valve may obstruct flow, causing chest pain or dyspnoea {725}. Embolic symptoms such as transient ischaemic attacks or stroke have been reported in as many as 33% of patients with papillary fibroelastomas found on imaging {2584}. Such embolic phenomena may be related to embolization of the tumour itself or most probably of adherent surface or entrapped thrombus {148,893}.
Echocardiography is the preferred imaging modality for visualization of papillary fibroelastomas, which typically manifest as small mobile masses attached to an endocardial surface, with independent motion and a contour that is either stippled or shimmering. The latter may be best appreciated on high-resolution or transoesophageal echocardiography.

Localization
By definition, papillary fibroelastomas arise from the endocardial surface, with most arising from the valves. In surgical series, the left-sided valves are most commonly involved, with the aortic valve being the usual site. Papillary fibroelastomas often arise from diseased valves (e.g. in degenerative stenosis or rheumatic valve disease). Less common sites of involvement include the right-sided valves, the cardiac chambers, and the papillary muscles; exceptional cases arising within the aortic sinus have also been reported {230,1370}.
Papillary fibroelastomas may occur singly or as multifocal lesions (which are particularly common in iatrogenic settings and rheumatic valve disease). Individual patients with > 40 discrete synchronous papillary fibroelastomas have been described {1830}.

Macroscopy
Grossly, excised papillary fibroelastomas often have a round, whitish appearance and a soft consistency. When placed in solution, multiple delicate fronds unfurl, giving the tumour what has been termed a sea anemone-like appearance. The tumours range in size from 2 to 50 mm, and are usually attached to the endocardium by a single stalk. Occasionally, the stalk and fronds can be matted together in a thrombus, fibrosis, or calcification {148,725}.

Histopathology
Papillary fibroelastomas consist of narrow avascular papillary fronds that often exhibit complex branching patterns. Histologically, the collagen and elastic fibre arrangement is reminiscent of the tendinous cords of the atrioventricular valves. An elastic stain is helpful to delineate

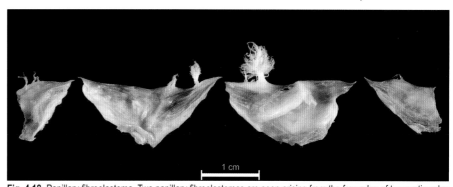

Fig. 4.18 Papillary fibroelastoma. Two papillary fibroelastomas are seen arising from the free edge of two aortic valve cusps; small Lambl excrescences that consist of simple, singular fronds can also be seen arising from the free edge of the cusps.

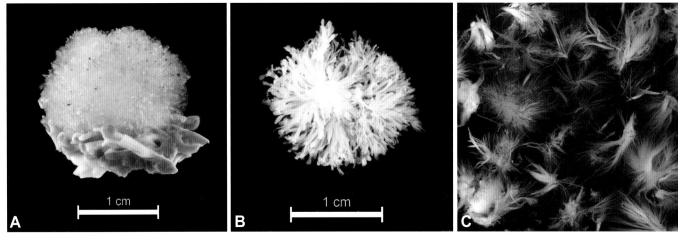

Fig. 4.19 Papillary fibroelastoma. **A** Papillary fibroelastoma arising from the left ventricle; the sea anemone-like quality of the tumour can be clearly seen. **B** Multiple fronds are visible, with complex branching. **C** Multiple (> 40) papillary fibroelastomas resected from the left ventricular outflow tract, 17 years after subaortic septal myectomy for hypertrophic obstructive cardiomyopathy.

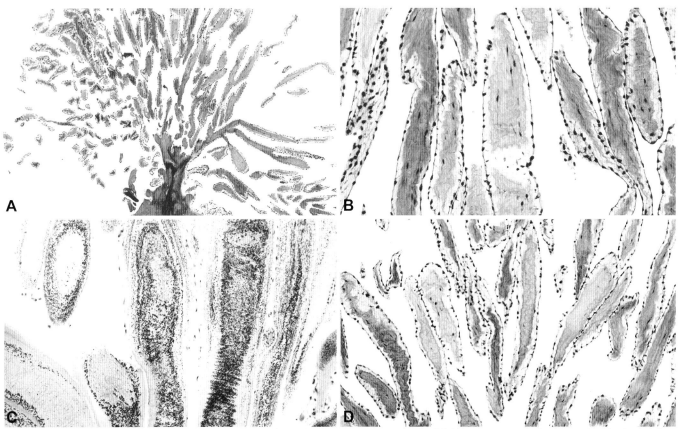

Fig. 4.20 Papillary fibroelastoma. **A** At low power; numerous arborizing fronds arise from a common central stalk. **B** At high power; avascular fronds, coated by bland endothelium, are prototypical of the lesion. **C** An elastic stain highlights the fibroelastic nature of the fronds. **D** Elastic fibres may be sparse or absent in the fronds, particularly at the tips.

the fibroelastic core, and a Movat pentachrome stain can highlight the rich mucopolysaccharide and proteoglycan matrix. The elastic fibres may be sparse or absent at the tips of the lesion. Occasionally, the fronds can fibrotically fuse together, but the fibroelastic fronds can still be visualized histologically. A single layer of endothelial cells coats the

fronds, and may have adherent surface thrombus.

Immunohistochemistry
Surface endothelial cells express factor VIII, CD34, and S100 protein {2218}. Less intense expression of factor VIII and CD31 compared to normal endocardial endothelial cells has been linked to

endothelial trauma and/or dysfunction. Some spindle cells within deeper layers may express S100 protein, possibly representing antigen-presenting dendritic cells.

Differential diagnosis
The differential diagnosis of papillary fibroelastoma includes cardiac myxoma,

thrombus, infective endocarditis vegetations, valvular strands, calcification (mural or valvular), and Lambl excrescences. Cardiac myxoma, particularly the papillary variety, can mimic a papillary fibroelastoma on imaging or gross evaluation. Although papillary fibroleastomas most commonly arise on the cardiac valves, it is very uncommon for myxomas to do so. Additionally, papillary fibroelastomas do not contain myxoma cells {24}, and have a characteristic fibroelastic core.

There is significant histological overlap between Lambl excrescences and papillary fibroelastomas. In fact, it is possible that the two processes represent a continuum of the same lesion. The term Lambl excrescence should only be applied to simple fronds (without branching) that are found on the closing surface of the valves (usually the aortic). Papillary fibroelastomas exhibit more complex branching patterns, and may arise on any endothelial surface.

Genetic profile
Given the relative paucicellularity of these tumours, detailed study of the genetics of papillary fibroelastoma is difficult. Two cases have been cytogenetically studied, showing heterogeneous translocations involving chromsomes 5, 21, and 15 in one case, and nullisomy Y with trisomies 12 and 20 in the other {2443,2814}.

Prognosis and predictive factors
Despite their benign histology, papillary fibroelastomas may have potentially devastating clinical sequelae, usually owing to their thromboembolic potential. Consequently, resection is recommended (particularly for left-sided lesions), and can often be done sparing the underlying cardiac structures. Anticoagulation may also be used if thromboembolic symptoms are present. Surgery provides excellent short- and long-term outcomes without significant recurrence, even when resection is incomplete {873,893,2512}. Regardless, follow-up echocardiography is often recommended after surgery.

Haemangioma

V. Thomas de Montpréville
J.J. Maleszewski

Definition
Cardiac haemangiomas are benign vascular tumours or malformations composed of mature blood vessels.

ICD-O codes
Haemangioma, NOS	9120/0
Capillary haemangioma	9131/0
Cavernous haemangioma	9121/0
Arteriovenous malformation	
Intramuscular haemangioma	9132/0

Synonyms
Cardiac angioma; cardiac vascular malformation

Epidemiology
Cardiac haemangiomas are rare, accounting for < 5% of benign tumours of the heart in recent published series {56,143,2628,2997}, and for 10% of benign tumours of the heart in a large multicentre surgical paediatric series {1954}. Haemangiomas can occur in patients of all ages, with a mean age at diagnosis in the fifth to sixth decade. There is no sex predominance.

Etiology
There is no known etiological factor in the formation of cardiac haemangioma. Most cardiac haemangiomas are sporadic.

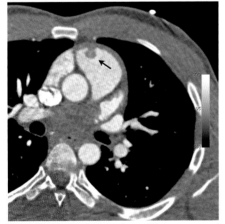

Fig. 4.21 Cardiac haemangioma. CT appearance of cardiac haemangioma; note the endocardial-based pedunculated mass in the anterior wall (arrow).

Clinical features

Signs and symptoms
Most cardiac haemangiomas are asymptomatic and found incidentally, although they may present with dyspnoea, palpitations, murmur, or (more rarely) thromboembolic events. These symptoms usually depend on tumour size and location. Intracavitary lesions may cause haemodynamic obstruction or valvular dysfunction. Arrhythmia and conduction disturbances may be related to an intramyocardial location. Pericardial involvement may lead to effusion, haemopericardium, or potentially tamponade {2429}. Congenital haemangiomas may be diagnosed in utero {193}, and are frequently associated with pericardial effusion {1383,1541}.
Large cardiac haemangiomas can result in thrombocytopenia and consumptive coagulopathy – the so-called Kasabach-Merritt syndrome {816}.

Imaging
Transthoracic echocardiography is a sensitive method for evaluating cardiac haemangioma {3942}. CT can show the heterogeneous appearance of these tumours, possible foci of calcification, and a typical avid enhancement {1021}. At MRI, haemangiomas are isointense to myocardium on T1-weighted images. High and prolonged enhancement after injection of gadolinium and high signal on T2-weighted spin echo are related to the important and slow blood flow {1021}. Distinction between haemangioma and highly vascular tumours such as paraganglioma may be difficult {193}. A typical tumour blush can be seen during coronary angiography {2169}.

Localization
Haemangiomas may arise from any cardiac layer: endocardium, myocardium, or pericardium {2628}. The ventricular free walls are the most common sites of involvement, with relatively equal distribution between the right and left {942}. Congenital haemangiomas most often involve the right atrium {1541}.

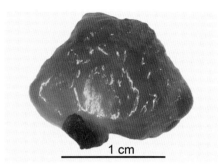

Fig. 4.22 Cardiac haemangioma. Gross photograph of a surgically excised cardiac haemangioma; the tumour has a cherry-red appearance; it arose as an intracavitary polypoid mass and was found on evaluation for chest palpitations.

Macroscopy
Cardiac haemangiomas form red to purple nodules that are usually solitary {942,1128}. Intramyocardial lesions are often poorly circumscribed, and merge with the adjacent myocardium. Endocardial haemangiomas manifest as sessile or polypoid intracavitary lesions. Tumours ranging in size from 1 to 8 cm have been described {942}.

Histopathology
Histologically, cardiac haemangiomas are composed of variably sized blood vessel-containing bland endothelial cells, similar to their extracardiac counterparts. There are several recognized morphological subtypes in the soft tissue, of which four (capillary, cavernous, intramuscular, and arteriovenous) occur in the heart. Many cases show features of multiple subtypes, and in the heart, the intramuscular and arteriovenous subtypes show overlapping histological features. Most tumours in the heart are of the capillary or cavernous type. Tumours with epithelioid features have also been described {280,1439}. Capillary and cavernous haemangiomas are typically endocardial-based tumours attached to the wall of the chamber by a broad base or small stalk, and do not infiltrate the myocardium. They often have a myxoid background, and if capillary, are frequently misdiagnosed as myxomas. The arteriovenous malformation type is intramural, and has some features of intramuscular haemangioma of skeletal muscle.

318   Tumours of the heart

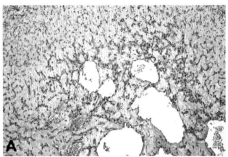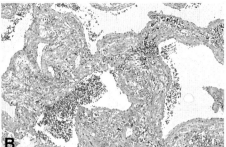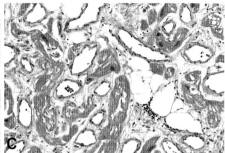

Fig. 4.23 Cardiac haemangioma. **A** Capillary-type haemangioma with a grouping of capillary-sized vessels around a central feeder vessel, in a myxoid background. **B** Cavernous-type haemangioma with large dilated vessels. **C** Intramuscular cardiac haemangioma with a mixture of vessels, fat, and entrapped cardiac myocytes.

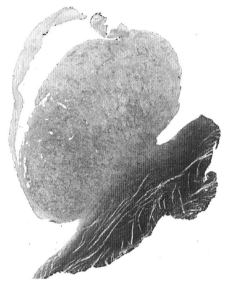

Fig. 4.24 Cardiac haemangioma, capillary type. Low-magnification view of endocardial cardiac haemangioma.

Capillary haemangiomas consist of small, thin-walled vessels arising from and clustered around a larger feeder vessel. Small capillary lumens may be difficult to immediately detect in cellular lesions. The intervening stroma may have a myxoid character, and scattered pericytes and fibroblasts may be seen. So-called infantile haemangiomas, which are considered a type of capillary haemangioma, contain back-to-back capillaries and no intervening fibrous tissue {1541}. In this type, mitoses may be numerous at the proliferative stage and immunohistochemical expression of GLUT1 is characteristic {1541}.

Cavernous types exhibit large, dilated vascular spaces, often situated within the myocardium itself. The vessels may be thin- or thick-walled, and pools of blood may be present throughout.

The arteriovenous type is characterized by arterial and venous structures, the latter of which often exhibit remodelling and arterialization, owing to the complex arterial anastomoses and exposure to systemic pressures.

The intramuscular type is characterized by entrapped myocytes. This variant often has fatty differentiation and fibrous tissue, similar to intramuscular haemangiomas of skeletal muscle. The vessels may be thin-walled, or resemble those of arteriovenous haemangioma.

Differential diagnosis

The differential diagnosis of haemangiomas consists of neoplastic and nonneoplastic entities. Blood cysts are congenital cysts often occurring along the lines of closure of heart valves. These endothelial-lined cysts are not connected to a feeder vessel and have no vessel wall. Cardiac varices, typically found in the right atrium, are dilated and thrombosed veins, considered by some to be a form of venous malformation/haemangioma {2195}. Organizing thrombi can occasionally mimic intracavitary haemangiomas, but usually contain more haemosiderin and fewer vessels. Cardiac myxomas may also be mistaken for haemangiomas, owing to their vascular nature. The latter, however, do not have the myxoma cells in the tumour or around the small vessels encountered in myxomas. Angiosarcomas may be difficult to distinguish from haemangioma in small biopsies. The diagnosis of angiosarcoma rests in cellular atypia, architectural features of anastomic channels, and other sarcomatous features.

Genetic profile

Cardiac haemangiomas are usually sporadic, without evidence of extracardiac visceral lesions. Neither molecular genetic nor cytogenetic studies of cardiac haemangiomas have been performed. However, extracardiac haemangiomas have been described in several syndromic contexts that may apply to a subset of cardiac haemangiomas. The malformation type of cardiac haemangioma has been rarely reported with syndromic association (in Klippel-Trenaunay syndrome) {1120}.

Prognosis and predictive factors

Cardiac haemangiomas are benign lesions that are usually resected with no recurrence. After a growth phase, infantile haemangiomas usually exhibit regression, either spontaneously or with pharmacotherapy {1438,1541,2653}. Therefore, when imaging studies suggest a benign vascular tumour, conservative management may be indicated, including steroid therapy, which may hasten regression {384}. Surgical excision is generally successful in alleviating symptoms in patients with cardiac haemangioma, even when necessitating extensive wall reconstruction {1383,1954,2474}.

Cardiac fibroma

K. Shibuya
A.P. Burke

Definition

Cardiac fibroma is a benign congenital mesenchymal tumour, composed of bland fibroblasts in a variably collagenized stroma.

ICD-O code   8810/0

Synonyms

Fibrous hamartoma; fibroelastic hamartoma; cardiac fibromatosis

Epidemiology

Cardiac fibroma is a tumour that primarily affects children. Most cases are detected in infants or in utero. They are the second most common benign cardiac tumour in children (after rhabdomyoma), as well as the second most common in fetuses, due to prenatal diagnosis {2660}. There is a slight male predominance.

Etiology

There is an increased risk of cardiac fibroma in patients with Gorlin syndrome {466,877,1328}. Cardiac fibromas are noted in < 14% of patients with the syndrome, but the association is not considered random {466,877,1328}. The etiology of sporadic cardiac fibroma is unknown. A patient with cardiac fibroma and multiple neural midline defects has also been described {545}.

Clinical features

The dimensions of the mass and its location are the main determinants of the clinical presentation. Although sometimes incidentally discovered in asymptomatic patients, cardiac fibromas more commonly cause ventricular arrhythmias and conduction disturbances. Occasionally, tumours may present as sudden death due to ventricular septal myocardium and conduction system involvement. When large and intramural, cardiac fibroma may protrude into the ventricular outflow tract and cause severe mechanical obstruction, together with contractile dysfunction and severe congestive heart failure {2628}.

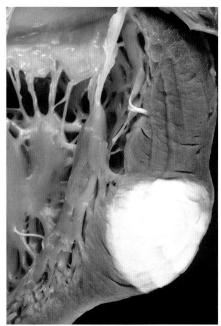

Fig. 4.25 Cardiac fibroma. The cut surface shows a homogeneous white circumscribed mass within the left ventricular free wall.

Cardiac imaging tools detect solid intramural masses that are homogeneously dense and may be either sharply marginated or infiltrative {193,2628}. Dystrophic calcification is common.

Because of their dense, fibrous nature, the tumours are usually homogeneous and hypointense on T2-weighted cardiac MRI, and isointense relative to muscle on T1-weighted images. Little or no contrast enhancement is usually detected {193}.

Localization

Most cardiac fibromas occur in the left ventricle, followed by the right ventricle, the ventricular septum, and the atria. They occur intramurally – within the ventricular wall or septum – as opposed to being intracavitary tumours, and bulge on cut section.

Macroscopy

Cardiac fibromas are well-circumscribed, firm, usually solitary, white masses, grossly resembling fibromatosis or uterine leiomyomas. Their appearance on cut section is typically whorled.

Histopathology

Cardiac fibroma is composed of monomorphic fibroblasts that demonstrate little or no atypia. The margins infiltrate into cardiac muscle. The degree of cellularity often decreases with the age of the patient, and the amount of collagen increases {287}. There can be a focally myxoid background. Mitoses are generally present only in tumours occurring in infants. There can be occasional perivascular aggregates of lymphocytes and histiocytes or sparse chronic inflammation at the junction of the tumour and uninvolved myocardium. Calcification is a common finding in fibromas from patients of all ages. Variable numbers of elastic fibres can be present, this finding is independent of age {287}. The presence of tumour at surgical margins has not been shown to increase the risk of recurrence.

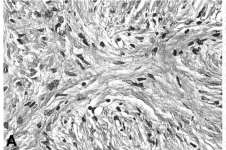
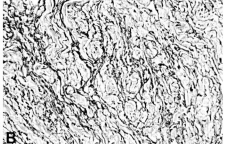

Fig. 4.26 Cardiac fibroma. A The tumour is composed of bland spindle cells in a collagenous matrix. B Elastic fibres are frequently present among the fibroblasts.

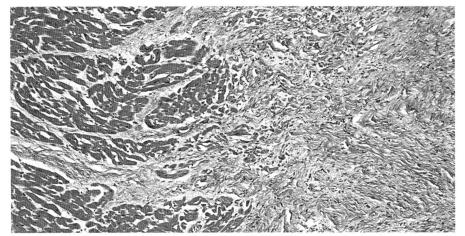
Fig. 4.27 Cardiac fibroma. The periphery of the tumour frequently interdigitates with cardiac muscle.

The tumour cells show myofibroblastic differentiation and are positive for vimentin and smooth muscle actin, whereas CD34, S100, and HMB45 are negative {50,550,2781,2791}.

In children, the differential diagnoses include well-differentiated fibrosarcoma, which is extraordinarily rare, and rhabdomyomas, which are histologically distinct. In adults, the differential diagnoses include fibrous lesions secondary to scarring, which do not form discrete masses.

Genetic profile
Mutations of the tumour suppressor gene *PTCH1* are the underlying cause of Gorlin syndrome {2291}. A suppressor gene role for *PTCH1* has also been found in non-syndromic cardiac fibroma {2291}.

Prognosis and predictive factors
Cardiac fibromas in infancy that are not surgically resectable because of size and extensive myocardial infiltration have a poor prognosis, and may require defibrillator implantation or cardiac transplantation {1954}. Tumours that can be resected (even incompletely) have a good prognosis. In one study, the median survival of patients with cardiac fibroma after successful surgery was 27 years {663}.

Lipoma

J.P. Veinot

Definition
Lipoma is a benign mesenchymal tumour of mature adipocytes (white fat cells).

ICD-O code   8850/0

Synonyms
Fibrolipoma; sclerosed lipoma

Epidemiology
Lipoma is a rare tumour in the heart, accounting for only 0.5–3% of all excised cardiac tumours. However, since lipomas do not usually require surgery, their surgical pathology prevalence is low. Additionally, the higher reported incidences in some publications may include lipomatous hypertrophy of the atrial septum {2769}. All ages are affected, and there is no sex predominance.

Etiology
These tumours can be part of diffuse lipomatosis or isolated neoplasms.

Clinical features
Many lipomas are clinically silent or indolent. The clinical presentation depends on the size and location of the mass. Pericardial lipomas may grow large and eventually present with a tamponade-like clinical picture. Lipomas may be associated with arrhythmias, sudden death, syncope, or signs of chamber enlargement {123,348,2414,2769}.
There is variable echogenicity by echocardiogram. CT and MRI allow characterization of the tissue type, and should facilitate the diagnosis {2114,2769}.

Localization
Lipomas are often located on the epicardial or endocardial surfaces. They

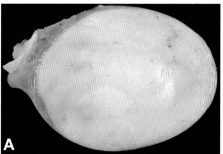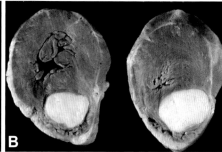

Fig. 4.28 Cardiac lipoma. **A** Gross appearance of a resected cardiac lipoma; note the rim of cardiac muscle at the left. **B** Cardiac lipoma at autopsy; round homogeneous fatty tumour within the myocardium.

may also occupy the pericardial space or be intracavitary. Rarely, they are intramyocardial. Fibrolipomas (sclerosed lipomas) have been described as small nodules on the cardiac valves {1611,2122,2414,2515,2769}.

Macroscopy
Lipomas are yellow, soft, smooth, well-circumscribed, encapsulated, usually solitary masses. They may be polypoid or pedunculated {2414,2769}.

Histopathology
The tumours consist of white fat with a fibrous capsule and some fibrous septa; a few entrapped cardiac myocytes at the periphery can be seen, but the fat cells often displace these. The fat cells have minimal to no atypia. Lipomas may be associated with fat necrosis, and the macrophages may resemble lipoblasts, but a lipoma does not have true lipoblasts.
Lipomas are S100 protein-positive.
The differential diagnoses are normal epicardial fat, lipomatous hypertrophy of the atrial septum, hibernoma, and liposarcoma. The distinction between hibernoma and lipomatous hypertrophy of the atrial septum may be difficult because of

overlapping histological features, namely the presence of brown fat {599,2481}. Lipomatous hypertrophy of the atrial septum is usually considered a non-neoplastic process. Rare reports of hibernoma (brown fat) have been described, but may represent lipomatous hypertrophy of the atrial septum.

Genetic profile
There are some reports of cardiac lipomas associated with tuberous sclerosis or Cowden syndrome. Cytogenetic studies have targeted candidate chromosomal loci that may be perturbed during cardiac lipoma pathogenesis {348,1117,1210,2764,2769}.

Prognosis and predictive factors
Prognosis depends on the size and location of the mass, and the clinical presentation. Usually lipomas do not represent an indication for surgery. Many can be resected with cure.

Cystic tumour of the atrioventricular node

J.P. Veinot

Definition
Cystic tumour of the atrioventricular node is a benign congenital mass located in the region of the atrioventricular node. This mass is not a tumour in the classical sense, but retains this designation for historical reasons and also because it forms a mass lesion. It is now thought to be an endodermal developmental rest {74,2769}.

ICD-O code   8454/0

Synonyms
Cystic tumour; ectopic heterotopia; endodermal heterotopia/inclusion/cyst {2628} Not recommended: lymphangioendothelioma; atrioventricular node mesothelioma; lymphangioma; endothelioma

Epidemiology
Cystic tumour of the atrioventricular node is considered to be a rare lesion, with fewer than 100 reported cases. However, the true incidence rate is unknown, because the mass is usually only discovered if the conduction system is examined at autopsy or transplantation {2628}.

The mean age at diagnosis is about 38 years, ranging from birth up to 95 years. Women are affected more often than men {74,1417,2769}.

Etiology
Cystic tumour of the atrioventricular node is thought to occur congenitally, as an embryonic rest related to development (choristoma). A rest of endoderm becomes included into the heart during cardiac folding and development. The mass is occasionally associated with other defects, including omphalocele, nasopharyngeal abnormalities, septum pellucidum absence, ectopic thyroid tissue, and thyroglossal duct cysts {74,311,2769}.

Clinical features
These tumours are most often discovered at autopsy of a patient with sudden death, when the conduction system is examined. They may also be detected by imaging. Clinically, they may be associated with variable degrees of atrioventricular conduction block (often complete block), and sometimes with congenital complete heart block {1417,2769}. The mass may be clinically silent or there may be signs and symptoms related to heart block. A pacemaker is often required.
A cystic lesion at the base of the atrial septum may be found by echocardiography and CT or MRI {1973}.

Macroscopy
A cystic tumour of the atrioventricular node may be apparent as a small bulge or swelling at the base of the atrial septum. Cysts may not be visible grossly.

Localization
The mass occurs in the region of the atrioventricular node in the right atrium near the base of the atrial septum, in the area of the membranous septum.

Histopathology
Cystic tumours of the atrioventricular node contain multiple variably sized cysts that may contain fluid. The atrioventricular node is displaced or absent. The mass does not invade into the myocardium or the membranous septum. The cyst walls are usually lined by columnar,

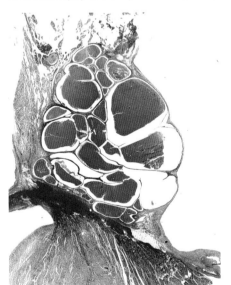

Fig. 4.29 Cystic tumour of the atrioventricular node. Panoramic view; atrioventricular node histology reveals a subendocardial mass that consists of multiple cysts varying in size and filled with mucoid material. Reprinted from Basso C et al. {147A}.

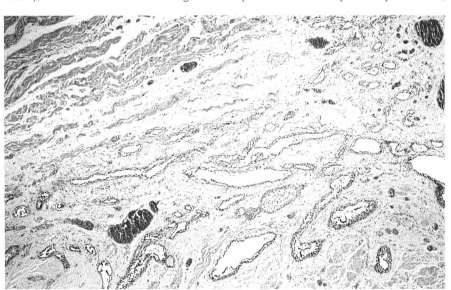

Fig. 4.30 Cystic tumour of the atrioventricular node. The tumour is composed of separated nests of epithelial cells (most forming cystic spaces) interspersed in the fibrous tissue, and myocytes in the atrial septum near the central fibrous body.

transitional, or squamous cells. Goblet cells and sebaceous cells have also been described. No cellular atypia is present. Mitotic figures are rare, but have been interpreted as evidence of growth after birth. The mass grows slowly, and may present clinically later in life {74,2769}.

The endodermal origin is reflected by positive staining for cytokeratin AE1/AE3, CK5, and carcinoembryonic antigen, and scattered cells may be positive for serotonin, chromogranin, and calcitonin. Mesothelial markers such as calretinin and HBME are negative. Endothelial and lymphatic markers are negative {74,311,1970}.

Differential diagnoses include simple cysts or bronchogenic cysts, which are rarely present in the atrial septum, and intracardiac teratoma {2769}.

Prognosis and predictive factors
The tumours are usually only apparent after development of conduction block or sudden death. Rare cases have been surgically excised, after which the individuals required a pacemaker {1417,1973}.

Granular cell tumour

A.P. Burke
V. Thomas de Montpréville
C.D.M. Fletcher
J.J. Maleszewski
F. Tavora
H. Tazelaar

Definition
Cardiac granular cell tumours are neoplasms of large, eosinophilic granular cells of Schwannian origin.

ICD-O code   9580/0

Synonyms
Granular cell schwannoma; granular cell myoblastoma (obsolete); granular cell nerve sheath tumour

Epidemiology
Most cardiac granular cell tumours occur in adults in the third to sixth decade of life. No sex predominance has been described.

Etiology
The precise etiology of cardiac granular cell tumours is unknown, but they are thought to be of neuroectodermal origin.

Clinical features
Most cardiac granular cell tumours are discovered incidentally at surgery or on autopsy. Multicentric granular cell tumours that occurred in more organs, including the heart, have also been reported {2100}.

Localization
Cardiac granular cell tumours usually arise epicardially, in regions of the heart that are rich in neural tissue, particularly the sinus node region {2802}.

Macroscopy
Cardiac granular cell tumours are firm, well-circumscribed epicardial masses.

Histopathology
The tumours are characterized by abundant collections of cells with eosinophilic, distinctly granular cytoplasm. They may appear to infiltrate the adjacent myocardial interstitium, despite their gross circumscription.

Tumour cells show reactivity with antibodies directed against S100 protein, neuron-specific enolase, CD68, and inhibin alpha. They are non-reactive for neurofilament and glial fibrillary acidic protein.

The differential diagnoses of cardiac granular cell tumour include histiocytic processes such as juvenile xanthogranuloma and Rosai-Dorfman disease {1445,1559}. The absence of giant cells, lack of emperipolesis, and reactivity with neuron-specific enolase can help to

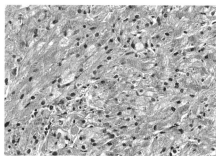

Fig. 4.31 Cardiac granular cell tumour. The tumour is characterized by a proliferation of bland cells, with an eosinophilic granular cytoplasm.

distinguish granular cell tumour from these lesions.

Genetic profile
No genetic data are available for cardiac granular cell tumour. However, multiple granular cell tumours have been reported in the context of LEOPARD syndrome, due to a mutation in the *PTPN11* gene {2307}.

Prognosis and predictive factors
To date, no malignant primary granular cell tumours of the heart have been described. However, involvement of the heart by metastases or disseminated congenital granular cell tumour has been reported {906,1992}.

Schwannoma

A.P. Burke
V. Thomas de Montpréville
C.D.M. Fletcher
J.J. Maleszewski
F. Tavora
H. Tazelaar

Definition
Schwannoma is a benign neoplasm differentiating as or originating from the Schwann cells of nerve fibres.

ICD-O code   9560/0

Synonyms
Neurilemmoma; neurinoma; neurolemmoma

Epidemiology
Cardiac schwannomas occur in adults, with a reported age range of 26–72 years, and a mean age of 53 years {213,850}. No cardiac schwannomas have occured in the paediatric age group. Women seem to be affected slightly more often than men – the female-to-male ratio is 3:2.

Etiology
No etiological factors have been identified, and none of the reported patients has had neurofibromatosis type 1.

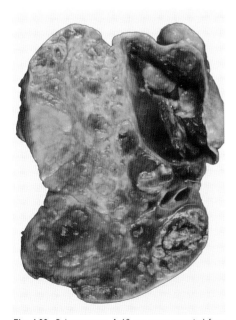

Fig. 4.32 Schwannoma. A 16 cm mass resected from a middle-aged woman with an abnormal chest X-ray; imaging showed an intrapericardial tumour located in the transverse sinus between the roof of the left atrium and the inferior surface of the left pulmonary artery; the cut surface shows solid and cystic areas.

Clinical features
Some patients report palpitation, shortness of breath, syncope, and atypical chest pain. Other patients are asymptomatic {2475}, with tumours identified during an evaluation for another disease {59} or at autopsy. Work-up of patients has identified the presence of murmurs and atrial fibrillation {194}.
Whether by CT, echocardiography, or MRI, schwannomas are described as heterogeneous, hypodense, and often cystic. They are rarely calcified. Tumour blush has been observed on angiography {2335}.

Localization
All four cardiac chambers have been the site of schwannoma growth, although there is a tendency for these tumours to arise in the right atrium. Within the right atrium, they typically arise near the septum, but they have also been found attached to the Eustachian valve, near the cavoatrial junction and the atrioventricular node.

Macroscopy
Schwannomas as small as 1.5 cm and as large as 10 cm in greatest dimension have been reported, with most cases in the range of 5 to 6 cm.
They have a variety of appearances; some look like classical schwannomas (tan-white to yellow with foci of cystic change), but degenerative changes may be present, so some schwannomas are red-brown and focally calcified.

Histopathology
Features of typical schwannomas characterize these tumours, most having Antoni

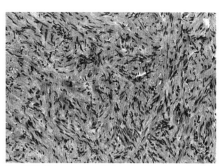

Fig. 4.33 Schwannoma. Cytological bland spindle cells with wavy nuclei, characteristic of schwannoma.

A and Antoni B areas {59}. The majority of cases are encapsulated, but at least one report describes a tumour as being extensively infiltrating. Most tumours are bland and clearly benign, but an occasional tumour may have foci of nuclear pleomorphism and hyperchromasia.
The tumour cells are reactive with antibodies for S100 protein, neuron-specific enolase, nerve growth factor receptor, and collagen IV {745}. They typically fail to react with antibodies for chromogranin, synaptophysin, desmin, factor VIII, or keratin. Weak reactivity of tumour cells with antibodies to CD34 has been reported.
Although clinically the tumours may be thought to be cardiac myxoma, microscopically the features are distinctive. Immunohistochemical evaluation with S100 protein and calretinin (positive in myxomas) can also be helpful.

Prognosis and predictive factors
The tumours are benign, and all patients who have undergone surgery for tumour removal have had a benign follow-up.

Tumours of uncertain behaviour and germ cell tumours

A.P. Burke
V. Thomas de Montpréville
C.D.M. Fletcher
J.J. Maleszewski
F. Tavora
H. Tazelaar

Inflammatory myofibroblastic tumour

Definition
Inflammatory myofibroblastic tumour is a low-grade neoplasm of mesenchymal cells, with smooth muscle and fibrocytic (myofibroblastic) differentiation in a chronic inflammatory background.

ICD-O code   8825/1

Synonyms
Inflammatory pseudotumour; pseudosarcomatous myofibroblastic proliferation; these terms are no longer recommended

Epidemiology
Cardiac inflammatory myofibroblastic tumour is rare, with fewer than 40 reported cases. There is no sex predominance.

Etiology
The etiology is unknown. One cardiac inflammatory myofibroblastic tumour arose after cardiac instrumentation {559}.

Clinical features
The mean patient age at presentation is 16 years, with a median age of 5.5 years and a range of 5 weeks {281} to 75 years {1825}. Clinical manifestations are related to heart failure, cyanosis, peripheral oedema, dyspnoea, and syncope. Because cardiac inflammatory myofibroblastic tumours are endocardial-based lesions, pericardial effusions are uncommon {598}, and systemic embolization

to the brain or lower extremities is relatively common {281}. Prolapse into the coronary arteries by lesions on the mitral or aortic valve can result in ischaemia, myocardial infarction, and sudden death {1364,1464,1629}. A few patients present with inflammatory symptoms – with fever, malaise, and elevated serum acute-phase reactants {664}. There is one reported case of inflammatory myofibroblastic tumour in a child with a cardiac fibroma {550}.

Localization
Cardiac inflammatory myofibroblastic tumours are endocardial-based. They most commonly occur on the mitral valve, followed by the right atrium, the right ventricle inflow portion and the tricuspid valve, the right ventricular outflow portion and the pulmonary valve, the aortic valve, the left atrium, the left ventricle, and the ventricular septum.

Macroscopy
Inflammatory myofibroblastic tumours are polypoid lesions of the endocardium that may resemble myxoma or papillary fibroelastoma.

Histopathology
Cardiac inflammatory myofibroblastic tumours are polypoid lesions, often with surface fibrin {281,550}. They are identical to inflammatory myofibroblastic tumours of soft tissue. Myofibroblast-like spindle cells, with abundant cytoplasm and open, vesicular nuclei, with myxoid

areas are visible. Mitotic figures are infrequent, and there are generally < 2 mitoses per 2 mm^2 {281}. Atypical mitotic figures are absent. There is variable inflammation, but lymphoid aggregates and germinal centres are uncommon. Immunohistochemical expression of ALK1 is observed in half of all cases.
The differential diagnoses include sarcomas, which in children are rare on the endocardial surface and which demonstrate mitotic activity and pleomorphism. Reported paediatric sarcomas with a benign outcome occurring on cardiac valves are likely cardiac inflammatory myofibroblastic tumours {1108,1436}.

Genetic profile
Like its soft tissue counterpart, cardiac inflammatory myofibroblastic tumour may demonstrate *ALK1* gene rearrangement {1825}.

Prognosis and predictive factors
To date, all reported cardiac inflammatory myofibroblastic tumours have been biologically benign. However, embolization may cause ischaemia, myocardial infarction, and sudden death.

Paraganglioma

Definition
Paraganglioma is a rare benign neuroendocrine neoplasm arising from paraganglion cells.

ICD-O code   8680/1

Synonyms
Phaeochromocytoma; extra-adrenal phaeochromocytoma; chemodectoma

Epidemiology
The mean patient age at paraganglioma presentation is in the fourth decade, and there is a slight female predominance {268}.

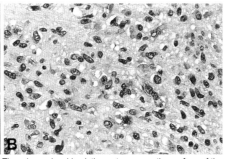

Fig. 4.34 Cardiac inflammatory myofibroblastic tumour. **A** There is a polypoid gelatinous tumour on the surface of the aortic valve and the intimal surface of the right sinus of Valsalva. **B** Immunohistochemical staining may demonstrate cytoplasmic expression of ALK1.

Etiology

Cardiac paraganglioma arises from intrinsic cardiac paraganglia, commonly located in the atria, along the atrioventricular groove, and near the root of the aorta and pulmonary artery {2344}. No specific environmental triggers are known. There is an uncommon association with multiple endocrine neoplasia syndromes.

Clinical features

About two thirds of cardiac paragangliomas are functionally active, and dissection of the lesions during surgery can result in episodes of hypertension {1243}. Other symptoms include palpitations, chest pain, headache, shortness of breath, murmurs, angina, and acute myocardial infarction {1050,2119,2556}. Tumours may infiltrate cardiac tissues, resulting in valve dysfunction or outflow tract obstruction, necessitating complex surgery or transplantation.

Echocardiography, CT, and MRI have been used to diagnose cardiac paragangliomas {46}. MRI is superior in delineating the extent of the tumour and its relation to surrounding structures {487}.

Although cardiac paraganglioma may be locally aggressive, distant metastasis is rare, and has not been extensively documented {2344}.

Localization

Cardiac paragangliomas are most commonly found in the atria (more often the left than the right), the atrioventricular groove, and the atrial septum. They tend to project into the pericardial space as opposed to intraluminally {1243}. Cardiac paragangliomas are rare in the ventricular walls {46,777,1516}.

Macroscopy

Paragangliomas are relatively well-defined masses that may invade into the surrounding tissue {76}. Left atrial paragangliomas can mimic myxomas, with an intraluminal growth.

Histopathology

Cardiac paragangliomas are histologically similar to those at other sites, and are characterized by epithelioid tumour cells arranged in cell nests, cords, and trabeculae. The stroma is highly vascular. Cytoplasmic clearing is often a prominent feature in cardiac paragangliomas. There are two cellular components: chief (or principal) cells and sustentacular cells. There may be cytological atypia, usually exhibited by scattered, enlarged, and pleomorphic cells. Mitotic figures are uncommon.

Sustentacular cells are S100-positive and glial fibrillary acidic protein-positive, and epithelioid (chief) cells are chromogranin-positive and synaptophysin-positive. Unlike in carcinoid tumours, epithelial markers are negative. Immunohistochemical staining for Ki-67 generally shows a low proliferative rate.

The differential diagnoses include carcinoid tumour, granular cell tumour, and rhabdomyoma. Carcinoid tumours occur only secondarily in the heart, usually in the right ventricle. Granular cell tumours occur on the epicardial surface (usually near the coronary arteries), and are histologically distinct. Metastatic tumours, particularly melanoma, can mimic cardiac paragangliomas histologically.

Genetic profile

Although paragangliomas are part of multiple endocrine neoplasia types 2A and 2B, primary cardiac tumours as part of the syndrome are rare {1077}. Genes related to extra-adrenal paragangliomas include the proto-oncogene *RET* (associated with multiple endocrine neoplasia type 2) and the tumour suppressor gene *VHL* (associated with von Hippel-Lindau disease). There has been one case of a cardiac paraganglioma in a child with Carney-Stratakis syndrome {2765}. *SDHB* gene mutations, which are associated with paraganglioma syndrome type 4, have been reported in cardiac paragangliomas {1072}.

Prognosis and predictive factors

Paraganglioma may be locally aggressive, with rare instances of metastatic spread. There are no histological criteria that predict aggressive behaviour in cardiac paragangliomas, but features that have been linked to aggressiveness include necrosis, mitoses, capsular invasion, and a high Ki-67 index {1271}. Long-term prognosis appears to be excellent if complete surgical excision is achieved; however, about 10% of cases cannot be completed removed {1243}.

Germ cell tumours

Definition

Cardiac germ cell tumours are neoplasms of germ cell origin that arise within the myocardium or cardiac chambers. A gonadal site or other site outside the pericardium is by definition absent. To date, all reported intracardiac germ cell tumours have been teratomas or yolk sac tumours.

ICD-O codes

Teratoma, mature	9080/0
Teratoma, immature	9080/3
Yolk sac tumour	9071/3

Synonyms

Intracardiac teratoma; intracardiac endodermal sinus tumour

Epidemiology

About 10 germ cell tumours arising within the myocardium have been reported; most were teratomas, and 3 were yolk sac tumours {518,895,1748,1998}.

Clinical features

Patients range in age from 2 to 20 years, with a female predominance. All reported yolk sac tumours have occurred in girls. The manifestations of the tumour depend on its location, and include heart block, right ventricular outflow tract obstruction with seizures, murmurs, and sudden

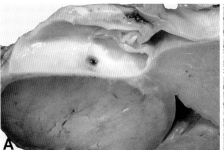
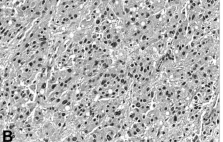

Fig. 4.35 Paraganglioma. **A** Gross appearance in an explanted heart; the unresectable tumour is located in close relationship to the ascending aorta; the right coronary ostium is evident. **B** Typical histological appearance of groups of cells in an organoid fashion, showing abundant eosinophilic cytoplasm and nuclei with random atypia.

death. One tumour in the atrial septum was incidentally found.

Localization
Intracardiac teratomas occur in the ventricular septum near the base of the heart, or less commonly in the atrial septum. Yolk sac tumours have been described in the right atrial and ventricular cavities, as well as in the left ventricle.

Macroscopy
Teratomas are commonly multicystic. Yolk sac tumours are typically lobulated, may be solid or cystic, and are soft, with relatively little fibrous tissue.

Histopathology
Intramyocardial teratomas are composed of various combinations of endodermal structures (e.g. gastrointestinal epithelium and respiratory epithelium), ectoderm (e.g. glial tissue, primitive neuroectoderm, and skin with sebaceous appendages and hair), and mesoderm (e.g. fat, cartilage, and primitive blastema). Yolk sac tumours contain interlacing papillary and tubular structures similar to those of their mediastinal counterparts. The differential diagnosis of intraventricular teratomas is cystic tumour of the atrioventricular node, which shows histological overlap; however, cystic tumours of the atrioventricular node do not contain mesodermal or ectodermal structures.

Prognosis and predictive factors
Intramyocardial teratoma has been shown to recur, and may cause sudden death. Intramyocardial yolk sac tumour responds to chemotherapy, but may result in death due to local disease burden in the heart {895,1748,1998}.

Malignant tumours
Angiosarcoma

J. Butany
R.M. Bohle
A.P. Burke
C.D.M. Fletcher

Definition
Cardiac angiosarcoma is a primary cardiac sarcoma with endothelial differentiation. There are two types, with distinctive histological and genetic features: angiosarcoma (high-grade sarcomas) and epithelioid haemangioendothelioma (low-grade sarcomas).

ICD-O code   9120/3

Epidemiology
Angiosarcomas are the most common primary cardiac malignancies with specific differentiation, accounting for approximately 40% of all cardiac sarcomas {284,300,1248,3016}. Cardiac angiosarcoma accounts for about 5% of biopsied or resected primary heart tumours. As a primary heart tumour, angiosarcoma is almost 50 times more common than epithelioid haemangioendothelioma, which accounts for only about 2% of primary cardiac malignant vascular tumours.

Clinical features
Cardiac angiosarcomas have a peak incidence in the fourth to fifth decade, and there may be a slight male predilection {284}. The most common initial manifestations are chest pain, dyspnoea related to pericardial and pleural effusions, recurrent pericarditis, and supraventricular

arrhythmias. In some cases, the diagnosis is made at autopsy after a period of clinical investigation for pericardial disease {2159,2724}. Because of the propensity for pericardial involvement, cardiac tamponade occurs more frequently than with other types of cardiac sarcomas {661,1250,2746}.

On MRI, angiosarcoma appears as a heterogeneous, nodular mass in the right atrium {75,562,1232,2786}. MRI sequences are sensitive for haemorrhage, and may show areas of nodularity on T1-weighted imaging {75,1545,2143}. After administration of intravenous contrast (gadolinium-diethylenetriaminepentacetate), enhancement along vascular lakes may be seen, which has been described as a sunray appearance.

Cardiac epithelioid haemangioendothelioma typically occurs in the atria, and may present as an incidental mass or embolic phenomena {2631,3016}.

Localization
Cardiac angiosarcoma most often arises in the right atrium near the atrioventricular groove (in 80% of cases), replacing the right atrial wall and protruding into the cavity. There is often involvement of the pericardium, which can be the predominant localization. After the right atrium and pericardium, the left atrium is the

third most common location {300,1014}. Invasion of the vena cava and tricuspid valve is common, but the atrial septum and pulmonary artery are usually spared.

Macroscopy
Angiosarcomas are typically dark brown or black haemorrhagic masses with unclear, infiltrating borders {2072}.

Cytology
Cytological examination of pericardial effusion has not proven very sensitive {1111,2159,2338}, although fine-needle aspiration biopsy may establish the diagnosis in some cases {195}.

Histopathology
Angiosarcoma typically infiltrates cardiac muscle, without distinct margins. The vascular channels are irregular, anastomosing, and sinusoidal, with pleomorphic lining cells showing frequent mitotic figures. There are often areas composed predominantly of anaplastic spindle cells. The epithelioid variant of angiosarcoma is characterized by rounded cells with abundant cytoplasm, and is unusual in the heart. Immunohistochemical staining for CD31 is positive in > 90% of cases of cardiac angiosarcoma. Immunohistochemical expression of ERG oncoprotein, an Ets family transcription

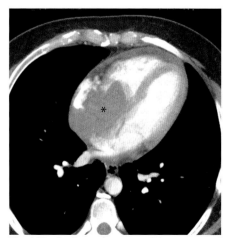

Fig. 4.36 Cardiac angiosarcoma. CT appearance of cardiac angiosarcoma of the right atrium showing an infiltrating tumour with irregular borders (asterisk).

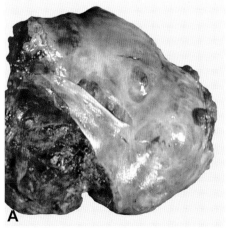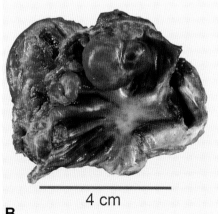

Fig. 4.37 Cardiac angiosarcoma. **A** A surgically excised specimen showing a haemorrhagic mass focally invested by pericardium. **B** A surgically excised specimen showing involvement of the right atrium, including the crista terminalis and pectinate muscles.

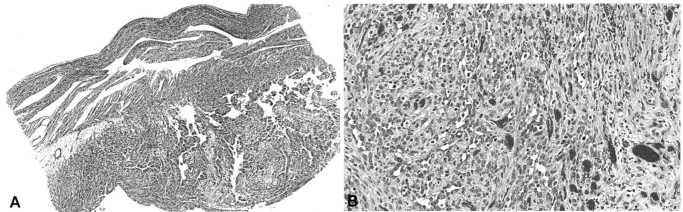

Fig. 4.38 Cardiac angiosarcoma. **A** A low-magnification view of a right atrial resection demonstrates endocardial tumour. **B** A higher-magnification view demonstrates typical features of angiosarcoma.

factor, is highly specific and sensitive for angiosarcoma {1670}.

Cardiac epithelioid haemangioendothelioma is quite distinctive histologically, and is similar to epithelioid haemangioendothelioma of the lung and soft tissue. It is composed of short strands or solid nests of round or oval epithelioid cells, which form small, intracellular lumina, and infiltrate the muscular walls of vessels. Antigenically, epithelioid haemangioendothelioma is similar to epithelioid angiosarcoma, and expresses endothelial markers CD31, CD34, and ERG oncoprotein , as well as cytokeratins (especially CK7 and CK18). Epithelioid haemangioendothelioma is more likely to express factor VIII than are less differentiated angiosarcomas.

Genetic profile

Familial angiosarcoma has been reported {1231,1524}. Cytogenetic analyses of cardiac angiosarcomas show no consistent chromosomal abnormality; however, a case of right atrial angiosarcoma demonstrated hyperdiploid clonal populations with changes in chromosome number, as follows: 55, XY, +der (1;17)(q10;q10), +2, +7, +8, +19, +20, +21, +22, and polysomy of chromosome 8 {2308}. Genetic alterations of *TP53* and *KRAS* have been documented in cardiac angiosarcomas in humans as well as animal models {1026,1791}. Epithelioid haemangioendothelioma at all locations has now been shown to harbour a specific *WWTR1-CAMTA1* gene fusion {683,2592}.

Prognosis and predictive factors

The survival of patients with angiosarcoma of the heart is poor {1774,2251}. One series showed a median survival of 13 months, with better survival among patients with localized disease {1508}. In another series, about 90% of patients died of disease by 38 months {1096}. The survival of angiosarcoma was shorter than that of other histological subtypes.

Undifferentiated pleomorphic sarcoma

H. Tazelaar
P.J. Zhang
A.P. Burke
C.D.M. Fletcher

Definition
Undifferentiated pleomorphic sarcomas are high-grade sarcomas showing no definable line of differentiation based on the currently available ancillary techniques.

ICD-O code   8830/3

Synonyms
Malignant fibrous histiocytoma (obsolete); undifferentiated sarcoma; intimal sarcoma

Epidemiology
Primary cardiac sarcomas account for approximately 10% of all primary cardiac tumours {279,2628}. Undifferentiated pleomorphic sarcoma is a common histological subtype of primary cardiac sarcoma, with a frequency similar to that of angiosarcoma, accounting for about a quarter to a third of all primary cardiac sarcomas {279}. The average patient age is 40–50 years {279}. Undifferentiated pleomorphic sarcomas occur in patients over a wide age range, from adolescents to elderly adults. There does not appear to be any sex predominance.

Clinical features
Approximately 65% of pleomorphic undifferentiated cardiac sarcomas occur in the left atrium {23,1896,2608} and cause signs and symptoms related to pulmonary congestion {143}, mitral stenosis, and pulmonary vein obstruction. Tumours may also present with metastases – the lungs, lymph nodes, kidneys, and skin are common sites. As with all cardiac tumours, the signs and symptoms are related to the site of origin and the extent of growth into adjacent cardiac structures and organs. Constitutional signs and symptoms may precede symptoms referable to the heart.

Diagnosis of undifferentiated pleomorphic sarcoma most often starts with echocardiography, when confusion with myxoma is quite common because of the common left atrial location. Cardiac MRI is helpful preoperatively to determine precise tumour size, location, invasion of adjacent normal tissues, and postoperatively for assessment of excision and recurrence {176}.

The tumours may metastasize to the lung, brain, bone, liver, skin, gastrointestinal tract, and other organs {279}.

Localization
Most undifferentiated pleomorphic sarcomas occur in the left atrium, where they most often present like cardiac myxomas; but unlike myxomas, they tend to arise away from the septum {279}. Other reported locations include the pericardial space, the right ventricle/pulmonary valve, the right atrium, and the left ventricle. The tumours often cause distension of the chamber in which they are growing, and extend into the pulmonary veins or lung parenchyma.

Macroscopy
Undifferentiated pleomorphic sarcoma typically presents as a polypoid endocardial-based tumour {176}. It may be sessile or pedunculated, simulating myxoma; but unlike myxoma, it may form multiple masses. The mass may distend the atrium and impinge on the mitral valve. Extension into the pulmonary veins and lung parenchyma may be present. The tumours may be uniform tan-white or variegated due to haemorrhage and necrosis {1932}. Calcification is uncommon.

Cytology
Intraoperative imprint cytological preparations have proven useful in guiding surgeons to do a more extensive resection than was originally planned {2703}. The imprints showed a cellular mesenchymal neoplasm.

Histopathology
Cardiac undifferentiated pleomorphic sarcoma forms a spectrum with myxofibrosarcoma (see *Myxofibrosarcoma*, p. 334), but is predominantly undifferentiated, with prominent pleomorphism. It shares histological features with intimal sarcomas of the aorta and pulmonary artery; namely, predominantly lateral spread along the intima and growth over

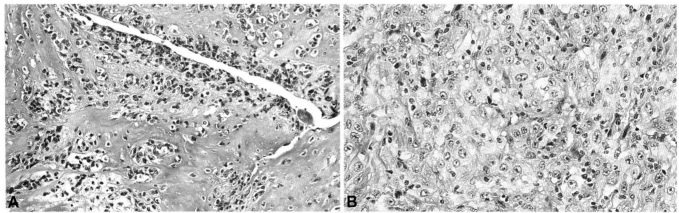

Fig. 4.39 Undifferentiated pleomorphic sarcoma. **A** In this example, the tumour cells are epithelioid, and are more prominent on the endoluminal surface. **B** The tumour is composed of undifferentiated pleomorphic cells with an epithelioid appearance.

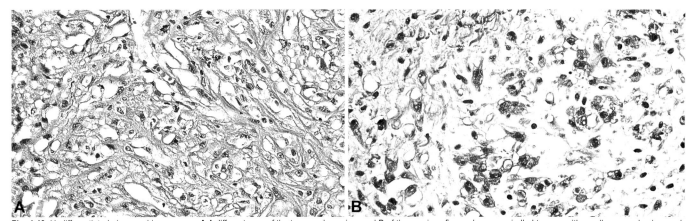
Fig. 4.40 Undifferentiated pleomorphic sarcoma. **A** A different area of the tumour shown in panel B of the previous figure shows a spindled tumour with a collagenous background. **B** This sarcoma has discohesive pleomorphic cells with abundant cytoplasm in a myxoid background; the patient was a 72-year-old woman with a left atrial mass and multiple lung nodules.

luminal thrombus. It often has storiform architecture and variable degrees of collagenized stroma, which may resemble myxofibrosarcoma in some areas. Other histological variants include myxoid round cell sarcoma and undifferentiated epithelioid sarcoma. Most contain some tumour giant cells. Mitotic activity and necrosis are usually easy to find. The stroma typically contains some chronic inflammatory cells, and may include collections of prominent foamy macrophages.

Rare cells may express cytokeratin, and smooth muscle actin is positive in up to 50% of tumours. Vimentin and CD34 may be positive, but have no discriminatory value. The primary distinction is from cardiac myxoma, which is also an endocardial-based tumour with frequent myxoid background. Myxoma lacks atypia and frequent mitotic figures, and expresses calretinin (unlike undifferentiated pleomorphic sarcoma). Other soft tissue sarcomas (e.g. angiosarcoma and synovial sarcoma) may be distinguished from undifferentiated pleomorphic sarcoma on the basis of a combination of morphology and immunohistochemistry. Unlike in myxofibrosarcoma, there is generally only a minor component of myxoid stroma in undifferentiated pleomorphic sarcoma.

Genetic profile
One study showed *MDM2* amplification by FISH in all 29 cases tested and overexpression in all 42 intimal sarcomas tested {1828}. In contrast MDM2 overexpression was found in 27% of undifferentiated pleomorphic sarcomas and no MDM2 amplification was found by FISH in 9 tumors {1828}. However, the distinction of intimal sarcoma from undifferentiated pleomorphic sarcoma is controversial {1560A}.

Prognosis and predictive factors
There are no specific prognostic factors except the completeness of surgical resection. Most patients die of disease within 2 years {1827,2583}. Causes of death are typically related to metastases, bulky intracardiac recurrences, or general debilitation. Some patients have undergone cardiac transplantation, but this does not usually provide any survival advantage.

Osteosarcoma

A.P. Burke
F. Tavora

Definition

Primary cardiac osteosarcoma is a sarcoma that originates in the heart and produces osteoid or bone, occasionally with chondroblastic differentiation. Cardiac osteosarcoma is a subset of extraskeletal osteosarcoma of soft tissue.

ICD-O code   9180/3

Synonyms

Osteogenic sarcoma; osteoblastic osteosarcoma; extraskeletal osteosarcoma

Epidemiology

Cardiac osteosarcomas account for approximately 10% of all primary cardiac sarcomas {279,289,3016}. In the past 10 years, there have been fewer than 15 cases reported {1209,2956}. Men and women are affected equally. Cardiac osteosarcomas occur most commonly between the second and fifth decades of life, with a mean patient age of 40 years {2572}. The youngest reported patient was 14 years old {1526}.

Etiology

Extraskeletal osteosarcomas are usually sporadic, with occasional cases related

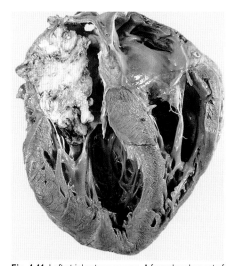

Fig. 4.41 Left atrial osteosarcoma. A four-chamber cut of a heart at autopsy shows a heterogeneous mass nearly filling the left atrium; the tumour contained mature bone that required extensive decalcification before sectioning.

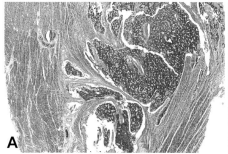 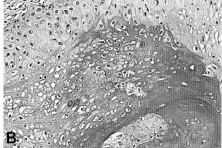

Fig. 4.42 A Primary cardiac osteosarcoma. Well-differentiated osteosarcoma infiltrating the left ventricular myocardium. **B** Primary cardiac osteosarcoma with chondrosarcoma. Areas of chondroid differentiation are common in osteosarcoma.

to prior radiation exposure, but this association has not been reported in primary cardiac osteosarcoma.

Clinical features

Due to the left atrial location, initial symptoms are most frequently related to mitral valve obstruction. Dyspnoea, chest pain, palpitations, dizziness, murmurs, and congestive heart failure have all been reported {143,1209,2572}.

Localization

Primary osteosarcomas, like other sarcomas (except angiosarcoma), arise most frequently in the left atrium, and may extend into the pulmonary veins or the mitral valve. The second most common location is the right atrium, with extension into the vena cava {609,1526}. Reports of right ventricular osteosarcoma indicate involvement of the pulmonary valve and pulmonary trunk, and these tumours are likely primary intimal sarcomas {2424,3013}.

Macroscopy

Cardiac osteosarcomas usually present as nodular masses with infiltrative, irregular margins. The cut surface is heterogeneous, firm, and white, with areas of haemorrhage, necrosis, and bone. Osteosarcomas have also been reported to occur as pedunculated masses projecting into the vascular lumina or cavities, causing obstructive symptoms {289,609}.

Histopathology

Cardiac osteosarcoma is similar to other extraskeletal osteosarcomas. The bone-forming areas range from well-differentiated trabeculated osteosarcoma to poorly differentiated sarcomas with stromal osteoid. Chondrosarcomatous areas are also present in about half of all cases {289}. There are usually extensive areas of undifferentiated pleomorphic sarcoma. Most tumours express smooth muscle actin, and S100 protein is expressed in chondroid areas. Epithelial membrane antigen can be focally positive in epithelioid areas {289,3013}.

Genetic profile

One case of a primary cardiac osteosarcoma revealed complex genetic alterations that included allelic losses involving chromosomes 1, 9, 10, 17, and 22, and structural abnormalities of chromosomes 1, 3, 9, and 17 {1999}. One case of *JAZF1/PHF1* translocation was reported in a primary ossifying cardiac sarcoma {2306}.

Prognosis and predictive factors

Prognosis of cardiac osteosarcoma is uniformly poor; survival beyond 1 year is unusual {609,2385}. The clinical course is aggressive, with early metastases to sites including the lungs, skin, skeleton, and thyroid. There is one report of a patient living for 7 years with local recurrence and distant metastasis {1999}.

Myxofibrosarcoma

J. Butany
C.D.M. Fletcher

Definition

Myxofibrosarcoma is a low-grade cardiac sarcoma composed of spindle cells in a myxoid matrix, which is usually endocardial-based. Fibrosarcoma denotes the proliferation of spindle cells with minimal pleomorphism in a fibrous background, without myxoid areas. The two patterns frequently coexist, and the single term myxofibrosarcoma should be used until further molecular characterization. There may be a minor component of pleomorphic epithelioid cells resembling undifferentiated pleomorphic sarcoma in either case.

ICD-O code   8811/3

Synonyms

Myxoid malignant fibrous histiocytoma (obsolete); fibromyxosarcoma; myxoid fibrosarcoma; intimal sarcoma (not recommended)

Epidemiology

Because of the various terms that have been used for this tumour in the heart, the precise incidence rate is uncertain, but myxofibrosarcoma probably accounts for about 10% of cardiac sarcomas, making it the fourth most common cardiac sarcoma (after angiosarcoma, undifferentiated pleomorphic sarcoma, and osteosarcoma) {279}. In a recent series,

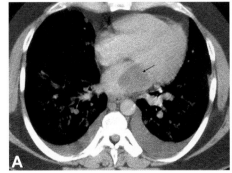 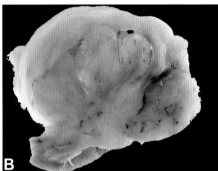

Fig. 4.44 A Myxofibrosarcoma. CT appearance of left atrial myxofibrosarcoma attached to the posterior wall and protruding into the mitral valve. **B** Cardiac myxofibrosarcoma. Gross appearance of resected cardiac myxofibrosarcoma with a glistening mucoid cut surface.

the diagnosis of myxofibrosarcoma was applied to 5 of 21 primary cardiac sarcomas in adults (24%) {3016}.

Clinical features

Cardiac myxofibrosarcomas have been described most frequently in the left atrium {1420}, typically causing obstruction and symptoms of mitral stenosis {985,1292}.

Localization

The most common location for cardiac myxofibrosarcoma is the left atrium, followed by the right atrium {149}, the right ventricle {1170}, and the ventricular septum {2365}.

Macroscopy

Myxofibrosarcoma is typically an endocardial-based, homogeneous tumour (with little necrosis or haemorrhage) that projects into the atrial cavity {279}.

Histopathology

Histologically, myxofibrosarcomas demonstrate spindle or rounded cells within a myxoid matrix, without significant pleomorphism. Necrosis is absent, and although there is a continuum with undifferentiated pleomorphic sarcoma, there is no storiform pattern or marked pleomorphism.

Immunohistochemical staining is not helpful in the diagnosis, except to exclude other tumours.

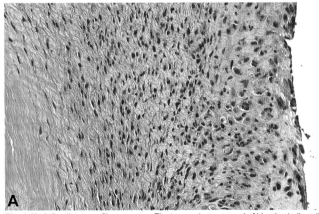 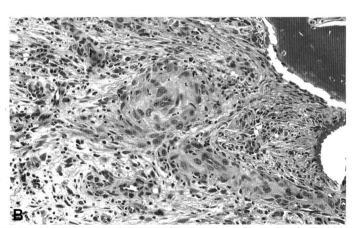

Fig. 4.43 A Cardiac myxofibrosarcoma. The tumour is composed of bland spindle cells in a collagenous matrix; towards the intimal surface, there is more pleomorphism (on the right). **B** Cardiac myxofibrosarcoma, osseous metastasis. The tumour shown in the previous figure metastasized to the thoracic spine 13 months after resection of the primary cardiac mass; this figure shows somewhat more pleomorphism than seen in the primary lesion.

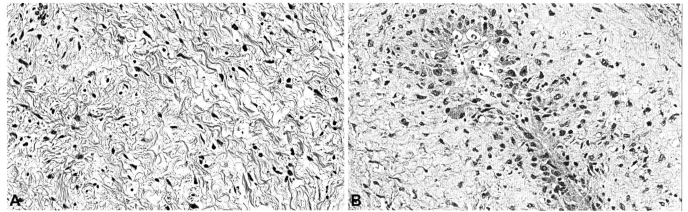

Fig. 4.45 Cardiac myxofibrosarcoma. **A** The tumour is composed of bland spindle cells in a collagenous myxoid matrix. **B** A different area of the same tumour shows moderate pleomorphism.

Myxoma may be confused with myxofibrosarcoma because of the proteoglycan-rich matrix. However, vasocentric tumour structures, haemosiderin macrophages, and calretinin expression are absent in myxofibrosarcoma. Because myxofibrosarcoma may be histologically bland, the absence of pleomorphism is not a distinguishing feature between myxoma and myxofibrosarcoma {279}. Myxoid tumours on heart valves, especially in children, are likely best classified as inflammatory myofibroblastic tumours.

Several reported cases of valvular sarcomas in children with a long-term benign course are likely inflammatory myofibroblastic tumour {163,1436,1629,3016}.

Genetic profile
Genetic studies of cardiac myxofibrosarcoma have not been published. However, in soft tissues they have been shown to have highly complex karyotypes with increase in cytogenetic aberrations with increased grade {735A}.

Prognosis and predictive factors
Although endocardial-based sarcomas have a slightly better prognosis than angiosarcomas of the heart, it is unclear whether there is a survival difference between cardiac myxofibrosarcoma and undifferentiated pleomorphic sarcoma. In one small series that included 3 adults with myxofibrosarcoma of the heart, all were alive and well at 12 months, 19 months, and 36 months, although 2 had recurrence and 1 had metastasis to the bone {3016}.

Leiomyosarcoma

A.P. Burke

Definition
Cardiac leiomyosarcoma is a sarcoma arising in the chambers or wall of the heart that shows smooth muscle cell differentiation.

ICD-O code   8890/3

Synonym
Epithelioid leiomyosarcoma

Epidemiology
In published series, leiomyosarcoma accounts for < 20% of primary cardiac sarcomas {615,1248,1885,2401,2482, 2631,3016}.

Clinical features
The mean patient age at presentation is 58 years (ranging from 45 to 71 years), with no sex predominance {127,238,615, 672,896,1197,1248,1885,2401,2482, 2631,3016}. Presenting symptoms relate to the site in the heart, and include peripheral oedema and ascites for right-sided tumours {3016}, and shortness of breath, dyspnoea, and haemoptysis for left atrial tumours {615}.

Localization
Most cardiac leiomyosarcomas occur in the left atrium, followed by the right atrium. They occasionally occur in the right ventricle {127,238,615,1248,2401,3016}. Cardiac leiomyosarcomas often form luminal masses, which may obstruct blood flow.

Macroscopy
Leiomyosarcomas are homogeneous, firm, white to tan masses with variable necrosis.

Histopathology
The histological features of cardiac leiomyosarcomas are identical to those of soft tissue. They are monomorphous tumours formed by fascicles of spindle cells that lack a collagenous background.

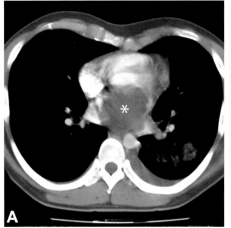 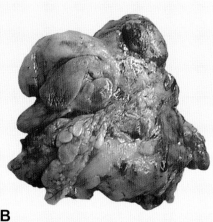

Fig. 4.46 Cardiac leiomyosarcoma. **A** Cardiac CT showing a large mass filling the left atrium (asterisk). **B** The excised tumour was shelled out of the left atrium; the endoluminal surface demonstrated multiple projections.

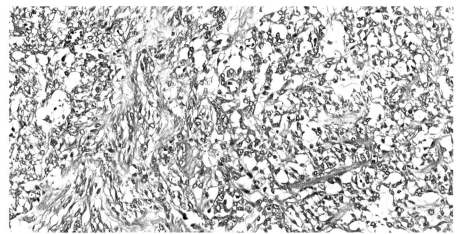

Fig. 4.47 Cardiac epithelioid leiomyosarcoma. A higher-magnification view demonstrates a cellular monomorphous tumour of epithelioid and spindle cells; immunohistochemical staining (not shown) confirmed myogenic origin.

Immunohistochemical expression of desmin is typically found. Cardiac leiomyosarcomas are mitotically active, with mitotic rates ranging from 4 to 18 mitoses per 2 mm^2 {615}. Most are grade II to III {615} according to the Fédération Nationale des Centres de Lutte Contre le Cancer (FNCLCC) grading criteria {2685}. More than half contain tumour necrosis {615}. Occasional epithelioid morphology has been described {576}.

Prognosis and predictive factors
There are few data regarding the prognosis of cardiac leiomyosarcoma. Most patients die of disease within 1 year {1248}, although a few have reportedly survived longer, one with a positive margin at surgery {238,615,1620}. Adjuvant chemotherapy and radiation therapy is of unclear benefit in primary cardiac sarcomas {3016}. The completeness of excision in general affects survival.

Rhabdomyosarcoma

J. Butany
C.D.M. Fletcher

Definition
Cardiac rhabdomyosarcoma is a primary sarcoma of the heart, with striated muscle differentiation.

ICD-O code
8900/3

Synonyms
Embryonal rhabdomyosarcoma; alveolar rhabdomyosarcoma; spindle cell rhabdomyosarcoma

Epidemiology
Primary cardiac rhabdomyosarcomas are extremely rare. Several series of heart sarcomas include no examples {127,615,1248,3016}, and several include only one {1197,1885,2401}. In series from the previous century, rhabdomyosarcoma is overrepresented, and not documented immunohistochemically {672}.

Clinical features
Cardiac rhabdomyosarcoma is a tumour predominantly of childhood and infancy {47,55,2706,2780}. The mean patient age at presentation is about 14 years. Clinical symptoms are diverse, and depend on the site of the tumour within the heart. Those arising in the left atrium may present with severe mitral stenosis, similar to undifferentiated pleomorphic sarcomas {341}. Embolization may result in stroke {94,97,108}.

Localization
All cardiac chambers may be involved, but there is a predilection for the left ventricle.

Macroscopy
Cardiac rhabdomyosarcomas are bosselated, solid, and whitish grey on cut surface {753}.

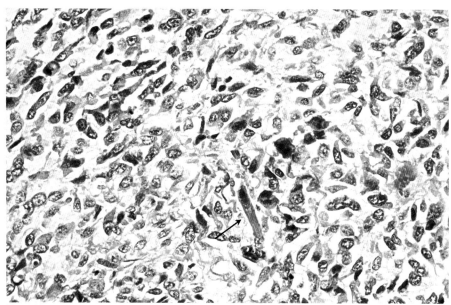

Fig. 4.48 Primary cardiac embryonal rhabdomyosarcoma. Spindled rhabdomyoblasts (arrow) are present, which suggests the diagnosis based on routine microscopy, confirmed by immunohistochemical staining for myogenic markers; the patient was a 19-year-old man with a right atrial sarcoma with multiple pulmonary metastases.

Cytology
Aspiration cytology shows spindle cells with moderate pleomorphism occurring in irregular sheets and singly, with granular pink cytoplasm and occasional rhabdomyoblasts with cross-striations {47,753}.

Histopathology
Most cardiac rhabdomyosarcomas are of the embryonal type. There are also a few instances of alveolar cardiac rhabdomyosarcoma – a poor-prognostic subtype {1933}. There are a few reports of cardiac rhabdomyosarcoma with a botryoid endocardial growth pattern {929,1051}. One case of spindle cell type has been reported in the myocardium of a child {753}. Immunohistochemical staining for rhabdomyosarcoma shows positivity for smooth muscle actin, desmin and myogenin {753}. The differential diagnoses include other small round blue cell tumours and undifferentiated pleomorphic sarcoma.

Genetic profile
The majority of extracardiac alveolar rhabdomyosarcomas carry the specific *PAX3/7-FKHR* translocation, corresponding cytogenetically to t(2; 13) or t(1; 13) translocations, respectively.

Prognosis and predictive factors
Overall survival is poor {1197,1885}, and distant metastases are possible, including to the brain and bone {47,94}. One young man with spindle cell cardiac rhabdomyosarcoma (a relatively favourable histological subtype) arising in the left atrium was alive at 14 months after chemotherapy {753}.

Synovial sarcoma

H. Tazelaar
C.D.M. Fletcher

Definition

Synovial sarcoma is a malignant mesenchymal tumour characterized by a specific X;18 chromosomal translocation, resulting in an *SS18-SSX* fusion gene. It may be biphasic (consisting of spindle cell and epithelial cell areas) or monophasic (consisting of spindle cells only).

ICD-O code   9040/3

Epidemiology

Synovial sarcomas account for 4% of all cardiac sarcomas. The male-to-female ratio is 3:1. The mean patient age at diagnosis is 37 years, ranging from 13 to 70 years {2803}.

Clinical features

Dyspnoea is the most common symptom, affecting 70% of patients. Signs are usually related to heart failure {2803}. CT and MRI show synovial sarcoma to be heterogeneous and slightly enhancing, with some calcification and cystic change {2313}.

Localization

The pericardium is the most common site of involvement, affected in 40% of patients {2803}. The right atrium is affected in 24% of patients. Other sites of involvement include the left atrium, the tricuspid and mitral valves, and the right and left ventricles.

Macroscopy

Synovial sarcomas are often polypoid and smooth-surfaced. They may be tan-white or red, with haemorrhagic, necrotic, or cystic foci, or they may be homogeneous, fleshy masses.

Cytology

Cytology can show the two populations. One population consists of small spindle to oval cells, which can be present in tight clusters or as single cells tethered along branched capillaries. The epithelial component consists of clusters of polygonal cells. The chromatin is fine and well dispersed in the spindle cells, and coarser in the epithelial cells. Nucleoli are more prominent in the epithelial components. The cytoplasm in both cell types is scant {2066}.

Histopathology

The only histological types of synovial sarcoma that occur in the heart are the monophasic spindle cell and biphasic variants. The spindle cell variant is most common. The spindle cell component consists of cells arranged in fascicles with uniform, compact, overlapping, tapering nuclei, but alternating cellular and oedematous areas are typical {3016}. The epithelioid cells form clusters and nests, and occasionally larger gland-like spaces that may show branching. Branching of somewhat gaping thin-walled blood vessels is also typical. Calcifications may be present. Both components are reactive with epithelial antibodies such as keratin and epithelial membrane antigen. In the spindle cell component, the reactivity is usually strong but focal, especially for epithelial membrane antigen

(which is more sensitive). Tumour cells also express CD99 and TLE1 (80%), but TLE1 is not specific, as it is also positive in some malignant peripheral nerve sheath sarcomas. Epithelial membrane antigen expression is more common than pancytokeratin, is more frequent in the epithelioid areas, and is more likely to be positive in larger resection specimens, as the expression is typically focal, not diffuse. S100 protein is focally positive in about 40% of cases. Synovial sarcomas are circumscribed, whereas mesothelioma tends to grow diffusely over the pericardium {412}. Additionally, the spindle cells of synovial sarcoma tend to be more monomorphic, cellular, and compact. Reactivity for calretinin has been described in both tumours. Solitary fibrous tumour is generally lower-grade, and tends to have alternating hyper- and hypocellular areas, often with prominent hyalinized stroma.

Genetic profile

Synovial sarcoma has the defining reciprocal translocation t(X;18)(p11.2;q11.2), resulting in fusion between the *SS18* gene (also called *SYT*) and one of the *SSX* genes on the X chromosome. The most common fusion gene is *SS18-SSX1*, but the specific fusion gene has no prognostic value.

Prognosis and predictive factors

Synovial sarcoma is high-grade. The median overall survival is approximately 24 months. Chemotherapy with or without radiotherapy seems to improve survival.

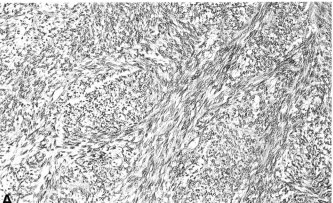
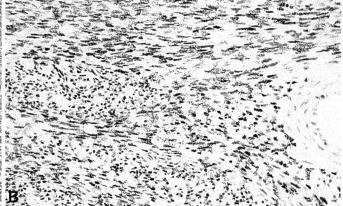

Fig. 4.49 Monophasic synovial sarcoma. **A** This tumour arose from the right atrium of a 15-year-old boy; note the long fascicles of compact spindle cells. **B** There is strong nuclear staining for TLE1.

Miscellaneous sarcomas

A.P. Burke

Definition
Rare primary cardiac sarcomas are defined by the nomenclature of their more common soft tissue counterparts. Miscellaneous sarcomas include malignant peripheral nerve sheath tumour (MPNST), liposarcoma, extraskeletal Ewing sarcoma/primitive neuroectodermal tumour/the Ewing family of tumours (EFTs), carcinosarcoma, desmoplastic small round cell tumour (DSRCT), extrarenal rhabdoid tumour/malignant extrarenal rhabdoid tumour (MERT), and chondrosarcoma.

Epidemiology
These are primary cardiac tumours with sarcomatous components that are rare in the heart and reported as individual cases.

There have been fewer than 20 well-documented reports of primary cardiac liposarcoma {1980} and rarer primary cardiac MPNST {433,3016}, EFTs, DSRCT, and MERT occurring as primary cardiac neoplasms.

Clinical features
Most of these rare cardiac sarcomas have a predilection for children, including EFTs, DSRCT, and MERT. Cardiac MPNST and liposarcoma have been described primarily in young adults. Symptoms are related to location in the heart, obstruction of cardiac blood flow, pericardial tamponade, and metastatic disease.

Macroscopy
The gross appearance varies by histological type; liposarcomas are bulky fatty lesions, whereas poorly differentiated or undifferentiated round cell sarcomas are often described as fleshy lobulated masses. MPNSTs have been described as yellow-white, glistening, and myxoid {433}.

Localization
The members of this heterogeneous group of neoplasms have been reported in all cardiac chambers, with a possible predilection for the ventricles and ventricular septum {397,433,1980,2118,2187,2411,3016}. Complete excision with intraoperative frozen margins has been described in cardiac MPNST {433}.

Histopathology
The histological features of these rare primary cardiac sarcomas are identical to those of their extracardiac soft tissue counterparts. Several of these entities fall under the small round blue cell tumour category (e.g. EFTs, small round blue cell tumour, and MERT). In the case of EFTs, immunohistochemical staining for neuroendocrine markers is helpful to distinguish these tumours from the more common (in the heart) undifferentiated type of synovial sarcoma {397}. FLI1 and NKX2-2 staining is also helpful. In the case of small round blue cell tumour, immunohistochemical staining for desmin and cytokeratin in a dot-like cytoplasmic distribution is helpful. The single carcinosarcoma of the heart was identified as adenocarcinoma with rhabdomyosarcoma, and arose from the atrial septum {2118}. Immunohistochemical expression of WT1 is negative in EFTs and DSRCT, unlike in rhabdomyosarcoma. Extraskeletal chondrosarcoma are classified as myxoid or mesenchymal, with respective molecular alterations. Although there have been several reports of primary cardiac chondrosarcomas, not all have been adequetely characterized from a molecular or histological standpoint.

Genetic profile
The genetic profiles of these rare cardiac sarcomas are identical to those of their extracardiac counterparts.

Prognosis and predictive factors
The prognosis for poorly differentiated small blue round cell tumours is poor {2118,2187,2411}, although some patients with cardiac MPNST may survive for extended periods {433,3016}.

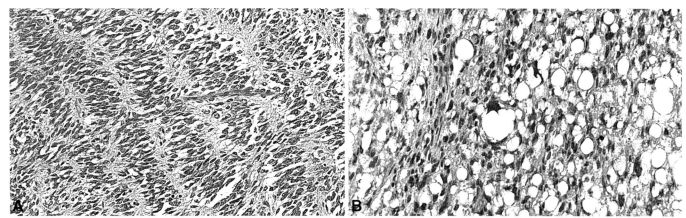

Fig. 4.50 A Cardiac malignant peripheral nerve sheath tumour. The tumour is composed of parallel spindle cells with alternating acellular areas; a 46-year-old man presented with chest pain; a right atrial/ventricular mass was seen on cardiac CT; the tumour cells expressed S100 protein, with focal positivity for CD34 and absence of staining for smooth muscle actin. **B** Cardiac liposarcoma. The tumour is composed of spindle cells with numerous lipoblastus; the patient was a 64-year-old man who was found to have an infiltrating right atrial mass after a painful metastatic lesion was found in the thoracic spine.

Cardiac lymphomas

J.J. Maleszewski
E.S. Jaffe

Definition

Primary cardiac lymphoma is an extranodal lymphoma, involving only the heart and/or the pericardium. More broadly, it may include processes that have limited extracardiac involvement, but the tumour resides primarily in the heart or presents with primarily cardiac manifestations.

Epidemiology

Primary cardiac lymphomas account for < 2% of primary cardiac neoplasms in surgical series {1144,2044}. However, their incidence is increasing due to increasingly sensitive imaging and diagnostic modalities. Primary cardiac lymphomas affect men twice as commonly as women {2044}. Although they more commonly present in older adults (with a median age of 63 years), they have been reported in patients as young as 9 years old {365}. Certain subtypes of primary cardiac lymphoma occur more frequently in an immunocompromised setting, especially in HIV disease – particularly primary effusion lymphoma (associated with human herpesvirus 8/Kaposi sarcoma-associated herpesvirus) and Burkitt lymphoma {182,299}.

Etiology

Although lymphoid tissue is not itself a normal constituent of the myocardium, the epicardial lymphatic drainage of the heart may be the source. Most primary cardiac lymphomas are of B-cell lineage – usually diffuse large B-cell lymphoma (DLBCL) – although there have also been reports of T-cell lymphomas. T-cell lymphoma can be associated with the retrovirus human T-lymphotropic virus type 1 (HTLV-1) {1882}, and invariably occurs in the setting of disseminated disease. Primary effusion lymphomas can develop within the pericardial space, and are associated with human herpesvirus 8/Kaposi sarcoma-associated herpesvirus. Cardiac lymphomas have also been reported to arise in association with implanted devices (e.g. prosthetic valves and pacemaker leads) and cardiac myxomas {122,229}. These cases are associated with the presence of EBV, and are

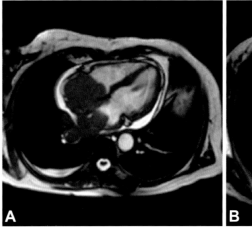
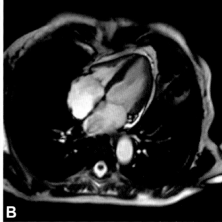

Fig. 4.51 Cardiac lymphoma. MRI of non-Hodgkin lymphoma. **A** A mass occupies both atria, extending to the pulmonary veins. **B** At last follow-up, 2 years later (after R-CHOP chemotherapy), there is complete remission. Reprinted from Lestuzzi C et al. {1456A}.

categorized as DLBCL associated with chronic inflammation {1509}, a tumour initially recognized in the setting of chronic long-standing pyothorax.

Clinical features

As with most cardiac tumours, the symptoms are variable, and are contingent on the size and location of the mass lesions. Dyspnoea, constitutional symptoms, and chest pain are frequently reported as the initial manifestations. Almost half of all patients meet the criteria for congestive heart failure at presentation {2044}. Pulmonary thromboembolism has also been reported {411,2406}.

Arrhythmias are also occasionally encountered, with abnormal atrial rhythms and atrioventricular block having been described. Treatment of the lymphoma, in at least some instances, has alleviated the underlying arrhythmia {1294}. Sudden cardiac death may be the first manifestation {425}.

Echocardiography is an excellent means of evaluating involvement of the myocardium by lymphoma, with transoesophageal echocardiography having superior diagnostic sensitivity versus transthoracic echocardiography {349}. Cardiac lymphoma usually manifests as hypoechogenic lesions infiltrating the myocardium, often with pericardial effusion {1144}. CT and MRI can provide additional detail

regarding the location and character of the tumour.

Endomyocardial biopsy is increasingly used to obtain histological diagnosis without thoracotomy, in order to plan the best therapeutic intervention {1433}.

Localization

The right side of the heart is usually involved, with the right atrium being the most common site. Less than 10% of cases have isolated left heart involvement. About a third of all cases involve the pericardium {2044}. Valvular involvement is rare, and likely a product of the limited lymphatic network present in the cardiac valves {3031}.

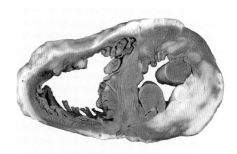

Fig. 4.52 Primary cardiac lymphoma. An infiltrative mass is noted primarily along the inferolateral left ventricle, with smaller satellite foci along the anterior aspect of the ventricle; the tumour involves the epicardium, myocardium, and endocardium.

Macroscopy

Grossly, primary cardiac lymphomas manifest as grey-white coalescing masses that extend along the epicardium and sometimes into the myocardium itself. The masses can track along and encase the great arteries as well as the epicardial coronary arteries. Occasionally, the vena cavae may be involved.

Cytology

Diagnosis may be made by cytological evaluation, particularly in cases with effusion necessitating pericardiocentesis {2186}. Ancillary testing such as cytogenetics and flow cytometry can aid in the diagnostic evaluation.

Histopathology

The histological features vary in accordance with the diagnosis. The most common subtype of primary cardiac lymphoma is DLBCL, accounting for > 75% of published reports {2044}. The tumour cells resemble centroblasts or immunoblasts. Other types that have been described include Burkitt lymphoma (endemic and sporadic forms), so-called Burkitt-like lymphoma (now an obsolete term), unspecified forms of T-cell lymphoma, and low-grade B-cell lymphomas (small lymphocytic lymphoma and follicular lymphoma) {837,837,1137,1444,1882}. The immunophenotype varies according to the precise diagnosis. DLBCLs are characterized by positivity for CD20, CD19, and CD79a, and variable expression of Bcl2, Bcl6, IRF4/MUM1, and CD10. The differential diagnoses for primary cardiac lymphoma include metastatic tumours to the heart/pericardium and primary cardiac sarcomas. Distinguishing between these entities is typically accomplished with the assistance of immunohistochemistry. Secondary cardiac involvement by a primary mediastinal large B-cell lymphoma must also be ruled out.

Genetic profile

B-cell neoplasms show clonal rearrangement of immunoglobulin genes.

Prognosis and predictive factors

The prognosis of primary cardiac lymphoma is typically poor. Unusual complications such as myocardial rupture have been reported {1701}. Anthracycline-based chemotherapy has been reported to result in a nearly 60% complete response rate (with a mean follow-up of 17 months, ranging from 3 to 40 months) {2044}. Lymphomas that arise in the setting of cardiac devices (also called fibrin-associated large B-cell lymphomas) do not appear to carry the same grave prognosis as other types of primary cardiac lymphomas, particularly with current-generation management strategies {905}.

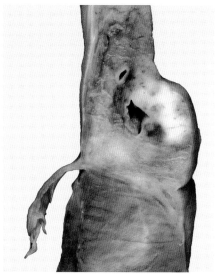

Fig. 4.53 Primary cardiac lymphoma. Primary cardiac lymphoma often exhibits striking epicardial involvement, sometimes with encasement of the epicardial vessels; the coronary sinus exhibits such encasement, with the circumflex coronary artery located just above.

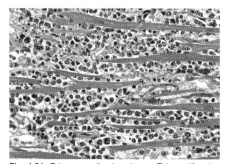

Fig. 4.54 Primary cardiac lymphoma. This proliferation of atypical, malignant B lymphocytes exhibits extensive interstitial infiltration with both atrophic and damaged cardiac myocytes.

Metastatic tumours

H. Tazelaar

Definition

A metastatic tumour in the heart is defined as the involvement of the heart by a malignant neoplasm arising from an organ or site other than the heart, typically by a haematogenous route, lymphatic route, or venous extension (i.e. the venae cavae or pulmonary veins).

Epidemiology

Metastatic tumours to the heart are at least 100 times more common than primary cardiac tumours when identified at autopsy, occurring in 1–3% of all autopsied patients {298}. Metastases to the heart are present in about 10% of all patients with widespread malignancy {296}, and approximately 15–20% of surgically resected tumours are metastatic {12,298,1389,1775}.

Tumours in the organs closest in anatomical proximity to the heart are the most common to metastasize to the heart; 30–35% of all metastases to the heart are from the lung, 30% in men are from the oesophagus, and 8% in women are from the breast. Lymphoma and leukaemias are also fairly common, accounting for 10–20% of tumours that secondarily involve the heart. Tumours of almost all organ sites have been reported to metastasize to the heart, but the most frequently reported primary sites after those listed above are the liver, pancreas, stomach, colon, skin (melanoma), and genitourinary tract (especially the kidney). Sarcomas of various types can also metastasize to the heart. The rate of cardiac involvement by metastatic disease appears to be stable, and does not seem to have been affected by advances in chemotherapy and radiation.

Etiology

There is no specific etiological factor known to predispose patients to developing metastases to the heart. A primary tumour's proximity to the heart, and its vascular and lymphatic system seem to play the biggest roles in putting a patient at risk for these metastases

Clinical features

The site of the tumour within the heart greatly affects the signs and symptoms. These can include symptoms related to pericardial effusions, arrhythmias, or congestive heart failure. If there is obstruction of the mitral or aortic valve, there may be syncope. Involvement of the right heart and tricuspid valves may give rise to right-sided failure.

Generalizing the imaging characteristics of metastatic tumours is very difficult, and they depend on testing modality, tumour type, and localization. On MRI, metastases to the heart typically show low signal intensity on T1-weighted images and high signal intensity on T2-weighted images. But melanoma is the exception to this generalization, with high T1- and low T2-weighted signal intensity. The tumours are typically heterogeneous after contrast enhancement {1760}.

Localization

Metastatic carcinomas most frequently involve the pericardium, followed by the myocardium. The right side of the myocardium is involved more often than the left (in 20–30% versus 10–30% of cases, respectively), and diffuse myocardial involvement occurs in 30–35% of cases. The endocardium is involved rarely, and the cardiac valves are almost never involved. The myocardium is involved in virtually all cases of metastatic melanoma, with less frequent infiltration of the epicardium and endocardium. Leukaemic and lymphomatous infiltrates are typically widespread, involving the epicardium (61%), and myocardium. The right and left ventricles tend to be equally involved. Metastatic sarcomas involve the myocardium (50%), the pericardium (33%), or both (17%).

Macroscopy

Carcinomas, such as those arising from lung or breast, may either show direct extension into the pericardium and/or myocardium, or may show lymphatic/ vascular myocardial involvement. Metastatic deposits can be large, solitary,

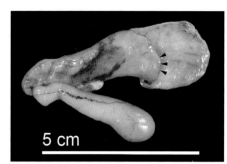

Fig. 4.55 Metastatic endometrial stromal sarcoma. A 43-year-old woman underwent resection of an obstructing metastatic endometrial stromal sarcoma in the inferior vena cava, right atrium, and right ventricle; the arrows show an indentation at the level of the tricuspid valve.

bulky masses; can consist of multiple smaller masses; or (rarely) can be present only microscopically. Sometimes metastatic carcinomas to the pericardium are indistinguishable from malignant mesotheliomas. Melanomas, renal tumours (including Wilms tumour and renal cell carcinoma), adrenal tumours, liver tumours, and uterine tumours may form intracavitary masses, sometimes spreading up the inferior vena cava directly into the right atrium or ventricle.

Cytology

Although cytopathological diagnosis of pericardial tumours is common, cytological diagnosis of tumours metastatic to the heart has not been reported. Transcutaneous needle aspiration via jugular approach is possible for atrial masses, and has been successful in primary lesions.

Histopathology

Among the more common carcinomas to metastasize, adenocarcinomas from a variety of organs (e.g. lung gastrointestinal tract, and breast) outweigh other subtypes {298}. Among the lung carcinomas to spread to the heart, adenocarcinomas account for about 35% of metastatic cancers; small cell carcinoma is the next most common subtype (27%), and squamous carcinomas of the lung constitute a smaller subset (13%).

Of all bone marrow-derived haematolymphoid malignancies, acute myelogenous

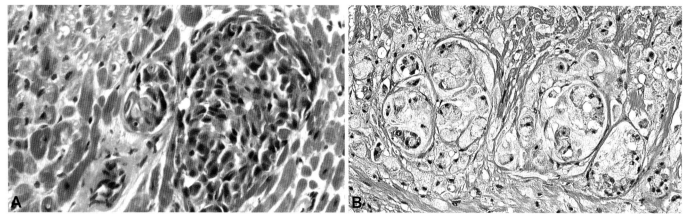

Fig. 4.56 A Metastatic breast carcinoma diagnosed on a right ventricular endomyocardial biopsy. Lymphatic carcinoma is evident. **B** Metastatic signet ring carcinoma, left ventricle. There is extensive lymphatic involvement by poorly differentiated adenocarcinoma.

leukaemia is the most common to involve the heart, accounting for 35% of cases {298}, followed by chronic myelogenous leukaemia (26%), other leukaemias, and multiple myeloma.

The histology of most metastases makes differential diagnosis from a primary cardiac tumour relatively easy. Metastatic sarcomas may be difficult to differentiate from primary cardiac sarcoma; the differential may have to depend on the clinical presentation and presence or absence of a tumour in a different organ. Most sarcomas arising in the left atrium are nearly always primary, although right-sided sarcomas other than angiosarcoma should raise the suspicion of metastasis.

Prognosis and predictive factors

The prognosis of cardiac metastasis is generally dismal. However, surgical resection of cardiac metastases may prolong life, especially in cases of solitary metastases that are extensions from pulmonary veins, and obstructive right-sided tumour deposits {959,2911,2943}.

Tumours of the pericardium

Solitary fibrous tumour

F. Tavora
W.D. Travis

Definition
Solitary fibrous tumour is a neoplasm of fibroblasts with a characteristic histological appearance; showing round to spindle cells, a fibrous matrix, and frequently haemangiopericytoma-like vasculature.

ICD-O codes
Solitary fibrous tumour   8815/1
Malignant solitary fibrous tumour   8815/3

Synonyms
Localized fibrous tumour; haemangiopericytoma

Epidemiology
Pericardial solitary fibrous tumours are extremely rare. Most cases are reported on the pericardial surface, and some within the pericardial sac or within the myocardium {54,199,1885,2732}.

Etiology
A fibroblastic origin with occasional myofibroblastic differentiation has been established.

Clinical features
Symptoms are related to a mass lesion within the pericardial cavity, including pericarditis and pericardial effusion. Intracardiac tumours have been reported to cause arrhythmias, tamponade, embolism, and heart failure {199}.
On CT, solitary fibrous tumours appear as homogeneous well-circumscribed lobulated masses, typically abutting the pericardial surface {1522}. On MRI, areas of low to intermediate signal intensity are more commonly seen on T1-weighted images, and areas of high signal intensity are demonstrated more frequently on T2-weighted images {2189}.

Localization
By definition, pericardial solitary fibrous tumours occur primarily within the pericardial cavity, with variable extension into the surrounding mediastinum. Intracardiac location is very rare {239,505,3021}.

Macroscopy
Solitary fibrous tumours are fibrous, firm, white tumours with a whorled appearance on cut surface. An attachment pedicle is rarely seen. The rare intracardiac tumours are also well-circumscribed, white-tan masses, with pushing borders and usually no clear invasion of the surrounding structures.

Histopathology
The tumour is characterized by a population of bland, oval to spindled cells with round nuclei and evenly distributed chromatin. The uncommon presence of necrosis, pleomorphism or increased mitoses raise concern for malignancy (see pleural Solitary fibrous tumour, p. 178). There is a variable amount of collagen content in the stroma. Myxoid change and degenerative changes can be seen. Solitary fibrous tumours are typically positive for CD34, Bcl2, and CD99, but these markers are not specific. Smooth muscle markers, epithelial and mesothelial markers, and S100 are usually negative. Nuclear cxpression of STAT6 is a specific and sensitive marker for solitary fibrous tumour {624}.
Leiomyomas and schwannomas are extremely rare in this location. Cardiac

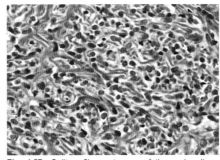

Fig. 4.57 Solitary fibrous tumour of the pericardium. High-power view showing round cells with minimal atypia in a stroma rich with ropy collagen.

fibroma is intracardiac, lacks CD34 and STAT6 expression, and is generally less cellular. Synovial sarcomas are more cellular, demonstrate mitotic activity and proliferation, lack collagenous stroma, and may show epithelial differentiation. Mesothelioma in its spindled form is generally more cellular, pleomorphic, and invasive. Occasionally, myxofibrosarcomas and low-grade myofibroblastic tumours can also histologically mimic solitary fibrous tumour.

Genetic profile
A fusion between the NAB2 and STAT6 genes has been identified as a consistent finding in solitary fibrous tumours from various sites. IGF2 overexpression is probably due to IGF2 imprinting {930}.

Prognosis and predictive factors
Most reported solitary fibrous tumours of the pericardium were benign, with one case of a malignant pleural tumour metastatic to the heart {508}. A malignant solitary fibrous tumour of the heart was reported, but without follow-up information, because the patient died postoperatively {3021}. Histologically, criteria that should raise suspicion of malignancy include necrosis, increased mitotic activity, and nuclear pleomorphism, but these criteria have not been tested in pericardial tumours.

Sarcomas

F. Tavora
C.D.M. Fletcher

Definition
Pericardial sarcomas are malignant mesenchymal lesions that are classified according to their line of differentiation.

ICD-O codes
Angiosarcoma   9120/3
Synovial sarcoma   9040/3

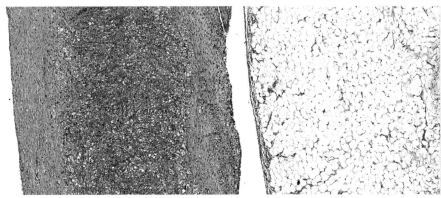

Fig. 4.58 Pericardial angiosarcoma. Tumour diffusely replaces the pericardial surface; the tumour is more cellular in the centre, and shows a desmoplastic reaction at the periphery. Benign pericardial fat on right.

Epidemiology
Pericardial sarcomas are rare tumours. The two most common types that arise within the pericardium are angiosarcoma and synovial sarcoma {284,412,2645}. Pericardial liposarcomas usually occur in close relationship with the atrial walls and epicardium, and may extend into the mediastinum {1496}. Leiomyosarcomas involving the pericardium are usually associated with cardiac or lung lesions {576}. Undifferentiated pleomorphic sarcomas have also been reported in the pericardium {284,1386}. Ewing sarcoma/primitive neuroectodermal tumour and myofibroblastic sarcoma in the pericardium are exceedingly rare.

Clinical features
Pericardial sarcomas arise in a younger population than do their soft tissue counterparts, with peak incidence in the fourth to fifth decade. There is no sex predilection. These tumours cause symptoms often related to pericardial effusion. Cough, dyspnoea, and chest pain can be the result of tumours extending into the cardiac chambers. The diagnosis is often first considered at transthoracic echocardiography, usually for the work-up of an associated effusion. CT is useful to determine the precise location of the tumour to guide the biopsy. Pericardial sarcomas are usually confined to the cavity at the time of diagnosis. Invasion into the myocardium and extension to the mediastinum usually occur later in the course of the disease.

Macroscopy
The pericardium is usually thickened by tumour infiltration, which may be diffuse, mimicking mesothelioma. Pericardial effusion can be massive. Pericardial synovial sarcomas are usually localized, solid tumours. Some tumours have been reported to be pedunculated, and others encapsulated {2982}.

Cytology
Since pericardial effusion is usually the first manifestation of the disease, cytological sampling may sometimes provide the first specimen.

Histopathology
The histologies of the specific types of pleural sarcomas are similar to those of their counterparts arising in the soft tissue. As noted above, the most common types are angiosarcoma and synovial sarcoma.
By immunohistochemistry, identification of endothelial differentiation (i.e. expression of CD31, ERG oncoprotein, FLI1, and other endothelial markers) may be helpful in the diagnosis of angiosarcoma, while epithelial membrane antigen and TLE1 are useful in identifying synovial sarcoma. The differential diagnosis will depend on specific sarcoma type. Mesothelioma is the most important tumour in the differential diagnosis of angiosarcoma and synovial sarcoma.

Genetic profile
Specific genetic alterations relate to the type of sarcoma. Synovial sarcomas demonstrate the presence of *SS18* (also called *SYT*) gene rearrangements in molecular cytogenetic assays {412}.

Prognosis and predictive factors
Since pericardial sarcomas are rare, there have been no large series comparing their histological features with prognosis. Surgical excision is the mainstay of treatment, and the only therapy that has been responsible for rare cases of extended follow-up, when complete resection can be performed {284,2645}. Response to radiation therapy has been documented, and adjuvant therapy is usually recommended {3016}.

Malignant mesothelioma

V. Roggli

Definition
Pericardial mesothelioma is a tumour that arises from mesothelial cells or demonstrates mesothelial differentiation, without a primary lesion in the pleura. As in the pleura, most pericardial mesotheliomas are diffuse malignant mesotheliomas. Low-grade or localized mesotheliomas, such as well-differentiated papillary mesothelioma and multicystic mesothelioma are exceedingly rare in the pericardium {1751,2270}.

ICD-O code   9050/3

Synonym
Diffuse malignant mesothelioma

Epidemiology
Malignant mesothelioma is the most common malignant tumour primary to the pericardium, but is rare overall {899,2006}. It accounts for about 3% of all cardiac and pericardial primary tumours, and for < 2% of all mesotheliomas. The mean patient age at presentation is in the fifth decade, with a male-to-female ratio of 2:1.

Etiology
Mesotheliomas arise from pluripotent mesothelial cells or mesothelial precursor cells in the submesothelial space {899,2006,2732}. The link between pericardial mesothelioma and asbestos exposure is weak {972,1654,2006,2183}. One review found that only 14% of patients had documented asbestos exposure {2633}.

Clinical features
Symptoms are related to a mass in the pericardium, which may cause compression of the heart. Pericardial effusion is often asymptomatic, with tamponade as the disease progresses.

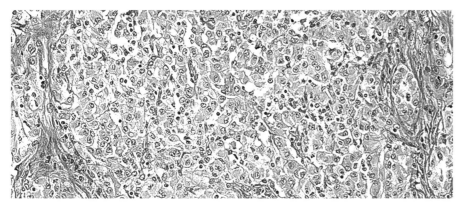

Fig. 4.59 Malignant mesothelioma of the pericardium. In a 51-year-old woman with shortness of breath and pericardial tamponade; there was a 7.5 cm lobulated spherical mass removed from the inner surface of the pericardium on the superior left ventricular free wall. The histology shows an epithelioid mesothelioma arranged in solid nests and cords.

Echocardiography and CT show cardiac enlargement, with thickened pleura with tumour nodules and associated effusion {2274}.

Mesotheliomas of the pericardium are locally aggressive tumours that may extend to the pleura and encase the heart and great vessels, with invasion of the mediastinum {2131}. Distant metastasis has not been reported.

Macroscopy
Pericardial mesotheliomas typically involve the pericardium diffusely, forming multiple nodules along its surface. Involvement of the great vessels is common. One well-differentiated papillary mesothelioma has been reported in the pericardium {2270}. Infiltration deep into the myocardium is not common {1003}.

Cytology
Effusion cytology is not particularly sensitive for this diagnosis {2633}, and shows similar features as those of pleural mesothelioma.

Histopathology
Pericardial mesotheliomas are either epithelioid or biphasic {997,2617}. The epithelioid types typically invade the surrounding fat and stroma, and often the myocardium. A deciduoid variant (poorly differentiated epithelioid mesothelioma with abundant eosinophilic cytoplasm and sheet-like growth) has also been reported in the pericardium {2131}. A single case of desmoplastic mesothelioma has been reported in the pericardium {1851}.

Immunohistocemical studies are indispensable in the diagnosis of pericardial

mesotheliomas, especially in the differential diagnosis of the far more common metastatic carcinomas. The profile is identical to that of pleural mesotheliomas. The main differential diagnosis is metastatic carcinoma, especially lung adenocarcinoma that also involves the pleura. Angiosarcomas may mimic mesothelioma, as they show an epithelioid configuration and grow along the pericardial lining. Synovial sarcomas may mimic sarcomatoid mesothelioma, but are usually more cellular and have distinct immunohistochemical and molecular characteristics. Malignant solitary fibrous tumours can also be confused with desmoplastic mesothelioma, but lack expression of keratins. Rarely, germ cell tumours may involve the pericardium and show a solid growth and histological features of malignant mesothelioma. Pleural mesotheliomas extending to the pericardium are

far more common than primary pericardial mesotheliomas, and this possibility should be excluded before the diagnosis is made.

Prognosis and predictive factors
Surgical resection is the treatment of choice for localized disease, but most cases present with diffuse disease. Even with therapy, the median survival from the onset of symptoms is only about 6 months {1225}. New chemotherapeutic regimens have been attempted with longer survival in pleural tumours {1234}.

Germ cell tumours

A.P. Burke
F. Tavora

Definition
Intrapericardial germ cell tumours are neoplasms of germ cell origin that arise within the pericardium. A gonadal site or other site outside the pericardium is by definition absent. To date, all reported intrapericardial germ cell tumours have been teratomas or yolk sac tumours.

ICD-O codes
Teratoma, mature	9080/0
Teratoma, immature	9080/3
Yolk sac tumour	9071/3

Synonyms
Teratoma; pericardial teratoma; dermoid cyst; yolk sac tumour; endodermal sinus tumour

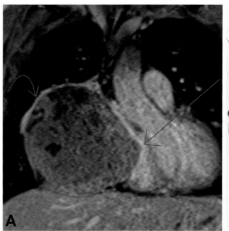 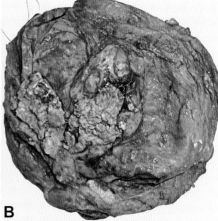

Fig. 4.60 Intrapericardial teratoma. **A** T1-weighted MRI (VIBE) post contrast coronal image shows heterogeneous internal debris (asterisk) with rim enhancement (curved arrow) and mass effect (straight arrow). **B** Gross photograph shows tumour that contained fat, hair, and calcification; the tumour was an incidental finding in a young woman who had a chest X-ray following a motor vehicle accident.

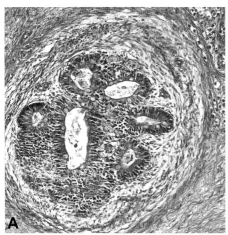 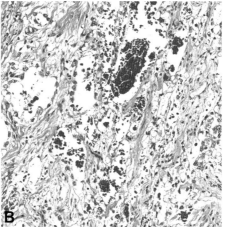

Fig. 4.61 **A** Pericardial teratoma. Endodermal-derived gastrointestinal-type mucosa with smooth muscle stroma. **B** Intrapericardial yolk sac tumour. These tumours have an appearance similar to that of their counterparts in the mediastinum and gonads.

Epidemiology

Fewer than 150 germ cell tumours arising within the pericardial sac or heart have been reported {382,427,496,895,1468, 1540,1748,1998,2407}. Approximately 90% are teratomas and the remainder are yolk sac tumours.

Clinical features

Intrapericardial germ cell tumours can occur from intrauterine life to the seventh decade, but most patients are infants or children {496,1540}. In adults, intrapericardial teratomas occur more frequently in men than in women. Intrapericardial yolk sac tumours are also predominantly seen in the paediatric group, and predominantly in girls. In children, symptoms are usually related to pericardial effusions or tamponade, or to compression of cardiac chambers. In adults, pericardial teratomas are usually discovered as an incidental radiographical finding. In fetuses, hydrops fetalis can occur. Sudden death is a rare complication.

Localization

Teratomas are usually attached by a pedicle to one of the great vessels with arterial supply directly from the aorta. They displace the heart and rotate it along its longitudinal axis, and often compress the right atrium and superior vena cava. Intrapericardial yolk sac tumours occur in the pericardial cavity, similar to teratomas, at the base of the heart. The tumours do not involve the myocardium.

Macroscopy

Teratomas are commonly multicystic, and may contain large solid areas and bone. They can grow as large as 15 cm. The surface is typically smooth. Yolk sac tumours are lobulated, smooth-surfaced tumours that are either homogeneous soft tumours, or partly cystic and haemorrhagic on cut section.

Histopathology

Intrapericardial teratomas have a predominance of immature elements in fetuses and newborns, with mature elements predominating in adults. Typically there are cysts lined by squamous epithelium, with foci of cartilage and stroma. There are variable amounts of respiratory, gastric, and intestinal mucosa. Uncommon tissues include glial, liver, and pancreatic islet tissue. Most reports of intrapericardial teratoma describe the presence of only one or two germ cell layers. If only cystic epithelial structures are present, the term bronchogenic or dermoid cyst is appropriate depending

whether glandular or squamous epithelium is present, respectively. The histological features of intrapericardial yolk sac tumour are similar to those of extrapericardial mediastinal yolk sac tumours {282,496,2350}.

Somatic malignancy may rarely be associated with pericardial teratoma {1048}.

A single case of yolk sac tumour that recurred as benign cystic teratoma after chemotherapy, as occurs with treated retroperitoneal tumours, has been described {1153}.

Prognosis and predictive factors

Pure teratomas are benign in the paediatric population. Surgical excision is the treatment of choice. Yolk sac tumours are predisposed to metastasis or bulky intrapericardial recurrence, although many patients remain well without recurrence after surgery and chemotherapy {1153}. One patient experienced recurrence with teratoma after treatment for yolk sac tumour {48}.

Metastatic tumours

J.J. Maleszewski

Definition

In the pericardium, a metastatic tumour is any malignant neoplasm of non-pericardial and non-cardiac origin.

Epidemiology

Up to 10% of all patients with advanced-stage cancer develop cardiac metastasis, with the majority of metastases (about 75%) involving the epicardium

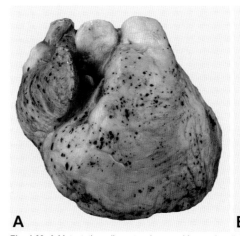 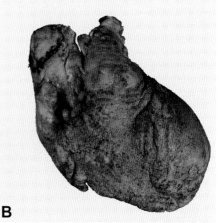

Fig. 4.62 **A** Metastatic malignant melanoma. Many epicardial nodules studding the surface of the heart. **B** Metastatic adenocarcinoma. Fibrinous pericarditis.

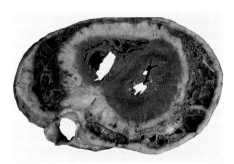

Fig. **4.63** Metastatic adenocarcinoma. Metastatic pulmonary adenocarcinoma directly involving the epicardium, with haemopericardium.

and/or pericardium {12,1277}. In a large autopsy series of more than 7000 cases, 622 metastatic tumours to the heart were found {296}.

Etiology

Metastatic tumours to the pericardium are most commonly epithelial tumours from the lung or breast, or melanoma {296,796}. Other primary sites include the gastrointestinal tract, kidney, thyroid, urinary bladder, ovary, endometrium, and thymus {533,692,1298,1411,2117, 2580}. Other non-epithelial metastases include lymphoma, angiosarcoma, and other metastatic sarcomas {71,145,1502, 1551,2272,2280,2702}.

Clinical features

Common symptoms include acute and chronic pericarditis, recurrent effusions, and enlargement of the heart shadow on imaging. The most common features reported are chest discomfort, dyspnoea on exertion, and associated pleural effusion {20}. Malignant pericardial fluid is usually haemorrhagic {1661}. Pericardial tamponade due to metastases is a common complication.

CT and echocardiogram are the most important modalities for the diagnosis of pericardial metastases. The most

common CT features (in order of decreasing frequency) include pericardial effusion, enlarged lymph nodes, thickening, enhancement, and nodules {2081}. Tumours may spread to involve the pericardium by lymphatics, haematogenous seeding, or direct extension {2146}.

Localization

Metastatic tumours are commonly located near the base of the heart. About two thirds of metastases to the heart involve the pericardium, one third the epicardium, one third the myocardium, and only 5% the endocardium {296}.

Macroscopy

The most common finding at surgery or autopsy is haemorrhagic, fibrinous exudates with nodules on the surface of the pericardium. Diffuse pericardial thickening without masses is a rare appearance that suggests the possibility of benign chronic fibrous pericarditis or malignant mesothelioma (either primary pericardial or spread from a pleural primary).

Cytology

Benign pericardial effusion is far more common than malignant effusions, but in series from large cancer centres, malignant diagnoses may account for up to 30% of cases, diagnosed most commonly in cytology specimens {137,625,2903}. Cytological evaluation of pericardiocentesis specimens provides a highly specific means of diagnosing malignant effusion, with sensitivity varying from 40% to 95% {1553,1661,2010}.

Histopathology

Metastatic tumours commonly appear in association with acute and chronic pericarditis. Epithelial tumours usually grow along the pericardial surface, with invasion and presence of

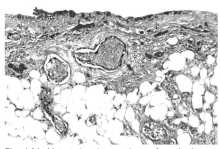

Fig. **4.64** Metastatic adenocarcinoma from the breast. Angiolymphatic involvement of the pericardium by metastatic adenocarcinoma of the breast.

tumour nests within the pericardial wall or angiolymphatics.

Immunohistochemistry can be very helpful in the distinction between metastatic disease and reactive mesothelial hyperplasia seen in organizing fibrinous pericarditis. It is also very useful in determining the primary site of a metastatic process.

Cancer patients may present with effusion, which can be neoplastic or secondary to treatment (especially radiation). The differential diagnosis in these cases involves metastatic carcinoma, reactive mesothelial hyperplasia, and malignant mesothelioma. In patients with breast cancer, effusions are most often benign; even in those with large symptomatic effusions, only 50% are malignant {273,625,2010}.

Genetic profile

The genetic profile depends on the biology of the primary tumour.

Prognosis and predictive factors

The majority of malignant effusions recur after pericardiocentesis, and the mean survival is poor, even after surgical drainage.

Contributors

Dr Abbas AGAIMY
Institute of Pathology
Universitätsklinikum Erlangen
Krankenhausstrasse 8–10
91054 Erlangen
GERMANY
Tel. +49 9131 85 22288
Fax + 49 9131 85 24745
abbas.agaimy@uk-erlangen.de

Dr Seena C. AISNER
Department of Pathology
Rutgers New Jersey Medical School
150 Bergen St, UH E 155
Newark, NJ 07103
USA
Tel. +1 973 972 5726
Fax +1 973 972 5724
aisnersc@njms.rutgers.edu

Dr Fouad AL-DAYEL
Department of Pathology
King Faisal Specialist Hospital
and Research Centre
Takhassussi Street, MBC-10
P.O. Box 3354
11211 Riyadh
SAUDI ARABIA
Tel. +966 11 442 7224
Fax +966 11 442 4280
dayelf@kfshrc.edu.sa

Dr Emilio ALVAREZ-FERNANDEZ
Department of Pathology
Hospital General Universitario Gregorio
Maranon
Dr. Esquerdo 46
28007 Madrid
SPAIN
Tel. +34 91 586 81 63
Fax +34 91 586 80 18
ealvarez@salud.madrid.org

Dr Richard ATTANOOS #
Department of Histopathology
Llandough Hospital
Penlan Road
Cardiff CF64 2XX
Wales
UNITED KINGDOM
Tel. +44 7812 083 396
Fax +44 1446 792 292
richard.attanoos@cardiffandvale.wales.nhs.uk

Dr Marie Christine AUBRY
Department of Pathology
Mayo Clinic
200 First Street NW
Rochester, MN 55905
USA
Tel. +1 507 284 1196
Fax +1 507 538 3267
aubry.mariechristine@mayo.edu

Dr John H.M. AUSTIN
Department of Radiology
Columbia University Medical Center
622 West 168th Street
New York, NY 10032
USA
Tel. +1 212 305 2639
Fax +1 212 305 2962
jha3@cumc.columbia.edu

Dr Chris BACON
Northern Institute for Cancer Research
Paul O'Gorman Bldg
Newcastle University
Framlington Place
Newcastle upon Tyne NE2 4HH
UNITED KINGDOM
Tel. +44 191 208 4404
Fax +44 191 208 4301
chris.bacon@ncl.ac.uk

Dr Sunil BADVE
Pathology and Lab Medicine
IU Health Pathology Laboratory
350 West 11th Street
Indianapolis, IN 46202-4108
USA
Tel. +1 317 491 6417
Fax +1 317 491 6419
sbadve@iupui.edu

Dr Cristina BASSO*
Cardiovascular Pathology Unit
Department of Cardiac, Thoracic
and Vascular Sciences
University of Padua
via A. Gabelli, 61
35121 Padua
ITALY
Tel. +39 049 827 2286
Fax +39 049 827 2284
cristina.basso@unipd.it

Dr Mary Beth BEASLEY*
Department of Pathology
Mount Sinai Hospital
Annenberg Building
15th Floor Room 50
1468 Madison Avenue
New York, NY 10029
USA
Tel. +1 212 241 5307
Fax +1 212 289 2899
mary.beasley@mountsinai.org

Dr Rainer M. BOHLE
Department of Pathology
University of Saarland
Kirrberger Strasse, Geb. 26
66421 Homburg/Saar
GERMANY
Tel. +49 6841 16 23850
Fax +49 6841 16 21802
rainer.bohle@uks.eu

Dr Alain BORCZUK*
Department of Pathology
Columbia University
630 W 168th St, VC14-237
New York, NY 10032
USA
Tel. +1 212 305 6719
Fax +1 212 305 2301
ab748@columbia.edu

Dr Elisabeth BRAMBILLA*
Centre Hospitalier Universitaire de Grenoble
Département d'Anatomie et
Cytologie Pathologiques
INSERM U823
Université Joseph Fourier
CS 10217 - 38043 Grenoble Cedex 09
FRANCE
Tel. +33 4 76 76 58 75
Fax +33 4 76 76 59 29
ebrambilla@chu-grenoble.fr

Dr Lukas BUBENDORF #
Institute for Pathology
University of Basel
Schönbeinstrasse 40
4031 Basel
SWITZERLAND
Tel. +41 61 265 28 51
Fax +41 61 265 20 28
lukas.bubendorf@usb.ch

* Indicates participation in the Working Group Meeting on the WHO Classification of Tumours of the Lung, Pleura, Thymus and Heart that was held in Lyon, France, April 24–26, 2014.
# Indicates disclosure of interests.

Dr Allen P. BURKE*
Department of Anatomic Pathology
University of Maryland School of Medicine
22 S Greene St, Rm NBW47
Baltimore, MD 21201
USA
Tel. +1 410 328 1346
Fax +1 410 328 5508
aburke@umm.edu

Dr Jagdish BUTANY
Department of Pathology, E11-444
Toronto General Hospital
200 Elizabeth Street
Toronto, ON M5G 2C4
CANADA
Tel. +1 416 340 3003
Fax +1 416 586 9901
jagdish.butany@uhn.ca

Dr Kelly J. BUTNOR
Department of Pathology and
Laboratory Medicine
The University of Vermont Medical Center
111 Colchester Ave, ACC Bldg, EP2-120
Burlington, VT 05401
USA
Tel. +1 802 847 8211
Fax +1 802 847 4155
kelly.butnor@vtmednet.org

Dr Philip CAGLE
Department of Pathology and
Genomic Medicine
Houston Methodist Hospital
6565 Fannin St, Room 227
Houston, TX 77030
USA
Tel. +1 713 441 6478
Fax +1 713 793 1603
pcagle@houstonMethodist.org

Dr Vera L. CAPELOZZI
Departamento de Patologia
Faculdade de Medicina, USP
Av. Dr. Arnaldo, 455, sala 1143
Cerqueira César
01296-903 São Paulo, SP
BRAZIL
Tel. +55 11 3061 7427
Fax +55 11 3064 2744
vcapelozzi@lim05.fm.usp.br

Dr Neil E. CAPORASO
Division of Cancer, Genetic Epidemiology
Branch, National Cancer Institute
National Institute of Health
9609 Medical Center Drive
Rockville, MD 20850
USA
Tel. +1 240 276 7228
Fax +1 240 276 7837
caporasn@mail.nih.gov
caporaso@nih.gov

Dr Lina CARVALHO #
Servico de Anatomia Patologica
Hospitais da Universidade de Coimbra
3000 Coimbra
PORTUGAL
Tel. +351 911 815 774
Fax +351 239 857 757
lcarvalho@huc.min-saude.pt

Dr Lara CHALABREYSSE
Centre de Pathologie Est
Hopital Louis Pradel
Groupement Hospitalier Est
59, Boulevard Pinel
69677 Bron Cedex
FRANCE
Tel. +33 4 72 12 95 96
Fax +33 4 72 35 70 67
lara.chalabreysse@chu-lyon.fr

Dr John K.C. CHAN
Department of Pathology
Queen Elizabeth Hospital
Wylie Road, Kowloon
HONG KONG SAR, CHINA
Tel. +852 3506 6830
Fax +852 2385 2455
jkcchan@ha.org.hk

Dr Yih-Leong CHANG
Department of Pathology
National Taiwan University Hospital
National Taiwan University
College of Medicine
Taipei
TAIWAN, CHINA
Tel. +886 223 123 456 ext 65460
Fax +886 223 934 172
ntuhylc@gmail.com

Dr Gang CHEN
Department of Pathology
Zhongshan Hospital
Fudan University
180 Fenglin Road
200032 Shanghai
CHINA
Tel. +86 21 6404 1990
Fax +86 21 6403 7269
chestpathology@126.com

Dr Lucian R. CHIRIEAC #
Department of Pathology
Harvard Medical School
Brigham and Women's Hospital
75 Francis St
Boston, MA 02115
USA
Tel. +1 617 732 8126
Fax +1 617 264 5118
lchirieac@partners.org

Dr Teh-Ying CHOU
Department of Pathology and
Laboratory Medicine
Taipei Veterans General Hospital
201, Section 2, Shipai Road
Taipei 112
TAIWAN, CHINA
Tel. +886 2 2875 7080
Fax +886 2 2875 7056
tehying@gmail.com

Dr Jin-Haeng CHUNG
Department of Pathology
and Respiratory Center
Seoul National University Bundang Hospital
300 Gumidong, Bundang-gu, Seongnam City
Gyeonggi-do 463-707
REPUBLIC OF KOREA
Tel. +82 31 787 7713
Fax +82 31 787 4012
chungjh@snu.ac.kr

Dr Andrew CHURG
Department of Pathology
University of British Columbia
2211 Westbrook Mall
Vancouver, BC V6T 2B5
CANADA
Tel. +1 604 822 7776
Fax +1 604 875 4797
achurg@interchange.ubc.ca

Dr Cheryl COFFIN
Department of Pathology, Microbiology, and
Immunology
Vanderbilt University School of Medicine
1161 21st Avenue South
Nashville, TN 37232
USA
Tel. +1 207 664 7414
ccoffin@hotmail.com

Dr Jean-Michel COINDRE
Department of Pathology
Institut Bergonié
33076 Bordeaux Cedex
FRANCE
Tel. +33 5 56 33 04 36
Fax +33 5 56 33 04 38
j.coindre@bordeaux.unicancer.fr

Dr Sanja DACIC*
Department of Pathology
Univ of Pittsburgh Medical Center
200 Lothrop Street, PUH-C608
Pittsburgh, PA 15213
USA
Tel. +1 412 647 8694
Fax +1 412 647 3455
dacics@upmc.edu

Dr Mercedes Liliana DALURZO #
Department of Pathology
Hospital Italiano de Buenos Aires
Peron 4190
C1181ACH Buenos Aires
ARGENTINA
Tel. +54 11 4949 0200 ext 9215
Fax +54 11 4959 0352
mercedes.dalurzo@hospitalitaliano.org.ar

Dr Laurence DE LEVAL
Institut Universitaire de Pathologie, CHUV
25 rue du Bugnon
CH 1011 Lausanne
SWITZERLAND
Tel. +41 21 314 7194
Fax +41 21 314 7202
laurence.deleval@chuv.ch

Dr Michael A. DEN BAKKER #
Department of Pathology
Maasstad Ziekenhuis
PO Box 9100
3007 AC Rotterdam
THE NETHERLANDS
Tel. +31 10 291 441
Fax +31 10 2913 801
bakkerma@maasstadziekenhuis.nl
m.denbakker@erasmusmc.nl

Dr Frank DETTERBECK
Department of Thoracic Surgery
Yale School of Medicine
330 Cedar St., BB205,
New Haven, CT 06520-8062
USA
Tel. +1 203 785 4931
Fax +1 203 737 2163
frank.detterbeck@yale.edu

Dr Susan S. DEVESA
Division of Cancer Epidemiology and
Genetics
National Cancer Institute
9609 Medical Center Drive, Room 7E580
Bethesda, MD 20892
USA
Tel. +1 240 276 7410
devesas@mail.nih.gov

Dr Edwina DUHIG*
Sullivan Nicolaides Pathology
John Flynn Hospital
42 Inland Ave
Tugun QLD 4224
AUSTRALIA
Tel. +61 7 5507 9709
Fax +61 7 5598 0777
Edwina_Duhig@snp.com.au

Dr Rafal DZIADZIUSZKO #
Department of Oncology/Radiotherapy
Medical University of Gdansk
7, Debinki St
Gdansk, 80-211
POLAND
Tel. +48 58 349 2979
Fax +48 58 349 2210
rafald@gumed.edu.pl

Dr Andrew W. ELBARDISSI
Department of Cardiothoracic Surgery
Stanford University
300 Pasteur Drive
Stanford, CA 94305
USA
Tel. +1 650 723 6661
Fax +1 650 725 3846
andrewel@stanford.edu

Dr Göran ELMBERGER #
Department of Laboratory Medicine,
Pathology
Örebro University Hospital
701 85 Örebro läns landsting
SWEDEN
Tel. +46 19 602 1035
Fax +46 19 602 1035
Goran.Elmberger@orebroll.se

Dr Christopher D.M. FLETCHER
Department of Pathology
Brigham and Women's Hospital
Boston, MA 02115
USA
Tel. +1 617 732 8558
Fax +1 617 566 3897
cfletcher@partners.org

Dr Douglas B. FLIEDER
Department of Pathology
Fox Chase Cancer Center
333 Cottman Ave
Philadelphia, PA 19111
USA
Tel. +1 215 728 4092
Fax +1 215 728 2899
Douglas.Flieder@fccc.edu

Dr Georgy A. FRANK
Department of Pathologic Anatomy
P.A. Herzen Research Oncological Institute
2nd Botkinsky proezd, 3
125284 Moscow
RUSSIAN FEDERATION
Tel. +7 903 720 0146
Fax +7 495 945 8644
georgyfrank1@gmail.com

Dr Wilbur A. FRANKLIN
Department of Pathology
University of Colorado Anschutz Medical
Campus
12801 East 17th Ave
PO Box 6511, Mailstop 8104
Aurora, CO 80045
USA
Tel. +1 303 724 3080
Fax +1 303 724 3096
Wilbur.Franklin@ucdenver.edu

Dr Teri J. FRANKS
Pulmonary and Mediastinal Pathology
The Joint Pathology Center
606 Stephen Sitter Ave.
Silver Spring, MD 20910
USA
Tel. +1 855 393 3904
Fax +1 301 295 5675
teri.j.franks.civ@mail.mil

Dr Aletta Ann FRAZIER
Department of Radiology
University of Maryland School of Medicine
Department of Diagnostic Radiology
22 South Greene Street
Baltimore, MD 21201
USA
Tel. +1 410 328 3477
Fax +1 301 585 0143
anniefrazier@mac.com

Dr Christopher A. FRENCH #
Department of Pathology
New Research Building #630G
77 Avenue Louis Pasteur
Boston, MA 02115
USA
Tel. +1 617 525 4415
Fax +1 617 525 4422
cfrench@partners.org

Dr Junya FUKUOKA
Department of Pathology
Nagasaki University Graduate School
of Biomedical Sciences
1-12-4, Sakamato
Nagasaki 852-8523
JAPAN
Tel. +81 95 819 7407
Fax +81 95 819 7564
fukuokaj@nagasaki-u.ac.jp

Dr Francoise GALATEAU-SALLE*
MESOPATH Reference Center
Department of Pathology
INSERM U 1086
CHU Caen
Avenue Cote de Nacre
14033 Caen Cedex
FRANCE
Tel. +33 2 31 06 44 07
Fax +33 2 31 06 50 63
galateausalle-f@chu-caen.fr

Dr Randy GASCOYNE #
Center for Lymphoid Cancers
BC Cancer Agency
675 West, 10th Avenue
Vancouver, BC V5Z 1L3
CANADA
Tel. +1 604 675 8025
Fax +1 604 675 8183
rgascoyn@bccancer.bc.ca

Dr Philippe GAULARD
Départment de Pathologie
Hopital Henri Mondor
51 av du Marechal de Lattre de Tassigny
90410 Créteil Cedex
FRANCE
Tel. +33 1 49 81 2743
Fax +33 1 49 81 2733
philippe.gaulard@hmn.aphp.fr

Dr Adi GAZDAR #
Hamon Cancer Center
UT Southwestern Medical Ctr.
5323 Harry Hines Blvd., Rm NB8-206
Dallas, TX 75235-8593
USA
Tel. +1 214 648 4921
Fax +1 214 648 4940
adi.gazdar@utsouthwestern.edu

Dr Kim GEISINGER #
Department of Pathology
University of Mississippi Medical Center
2500 N. State Street
Jackson, MS 39216
USA
Tel. +1 601 984 1530
Fax +1 601 984 1531
krgeisin@yahoo.com

Dr Allen GIBBS #
Department of Histopathology
Llandough Hospital
Penlan Road, Penarth, South Glamorgan
Cardiff, CF642XX
Wales
UNITED KINGDOM
Tel. +44 29 20 744273
Fax +44 29 20 742701
allenrg@btinternet.com

Dr Nicolas GIRARD*
Respiratory Medicine
Thoracic Oncology Department
Hôpital Louis Pradel
Hospices Civils de Lyon
28 avenue doyen Lépine
69677 Lyon (Bron) Cedex
FRANCE
Tel. +33 4 72 35 76 44
Fax +33 4 72 35 76 53
nicolas.girard@chu-lyon.fr

Dr Sergio GONZALEZ
Department of Anatomic Pathology
Pontificia Universidad Católica de Chile
Marcoleta 377, 10th floor
Santiago
CHILE
Tel. +56 2 2354 3206
Fax +56 2 2639 5871
sgonzale@med.puc.cl

Dr John R. GOSNEY
Department of Pathology
Royal Liverpool University Hospital
Duncan Building, Daulby Street
Liverpool, L69 3GA
UNITED KINGDOM
Tel. +44 151 706 4490
Fax +44 151 706 5859
J.Gosney@rlbuht.nhs.uk

Dr Donald GUINEE #
Department of Pathology
Virginia Mason Medical Center
1100 Ninth Avenue, C6-PTH
Seattle, WA 98111
USA
Tel. +1 206 223 6861
Fax +1 206 341 0525
Donald.Guinee@vmmc.org

Dr Pierre HAINAUT #
Institut Albert Bonniot
Université Joseph Fourier
CRI INSERM/UJF U823
Rond-point de la Chantourne
38706 La Tronche Cedex
FRANCE
Tel. +33 4 76 54 94 63
Fax +33 4 76 54 94 54
pierre.hainaut@ujf-grenoble.fr

Dr Samuel HAMMAR #
Diagnostic Specialties Laboratory
700 Lebo Blvd
Bremerton, WA 98310
USA
Tel. +1 360 479 7707
Fax +1 360 479 7886
sam@samhammarmd.com

Dr Nancy L. HARRIS
Department of Pathology
Massachusetts General Hospital
55 Fruit Street
Boston, MA 02114
USA
Tel. +1 617 724 1406
Fax +1 617 726 5626
nlharris@partners.org

Dr Philip HASLETON
Department of Inflammation and Repair
University of Manchester
Wythenshawe Hospital
Southmoor Road
Manchester, M23 9LT
UNITED KINGDOM
Tel. +44 161 428 2797
philiphasleton@gmail.com

Dr Elizabeth HENSKE #
Center for LAM Research and Clinical Care
Brigham and Women's Hospital
Harvard Medical School
1 Blackfan Circle
Boston, MA 02115
USA
Tel. +1 617 355 9049
Fax +1 617 355 9016
ehenske@partners.org

Dr Kenzo HIROSHIMA
Department of Pathology
Tokyo Women's Medical University
Yachiyo Medical Center
477-96 Owada-Shinden, Yachiyo
Chiba 276-8524
JAPAN
Tel. +81 47 450 6000
Fax +81 47 458 7047
hiroshima.kenzo@twmu.ac.jp

Dr Fred R. HIRSCH*
University of Colorado Cancer Center
RC1-South Tower, 8th Floor
12801 East Seventeenth Ave
Mail Stop #8111, PO Box 6511
Aurora, CO 80045
USA
Tel. +1 303 724 3858
Fax +1 303 724 0714
Fred.hirsch@ucdenver.edu

Dr Aliya N. HUSAIN
Department of Pathology, MC6101
University of Chicago Medical Center
5841 S. Maryland Ave, Room S-627
Chicago, IL 60637
USA
Tel. +1 773 834 8397
Fax +1 773 834 7664
Aliya.Husain@uchospitals.edu

Dr Hiroshi INAGAKI
Department of Pathology
Graduate School of Medical Sciences
Nagoya City University
Nagoya 467-8601
JAPAN
Tel. +81 52 853 8161
Fax +81 52 851 4166
hinagaki@med.nagoya-cu.ac.jp

Dr Kouki INAI
Pathological Diagnostic Center, Inc.
7-1 Mikawa-cho, Naka-Ku
Hiroshima 730-0029
JAPAN
Tel. +81 82 248 0101
Fax +81 82 248 0103
koinai@hiroshima-u.ac.jp

Dr Yuichi ISHIKAWA*
Department of Pathology
The JFCR Cancer Institute
3-8-31 Ariake, Koto-ku
Tokyo 135-8550
JAPAN
Tel. +81 3 3570 0448
Fax +81 3 3570 0558
ishikawa@jfcr.or.jp

Dr Elaine S. JAFFE*
Hematopathology Section,
Laboratory of Pathology
Center for Cancer Research
National Cancer Institute
10 Center Drive
Bethesda, MA 20892
USA
Tel. +1 301 496 0184
Fax +1 301 402 2415
elainejaffe@nih.gov

Dr Deepali JAIN
Department of Pathology
All India Institute of Medical Sciences
Ansari Nagar
New Delhi, 110029
INDIA
Tel. +91 11 2659 4774
Fax +91 11 2658 8663
deepalijain76@gmail.com

Dr Robert JAKOB*
Classifications, Terminology and
Standards Unit
World Health Organization
20 Avenue Appia
1211 Geneva 27
SWITZERLAND
Tel. +41 22 791 5877
jakobr@who.int

Dr Nirmala A. JAMBHEKAR
Department of Pathology
Tata Memorial Hospital
Dr E.B. Road
Parel, Mumbai, 400012
INDIA
Tel. +91 22 2417 7000 (ext 7271)
Fax +91 22 2414 6937
najambhekar@rediffmail.com
najambehkar12@gmail.com

Dr Jin JEN
Department of Laboratory Medicine and
Pathology
Mayo Clinic
200 First Street, SW
Rochester, MN 55905
USA
Tel. +1 507 284 0526
Fax +1 507 266 0340
Jen.Jin@mayo.edu

Dr James JETT #
National Jewish Health
1400 Jackson Street, J229
Denver, CO 80206
USA
Tel. +1 507 358 0585
Fax +1 303 398 1476
jettj@njhealth.org

Dr Keith M. KERR*
Department of Pathology
Aberdeen Royal Infirmary
Aberdeen University Medical School
Foresterhill, Aberdeen
Scotland, AB25 2ZD
UNITED KINGDOM
Tel. +44 1224 550 948
Fax +44 1224 663 002
k.kerr@abdn.ac.uk

Dr Wolfram KLAPPER
Institute of Pathology
Kiel University
Michaelsstrasse 11
24105 Kiel
GERMANY
Tel. +49 431 1597 3399
Fax +49 431 1597 4129
wklapper@path.uni-kiel.de

Dr Michael N. KOSS
Department of Pathology
Keck School of Medicine
University of Southern California
2011 Zonal Ave, HMR 209
Los Angeles, CA 90333
USA
Tel. +1 323 442 8591
Fax +1 323 442 9993
mnkoss@earthlink.net

Dr Michael O. KURRER
Gemeinschaftspraxis für Pathologie
Cäcilientrasse 3
Postfach 1520
8032 Zurich
SWITZERLAND
Tel. +41 44 251 4890
Fax +41 44 251 4893
michael.kurrer@hin.ch

Dr Marc LADANYI*
Department of Pathology
Memorial Sloan Kettering Cancer Center
1275 York Ave
New York, NY 10065
USA
Tel. +1 212 639 6369
Fax +1 212 717 3515
ladanyim@mskcc.org

Dr Stephen LAM
BC Cancer Agency
Room 10-111, 675 West 10th Ave
Vancouver, BC V5Z 1L3
CANADA
Tel. +1 604 675 8090
Fax +1 604 675 8099
slam2@bccancer.bc.ca

Dr Laurence LAMANT
Department of Pathology
Institut Universitaire du Cancer
1, Avenue Irène Joliot-Curie
31059 Toulouse
FRANCE
Tel. +33 5 31 15 61 97
Fax +33 5 31 15 65 94
lamant.l@chu-toulouse.fr

Dr Sylvie LANTUEJOUL
Département d'Anatomie et Cytologie
Centre Hospitalier Universitaire de Grenoble
B.P. 217
38043 Grenoble
FRANCE
Tel. +33 4 76 76 73 77
Fax +33 4 76 76 59 29
SLantuejoul@chu-grenoble.fr

Dr Leendert H.J. LOOIJENGA*
Department of Pathology, Erasmus MC
Josephine Nefkens Institute
Laboratory of Experimental Patho-Oncology
3000 CA Rotterdam
THE NETHERLANDS
Tel. +31 10 704 4329
Fax +31 10 704 4365
l.looijenga@erasmusmc.nl

Dr Joseph J. MALESZEWSKI*
Department of Pathology
Mayo Clinic
200 1st Street SW
Rochester, MN 55905
USA
Tel. +1 507 266 4010
Fax +1 507 284 1875
maleszewski.joseph@mayo.edu

Dr Alberto M. MARCHEVSKY*
Department of Pathology
and Laboratory Medicine
Cedars-Sinai Medical Center
8700 Beverly Blvd
Los Angeles, CA 90048
USA
Tel. +1 310 423 6629
Fax +1 310 423 1071
alberto.marchevsky@cshs.org

Dr Mirella MARINO
Department of Pathology
Regina Elena National Cancer Institute
Via Elio Chianesi, 53
00144 Rome
ITALY
Tel. +39 065 2665 195
Fax +39 065 2665 523
mirellamarino@inwind.it
marino@ifo.it

Dr Edith M. MAROM
Professor of Radiology
Head of Thoracic Imaging
Department of Diagnostic Imaging
The Chaim Sheba Medical Center
Tel Hashomer 5265601
ISRAEL
Tel. +972 3 530 5203
Fax +972 3 535 7315
edith.marom@gmail.com

Dr Alexander MARX*
Department of Pathology
University Medical Centre Mannheim
Theodor-Kutzer-Ufer 1-3
68167 Mannheim
GERMANY
Tel. +49 621 383 2275
Fax +49 621 383 2005
alexander.marx@umm.de

Dr Yoshihiro MATSUNO
Department of Surgical Pathology
Hokkaido University Hospital
Sapporo
Hokkaido 060-8648
JAPAN
Tel. +81 11 706 5716
Fax +81 11 707 5116
ymatsuno@med.hokudai.ac.jp

Dr Matthew MEYERSON #
Department of Pathology
Dana-Farber Cancer Institute
44 Binney St, Mayer 446
Boston, MA 02115
USA
Tel. +1 617 632 4768
Fax +1 617 582 7880
matthew_meyerson@dfci.harvard.edu

Dr Hiroshi MINATO
Professor of Clinical Pathology
Medical College of Kanazawa
1-1 Daigaku, Uchinada-cho, Kahoku-gun,
Ishikawa-pref, 920-0293
JAPAN
Tel. +81 76 218 8017
Fax +81 76 218 8440
hminato@kanazawa-med.ac.jp

Dr Mari MINO-KENUDSON
Department of Pathology
Massachusetts General Hospital
55 Fruit St, Warren 122
Boston, MA 02214
USA
Tel. +1 617 726 8026
Fax +1 617 726 7474
mminokenudson@partners.org

Dr Thierry J. MOLINA #
Department of Pathology
Hôpital Necker, AP-HP
Université Paris Descartes
149 rue de Sèvres
75743 Paris Cedex 15
FRANCE
Tel. +33 1 44 49 49 94
Fax +33 1 44 49 49 99
thierry.molina@nck.aphp.fr

Dr Peter MÖLLER
Institute of Pathology
University of Ulm
Albert-Einstein-Allee 23
89070 Ulm
GERMANY
Tel. +49 731 500 56321
Fax +49 731 500 56384
elke.carter@uniklinik-ulm.de

Dr Andre L. MOREIRA*
Department of Pathology
Memorial Sloan Kettering Cancer Center
1275 York Ave
New York, NY 10065
USA
Tel. +212 639 2249
Fax +212 639 6318
moreiraa@mskcc.org

Dr Kiyoshi MUKAI
Department of Diagnostic Pathology
Saiseikai Central Hospital
Mita 1-4-17, Minato-ku
Tokyo
JAPAN
Tel. +81 3 3451 8211 ext 3665
Fax +81 3 3451 6102
kmukai@saichu.jp

Dr David NAIDICH
Department of Radiology
NYU Langone Medical Center
560 First Ave
New York, NY 10016
USA
Tel. +1 212 263 5229
Fax +1 212 263 0390
david.naidich@nyumc.org

Dr Shigeo NAKAMURA
Department of Pathology
and Laboratory Medicine
Nagoya University Hospital
65 Tsuyumai-cho, Showa-ku
Nagoya 466-8550
JAPAN
Tel. +81 52 744 2896
Fax +81 52 744 2897
snakamur@med.nagoya-u.ac.jp

Dr Yukio NAKATANI
Department of Diagnostic Pathology
Chiba University Graduate School of Medicine
Chiba University Hospital
1-8-1 Inohana, Chuo-ku
Chiba 260-8670
JAPAN
Tel. +81 43 222 7171
Fax +81 43 226 2013
nakatani@faculty.chiba-u.jp

Dr Andrew G. NICHOLSON*
Department of Histopathology
Royal Brompton and Harefield
NHS Foundation Trust
Sydney St.
London SW3 6NP
UNITED KINGDOM
Tel. +44 207 351 8423
Fax +44 207 351 8293
a.nicholson@rbht.nhs.uk

Dr Siobhan NICHOLSON
Department of Histopathology
St. James's Hospital
James's Street
Dublin 8
IRELAND
Tel. +353 1 416 2903
Fax +353 1 410 3514
snicholson@stjames.ie

Dr Masayuki NOGUCHI*
Department of Pathology
Institute of Basic Medical Sciences
University of Tsukuba
Tsukuba-shi
Ibaraki 305-8575
JAPAN
Tel. +81 29 853 3750
Fax +81 29 853 3150
nmasayuk@md.tsukuba.ac.jp

Dr Daisuke NONAKA
Department of Histopathology
The Christie Hospital
Institute of Cancer Sciences
Manchester University
550 Wilmslow Road
Manchester M20 4BX
UNITED KINGDOM
Tel. +44 161 446 3292
Fax +44 161 446 3300
dnonaka@msn.com

Dr Hiroko OHGAKI*
Section of Molecular Pathology
International Agency for Research on Cancer
150 cours Albert Thomas
69372 Lyon Cedex 08
FRANCE
Tel. +33 4 72 73 85 34
Fax +33 4 72 73 86 98
ohgaki@iarc.fr

Dr Wlodzimierz OLSZEWSKI #
Department of Pathology
Institute of Oncology
5, Roentgena Street
02-781 Warsaw
POLAND
Tel. +48 506 160 331
Fax +48 22 5426 29 84
wtolszewski@coi.waw.pl

Dr Attilio ORAZI
Department of Pathology and
Laboratory Medicine
Weill Cornell Medical College
525 East 68th Street
New York Presbyterian Hospital
New York, NY 10065
USA
Tel. +1 212 746 2050
Fax +1 212 746 2009
ato9002@med.cornell.edu

Dr Nelson G. ORDÓÑEZ
Department of Pathology
MD Anderson Cancer Center
1515 Holcombe Blvd
Houston, TX 77030
USA
Tel. +1 713 792 3167
Fax +1 713 792 3696
nordonez@mdanderson.org

Dr Mauro PAPOTTI #
Division of Pathology
University of Turin at San Luigi Hospital
Regione Gonzole 10
10043 Orbassano, Torino
ITALY
Tel. +39 011 670 5432
    +39 335 782 9605
Fax +39 011 670 5432
mauro.papotti@unito.it

Dr Giuseppe PELOSI*
Department of Pathology and
Laboratory Medicine
Fondazione IRCCS Istituto Nazionale dei
Tumori, Università degli Studi di Milano
Via G. Venezian, 1
20133 Milan
ITALY
Tel. +39 02 2390 2260 /2876 /3017
Fax +39 02 2390 2877
giuseppe.pelosi@unimi.it

Dr Iver PETERSEN
Institute of Pathology
Universitätsklinikum
Friedrich-Schiller-University Jena
Ziegelmühlenweg 1
07743 Jena
GERMANY
Tel. +49 3641 933 120
Fax +49 3641 933 111
iver.petersen@med.uni-jena.de

Dr Stefano A. PILERI
Department of Experimental, Diagnostic and
Speciality Medicine
Bologna University School of Medicine
Bologna 40138
ITALY
Tel. +39 051 636 3044
Fax +39 051 636 3606
stefano.pileri@unibo.it
stefano.pileri@aosp.bo.it

Dr Charles A. POWELL #
Division of Pulmonary Critical Care and
Sleep Medicine
Ichan School of Medicine at Mt Sinai
One Gustave Levy Place, Box 1232
New York, NY 10029
USA
Tel. +1 212 241 4280
Fax +1 212 876 5519
charles.powell@mssm.edu

Dr Ramon RAMI-PORTA
Thoracic Surgery Service
Hospital Univeritari Mutua Terrassa
Plaza Dr. Robert 5
08221 Terrassa, Barcelona
SPAIN
Tel. +34 93 736 50 50
Fax +34 93 736 50 59
rramip@yahoo.es

Dr Natasha REKHTMAN
Department of Pathology
Memorial Sloan Kettering Cancer Center
1275 York Ave
New York, NY 10065
USA
Tel. +1 212 639 5905
Fax +1 212 639 6318
rekhtman@mskcc.org

Dr David C. RICE
Department of Thoracic and
Cardiovascular Surgery
MD Anderson Cancer Center
1515 Holcombe Boulevard, Unit 1489
Houston, TX 77030
USA
Tel. +1 713 794 1477
Fax +1 713 794 4901
drice@mdanderson.org

Dr Ralf J. RIEKER
Institute for Pathology
University Hospital Erlangen
Krankenhausstrasse 8-10
91054 Erlangen
GERMANY
Tel. +49 9131 852 2868
Fax +49 9131 852 4745
ralf.rieker@uk-erlangen.de

Dr Gregory RIELY #
Thoracic Oncology Service
Memorial Sloan Kettering Cancer Center
300 E 66th St
New York, NY 10065
USA
Tel. +1 646 888 4199
Fax +1 212 794 4357
rielyg@mskcc.org

Dr Victor ROGGLI #
Department of Pathology
Duke University Medical Center
M255 Davidson Bld; 200 Trent Dr
Durham NC 27710
USA
Tel. +1 919 668 5440
Fax +1 919 681 1658
roggl002@mc.duke.edu

Dr Andreas ROSENWALD
Institute of Pathology
University of Würzburg
Josef-Schneider-Str. 2
97080 Würzburg
GERMANY
Tel. +49 931 318 1199
Fax +49 931 318 1224
rosenwald@mail.uni-wuerzburg.de

Dr Giulio ROSSI
Anatomia Patologica
Azienda Ospedaliera
Universitaria Policlinico di Modena
Via del Pozzo, 71
41123 Modena
ITALY
Tel. +39 338 3128 985
Fax +39 059 4224 820
giurossi68@gmail.com

Dr Brian ROUS*
Eastern Cancer Registry and
Information Centre
Unit C - Magog Court
Shelford Bottom, Hinton Way
Cambridge CB22 3AD
UNITED KINGDOM
Tel. +1 223 213 625
Fax +1 223 213 571
brian.rous@ecric.nhs.uk

Dr Prudence RUSSELL
Department of Pathology
St. Vincent's Hospital
41 Victoria Parade
Fitzroy VIC 3065
AUSTRALIA
Tel. +61 3 9288 2254
Fax +61 3 9288 4580
prue.russell@svhm.org.au

Dr Jonathan SAMET
USC Institute for Global Health
Department of Preventive Medicine
Keck School of Medicine
University of Southern California, Suite #330
2001 Soto Street (SSB)
Los Angeles, CA 90032
USA
Tel. +1 323 865 0803
Fax +1 323 865 0854
jsamet@usc.edu

Dr Giorgio SCAGLIOTTI
University of Torino
Department of Oncology
S. Luigi Hospital
Regione Gonzole, 10
10043 Orbassano, Torino
ITALY
Tel. +39 011 9026 414
Fax +39 011 9015 184
giorgio.scagliotti@unito.it

Dr Sven SEIWERTH #
Institute of Pathology Medical Faculty
School of Medicine University of Zagreb
Clinical Center Zagreb
Salata 10
10000 Zagreb
CROATIA
Tel. +385 1 456 6980 /977
Fax +385 1 492 1151
seiwerth@mef.hr

Dr Michael T. SHEAFF
Department of Cellular Pathology
Barts Health NHS Trust
80 Newark Street
London E1 2ES
UNITED KINGDOM
Tel. + 44 20 3246 0214
Fax + 44 20 3246 0202
michael.sheaff@bartshealth.nhs.uk

Dr Bahig M. SHEHATA #
Department of Pathology
Emory University School of Medicine
1405 Clifton Rd
Atlanta, GA 30322
USA
Tel. +1 404 785 1390
Fax +1 404 785 1370
bshehat@emory.edu

Dr Kazutoshi SHIBUYA #
Department of Surgical Pathology
Toho University School of Medicine
6-11-1 Omori-Nishi, Ota-Ku
Tokyo 143-8541
JAPAN
Tel. +81 3 3762 4151 Ext. 6811 3451
Fax +81 3 3767 1567
kaz@med.toho-u.ac.jp

Dr Lynette SHOLL #
Department of Pathology
Brigham and Women's Hospital
75 Francis Street
Boston, MA 02115
USA
Tel. +1 617 732 5985
Fax +1 617 264 5118
lmsholl@partners.org

Dr Thomas STRECKER
Center of Cardiac Surgery
Friedrich-Alexander-University
Erlangen-Nuremberg
Krankenhausstrasse 12
91054 Erlangen
GERMANY
Tel. +49 9131 85 33985
Fax +49 9131 85 36088
thomas.strecker@uk-erlangen.de

Dr Philipp STRÖBEL*
Institute of Pathology
University Medical Center Göttingen
Robert-Koch-Str. 40
37075 Göttingen
GERMANY
Tel. +49 551 39 6858
Fax +49 551 39 8627
philipp.stroebel@med.uni-goettingen.de

Dr Angela TAKANO
Department of Pathology
Singapore General Hospital
The Academia, 20 College Road #10-11
Singapore 169856
SINGAPORE
Tel. +65 6326 5386
Fax +65 6227 6562
angela.takano@sgh.com.sg

Dr Hisashi TATEYAMA
Department of Pathology
Kasugai Municipal Hospital
1-1-1 Takagi-cho, Kasugai
Aichi 486-8510
JAPAN
Tel. +81 568 57 0057
Fax +81 568 81 2128
htateyama@hospital.kasugai.aichi.jp

Dr Fabio TAVORA*
Department of Pathology, Argos Laboratory
Messejana Heart and Lung Hospital
Av Frei Cirilo, 3480
60846-190 Fortaleza, CE
BRAZIL
Tel. +55 85 970 82600
Fax +55 85 326 58392
ftavora@gmail.com

Dr Henry TAZELAAR
Department of Pathology
Mayo Clinic Arizona
13400 East Shea Blvd.
Scottsdale, AZ 85259
USA
Tel. +1 480 301 5530
Fax +1 480 301 8372
tazelaar.henry@mayo.edu

Dr Vincent THOMAS DE MONTPRÉVILLE
Department of Pathology
Centre Chirurgical Marie Lanelongue
133 Ave. de la Resistance
92350 Le Plessis Robinson
FRANCE
Tel. +33 1 40 94 87 05
Fax +33 1 40 94 87 07
v.thomasdemontprevil@ccml.com

Dr Erik THUNNISSEN #
Department of Pathology
VU University Hospital
De Boelelaan 1117
1081 HV Amsterdam
THE NETHERLANDS
Tel. +31 20 444 4048
Fax +31 20 444 4586
e.thunnissen@vumc.nl

Dr Ka-Fai TO
Department of Anatomical
and Cellular Pathology
The Chinese University of Hong Kong
Prince of Wales Hospital
Shatin
HONG KONG SAR, CHINA
Tel. +1 852 2632 3335
Fax +1 852 2637 6274
kfto@cuhk.edu.hk

Dr Joseph F. TOMASHEFSKI
Department of Pathology
MetroHealth Medical Center
2500 MetroHealth Dr
Cleveland, OH 44109
USA
Tel. +1 216 778 5181
Fax +1 216 778 7112
jtomashefski@metrohealth.org

Dr William D. TRAVIS*
Department of Pathology
Memorial Sloan Kettering Cancer Center
1275 York Avenue
New York, NY 10065
USA
Tel. +1 212 639 3325
Fax +1 212 717 3576
travisw@mskcc.org

Dr Ming-Sound TSAO*
Department of Laboratory Medicine and
Pathobiology, University of Toronto
University Health Network
Princess Margaret Cancer Centre
200 Elizabeth Street
Toronto, ON M5G 2C4
CANADA
Tel. +1 416 340 4737
Fax +1 416 340 5517
ming.tsao@uhn.ca

Dr Koji TSUTA
Pathology and Clinical Laboratory Division
National Cancer Center Hospital
5-1-1 Tsukiji, Chuo-ku
104-0045 Tokyo
JAPAN
Tel. +81 3 3542 2511
Fax +81 3 3545 3567
ktsuta@ncc.go.jp

Dr Thomas M. ULBRIGHT
Health Pathology Laboratory
Indiana University School of Medicine
350 West 11th Street, Room 4078
Indianapolis, IN 46202-4108
USA
Tel. +1 317 491 6498
Fax +1 317 491 6419
tulbrigh@iupui.edu

Dr Jan VAN MEERBEECK
MOCA/Thoraxoncologie
Antwerp University Hospital
Wilrijkstraat 10
2650 Edegem
BELGIUM
Tel. +32 3 821 3107
Fax +32 3 821 4121
Jan.Van.Meerbeeck@uza.be

Dr Paul VAN SCHIL*
Thoracic Surgery
Antwerp University Hospital
Wilrijkstraat 10
2650 Edegem
BELGIUM
Tel. +32 3 821 4360
Fax +32 3 821 4396
paul.van.schil@uza.be

Dr John P. VEINOT
Department of Pathology
and Laboratory Medicine
University of Ottawa
CCW Room 4121
501 Smyth Road
Ottawa, ON K1H 8L6
CANADA
Tel. +1 613 737 8294
Fax +1 613 738 8712
jpveinot@ottawahospital.on.ca

Dr Arne WARTH
Institute of Pathology
University Hospital Heidelberg
Im Neuenheimer Feld 224
D 69120 Heidelberg
GERMANY
Tel. +49 6221 56 39968
Fax +49 6221 56 5251
arne.warth@med.uni-heidelberg.de

Dr Mark WICK
Department of Pathology
University of Virginia Health System
University of Virginia Hospital
Room 3020, 1215 Lee Street
Charlottesville, VA 22908-0214
USA
Tel. +1 434 924 9038
Fax +1 434 924 9617
mrw9c@virginia.edu

Dr Ignacio I. WISTUBA*
Department of Translational Molecular
Pathology, The University of Texas - MD
Anderson Cancer Center
2130 W. Holcombe Blvd.
Life Science Plaza 9, 4029, Unit 2951
Houston, TX 77030
USA
Tel. +1 713 834 6029
Fax +1 713 834 6082
iiwistuba@mdanderson.org

Dr Ping YANG
Health Sciences Research
Mayo Clinic
200 First Street SW
Rochester, MN 55905
USA
Tel. +1 507 266 5369
Fax +1 507 266 2478
Yang.Ping@mayo.edu

Dr Woo Ick YANG
Department of Pathology
Yonsei University College of Medicine
250 Seongsanno, Seodaemun-gu
Seoul, 120-752
REPUBLIC OF KOREA
Tel. +82 2 2228 1765
Fax +82 2 362 0860
wiyang9660@yuhs.ac

Dr David YANKELEVITZ #
Early Lung and Cardiac Action Program
Icahn School of Medicine at Mount Sinai
One Gustave L. Levy Place, Box 1234
New York, NY 10029
USA
Tel. +1 212 241 2420
Fax +1 212 241 9655
DFYank@gmail.com

Dr Yasushi YATABE*
Department of Pathology
and Molecular Diagnostics
Aichi Cancer Center
1-1 Kanokoden, Chikusa-ku
Nagoya 464-8681
JAPAN
Tel. +81 52 764 9898
Fax +81 52 757 4810
yyatabe@aichi-cc.jp

Dr Eunhee S. YI
Department of Pathology
Mayo Clinic
200 First Street SW
Rochester, MN 55905
USA
Tel. +1 507 284 2656
Fax +1 507 284 1875
yi.joanne@mayo.edu

Dr Paul J. ZHANG
Department of Pathology and
Laboratory Medicine
Hospital of the University of Pennsylvania
3400 Spruce Street, 6 Founders
Philadelphia, PA 19104
USA
Tel. +1 215 662 6503
Fax +1 215 349 5910
pjz@mail.med.upenn.edu

Declaration of interest statements

Dr Attanoos reports receiving personal fees for medico-legal work undertaken in a variety of occupational liability cases for both claimants and defendants and for testifying as an expert witness in asbestos-related litigation. Dr Attanoos reports investment interests in APC Pathology Ltd.

Dr Bubendorf reports receiving personal speaker's fees and consultancy fees from Pfizer, Roche, Boehringer, and AstraZeneca. Dr Bubendorf reports owning shares in Roche. Dr Bubendorf reports receiving research funding from Abbott Molecular Inc.

Dr Carvalho reports receiving personal speaker's fees from Roche. Dr Carvalho reports giving unremunerated lectures for Pfizer.

Dr Chirieac reports he received personal consultancy fees from Infinity Pharmaceuticals. Dr Chirieac reports receiving personal consultancy fees for medico-legal work for law firms representing defendants in tobacco and mesothelioma litigation.

Dr Dalurzo reports she received personal speaker's fees and consultancy fees from Pfizer and AstraZeneca.

Dr den Bakker reports that the Department of Pathology at the Maasstad Ziekenhuis received research funding from SKMS (Stichting Kwaliteitsgelden Medisch Specialisten).

Dr Dziadziuszko reports receiving personal consultancy fees from Pfizer and Boehringer Ingelheim. Dr Dziadziuszko reports receiving personal speaker's fees from Pfizer, Boehringer Ingelheim, and AstraZeneca.

Dr Elmberger reports receiving personal consultancy fees from Pfizer and Qiagen.

Dr French reports receiving personal consultancy fees from GlaxoSmithKline and Ono Pharmaceutical.

Dr Gascoyne reports receiving personal consultancy fees from Celgene, Seattle Genetics, Genentech, and Roche. Dr Gascoyne reports receiving personal speaker's fees from Seattle Genetics.

Dr Gazdar reports receiving personal speaker's fees and consultancy fees from AstraZeneca, Genentech, and GlaxoSmithKline.

Dr Geisinger reports receiving personal consultancy fees for medico-legal work and for testifying as an expert witness for a law firm representing defendants in tobacco litigation.

Dr Gibbs reports receiving personal consultancy fees for medico-legal work for law firms representing plaintiffs and defendants, on a variety of occupational liability cases, including asbestos-related litigation.

Dr Guinee reports owning shares in Pfizer, Novartis, Merck, ARIAD Pharmaceuticals, and Generex Biotechnology.

Dr Hainaut reports being part of a consortium receiving unrestricted research funding from Sanofi-Aventis.

Dr Hammar reports owning Diagnostic Specialties Laboratory, Inc. P.S., a consultancy firm that undertakes medico-legal work for both plaintiffs and defendants, mostly in asbestos-related litigation.

Dr Henske reports having received personal consultancy fees from LAM Therapeutics, Genzyme, and BioMarin.

Dr Jett reports that his unit at National Jewish Health benefits from research funding from Oncimmune and Metabolomx. Dr Jett reports receiving personal consultancy fees from Quest Diagnostics and Varian Medical Systems. Dr Jett reports benefiting from support for travel and accommodation from Varian Medical Systems and Oncimmune.

Dr Meyerson reports receiving personal consultancy fees from Novartis and Foundation Medicine. Dr Meyerson reports receiving research funding from Novartis and Bayer. Dr Meyerson reports owning shares in Foundation Medicine. Dr Meyerson reports holding IP rights in a patent licensed by Dana-Farber Cancer Institute to LabCorp.

Dr Molina reports receiving personal consultancy fees from Merck.

Dr Olszewski reports receiving personal speaker's fees from Roche, Lilly, Abbott, and Boehringer Ingelheim.

Dr Papotti reports that his unit at the University of Turin benefits from research funding from Novartis. Dr Papotti reports receiving personal speaker's fees from Novartis.

Dr Powell reports having received personal consultancy fees from Pfizer.

Dr Riely reports having received personal consultancy fees from Boehringer Ingelheim, Chugai Pharmaceutical Co., ARIAD Pharmaceuticals, Daiichi Sankyo, Novartis, Abbott, Foundation Medicine, and Celgene. Dr Riely reports that his unit at the Memorial Sloan Kettering Cancer Center receives research funding from Bristol-Myers Squibb, Novartis, Pfizer, Chugai Pharmaceutical Co., GlaxoSmithKline, Infinity Pharmaceuticals, Merck, Millennium Pharmaceuticals, and Astellas.

Dr Roggli reports receiving personal fees for medico-legal work and for testifying as an expert witness for both plaintiffs and defendants in asbestos litigation for various law firms.

Dr Seiwerth reports that his research unit at the University of Zagreb benefited from non-financial research support from Lilly and Pfizer. Dr Seiwerth reports receiving speaker's fees and benefiting from support for travel from Lilly and Pfizer.

Dr Shehata reports holding IP rights in a patent owned by Emory University.

Dr Shibuya reports receiving research funding from Pfizer, Dainippon Sumitomo Pharma, and Astellas Pharma Inc. Dr Shibuya reports receiving personal speaker's fees from Pfizer, Dainippon Sumitomo Pharma, MSD KK, Astellas Pharma Inc., and Chugai Pharmaceutical Co., Ltd.

Dr Sholl reports receiving personal consultancy fees from Genentech. Dr Sholl reports that her research group benefits from non-financial research support from Ventana Medical Systems, Inc.

Dr Thunnissen reports that his unit at VU University Hospital receives research funding from Boehringer Ingelheim, Pfizer, Lilly, and Merck. Dr Thunnissen reports that his research unit at VU Medical Center receives research funding from Pfizer and AstraZeneca. Dr Thunnissen reports receiving personal speaker's fees and consultancy fees from Pfizer, Lilly, and Merck.

Dr Yankelevitz reports holding IP rights in multiple patents owned by the Cornell Research Foundation, some of which are non-exclusively licensed to General Electric, from which Dr Yankelevitz reports receiving revenue.

IARC/WHO Committee for the International Classification of Diseases for Oncology (ICD-O)

Dr Freddie BRAY
Section of Cancer Surveillance
International Agency for
Research on Cancer
150 cours Albert Thomas
69372 Lyon Cedex 08
FRANCE
Tel. +33 4 72 73 84 53
Fax +33 4 72 73 86 96
brayf@iarc.fr

Dr David FORMAN
Section of Cancer Surveillance
International Agency for
Research on Cancer
150 cours Albert Thomas
69372 Lyon Cedex 08
FRANCE
Tel. +33 4 72 73 80 09
Fax +33 4 72 73 86 96
formand@iarc.fr

Mrs April FRITZ
A. Fritz and Associates, LLC
21361 Crestview Road
Reno, NV 89521
USA
Tel. +1 775 636 7243
Fax +1 888 891 3012
april@afritz.org

Dr Robert JAKOB
Classifications, Terminology
and Standards Unit
World Health Organization
20 Avenue Appia
1211 Geneva 27
SWITZERLAND
Tel. +41 22 791 58 77
Fax +41 22 791 48 94
jakobr@who.int

Dr Paul KLEIHUES
Medical Faculty
University of Zurich
Pestalozzistrasse 5
8032 Zurich
SWITZERLAND
Tel. +41 44 362 21 10
Fax +41 44 251 06 65
kleihues@pathol.uzh.ch

Dr Alexander MARX
Department of Pathology
University Medical Center Mannheim
Theodor-Kutzer-Ufer 1-3
68167 Mannheim
GERMANY
Tel. +49 621 383 2275
Fax +49 621 383 2005
alexander.marx@umm.de

Dr Hiroko OHGAKI
Section of Molecular Pathology
International Agency for
Research on Cancer
150 cours Albert Thomas
69372 Lyon Cedex 08
FRANCE
Tel. +33 4 72 73 85 34
Fax +33 4 72 73 86 98
ohgaki@iarc.fr

Dr Brian ROUS
Eastern Cancer Registry and
Information Centre
Unit C - Magog Court
Shelford Bottom, Hinton Way
Cambridge CB22 3AD
UNITED KINGDOM
Tel. +1 223 213 625
Fax +1 223 213 571
brian.rous@ecric.nhs.uk

Dr Leslie H. SOBIN
Frederick National Laboratory for
Cancer Research
The Cancer Human Biobank
National Cancer Institute
6110 Executive Blvd, Suite 250
Rockville, MD 20852
USA
Tel. +1 301 443 7947
Fax +1 301 402 9325
leslie.sobin@nih.gov

Dr William D. TRAVIS
Department of Pathology
Memorial Sloan Kettering
Cancer Center
1275 York Avenue
New York, NY 10065
USA
Tel. +1 212 639 3325
Fax +1 212 717 3576
travisw@mskcc.org

Sources of figures and tables

Sources of figures

1.01	Reprinted from: Rusch VW, Asamura H, Watanabe H, et al; Members of IASLC Staging Committee. The IASLC lung cancer staging project: a proposal for a new international lymph node map in the forthcoming seventh edition of the TNM classification for lung cancer. J Thorac Oncol. 2009 May;4(5):568–77. With permission from Wolters Kluwer Health.
1.02A–C	Travis W.D.
1.03	Travis W.D.
1.04A–C	Travis W.D.
1.05A–D	Travis W.D.
1.06	Reprinted from: Travis WD, Brambilla E, Noguchi M, et al. (2011) International Association for the Study of Lung Cancer/American Thoracic Society/European Respiratory Society International multidisciplinary classification of lung adenocarcinoma. J Thorac Oncol. 6:244–85. With permission from Wolters Kluwer Health.
1.07	Wang L. Department of Pathology Memorial Sloan Kettering Cancer Center New York, NY, USA
1.08A,B	Yatabe Y.
1.08C	Mino-Kenudson M.
1.08D	Lukas Bubendorf
1.09	Yatabe Y., Ladanyi M.
1.10	Yatabe Y.
1.11	Devesa S.
1.12	Devesa S.
1.13	Garg K. Department of Radiology University of Colorado Aurora, CO, USA
1.14	See above (1.13).
1.15	Yatabe Y.
1.16A–C	Rekhtman N.
1.17A,B	Travis W.D.
1.18A	Yatabe Y.
1.18B	Travis W.D.
1.19A,B	Travis W.D.
1.20A,B	Travis W.D.
1.21A–D	Travis W.D.
1.22A,B	Travis W.D.
1.23	Reprinted with permission from: Macmillan Publishers Ltd:

	Nature, Cancer Genome Atlas Research Network (2014) Comprehensive molecular profiling of lung adenocarcinoma. Nature. 511(7511):543–50. Copyright 2014.
1.24	Naidich D.
1.25	Travis W.D.
1.26A	Rekhtman N.
1.26B–D	Travis W.D.
1.27	Yatabe Y.
1.28	Yatabe Y.
1.29	Rekhtman N.
1.30A,B	Rossi G.
1.31A	Travis W.D.
1.31B	Yoshida A. Department of Pathology National Cancer Center Tokyo, Japan
1.32	Nakatani Y.
1.33	Travis W.D.
1.34	Travis W.D.
1.35	See above (1.13).
1.36	Yatabe Y.
1.37	Travis W.D.
1.38A,B	Travis W.D.
1.39	Reprinted from: Travis WD, Brambilla E, Noguchi M, et al. (2011). International Association for the Study of Lung Cancer/American Thoracic Society/European Respiratory Society International multidisciplinary classification of lung adenocarcinoma. J Thorac Oncol. 6:244–85. With permission from Wolters Kluwer Health.
1.40	Naidich D.
1.41	Noguchi M.
1.42A,B	Travis W.D.
1.43	Yatabe Y.
1.44	Naidich D.
1.45A	Noguchi M.
1.45B	Rekhtman N.
1.46A,B	Noguchi M.
1.46C,D	Reprinted from: Travis WD, Brambilla E, Noguchi M, et al. (2011). International Association for the Study of Lung Cancer/American Thoracic Society/European Respiratory Society International multidisciplinary classification of lung adenocarcinoma. J Thorac Oncol. 6:244–85. With permission from Wolters Kluwer Health.

1.47A,C	Fernandez E.A. Departamento de Anatomía Patológica, Hospital General Gregorio Marañón, Madrid, Spain
1.47B	Vogt P. Department of Pathology University Hospital Zurich, Switzerland
1.47D	Kerr K.M.
1.48A,B	Kerr K.M.
1.49A,B	Reprinted from: Travis WD, Rekhtman N. (2011) Pathological diagnosis and classification of lung cancer in small biopsies and cytology: strategic management of tissue for molecular testing. Semin Respir Crit Care Med. 32:22–31. With permission from Thieme Publishing Group.
1.50A-C	Reprinted from: Travis WD, Colby TV, Corrin B, et al. (1999). Histological Typing of Lung and Pleural Tumours. WHO International Histological Classification of Tumours 3rd ed. Springer-Verlag: Berlin. With kind permission of Springer Science+Business Media.
1.51A,B	Reprinted from: Drilon A, Rekhtman N, Ladanyi M, Paik P. (2012). Squamous-cell carcinomas of the lung: emerging biology, controversies, and the promise of targeted therapy. Lancet Oncol. 13(10):e418–26. © 2012 With permission from Elsevier.
1.52	Reprinted from: Cancer Genome Atlas Research Network. Comprehensive genomic characterization of squamous cell lung cancers. Nature. 489:519–25. With permission from Macmillan Publishers Ltd. © 2012.
1.53	See above (1.52)
1.54	Brambilla E.
1.55A	Travis W.D.
1.55B	Brambilla E.
1.56A	Brambilla E.
1.56B	Travis W.D.
1.57	Travis W.D.
1.58	Brambilla E.
1.59	Lam S.
1.60	Mueller K.M. Gerhard-Domagkinstitut für Pathologie,

Universitätskliniken Münster (UKM), Münster, Germany
1.61   Franklin W.A.
1.62   Modified with permission from: Kadara, H. and Wistuba, I. I. (2014). Molecular Biology of Lung Preneoplasia. In: Roth J.A., Hong W.K., Komaki R.U., et al., eds. Lung Cancer, 4th ed. John Wiley & Sons, Inc., Hoboken, NJ, USA. Copyright © 2014 by John Wiley & Sons, Inc. All rights reserved. With permission from John Wiley & Sons, Inc.
1.63A–C   Austin J.H.M.
1.64A   Travis W.D.
1.64B   Capelozzi V.L.
1.65A,B   Nicholson S.
1.66A,B   Travis W.D.
1.67A–D   Travis W.D.
1.68A   Pelosi G.
1.68B   Travis W.D.
1.69A,B   Pelosi G.
1.70   Travis W.D.
1.71   Reprinted from: Peifer M, Fernández-Cuesta L, Sos ML, et al. (2012) Integrative genome analyses identify key somatic driver mutations of small-cell lung cancer. Nat Genet. 44:1104–10. With permission from Macmillan Publishers Ltd. © 2012.
1.72   Pelosi G.
1.73   Nicholson S.
1.74A–C   Pelosi G.
1.75A–C   Brambilla E.
1.76   Reprinted from: Travis WD, Colby TV, Corrin B et al. (1999). Histological Typing of Lung and Pleural Tumours. WHO International Histological Classification of Tumours 3rd ed. Springer-Verlag: Berlin. With kind permission of Springer Science + Business Media.
1.77   Travis W.D.
1.78A,B   Hasleton P.S.
1.78C   Vogt P. Department of Pathology University Hospital Zurich, Switzerland
1.78D   Travis W.D.
1.79A,B   Nicholson S.
1.80A–D   See above (1.76)
1.81A–C   See above (1.76)
1.82A,B   Pelosi G.
1.83A–C   Pelosi G.
1.84A,B   See above (1.76)
1.85   Reprinted from: Fernandez-Cuesta L, Peifer M, Lu X, et al. (2014). Frequent mutations in chromatin-remodelling genes in pulmonary carcinoids. Nat Commun 5:3518. Reprinted with permission from Macmillan Publishers Ltd. © 2014.

1.86A,B   Webb R. Department of Radiology and Biomedical Imaging, University of California, San Francisco, CA, USA
1.87   Gosney J.R.
1.88A,B   Gosney J.R.
1.89   Gosney J.R.
1.90   Rekhtman N.
1.91A   See above (1.76)
1.91B   Brambilla E.
1.92A–I   Sholl L.
1.93   Reprinted from: Clinical Lung Cancer Genome Project (CLCGP); Network Genomic Medicine (NGM). (2013) A genomics-based classification of human lung tumors. *Sci Transl Med* 5(209):209ra153. With permission from AAAS.
1.94   See above (1.93)
1.95   Yatabe Y.
1.96A-C   Yatabe Y.
1.97   Kerr K.M.
1.98A   Rossi G.
1.98B   Jambhekar N.A.
1.98C,D   Kerr K.M.
1.99A,B   Kerr K.M.
1.100A   Koss M.N.
1.100B   Travis W.D.
1.101A–C   Travis W.D.
1.102A,B   Nakatani Y.
1.103A,B   Koss M.N.
1.103C,D   See above (1.76)
1.104A–C   Chirieac L.R.
1.105   Chirieac L.R.
1.106   Chirieac L.R.
1.107   Sholl L.
1.108   French C.A.
1.109A   Sholl L.
1.109B   French C.A.
1.110A,B   Ishikawa Y.
1.111A,B   Travis W.D.
1.112A   Ishikawa Y.
1.112B   Dacic S.
1.113A,C   Travis W.D.
1.113B   Ishikawa Y.
1.114A   Vogt P. Department of Pathology University Hospital Zurich, Switzerland
1.114B   Travis W.D.
1.115A,B   Thivolet-Béjui F. Centre de Pathologie Est Groupement hospitalier est Bron, France
1.116   Ishikawa Y.
1.117   Ishikawa Y.
1.118   Travis W.D.
1.119A–C   Travis W.D.
1.120   Travis W.D.
1.121A–C   Flieder D.B.
1.122A,B   Flieder D.B.
1.123A,B   Reprinted from: Flieder DB, Koss MN, Nicholson A, et al. (1998). Solitary pulmonary papillomas in adults: a clinicopathologic and in situ

hybridization study of 14 cases combined with 27 cases in the literature. Am J Surg Pathol. 22:1328–42. With permission from Wolters Kluwer Health.
  Reprinted from: Travis WD, Colby TV, Corrin B, et al. (1999). Histological Typing of Lung and Pleural Tumours. WHO International Histological Classification of Tumours 3rd ed. Springer-Verlag: Berlin. With kind permission of Springer Science + Business Media.
1.124   Travis W.D.
1.125   Flieder D.B.
1.126A   Devouassoux-Shisheboran M.N. Department d'Anatomie et Cytologie Pathologiques Hopital de la Croix Rousse Lyon, France
1.126B   See above (1.76)
1.127   See above (1.76)
1.128A   Beasley M.B.
1.128B,C   See above (1.126A)
1.129A–D   Travis W.D.
1.130   See above (1.76)
1.131   See above (1.76)
1.132A-D   See above (1.76)
1.133A–D   Tomashefski J.F.
1.134A   Tomashefski J.F.
1.134B   Nicholson A.G.
1.135A–C   Aubry M.C.
1.136   Nicholson A.G.
1.137   Nicholson A.G.
1.138   Nicholson A.G.
1.139   Nicholson A.G.
1.140A,B   Dehner L.P. Department of Pathology & Immunology Washington University School of Medicine St. Louis, MO, USA
1.141A,B   See above (1.76)
1.141C,D   Travis W.D.
1.142A   See above (1.76)
1.142B   Yi E.S.
1.143A,B   Fletcher C.D.M.
1.144   Travis W.D.
1.145A,B   Cagle P.
1.146A,B   Antonescu C. Department of Pathology Memorial Sloan Kettering Cancer Center New York, NY, USA
1.147A   Nicholson A.G.
1.147B,C   Reprinted from: Travis WD, Colby TV, Corrin B et al. (1999). Histological Typing of Lung and Pleural Tumours. WHO International Histological Classification of Tumours 3rd ed. Springer-Verlag: Berlin. With kind permission of Springer Science + Business Media.
1.148   Nicholson A.G.
1.149A,B   Nicholson A.G.
1.150A,B   Nicholson A.G.

1.151A,B   Travis W.D.
1.152   Burke A.P.
1.153A,B   Burke A.P.
1.154A   Nicholson A.G.
1.154B,C   Reprinted from:
Thway K, Nicholson AG, Lawson K, et al. (2011). Primary pulmonary myxoid sarcoma with EWSR1-CREB1 fusion: a new tumor entity. Am J Surg Pathol. 35:1722–32. With permission from Wolters Kluwer Health.
1.155   Nicholson A.G.
1.156   Reprinted from:
Sarkaria IS, DeLair D, Travis WD, et al. (2011). Primary myoepithelial carcinoma of the lung: a rare entity treated with parenchymal sparing resection. Reprinted from: J Cardiothorac Surg. 6:27. This article is licensed under a Creative Commons License (http://creativecommons.org/licenses/by/2.0).
1.157   Travis W.D.
1.158A,B   Travis W.D.
1.159A–C   Dacic S.
1.160A,B   Reprinted from:
Chen G, Folpe AL, Colby TV, et al. (2011). Angiomatoid fibrous histiocytoma: unusual sites and unusual morphology. Mod Pathol. 24:1560–70. With permission from Macmillan Publishers Ltd. © 2011.
1.161   Nicholson A.G.
1.162   Nicholson A.G.
1.163   Nicholson A.G.
1.164A,C   Nicholson A.G.
1.164B   Travis W.D.
1.165A–C   Nicholson A.G.
1.166   Reprinted from:
Guinee D Jr, Jaffe E, Kingma D, et al. (1994). Pulmonary lymphomatoid granulomatosis. Evidence for a proliferation of Epstein-Barr virus infected B-lymphocytes with a prominent T-cell component and vasculitis. Am J Surg Pathol. 18(8):753–64. With permission from Wolters Kluwer Health.
1.167   Jaffe E.S.
1.168   Jaffe E.S.
1.169   Jaffe E.S.
1.170A,B   Jaffe E.S.
1.171A,B   Nicholson A.G.
1.172   Nicholson A.G.
1.173A,B   Nicholson A.G.
1.174A,B   Nicholson A.G.
1.175A   Duhig E.
1.175B   Nicholson A.G.
1.176A,B   Nicholson A.G.
1.177A,B   Reprinted with permission from:
Colby TV, Koss M, Travis WD (1995). Tumors of the Lower Respiratory Tract. 3rd ed. Volume 13. Armed Forces Institute of Pathology: Washington, DC.
And from:
Travis WD, Colby TV, Corrin B, et al. (1999). Histological Typing of Lung and Pleural Tumours. WHO International Histological Classification of Tumours 3rd ed. Springer-Verlag: Berlin. With kind permission of Springer Science + Business Media.
1.178A,B   See above (1.76)
1.179A,B   See above (1.177)
1.180A   Duhig E.
1.180B   Geisinger K.
1.181   Nicholson A.G.
1.182   Hiroshima K.
1.183   Hiroshima K.
1.184   Hiroshima K.
1.185A,B   Fukuoka J.
1.186   Hiroshima K.
1.187A,B   Hiroshima K.
1.187C,D   Pelosi G.
1.188A   Hiroshima K.
1.188B   Pelosi G.

2.01   SEER 9 areas.
Rates are age-adjusted to the 2000 US Std Population (19 age groups - Census P25-1103). Regression lines are calculated using the Joinpoint Regression Program Version 3.5, April 2011, National Cancer Institute.
2.02   Kleihues P.
2.03A,B   Naidich D.
2.04   Galateau-Salle F.
2.05A   Reprinted from:
Galateau-Salle F (Ed.) (2006). Pathology of Malignant Mesothelioma. Springer: London. With kind permission of Springer Science + Business Media.
2.05B   Vogt P.
Department of Pathology University Hospital Zurich, Switzerland
2.06   Reprinted from:
Churg A, Galateau-Salle F. (2012). The separation of benign and malignant mesothelial proliferations. Arch Pathol Lab Med. 136(10):1217–26. © College of American Pathologists.
2.07   Galateau-Salle F.
2.08   See above (1.76)
2.09A   Travis W.D.
2.09B   See above (1.76)
2.09C   Galateau-Salle F.
2.10A   Galateau-Salle F.
2.10B   Travis W.D.
2.11A   See above (2.05A)
2.11B–D   Galateau-Salle F.
2.12A,C,D   Travis W.D.
2.12B   Galateau-Salle F.
2.13   Dacic S.
2.14A,B   Galateau-Salle F.
2.14C   See above (2.05A)
2.14D   Travis W.D.

2.15A,B   Galateau-Salle F.
2.16A   Galateau-Salle F.
2.16B   Travis W.D.
2.17A,B   Travis W.D.
2.18   Travis W.D.
2.19A,B   Galateau-Salle F.
2.20A   Galateau-Salle F.
2.20B   Borczuk A.
2.21   Inai K.
2.22A   Jaffe E.S.
2.22B   Bacon C.
2.23A,B   Bacon C.
2.24   Aozasa K.
Department of Pathology Osaka University Graduate School of Medicine Osaka, Japan
2.25A,B   Jaffe E.S.
2.26   Fletcher C.D.M.
2.27   Fletcher C.D.M.
2.28   Fletcher C.D.M.
2.29A,B   Fletcher C.D.M.
2.30A   Fletcher C.D.M.
2.30B   Travis W.D.
2.31A,B   Fletcher C.D.M.
2.32   Fletcher C.D.M.
2.33A,B   Dacic S.

3.01A,B   Modified with permission from:
Williamson SR, Ulbright TM (2014) Germ Cell Tumors of the Mediastinum. In: Pathology of the Mediastinum. Marchevsky A.M. Wick M.R. (Eds). © Cambridge University Press 2014
3.02   Detterbeck F.
3.03A   Marom E.M.
3.03B   Nicholson A.G.
3.03C   Moreira A.L.
3.04A   Marx A.
3.04B   Reprinted from:
Marx A, Ströbel P, Badve SS, et al. (2014). ITMIG consensus statement on the use of the WHO histological classification of thymoma and thymic carcinoma: refined definitions, histological criteria, and reporting. J Thorac Oncol. 9:596–611 Copyright with permission from Wolters Kluwer Health.
3.05A–D   See above (3.04B)
3.06A   Marx A.
3.06B   Mukai K.
3.07A–D   Marx A.
3.08   Marom E.M.
3.09   Ströbel P.
3.10   Thomas de Montpréville V.
3.11A,B   Ströbel P.
3.12A,B   Ströbel P.
3.13A,B   Marx A.
3.14A,B   See above (3.04B)
3.15   Marom E.M.
3.16   Marom E.M.
3.17A   Capelozzi V.L.
3.17B   den Bakker M.A.
3.18A   Chan J.K.C.
3.18B   Marx A.

3.19A–C	See above (3.04B)
3.20A	See above (3.04B)
3.20B	Chan J.K.C.
3.21	Marchevsky A.M.
3.22	Moreira A.L.
3.23A	Marchevsky A.M.
3.23B	Marx A.
3.24A	Marx A.
3.24B	Mukai K.
3.25A	Marx A.
3.25B	Mukai K.
3.26A,C	Marchevsky A.M.
3.26B,D–F	Marx A.
3.27A,B	Marom E.M.
3.28	Moreira A.L.
3.29	Thomas de Montpréville V.
3.30A,B,D	Mukai K.
3.30C	Marx A.
3.31A	Chan J.K.C.
3.31B,C	Marx A.
3.32A,B	Marx A.
3.33	Marom E.M.
3.34	Travis W.D.
3.35A,B	Tateyama H.
3.36A,B	Tateyama H.
3.36C	Mukai K.
3.37	Thomas de Montpréville V.
3.38A,B	Chan J.K.C.
3.39A–D	Chan J.K.C.
3.40A–C	Chan J.K.C.
3.41	Ströbel P.
3.42	Marx A.
3.43A	Chen G.
3.43B,C	Marx A.
3.44	Chen G.
3.45A,B	Chen G.
3.46	Marom E.M.
3.47	Marom E.M.
3.48	Thomas de Montpréville V.
3.49A–D	Chan J.K.C.
3.50	Chan J.K.C.
3.51A–D	Chan J.K.C.
3.52	Chan J.K.C.
3.53A–D	Chan J.K.C.
3.54A,B	Zettl A.
	FMH Pathologie Viollier AG
	Allschwil, Switzerland
3.55A,B	Chan J.K.C.
3.56	Chan J.K.C.
3.57A	Papotti M.
3.57B	Chan J.K.C.
3.58A,B	Chan J.K.C.
3.59A–D	Chan J.K.C.
3.60	Chan J.K.C.
3.61	Marom E.M.
3.62	Marom E.M.
3.63	Kuo T.T.
	Department of Pathology
	Chang Gung Memorial Hospital
	Taipei, Taiwan, China
3.64A	Marx A.
3.64B–D	Chan J.K.C.
3.65A,B	Chan J.K.C.
3.66	Chan J.K.C.
3.67A,B	Chan J.K.C.
3.68A–D	Chan J.K.C.
3.69A–C	Chan J.K.C.
3.70	Marom E.M.

3.71	Kurrer M.O.
3.72A–C	Chan J.K.C.
3.73A,B	Chan J.K.C.
3.74A,B	Chan J.K.C.
3.75A,B	French C.A.
3.76	French C.A.
3.77	Adapted by permission from Macmillan Publishers Ltd: Oncogene. French CA, Ramirez CL, et al. (2008). BRD-NUT oncoproteins: a family of closely related nuclear proteins that block epithelial differentiation and maintain the growth of carcinoma cells. ;27(15):2237-42. © 2008. Reproduced from: J Clin Pathol. French CA. (2008). Demystified molecular pathology of NUT midline carcinomas;63(6):492-6. © 2008, with permission from BMJ Publishing Group Ltd. Adapted from: French CA. (2012). Pathogenesis of NUT midline carcinoma. AnnuRev Pathol. 7:247–65.
3.78A–D	French C.A.
3.79	Adapted from: French CA. (2012). Pathogenesis of NUT midline carcinoma. AnnuRev Pathol. 7:247–65. And courtesy of Drs Y. Tanaka, M. Tanaka, T. Horisawa and Y. Saikawa, Division of Pathology, Kanazawa Children's Medical Center, Yokohama, Japan
3.80	Adapted from: French CA. (2012). Pathogenesis of NUT midline carcinoma. AnnuRev Pathol. 7:247–65.
3.81	See above (3.80), and courtesy of Dr S Gollin, Department of Human Genetics, University of Pittsburgh, Pittsburgh, PA, USA.
3.82	Thomas de Montpréville V.
3.83A,B	Marx A.
3.84	Marx A.
3.85A,B	Marx A.
3.86A,B	Marom E.M.
3.87A,B	Chan J.K.C.
3.88	Ströbel P.
3.89A,B	Ströbel P.
3.90A–D	Ströbel P.
3.91A–D	Ströbel P.
3.92A,B	Marx A.
3.93A–C	Marx A.
3.94A	Zettl A.
	FMH Pathologie Viollier AG
	Allschwil, Switzerland
3.94B	Reprinted from: Ströbel P, Zettl A, Shilo K, et al. (2014). Tumor genetics and survival of thymic neuroendocrine neoplasms: A multi-institutional clinicopathologic study. Genes Chromosomes Cancer. 2014 53(9):738–49. © 2014 With permission from John Wiley & Sons, Inc.

3.95A,C	Chan J.K.C.
3.95B,D	Wick M.
3.96	Marx A.
3.97A,B	Chan J.K.C.
3.98	Chan J.K.C.
3.99A–C	Reprinted from: Williamson SR, Ulbright TM (2014). Germ Cell Tumors of the Mediastinum. In: Pathology of the Mediastinum. Marchevsky AM Wick MR (Eds). Cambridge University Press: Cambridge. © Cambridge University Press 2014, reproduced with permission.
3.100	Moreira A.L.
3.101	Moreira A.L.
3.102A	Moreira A.L.
3.102B	Ströbel P.
3.103A	Zaloudek C.J.
	Department of Pathology
	UCSF School of Medicine
	San Francisco, CA, USA
3.103B	Moreira A.L.
3.104	Moreira A.L.
3.105A,B	Chan J.K.C.
3.106A–D	Chan J.K.C.
3.107A–C	Chan J.K.C.
3.108	Marom E.M.
3.109	Moreira A.L.
3.110	Perlman E.J.
	Department of Pathology and Laboratory Medicine
	Children's Hospital of Chicago
	Chicago, IL, USA
3.111A,B	Ulbright T.M.
3.111C	Chan J.K.C.
3.112A	Chan J.K.C.
3.112B	Marx A.
3.113A–C	Marx A.
3.114A	Chan J.K.C.
3.114B	Ulbright T.M.
3.115	Ströbel P.
3.116	Moreira A.L.
3.117	Moreira A.L.
3.118A–C	Moreira A.L.
3.118D	Reuter V.
	Department of Pathology,
	Memorial Sloan Kettering Cancer,
	New York, NY, USA
3.119	Thomas de Montpréville V.
3.120A–C	Chan J.K.C.
3.121A,B	Chan J.K.C.
3.122	Travis W.D.
3.123A,B	Ströbel P.
3.124A,B	Orazi A.
3.125A,B	Orazi A.
3.126	Möller P.
3.127A	Möller P.
3.127B	Ströbel P.
3.128A–D	Möller P.
3.129	Jaffe E.S.
3.130A–D	Möller P.
3.131	Inagaki H.
3.132	Inagaki H.
3.133A,B	Inagaki H.
3.134	Nakamura S.
3.135A,B	Ströbel P.
3.136	Marx A., Ströbel P.

3.137A,B	Ströbel P.			4.34A,B	Burke A.P.
3.138	Jaffe E.S.			4.35A	Burke A.P.
3.139A,B	Jaffe E.S.			4.35B	Tavora F.
3.140A–C	Lamant L.			4.36	Frazier A.A.

3.137A,B   Ströbel P.
3.138   Jaffe E.S.
3.139A,B   Jaffe E.S.
3.140A–C   Lamant L.
3.141A,B   Nakamura S.
3.142   Nakamura S.
3.143A   Nakamura S.
3.143B   Jaffe E.S.
3.144   Nakamura S.
3.145   Jaffe E.S.
3.146A–D   Jaffe E.S.
3.147A   Chan J.K.C.
3.147B   Marx A.
3.148   Chan J.K.C.
3.149A,B   Chan J.K.C.
3.150A–D   Chan J.K.C.
3.151A,B   Chan J.K.C.
3.152A–C   Chan J.K.C.
3.153A,B   Chan J.K.C.
3.154   Orazi A.
3.155A   Reprinted with permission from: Shimosato Y, Mukai K (1997). Tumors of the Mediastinum. AFIP Atlas of tumour pathology. 3rd Edition. Washington: American Registry of Pathology.
3.155B   Marx A.
3.156A,B   Rieker R.J.
3.157A,B   Rieker R.J.
3.158A,B   Coindre J.M.
3.159   Chen W.J.
Department of Pathology
Chang Gung Memorial Hospital
Kaohsiung, Taiwan, China
3.160A   Coindre J.M.
3.160B   Chan J.K.C.
3.161A-C   Chiarle R.
Department of Pathology
Boston Children's Hospital
Boston, MA, USA
3.162A,B   Chan J.K.C.
3.163A–D   Chan J.K.C.
3.164   Ueda Y.
Department of Thoracic Surgery and Pathology Tauzuke Kofukai Medical Research Institute Kitano Hospital
Osaka, Japan
3.165A   See above (3.164)
3.165B   Leuschner I.
Institute of Pathology
University Medical Center
Schleswig-Holstein
Kiel, Germany
3.166A,B   Marx A.
3.167   Chan J.K.C.
3.168A,B   Chan J.K.C.
3.169A–C   Travis W.D.
3.170A,B   Ströbel P.

4.01A,B   Reprinted from:
Padalino MA, Vida VL, Bhattarai A, et al. (2011). Giant intramural left ventricular rhabdomyoma in a newborn. Circulation. 124:2275–7. With permission from Wolters Kluwer Health.
4.01C   Geva T.

Department of Cardiology
Children's Hospital
Harvard Medical School
Boston, MA, USA
4.02   See above (4.01A,B)
4.03A   Basso C.
4.03B   See above (4.01A,B)
4.04A   Basso C.
4.04B,C   See above (4.01A,B)
4.05A,B   Shehata B.M.
4.06   Shehata B.M.
4.07A,B   Shehata B.M.
4.08   Reprinted from:
Rizzo S, Basso C, Buja G, et al. (2014). Multifocal Purkinje-like hamartoma and junctional ectopic tachycardia with a rapidly fatal outcome in a newborn. Heart Rhythm. 11:1264–6. Copyright (2014) with permission from Elsevier.
4.09   Shehata B.M.
4.10   Shehata B.M.
4.11A–C   Maleszewski J.J.
4.12   Burke A.P.
4.13   Burke A.P.
4.14A   Reprinted from:
Thiene G, Valente M, Basso C (2013). Cardiac Tumors: From Autoptic Observations to Surgical Pathology in the Era of Advanced Cardiac Imaging. In: Cardiac Tumor Pathology. Basso C, Valente M, Thiene G (Eds). New York: Springer, pp 1–22, with kind permission from Springer Science + Business Media.
4.14B,C   Maleszewski J.J.
4.15A–C   Maleszewski J.J.
4.16A–C   Maleszewski J.J.
4.17A,B   Maleszewski J.J.
4.18   Maleszewski J.J.
4.19A,B   Maleszewski J.J.
4.19C   Tazelaar H.
4.20A–D   Maleszewski J.J.
4.21   Burke A.P.
4.22   Thomas de Montpréville V.
4.23A–C   Thomas de Montpréville V.
4.24   Burke A.P.
4.25   Burke A.P.
4.26A,B   Burke A.P.
4.27   Burke A.P.
4.28A   Maleszewski J.J.
4.28B   Burke A.P.
4.29   Reprinted from:
Basso C, Bottio T, Thiene G, Valente M, Gerosa G (2013). Other Benign Cardiac Tumors. In: Cardiac Tumor Pathology. Basso C, Valente M, Thiene G (Eds). New York: Springer, pp 45–58, with kind permission from Springer Science + Business Media.
4.30   Burke A.P.
4.31   Maleszewski J.
4.32   Burke A.P.
4.33   Burke A.P.

4.34A,B   Burke A.P.
4.35A   Burke A.P.
4.35B   Tavora F.
4.36   Frazier A.A.
4.37A   Burke A.P.
4.37B   Maleszewski J.J.
4.38A,B   Burke A.P.
4.39A,B   Burke A.P.
4.40A,B   Burke A.P.
4.41   Burke A.P.
4.42A,B   Burke A.P.
4.43A,B   Burke A.P.
4.44A,B   Burke A.P.
4.45A,B   Burke A.P.
4.46A,B   Burke A.P.
4.47   Burke A.P.
4.48   Burke A.P.
4.49A,B   Tazelaar H.
4.50A,B   Burke A.P.
4.51A,B   Reprinted from:
Lestuzzi C, Miolo G, De Paoli A (2013) Systemic Therapy, Radiotherapy, and Cardiotoxicity. In: Cardiac Tumor Pathology. Basso C, Valente M, Thiene G (Eds). New York: Springer, pp 165-182, with kind permission from Springer Science + Business Media.
4.52   Maleszewski J.J.
4.53   Maleszewski J.J.
4.54   Maleszewski J.J.
4.55   Tazelaar H.
4.56A   Tazelaar H.
4.56B   Burke A.P.P.
4.57   Tavora F.
4.58   Burke A.P.
4.59   Tavora F.
4.60A,B   Frazier A.A.
4.61A,B   Burke A.P.
4.62A,B   Maleszewski J.J.
4.63   Maleszewski J.J.
4.64   Maleszewski J.J.

Sources of figures for front cover

Top left   Maleszewski J.J.
Top center   Marom E.M.
Top right   Vogt P.
Department of Pathology
University Hospital
Zurich, Switzerland
Middle left   Chan J.K.C.
Middle center   Travis W.D.
Middle right   Galateau-Salle F.
Bottom left   Dacic S.
Bottom center   Reprinted from:
Clinical Lung Cancer Genome Project (CLCGP); Network Genomic Medicine (NGM). (2013) A genomics-based classification of human lung tumors. Sci Transl Med 5(209):209ra153. With permission from AAAS.
Bottom right   Zettl A.
FMH Pathologie Viollier AG
Allschwil, Switzerland

Sources of tables

1.01   Reprinted with permission from: Rusch VW, Asamura H, Watanabe H, et al. (2009). The IASLC lung cancer staging project: a proposal for a new international lymph node map in the forthcoming seventh edition of the TNM classification for lung cancer. J Thorac Oncol. 4: 568–577.

1.02   Reprinted with permission from: Sobin LH, Gospodarowicz MK, Wittekind C, eds (2009). TNM Classification of Malignant Tumours. 7th ed. Hoboken (NJ): Wiley-Blackwell.

1.03   Reprinted from: Travis WD, Brambilla E, Noguchi M, et al. (2013). Diagnosis of lung cancer in small biopsies and cytology: implications of the 2011 International Association for the Study of Lung Cancer/ American Thoracic Society/ European Respiratory Society classification. Arch Pathol Lab Med. 137:668â84. © College of American Pathologists.
And from: Travis WD, Brambilla E, Noguchi M, et al. (2011). International Association for the Study of Lung Cancer/American Thoracic Society/European Respiratory Society international multidisciplinary classification of lung adenocarcinoma. J Thorac Oncol. 6:244–85. With permission from Wolters Kluwer Health.

1.04   See above (1.03)

1.05   See above (1.03)

1.06   Nicholson A.G.

1.07   Meyerson M, Yatabe Y and Takahashi T, Department of Molecular Carcinogenesis, Nagoya University Graduate School of Medicine, Nagoya, Japan

1.08   http://monographs.iarc.fr/

1.09   Modified from: Colby TV, Koss MN, Travis WD (1995). Tumors of the Lower Respiratory Tract. AFIP Atlas of Tumor Pathology. 3rd ed. Volume 13. Washington, DC: American Registry of Pathology.

1.10   Yatabe Y.

1.11   Yatabe Y.

1.12   Reprinted from: Travis WD, Brambilla E, Noguchi M, et al. (2011). International Association for the Study of Lung Cancer/American Thoracic Society/European Respiratory Society International multidisciplinary classification of lung adenocarcinoma. J Thorac Oncol. 6:244–85. With permission from Wolters Kluwer Health.

1.13   Reprinted from: Travis WD, Brambilla E, Noguchi M, et al. (2013). Diagnosis of lung adenocarcinoma in resected specimens: implications of the 2011 International Association for the Study of Lung Cancer/ American Thoracic Society/ European Respiratory Society classification. Arch Pathol Lab Med. 137:685–705. © 2010 College of American Pathologists.

1.14   See above (1.13)

1.15   Reprinted from: Travis WD, Brambilla E, Muller-Hermelink HK, et al., eds. (2004). WHO Classification of Tumours. Pathology and Genetics of Tumours of the Lung, Pleura, Thymus and Heart. 3rd ed. Lyon: IARC.

1.16   Brambilla E, Beasley MB, Austin JHM. Capelozzi VL, Chirieac LR, Devesa SS, Frank GA, Gazdar A, Ishikawa Y, Jen J, Jett J, Marchevsky AM, Nicholson S, Pelosi G, Powell CA, Rami-Porta R, Scagliotti G, Thunnissen E, Travis WD, van Schil P, Yang P

1.17   Reprinted from: Travis WD, Colby TV, Corrin B, et al. (1999). Histological Typing of Lung and Pleural Tumours. WHO International Histological Classification of Tumours 3rd ed. Springer-Verlag: Berlin. With kind permission of Springer Science + Business Media.

1.18   Reprinted from: Brambilla E, Travis WD, Brennan P, Harris C (2014). Lung Cancer. In: World Cancer Report. Stewart B.W, Wild C.P. (Eds). IARC: Lyon; pp. 350–362.

1.19   Nicholson A.G.

1.20   Nicholson A.G.

1.21   Reprinted from: Louis DN, Ohgaki H, Wiestler OD, Cavenee WK (Eds.): World Health Organization Classification of Tumours of the Nervous System (4th edition). IARC: Lyon 2007

1.22   Fukuoka J.

2.01   Galateau-Salle F., Marchevsky A.M., Borczuk A

2.02   Modified with permission from: Churg A, Colby TV, Cagle P, et al. (2000). The separation of benign and malignant mesothelial proliferations. Am J Surg Pathol. 24:1183–200.

2.03   Reprinted from: Jean D, Daubriac J, Le Pimpec-Barthes F, et al. (2012). Molecular changes in mesothelioma with an impact on prognosis and treatment. Arch Pathol Lab Med. 136:277–93. © College of American Pathologists.

2.04   Galateau-Salle F., Borczuk A., Marchevsky A.M.

2.05   Galateau-Salle F., Marchevsky A.M., Borczuk A.

3.01   Marx A.

3.02   Marx A.

3.03   Marx A.

3.04   Marx A.

3.05   Marx A.

3.06   Chan J.K.C.

3.07   Ströbel P.

3.08   Moreira A.L.

3.09   Moreira A.L.

3.10   Moreira A.L.

3.11   Nakamura S.

3.12   Nakamura S.

4.01   Thomas de Monpréville V.

4.02   Reprinted from: Stratakis CA, Kirschner LS, Carney JA. (2001) Clinical and molecular features of the Carney complex: diagnostic criteria and recommendations for patient evaluation. J Clin Endocrinol Metab. 86:4041–6. Permission conveyed through Copyright Clearance Center, Inc.

4.03   Maleszewski J.J.

References

1. Ab' Saber AM, Massoni Neto LM, Bianchi CP et al. (2004). Neuroendocrine and biologic features of primary tumors and tissue in pulmonary large cell carcinomas. Ann Thorac Surg. 77:1883–90.

2. Abad C, De la Rosa P (2008). Right atrial papillary fibroelastoma associated with atrial septal defect, persistent superior vena cava, and coronary artery disease. J Thorac Cardiovasc Surg. 136:538.

3. Abad C, de Varona S, Limeres MA, et al. (2008). Resection of a left atrial hemangioma. Report of a case and overview of the literature on resected cardiac hemangiomas. Tex Heart Inst J. 35:69–72.

4. Abbondanzo SL, Rush W, Bijwaard KE, et al. (2000). Nodular lymphoid hyperplasia of the lung: a clinicopathologic study of 14 cases. Am J Surg Pathol. 24:587–97.

5. Abdel-Rahman U, Ozaslan F, Esmaeili A, et al. (2005). A giant rhabdomyoma with left ventricular inflow occlusion and univentricular physiology. Thorac Cardiovasc Surg. 53:259–60.

6. Abdul-Ghafar J, Yong SJ, Kwon W, et al. (2012). Primary thymic mucinous adenocarcinoma: a case report. Korean J Pathol. 46:377–81.

7. Abe A, Sugiyama Y, Furuta R, et al. (2013). Usefulness of intraoperative imprint cytology in ovarian germ cell tumors. Acta Cytol. 57:171–6.

8. Abiko K, Mandai M, Hamanishi J, et al. (2010). Oct4 expression in immature teratoma of the ovary: relevance to histologic grade and degree of differentiation. Am J Surg Pathol. 34:1842–8.

9. Abiko T, Koizumi S, Takanami I, et al. (2011). 18F-FDG-PET/CT findings in primary pulmonary mixed squamous cell and glandular papilloma. Ann Nucl Med. 25:227–9.

10. Ablin AR, Krailo MD, Ramsay NK, et al. (1991). Results of treatment of malignant germ cell tumors in 93 children: a report from the Childrens Cancer Study Group. J Clin Oncol. 9:1782–92.

11. Aboualfa K, Calandriello L, Dusmet M, et al. (2011). Benign metastasizing leiomyoma presenting as cystic lung disease: a diagnostic pitfall. Histopathology. 59:796–9.

12. Abraham KP, Reddy V, Gattuso P (1990). Neoplasms metastatic to the heart: review of 3314 consecutive autopsies. Am J Cardiovasc Pathol. 3:195–8.

13. Acebo E, Val-Bernal JF, Gomez-Roman JJ (2001). Thrombomodulin, calretinin and c-kit (CD117) expression in cardiac myxoma. Histol Histopathol. 16:1031–6.

14. Achcar Rde O, Nikiforova MN, Dacic S, et al. (2009). Mammalian mastermind like 2 11q21 gene rearrangement in bronchopulmonary mucoepidermoid carcinoma. Hum Pathol. 40:854–60.

15. Acikel S, Aksoy MM, Kilic H, et al. (2012). Cystic and hemorrhagic giant left atrial myxoma in a patient presenting with exertional angina and dyspnea. Cardiovasc Pathol. 21:e15–8.

16. Adachi Y, Okamura M, Yasumizu R, et al. (1995). [An autopsy case of immature teratoma with choriocarcinoma in the mediastinum]. Kyobu Geka. 48:829–32.

17. Adam P, Hakroush S, Hofmann I, et al. (2014). Thymoma with loss of keratin expression (and giant cells): a potential diagnostic pitfall. Virchows Arch. 465:313–20.

18. Adam T, Giry M, Boquet P, et al. (1996). Rho-dependent membrane folding causes Shigella entry into epithelial cells. EMBO J. 15:3315–21.

19. Addis BJ, Isaacson PG (1986). Large cell lymphoma of the mediastinum: a B-cell tumour of probable thymic origin. Histopathology. 10:379–90.

20. Adenle AD, Edwards JE (1982). Clinical and pathologic features of metastatic neoplasms of the pericardium. Chest. 81:166–9.

21. Afifi HY, Bosl GJ, Burt ME (1997). Mediastinal growing teratoma syndrome. Ann Thorac Surg. 64:359–62.

22. Agackiran Y, Ozcan A, Akyurek N, et al. (2012). Desmoglein-3 and Napsin A double stain, a useful immunohistochemical marker for differentiation of lung squamous cell carcinoma and adenocarcinoma from other subtypes. Appl Immunohistochem Mol Morphol. 20:350–5.

23. Agaimy A, Rosch J, Weyand M, et al. (2012). Primary and metastatic cardiac sarcomas: a 12-year experience at a German heart center. Int J Clin Exp Pathol. 5:928–38.

24. Agaimy A, Strecker T (2011). Left atrial myxoma with papillary fibroelastoma-like features. Int J Clin Exp Pathol. 4:307–11.

25. Agrons GA, Rosado-de-Christenson ML, Kirejczyk WM, et al. (1998). Pulmonary inflammatory pseudotumor: radiologic features. Radiology. 206:511–8.

26. Aguayo SM, Miller YE, Waldron JA Jr, et al. (1992). Brief report: idiopathic diffuse hyperplasia of pulmonary neuroendocrine cells and airways disease. N Engl J Med. 327:1285–8.

27. Ahmad I, Singh LB, Foth M, et al. (2011). K-Ras and beta-catenin mutations cooperate with Fgfr3 mutations in mice to promote tumorigenesis in the skin and lung, but not in the bladder. Dis Model Mech. 4:548–55.

28. Ahmad U, Yao X, Detterbeck F, et al. (2014). Outcomes of Thymic Carcinoma: A Joint Analysis of the International Thymic Malignancy Interest Group and European Society of Thoracic Surgeons Databases. J Thorac Cardiovasc Surg. 149:95–101.

29. Ahmed MA, Fouda R, Ammar H, et al. (2012). Massive pericardial effusion and multiple pericardial masses due to an anterior mediastinal teratoma rupturing in pericardial sac. BMJ Case Rep 2012:

30. Ahmed T, Bosl GJ, Hajdu SI (1985). Teratoma with malignant transformation in germ cell tumors in men. Cancer. 56:860–3.

31. Ahn C, Harvey JC (1990). Mediastinal hibernoma, a rare tumor. Ann Thorac Surg. 50:828–30.

32. Ahn S, Lee JJ, Ha SY, et al. (2012). Clinicopathological analysis of 21 thymic neuroendocrine tumors. Korean J Pathol. 46:221–5.

33. Aida S, Ohara I, Shimazaki H, et al. (2008). Solitary peripheral ciliated glandular papillomas of the lung: a report of 3 cases. Am J Surg Pathol. 32:1489–94.

34. Aigelsreiter A, Gerlza T, Deutsch AJ, et al. (2011). Chlamydia psittaci Infection in non-gastrointestinal extranodal MALT lymphomas and their precursor lesions. Am J Clin Pathol. 135:70–5.

35. Aizawa K, Endo S, Yamamoto S, et al. (2004). [Chest wall epithelioid sarcoma]. Kyobu Geka. 57:957–60.

36. Akata S, Okada S, Maeda J, et al. (2007). Computed tomographic findings of large cell neuroendocrine carcinoma of the lung. Clin Imaging. 31:379–84.

37. Akhtar M, al Dayel F (1997). Is it feasible to diagnose germ-cell tumors by fine-needle aspiration biopsy? Diagn Cytopathol. 16:72–7.

38. Akira M, Atagi S, Kawahara M, et al. (1999). High-resolution CT findings of diffuse bronchioloalveolar carcinoma in 38 patients. AJR Am J Roentgenol. 173:1623–9.

39. Akyuz C, Koseoglu V, Gogus S, et al. (1997). Germ cell tumours in a brother and sister. Acta Paediatr. 86:668–9.

40. Alahwal MS, Maniyar IH, Saleem F, et al. (2012). Pulmonary blastoma: a rare primary lung malignancy. Case Rep Med. 2012:471613.

41. Albany C, Einhorn LH (2013). Extragonadal germ cell tumors: clinical presentation and management. Curr Opin Oncol. 25:261–5.

42. Alberg AJ, Brock MV, Ford JG, et al. (2013). Epidemiology of lung cancer: Diagnosis and management of lung cancer, 3rd ed: American College of Chest Physicians evidence-based clinical practice guidelines. Chest 143: e1S–29S.

43. Jennings TA, Axiotis CA, Kress Y, Carter D (1990). Primary malignant melanoma of the lower respiratory tract. Report of a case and literature review. Am J Clin Pathol. 94:649–55.

44. Alexanian S, Said J, Lones M, et al. (2013). KSHV/HHV8-negative effusion-based lymphoma, a distinct entity associated with fluid overload states. Am J Surg Pathol. 37:241–9.

45. Alexiev BA, Drachenberg CB, Burke AP (2007). Thymomas: a cytological and immunohistochemical study, with emphasis on lymphoid and neuroendocrine markers. Diagn Pathol. 2:13.

46. Alghamdi AA, Sheth T, Manowski Z, et al. (2009). Utility of cardiac CT and MRI for the diagnosis and preoperative assessment of cardiac paraganglioma. J Card Surg. 24:700–1.

47. Ali SZ, Smilari TF, Teichberg S, et al. (1995). Pleomorphic rhabdomyosarcoma of the heart metastatic to bone. Report of a case with fine needle aspiration biopsy findings. Acta Cytol. 39:555–8.

48. Ali SZ, Susin M, Kahn E, et al. (1994). Intracardiac teratoma in a child simulating an atrioventricular nodal tumor. Pediatr Pathol. 14:913–7.

49. Aliotta PJ, Castillo J, Englander LS, et al. (1988). Primary mediastinal germ cell tumors. Histologic patterns of treatment failures at autopsy. Cancer. 62:982–4.

50. Aliperta A, De Rosa N, Aliperta M, et al. (1996). [Double cardiac fibroma in a newborn infant]. Minerva Cardioangiol. 44:623–9.

51. Allan BJ, Thorson CM, Davis JS, et al. (2013). An analysis of 73 cases of pediatric malignant tumors of the thymus. J Surg Res. 184:397–403.

52. Allen TC, Cagle PT, Churg AM, et al. (2005). Localized malignant mesothelioma. Am J Surg Pathol. 29:866–73.

53. Alobeid B, Beneck D, Sreekantaiah C, et al. (1997). Congenital pulmonary myofibroblastic tumor: a case report with cytogenetic analysis and review of the literature. Am J Surg Pathol. 21:610–4.

54. Altavilla G, Blandamura S, Gardiman M, et al. (1995). [Solitary fibrous tumor of the pericardium]. Pathologica. 87:82–6.

55. Altunbasak S, Demirtas M, Tunali N, et al. (1996). Primary rhabdomyosarcoma of the heart presenting with increased intracranial pressure. Pediatr Cardiol. 17:260–4.

56. Amano J, Nakayama J, Yoshimura Y, et al. (2013). Clinical classification of cardiovascular tumors and tumor-like lesions, and its incidences. Gen Thorac Cardiovasc Surg. 61:435–47.

57. Amin RM, Hiroshima K, Miyagi Y, et al. (2008). Role of the PI3K/Akt, mTOR, and STK11/LKB1 pathways in the tumorigenesis of sclerosing hemangioma of the lung. Pathol Int. 58:38–44.

58. Ammari ZA, Mollberg NM, Abdelhady K, et al. (2013). Diagnosis and management of primary effusion lymphoma in the immunocompetent and immunocompromised hosts. Thorac Cardiovasc Surg. 61:343–9.

59. Anderson CD, Hashimi S, Brown T, et al. (2011). Primary benign interatrial schwannoma encountered during aortic valve replacement. J Card Surg. 26:63–5.

60. Anderson M, Sladon S, Michels R, et al. (1996). Examination of p53 alterations and cytokeratin expression in sputa collected from patients prior to histological diagnosis of squamous cell carcinoma. J Cell Biochem Suppl. 25:185–90.

61. Anderson MB, Kriett JM, Kapelanski DP, et al. (1995). Primary pulmonary artery sarcoma: a report of six cases. Ann Thorac Surg. 59:1487–90.

61A. Anderson T, Zhang L, Hameed M, et al. (2015). Thoracic Epithelioid Malignant Vascular Tumors: A Clinicopathologic Study of 52 Cases With Emphasis on Pathologic Grading and Molecular Studies of WWTR1-CAMTA1 Fusions. Am J Surg Pathol. 39:132–9.

62. Andino L, Cagle PT, Murer B, et al. (2006). Pleuropulmonary desmoid tumors: immunohistochemical comparison with solitary fibrous tumors and assessment of beta-catenin and cyclin D1 expression. Arch Pathol Lab Med. 130:1503–9.

63. Andre F, Fizazi K, Culine S, et al. (2000). The growing teratoma syndrome: results of therapy and long-term follow-up of 33 patients. Eur J Cancer. 36:1389–94.

64. Andreu AL, Checcarelli N, Iwata S, et al. (2000). A missense mutation in the mitochondrial cytochrome b gene in a revisited case with histiocytoid cardiomyopathy. Pediatr Res. 48:311–4.

65. Andriko JW, Kaldjian EP, Tsokos M, et al. (1998). Reticulum cell neoplasms of lymph nodes: a clinicopathologic study of 11 cases with recognition of a new subtype derived from fibroblastic reticular cells. Am J Surg Pathol. 22:1048–58.

66. Annema JT, van Meerbeeck JP, Rintoul RC, et al. (2010). Mediastinoscopy vs endosonography for mediastinal nodal staging of lung cancer: a randomized trial. JAMA. 304:2245–52.

67. Annessi V, Paci M, De Franco S, et al. (2003). Diagnosis of anterior mediastinal masses with ultrasonically guided core needle biopsy. Chir Ital. 55:379–84.

68. Antonescu CR, Kawai A, Leung DH, et al. (2000). Strong association of SYT-SSX fusion type and morphologic epithelial differentiation in synovial sarcoma. Diagn Mol Pathol. 9:1–8.

69. Antonescu CR, Le Loarer F, Mosquera JM, et al. (2013). Novel YAP1-TFE3 fusion defines a distinct subset of epithelioid hemangioendothelioma. Genes Chromosomes Cancer. 52:775–84.

70. Antonescu CR, Zhang L, Chang NE, et al.

(2010). EWSR1-POU5F1 fusion in soft tissue myoepithelial tumors. A molecular analysis of sixty-six cases, including soft tissue, bone, and visceral lesions, showing common involvement of the EWSR1 gene. Genes Chromosomes Cancer. 49:1114–24.

71. Aoyama A, Isowa N, Chihara K, et al. (2005). Pericardial metastasis of myxoid liposarcoma causing cardiac tamponade. Jpn J Thorac Cardiovasc Surg. 53:193–5.

72. Aozasa K (2006). Pyothorax-associated lymphoma. J Clin Exp Hematop. 46:5–10.

73. Aozasa K, Takakuwa T, Nakatsuka S (2005). Pyothorax-associated lymphoma: a lymphoma developing in chronic inflammation. Adv Anat Pathol. 12:324–31.

74. Arai T, Kurashima C, Wada S, et al. (1998). Histological evidence for cell proliferation activity in cystic tumor (endodermal heterotopia) of the atrioventricular node. Pathol Int. 48:917–23.

75. Araoz PA, Eklund HE, Welch TJ, et al. (1999). CT and MR imaging of primary cardiac malignancies. Radiographics. 19:1421–34.

76. Aravot DJ, Banner NR, Cantor AM, et al. (1992). Location, localization and surgical treatment of cardiac pheochromocytoma. Am J Cardiol. 69:283–5.

77. Archie PH, Beasley MB, Ross HJ (2008). Biphasic pulmonary blastoma with germ cell differentiation in a 36-year-old man. J Thorac Oncol. 3:1185–7.

78. Arcila ME, Chaft JE, Nafa K, et al. (2012). Prevalence, clinicopathologic associations, and molecular spectrum of ERBB2 (HER2) tyrosine kinase mutations in lung adenocarcinomas. Clin Cancer Res. 18:4910–8.

79. Arcila ME, Nafa K, Chaft JE, et al. (2013). EGFR exon 20 insertion mutations in lung adenocarcinomas: prevalence, molecular heterogeneity, and clinicopathologic characteristics. Mol Cancer Ther. 12:220–9.

79A. Argani P, Aulmann S, Illei PB, et al. (2010). A distinctive subset of PEComas harbors TFE3 gene fusions. Am J Surg Pathol. 34:1395–406.

80. Argani P, de Chiocca I, Rosai J (1998). Thymoma arising with a thymolipoma. Histopathology. 32:573–4.

81. Argani P, Erlandson RA, Rosai J (1997). Thymic neuroblastoma in adults: report of three cases with special emphasis on its association with the syndrome of inappropriate secretion of antidiuretic hormone. Am J Clin Pathol. 108:537–43.

82. Arif F, Wu S, Andaz S, et al. (2012). Primary epithelial myoepithelial carcinoma of lung, reporting of a rare entity, its molecular histogenesis and review of the literature. Case Rep Pathol. 2012:319434.

83. Ariizumi Y, Koizumi H, Hoshikawa M, et al. (2012). A primary pulmonary glomus tumor: a case report and review of the literature. Case Rep Pathol. 2012:782304.

84. Ariza-Heredia EJ, Razonable RR (2011). Human herpes virus 8 in solid organ transplantation. Transplantation. 92:837–44.

85. Arkenau HT, Gordon C, Cunningham D, et al. (2007). Mucosa associated lymphoid tissue lymphoma of the lung: the Royal Marsden Hospital experience. Leuk Lymphoma. 48:547–50.

86. Arnaud L, Hervier B, Neel A, et al. (2011). CNS involvement and treatment with interferon-alpha are independent prognostic factors in Erdheim-Chester disease: a multicenter survival analysis of 53 patients. Blood. 117:2778–82.

87. Arnaud L, Pierre I, Beigelman-Aubry C, et al. (2010). Pulmonary involvement in Erdheim-Chester disease: a single-center study of thirty-four patients and a review of the literature. Arthritis Rheum. 62:3504–12.

88. Asada Y, Marutsuka K, Mitsukawa T, et al. (1996). Ganglioneuroblastoma of the thymus: an adult case with the syndrome of inappropriate secretion of antidiuretic hormone. Hum Pathol. 27:506–9.

89. Asakura S, Tezuka N, Inoue S, et al. (2001). Angiomatoid fibrous histiocytoma in mediastinum. Ann Thorac Surg. 72:283–5.

90. Asamura H, Goya T, Koshiishi Y, et al. (2008). A Japanese Lung Cancer Registry study: prognosis of 13,010 resected lung cancers. J Thorac Oncol. 3:46–52.

91. Asano S, Hoshikawa Y, Yamane Y, et al. (2000). An intrapulmonary teratoma associated with bronchiectasia containing various kinds of primordium: a case report and review of the literature. Virchows Arch. 436:384–8.

92. Ascoli V, Scalzo CC, Danese C, et al. (1999). Human herpes virus-8 associated primary effusion lymphoma of the pleural cavity in HIV-negative elderly men. Eur Respir J. 14:1231–4.

93. Ashby MA, Williams CJ, Buchanan RB, et al. (1986). Mediastinal germ cell tumour associated with malignant histiocytosis and high rubella titres. Hematol Oncol. 4:183–94.

94. Ashraf T, Day TG, Marek J, et al. (2013). A triad: cardiac rhabdomyosarcoma, stroke and tamponade. Pediatr Cardiol. 34:771–3.

95. Asirvatham JR, Esposito MJ, Bhuiya TA (2014). Role of PAX-8, CD5, and CD117 in distinguishing thymic carcinoma from poorly differentiated lung carcinoma. Appl Immunohistochem Mol Morphol. 22:372–6.

96. Athanasiou A, Vanel D, El Mesbahi O, et al. (2009). Non-germ cell tumours arising in germ cell tumours (teratoma with malignant transformation) in men: CT and MR findings. Eur J Radiol. 69:230–5.

97. Attanasio A, Romitelli S, Mauriello A, et al. (1998). Cardiac rhabdomyosarcoma: a clinicopathologic and electron microscopy study. G Ital Cardiol. 28:383–6.

98. Attanoos RL, Dojcinov SD, Webb R, et al. (2000). Anti-mesothelial markers in sarcomatoid mesothelioma and other spindle cell neoplasms. Histopathology. 37:224–31.

99. Attanoos RL, Suvarna SK, Rhead E, et al. (2000). Malignant vascular tumours of the pleura in "asbestos" workers and endothelial differentiation in malignant mesothelioma. Thorax. 55:860–3.

100. Attina D, Niro F, Tchouante P, et al. (2013). Pulmonary artery intimal sarcoma. Problems in the differential diagnosis. Radiol Med (Torino). 118:1259–68.

101. Aubry MC, Bridge JA, Wickert R, et al. (2001). Primary monophasic synovial sarcoma of the pleura: five cases confirmed by the presence of SYT-SSX fusion transcript. Am J Surg Pathol. 25:776–81.

102. Aubry MC, Heinrich MC, Molina J, et al. (2007). Primary adenoid cystic carcinoma of the lung: absence of KIT mutations. Cancer. 110:2507–10.

103. Aubry MC, Myers JL, Colby TV, et al. (2002). Endometrial stromal sarcoma metastatic to the lung: a detailed analysis of 16 patients. Am J Surg Pathol. 26:440–9.

104. Auger M, Katz RL, Johnston DA (1997). Differentiating cytological features of bronchioloalveolar carcinoma from adenocarcinoma of the lung in fine-needle aspirations: a statistical analysis of 27 cases. Diagn Cytopathol. 16:253–7.

105. Austin JH, Garg K, Aberle D, et al. (2013). Radiologic implications of the 2011 classification of adenocarcinoma of the lung. Radiology. 266:62–71.

106. Austin JH, Yip R, D'Souza BM, et al. (2012). Small-cell carcinoma of the lung detected by CT screening: stage distribution and curability. Lung Cancer. 76:339–43.

107. Aviel-Ronen S, Coe BP, Lau SK, et al. (2008). Genomic markers for malignant progression in pulmonary adenocarcinoma with bronchioloalveolar features. Proc Natl Acad Sci USA. 105:10155–60.

108. Awad M, Dunn B, al Halees Z, et al. (1992). Intracardiac rhabdomyosarcoma: transesophageal echocardiographic findings and diagnosis. J Am Soc Echocardiogr. 5:199–202.

109. Ayabe E, Kaira K, Takahashi T, et al. (2009). Thymic squamous cell carcinoma producing granulocyte colony-stimulating factor associated with a high serum level of interleukin 6. Int J Clin Oncol. 14:534–6.

110. Ayadi-Kaddour A, Bacha D, Smati B, et al. (2009). [Primary thymic carcinomas. Three cases and a review of the literature]. Rev Pneumol Clin. 65:113–7.

111. Azizkhan RG, Caty MG (1996). Teratomas in childhood. Curr Opin Pediatr. 8:287–92.

112. Baba M, Iyoda A, Nomoto Y, et al. (2007). Cytological findings of pre-invasive bronchial lesions detected by light-induced fluorescence endoscopy in a lung cancer screening system. Oncol Rep. 17:579–83.

113. Babakoohi S, Fu P, Yang M, et al. (2013). Combined SCLC clinical and pathologic characteristics. Clin Lung Cancer. 14:113–9.

114. Bacha EA, Wright CD, Grillo HC, et al. (1999). Surgical treatment of primary pulmonary sarcomas. Eur J Cardiothorac Surg. 15:456–60.

115. Badalian-Very G, Vergilio JA, Degar BA, et al. (2010). Recurrent BRAF mutations in Langerhans cell histiocytosis. Blood. 116:1919–23.

116. Bader RS, Chitayat D, Kelly E, et al. (2003). Fetal rhabdomyoma: prenatal diagnosis, clinical outcome, and incidence of associated tuberous sclerosis complex. J Pediatr. 143:620–4.

117. Bae YA, Lee KS, Han J, et al. (2008). Marginal zone B-cell lymphoma of bronchus-associated lymphoid tissue: imaging findings in 21 patients. Chest. 133:433–40.

118. Baez-Giangreco A, Afzal M, Hamdy MG, et al. (1997). Pleuropulmonary blastoma of the lung presenting as posterior mediastinal mass: a case report. Pediatr Hematol Oncol. 14:475–81.

119. Bagan P, Hassan M, Le Pimpec-Barthes F, et al. (2006). Prognostic factors and surgical indications of pulmonary epithelioid hemangioendothelioma: a review of the literature. Ann Thorac Surg. 82:2010–3.

120. Baghai-Wadji M, Sianati M, Nikpour H, et al. (2006). Pleomorphic adenoma of the trachea in an 8-year-old boy: a case report. J Pediatr Surg. 41:e23–6.

121. Bagheri R, Mashhadi M, Haghi SZ, et al. (2011). Tracheobronchopulmonary carcinoid tumors: analysis of 40 patients. Ann Thorac Cardiovasc Surg. 17:7–12.

122. Bagwan IN, Desai S, Wotherspoon A, et al. (2009). Unusual presentation of primary cardiac lymphoma. Interact Cardiovasc Thorac Surg. 9:127–9.

123. Bagwan IN, Sheppard MN (2009). Cardiac lipoma causing sudden cardiac death. Eur J Cardiothorac Surg. 35:727.

124. Bahadori M, Liebow AA (1973). Plasma cell granulomas of the lung. Cancer. 31:191–208.

125. Bahrami A, Allen TC, Cagle PT (2008). Pulmonary epithelioid hemangioendothelioma mimicking mesothelioma. Pathol Int. 58:730–4.

126. Bai S, Wei S, Pasha TL, et al. (2013). Immunohistochemical studies of metastatic germ-cell tumors in retroperitoneal dissection specimens: a sensitive and specific panel. Int J Surg Pathol. 21:342–51.

127. Bakaeen FG, Reardon MJ, Coselli JS, et al. (2003). Surgical outcome in 85 patients with primary cardiac tumors. Am J Surg. 186:641–7.

129. Baleydier F, Decouvelaere AV, Bergeron J, et al. (2008). T cell receptor genotyping and HOXA/TLX1 expression define three T lymphoblastic lymphoma subsets which might affect clinical outcome. Clin Cancer Res. 14:692–700.

130. Ball A, Bromley A, Glaze S, et al. (2012). A rare case of NUT midline carcinoma. Gynecol Oncol Case Rep. 3:1–3.

131. Ballestas ME, Kaye KM (2011). The latency-associated nuclear antigen, a multifunctional protein central to Kaposi's sarcoma-associated herpesvirus latency. Future Microbiol. 6:1399–413.

132. Ballouhey Q, Galinier P, Abbo O, et al. (2012). The surgical management and outcome of congenital mediastinal malformations. Interact Cardiovasc Thorac Surg. 14:754–9.

133. Baranzelli MC, Kramar A, Bouffet E, et al. (1999). Prognostic factors in children with localized malignant nonseminomatous germ cell tumors. J Clin Oncol. 17:1212.

134. Barbareschi M, Cantaloni C, Del Vescovo V, et al. (2011). Heterogeneity of large cell carcinoma of the lung: an immunophenotypic and miRNA-based analysis. Am J Clin Pathol. 136:773–82.

135. Barbareschi M, Murer B, Colby TV, et al. (2003). CDX-2 homeobox gene expression is a reliable marker of colorectal adenocarcinoma metastases to the lungs. Am J Surg Pathol. 27:141–9.

136. Barcena C, Oliva E (2011). WT1 expression in the female genital tract. Adv Anat Pathol. 18:454–65.

137. Bardales RH, Stanley MW, Schaefer RF, et al. (1996). Secondary pericardial malignancies: a critical appraisal of the role of cytology, pericardial biopsy, and DNA ploidy analysis. Am J Clin Pathol. 106:29–34.

138. Baresova P, Pitha PM, Lubyova B (2013). Distinct roles of Kaposi's sarcoma-associated herpesvirus-encoded viral interferon regulatory factors in inflammatory response and cancer. J Virol. 87:9398–410.

139. Bari MF, Brown H, Nicholson AG, et al. (2014). BAI3, CDX2 and VIL1: a panel of three antibodies to distinguish small cell from large cell neuroendocrine lung carcinomas. Histopathology. 64:547–56.

140. Baris YI, Grandjean P (2006). Prospective study of mesothelioma mortality in Turkish villages with exposure to fibrous zeolite. J Natl Cancer Inst. 98:414–7.

141. Barksdale EM Jr, Obokhare I (2009). Teratomas in infants and children. Curr Opin Pediatr. 21:344–9.

142. Barnholtz-Sloan JS, Sloan AE, Davis FG, et al. (2004). Incidence proportions of brain metastases in patients diagnosed (1973 to 2001) in the Metropolitan Detroit Cancer Surveillance System. J Clin Oncol. 22:2865–72.

143. Barreiro M, Renilla A, Jimenez JM, et al. (2013). Primary cardiac tumors: 32 years of experience from a Spanish tertiary surgical center. Cardiovasc Pathol. 22:424–7.

144. Barton AD (1997). T-cell lymphocytosis associated with lymphocyte-rich thymoma. Cancer. 80:1409–17.

145. Basarici I, Demir I, Yilmaz H, et al. (2006). Obstructive metastatic malignant melanoma of the heart: Imminent pulmonary arterial occlusion caused by right ventricular metastasis with unknown origin of the primary tumor. Heart Lung. 35:351–4.

146. Basile A, Gregoris A, Antoci B, et al. (1989). Malignant change in a benign pulmonary hamartoma. Thorax. 44:232–3.

147. Bass AJ, Watanabe H, Mermel CH, et al. (2009). SOX2 is an amplified lineage-survival oncogene in lung and esophageal squamous cell carcinomas. Nat Genet. 41:1238–42.

147A. Basso C, Bottio T, Thiene G, Valente M, Gerosa G (2013). Other Benign Cardiac Tumors. In: Cardiac Tumor Pathology. Basso C, Valente M, Thiene G (Eds). New York: Springer, pp 45–58.

148. Basso C, Bottio T, Valente M, et al. (2003). Primary cardiac valve tumours. Heart. 89:1259–60.

149. Basso C, Stefani A, Calabrese F, et al. (1996). Primary right atrial fibrosarcoma diagnosed by endocardial biopsy. Am Heart J. 131:399–402.

150. Basso C, Valente M, Casarotto D, et al. (1997). Cardiac lithomyxoma. Am J Cardiol. 80:1249–51.

151. Basso K, Mussolin L, Lettieri A, et al. (2011). T-cell lymphoblastic lymphoma shows differences and similarities with T-cell acute lymphoblastic leukemia by genomic and gene expression analyses. Genes Chromosomes Cancer. 50:1063–75.
152. Batra S, Shi Y, Kuchenbecker KM, et al. (2006). Wnt inhibitory factor-1, a Wnt antagonist, is silenced by promoter hypermethylation in malignant pleural mesothelioma. Biochem Biophys Res Commun. 342:1228–32.
153. Battafarano RJ, Fernandez FG, Ritter J, et al. (2005). Large cell neuroendocrine carcinoma: an aggressive form of non-small cell lung cancer. J Thorac Cardiovasc Surg. 130:166–72.
154. Bauer DE, Mitchell CM, Strait KM, et al. (2012). Clinicopathologic features and long-term outcomes of NUT midline carcinoma. Clin Cancer Res. 18:5773–9.
156. Bavikatty NR, Michael CW (2003). Cytologic features of small-cell carcinoma on ThinPrep. Diagn Cytopathol. 29:8–12.
157. Bean J, Brennan C, Shih JY, et al. (2007). MET amplification occurs with or without T790M mutations in EGFR mutant lung tumors with acquired resistance to gefitinib or erlotinib. Proc Natl Acad Sci USA. 104:20932–7.
158. Beasley MB, Lantuejoul S, Abbondanzo S, et al. (2003). The P16/cyclin D1/Rb pathway in neuroendocrine tumors of the lung. Hum Pathol. 34:136–42.
159. Beasley MB, Thunnissen FB, Brambilla E, et al. (2000). Pulmonary atypical carcinoid: predictors of survival in 106 cases. Hum Pathol. 31:1255–65.
160. Beasley SW, Tiedemann K, Howat A, et al. (1987). Precocious puberty associated with malignant thoracic teratoma and malignant histiocytosis in a child with Klinefelter's syndrome. Med Pediatr Oncol. 15:277–80.
161. Beaty MW, Toro J, Sorbara L, et al. (2001). Cutaneous lymphomatoid granulomatosis: correlation of clinical and biologic features. Am J Surg Pathol. 25:1111–20.
162. Becker AE (2000). Primary heart tumors in the pediatric age group: a review of salient pathologic features relevant for clinicians. Pediatr Cardiol. 21:317–23.
163. Becker AE, van der Wal AC (1998). Leiomyosarcoma on an infant's mitral valve. Pediatr Cardiol. 19:193.
164. Bedi HS, Sharma VK, Mishra M, et al. (1995). Papillary fibroelastoma of the mitral valve associated with rheumatic mitral stenosis. Eur J Cardiothorac Surg. 9:54–5.
165. Beghetti M, Gow RM, Haney I, et al. (1997). Pediatric primary benign cardiac tumors: a 15-year review. Am Heart J. 134:1107–14.
166. Begin LR, Eskandari J, Joncas J, et al. (1987). Epstein-Barr virus related lymphoepithelioma-like carcinoma of lung. J Surg Oncol. 36:280–3.
167. Begueret H, Galateau-Salle F, Guillou L, et al. (2005). Primary intrathoracic synovial sarcoma: a clinicopathologic study of 40 t(X-;18)-positive cases from the French Sarcoma Group and the Mesopath Group. Am J Surg Pathol. 29:339–46.
168. Begueret H, Vergier B, Parrens M, et al. (2002). Primary Lung Small B-Cell Lymphoma versus Lymphoid Hyperplasia: Evaluation of Diagnostic Criteria in 26 Cases. Am J Surg Pathol. 26:76–81.
169. Belge C, Renckens I, Van Puijenbroek R, et al. (2011). Intima sarcoma of the pulmonary artery mimicking takayasu disease. Case Rep Vasc Med. 2011:510708.
170. Belinsky SA, Nikula KJ, Palmisano WA, et al. (1998). Aberrant methylation of p16(INK4a) is an early event in lung cancer and a potential biomarker for early diagnosis. Proc Natl Acad Sci USA. 95:11891–6.
171. Belinsky SA, Palmisano WA, Gilliland FD, et al. (2002). Aberrant promoter methylation in bronchial epithelium and sputum from current and former smokers. Cancer Res. 62:2370–7.
172. Bell DA, Greco MA (1981). Cardiac myxoma with chondroid features: a light and electron microscopic study. Hum Pathol. 12:370–4.
173. Bell DW, Gore I, Okimoto RA, et al. (2005). Inherited susceptibility to lung cancer may be associated with the T790M drug resistance mutation in EGFR. Nat Genet. 37:1315–6.
174. Bell DW, Lynch TJ, Haserlat SM, et al. (2005). Epidermal growth factor receptor mutations and gene amplification in non-small-cell lung cancer: molecular analysis of the IDEAL/INTACT gefitinib trials. J Clin Oncol. 23:8081–92.
175. Bellizzi AM, Bruzzi C, French CA, et al. (2009). The cytologic features of NUT midline carcinoma. Cancer. 117:508–15.
176. Bendel EC, Maleszewski JJ, Araoz PA (2011). Imaging sarcomas of the great vessels and heart. Semin Ultrasound CT MR. 32:377–404.
177. Benjamin H, Lebanony D, Rosenwald S, et al. (2010). A diagnostic assay based on microRNA expression accurately identifies malignant pleural mesothelioma. J Mol Diagn. 12:771–9.
178. Bennett AK, Mills SE, Wick MR (2003). Salivary-type neoplasms of the breast and lung. Semin Diagn Pathol. 20:279–304.
179. Bennett WP, Colby TV, Travis WD, et al. (1993). p53 protein accumulates frequently in early bronchial neoplasia. Cancer Res. 53:4817–22.
180. Bentz M, Barth TF, Bruderlein S, et al. (2001). Gain of chromosome arm 9p is characteristic of primary mediastinal B-cell lymphoma (MBL): comprehensive molecular cytogenetic analysis and presentation of a novel MBL cell line. Genes Chromosomes Cancer. 30:393–401.
181. Benveniste MF, Moran CA, Mawlawi O, et al. (2013). FDG PET-CT aids in the preoperative assessment of patients with newly diagnosed thymic epithelial malignancies. J Thorac Oncol. 8:502–10.
182. Beral V, Peterman T, Berkelman R, et al. (1991). AIDS-associated non-Hodgkin lymphoma. Lancet. 337:805–9.
183. Beresford L, Fernandez CV, Cummings E, et al. (2003). Mediastinal polyembryoma associated with Klinefelter syndrome. J Pediatr Hematol Oncol. 25:321–3.
184. Berezowski K, Grimes MM, Gal A, et al. (1996). CD5 immunoreactivity of epithelial cells in thymic carcinoma and CASTLE using paraffin-embedded tissue. Am J Clin Pathol. 106:483–6.
185. Berger MD, Schneider J, Ballmer PE, et al. (2013). Mucin-producing adenocarcinoma arising in an atrial myxoma. Ann Diagn Pathol. 17:104–7.
186. Bergethon K, Shaw AT, Ou SH, et al. (2012). ROS1 rearrangements define a unique molecular class of lung cancers. J Clin Oncol. 30:863–70.
187. Berkow RL, Kelly DR (1995). Isolated CNS metastasis as the first site of recurrence in a child with germ cell tumor of the mediastinum. Med Pediatr Oncol. 24:36–9.
188. Berman DW, Crump KS (2008). Update of potency factors for asbestos-related lung cancer and mesothelioma. Crit Rev Toxicol. 38 Suppl 1:1–47.
189. Bernard A, Boumsell L, Reinherz EL, et al. (1981). Cell surface characterization of malignant T cells from lymphoblastic lymphoma using monoclonal antibodies: evidence for phenotypic differences between malignant T cells from patients with acute lymphoblastic leukemia and lymphoblastic lymphoma. Blood. 57:1105–10.
190. Bernard J, Yi ES (2007). Pulmonary thromboendarterectomy: a clinicopathologic study of 200 consecutive pulmonary thromboendarterectomy cases in one institution. Hum Pathol. 38:871–7.
191. Bernheim A, Toujani S, Saulnier P, et al. (2008). High-resolution array comparative genomic hybridization analysis of human bronchial and salivary adenoid cystic carcinoma. Lab Invest. 88:464–73.
192. Bernheim J, Griffel B, Versano S, et al. (1980). Mediastinal leiomyosarcoma in the wall of a bronchial cyst. Arch Pathol Lab Med. 104:221.
193. Beroukhim RS, Prakash A, Buechel ER, et al. (2011). Characterization of cardiac tumors in children by cardiovascular magnetic resonance imaging: a multicenter experience. J Am Coll Cardiol. 58:1044–54.
194. Betancourt B, Defendini EA, Johnson C, et al. (1979). Severe right ventricular outflow tract obstruction caused by an intracavitary cardiac neurilemoma: succesful surgical removal and postoperative diagnosis. Chest. 75:522–4.
195. Bhalla R, Nassar A (2007). Cardiac angiosarcoma: report of a case diagnosed by echocardiographic-guided fine-needle aspiration. Diagn Cytopathol. 35:164–6.
196. Bialas M, Szczepanski W, Szpor J, et al. (2010). Adenomatoid tumour of the adrenal gland: a case report and literature review. Pol J Pathol. 61:97–102.
197. Bian Y, Jordan AG, Rupp M, et al. (1993). Effusion cytology of desmoplastic small round cell tumor of the pleura. A case report. Acta Cytol. 37:77–82.
198. Bianchi AB, Mitsunaga SI, Cheng JQ, et al. (1995). High frequency of inactivating mutations in the neurofibromatosis type 2 gene (NF2) in primary malignant mesotheliomas. Proc Natl Acad Sci USA. 92:10854–8.
199. Bianchi G, Ferrarini M, Matteucci M, et al. (2013). Giant solitary fibrous tumor of the epicardium causing reversible heart failure. Ann Thorac Surg. 96:e49–51.
200. Bicakcioglu P, Demirag F, Yazicioglu A, et al. (2014). Intrathoracic neurogenic tumors. Thorac Cardiovasc Surg. 62:147–52.
201. Bielefeld KJ, Moller JH (2013). Cardiac tumors in infants and children: study of 120 operated patients. Pediatr Cardiol. 34:125–8.
202. Bigot P, Campillo B, Orsat M, et al. (2010). [Teaching and perception of urology by medical students at the end of the second cycle: an appraisal]. Prog Urol. 20:375–81.
203. Billmire D, Vinocur C, Rescorla F, et al. (2001). Malignant mediastinal germ cell tumors: an intergroup study. J Pediatr Surg. 36:18–24.
204. Binh MB, Sastre-Garau X, Guillou L, et al. (2005). MDM2 and CDK4 immunostainings are useful adjuncts in diagnosing well-differentiated and dedifferentiated liposarcoma subtypes: a comparative analysis of 559 soft tissue neoplasms with genetic data. Am J Surg Pathol. 29:1340–7.
205. Bini RM, Westaby S, Bargeron LM Jr, et al. (1983). Investigation and management of primary cardiac tumors in infants and children. J Am Coll Cardiol. 2:351–7.
206. Bird LM, Krous HF, Eichenfield LF, et al. (1994). Female infant with oncocytic cardiomyopathy and microphthalmia with linear skin defects (MLS): a clue to the pathogenesis of oncocytic cardiomyopathy? Am J Med Genet. 53:141–8.
207. Bireta C, Popov AF, Schotola H, et al. (2011). Carney-Complex: multiple resections of recurrent cardiac myxoma. J Cardiothorac Surg. 6:12.
208. Bishop JA, Ogawa T, Chang X, et al. (2012). HPV analysis in distinguishing second primary tumors from lung metastases in patients with head and neck squamous cell carcinoma. Am J Surg Pathol. 36:142–8.
209. Bishop JA, Teruya-Feldstein J, Westra WH, et al. (2012). p40 (DeltaNp63) is superior to p63 for the diagnosis of pulmonary squamous cell carcinoma. Mod Pathol. 25:405–15.
210. Bisig B, de Reynies A, Bonnet C, et al. (2013). CD30-positive peripheral T-cell lymphomas share molecular and phenotypic features. Haematologica. 98:1250–8.
211. Bisogno G, Brennan B, Orbach D, et al. (2014). Treatment and prognostic factors in pleuropulmonary blastoma: an EXPeRT report. Eur J Cancer. 50:178–84.
212. Bitar FF, el-Zein C, Tawil A, et al. (1998). Intrapericardial teratoma in an adult: a rare presentation. Med Pediatr Oncol. 30:249–51.
213. Bizzarri F, Mondillo S, Tanganelli P, et al. (2001). A primary intracavitary right atrial neurilemoma. J Cardiovasc Surg (Torino). 42:777–9.
214. Blanco LZ, Heagley DE, Montebelli F, et al. (2013). Cytologic features of sclerosing hemangioma of the lung on crush preparations. Diagn Cytopathol. 41:242–6.
215. Blaukovitsch M, Halbwedl I, Kothmaier H, et al. (2006). Sarcomatoid carcinomas of the lung--are these histogenetically heterogeneous tumors? Virchows Arch. 449:455–61.
216. Bockmuhl U, Wolf G, Schmidt S, et al. (1998). Genomic alterations associated with malignancy in head and neck cancer. Head Neck. 20:145–51.
217. Boddaert G, Grand B, Le Pimpec-Barthes F, et al. (2012). Bronchial carcinoid tumors causing Cushing's syndrome: more aggressive behavior and the need for early diagnosis. Ann Thorac Surg. 94:1823–9.
218. Bode-Lesniewska B, Zhao J, Speel EJ, et al. (2001). Gains of 12q13-14 and overexpression of mdm2 are frequent findings in intimal sarcomas of the pulmonary artery. Virchows Arch. 438:57–65.
219. Bodner SM, Koss MN (1996). Mutations in the p53 gene in pulmonary blastomas: immunohistochemical and molecular studies. Hum Pathol. 27:1117–23.
220. Bofill M, Janossy G, Willcox N, et al. (1985). Microenvironments in the normal thymus and the thymus in myasthenia gravis. Am J Pathol. 119:462–73.
221. Bokemeyer C, Droz JP, Horwich A, et al. (2001). Extragonadal seminoma: an international multicenter analysis of prognostic factors and long term treatment outcome. Cancer. 91:1394–401.
222. Bokemeyer C, Hartmann JT, Fossa SD, et al. (2003). Extragonadal germ cell tumors: relation to testicular neoplasia and management options. APMIS. 111:49–59.
223. Bokemeyer C, Nichols CR, Droz JP, et al. (2002). Extragonadal germ cell tumors of the mediastinum and retroperitoneum: results from an international analysis. J Clin Oncol. 20:1864–73.
224. Boland JM, Colby TV, Folpe AL (2012). Liposarcomas of the mediastinum and thorax: a clinicopathologic and molecular cytogenetic study of 24 cases, emphasizing unusual and diverse histologic features. Am J Surg Pathol. 36:1395–403.
225. Boland JM, Tazelaar HD, Colby TV, et al. (2012). Diffuse pulmonary lymphatic disease presenting as interstitial lung disease in adulthood: report of 3 cases. Am J Surg Pathol. 36:1548–54.
226. Boman F, Hill DA, Williams GM, et al. (2006). Familial association of pleuropulmonary blastoma with cystic nephroma and other renal tumors: a report from the International Pleuropulmonary Blastoma Registry. J Pediatr. 149:850–4.
227. Bonato M, Cerati M, Pagani A, et al. (1992). Differential diagnostic patterns of lung neuroendocrine tumours. A clinico-pathological and immunohistochemical study of 122 cases. Virchows Arch A Pathol Anat Histopathol. 420:201–11.
228. Bonn BR, Rohde M, Zimmermann M, et al. (2013). Incidence and prognostic relevance of genetic variations in T-cell lymphoblastic lymphoma in childhood and adolescence. Blood. 121:3153–60.
229. Bonnichsen CR, Dearani JA, Maleszewski JJ, et al. (2013). Recurrent Epstein-Barr

virus-associated diffuse large B-cell lymphoma in an ascending aorta graft. Circulation. 128:1481–3.
230. Boone S, Higginson LA, Walley VM (1992). Endothelial papillary fibroelastomas arising in and around the aortic sinus, filling the ostium of the right coronary artery. Arch Pathol Lab Med. 116:135–7.
231. Borczuk AC, Kim HK, Yegen HA, et al. (2005). Lung adenocarcinoma global profiling identifies type II transforming growth factor-beta receptor as a repressor of invasiveness. Am J Respir Crit Care Med. 172:729–37.
232. Borczuk AC, Qian F, Kazeros A, et al. (2009). Invasive size is an independent predictor of survival in pulmonary adenocarcinoma. Am J Surg Pathol. 33:462–9.
233. Bordalo AD, Alves I, Nobre AL, et al. (2012). [New clinical aspects of cardiac myxomas: a clinical and pathological reappraisal]. Rev Port Cardiol. 31:567–75.
234. Borie R, Wislez M, Antoine M, et al. (2011). Clonality and phenotyping analysis of alveolar lymphocytes is suggestive of pulmonary MALT lymphoma. Respir Med. 105:1231–7.
235. Borie R, Wislez M, Thabut G, et al. (2009). Clinical characteristics and prognostic factors of pulmonary MALT lymphoma. Eur Respir J. 34:1408–16.
236. Boroumand N, Ly TL, Sonstein J, et al. (2012). Microscopic diffuse large B-cell lymphoma (DLBCL) occurring in pseudocysts: do these tumors belong to the category of DLBCL associated with chronic inflammation? Am J Surg Pathol. 36:1074–80.
237. Bosi G, Lintermans JP, Pellegrino PA, et al. (1996). The natural history of cardiac rhabdomyoma with and without tuberous sclerosis. Acta Paediatr. 85:928–31.
238. Bossert T, Gummert JF, Battellini R, et al. (2005). Surgical experience with 77 primary cardiac tumors. Interact Cardiovasc Thorac Surg. 4:311–5.
239. Bothe W, Goebel H, Kunze M, et al. (2005). Right atrial solitary fibrous tumor - a new cardiac neoplasm? Interact Cardiovasc Thorac Surg. 4:396–7.
240. Bott M, Brevet M, Taylor BS, et al. (2011). The nuclear deubiquitinase BAP1 is commonly inactivated by somatic mutations and 3p21.1 losses in malignant pleural mesothelioma. Nat Genet. 43:668–72.
241. Bott MJ, Wang H, Travis W, et al. (2011). Management and outcomes of relapse after treatment for thymoma and thymic carcinoma. Ann Thorac Surg. 92:1984–91.
242. Boucheix C, David B, Sebban C, et al. (1994). Immunophenotype of adult acute lymphoblastic leukemia, clinical parameters, and outcome: an analysis of a prospective trial including 562 tested patients (LALA87). French Group on Therapy for Adult Acute Lymphoblastic Leukemia. Blood. 84:1603–12.
243. Boukhris AA, Baccari S, Kamoun NS, et al. (2002). [Pulmonary papillary adenoma: report of two cases]. Ann Pathol. 22:497–8.
244. Boulanger E, Gerard L, Gabarre J, et al. (2005). Prognostic factors and outcome of human herpesvirus 8-associated primary effusion lymphoma in patients with AIDS. J Clin Oncol. 23:4372–80.
245. Boulanger E, Hermine O, Fermand JP, et al. (2004). Human herpesvirus 8 (HHV-8)-associated peritoneal primary effusion lymphoma (PEL) in two HIV-negative elderly patients. Am J Hematol. 76:88–91.
246. Boulanger E, Marchio A, Hong SS, et al. (2009). Mutational analysis of TP53, PTEN, PIK3CA and CTNNB1/beta-catenin genes in human herpesvirus 8-associated primary effusion lymphoma. Haematologica. 94:1170–4.
247. Bourke SC, Nicholson AG, Gibson GJ (2003). Erdheim-Chester disease: pulmonary infiltration responding to cyclophosphamide and prednisolone. Thorax. 58:1004–5.
248. Bove KE, Hurtubise P, Wong KY (1985). Thymus in untreated systemic histiocytosis X. Pediatr Pathol. 4:99–115.
249. Bower M, Pria AD, Coyle C, et al. (2014). Diagnostic criteria schemes for multicentric Castleman disease in 75 cases. J Acquir Immune Defic Syndr. 65:e80–2.
250. Boyer MW, Moertel CL, Priest JR, et al. (1995). Use of intracavitary cisplatin for the treatment of childhood solid tumors in the chest or abdominal cavity. J Clin Oncol. 13:631–6.
251. Boylan E, Wyers M, Jaffar R (2011). A rare case of thymoma in a 15-month-old girl. Pediatr Radiol. 41:1469–71.
252. Bradshaw SH, Hendry P, Boodhwani M, et al. (2011). Left ventricular mesenchymal hamartoma, a new hamartoma of the heart. Cardiovasc Pathol. 20:307–14.
253. Brahmer JR (2013). Harnessing the immune system for the treatment of non-small-cell lung cancer. J Clin Oncol. 31:1021–8.
254. Braman SS, Mark EJ (1984). Case records of the Massachusetts General Hospital. Weekly clinicopathological exercises. Case 3-1984. A 58-year-old man with an enlarging nodule in the left upper lobe. N Engl J Med. 310:178–87.
255. Brambilla E, Gazzeri S, Lantuejoul S, et al. (1998). p53 mutant immunophenotype and deregulation of p53 transcription pathway (Bcl2, Bax, and Waf1) in precursor bronchial lesions of lung cancer. Clin Cancer Res. 4:1609–18.
256. Brambilla E, Gazzeri S, Moro D, et al. (1999). Alterations of Rb pathway (Rb-p16INK4-cyclin D1) in preinvasive bronchial lesions. Clin Cancer Res. 5:243–50.
256A. Brambilla CG, Laffaire J, Lantuejoul S, Moro-Sibilot D, Nagy-Mignotte H, Arbib F, Toffart AC, Petel F, Hainaut P, Rousseaux S, Khochbin S, DE Reynies A, Brambilla E (2014). Lung squamous cell carcinomas with basaloid histology represent a specific molecular entity. Clin Cancer Res. 20:5777–86.
257. Brambilla E, Moro D, Gazzeri S, et al. (1991). Cytotoxic chemotherapy induces cell differentiation in small-cell lung carcinoma. J Clin Oncol. 9:50–61.
258. Brambilla E, Moro D, Veale D, et al. (1992). Basal cell (basaloid) carcinoma of the lung: a new morphologic and phenotypic entity with separate prognostic significance. Hum Pathol. 23:993–1003.
259. Brambilla E, Negoescu A, Gazzeri S, et al. (1996). Apoptosis-related factors p53, Bcl2, and Bax in neuroendocrine lung tumors. Am J Pathol. 149:1941–52.
259A. Brambilla E, Travis WD, Brennan P, Harris C (2014). Lung Cancer. In: World Cancer Report. Stewart B.W, Wild C.P. eds. Lyon: IARC; pp. 350-362.
260. Bramwell NH, Burns BF (1986). Histiocytosis X of the thymus in association with myasthenia gravis. Am J Clin Pathol. 86:224–7.
261. Brandal P, Panagopoulos I, Bjerkehagen B, et al. (2008). Detection of a t(1;22)(q23;q12) translocation leading to an EWSR1-PBX1 fusion gene in a myoepithelioma. Genes Chromosomes Cancer. 47:558–64.
262. Breuer RH, Pasic A, Smit EF, et al. (2005). The natural course of preneoplastic lesions in bronchial epithelium. Clin Cancer Res. 11:537–43.
263. Brevet M, Shimizu S, Bott MJ, et al. (2011). Coactivation of receptor tyrosine kinases in malignant mesothelioma as a rationale for combination targeted therapy. J Thorac Oncol. 6:864–74.
263A. Brevet M, Arcila M, Ladanyi M. (2010). Assessment of EGFR mutation status in lung adenocarcinoma by immunohistochemistry using antibodies specific to the two major forms of mutant EGFR. J Mol Diagn. 2:169–76.
264. Brodeur GM, Pritchard J, Berthold F, et al. (1993). Revisions of the international criteria for neuroblastoma diagnosis, staging, and response to treatment. J Clin Oncol. 11:1466–77.
265. Brose MS, Volpe P, Feldman M, et al. (2002). BRAF and RAS mutations in human lung cancer and melanoma. Cancer Res. 62:6997–7000.
266. Brown AF, Sirohi D, Fukuoka J, et al. (2013). Tissue-preserving antibody cocktails to differentiate primary squamous cell carcinoma, adenocarcinoma, and small cell carcinoma of lung. Arch Pathol Lab Med. 137:1274–81.
267. Brown JG, Familiari U, Papotti M, et al. (2009). Thymic basaloid carcinoma: a clinicopathologic study of 12 cases, with a general discussion of basaloid carcinoma and its relationship with adenoid cystic carcinoma. Am J Surg Pathol. 33:1113–24.
268. Brown ML, Zayas GE, Abel MD, et al. (2008). Mediastinal paragangliomas: the mayo clinic experience. Ann Thorac Surg. 86:946–51.
269. Brugieres L, Deley MC, Pacquement H, et al. (1998). CD30(+) anaplastic large-cell lymphoma in children: analysis of 82 patients enrolled in two consecutive studies of the French Society of Pediatric Oncology. Blood. 92:3591–8.
270. Brun AL, Touitou-Gottenberg D, Haroche J, et al. (2010). Erdheim-Chester disease: CT findings of thoracic involvement. Eur Radiol. 20:2579–87.
271. Bruse S, Petersen H, Weissfeld J, et al. (2014). Increased methylation of lung cancer-associated genes in sputum DNA of former smokers with chronic mucous hypersecretion. Respir Res. 15:2.
273. Buck M, Ingle JN, Giuliani ER, et al. (1987). Pericardial effusion in women with breast cancer. Cancer. 60:263–9.
274. Bukowski RM (1993). Management of advanced and extragonadal germ-cell tumors. Urol Clin North Am. 20:153–60.
275. Bukowski RM, Wolf M, Kulander BG, et al. (1993). Alternating combination chemotherapy in patients with extragonadal germ cell tumors. A Southwest Oncology Group study. Cancer. 71:2631–8.
276. Buksa M, Gerc V, Dilic M, et al. (2009). Clinical, echocardiographic and echophonocardiographic characteristics of the atrial myxomas in 22 years period. Med Arh. 63:320–2.
277. Bull JC Jr, Grimes OF (1974). Pulmonary carcinosarcoma. Chest. 65:9–12.
278. Bulman W, Saqi A, Powell CA (2012). Acquisition and processing of endobronchial ultrasound-guided transbronchial needle aspiration specimens in the era of targeted lung cancer chemotherapy. Am J Respir Crit Care Med. 185:606–11.
279. Burke A (2008). Primary malignant cardiac tumors. Semin Diagn Pathol. 25:39–46.
280. Burke A, Johns JP, Virmani R (1990). Hemangiomas of the heart. A clinicopathologic study of ten cases. Am J Cardiovasc Pathol. 3:283–90.
281. Burke A, Li L, Kling E, et al. (2007). Cardiac inflammatory myofibroblastic tumor: a "benign" neoplasm that may result in syncope, myocardial infarction, and sudden death. Am J Surg Pathol. 31:1115–22.
282. Burke A, Virmani R (1996). Tumors of the Heart and Great Vessels. Atlas of Tumor Pathology. 3rd ed. Volume 16. Washington, DC: American Registry of Pathology.
283. Burke A, Virmani R (2008). Pediatric heart tumors. Cardiovasc Pathol. 17:193–8.
284. Burke AP, Cowan D, Virmani R (1992). Primary sarcomas of the heart. Cancer. 69:387–95.
285. Burke AP, Gatto-Weis C, Griego JE, et al. (2002). Adult cellular rhabdomyoma of the heart: a report of 3 cases. Hum Pathol. 33:1092–7.
286. Burke AP, Ribe JK, Bajaj AK, et al. (1998). Hamartoma of mature cardiac myocytes. Hum Pathol. 29:904–9.
287. Burke AP, Rosado-de-Christenson M, Templeton PA, et al. (1994). Cardiac fibroma: clinicopathologic correlates and surgical treatment. J Thorac Cardiovasc Surg. 108:862–70.
288. Burke AP, Tavora F (2010). Practical Cardiovascular Pathology. 1st ed. Philadelphia: Lippincott Williams & Wilkins.
289. Burke AP, Virmani R (1991). Osteosarcomas of the heart. Am J Surg Pathol. 15:289–95.
290. Burke AP, Virmani R (1993). Cardiac myxoma. A clinicopathologic study. Am J Clin Pathol. 100:671–80.
291. Burke LM, Rush WI, Khoor A, et al. (1999). Alveolar adenoma: a histochemical, immunohistochemical, and ultrastructural analysis of 17 cases. Hum Pathol. 30:158–67.
292. Burkhardt B (2010). Paediatric lymphoblastic T-cell leukaemia and lymphoma: one or two diseases? Br J Haematol. 149:653–68.
293. Burkhardt B, Bruch J, Zimmermann M, et al. (2006). Loss of heterozygosity on chromosome 6q14-q24 is associated with poor outcome in children and adolescents with T-cell lymphoblastic lymphoma. Leukemia. 20:1422–9.
294. Burns TR, Underwood RD, Greenberg SD, et al. (1989). Cytomorphometry of large cell carcinoma of the lung. Anal Quant Cytol Histol. 11:48–52.
295. Busam KJ, Jungbluth AA, Rekthman N, et al. (2009). Merkel cell polyomavirus expression in merkel cell carcinomas and its absence in combined tumors and pulmonary neuroendocrine carcinomas. Am J Surg Pathol. 33:1378–85.
296. Bussani R, De-Giorgio F, Abbate A, et al. (2007). Cardiac metastases. J Clin Pathol. 60:27–34.
297. Bussey KJ, Lawce HJ, Olson SB, et al. (1999). Chromosome abnormalities of eighty-one pediatric germ cell tumors: sex-, age-, site-, and histopathology-related differences--a Children's Cancer Group study. Genes Chromosomes Cancer. 25:134–46.
298. Butany J, Leong SW, Carmichael K, et al. (2005). A 30-year analysis of cardiac neoplasms at autopsy. Can J Cardiol. 21:675–80.
299. Butany J, Nair V, Naseemuddin A, et al. (2005). Cardiac tumours: diagnosis and management. Lancet Oncol. 6:219–28.
300. Butany J, Yu W (2000). Cardiac angiosarcoma: two cases and a review of the literature. Can J Cardiol. 16:197–205.
301. Butnor KJ, Burchette JL (2013). p40 (DeltaNp63) and keratin 34betaE12 provide greater diagnostic accuracy than p63 in the evaluation of small cell lung carcinoma in small biopsy samples. Hum Pathol. 44:1479–86.
302. Butnor KJ, Sporn TA, Hammar SP, et al. (2001). Well-differentiated papillary mesothelioma. Am J Surg Pathol. 25:1304–9.
303. Butrynski JE, D'Adamo DR, Hornick JL, et al. (2010). Crizotinib in ALK-rearranged inflammatory myofibroblastic tumor. N Engl J Med. 363:1727–33.
304. Byers LA, Wang J, Nilsson MB, et al. (2012). Proteomic profiling identifies dysregulated pathways in small cell lung cancer and novel therapeutic targets including PARP1. Cancer Discov. 2:798–811.
305. Cagini L, Nicholson AG, Horwich A, et al. (1998). Thoracic metastasectomy for germ cell tumours: long term survival and prognostic factors. Ann Oncol. 9:1185–91.
306. Cai JN, Shi M, Wang J (2011). [Perivascular epithelioid cell tumor, not otherwise specified: a clinicopathologic and immunohistochemical analysis of 31 cases]. Zhonghua Bing Li Xue Za Zhi. 40:240–5.
307. Calaminici M, Piper K, Lee AM, et al. (2004). CD23 expression in mediastinal large B-cell lymphomas. Histopathology. 45:619–24.
308. Callens C, Baleydier F, Lengline E, et al. (2012). Clinical impact of NOTCH1 and/or FBXW7 mutations, FLASH deletion, and TCR status in pediatric T-cell lymphoblastic lymphoma. J Clin Oncol. 30:1966–73.

309. Calvo-Garcia MA, Lim FY, Stanek J, et al. (2014). Congenital peribronchial myofibroblastic tumor: prenatal imaging clues to differentiate from other fetal chest lesions. Pediatr Radiol. 44:479–83.

310. Cameron SE, Alsharif M, McKeon D, et al. (2008). Cytology of metastatic thymic well-differentiated neuroendocrine carcinoma (thymic carcinoid) in pleural fluid: report of a case. Diagn Cytopathol. 36:333–7.

311. Cameselle-Teijeiro J, Abdulkader I, Soares P, et al. (2005). Cystic tumor of the atrioventricular node of the heart appears to be the heart equivalent of the solid cell nests (ultimobranchial rests) of the thyroid. Am J Clin Pathol. 123:369–75.

312. Camiade E, Gramond C, Jutand MA, et al. (2013). Characterization of a French series of female cases of mesothelioma. Am J Ind Med. 56:1307–16.

313. Camidge DR, Kono SA, Lu X, et al. (2011). Anaplastic lymphoma kinase gene rearrangements in non-small cell lung cancer are associated with prolonged progression-free survival on pemetrexed. J Thorac Oncol. 6:774–80.

314. Camilo R, Capelozzi VL, Siqueira SA, et al. (2006). Expression of p63, keratin 5/6, keratin 7, and surfactant-A in non-small cell lung carcinomas. Hum Pathol. 37:542–6.

315. Campos-Parra AD, Aviles A, Contreras-Reyes S, et al. (2014). Relevance of the novel IASLC/ATS/ERS classification of lung adenocarcinoma in advanced disease. Eur Respir J. 43:1439–47.

316. Camps C, Sirera R, Bremnes RM, et al. (2006). Analysis of c-kit expression in small cell lung cancer: prevalence and prognostic implications. Lung Cancer. 52:343–7.

317. Candes FP, Ajinkya MS (1987). Primary mediastinal choriocarcinoma (a case report). J Postgrad Med. 33:219–21.

318. Canty TG, Siemens R (1978). Malignant mediastinal teratoma in a 15-year-old girl. Cancer. 41:1623–6.

319. Cao C, Yan TD, Kennedy C, et al. (2011). Bronchopulmonary carcinoid tumors: long-term outcomes after resection. Ann Thorac Surg. 91:339–43.

320. Cao D, Allan RW, Cheng L, et al. (2011). RNA-binding protein LIN28 is a marker for testicular germ cell tumors. Hum Pathol. 42:710–8.

321. Cao D, Humphrey PA, Allan RW (2009). SALL4 is a novel sensitive and specific marker for metastatic germ cell tumors, with particular utility in detection of metastatic yolk sac tumors. Cancer. 115:2640–51.

322. Cao D, Li J, Guo CC, et al. (2009). SALL4 is a novel diagnostic marker for testicular germ cell tumors. Am J Surg Pathol. 33:1065–77.

323. Cao D, Liu A, Wang F, et al. (2011). RNA-binding protein LIN28 is a marker for primary extragonadal germ cell tumors: an immunohistochemical study of 131 cases. Mod Pathol. 24:288–96.

324. Cao M, Eshoa C, Schultz C, et al. (2007). Primary central nervous system histiocytic sarcoma with relapse to mediastinum: a case report and review of the literature. Arch Pathol Lab Med. 131:301–5.

325. Cappell MS, Lapin S, Rose M (2008). Large right atrial myxoma containing gastric heterotopia presenting with dyspnea and bilateral leg edema due to pulmonary emboli and cardiovascular obstruction: the first known report of gastric heterotopia in the cardiovascular system. Dig Dis Sci. 53:405–9.

326. Caraway NP, Fanning CV, Amato RJ, et al. (1995). Fine-needle aspiration cytology of seminoma: a review of 16 cases. Diagn Cytopathol. 12:327–33.

327. Carbone A, Gloghini A, Vaccher E, et al. (2005). Kaposi's sarcoma-associated herpesvirus/human herpesvirus type 8-positive solid lymphomas: a tissue-based variant of primary effusion lymphoma. J Mol Diagn. 7:17–27.

328. Carbone A, Gloghini A, Vaccher E, et al. (1996). Kaposi's sarcoma-associated herpesvirus DNA sequences in AIDS-related and AIDS-unrelated lymphomatous effusions. Br J Haematol. 94:533–43.

329. Carbone M, Baris YI, Bertino P, et al. (2011). Erionite exposure in North Dakota and Turkish villages with mesothelioma. Proc Natl Acad Sci USA. 108:13618–23.

330. Cardarella S, Ogino A, Nishino M, et al. (2013). Clinical, pathologic, and biologic features associated with BRAF mutations in non-small cell lung cancer. Clin Cancer Res. 19:4532–40.

331. Cardillo G, Treggiari S, Paul MA, et al. (2010). Primary neuroendocrine tumours of the thymus: a clinicopathologic and prognostic study in 19 patients. Eur J Cardiothorac Surg. 37:814–8.

332. Carlson JW, Fletcher CD (2007). Immunohistochemistry for beta-catenin in the differential diagnosis of spindle cell lesions: analysis of a series and review of the literature. Histopathology. 51:509–14.

333. Carney JA (2009). Carney triad: a syndrome featuring paraganglionic, adrenocortical, and possibly other endocrine tumors. J Clin Endocrinol Metab. 94:3656–62.

334. Carretta A, Libretti L, Taccagni G, et al. (2004). Salivary gland-type mixed tumor (pleomorphic adenoma) of the lung. Interact Cardiovasc Thorac Surg. 3:663–5.

335. Carsillo T, Astrinidis A, Henske EP (2000). Mutations in the tuberous sclerosis complex gene TSC2 are a cause of sporadic pulmonary lymphangioleiomyomatosis. Proc Natl Acad Sci USA. 97:6085–90.

336. Casali C, Rossi G, Marchioni A, et al. (2010). A single institution-based retrospective study of surgically treated bronchioloalveolar adenocarcinoma of the lung: clinicopathologic analysis, molecular features, and possible pitfalls in routine practice. J Thorac Oncol. 5:830–6.

337. Casali C, Stefani A, Rossi G, et al. (2004). The prognostic role of c-kit protein expression in resected large cell neuroendocrine carcinoma of the lung. Ann Thorac Surg. 77:247–52.

338. Casiraghi M, De Pas T, Maisonneuve P, et al. (2011). A 10-year single-center experience on 708 lung metastasectomies: the evidence of the "international registry of lung metastases". J Thorac Oncol. 6:1373–8.

339. Castillo JJ, Shum H, Lahijani M, et al. (2012). Prognosis in primary effusion lymphoma is associated with the number of body cavities involved. Leuk Lymphoma. 53:2378–82.

340. Castillo JJ, Winer ES, Olszewski AJ (2014). Sites of extranodal involvement are prognostic in patients with diffuse large B-cell lymphoma in the rituximab era: an analysis of the Surveillance, Epidemiology and End Results database. Am J Hematol. 89:310–4.

341. Castorino F, Masiello P, Quattrocchi E, et al. (2000). Primary cardiac rhabdomyosarcoma of the left atrium: an unusual presentation. Tex Heart Inst J. 27:206–8.

342. Castro CY, Ostrowski ML, Barrios R, et al. (2001). Relationship between Epstein-Barr virus and lymphoepithelioma-like carcinoma of the lung: a clinicopathologic study of 6 cases and review of the literature. Hum Pathol. 32:863–72.

343. Cavalli G, Guglielmi B, Berti A, et al. (2013). The multifaceted clinical presentations and manifestations of Erdheim-Chester disease: comprehensive review of the literature and of 10 new cases. Ann Rheum Dis. 72:1691–5.

344. Cavazza A, Colby TV, Tsokos M, et al. (1996). Lung tumors with a rhabdoid phenotype. Am J Clin Pathol. 105:182–8.

345. Cavazza A, Paci M, De Marco L, et al. (2004). Alveolar adenoma of the lung: a clinicopathologic, immunohistochemical, and molecular study of an unusual case. Int J Surg Pathol. 12:155–9.

346. Cazals-Hatem D, Lepage E, Brice P, et al. (1996). Primary mediastinal large B-cell lymphoma. A clinicopathologic study of 141 cases compared with 916 nonmediastinal large B-cell lymphomas, a GELA ("Groupe d'Etude des Lymphomes de l'Adulte") study. Am J Surg Pathol. 20:877–88.

347. Centofanti P, Di Rosa E, Deorsola L, et al. (1999). Primary cardiac tumors: early and late results of surgical treatment in 91 patients. Ann Thorac Surg. 68:1236–41.

348. Ceresa F, Calarco G, Franzi E, et al. (2010). Right atrial lipoma in patient with Cowden syndrome. Interact Cardiovasc Thorac Surg. 11:803–4.

349. Ceresoli GL, Ferreri AJ, Bucci E, et al. (1997). Primary cardiac lymphoma in immunocompetent patients: diagnostic and therapeutic management. Cancer. 80:1497–506.

350. Cerfolio RJ, Allen MS, Nascimento AG, et al. (1999). Inflammatory pseudotumors of the lung. Ann Thorac Surg. 67:933–6.

351. Cerny T, Martinelli G, Goldhirsch A, et al. (1991). Continuous 5-day infusion of ifosfamide with mesna in inoperable pancreatic cancer patients: a phase II study. J Cancer Res Clin Oncol. 117 Suppl 4:S135–8.

352. Cerroni L, Massone C, Kutzner H, et al. (2008). Intravascular large T-cell or NK-cell lymphoma: a rare variant of intravascular large cell lymphoma with frequent cytotoxic phenotype and association with Epstein-Barr virus infection. Am J Surg Pathol. 32:891–8.

353. Cesarman E (2014). Gammaherpesviruses and lymphoproliferative disorders. Annu Rev Pathol. 9:349–72.

354. Cesarman E, Chang Y, Moore PS, et al. (1995). Kaposi's sarcoma-associated herpesvirus-like DNA sequences in AIDS-related body-cavity-based lymphomas. N Engl J Med. 332:1186–91.

355. Cessna MH, Zhou H, Sanger WG, et al. (2002). Expression of ALK1 and p80 in inflammatory myofibroblastic tumor and its mesenchymal mimics: a study of 135 cases. Mod Pathol. 15:931–8.

356. Cetin G, Gursoy M, Ugurlucan M, et al. (2010). Single-institutional 22 years experience on cardiac myxomas. Angiology. 61:504–9.

357. Cha MJ, Lee HY, Lee KS, et al. (2014). Micropapillary and solid subtypes of invasive lung adenocarcinoma: clinical predictors of histopathology and outcome. J Thorac Cardiovasc Surg. 147:921–8.

358. Chabchoub Ben Abdallah R, Maalej B, Abdelmoulla S, et al. (2011). [Thymoma in children: a report of one case]. Arch Pediatr. 18:745–9.

359. Chadburn A, Hyjek E, Mathew S, et al. (2004). KSHV-positive solid lymphomas represent an extra-cavitary variant of primary effusion lymphoma. Am J Surg Pathol. 28:1401–16.

360. Chadburn A, Hyjek EM, Tam W, et al. (2008). Immunophenotypic analysis of the Kaposi sarcoma herpesvirus (KSHV; HHV-8)-infected B cells in HIV+ multicentric Castleman disease (MCD). Histopathology. 53:513–24.

361. Chaft JE, Rekhtman N, Ladanyi M, et al. (2012). ALK-rearranged lung cancer: adenosquamous lung cancer masquerading as pure squamous carcinoma. J Thorac Oncol. 7:768–9.

362. Chaft JE, Sima CS, Ginsberg MS, et al. (2012). Clinical outcomes with perioperative chemotherapy in sarcomatoid carcinomas of the lung. J Thorac Oncol. 7:1400–5.

363. Chaganti RS, Ladanyi M, Samaniego F, et al. (1989). Leukemic differentiation of a mediastinal germ cell tumor. Genes Chromosomes Cancer. 1:83–7.

364. Chaganti RS, Rodriguez E, Mathew S (1994). Origin of adult male mediastinal germ-cell tumours. Lancet. 343:1130–2.

365. Chalabreysse L, Berger F, Loire R, et al. (2002). Primary cardiac lymphoma in immunocompetent patients: a report of three cases and review of the literature. Virchows Arch. 441:456–61.

366. Chalabreysse L, Etienne-Mastroianni B, Adeleine P, et al. (2004). Thymic carcinoma: a clinicopathological and immunohistological study of 19 cases. Histopathology. 44:367–74.

367. Chalabreysse L, Gengler C, Sefiani S, et al. (2005). [Thymic neuroendocrine tumors: report on 6 cases]. Ann Pathol. 25:205–10.

368. Chalabreysse L, Orsini A, Vial C, et al. (2007). Microscopic thymoma. Interact Cardiovasc Thorac Surg. 6:133–5.

369. Chalabreysse L, Roy P, Cordier JF, et al. (2002). Correlation of the WHO schema for the classification of thymic epithelial neoplasms with prognosis: a retrospective study of 90 tumors. Am J Surg Pathol. 26:1605–11.

370. Chan AC, Chan JK (2000). Pulmonary sclerosing hemangioma consistently expresses thyroid transcription factor-1 (TTF-1): a new clue to its histogenesis. Am J Surg Pathol. 24:1531–6.

371. Chan AC, Chan JK (2002). Can pulmonary sclerosing haemangioma be accurately diagnosed by intra-operative frozen section? Histopathology. 41:392–403.

372. Chan AC, Chan KW, Chan JK, et al. (2001). Development of follicular dendritic cell sarcoma in hyaline-vascular Castleman's disease of the nasopharynx: tracing its evolution by sequential biopsies. Histopathology. 38:510–8.

373. Chan AC, Serrano-Olmo J, Erlandson RA, et al. (2000). Cytokeratin-positive malignant tumors with reticulum cell morphology: a subtype of fibroblastic reticulum cell neoplasm? Am J Surg Pathol. 24:107–16.

374. Chan ACL, Chan JKC, Eimoto T, et al. (2004). Sarcomatoid carcinoma. In: Travis WD, Brambilla E, Muller-Hermelink HK, Harris CC, eds. WHO Classification of Tumours. Pathology and Genetics of Tumours of the Lung, Pleura, Thymus and Heart. 3rd ed. Lyon: IARC; pp 179–181.

375. Chan ES, Alexander J, Swanson PE, et al. (2012). PDX-1, CDX-2, TTF-1, and CK7: a reliable immunohistochemical panel for pancreatic neuroendocrine neoplasms. Am J Surg Pathol. 36:737–43.

376. Chan JK (2013). Newly available antibodies with practical applications in surgical pathology. Int J Surg Pathol. 21:553–72.

377. Chan JK, Fletcher CD, Nayler SJ, et al. (1997). Follicular dendritic cell sarcoma. Clinicopathologic analysis of 17 cases suggesting a malignant potential higher than currently recognized. Cancer. 79:294–313.

378. Chan JK, Hui PK, Tsang WY, et al. (1995). Primary lymphoepithelioma-like carcinoma of the lung. A clinicopathologic study of 11 cases. Cancer. 76:413–22.

379. Chan JK, Sin VC, Wong KF, et al. (1997). Nonnasal lymphoma expressing the natural killer cell marker CD56: a clinicopathologic study of 49 cases of an uncommon aggressive neoplasm. Blood. 89:4501–13.

380. Chan JK, Suster S, Wenig BM, et al. (1997). Cytokeratin 20 immunoreactivity distinguishes Merkel cell (primary cutaneous neuroendocrine) carcinomas and salivary gland small cell carcinomas from small cell carcinomas of various sites. Am J Surg Pathol. 21:226–34.

381. Chan NG, Melega DE, Inculet RI, et al. (2003). Pulmonary sclerosing hemangioma with lymph node metastases. Can Respir J. 10:391–2.

382. Chandrashekar G (1995). Choriocarcinoma presenting as intracardiac (intracavitary) tumour. Int J Cardiol. 50:197.

383. Chang A, Amin A, Gabrielson E, et al. (2012). Utility of GATA3 immunohistochemistry in differentiating urothelial carcinoma from prostate adenocarcinoma and squamous cell carcinomas of the uterine cervix, anus, and lung. Am J Surg Pathol. 36:1472–6.

384. Chang JS, Young ML, Chuu WM, et al. (1992). Infantile cardiac hemangioendothelioma. Pediatr Cardiol. 13:52–5.

385. Chang T, Husain AN, Colby T, et al. (2007). Pneumocytic adenomyoepithelioma: a distinctive lung tumor with epithelial, myoepithelial, and pneumocytic differentiation. Am J Surg Pathol. 31:562–8.

386. Chang YL, Lee YC, Shih JY, et al. (2001). Pulmonary pleomorphic (spindle) cell carcinoma: peculiar clinicopathologic manifestations different from ordinary non-small cell carcinoma. Lung Cancer. 34:91–7.

387. Chang YL, Wu CT, Lee YC (2006). Mediastinal and retroperitoneal teratoma with focal gastrointestinal adenocarcinoma. J Thorac Oncol. 1:729–31.

388. Chang YL, Wu CT, Shih JY, et al. (2002). New aspects in clinicopathologic and oncogene studies of 23 pulmonary lymphoepithelioma-like carcinomas. Am J Surg Pathol. 26:715–23.

389. Chang YL, Wu CT, Shih JY, et al. (2011). EGFR and p53 status of pulmonary pleomorphic carcinoma: implications for EGFR tyrosine kinase inhibitors therapy of an aggressive lung malignancy. Ann Surg Oncol. 18:2952–60.

390. Chang YL, Wu CT, Shih JY, et al. (2011). Unique p53 and epidermal growth factor receptor gene mutation status in 46 pulmonary lymphoepithelioma-like carcinomas. Cancer Sci. 102:282–7.

391. Chanudet E, Adam P, Nicholson AG, et al. (2007). Chlamydiae and Mycoplasma infections in pulmonary MALT lymphoma. Br J Cancer. 97:949–51.

392. Chanudet E, Ye H, Ferry J, et al. (2009). A20 deletion is associated with copy number gain at the TNFA/B/C locus and occurs preferentially in translocation-negative MALT lymphoma of the ocular adnexa and salivary glands. J Pathol. 217:420–30.

393. Chao TY, Nieh S, Huang SH, et al. (1997). Cytology of fine needle aspirates of primary extragonadal germ cell tumors. Acta Cytol. 41:497–503.

394. Chapeau MC, Bui AD, Eugene F, et al. (1987). [Clear cell carcinoma of the thymus. Observation of a case of this exceptional variety of malignant thymoma]. Arch Anat Cytol Pathol. 35:179–82.

395. Chapman AD, Kerr KM (2000). The association between atypical adenomatous hyperplasia and primary lung cancer. Br J Cancer. 83:632–6.

396. Chariot P, Monnet I, Gaulard P, et al. (1993). Systemic mastocytosis following mediastinal germ cell tumor: an association confirmed. Hum Pathol. 24:111–2.

397. Charney DA, Charney JM, Ghali VS, et al. (1996). Primitive neuroectodermal tumor of the myocardium: a case report, review of the literature, immunohistochemical, and ultrastructural study. Hum Pathol. 27:1365–9.

398. Chaudary IU, Bojal SA, Attia A, et al. (2011). Mediastinal endodermal sinus tumor associated with fatal hemophagocytic syndrome. Hematol Oncol Stem Cell Ther. 4:138–41.

399. Chen B, Gao J, Chen H, et al. (2013). Pulmonary sclerosing hemangioma: a unique epithelial neoplasm of the lung (report of 26 cases). World J Surg Oncol. 11:85.

400. Chen F, Zhang S (2009). Diagnosis and treatment of the primary malignant meningioma in mediastinum: a case report. South Med J. 102:1164–6.

401. Chen G, Folpe AL, Colby TV, et al. (2011). Angiomatoid fibrous histiocytoma: unusual sites and unusual morphology. Mod Pathol. 24:1560–70.

402. Chen G, Marx A, Chen WH, et al. (2002). New WHO histologic classification predicts prognosis of thymic epithelial tumors: a clinicopathologic study of 200 thymoma cases from China. Cancer. 95:420–9.

403. Chen KT (1984). Squamous carcinoma of the thymus. J Surg Oncol. 25:61–3.

404. Chen M, Agrawal R, Nasseri-Nik N, et al. (2012). Indeterminate cell tumor of the spleen. Hum Pathol. 43:307–11.

405. Chen PC, Pan CC, Yang AH, et al. (2002). Detection of Epstein-Barr virus genome within thymic epithelial tumours in Taiwanese patients by nested PCR, PCR in situ hybridization, and RNA in situ hybridization. J Pathol. 197:684–8.

406. Chen TJ, Chiou CC, Chen CH, et al. (2008). Metastasis of mediastinal epithelioid angiosarcoma to the finger. Am J Clin Dermatol. 9:181–3.

407. Chen W, Chan CW, Mok C (1982). Malignant fibrous histiocytoma of the mediastinum. Cancer. 50:797–800.

408. Chen W, Lau SK, Fong D, et al. (2009). High frequency of clonal immunoglobulin receptor gene rearrangements in sporadic histiocytic/dendritic cell sarcomas. Am J Surg Pathol. 33:863–73.

409. Chen YB, Guo LC, Huang JA, et al. (2014). Clear cell tumor of the lung: a retrospective analysis. Am J Med Sci. 347:50–3.

410. Chen YB, Rahemtullah A, Hochberg E (2007). Primary effusion lymphoma. Oncologist. 12:569–76.

410A. Chen Z, Liu HB, Yu CH, et al. (2014). Diagnostic value of mutation specific antibodies for immunohistochemical detection of epidermal growth factor receptor mutations in non-small cell lung cancer: a meta-analysis. PLOS One 9:e105940.

411. Cheng JQ, Jhanwar SC, Klein WM, et al. (1994). p16 alterations and deletion mapping of 9p21-p22 in malignant mesothelioma. Cancer Res. 54:5547–51.

412. Cheng Y, Sheng W, Zhou X, et al. (2012). Pericardial synovial sarcoma, a potential for misdiagnosis: clinicopathologic and molecular cytogenetic analysis of three cases with literature review. Am J Clin Pathol. 137:142–9.

413. Chetritt J, Paradis V, Dargere D, et al. (1999). Chester-Erdheim disease: a neoplastic disorder. Hum Pathol. 30:1093–6.

414. Chetty R, Batitang S, Govender D (1997). Large cell neuroendocrine carcinoma of the thymus. Histopathology. 31:274–6.

415. Chetty R, Bhana B, Batitang S, et al. (1997). Lung carcinomas composed of rhabdoid cells. Eur J Surg Oncol. 23:432–4.

416. Cheuk W, Chan AC, Chan JK, et al. (2005). Metallic implant-associated lymphoma: a distinct subgroup of large B-cell lymphoma related to pyothorax-associated lymphoma? Am J Surg Pathol. 29:832–6.

417. Cheuk W, Cheung FY, Lee KC, et al. (2009). Cutaneous indeterminate dendritic cell tumor with a protracted relapsing clinical course. Am J Surg Pathol. 33:1261–3.

418. Cheuk W, Kwan MY, Suster S, et al. (2001). Immunostaining for thyroid transcription factor 1 and cytokeratin 20 aids the distinction of small cell carcinoma from Merkel cell carcinoma, but not pulmonary from extrapulmonary small cell carcinomas. Arch Pathol Lab Med. 125:228–31.

419. Cheuk W, Tsang WY, Chan JK (2005). Microthymoma: definition of the entity and distinction from nodular hyperplasia of the thymic epithelium (so-called microscopic thymoma). Am J Surg Pathol. 29:415–9.

420. Cheung M, Talarchek J, Schindeler K, et al. (2013). Further evidence for germline BAP1 mutations predisposing to melanoma and malignant mesothelioma. Cancer Genet. 206:206–10.

421. Chhatwal I, Dreyer F (1992). Isolation and characterization of dracotoxin from the venom of the greater weever fish Trachinus draco. Toxicon. 30:87–93.

422. Chhieng DC, Rose D, Ludwig ME, et al. (2000). Cytology of thymomas: emphasis on morphology and correlation with histologic subtypes. Cancer. 90:24–32.

423. Chick JF, Chauhan NR, Madan R (2013). Solitary fibrous tumors of the thorax: nomenclature, epidemiology, radiologic and pathologic findings, differential diagnoses, and management. AJR Am J Roentgenol. 200:W238–48.

424. Chilosi M, Zamo A, Brighenti A, et al. (2003). Constitutive expression of DeltaN-p63alpha isoform in human thymus and thymic epithelial tumours. Virchows Arch. 443:175–83.

425. Chinen K, Izumo T (2005). Cardiac involvement by malignant lymphoma: a clinicopathologic study of 25 autopsy cases based on the WHO classification. Ann Hematol. 84:498–505.

426. Chinen K, Tokuda Y, Fujiwara M, et al. (2010). Pulmonary tumor thrombotic microangiopathy in patients with gastric carcinoma: an analysis of 6 autopsy cases and review of the literature. Pathol Res Pract. 206:682–9.

427. Chintala K, Bloom DA, Walters HL 3rd, et al. (2004). Images in cardiology: Pericardial yolk sac tumor presenting as cardiac tamponade in a 21-month-old child. Clin Cardiol. 27:411.

428. Chiosea S, Krasinskas A, Cagle PT, et al. (2008). Diagnostic importance of 9p21 homozygous deletion in malignant mesotheliomas. Mod Pathol. 21:742–7.

429. Chiosea SI, Miller M, Seethala RR (2014). HRAS mutations in epithelial-myoepithelial carcinoma. Head Neck Pathol. 8:146–50.

430. Chirieac LR, Barletta JA, Yeap BY, et al. (2013). Clinicopathologic characteristics of malignant mesotheliomas arising in patients with a history of radiation for Hodgkin and non-Hodgkin lymphoma. J Clin Oncol. 31:4544–9.

431. Chirieac LR, Pinkus GS, Pinkus JL, et al. (2011). The immunohistochemical characterization of sarcomatoid malignant mesothelioma of the pleura. Am J Cancer Res. 1:14–24.

432. Chng WJ, Remstein ED, Fonseca R, et al. (2009). Gene expression profiling of pulmonary mucosa-associated lymphoid tissue lymphoma identifies new biologic insights with potential diagnostic and therapeutic applications. Blood. 113:635–45.

433. Cho WC, Jung SH, Lee SH, et al. (2012). Malignant peripheral nerve sheath tumor arising from the left ventricle. J Card Surg. 27:567–70.

434. Choi CH, Park CH, Kim JS, et al. (2013). Giant biatrial myxoma nearly obstructing the orifice of the inferior vena cava. J Cardiothorac Surg. 8:148.

435. Choi HS, Seol H, Heo IY, et al. (2012). Fine-needle aspiration cytology of pleomorphic carcinomas of the lung. Korean J Pathol. 46:576–82.

436. Choi JS, Choi JS, Kim EJ (2009). Primary pulmonary rhabdomyosarcoma in an adult with neurofibromatosis-1. Ann Thorac Surg. 88:1356–8.

437. Choi PC, To KF, Lai FM, et al. (2000). Follicular dendritic cell sarcoma of the neck: report of two cases complicated by pulmonary metastases. Cancer. 89:664–72.

438. Choi WW, Lui YH, Lau WH, et al. (2003). Adenocarcinoma of the thymus: report of two cases, including a previously undescribed mucinous subtype. Am J Surg Pathol. 27:124–30.

439. Choi WW, Weisenburger DD, Greiner TC, et al. (2009). A new immunostain algorithm classifies diffuse large B-cell lymphoma into molecular subtypes with high accuracy. Clin Cancer Res. 15:5494–502.

440. Choi YD, Kim JH, Nam JH, et al. (2008). Aggressive angiomyxoma of the lung. J Clin Pathol. 61:962–4.

441. Chou ST, Arkles LB, Gill GD, et al. (1983). Primary lymphoma of the heart. A case report. Cancer. 52:744–7.

442. Chow MB, Lim TC (2014). Massive mediastinal teratoma mimicking a pleural effusion on computed tomography. Singapore Med J. 55:e67–8.

443. Christensen BC, Godleski JJ, Marsit CJ, et al. (2008). Asbestos exposure predicts cell cycle control gene promoter methylation in pleural mesothelioma. Carcinogenesis. 29:1555–9.

444. Christie BI, Moremen JR (2012). Thymic carcinoma: incidence, classification and treatment strategies of a rare tumor. Am Surg. 78:E335–7.

445. Christodoulou J, Schoch C, Schnittger S, et al. (2004). Myelodysplastic syndrome (RARS) with +i(12p) abnormality in a patient 10 months after diagnosis and successful treatment of a mediastinal germ cell tumor (MGCT). Ann Hematol. 83:386–9.

446. Chu P, Wu E, Weiss LM (2000). Cytokeratin 7 and cytokeratin 20 expression in epithelial neoplasms: a survey of 435 cases. Mod Pathol. 13:962–72.

447. Chu PG, Schwarz RE, Lau SK, et al. (2005). Immunohistochemical staining in the diagnosis of pancreatobiliary and ampulla of Vater adenocarcinoma: application of CDX2, CK17, MUC1, and MUC2. Am J Surg Pathol. 29:359–67.

448. Chu PH, Yeh HI, Jung SM, et al. (2004). Irregular connexin43 expressed in a rare cardiac hamartoma containing adipose tissue in the crista terminalis. Virchows Arch. 444:383–6.

449. Chuang SC, Scelo G, Lee YC, et al. (2010). Risks of second primary cancer among patients with major histological types of lung cancers in both men and women. Br J Cancer. 102:1190–5.

450. Chubachi A, Miura I, Takahashi N, et al. (1993). Acute myelogenous leukemia associated with a mediastinal tumor. Leuk Lymphoma. 12:143–6.

451. Chun YS, Wang L, Nascimento AG, et al. (2005). Pediatric inflammatory myofibroblastic tumor: anaplastic lymphoma kinase (ALK) expression and prognosis. Pediatr Blood Cancer. 45:796–801.

452. Chung DA (2000). Thymic carcinoma--analysis of nineteen clinicopathological studies. Thorac Cardiovasc Surg. 48:114–9.

453. Chung JH, Choe G, Jheon S, et al. (2009). Epidermal growth factor receptor mutation and pathologic-radiologic correlation between multiple lung nodules with ground-glass opacity differentiates multicentric origin from intrapulmonary spread. J Thorac Oncol. 4:1490–5.

454. Church TR, Black WC, Aberle DR, et al. (2013). Results of initial low-dose computed tomographic screening for lung cancer. N Engl J Med. 368:1980–91.

455. Churg A, Allen T, Borczuk AC, et al. (2014). Well-differentiated Papillary Mesothelioma With Invasive Foci. Am J Surg Pathol. 38:990–8.

456. Churg A, Cagle P, Colby TV, et al. (2011). The fake fat phenomenon in organizing pleuritis: a source of confusion with desmoplastic malignant mesotheliomas. Am J Surg Pathol. 35:1823–9.

457. Churg A, Cagle PT, Roggli VL (2006). Tumors of the Serosal Membranes. AFIP Atlas of Tumor Pathology. 4th ed. Volume 3. Washington, DC: American Registry of Pathology.

458. Churg A, Colby TV, Cagle P, et al. (2000). The separation of benign and malignant mesothelial proliferations. Am J Surg Pathol. 24:1183–200.

459. Churg A, Galateau-Salle F (2012). The separation of benign and malignant mesothelial proliferations. Arch Pathol Lab Med. 136:1217–26.

460. Citterio A, Beghi E, Millul A, et al. (2009). Risk factors for tumor occurrence in patients with myasthenia gravis. J Neurol. 256:1221–7.

461. Clark OH (1988). Mediastinal parathyroid tumors. Arch Surg. 123:1096–100.

462. Clavel J, Steliarova-Foucher E, Berger C, et al. (2006). Hodgkin's disease incidence and survival in European children and adolescents (1978-1997): report from the Automated

Cancer Information System project. Eur J Cancer. 42:2037–49.
463. Clement PB, Young RH, Scully RE (1987). Endometrioid-like variant of ovarian yolk sac tumor. A clinicopathological analysis of eight cases. Am J Surg Pathol. 11:767–78.
464. Clin B, Andujar P, Abd Al Samad I, et al. (2012). Pulmonary carcinoid tumors and asbestos exposure. Ann Occup Hyg. 56:789–95.
465. Coe BP, Lee EH, Chi B, et al. (2006). Gain of a region on 7p22.3, containing MAD1L1, is the most frequent event in small-cell lung cancer cell lines. Genes Chromosomes Cancer. 45:11–9.
466. Coffin CM (1992). Congenital cardiac fibroma associated with Gorlin syndrome. Pediatr Pathol. 12:255–62.
467. Coffin CM, Hornick JL, Fletcher CD (2007). Inflammatory myofibroblastic tumor: comparison of clinicopathologic, histologic, and immunohistochemical features including ALK expression in atypical and aggressive cases. Am J Surg Pathol. 31:509–20.
468. Coffin CM, Jaszcz W, O'Shea PA, et al. (1994). So-called congenital-infantile fibrosarcoma: does it exist and what is it? Pediatr Pathol. 14:133–50.
469. Coffin CM, Patel A, Perkins S, et al. (2001). ALK1 and p80 expression and chromosomal rearrangements involving 2p23 in inflammatory myofibroblastic tumor. Mod Pathol. 14:569–76.
470. Cohen MB, Friend DS, Molnar JJ, et al. (1987). Gonadal endodermal sinus (yolk sac) tumor with pure intestinal differentiation: a new histologic type. Pathol Res Pract. 182:609–16.
471. Cohen R, Mirrer B, Loarte P, et al. (2013). Intrapericardial mature cystic teratoma in an adult: case presentation. Clin Cardiol. 36:6–9.
472. Cohen RE, Weaver MG, Montenegro HD, et al. (1990). Pulmonary blastoma with malignant melanoma component. Arch Pathol Lab Med. 114:1076–8.
473. Cohn SL, Pearson AD, London WB, et al. (2009). The International Neuroblastoma Risk Group (INRG) classification system: an INRG Task Force report. J Clin Oncol. 27:289–97.
474. Colby TV (1995). Malignancies in the lung and pleura mimicking benign processes. Semin Diagn Pathol. 12:30–44.
475. Colby TV (1999). Benign mesothelial cells in lymph node. Adv Anat Pathol. 6:41–8.
476. Colby TV (2012). Current histological diagnosis of lymphomatoid granulomatosis. Mod Pathol. 25 Suppl 1:S39–42.
477. Colby TV, Koss MN, Travis WD (1995). Tumors of the Lower Respiratory Tract. AFIP Atlas of Tumor Pathology. 3rd ed. Volume 13. Washington, DC: American Registry of Pathology.
478. Collins BT, Cramer HM (1996). Fine needle aspiration cytology of carcinoid tumors. Acta Cytol. 40:695–707.
479. Collins BT, Janney CG, Ong M, et al. (2009). Fine needle aspiration biopsy of monophasic spindle synovial sarcoma of lung with fluorescence in situ hybridization identification of t(x;18) translocation: a case report. Acta Cytol. 53:105–8.
480. Collins KA, Geisinger KR, Wakely PE Jr, et al. (1995). Extragonadal germ cell tumors: a fine-needle aspiration biopsy study. Diagn Cytopathol. 12:223–9.
481. Colombo C, Miceli R, Lazar AJ, et al. (2013). CTNNB1 45F mutation is a molecular prognosticator of increased postoperative primary desmoid tumor recurrence: an independent, multicenter validation study. Cancer. 119:3696–702.
482. Comiter CV, Kibel AS, Richie JP, et al. (1998). Prognostic features of teratomas with malignant transformation: a clinicopathological study of 21 cases. J Urol. 159:859–63.
483. Compton CC, Byrd DR, Garcia-Aguilar J, et al. (2012). AJCC Cancer Staging Atlas. A Companion to the Seventh Edition of the AJCC Cancer Staging Manual and Handbook. 2nd ed. New York: Springer.
484. Conlan AA, Payne WS, Woolner LB, et al. (1978). Adenoid cystic carcinoma (cylindroma) and mucoepidermoid carcinoma of the bronchus. Factors affecting survival. J Thorac Cardiovasc Surg. 76:369–77.
485. Conn JM, Goncalves MA, Mansour KA, et al. (1991). The mediastinal parathyroid. Am Surg. 57:62–6.
486. Connors JM (2011). Positron emission tomography in the management of Hodgkin lymphoma. Hematology (Am Soc Hematol Educ Program). 2011:317–22.
487. Conti VR, Saydjari R, Amparo EG (1986). Paraganglioma of the heart. The value of magnetic resonance imaging in the preoperative evaluation. Chest. 90:604–6.
488. Contreras AL, Punar M, Tamboli P, et al. (2010). Mediastinal germ cell tumors with an angiosarcomatous component: a report of 12 cases. Hum Pathol. 41:832–7.
489. Copie-Bergman C, Gaulard P, Maouche-Chretien L, et al. (1999). The MAL gene is expressed in primary mediastinal large B-cell lymphoma. Blood. 94:3567–75.
490. Copie-Bergman C, Plonquet A, Alonso MA, et al. (2002). MAL expression in lymphoid cells: further evidence for MAL as a distinct molecular marker of primary mediastinal large B-cell lymphomas. Mod Pathol. 15:1172–80.
491. Corbett R, Carter R, MacVicar D, et al. (1994). Embryonal rhabdomyosarcoma arising in a germ cell tumour. Med Pediatr Oncol. 23:497–502.
492. Cornea R, Lazar E, Dema A, et al. (2009). A nodular hyperplasia of the thymic epithelium (so-called microscopic thymoma). Rom J Morphol Embryol. 50:729–31.
493. Cornejo KM, Shi M, Akalin A, et al. (2013). Pulmonary papillary adenoma: a case report and review of the literature. J Bronchology Interv Pulmonol. 20:52–7.
494. Corrin B, Symmers WStC (2014). Systemic Pathology: The Lungs. Volume 5. 3rd ed. London: Churchill Livingstone.
495. Cosio BG, Villena V, Echave-Sustaeta J, et al. (2002). Endobronchial hamartoma. Chest. 122:202–5.
496. Coskun U, Gunel N, Yildirim Y, et al. (2002). Primary mediastinal yolk sac tumor in a 66-year-old woman. Med Princ Pract. 11:218–20.
497. Cote ML, Wenzlaff AS, Philip PA, et al. (2006). Secondary cancers after a lung carcinoid primary: a population-based analysis. Lung Cancer. 52:273–9.
498. Coupland SE, Charlotte F, Mansour G, et al. (2005). HHV-8-associated T-cell lymphoma in a lymph node with concurrent peritoneal effusion in an HIV-positive man. Am J Surg Pathol. 29:647–52.
499. Coustan-Smith E, Mullighan CG, Onciu M, et al. (2009). Early T-cell precursor leukaemia: a subtype of very high-risk acute lymphoblastic leukaemia. Lancet Oncol. 10:147–56.
500. Crespo C, Navarro M, Gonzalez I, et al. (2001). Intracranial and mediastinal inflammatory myofibroblastic tumour. Pediatr Radiol. 31:600–2.
501. Crispi S, Calogero RA, Santini M, et al. (2009). Global gene expression profiling of human pleural mesotheliomas: identification of matrix metalloproteinase 14 (MMP-14) as potential tumour target. PLoS ONE. 4:e7016.
502. Crispi S, Fagliarone C, Biroccio A, et al. (2010). Antiproliferative effect of Aurora kinase targeting in mesothelioma. Lung Cancer. 70:271–9.
503. Crona J, Bjorklund P, Welin S, et al. (2013). Treatment, prognostic markers and survival in thymic neuroendocrine tumours. a study from a single tertiary referral centre. Lung Cancer. 79:289–93.
504. Cross SF, Arbuckle S, Priest JR, et al. (2010). Familial pleuropulmonary blastoma in Australia. Pediatr Blood Cancer. 55:1417–9.
505. Croti UA, Braile DM, Moscardini AC, et al. (2008). [Solitary fibrous tumor in a child's heart]. Rev Bras Cir Cardiovasc. 23:139–41.
506. Crotty EJ, McAdams HP, Erasmus JJ, et al. (2000). Epithelioid hemangioendothelioma of the pleura: clinical and radiologic features. AJR Am J Roentgenol. 175:1545–9.
507. Crotty TB, Myers JL, Katzenstein AL, et al. (1994). Localized malignant mesothelioma. A clinicopathologic and flow cytometric study. Am J Surg Pathol. 18:357–63.
508. Cuadrado M, Garcia-Camarero T, Exposito V, et al. (2007). Cardiac intracavitary metastasis of a malignant solitary fibrous tumor: case report and review of the literature on sarcomas with left intracavitary extension. Cardiovasc Pathol. 16:241–7.
509. Cummings NM, Desai S, Thway K, et al. (2010). Cystic primary pulmonary synovial sarcoma presenting as recurrent pneumothorax: report of 4 cases. Am J Surg Pathol. 34:1176–9.
510. Cunningham-Rundles C, Cooper DL, Duffy TP, et al. (2002). Lymphomas of mucosal-associated lymphoid tissue in common variable immunodeficiency. Am J Hematol. 69:171–8.
511. Curry WA, McKay CE, Richardson RL, et al. (1981). Klinefelter's syndrome and mediastinal germ cell neoplasms. J Urol. 125:127–9.
512. Cushing B, Bhanot PK, Watts FB Jr, et al. (1983). Rhabdomyosarcoma and benign teratoma. Pediatr Pathol. 1:345–8.
513. Cushing B, Giller R, Cullen JW, et al. (2004). Randomized comparison of combination chemotherapy with etoposide, bleomycin, and either high-dose or standard-dose cisplatin in children and adolescents with high-risk malignant germ cell tumors: a pediatric intergroup study--Pediatric Oncology Group 9049 and Children's Cancer Group 8882. J Clin Oncol. 22:2691–700.
514. D'Angelo SP, Pietanza MC (2010). The molecular pathogenesis of small cell lung cancer. Cancer Biol Ther. 10:1–10.
515. D'Armiento J, Imai K, Schiltz J, et al. (2007). Identification of the benign mesenchymal tumor gene HMGA2 in lymphangiomyomatosis. Cancer Res. 67:1902–9.
516. da Cunha Santos G, Lai SW, Saieg MA, et al. (2012). Cyto-histologic agreement in pathologic subtyping of non small cell lung carcinoma: review of 602 fine needle aspirates with follow-up surgical specimens over a nine year period and analysis of factors underlying failure to subtype. Lung Cancer. 77:501–6.
517. da Silva SP, Resnick E, Lucas M, et al. (2011). Lymphoid proliferations of indeterminate malignant potential arising in adults with common variable immunodeficiency disorders: unusual case studies and immunohistological review in the light of possible causative events. J Clin Immunol. 31:784–91.
518. Dabbs CH, Peirce EC, Rawson FL (1957). Intrapericardial interatrial teratoma (bronchogenic cyst): report of a case correctly diagnosed and successfully removed. N Engl J Med. 256:541–6.
519. Dacic S, Finkelstein SD, Sasatomi E, et al. (2002). Molecular pathogenesis of pulmonary carcinosarcoma as determined by microdissection-based allelotyping. Am J Surg Pathol. 26:510–6.
520. Dacic S, Kothmaier H, Land S, et al. (2008). Prognostic significance of p16/cdkn2a loss in pleural malignant mesotheliomas. Virchows Arch. 453:627–35.
521. Dacic S, Sasatomi E, Swalsky PA, et al. (2004). Loss of heterozygosity patterns of sclerosing hemangioma of the lung and bronchioloalveolar carcinoma indicate a similar molecular pathogenesis. Arch Pathol Lab Med. 128:880–4.
522. Daddi N, Schiavon M, Filosso PL, et al. (2014). Prognostic factors in a multicentre study of 247 atypical pulmonary carcinoids. Eur J Cardiothorac Surg. 45:677–86.
523. Dainese E, Pozzi B, Milani M, et al. (2010). Primary pleural epithelioid angiosarcoma. A case report and review of the literature. Pathol Res Pract. 206:415–9.
524. Dal Cin P, De Wolf-Peeters C, Aly MS, et al. (1993). Ring chromosome 6 as the only change in a thymoma. Genes Chromosomes Cancer. 6:243–4.
525. Dal Cin P, De Wolf-Peeters C, Deneffe G, et al. (1996). Thymoma with a t(15;22)(p11;q11). Cancer Genet Cytogenet. 89:181–3.
526. Dal Cin P, Kools P, De Jonge I, et al. (1993). Rearrangement of 12q14-15 in pulmonary chondroid hamartoma. Genes Chromosomes Cancer. 8:131–3.
527. Dalal U, Jora MS, Dalal AK, et al. (2014). Primary germ cell tumor of the mediastinum - presenting as a huge mass. Int J Prev Med. 5:230–2.
528. Damadoglu E, Salturk C, Takir HB, et al. (2007). Mediastinal thymolipoma: an analysis of 10 cases. Respirology. 12:924–7.
529. Daniels CE, Myers JL, Utz JP, et al. (2007). Organizing pneumonia in patients with hematologic malignancies: a steroid-responsive lesion. Respir Med. 101:162–8.
530. Darvishian F, Farmer P (2001). Papillary fibroelastoma of the heart: report of two cases and review of the literature. Ann Clin Lab Sci. 31:291–6.
531. Dasanu CA, Shimanovsky A, Jain K, et al. (2013). Mediastinal choriocarcinoma presenting with syncope. Conn Med. 77:473–5.
532. Dasgupta A, Mahapatra M, Saxena R (2013). Flow cytometric immunophenotyping of regulatory T cells in chronic lymphocytic leukemia: comparative assessment of various markers and use of novel antibody panel with CD127 as alternative to transcription factor FoxP3. Leuk Lymphoma. 54:778–89.
533. Dauplat J, Hacker NF, Nieberg RK, et al. (1987). Distant metastases in epithelial ovarian carcinoma. Cancer. 60:1561–6.
534. Davies H, Bignell GR, Cox C, et al. (2002). Mutations of the BRAF gene in human cancer. Nature. 417:949–54.
535. Davies SJ, Gosney JR, Hansell DM, et al. (2007). Diffuse idiopathic pulmonary neuroendocrine cell hyperplasia: an under-recognised spectrum of disease. Thorax. 62:248–52.
537. Davis SD (1991). CT evaluation for pulmonary metastases in patients with extrathoracic malignancy. Radiology. 180:1–12.
538. Daya SK, Gowda RM, Gowda MR, et al. (2004). Thoracic cystic lymphangioma (cystic hygroma): a chest pain syndrome--a case report. Angiology. 55:561–4.
539. De Bruin ML, Burgers JA, Baas P, et al. (2009). Malignant mesothelioma after radiation treatment for Hodgkin lymphoma. Blood. 113:3679–81.
540. De Dominicis E, Frigiola A, Thiene G, et al. (1989). Subaortic stenosis by solitary rhabdomyoma. Successful excision in an infant following 2D echocardiogram and Doppler diagnosis. Chest. 95:470–2.
541. de Jong D, Richel DJ, Schenkeveld C, et al. (1997). Oligoclonal peripheral T-cell lymphocytosis as a result of aberrant T-cell development in a cortical thymoma. Diagn Mol Pathol. 6:244–8.
542. de Jong J, Stoop H, Gillis AJ, et al. (2008). Differential expression of SOX17 and SOX2 in germ cells and stem cells has biological and clinical implications. J Pathol. 215:21–30.
543. de Jong WK, Blaauwgeers JL, Schaapveld M, et al. (2008). Thymic epithelial tumours: a population-based study of the incidence, diagnostic procedures and therapy. Eur J Cancer. 44:123–30.
544. de Krijger RR, Claessen SM, van der Ham F, et al. (2007). Gain of chromosome 8q is a frequent finding in pleuropulmonary blastoma. Mod Pathol. 20:1191–9.

545. de Leon GA, Zaeri N, Donner RM, et al. (1990). Cerebral rhinocele, hydrocephalus, and cleft lip and palate in infants with cardiac fibroma. J Neurol Sci. 99:27–36.

546. de Leval L, Ferry JA, Falini B, et al. (2001). Expression of bcl-6 and CD10 in primary mediastinal large B-cell lymphoma: evidence for derivation from germinal center B cells? Am J Surg Pathol. 25:1277–82.

547. De Leyn P, Dooms C, Kuzdzal J, et al. (2014). Revised ESTS guidelines for preoperative mediastinal lymph node staging for non-small-cell lung cancer. Eur J Cardiothorac Surg. 45:787–98.

548. De Leyn P, Lardinois D, Van Schil PE, et al. (2007). ESTS guidelines for preoperative lymph node staging for non-small cell lung cancer. Eur J Cardiothorac Surg. 32:1–8.

549. de Montpreville V, Macchiarini P, Dulmet E (1996). Thymic neuroendocrine carcinoma (carcinoid): a clinicopathologic study of fourteen cases. J Thorac Cardiovasc Surg. 111:134–41.

550. de Montpreville V, Serraf A, Aznag H, et al. (2001). Fibroma and inflammatory myofibroblastic tumor of the heart. Ann Diagn Pathol. 5:335–42.

551. de Montpreville V, Zemoura L, Vaksmann G, et al. (2004). Endocardial location of familial myofibromatosis revealed by cerebral embolization: cardiac counterpart of the frequent intravascular growth of the disease? Virchows Arch. 444:300–3.

552. De Nictolis M, Goteri G, Campanati G, et al. (1995). Elastofibrolipoma of the mediastinum. A previously undescribed benign tumor containing abnormal elastic fibers. Am J Surg Pathol. 19:364–7.

553. De Oliveira Duarte Achcar R, Nikiforova MN, Yousem SA (2009). Micropapillary lung adenocarcinoma: EGFR, K-ras, and BRAF mutational profile. Am J Clin Pathol. 131:694–700.

554. de Perrot M, Spiliopoulos A, Fischer S, et al. (2002). Neuroendocrine carcinoma (carcinoid) of the thymus associated with Cushing's syndrome. Ann Thorac Surg. 73:675–81.

555. de Queiroga EM, Chikota H, Bacchi CE, et al. (2004). Rhabdomyomatous carcinoma of the thymus. Am J Surg Pathol. 28:1245–50.

556. De Rosa N, Maiorino A, De Rosa I, et al. (2012). CD34 Expression in the Stromal Cells of Alveolar Adenoma. Case Rep Med. 2012:913517.

557. De Santis M, Bokemeyer C, Becherer A, et al. (2001). Predictive impact of 2-18fluoro-2-deoxy-D-glucose positron emission tomography for residual postchemotherapy masses in patients with bulky seminoma. J Clin Oncol. 19:3740–4.

558. de Wilt JH, Farmer SE, Scolyer RA, et al. (2005). Isolated melanoma in the lung where there is no known primary site: metastatic disease or primary lung tumour? Melanoma Res. 15:531–7.

559. de Winkel N, Becker K, Vogt M (2010). Echogenic mass in the right atrium after surgical ventricular septal defect closure: thrombus or tumour? Cardiol Young. 20:86–8.

560. Debelenko LV, Brambilla E, Agarwal SK, et al. (1997). Identification of MEN1 gene mutations in sporadic carcinoid tumors of the lung. Hum Mol Genet. 6:2285–90.

561. Debelenko LV, Swalwell JI, Kelley MJ, et al. (2000). MEN1 gene mutation analysis of high-grade neuroendocrine lung carcinoma. Genes Chromosomes Cancer. 28:58–65.

562. Deetjen AG, Conradi G, Mollmann S, et al. (2006). Cardiac angiosarcoma diagnosed and characterized by cardiac magnetic resonance imaging. Cardiol Rev. 14:101–3.

563. Degan S, Lopez GY, Kevill K, et al. (2008). Gastrin-releasing peptide, immune responses, and lung disease. Ann N Y Acad Sci. 1144:136–47.

564. Dehner LP (1990). Germ cell tumors of the mediastinum. Semin Diagn Pathol. 7:266–84.

565. Dei Tos AP (2006). Classification of pleomorphic sarcomas: where are we now? Histopathology. 48:51–62.

566. Delaney SE, Wermers RA, Thompson GB, et al. (1999). Mediastinal parathyroid carcinoma. Endocr Pract. 5:133–6.

567. DeLellis RA, Lloyd RV, Heitz PU, et al., eds. (2004). WHO Classification of Tumours. Pathology and Genetics of Tumours of Endocrine Organs. 3rd ed. Lyon: IARC.

568. Dell'Amore A, Lanzanova G, Silenzi A, et al. (2011). Hamartoma of mature cardiac myocytes: case report and review of the literature. Heart Lung Circ. 20:336–40.

569. Delpiano C, Claren R, Sironi M, et al. (2000). Cytological appearance of papillary mucous gland adenoma of the left lobar bronchus with histological confirmation. Cytopathology. 11:193–6.

570. DeMent SH, Eggleston JC, Spivak JL (1985). Association between mediastinal germ cell tumors and hematologic malignancies. Report of two cases and review of the literature. Am J Surg Pathol. 9:23–30.

571. Demir HA, Yalcin B, Buyukpamukcu N, et al. (2010). Thoracic neuroblastic tumors in childhood. Pediatr Blood Cancer. 54:885–9.

572. den Bakker MA, Beverloo BH, van den Heuvel-Eibrink MM, et al. (2009). NUT midline carcinoma of the parotid gland with mesenchymal differentiation. Am J Surg Pathol. 33:1253–8.

573. den Bakker MA, Oosterhuis JW (2009). Tumours and tumour-like conditions of the thymus other than thymoma; a practical approach. Histopathology. 54:69–89.

574. den Bakker MA, Thunnissen FB (2013). Neuroendocrine tumours--challenges in the diagnosis and classification of pulmonary neuroendocrine tumours. J Clin Pathol. 66:862–9.

575. den Bakker MA, Willemsen S, Grunberg K, et al. (2010). Small cell carcinoma of the lung and large cell neuroendocrine carcinoma interobserver variability. Histopathology. 56:356–63.

576. Deora S, Gurmukhani S, Shah S, et al. (2013). Cardiac epithelioid leiomyosarcoma as both intracardiac and pericardial mass with massive pericardial effusion: a rare presentation. J Am Coll Cardiol. 62:e25.

577. DePond W, Said JW, Tasaka T, et al. (1997). Kaposi's sarcoma-associated herpesvirus and human herpesvirus 8 (KSHV/HHV8)-associated lymphoma of the bowel. Report of two cases in HIV-positive men with secondary effusion lymphomas. Am J Surg Pathol. 21:719–24.

578. Derenoncourt AN, Castro-Magana M, Jones KL (1995). Mediastinal teratoma and precocious puberty in a boy with mosaic Klinefelter syndrome. Am J Med Genet. 55:38–42.

579. Derkay CS, Wiatrak B (2008). Recurrent respiratory papillomatosis: a review. Laryngoscope. 118:1236–47.

580. Desai SB, Pradhan SA, Chinoy RF (2000). Mediastinal Castleman's disease complicated by follicular dendritic cell tumour. Indian J Cancer. 37:129–32.

581. Desai TJ, Brownfield DG, Krasnow MA (2014). Alveolar progenitor and stem cells in lung development, renewal and cancer. Nature. 507:190–4.

582. Dessy E, Braidotti P, Del Curto B, et al. (2000). Peripheral papillary tumor of type-II pneumocytes: a rare neoplasm of undetermined malignant potential. Virchows Arch. 436:289–95.

583. Detterbeck F, Youssef S, Ruffini E, et al. (2011). A review of prognostic factors in thymic malignancies. J Thorac Oncol. 6:S1698–704.

584. Detterbeck FC (2006). Clinical value of the WHO classification system of thymoma. Ann Thorac Surg. 81:2328–34.

585. Detterbeck FC, Nicholson AG, Kondo K, et al. (2011). The Masaoka-Koga stage classification for thymic malignancies: clarification and definition of terms. J Thorac Oncol. 6:S1710–6.

586. Detterbeck FC, Parsons AM (2004). Thymic tumors. Ann Thorac Surg. 77:1860–9.

586A. Detterbeck F, Stratton K, Giroux D, et al. (2014). The IASLC/ITMIG Thymic Epithelial Tumors Staging Project: Proposal for an Evidence-Based Stage Classification System for the Forthcoming (8th) Edition of the TNM Classification of Malignant Tumors. J Thorac Oncol. 9(9 Suppl 2):S65–72.

587. Dettmer P, Beck M, Eufinger H, et al. (2009). Bilateral cystic pulmonary glial heterotopia and palatinal teratoma causing respiratory distress in an infant. J Pediatr Surg. 44:2206–10.

588. Dettrick A, Meikle A, Fong KM (2014). Fine-needle aspiration diagnosis of sclerosing hemangioma (pneumocytoma): report of a case and review of the literature. Diagn Cytopathol. 42:242–6.

589. Deutsch M, Land SR, Begovic M, et al. (2007). An association between postoperative radiotherapy for primary breast cancer in 11 National Surgical Adjuvant Breast and Bowel Project (NSABP) studies and the subsequent appearance of pleural mesothelioma. Am J Clin Oncol. 30:294–6.

590. Devarakonda S, Morgensztern D, Govindan R (2013). Clinical applications of The Cancer Genome Atlas project (TCGA) for squamous cell lung carcinoma. Oncology (Williston Park). 27:899–906.

591. Devesa SS, Bray F, Vizcaino AP, et al. (2005). International lung cancer trends by histologic type: male:female differences diminishing and adenocarcinoma rates rising. Int J Cancer. 117:294–9.

592. Devouassoux-Shisheboran M, de la Fouchardiere A, Thivolet-Bejui F, et al. (2004). Endobronchial variant of sclerosing hemangioma of the lung: histological and cytological features on endobronchial material. Mod Pathol. 17:252–7.

593. Devouassoux-Shisheboran M, Hayashi T, Linnoila RI, et al. (2000). A clinicopathologic study of 100 cases of pulmonary sclerosing hemangioma with immunohistochemical studies: TTF-1 is expressed in both round and surface cells, suggesting an origin from primitive respiratory epithelium. Am J Surg Pathol. 24:906–16.

594. Dewaele B, Floris G, Finalet-Ferreiro J, et al. (2010). Coactivated platelet-derived growth factor receptor {alpha} and epidermal growth factor receptor are potential therapeutic targets in intimal sarcoma. Cancer Res. 70:7304–14.

595. Dexeus FH, Logothetis CJ, Chong C, et al. (1988). Genetic abnormalities in men with germ cell tumors. J Urol. 140:80–4.

596. Deyrup AT, Miettinen M, North PE, et al. (2009). Angiosarcomas arising in the viscera and soft tissue of children and young adults: a clinicopathologic study of 15 cases. Am J Surg Pathol. 33:264–9.

597. Di Cataldo A, Villari L, Milone P, et al. (2000). Thymic carcinoma, systemic lupus erythematosus, and hypertrophic pulmonary osteoarthropathy in an 11-year-old boy: a novel association. Pediatr Hematol Oncol. 17:701–6.

598. Di Maria MV, Campbell DN, Mitchell MB, et al. (2008). Successful orthotopic heart transplant in an infant with an inflammatory myofibroblastic tumor of the left ventricle. J Heart Lung Transplant. 27:792–6.

599. Di Tommaso L, Chiesa G, Arena V, et al. (2012). Cardiac hibernoma: a case report. Histopathology. 61:985–7.

600. Di Tommaso L, Kuhn E, Kurrer M, et al. (2007). Thymic tumor with adenoid cystic carcinomalike features: a clinicopathologic study of 4 cases. Am J Surg Pathol. 31:1161–7.

601. Dijkhuizen T, de Jong B, Meuzelaar JJ, et al. (2001). No cytogenetic evidence for involvement of gene(s) at 2p16 in sporadic cardiac myxomas: cytogenetic changes in ten sporadic cardiac myxomas. Cancer Genet Cytogenet. 126:162–5.

602. Dikensoy O (2008). Mesothelioma due to environmental exposure to erionite in Turkey. Curr Opin Pulm Med. 14:322–5.

603. Dillon KM, Hill CM, Cameron CH, et al. (2002). Mediastinal mixed dendritic cell sarcoma with hybrid features. J Clin Pathol. 55:791–4.

604. Dishop MK, McKay EM, Kreiger PA, et al. (2010). Fetal lung interstitial tumor (FLIT): A proposed newly recognized lung tumor of infancy to be differentiated from cystic pleuropulmonary blastoma and other developmental pulmonary lesions. Am J Surg Pathol. 34:1762–72.

605. Disibio G, French SW (2008). Metastatic patterns of cancers: results from a large autopsy study. Arch Pathol Lab Med. 132:931–9.

606. Dogan S, Shen R, Ang DC, et al. (2012). Molecular epidemiology of EGFR and KRAS mutations in 3,026 lung adenocarcinomas: higher susceptibility of women to smoking-related KRAS-mutant cancers. Clin Cancer Res. 18:6169–77.

607. Doglioni C, Bontempini L, Iuzzolino P, et al. (1988). Ependymoma of the mediastinum. Arch Pathol Lab Med. 112:194–6.

608. Doglioni C, Dell'Orto P, Zanetti G, et al. (1990). Cytokeratin-immunoreactive cells of human lymph nodes and spleen in normal and pathological conditions. An immunocytochemical study. Virchows Arch A Pathol Anat Histopathol. 416:479–90.

609. Dohi T, Ohmura H, Daida H, et al. (2009). Primary right atrial cardiac osteosarcoma with congestive heart failure. Eur J Cardiothorac Surg. 35:544–6.

610. Dojcinov SD, Venkataraman G, Pittaluga S, et al. (2011). Age-related EBV-associated lymphoproliferative disorders in the Western population: a spectrum of reactive lymphoid hyperplasia and lymphoma. Blood. 117:4726–35.

611. Domingo A, Romagosa V, Callis M, et al. (1989). Mediastinal germ cell tumor and acute megakaryoblastic leukemia. Ann Intern Med. 111:539.

612. Dominguez-Malagon H, Guerrero-Medrano J, Suster S (1995). Ectopic poorly differentiated (insular) carcinoma of the thyroid. Report of a case presenting as an anterior mediastinal mass. Am J Clin Pathol. 104:408–12.

613. Domont J, Salas S, Lacroix L, et al. (2010). High frequency of beta-catenin heterozygous mutations in extra-abdominal fibromatosis: a potential molecular tool for disease management. Br J Cancer. 102:1032–6.

614. Donadio AC, Motzer RJ, Bajorin DF, et al. (2003). Chemotherapy for teratoma with malignant transformation. J Clin Oncol. 21:4285–91.

615. Donsbeck AV, Ranchere D, Coindre JM, et al. (1999). Primary cardiac sarcomas: an immunohistochemical and grading study with long-term follow-up of 24 cases. Histopathology. 34:295–304.

616. Dorfman DM, Shahsafaei A, Chan JK (1997). Thymic carcinomas, but not thymomas and carcinomas of other sites, show CD5 immunoreactivity. Am J Surg Pathol. 21:936–40.

617. Doros L, Yang J, Dehner L, et al. (2012). DICER1 mutations in embryonal rhabdomyosarcomas from children with and without familial PPB-tumor predisposition syndrome. Pediatr Blood Cancer. 59:558–60.

618. Dosaka-Akita H, Cagle PT, Hiroumi H, et al. (2000). Differential retinoblastoma and p16(INK4A) protein expression in neuroendocrine tumors of the lung. Cancer. 88:550–6.

619. Dotto J, Pelosi G, Rosai J (2007). Expression of p63 in thymomas and normal thymus. Am J Clin Pathol. 127:415–20.

620. Downes MR, Torlakovic EE, Aldaoud N, et al. (2013). Diagnostic utility of androgen receptor expression in discriminating poorly differentiated urothelial and prostate carcinoma. J Clin Pathol. 66:779–86.

621. Downie PA, Vogelzang NJ, Moldwin RL, et al. (1994). Establishment of a leukemia cell line with i(12p) from a patient with a mediastinal germ cell tumor and acute lymphoblastic leukemia. Cancer Res. 54:4999–5004.
622. Doyle CT, Bolster MA (1992). The medico-legal organization of a mass disaster--the Air India crash 1985. Med Sci Law. 32:5–8.
623. Doyle LA, Fletcher CD (2013). Predicting behavior of solitary fibrous tumor: are we getting closer to more accurate risk assessment? Ann Surg Oncol. 20:4055–6.
624. Doyle LA, Vivero M, Fletcher CD, et al. (2014). Nuclear expression of STAT6 distinguishes solitary fibrous tumor from histologic mimics. Mod Pathol. 27:390–5.
625. Dragoescu EA, Liu L (2013). Pericardial fluid cytology: an analysis of 128 specimens over a 6-year period. Cancer Cytopathol. 121:242–51.
626. Drexler HG, Gignac SM, von Wasielewski R, et al. (2000). Pathobiology of NPM-ALK and variant fusion genes in anaplastic large cell lymphoma and other lymphomas. Leukemia. 14:1533–59.
626A. Drilon A, Rekhtman N, Ladanyi M, et al. (2012). Squamous-cell carcinomas of the lung: emerging biology, controversies, and the promise of targeted therapy. Lancet Oncol. 13:e418–26.
627. Drilon A, Wang L, Hasanovic A, et al. (2013). Response to Cabozantinib in patients with RET fusion-positive lung adenocarcinomas. Cancer Discov. 3:630–5.
628. Drut R, Pollono D (1998). Pleuropulmonary blastoma: diagnosis by fine-needle aspiration cytology: a case report. Diagn Cytopathol. 19:303–5.
629. Du EZ, Goldstraw P, Zacharias J, et al. (2004). TTF-1 expression is specific for lung primary in typical and atypical carcinoids: TTF-1-positive carcinoids are predominantly in peripheral location. Hum Pathol. 35:825–31.
630. Duarte IG, Gal AA, Mansour KA (1998). Primary malignant melanoma of the trachea. Ann Thorac Surg. 65:559–60.
631. Dubois SG, London WB, Zhang Y, et al. (2008). Lung metastases in neuroblastoma at initial diagnosis: A report from the International Neuroblastoma Risk Group (INRG) project. Pediatr Blood Cancer. 51:589–92.
631A. Ducassou S, Seyrig F, Thomas C, et al. (2013). Thymus and mediastinal node involvement in childhood Langerhans cell histiocytosis: long-term follow-up from the French national cohort. Pediatr Blood Cancer. 60:1759–65.
632. Dudgeon DL, Haller JA Jr (1984). Pediatric lipoblastomatosis: two unusual cases. Surgery. 95:371–3.
633. Dugan JM (1995). Cytologic diagnosis of basal cell (basaloid) carcinoma of the lung. A report of two cases. Acta Cytol. 39:539–42.
634. Dulmet EM, Macchiarini P, Suc B, et al. (1993). Germ cell tumors of the mediastinum. A 30-year experience. Cancer. 72:1894–901.
635. Dulmet-Brender E, Jaubert F, Huchon G (1986). Exophytic endobronchial epidermoid carcinoma. Cancer. 57:1358–64.
636. Dundr P, Fischerova D, Povysil C, et al. (2008). Primary pure large-cell neuroendocrine carcinoma of the ovary. Pathol Res Pract. 204:133–7.
637. Dungo RT, Keating GM (2013). Afatinib: first global approval. Drugs. 73:1503–15.
638. Dunleavy K, Grant C, Eberle FC, et al. (2012). Gray zone lymphoma: better treated like hodgkin lymphoma or mediastinal large B-cell lymphoma? Curr Hematol Malig Rep. 7:241–7.
639. Dunleavy K, Pittaluga S, Maeda LS, et al. (2013). Dose-adjusted EPOCH-rituximab therapy in primary mediastinal B-cell lymphoma. N Engl J Med. 368:1408–16.
640. Dunleavy K, Roschewski M, Wilson WH (2012). Lymphomatoid granulomatosis and other Epstein-Barr virus associated lymphoproliferative processes. Curr Hematol Malig Rep. 7:208–15.
641. Dunn PJ (1984). Pancreatic endocrine tissue in benign mediastinal teratoma. J Clin Pathol. 37:1105–9.
642. Dupin N, Fisher C, Kellam P, et al. (1999). Distribution of human herpesvirus-8 latently infected cells in Kaposi's sarcoma, multicentric Castleman's disease, and primary effusion lymphoma. Proc Natl Acad Sci USA. 96:4546–51.
643. Dursun AB, Demirag F, Bayiz H, et al. (2005). Endobronchial metastases: a clinicopathological analysis. Respirology. 10:510–4.
644. Dutta R, Kumar A, Julka PK, et al. (2010). Thymic neuroendocrine tumour (carcinoid): clinicopathological features of four patients with different presentation. Interact Cardiovasc Thorac Surg. 11:732–6.
645. Duwe BV, Sterman DH, Musani AI (2005). Tumors of the mediastinum. Chest. 128:2893–909.
646. Dy GK, Miller AA, Mandrekar SJ, et al. (2005). A phase II trial of imatinib (ST1571) in patients with c-kit expressing relapsed small-cell lung cancer: a CALGB and NCCTG study. Ann Oncol. 16:1811–6.
647. Eberhard DA, Johnson BE, Amler LC, et al. (2005). Mutations in the epidermal growth factor receptor and in KRAS are predictive and prognostic indicators in patients with non-small-cell lung cancer treated with chemotherapy alone and in combination with erlotinib. J Clin Oncol. 23:5900–9.
648. Eberle FC, Mani H, Jaffe ES (2009). Histopathology of Hodgkin's lymphoma. Cancer J. 15:129–37.
649. Eberle FC, Rodriguez-Canales J, Wei L, et al. (2011). Methylation profiling of mediastinal gray zone lymphoma reveals a distinctive signature with elements shared by classical Hodgkin's lymphoma and primary mediastinal large B-cell lymphoma. Haematologica. 96:558–66.
650. Eberle FC, Salaverria I, Steidl C, et al. (2011). Gray zone lymphoma: chromosomal aberrations with immunophenotypic and clinical correlations. Mod Pathol. 24:1586–97.
651. Eberle MC, Boudousq V, Becassis P, et al. (2002). Cardiac rhabdomyoma in an adult: an aspect of Tc-99m sestamibi myocardial perfusion. J Nucl Cardiol. 9:131–2.
652. Economopoulos GC, Lewis JW Jr, Lee MW, et al. (1990). Carcinoid tumors of the thymus. Ann Thorac Surg. 50:58–61.
652A. Edge S, Byrd DR, Compton CC, Fritz AG, Greene FL, Trotti A, eds. (2010). AJCC Cancer Staging Manual. 7th ed. New York (NY): Springer.
653. Edge SB, Byrd DR, Compton CC, et al. (2010). Pleural Mesothelioma. In: Edge S, Byrd DR, Compton CC, Fritz AG, Greene FL, Trotti A, eds. AJCC Cancer Staging Manual, 7th ed. New York (NY): Springer; pp. 271–7.
654. Edge SB, Compton CC (2010). The American Joint Committee on Cancer: the 7th edition of the AJCC cancer staging manual and the future of TNM. Ann Surg Oncol. 17: 1471–1474.
655. Edwards FH, Hale D, Cohen A, et al. (1991). Primary cardiac valve tumors. Ann Thorac Surg. 52:1127–31.
656. Egan AJ, Boardman LA, Tazelaar HD, et al. (1999). Erdheim-Chester disease: clinical, radiologic, and histopathologic findings in five patients with interstitial lung disease. Am J Surg Pathol. 23:17–26.
657. Eimoto T, Kitaoka M, Ogawa H, et al. (2002). Thymic sarcomatoid carcinoma with skeletal muscle differentiation: report of two cases, one with cytogenetic analysis. Histopathology. 40:46–57.
658. Eini R, Stoop H, Gillis AJ, et al. (2014). Role of SOX2 in the etiology of embryonal carcinoma, based on analysis of the NCCIT and NT2 cell lines. PLoS ONE. 9:e83585.
659. Ejaz S, Vassilopoulou-Sellin R, Busaidy NL, et al. (2011). Cushing syndrome secondary to ectopic adrenocorticotropic hormone secretion: the University of Texas MD Anderson Cancer Center Experience. Cancer. 117:4381–9.
660. El Hajj L, Mazieres J, Rouquette I, et al. (2005). Diagnostic value of bronchoscopy, CT and transbronchial biopsies in diffuse pulmonary lymphangiomatosis: case report and review of the literature. Clin Radiol. 60:921–5.
661. El-Osta HE, Yammine YS, Chehab BM, et al. (2008). Unexplained hemopericardium as a presenting feature of primary cardiac angiosarcoma: a case report and a review of the diagnostic dilemma. J Thorac Oncol. 3:800–2.
662. Elbardissi AW, Dearani JA, Daly RC, et al. (2008). Analysis of benign ventricular tumors: long-term outcome after resection. J Thorac Cardiovasc Surg. 135:1061–8.
663. Elbardissi AW, Dearani JA, Daly RC, et al. (2008). Survival after resection of primary cardiac tumors: a 48-year experience. Circulation. 118:S7–15.
664. Elkiran O, Karakurt C, Erdil N, et al. (2013). An unexpected cause of respiratory distress and cyanosis: cardiac inflammatory myofibroblastic tumor. Congenit Heart Dis. 8:E174–7.
665. Ellis PM, Blais N, Soulieres D, et al. (2011). A systematic review and Canadian consensus recommendations on the use of biomarkers in the treatment of non-small cell lung cancer. J Thorac Oncol. 6:1379–91.
666. Elmes PC, Simpson JC (1976). The clinical aspects of mesothelioma. Q J Med. 45:427–49.
667. Elnayal A, Moran CA, Fox PS, et al. (2013). Primary salivary gland-type lung cancer: imaging and clinical predictors of outcome. AJR Am J Roentgenol. 201:W57–63.
668. Elouazzani H, Zouaidia F, Jahid A, et al. (2012). Primary endobronchial leiomyosarcoma of the lung: clinical, gross and microscopic findings of two cases. J Clin Imaging Sci. 2:35.
669. Ema T, Kawano R (2014). Myelolipoma of the posterior mediastinum: report of a case. Gen Thorac Cardiovasc Surg. Gen Thorac Cardiovasc Surg. 62:241–3.
670. Emerson LL, Layfield LJ (2012). Solitary peripheral pulmonary papilloma evaluation on frozen section: a potential pitfall for the pathologist. Pathol Res Pract. 208:726–9.
671. En-Nafaa I, El Ounani F, Latib R, et al. (2010). [Ewing sarcoma of the anterior mediastinum: a rare tumor localization]. J Radiol. 91:1287–8.
672. Endo A, Ohtahara A, Kinugawa T, et al. (1997). Characteristics of 161 patients with cardiac tumors diagnosed during 1993 and 1994 in Japan. Am J Cardiol. 79:1708–11.
673. Endo A, Ohtahara A, Kinugawa T, et al. (2002). Characteristics of cardiac myxoma with constitutional signs: a multicenter study in Japan. Clin Cardiol. 25:367–70.
674. Engel PJ (2000). Absence of latent Epstein-Barr virus in thymic epithelial tumors as demonstrated by Epstein-Barr-encoded RNA(EBER) in situ hybridization. APMIS. 108:393–7.
675. Engel PJ, Sabroe S (1997). [Thymomoa in Denmark]. Ugeskr Laeger. 159:3155–9.
676. Engelman JA, Zejnullahu K, Mitsudomi T, et al. (2007). MET amplification leads to gefitinib resistance in lung cancer by activating ERBB3 signaling. Science. 316:1039–43.
677. Engels EA (2010). Epidemiology of thymoma and associated malignancies. J Thorac Oncol. 5:S260–5.
678. England DM, Hochholzer L (1995). Truly benign "bronchial adenoma". Report of 10 cases of mucous gland adenoma with immunohistochemical and ultrastructural findings. Am J Surg Pathol. 19:887–99.
679. England DM, Hochholzer L, McCarthy MJ (1989). Localized benign and malignant fibrous tumors of the pleura. A clinicopathologic review of 223 cases. Am J Surg Pathol. 13:640–58.
680. Engleson J, Soller M, Panagopoulos I, et al. (2006). Midline carcinoma with t(15;19) and BRD4-NUT fusion oncogene in a 30-year-old female with response to docetaxel and radiotherapy. BMC Cancer. 6:69.
681. Erlander MG, Ma XJ, Kesty NC, et al. (2011). Performance and clinical evaluation of the 92-gene real-time PCR assay for tumor classification. J Mol Diagn. 13:493–503.
682. Errani C, Sung YS, Zhang L, et al. (2012). Monoclonality of multifocal epithelioid hemangioendothelioma of the liver by analysis of WWTR1-CAMTA1 breakpoints. Cancer Genet. 205:12–7.
683. Errani C, Zhang L, Sung YS, et al. (2011). A novel WWTR1-CAMTA1 gene fusion is a consistent abnormality in epithelioid hemangioendothelioma of different anatomic sites. Genes Chromosomes Cancer. 50:644–53.
684. Ertel V, Fruh M, Guenther A, et al. (2013). Thymoma with molecularly verified "conversion" to T lymphoblastic leukemia/lymphoma over 9 years. Leuk Lymphoma. 54:2765–8.
685. Ertugrul T, Dindar A, Elmaci TT, et al. (2001). An intrapericardial teratoma with endocrine function. J Cardiovasc Surg (Torino). 42:781–3.
686. Essary LR, Vargas SO, Fletcher CD (2002). Primary pleuropulmonary synovial sarcoma: reappraisal of a recently described anatomic subset. Cancer. 94:459–69.
687. Estrozi B, Queiroga E, Bacchi CE, et al. (2006). Myxopapillary ependymoma of the posterior mediastinum. Ann Diagn Pathol. 10:283–7.
688. Etienne-Mastroianni B, Falchero L, Chalabreysse L, et al. (2002). Primary sarcomas of the lung: a clinicopathologic study of 12 cases. Lung Cancer. 38:283–9.
689. Evans AG, French CA, Cameron MJ, et al. (2012). Pathologic characteristics of NUT midline carcinoma arising in the mediastinum. Am J Surg Pathol. 36:1222–7.
690. Ewing CA, Zakowski MF, Lin O (2004). Monophasic synovial sarcoma: a cytologic spectrum. Diagn Cytopathol. 30:19–23.
691. Eymin B, Gazzeri S, Brambilla C, et al. (2001). Distinct pattern of E2F1 expression in human lung tumours: E2F1 is upregulated in small cell lung carcinoma. Oncogene. 20:1678–87.
692. Fabozzi SJ, Newton JR Jr, Moriarty RP, et al. (1995). Malignant pericardial effusion as initial solitary site of metastasis from transitional cell carcinoma of the bladder. Urology. 45:320–2.
693. Fabre D, Fadel E, Singhal S, et al. (2009). Complete resection of pulmonary inflammatory pseudotumors has excellent long-term prognosis. J Thorac Cardiovasc Surg. 137:435–40.
694. Faerber EN, Balsara RK, Schidlow DV, et al. (1990). Thymolipoma: computed tomographic appearances. Pediatr Radiol. 20:196–7.
695. Fais F, Gaidano G, Capello D, et al. (1999). Immunoglobulin V region gene use and structure suggest antigen selection in AIDS-related primary effusion lymphomas. Leukemia. 13:1093–9.
696. Falini B, Agostinelli C, Bigerna B, et al. (2012). IRTA1 is selectively expressed in nodal and extranodal marginal zone lymphomas. Histopathology. 61:930–41.
697. Fallone E, Bourne PA, Watson TJ, et al. (2009). Ectopic (mediastinal) parathyroid adenoma with prominent lymphocytic infiltration. Appl Immunohistochem Mol Morphol. 17:82–4.
698. Fan W, Bubman D, Chadburn A, et al. (2005). Distinct subsets of primary effusion lymphoma can be identified based on their cellular gene expression profile and viral association. J Virol. 79:1244–51.
699. Fantone JC, Geisinger KR, Appelman HD (1982). Papillary adenoma of the lung with lamellar and electron dense granules. An ultrastructural study. Cancer. 50:2839–44.
700. Farley MN, Schmidt LS, Mester JL, et al. (2013). A novel germline mutation in BAP1

predisposes to familial clear-cell renal cell carcinoma. Mol Cancer Res. 11:1061–71.
701. Farrell DJ, Cooper PN, Malcolm AJ (1995). Carcinosarcoma of lung associated with asbestosis. Histopathology. 27:484–6.
702. Farrell DJ, Kashyap AP, Ashcroft T, et al. (1996). Primary malignant melanoma of the bronchus. Thorax. 51:223–4.
703. Fasching K, Panzer S, Haas OA, et al. (2000). Presence of clone-specific antigen receptor gene rearrangements at birth indicates an in utero origin of diverse types of early childhood acute lymphoblastic leukemia. Blood. 95:2722–4.
704. Fassina A, Marino F, Poletti A, et al. (2001). Follicular dendritic cell tumor of the mediastinum. Ann Diagn Pathol. 5:361–7.
705. Fauci AS, Haynes BF, Costa J, et al. (1982). Lymphomatoid Granulomatosis. Prospective clinical and therapeutic experience over 10 years. N Engl J Med. 306:68–74.
706. Fealey ME, Edwards WD, Miller DV, et al. (2008). Hamartomas of mature cardiac myocytes: report of 7 new cases and review of literature. Hum Pathol. 39:1064–71.
707. Fedyanin M, Tryakin A, Mosyakova Y, et al. (2014). Prognostic factors and efficacy of different chemotherapeutic regimens in patients with mediastinal nonseminomatous germ cell tumors. J Cancer Res Clin Oncol. 140:311–8.
708. Feigin GA, Robinson B, Marchevsky A (1986). Mixed tumor of the mediastinum. Arch Pathol Lab Med. 110:80–1.
709. Feldman AL, Arber DA, Pittaluga S, et al. (2008). Clonally related follicular lymphomas and histiocytic/dendritic cell sarcomas: evidence for transdifferentiation of the follicular lymphoma clone. Blood. 111:5433–9.
710. Feldman AL, Dogan A, Smith DI, et al. (2011). Discovery of recurrent t(6;7)(p25.3;q32.3) translocations in ALK-negative anaplastic large cell lymphomas by massively parallel genomic sequencing. Blood. 117:915–9.
711. Feltkamp CA, van Heerde P, Feltkamp-Vroom TM, et al. (1981). A malignant tumor arising from interdigitating cells; light microscopical, ultrastructural, immuno-and enzyme-histochemical characteristics. Virchows Arch A Pathol Anat Histol. 393:183–92.
712. Fernandez AL, Vega M, El-Diasty MM, et al. (2012). Myxoma of the aortic valve. Interact Cardiovasc Thorac Surg. 15:560–2.
713. Fernandez FG, Battafarano RJ (2006). Large-cell neuroendocrine carcinoma of the lung. Cancer Contr. 13:270–5.
714. Fernandez-Cuesta L, Peifer M, Lu X, et al. (2014). Cross-entity mutation analysis of lung neuroendocrine tumors sheds light into their molecular origin and identifies new therapeutic targets. Abstract nr 1531. Proceedings of the 105th Annual Meeting of the American Association for Cancer Research, Apr 5-9; 2014 San Diego, CA. Philadelphia (PA) : AACR.
715. Fernandez-Cuesta L, Peifer M, Lu X, et al. (2014). Frequent mutations in chromatin-remodelling genes in pulmonary carcinoids. Nat Commun. 5:3518.
716. Fernandez-Cuesta L, Plenker D, Osada H, et al. (2014). CD74-NRG1 Fusions in Lung Adenocarcinoma. Cancer Discov. 4:415–22.
717. Ferolla P, Falchetti A, Filosso P, et al. (2005). Thymic neuroendocrine carcinoma (carcinoid) in multiple endocrine neoplasia type 1 syndrome: the Italian series. J Clin Endocrinol Metab. 90:2603–9.
718. Ferreri AJ, Dognini GP, Bairey O, et al. (2008). The addition of rituximab to anthracycline-based chemotherapy significantly improves outcome in 'Western' patients with intravascular large B-cell lymphoma. Br J Haematol. 143:253–7.
719. Ferreri AJ, Dognini GP, Campo E, et al. (2007). Variations in clinical presentation, frequency of hemophagocytosis and clinical behavior of intravascular lymphoma diagnosed in different geographical regions. Haematologica. 92:486–92.
720. Ferry JA, Sohani AR, Longtine JA, et al. (2009). HHV8-positive, EBV-positive Hodgkin lymphoma-like large B-cell lymphoma and HHV8-positive intravascular large B-cell lymphoma. Mod Pathol. 22:618–26.
721. Feuerhake F, Kutok JL, Monti S, et al. (2005). NFkappaB activity, function, and target-gene signatures in primary mediastinal large B-cell lymphoma and diffuse large B-cell lymphoma subtypes. Blood. 106:1392–9.
722. Feyma T, Carter GT, Weiss MD (2008). Myotonic dystrophy type 1 coexisting with myasthenia gravis and thymoma. Muscle Nerve. 38:916–20.
723. Filosso PL, Galassi C, Ruffini E, et al. (2013). Thymoma and the increased risk of developing extrathymic malignancies: a multicentre study. Eur J Cardiothorac Surg. 44:219–24.
724. Finberg KE, Sequist LV, Joshi VA, et al. (2007). Mucinous differentiation correlates with absence of EGFR mutation and presence of KRAS mutation in lung adenocarcinomas with bronchioloalveolar features. J Mol Diagn. 9:320–6.
725. Fine NM, Foley DA, Breen JF, et al. (2013). Multimodality imaging of a giant aortic valve papillary fibroelastoma. Case Rep Med. 2013:705101.
726. Fink G, Krelbaum T, Yellin A, et al. (2001). Pulmonary carcinoid: presentation, diagnosis, and outcome in 142 cases in Israel and review of 640 cases from the literature. Chest. 119:1647–51.
727. Finsterer J (2008). Histiocytoid cardiomyopathy: a mitochondrial disorder. Clin Cardiol. 31:225–7.
728. Fiorella RM, Lavin M, Dubey S, et al. (1997). Malignant thymoma in a patient with HIV positivity: a case report with a review of the differential cytologic diagnoses. Diagn Cytopathol. 16:267–9.
729. Fischer DR, Beerman LB, Park SC, et al. (1984). Diagnosis of intracardiac rhabdomyoma by two-dimensional echocardiography. Am J Cardiol. 53:978–9.
730. Fischer JR, Ohnmacht U, Rieger N, et al. (2006). Promoter methylation of RASSF1A, RARbeta and DAPK predict poor prognosis of patients with malignant mesothelioma. Lung Cancer. 54:109–16.
731. Fishback NF, Travis WD, Moran CA, et al. (1994). Pleomorphic (spindle/giant cell) carcinoma of the lung. A clinicopathologic correlation of 78 cases. Cancer. 73:2936–45.
732. Fizazi K, Culine S, Droz JP, et al. (1998). Primary mediastinal nonseminomatous germ cell tumors: results of modern therapy including cisplatin-based chemotherapy. J Clin Oncol. 16:725–32.
733. Fizazi K, Tjulandin S, Salvioni R, et al. (2001). Viable malignant cells after primary chemotherapy for disseminated nonseminomatous germ cell tumors: prognostic factors and role of postsurgery chemotherapy--results from an international study group. J Clin Oncol. 19:2647–57.
734. Flavin RJ, Cook J, Fiorentino M, et al. (2011). beta-Catenin is a useful adjunct immunohistochemical marker for the diagnosis of pulmonary lymphangioleiomyomatosis. Am J Clin Pathol. 135:776–82.
735. Fletcher CDM, Antonescu CR, Heim S, et al. (2013). Myoepithelioma/myoepithelial carcinoma/mixed tumour. In: Fletcher CDM, Bridge JA, Hogendoorn PCW, Mertens F, eds. WHO Classification of Tumours of Soft Tissue and Bone. 4th ed. Lyon: IARC; pp. 208–9.
735A. Fletcher CDM, Bridge JA, Hogendoorn PCW, Mertens F, eds. (2013). WHO Classification of Tumours of Soft Tissue and Bone. 4th ed. Lyon: IARC.
736. Fletcher CDM, Bridge JA, Hogendoorn PCW, et al., eds. (2013). Nerve sheath tumours. In: WHO Classification of Tumours of Soft Tissue and Bone. 4th ed. Lyon: IARC; pp. 169–91.
737. Fletcher JA, Longtine J, Wallace K, et al. (1995). Cytogenetic and histologic findings in 17 pulmonary chondroid hamartomas: evidence for a pathogenetic relationship with lipomas and leiomyomas. Genes Chromosomes Cancer. 12:220–3.
738. Flieder DB (2003). Screen-detected adenocarcinoma of the lung. Practical points for surgical pathologists. Am J Clin Pathol. 119 Suppl:S39–57.
739. Flieder DB, Koss MN, Nicholson A, et al. (1998). Solitary pulmonary papillomas in adults: a clinicopathologic and in situ hybridization study of 14 cases combined with 27 cases in the literature. Am J Surg Pathol. 22:1328–42.
740. Flieder DB, Moran CA, Suster S (1997). Primary alveolar soft-part sarcoma of the mediastinum: a clinicopathological and immunohistochemical study of two cases. Histopathology. 31:469–73.
741. Flieder DB, Travis WD (1997). Clear cell "sugar" tumor of the lung: association with lymphangioleiomyomatosis and multifocal micronodular pneumocyte hyperplasia in a patient with tuberous sclerosis. Am J Surg Pathol. 21:1242–7.
742. Flores RM, Routledge T, Seshan VE, et al. (2008). The impact of lymph node station on survival in 348 patients with surgically resected malignant pleural mesothelioma: implications for revision of the American Joint Committee on Cancer staging system. J Thorac Cardiovasc Surg. 136:605–10.
743. Fong Y, Coit DG, Woodruff JM, et al. (1993). Lymph node metastasis from soft tissue sarcoma in adults. Analysis of data from a prospective database of 1772 sarcoma patients. Ann Surg. 217:72–7.
744. Fontanini G, Calcinai A, Boldrini L, et al. (1999). Modulation of neoangiogenesis in bronchial preneoplastic lesions. Oncol Rep. 6:813–7.
745. Forbes AD, Schmidt RA, Wood DE, et al. (1994). Schwannoma of the left atrium: diagnostic evaluation and surgical resection. Ann Thorac Surg. 57:743–6.
746. Forman D, Bray F, Brewster DH, et al., eds. (electronic version). Cancer Incidence in Five Continents. Volume X. Lyon: IARC; Available from: http://ci5.iarc.fr
747. Foroulis CN, Iliadis KH, Mauroudis PM, et al. (2002). Basaloid carcinoma, a rare primary lung neoplasm: report of a case and review of the literature. Lung Cancer. 35:335–8.
748. Forquer JA, Rong N, Fakiris AJ, et al. (2010). Postoperative radiotherapy after surgical resection of thymoma: differing roles in localized and regional disease. Int J Radiat Oncol Biol Phys. 76:440–5.
749. Franke A, Strobel P, Fackeldey V, et al. (2004). Hepatoid thymic carcinoma: report of a case. Am J Surg Pathol. 28:250–6.
750. Franke WW, Moll R (1987). Cytoskeletal components of lymphoid organs. I. Synthesis of cytokeratins 8 and 18 and desmin in subpopulations of extrafollicular reticulum cells of human lymph nodes, tonsils, and spleen. Differentiation. 36:145–63.
751. Franklin WA, Veve R, Hirsch FR, et al. (2002). Epidermal growth factor receptor family in lung cancer and premalignancy. Semin Oncol. 29:3–14.
752. Franklin WA, Waintrub M, Edwards D, et al. (1994). New anti-lung-cancer antibody cluster 12 reacts with human folate receptors present on adenocarcinoma. Int J Cancer Suppl. 8:89–95.
753. Fraternali Orcioni G, Ravetti JL, Gaggero G, et al. (2010). Primary embryonal spindle cell cardiac rhabdomyosarcoma: case report. Pathol Res Pract. 206:325–30.
754. Frazier AA, Franks TJ, Pugatch RD, et al. (2006). From the archives of the AFIP: Pleuropulmonary synovial sarcoma. Radiographics. 26:923–40.
755. Freedom RM, Lee KJ, MacDonald C, et al. (2000). Selected aspects of cardiac tumors in infancy and childhood. Pediatr Cardiol. 21:299–316.
755B. French CA (2010). Demystified molecular pathology of NUT midline carcinomas. J Clin Pathol. 63(6):492-6.
756. French CA (2012). Pathogenesis of NUT midline carcinoma. Annu Rev Pathol. 7:247–65.
757. French CA (2013). The importance of diagnosing NUT midline carcinoma. Head Neck Pathol. 7:11–6.
758. French CA, Kutok JL, Faquin WC, et al. (2004). Midline carcinoma of children and young adults with NUT rearrangement. J Clin Oncol. 22:4135–9.
759. French CA, Miyoshi I, Kubonishi I, et al. (2003). BRD4-NUT fusion oncogene: a novel mechanism in aggressive carcinoma. Cancer Res. 63:304–7.
759A. French CA, Rahman S, Walsh EM, et al. (2014) NSD3-NUT fusion oncoprotein in NUT midline carcinoma: implications for a novel oncogenic mechanism. Cancer Discov. 4:928–41.
760. French CA, Ramirez CL, Kolmakova J, et al. (2008). BRD-NUT oncoproteins: a family of closely related nuclear proteins that block epithelial differentiation and maintain the growth of carcinoma cells. Oncogene. 27:2237–42.
761. Friedberg M, Silverman NH (2005). Right ventricular outflow tract obstruction in an infant. Heart. 91:748.
762. Friedel G, Pastorino U, Ginsberg RJ, et al. (2002). Results of lung metastasectomy from breast cancer: prognostic criteria on the basis of 467 cases of the International Registry of Lung Metastases. Eur J Cardiothorac Surg. 22:335–44.
763. Fritz A, Percy C, Jack A, et al. (2000). International Classification of Diseases for Oncology. 3rd ed. Geneva: WHO Press.
764. Fritzsche FR, Kristiansen G, Frauenfelder T, et al. (2009). Large mixed germ cell tumor in a young patient presenting as an intrapulmonary mass. Pathol Res Pract. 205:572–8.
765. Fu K, Moran CA, Suster S (2002). Primary mediastinal giant cell tumors: a clinicopathologic and immunohistochemical study of two cases. Ann Diagn Pathol. 6:100–5.
766. Fujii T, Kawai T, Saito K, et al. (1993). EBER-1 expression in thymic carcinoma. Acta Pathol Jpn. 43:107–10.
767. Fujita Y, Shimizu T, Yamazaki K, et al. (2000). Bronchial brushing cytology features of primary malignant fibrous histiocytoma of the lung. A case report. Acta Cytol. 44:227–31.
768. Fukai I, Masaoka A, Fujii Y, et al. (1999). Thymic neuroendocrine tumor (thymic carcinoid): a clinicopathologic study in 15 patients. Ann Thorac Surg. 67:208–11.
769. Fukai I, Masaoka A, Hashimoto T, et al. (1992). The distribution of epithelial membrane antigen in thymic epithelial neoplasms. Cancer. 70:2077–81.
770. Fukayama M, Maeda Y, Funata N, et al. (1988). Pulmonary and pleural thymoma. Diagnostic application of lymphocyte markers to the thymoma of unusual site. Am J Clin Pathol. 89:617–21.
771. Fuks L, Kramer MR, Shitrit D, et al. (2014). Pulmonary Langerhans cell histiocytosis and diabetes insipidus in pregnant women: our experience. Lung. 192:285–7.
772. Fukumoto K, Taniguchi T, Ishikawa Y, et al. (2012). The utility of [18F]-fluorodeoxyglucose positron emission tomography-computed tomography in thymic epithelial tumours. Eur J Cardiothorac Surg. 42:e152–6.
773. Fulford LG, Kamata Y, Okudera K, et al. (2001). Epithelial-myoepithelial carcinomas of the bronchus. Am J Surg Pathol.

25:1508–14.
774. Funai K, Yokose T, Ishii G, et al. (2003). Clinicopathologic characteristics of peripheral squamous cell carcinoma of the lung. Am J Surg Pathol. 27:978–84.
775. Furtado A, Nogueira R, Ferreira D, et al. (2010). Papillary adenocarcinoma of the thymus: case report and review of the literature. Int J Surg Pathol. 18:530–3.
776. Furuya K, Murayama S, Soeda H, et al. (1999). New classification of small pulmonary nodules by margin characteristics on high-resolution CT. Acta Radiol. 40:496–504.
777. Gabhane SK, Gangane NM, Sinha RT (2009). Pentalogy of Fallot and cardiac paraganglioma: a case report. Cases J. 2:9392.
778. Gadalla SM, Rajan A, Pfeiffer R, et al. (2011). A population-based assessment of mortality and morbidity patterns among patients with thymoma. Int J Cancer. 128:2688–94.
779. Gaertner E, Zeren EH, Fleming MV, et al. (1996). Biphasic synovial sarcomas arising in the pleural cavity. A clinicopathologic study of five cases. Am J Surg Pathol. 20:36–45.
780. Gaffey MJ, Mills SE, Askin FB, et al. (1990). Clear cell tumor of the lung. A clinicopathologic, immunohistochemical, and ultrastructural study of eight cases. Am J Surg Pathol. 14:248–59.
781. Gaidano G, Capello D, Cilia AM, et al. (1999). Genetic characterization of HHV-8/KSHV-positive primary effusion lymphoma reveals frequent mutations of BCL6: implications for disease pathogenesis and histogenesis. Genes Chromosomes Cancer. 24:16–23.
782. Gainor JF, Varghese AM, Ou SH, et al. (2013). ALK rearrangements are mutually exclusive with mutations in EGFR or KRAS: an analysis of 1,683 patients with non-small cell lung cancer. Clin Cancer Res. 19:4273–81.
783. Gal AA, Kornstein MJ, Cohen C, et al. (2001). Neuroendocrine tumors of the thymus: a clinicopathological and prognostic study. Ann Thorac Surg. 72:1179–82.
784. Gal AA, Nassar VH, Miller JI (2002). Cytopathologic diagnosis of pulmonary sclerosing hemangioma. Diagn Cytopathol. 26:163–6.
785. Galateau-Salle F (2006). Pathology of Malignant Mesothelioma. London: Springer.
786. Galateau-Salle F, Attanoos R, Gibbs AR, et al. (2007). Lymphohistiocytoid variant of malignant mesothelioma of the pleura: a series of 22 cases. Am J Surg Pathol. 31:711–6.
787. Galateau-Salle F, Vignaud JM, Burke L, et al. (2004). Well-differentiated papillary mesothelioma of the pleura: a series of 24 cases. Am J Surg Pathol. 28:534–40.
788. Galateau-Salle FB, Luna RE, Horiba K, et al. (2000). Matrix metalloproteinases and tissue inhibitors of metalloproteinases in bronchial squamous preinvasive lesions. Hum Pathol. 31:296–305.
789. Galbis Caravajal JM, Sales Badia JG, Trescoli SC, et al. (2008). Endotracheal metastases from colon adenocarcinoma. Clin Transl Oncol. 10:676–8.
790. Gandhi SA, Mufti G, Devereux S, et al. (2011). Primary effusion lymphoma in an HIV-negative man. Br J Haematol. 155:411.
791. Ganjoo KN, Rieger KM, Kesler KA, et al. (2000). Results of modern therapy for patients with mediastinal nonseminomatous germ cell tumors. Cancer. 88:1051–6.
792. Gao ZH, Urbanski SJ (2005). The spectrum of pulmonary mucinous cystic neoplasia: a clinicopathologic and immunohistochemical study of ten cases and review of literature. Am J Clin Pathol. 124:62–70.
793. Garber ME, Troyanskaya OG, Schluens K, et al. (2001). Diversity of gene expression in adenocarcinoma of the lung. Proc Natl Acad Sci USA. 98:13784–9.
794. Garces-Inigo EF, Leung R, Sebire NJ, et al. (2009). Extrarenal rhabdoid tumours outside the central nervous system in infancy. Pediatr Radiol. 39:817–22.
795. Garcia-Escudero A, Gonzalez-Campora R, Villar-Rodriguez JL, et al. (2004). Thyroid transcription factor-1 expression in pulmonary blastoma. Histopathology. 44:507–8.
796. Garcia-Riego A, Cuinas C, Vilanova JJ (2001). Malignant pericardial effusion. Acta Cytol. 45:561–6.
797. Garnick MB, Griffin JD (1983). Idiopathic thrombocytopenia in association with extragonadal germ cell cancer. Ann Intern Med. 98:926–7.
798. Garson A Jr, Moak JP, Friedman RA, et al. (1989). Surgical treatment of arrhythmias in children. Cardiol Clin. 7:319–29.
799. Gartner LA, Voorhess ML (1993). Adrenocorticotropic hormone--producing thymic carcinoid in a teenager. Cancer. 71:106–11.
800. Gaspar LE, McNamara EJ, Gay EG, et al. (2012). Small-cell lung cancer: prognostic factors and changing treatment over 15 years. Clin Lung Cancer. 13:115–22.
801. Gatta G, Botta L, Rossi S, et al. (2014). Childhood cancer survival in Europe 1999-2007: results of EUROCARE-5--a population-based study. Lancet Oncol. 15:35–47.
802. Gaude GS, Patil P, Malur PR, et al. (2013). Primary mediastinal choriocarcinoma. South Asian J Cancer. 2:79.
803. Gaur P, Leary C, Yao JC (2010). Thymic neuroendocrine tumors: a SEER database analysis of 160 patients. Ann Surg. 251:1117–21.
804. Gautschi O, Pauli C, Strobel K, et al. (2012). A patient with BRAF V600E lung adenocarcinoma responding to vemurafenib. J Thorac Oncol. 7:e23–4.
805. Gawrychowski J, Brulinski K, Malinowski E, et al. (2005). Prognosis and survival after radical resection of primary adenosquamous lung carcinoma. Eur J Cardiothorac Surg. 27:686–92.
806. Gazdar A, Robinson L, Oliver D, et al. (2014). Hereditary lung cancer syndrome targets never smokers with germline EGFR gene T790M mutations. J Thorac Oncol. 9:456–63.
807. Gazzeri S, Brambilla E, Caron de Fromentel C, et al. (1994). p53 genetic abnormalities and myc activation in human lung carcinoma. Int J Cancer. 58:24–32.
808. Gazzeri S, Brambilla E, Chauvin C, et al. (1990). Analysis of the activation of the myc family oncogene and of its stability over time in xenografted human lung carcinomas. Cancer Res. 50:1566–70.
809. Gazzeri S, Della Valle V, Chaussade L, et al. (1998). The human p19ARF protein encoded by the beta transcript of the p16INK4a gene is frequently lost in small cell lung cancer. Cancer Res. 58:3926–31.
810. Ge Y, Ro JY, Kim D, et al. (2011). Clinicopathologic and immunohistochemical characteristics of adult primary cardiac angiosarcomas: analysis of 10 cases. Ann Diagn Pathol. 15:262–7.
811. Gee GV, Stanifer ML, Christensen BC, et al. (2010). SV40 associated miRNAs are not detectable in mesotheliomas. Br J Cancer. 103:885–8.
812. Geisinger KR, Stanley MW, Raab SS, et al. (2003). Modern Cytopathology. Philadelphia: Churchill Livingstone.
813. Geisinger KR, Travis WD, Perkins LA, et al. (2010). Aspiration cytomorphology of fetal adenocarcinoma of the lung. Am J Clin Pathol. 134:894–902.
814. Oechsle K, Bokemeyer C, Kollmannsberger C, et al. (2012). Bone metastases in germ cell tumor patients. J Cancer Res Clin Oncol. 138:947–52.
815. Gelinas JF, Manoukian J, Cote A (2008). Lung involvement in juvenile onset recurrent respiratory papillomatosis: a systematic review of the literature. Int J Pediatr Otorhinolaryngol. 72:433–52.
816. Gengenbach S, Ridker PM (1991). Left ventricular hemangioma in Kasabach-Merritt syndrome. Am Heart J. 121:202–3.
817. Geoerger B, Hero B, Harms D, et al. (2001). Metabolic activity and clinical features of primary ganglioneuromas. Cancer. 91:1905–13.
818. George RE, London WB, Cohn SL, et al. (2005). Hyperdiploidy plus nonamplified MYCN confers a favorable prognosis in children 12 to 18 months old with disseminated neuroblastoma: a Pediatric Oncology Group study. J Clin Oncol. 23:6466–73.
819. Georgin-Lavialle S, Darmon M, Galicier L, et al. (2009). Intravascular lymphoma presenting as a specific pulmonary embolism and acute respiratory failure: a case report. J Med Case Reports. 3:7253.
820. Geradts J, Fong KM, Zimmerman PV, et al. (2000). Loss of Fhit expression in non-small-cell lung cancer: correlation with molecular genetic abnormalities and clinicopathological features. Br J Cancer. 82:1191–7.
821. Gerald WL, Ladanyi M, de Alava E, et al. (1998). Clinical, pathologic, and molecular spectrum of tumors associated with t(11;22)(p13;q12): desmoplastic small round-cell tumor and its variants. J Clin Oncol. 16:3028–36.
822. Gerrard JW, Vickers P, Gerrard CD (1976). The familial incidence of allergic disease. Ann Allergy. 36:10–5.
823. Geurts TW, Nederlof PM, van den Brekel MW, et al. (2005). Pulmonary squamous cell carcinoma following head and neck squamous cell carcinoma: metastasis or second primary? Clin Cancer Res. 11:6608–14.
824. Geurts TW, van Velthuysen ML, Broekman F, et al. (2009). Differential diagnosis of pulmonary carcinoma following head and neck cancer by genetic analysis. Clin Cancer Res. 15:980–5.
825. Gezelius C, Eriksson A (1988). Neoplastic disease in a medicolegal autopsy material. A retrospective study in northern Sweden. Z Rechtsmed. 101:115–30.
826. Gharagozloo F, Porter CJ, Tazelaar HD, et al. (1994). Multiple myocardial hamartomas causing ventricular tachycardia in young children: combined surgical modification and medical treatment. Mayo Clin Proc. 69:262–7.
827. Giaccone G, Rajan A, Ruijter R, et al. (2009). Imatinib mesylate in patients with WHO B3 thymomas and thymic carcinomas. J Thorac Oncol. 4:1270–3.
828. Giaj Levra M, Novello S, Scagliotti GV, et al. (2012). Primary pleuropulmonary sarcoma: a rare disease entity. Clin Lung Cancer. 13:399–407.
829. Giancotti A, La Torre R, Bevilacqua E, et al. (2012). Mediastinal masses: a case of fetal teratoma and literature review. Clin Exp Obstet Gynecol. 39:384–7.
830. Giangreco A, Reynolds SD, Stripp BR (2002). Terminal bronchioles harbor a unique airway stem cell population that localizes to the bronchoalveolar duct junction. Am J Pathol. 161:173–82.
831. Gibbs AR, Johnson NF, Giddings JC, et al. (1984). Primary angiosarcoma of the mediastinum: light and electron microscopic demonstration of Factor VIII-related antigen in neoplastic cells. Hum Pathol. 15:687–91.
832. Gibbs GW, Berry G (2008). Mesothelioma and asbestos. Regul Toxicol Pharmacol. 52:S223–31.
833. Gibril F, Chen YJ, Schrump DS, et al. (2003). Prospective study of thymic carcinoids in patients with multiple endocrine neoplasia type 1. J Clin Endocrinol Metab. 88:1066–81.
834. Giffin L, Damania B (2014). KSHV: pathways to tumorigenesis and persistent infection. Adv Virus Res. 88:111–59.
835. Gilbert-Barness E, Barness LA (1999). Nonmalformative cardiovascular pathology in infants and children. Pediatr Dev Pathol. 2:499–530.
836. Gilcrease MZ, Rajan B, Ostrowski ML, et al. (1997). Localized thymic Langerhans' cell histiocytosis and its relationship with myasthenia gravis. Immunohistochemical, ultrastructural, and cytometric studies. Arch Pathol Lab Med. 121:134–8.
837. Gill PS, Chandraratna PA, Meyer PR, et al. (1987). Malignant lymphoma: cardiac involvement at initial presentation. J Clin Oncol. 5:216–24.
838. Gilligan TD, Seidenfeld J, Basch EM, et al. (2010). American Society of Clinical Oncology Clinical Practice Guideline on uses of serum tumor markers in adult males with germ cell tumors. J Clin Oncol. 28:3388–404.
839. Gillis AJ, Stoop H, Biermann K, et al. (2011). Expression and interdependencies of pluripotency factors LIN28, OCT3/4, NANOG and SOX2 in human testicular germ cells and tumours of the testis. Int J Androl. 34:e160–74.
840. Gilman G, Wright RS, Glockner JF, et al. (2005). Ventricular septal hamartoma mimicking hypertrophic cardiomyopathy in a 41-year-old woman presenting with paroxysmal supraventricular tachycardia. J Am Soc Echocardiogr. 18:272–4.
841. Girard N (2012). Chemotherapy and targeted agents for thymic malignancies. Expert Rev Anticancer Ther. 12:685–95.
842. Girard N, Deshpande C, Lau C, et al. (2009). Comprehensive histologic assessment helps to differentiate multiple lung primary nonsmall cell carcinomas from metastases. Am J Surg Pathol. 33:1752–64.
843. Girard N, Ostrovnaya I, Lau C, et al. (2009). Genomic and mutational profiling to assess clonal relationships between multiple non-small cell lung cancers. Clin Cancer Res. 15:5184–90.
844. Girard N, Shen R, Guo T, et al. (2009). Comprehensive genomic analysis reveals clinically relevant molecular distinctions between thymic carcinomas and thymomas. Clin Cancer Res. 15:6790–9.
845. Girard P, Spaggiari L, Baldeyrou P, et al. (1997). Should the number of pulmonary metastases influence the surgical decision? Eur J Cardiothorac Surg. 12:385–91.
846. Giuseppucci C, Boglione M, Cadario M, et al. (2012). [Myofibroblastic tumor of the lung: clinical features and results in 9 children]. Cir Pediatr. 25:35–9.
847. Gladish GW, Sabloff BM, Munden RF, et al. (2002). Primary thoracic sarcomas. Radiographics. 22:621–37.
848. Gleason BC, Fletcher CD (2008). Deep "benign" fibrous histiocytoma: clinicopathologic analysis of 69 cases of a rare tumor indicating occasional metastatic potential. Am J Surg Pathol. 32:354–62.
849. Gleason BC, Hornick JL (2008). Inflammatory myofibroblastic tumours: where are we now? J Clin Pathol. 61:428–37.
850. Gleason TH, Dillard DH, Gould VE (1972). Cardiac neurilemoma. N Y State J Med. 72:2435–6.
851. Gleeson T, Thiessen R, Hannigan A, et al. (2013). Pulmonary hamartomas: CT pixel analysis for fat attenuation using radiologic-pathologic correlation. J Med Imaging Radiat Oncol. 57:534–43.
852. Glinsky GV, Berezovska O, Glinskii AB (2005). Microarray analysis identifies a death-from-cancer signature predicting therapy failure in patients with multiple types of cancer. J Clin Invest. 115:1503–21.
853. Go C, Schwartz MR, Donovan DT (2003). Molecular transformation of recurrent respiratory papillomatosis: viral typing and p53 overexpression. Ann Otol Rhinol Laryngol. 112:298–302.
854. Go H, Cho HJ, Paik JH, et al. (2011). Thymic extranodal marginal zone B-cell lymphoma of mucosa-associated lymphoid tissue: a clinicopathological and genetic analysis of six cases. Leuk Lymphoma. 52:2276–83.

855. Gobel U, Schneider DT, Calaminus G, et al. (2000). Germ-cell tumors in childhood and adolescence. GPOH MAKEI and the MAHO study groups. Ann Oncol. 11:263–71.
856. Gobel U, Schneider DT, Teske C, et al. (2010). Brain metastases in children and adolescents with extracranial germ cell tumor - data of the MAHO/MAKEI-registry. Klin Padiatr. 222:140–4.
857. Gobel U, von Kries R, Teske C, et al. (2013). Brain metastases during follow-up of children and adolescents with extracranial malignant germ cell tumors: risk adapted management decision tree analysis based on data of the MAHO/MAKEI-registry. Pediatr Blood Cancer. 60:217–23.
858. Goetz SP, Robinson RA, Landas SK (1992). Extraskeletal myxoid chondrosarcoma of the pleura. Report of a case clinically simulating mesothelioma. Am J Clin Pathol. 97:498–502.
859. Gokmen-Polar Y, Sanders KL, Goswami CP, et al. (2012). Establishment and characterization of a novel cell line derived from human thymoma AB tumor. Lab Invest. 92:1564–73.
860. Goldberg J, Azizad S, Bandovic J, et al. (2009). Primary mediastinal giant cell tumor. Rare Tumors. 1:e45.
861. Goldberg JM, Silverman LB, Levy DE, et al. (2003). Childhood T-cell acute lymphoblastic leukemia: the Dana-Farber Cancer Institute acute lymphoblastic leukemia consortium experience. J Clin Oncol. 21:3616–22.
862. Goldberg M, Imbernon E, Rolland P, et al. (2006). The French National Mesothelioma Surveillance Program. Occup Environ Med. 63:390–5.
863. Goldin LR, Pfeiffer RM, Gridley G, et al. (2004). Familial aggregation of Hodgkin lymphoma and related tumors. Cancer. 100:1902–8.
864. Goldsmith JD, Pawel B, Goldblum JR, et al. (2002). Detection and diagnostic utilization of placental alkaline phosphatase in muscular tissue and tumors with myogenic differentiation. Am J Surg Pathol. 26:1627–33.
865. Goldstein MG, Siegel R (2009). Thymoma developing 30 years after mantle radiation for Hodgkin's lymphoma. Conn Med. 73:521–3.
866. Goldstraw P, Crowley J, Chansky K, et al. (2007). The IASLC Lung Cancer Staging Project: proposals for the revision of the TNM stage groupings in the forthcoming (seventh) edition of the TNM Classification of malignant tumours. J Thorac Oncol. 2:706–14.
867. Gollard R, Jhatakia S, Elliott M, et al. (2010). Large cell/neuroendocrine carcinoma. Lung Cancer. 69:13–8.
868. Gomez-Aracil V, Mayayo E, Alvira R, et al. (2002). Fine needle aspiration cytology of primary pulmonary meningioma associated with minute meningotheliallike nodules. Report of a case with histologic, immunohistochemical and ultrastructural studies. Acta Cytol. 46:899–903.
869. Gong L, He XL, Li YH, et al. (2009). Clonal status and clinicopathological feature of Erdheim-Chester disease. Pathol Res Pract. 205:601–7.
870. Gong L, Li YH, He XL, et al. (2009). Primary intrapulmonary thymomas: case report and review of the literature. J Int Med Res. 37:1252–7.
871. Gonzalez ET, Sanchez-Yuste R, Jimenez-Heffernan JA (2008). Cytologic features of pulmonary alveolar adenoma. Acta Cytol. 52:739–40.
872. Gonzalez-Vela JL, Savage PD, Manivel JC, et al. (1990). Poor prognosis of mediastinal germ cell cancers containing sarcomatous components. Cancer. 66:1114–6.
873. Gopaldas RR, Atluri PV, Blaustein AS, et al. (2009). Papillary fibroelastoma of the aortic valve: operative approaches upon incidental discovery. Tex Heart Inst J. 36:160–3.
874. Gordon GJ, Dong L, Yeap BY, et al. (2009). Four-gene expression ratio test for survival in patients undergoing surgery for mesothelioma. J Natl Cancer Inst. 101:678–86.
875. Gordon GJ, Jensen RV, Hsiao LL, et al. (2003). Using gene expression ratios to predict outcome among patients with mesothelioma. J Natl Cancer Inst. 95:598–605.
876. Gordon GJ, Rockwell GN, Godfrey PA, et al. (2005). Validation of genomics-based prognostic tests in malignant pleural mesothelioma. Clin Cancer Res. 11:4406–14.
877. Gorlin RJ (2004). Nevoid basal cell carcinoma (Gorlin) syndrome. Genet Med. 6:530–9.
878. Gorshtein A, Gross DJ, Barak D, et al. (2012). Diffuse idiopathic pulmonary neuroendocrine cell hyperplasia and the associated lung neuroendocrine tumors: clinical experience with a rare entity. Cancer. 118:612–9.
879. Gosev I, Paic F, Duric Z, et al. (2013). Cardiac myxoma the great imitators: comprehensive histopathological and molecular approach. Int J Cardiol. 164:7–20.
880. Gosney JR (2013). Neuroendocrine tumors and other neuroendocrine proliferations of the lung. In: Hasleton P, Flieder DB, eds. Spencer's Pathology of the Lung. Cambridge: Cambridge University Press; pp. 1151–85.
881. Gosney JR, Williams IJ, Dodson AR, et al. (2011). Morphology and antigen expression profile of pulmonary neuroendocrine cells in reactive proliferations and diffuse idiopathic pulmonary neuroendocrine cell hyperplasia (DIPNECH). Histopathology. 59:751–62.
882. Goss PE, Schwertfeger L, Blackstein ME, et al. (1994). Extragonadal germ cell tumors. A 14-year Toronto experience. Cancer. 73:1971–9.
883. Goto K, Kodama T, Matsuno Y, et al. (2001). Clinicopathologic and DNA cytometric analysis of carcinoid tumors of the thymus. Mod Pathol. 14:985–94.
884. Goudet P, Murat A, Cardot-Bauters C, et al. (2009). Thymic neuroendocrine tumors in multiple endocrine neoplasia type 1: a comparative study on 21 cases among a series of 761 MEN1 from the GTE (Groupe des Tumeurs Endocrines). World J Surg. 33:1197–207.
885. Gould VE, Bloom KJ, Franke WW, et al. (1995). Increased numbers of cytokeratin-positive interstitial reticulum cells (CIRC) in reactive, inflammatory and neoplastic lymphadenopathies: hyperplasia or induced expression? Virchows Arch. 425:617–29.
886. Gould VE, Linnoila RI, Memoli VA, et al. (1983). Neuroendocrine components of the bronchopulmonary tract: hyperplasias, dysplasias, and neoplasms. Lab Invest. 49:519–37.
887. Gould VE, Warren WH, Faber LP, et al. (1990). Malignant cells of epithelial phenotype limited to thoracic lymph nodes. Eur J Cancer. 26:1121–6.
888. Gouttefangeas C, Bensussan A, Boumsell L (1990). Study of the CD3-associated T-cell receptors reveals further differences between T-cell acute lymphoblastic lymphoma and leukemia. Blood. 75:931–4.
889. Gouyer V, Gazzeri S, Bolon I, et al. (1998). Mechanism of retinoblastoma gene inactivation in the spectrum of neuroendocrine lung tumors. Am J Respir Cell Mol Biol. 18:188–96.
890. Gouyer V, Gazzeri S, Brambilla E, et al. (1994). Loss of heterozygosity at the RB locus correlates with loss of RB protein in primary malignant neuro-endocrine lung carcinomas. Int J Cancer. 58:818–24.
891. Govender D, Pillay SV (2002). Mediastinal immature teratoma with yolk sac tumor and myelomonocytic leukemia associated with Klinefelter's syndrome. Int J Surg Pathol. 10:157–62.
892. Govindan R, Ding L, Griffith M, et al. (2012). Genomic landscape of non-small cell lung cancer in smokers and never-smokers. Cell. 150:1121–34.
893. Gowda RM, Khan IA, Nair CK, et al. (2003). Cardiac papillary fibroelastoma: a comprehensive analysis of 725 cases. Am Heart J. 146:404–10.
894. Goya T, Asamura H, Yoshimura H, et al. (2005). Prognosis of 6644 resected non-small cell lung cancers in Japan: a Japanese lung cancer registry study. Lung Cancer. 50:227–34.
895. Graf M, Blaeker H, Schnabel P, et al. (1999). Intracardiac yolk sac tumor in an infant girl. Pathol Res Pract. 195:193–7.
896. Grande AM, Ragni T, Vigano M (1993). Primary cardiac tumors. A clinical experience of 12 years. Tex Heart Inst J. 20:223–30.
897. Gray SG, Fennell DA, Mutti L, et al. (2009). In arrayed ranks: array technology in the study of mesothelioma. J Thorac Oncol. 4:411–25.
898. Greaves P, Clear A, Owen A, et al. (2013). Defining characteristics of classical Hodgkin lymphoma microenvironment T-helper cells. Blood. 122:2856–63.
899. Grebenc ML, Rosado de Christenson ML, Burke AP, et al. (2000). Primary cardiac and pericardial neoplasms: radiologic-pathologic correlation. Radiographics. 20:1073–103.
899A. Green AC, Marx A, Ströbel P, et al. (2014). Type A and AB thymomas: histological features associated with increased stage. Histopathology. Forthcoming.
900. Greulich H, Kaplan B, Mertins P, et al. (2012). Functional analysis of receptor tyrosine kinase mutations in lung cancer identifies oncogenic extracellular domain mutations of ERBB2. Proc Natl Acad Sci USA. 109:14476–81.
901. Griffin CA, Hawkins AL, Dvorak C, et al. (1999). Recurrent involvement of 2p23 in inflammatory myofibroblastic tumors. Cancer Res. 59:2776–80.
902. Griffin N, Devaraj A, Goldstraw P, et al. (2008). CT and histopathological correlation of congenital cystic pulmonary lesions: a common pathogenesis? Clin Radiol. 63:995–1005.
903. Grizzard JD, Ang GB (2007). Magnetic resonance imaging of pericardial disease and cardiac masses. Magn Reson Imaging Clin N Am. 15:579–607. [vi.]
904. Grogg KL, Aubry MC, Vrana JA, et al. (2013). Nodular pulmonary amyloidosis is characterized by localized immunoglobulin deposition and is frequently associated with an indolent B-cell lymphoproliferative disorder. Am J Surg Pathol. 37:406–12.
904A. Gruver AM, Amin MB, Luthringer DJ, et al. (2012). Selective immunohistochemical markers to distinguish between metastatic high-grade urothelial carcinoma and primary poorly differentiated invasive squamous cell carcinoma of the lung. Arch Pathol Lab Med. 136:1339–46.
905. Gruver AM, Huba MA, Dogan A, et al. (2012). Fibrin-associated large B-cell lymphoma: part of the spectrum of cardiac lymphomas. Am J Surg Pathol. 36:1527–37.
906. Gualis J, Carrascal Y, de la Fuente L, et al. (2007). Heart transplantation treatment for a malignant cardiac granular cell tumor: 33 months of survival. Interact Cardiovasc Thorac Surg. 6:679–81.
907. Guan Y, Chen G, Zhang W, et al. (2012). Computed tomography appearance of inflammatory myofibroblastic tumor in the mediastinum. J Comput Assist Tomogr. 36:654–8.
908. Guardiola T, Horton E, Lopez-Camarillo L, et al. (2004). Cardiac myxoma: a cytogenetic study of two cases. Cancer Genet Cytogenet. 148:145–7.
909. Guasparri I, Keller SA, Cesarman E (2004). KSHV vFLIP is essential for the survival of infected lymphoma cells. J Exp Med. 199:993–1003.
910. Guibert N, Attias D, Pontier S, et al. (2011). Mediastinal teratoma and trichoptysis. Ann Thorac Surg. 92:351–3.
911. Guibert N, Brouchet L, Rouquette I, et al. (2012). Thymoma and solid-organ transplantation. Lung Cancer. 77:232–4.
912. Guimaraes AR, Wain JC, Mark EJ, et al. (2004). Mucinous cystadenoma of the lung. AJR Am J Roentgenol. 183:282.
913. Guimaraes MD, Benveniste MF, Bitencourt AG, et al. (2013). Thymoma originating in a giant thymolipoma: a rare intrathoracic lesion. Ann Thorac Surg. 96:1083–5.
914. Guinee D Jr, Jaffe E, Kingma D, et al. (1994). Pulmonary lymphomatoid granulomatosis. Evidence for a proliferation of Epstein-Barr virus infected B-lymphocytes with a prominent T-cell component and vasculitis. Am J Surg Pathol. 18:753–64.
915. Guinee DG Jr, Fishback NF, Koss MN, et al. (1994). The spectrum of immunohistochemical staining of small-cell lung carcinoma in specimens from transbronchial and open-lung biopsies. Am J Clin Pathol. 102:406–14.
916. Guinee DG Jr, Franks TJ, Gerbino AJ, et al. (2013). Pulmonary nodular lymphoid hyperplasia (pulmonary pseudolymphoma): the significance of increased numbers of IgG4-positive plasma cells. Am J Surg Pathol. 37:699–709.
917. Guinee DG Jr, Perkins SL, Travis WD, et al. (1998). Proliferation and cellular phenotype in lymphomatoid granulomatosis: implications of a higher proliferation index in B cells. Am J Surg Pathol. 22:1093–100.
917A. Guinee DG Jr, Thornberry DS, Azumi N, et al. (1995). Unique pulmonary presentation of an angiomyolipoma. Analysis of clinical, radiographic, and histopathologic features. Am J Surg Pathol. 19:476–80.
918. Gulmann C, Paner GP, Parakh RS, et al. (2013). Immunohistochemical profile to distinguish urothelial from squamous differentiation in carcinomas of urothelial tract. Hum Pathol. 44:164–72.
919. Gunaldi M, Oguz K, I, Duman BB, et al. (2012). Primary intrapulmonary thymoma associated with myasthenia gravis. Gen Thorac Cardiovasc Surg. 60:610–3.
920. Gunawardana J, Chan FC, Telenius A, et al. (2014). Recurrent somatic mutations of PTPN1 in primary mediastinal B cell lymphoma and Hodgkin lymphoma. Nat Genet. 46:329–35.
921. Guo HR, Wang NS, Hu H, et al. (2004). Cell type specificity of lung cancer associated with arsenic ingestion. Cancer Epidemiol Biomarkers Prev. 13:638–43.
922. Gupta R, Marchevsky AM, McKenna RJ, et al. (2008). Evidence-based pathology and the pathologic evaluation of thymomas: transcapsular invasion is not a significant prognostic feature. Arch Pathol Lab Med. 132:926–30.
923. Gupta R, Mathur SR, Arora VK, et al. (2008). Cytologic features of extragonadal germ cell tumors: a study of 88 cases with aspiration cytology. Cancer. 114:504–11.
924. Gururangan S, Bowman LC, Parham DM, et al. (1993). Primary extracranial rhabdoid tumors. Clinicopathologic features and response to ifosfamide. Cancer. 71:2653–9.
925. Haack H, Johnson LA, Fry CJ, et al. (2009). Diagnosis of NUT midline carcinoma using a NUT-specific monoclonal antibody. Am J Surg Pathol. 33:984–91.
926. Hahn HP, Fletcher CD (2007). Primary mediastinal liposarcoma: clinicopathologic analysis of 24 cases. Am J Surg Pathol. 31:1868–74.
927. Hailemariam S, Engeler DS, Bannwart F, et al. (1997). Primary mediastinal germ cell tumor with intratubular germ cell neoplasia of the testis--further support for germ cell origin of these tumors: a case report. Cancer. 79:1031–6.
928. Hainsworth JD, Greco FA (2001). Germ cell neoplasms and other malignancies of the mediastinum. Cancer Treat Res. 105:303–25.
929. Hajar R, Roberts WC, Folger GM Jr (1986). Embryonal botryoid rhabdomyosarcoma of the mitral valve. Am J Cardiol. 57:376.
930. Hajdu M, Singer S, Maki RG, et al. (2010). IGF2 over-expression in solitary fibrous tumours is independent of anatomical location and is related to loss of imprinting. J Pathol.

221:300–7.
931. Halicek F, Rosai J (1984). Histioeosinophilic granulomas in the thymuses of 29 myasthenic patients: a complication of pneumomediastinum. Hum Pathol. 15:1137–44.
932. Halliday BE, Slagel DD, Elsheikh TE, et al. (1998). Diagnostic utility of MIC-2 immunocytochemical staining in the differential diagnosis of small blue cell tumors. Diagn Cytopathol. 19:410–6.
933. Hamaji M, Vanderlaan PA, Sugarbaker DJ, et al. (2013). A microthymoma and no germinal centre in myasthenia gravis. Eur J Cardiothorac Surg. 44:1146–7.
934. Hamaratoglu F, Willecke M, Kango-Singh M, et al. (2006). The tumour-suppressor genes NF2/Merlin and Expanded act through Hippo signalling to regulate cell proliferation and apoptosis. Nat Cell Biol. 8:27–36.
935. Hammar S, Mennemeyer R (1976). Lymphomatoid granulomatosis in a renal transplant recipient. Hum Pathol. 7:111–6.
936. Hammerman PS, Lawrence MS, Voet D, et al. (2012). Comprehensive genomic characterization of squamous cell lung cancers. Nature. 489:519–25.
937. Hamoudi R, Diss TC, Oksenhendler E, et al. (2004). Distinct cellular origins of primary effusion lymphoma with and without EBV infection. Leuk Res. 28:333–8.
938. Han AJ, Xiong M, Gu YY, et al. (2001). Lymphoepithelioma-like carcinoma of the lung with a better prognosis. A clinicopathologic study of 32 cases. Am J Clin Pathol. 115:841–50.
939. Han AJ, Xiong M, Zong YS (2000). Association of Epstein-Barr virus with lymphoepithelioma-like carcinoma of the lung in southern China. Am J Clin Pathol. 114:220–6.
940. Han HJ, Park SJ, Min KH, et al. (2011). Whole-body magnetic resonance imaging for staging metastatic thymic carcinoma. Am J Respir Crit Care Med. 183:1573–4.
941. Han SW, Kim HP, Jeon YK, et al. (2008). Mucoepidermoid carcinoma of lung: potential target of EGFR-directed treatment. Lung Cancer. 61:30–4.
942. Han Y, Chen X, Wang X, et al. (2014). Cardiac capillary hemangioma: a case report and brief review of the literature. J Clin Ultrasound. 42:53–6.
943. Hannah CD, Oliver DH, Liu J (2007). Fine needle aspiration biopsy and immunostaining findings in an aggressive inflammatory myofibroblastic tumor of the lung: a case report. Acta Cytol. 51:239–43.
944. Haque AK, Myers JL, Hudnall SD, et al. (1998). Pulmonary lymphomatoid granulomatosis in acquired immunodeficiency syndrome: lesions with Epstein-Barr virus infection. Mod Pathol. 11:347–56.
945. Hara M, Iida A, Tohyama J, et al. (2001). FDG-PET findings in sclerosing hemangioma of the lung: a case report. Radiat Med. 19:215–8.
946. Hara M, Sato Y, Kitase M, et al. (2001). CT and MR findings of a pleomorphic adenoma in the peripheral lung. Radiat Med. 19:111–4.
947. Harada H, Miura K, Tsutsui Y, et al. (2000). Solitary squamous cell papilloma of the lung in a 40-year-old woman with recurrent laryngeal papillomatosis. Pathol Int. 50:431–9.
948. Harari S, Torre O, Cassandro R, et al. (2012). Bronchoscopic diagnosis of Langerhans cell histiocytosis and lymphangioleiomyomatosis. Respir Med. 106:1286–92.
949. Harding CO, Pagon RA (1990). Incidence of tuberous sclerosis in patients with cardiac rhabdomyoma. Am J Med Genet. 37:443–6.
950. Harigae H, Ichinohasama R, Miura I, et al. (2002). Primary marginal zone lymphoma of the thymus accompanied by chromosomal anomaly 46,X,dup(X)(p11p22). Cancer Genet Cytogenet. 133:142–7.
951. Hariri LP, Applegate MB, Mino-Kenudson M, et al. (2013). Volumetric optical frequency domain imaging of pulmonary pathology with precise correlation to histopathology. Chest. 143:64–74.
952. Harnath T, Marx A, Strobel P, et al. (2012). Thymoma-a clinico-pathological long-term study with emphasis on histology and adjuvant radiotherapy dose. J Thorac Oncol. 7:1867–71.
953. Haroche J, Charlotte F, Arnaud L, et al. (2012). High prevalence of BRAF V600E mutations in Erdheim-Chester disease but not in other non-Langerhans cell histiocytoses. Blood. 120:2700–3.
954. Haroche J, Cohen-Aubart F, Emile JF, et al. (2013). Dramatic efficacy of vemurafenib in both multisystemic and refractory Erdheim-Chester disease and Langerhans cell histiocytosis harboring the BRAF V600E mutation. Blood. 121:1495–500.
955. Harris NL (1999). Hodgkin's disease: classification and differential diagnosis. Mod Pathol. 12:159–75.
956. Harris NL, Jaffe ES, Stein H, et al. (1994). A revised European-American classification of lymphoid neoplasms: a proposal from the International Lymphoma Study Group. Blood. 84:1361–92.
957. Hartel PH, Fanburg-Smith JC, Frazier AA, et al. (2007). Primary pulmonary and mediastinal synovial sarcoma: a clinicopathologic study of 60 cases and comparison with five prior series. Mod Pathol. 20:760–9.
958. Hartert M, Strobel P, Dahm M, et al. (2010). A follicular dendritic cell sarcoma of the mediastinum with immature T cells and association with myasthenia gravis. Am J Surg Pathol. 34:742–5.
959. Harting MT, Messner GN, Gregoric ID, et al. (2004). Sarcoma metastatic to the right ventricle: surgical intervention followed by prolonged survival. Tex Heart Inst J. 31:93–5.
960. Hartmann CA, Roth C, Minck C, et al. (1990). Thymic carcinoma. Report of five cases and review of the literature. J Cancer Res Clin Oncol. 116:69–82.
961. Hartmann JT, Einhorn L, Nichols CR, et al. (2001). Second-line chemotherapy in patients with relapsed extragonadal nonseminomatous germ cell tumors: results of an international multicenter analysis. J Clin Oncol. 19:1641–8.
962. Hartmann JT, Fossa SD, Nichols CR, et al. (2001). Incidence of metachronous testicular cancer in patients with extragonadal germ cell tumors. J Natl Cancer Inst. 93:1733–8.
963. Hartmann JT, Nichols CR, Droz JP, et al. (2000). The relative risk of second nongerminal malignancies in patients with extragonadal germ cell tumors. Cancer. 88:2629–35.
964. Hartmann JT, Nichols CR, Droz JP, et al. (2000). Hematologic disorders associated with primary mediastinal nonseminomatous germ cell tumors. J Natl Cancer Inst. 92:54–61.
965. Hartmann JT, Nichols CR, Droz JP, et al. (2002). Prognostic variables for response and outcome in patients with extragonadal germ-cell tumors. Ann Oncol. 13:1017–28.
966. Hasegawa T, Matsuno Y, Shimoda T, et al. (2001). Proximal-type epithelioid sarcoma: a clinicopathologic study of 20 cases. Mod Pathol. 14:655–63.
967. Hasleton P, Flieder DB (2013). Spencer's Pathology of the Lung. 6th ed. Cambridge: Cambridge University Press.
968. Hasle H, Jacobsen BB (1995). Origin of male mediastinal germ-cell tumours. Lancet. 345:1046.
969. Hasle H, Jacobsen BB, Asschenfeldt P, et al. (1992). Mediastinal germ cell tumour associated with Klinefelter syndrome. A report of case and review of the literature. Eur J Pediatr. 151:735–9.
970. Hasle H, Mellemgaard A, Nielsen J, et al. (1995). Cancer incidence in men with Klinefelter syndrome. Br J Cancer. 71:416–20.
971. Hasleton PS (1994). Histopathology and prognostic factors in bronchial carcinoid tumours. Thorax. 49 Suppl:S56–62.
972. Hassan R, Alexander R (2005). Nonpleural mesotheliomas: mesothelioma of the peritoneum, tunica vaginalis, and pericardium. Hematol Oncol Clin North Am. 19:1067–87. [vi.]
973. Hasserjian RP, Klimstra DS, Rosai J (1995). Carcinoma of the thymus with clear-cell features. Report of eight cases and review of the literature. Am J Surg Pathol. 19:835–41.
974. Hata A, Katakami N, Fujita S, et al. (2010). Frequency of EGFR and KRAS mutations in Japanese patients with lung adenocarcinoma with features of the mucinous subtype of bronchioloalveolar carcinoma. J Thorac Oncol. 5:1197–200.
975. Hayashi A, Fumon T, Miki Y, et al. (2013). The evaluation of immunohistochemical markers and thymic cortical microenvironmental cells in distinguishing thymic carcinoma from type b3 thymoma or lung squamous cell carcinoma. J Clin Exp Hematop. 53:9–19.
976. Hayashi A, Takamori S, Tayama K, et al. (1997). Thymolipoma: clinical and pathological features--report of three cases and review of literature. Kurume Med J. 44:141–6.
977. Hayashi T, Haba R, Tanizawa J, et al. (2012). Cytopathologic features and differential diagnostic considerations of primary lymphoepithelioma-like carcinoma of the lung. Diagn Cytopathol. 40:820–5.
978. Hayashida M, Seyama K, Inoue Y, et al. (2007). The epidemiology of lymphangioleiomyomatosis in Japan: a nationwide cross-sectional study of presenting features and prognostic factors. Respirology. 12:523–30.
979. Heard BE, Corrin B, Dewar A (1985). Pathology of seven mucous cell adenomas of the bronchial glands with particular reference to ultrastructure. Histopathology. 9:687–701.
980. Hecht SS, Szabo E (2014). Fifty years of tobacco carcinogenesis research: from mechanisms to early detection and prevention of lung cancer. Cancer Prev Res (Phila). 7:1–8.
981. Heenan PJ, Maize JC, Cook MG, et al. (2006). Persistent melanoma and local metastasis of melanoma. In: LeBoit PE, Burg G, Weedon D, Sarasin A, eds. WHO Classification of Tumours. Pathology and Genetics of Skin Tumours. 3rd ed. Lyon: IARC; pp 90–92.
982. Hegg CA, Flint A, Singh G (1992). Papillary adenoma of the lung. Am J Clin Pathol. 97:393–7.
983. Heitmiller RF, Mathisen DJ, Ferry JA, et al. (1989). Mucoepidermoid lung tumors. Ann Thorac Surg. 47:394–9.
984. Hekimgil M, Hamulu F, Cagirici U, et al. (2001). Small cell neuroendocrine carcinoma of the thymus complicated by Cushing's syndrome. Report of a 58-year-old woman with a 3-year history of hypertension. Pathol Res Pract. 197:129–33.
985. Heletz I, Abramson SV (2009). Large obstructive cardiac myxofibrosarcoma is nearly invisible on transthoracic echocardiogram. Echocardiography. 26:847–51.
986. Hemachandran M, Kakkar N, Khandelwal N (2003). Giant-cell-rich myxoma of right atrium. An ultrastructural analysis. Cardiovasc Pathol. 12:287–9.
987. Hemminki K, Li X (2001). Incidence trends and risk factors of carcinoid tumors: a nationwide epidemiologic study from Sweden. Cancer. 92:2204–10.
988. Henley JD, Cummings OW, Loehrer PJ Sr (2004). Tyrosine kinase receptor expression in thymomas. J Cancer Res Clin Oncol. 130:222–4.
989. Heravi-Moussavi A, Anglesio MS, Cheng SW, et al. (2012). Recurrent somatic DICER1 mutations in nonepithelial ovarian cancers. N Engl J Med. 366:234–42.
989A. Herbst RS, Soria JC, Kowanetz M, et al. (2014). Predictive correlates of response to the anti-PD-L1 antibody MPDL3280A in cancer patients. Nature. 515:563–7.
990. Herbst WM, Kummer W, Hofmann W, et al. (1987). Carcinoid tumors of the thymus. An immunohistochemical study. Cancer. 60:2465–70.
991. Hernandez A, Gill FI, Aventura E, et al. (2012). Mediastinal pleomorphic sarcoma in an immunodeficient patient: case report and review of the literature. J La State Med Soc. 164:21–5.
992. Herth FJ, Eberhardt R, Anantham D, et al. (2009). Narrow-band imaging bronchoscopy increases the specificity of bronchoscopic early lung cancer detection. J Thorac Oncol. 4:1060–5.
993. Higashiyama M, Doi O, Kodama K, et al. (1995). Lymphoepithelioma-like carcinoma of the lung: analysis of two cases for Epstein-Barr virus infection. Hum Pathol. 26:1278–82.
994. Higgins JP, Warnke RA (1999). CD30 expression is common in mediastinal large B-cell lymphoma. Am J Clin Pathol. 112:241–7.
995. Hill DA, Ivanovich J, Priest JR, et al. (2009). DICER1 mutations in familial pleuropulmonary blastoma. Science. 325:965.
996. Hill DA, Jarzembowski JA, Priest JR, et al. (2008). Type I pleuropulmonary blastoma: pathology and biology study of 51 cases from the international pleuropulmonary blastoma registry. Am J Surg Pathol. 32:282–95.
997. Hillerdal G (1983). Malignant mesothelioma 1982: review of 4710 published cases. Br J Dis Chest. 77:321–43.
998. Hinterberger M, Reineke T, Storz M, et al. (2007). D2-40 and calretinin - a tissue microarray analysis of 341 malignant mesotheliomas with emphasis on sarcomatoid differentiation. Mod Pathol. 20:248–55.
999. Hirabayashi H, Fujii Y, Sakaguchi M, et al. (1997). p16INK4, pRB, p53 and cyclin D1 expression and hypermethylation of CDKN2 gene in thymoma and thymic carcinoma. Int J Cancer. 73:639–44.
1000. Hirai T, Yamanaka A, Fujimoto T, et al. (2001). Multiple thymoma with myotonic dystrophy. Jpn J Thorac Cardiovasc Surg. 49:457–60.
1001. Hiraiwa H, Hamazaki M, Tsuruta S, et al. (1998). Infantile hemangioendothelioma of the thymus with massive pleural effusion and Kasabach--Merritt syndrome: histopathological, flow cytometrical analysis of the tumor. Acta Paediatr Jpn. 40:604–7.
1002. Hirakata K, Nakata H, Nakagawa T (1995). CT of pulmonary metastases with pathological correlation. Semin Ultrasound CT MR. 16:379–94.
1003. Hirano H, Maeda T, Tsuji M, et al. (2002). Malignant mesothelioma of the pericardium: case reports and immunohistochemical studies including Ki-67 expression. Pathol Int. 52:669–76.
1004. Hirao T, Bueno R, Chen CJ, et al. (2002). Alterations of the p16(INK4) locus in human malignant mesothelial tumors. Carcinogenesis. 23:1127–30.
1005. Hirata J, Ohya M (2013). Cardiac tamponade following traumatic rupture of a mediastinal mature teratoma. BMJ Case Rep 2013:
1006. Hirsch FR, Bunn PA Jr (2014). Progress in research on screening and genetics in lung cancer. Lancet Respir Med. 2:19–21.
1007. Hirsch FR, Franklin WA, Gazdar AF, et al. (2001). Early detection of lung cancer: clinical perspectives of recent advances in biology and radiology. Clin Cancer Res. 7:5–22.
1008. Hirsch FR, Prindiville SA, Miller YE, et al. (2001). Fluorescence versus white-light bronchoscopy for detection of preneoplastic lesions: a randomized study. J Natl Cancer Inst. 93:1385–91.
1009. Hirsch FR, Wynes MW, Gandara DR, et al. (2010). The tissue is the issue: personalized medicine for non-small cell lung cancer. Clin Cancer Res. 16:4909–11.
1010. Hishida T, Yoshida J, Nishimura M, et al. (2009). Extraskeletal osteosarcoma arising in anterior mediastinum: brief report with a review of the literature. J Thorac Oncol. 4:927–9.

1011. Hishima T, Fukayama M, Fujisawa M, et al. (1994). CD5 expression in thymic carcinoma. Am J Pathol. 145:268–75.
1012. Hishima T, Fukayama M, Hayashi Y, et al. (1998). Neuroendocrine differentiation in thymic epithelial tumors with special reference to thymic carcinoma and atypical thymoma. Hum Pathol. 29:330–8.
1013. Hishima T, Fukayama M, Hayashi Y, et al. (2000). CD70 expression in thymic carcinoma. Am J Surg Pathol. 24:742–6.
1014. Ho CK, Wang E, Au WK, et al. (2009). Primary cardiac angiosarcoma of left atrium. J Card Surg. 24:524–5.
1015. Ho FC, Ho JC (1977). Pigmented carcinoid tumour of the thymus. Histopathology. 1:363–9.
1016. Ho JC, Wong MP, Lam WK (2006). Lymphoepithelioma-like carcinoma of the lung. Respirology. 11:539–45.
1017. Hoang CD, Zhang X, Scott PD, et al. (2004). Selective activation of insulin receptor substrate-1 and -2 in pleural mesothelioma cells: association with distinct malignant phenotypes. Cancer Res. 64:7479–85.
1017A. Hoang LL, Tacha DE, Qi W, et al. (2014). A newly developed uroplakin II antibody with increased sensitivity in urothelial carcinoma of the bladder. Arch Pathol Lab Med. 138:943–9.
1018. Hochberg J, Waxman IM, Kelly KM, et al. (2009). Adolescent non-Hodgkin lymphoma and Hodgkin lymphoma: state of the science. Br J Haematol. 144:24–40.
1019. Hodgson JT, Darnton A (2000). The quantitative risks of mesothelioma and lung cancer in relation to asbestos exposure. Ann Occup Hyg. 44:565–601.
1020. Hodgson JT, McElvenny DM, Darnton AJ, et al. (2005). The expected burden of mesothelioma mortality in Great Britain from 2002 to 2050. Br J Cancer. 92:587–93.
1021. Hoey ET, Mankad K, Puppala S, et al. (2009). MRI and CT appearances of cardiac tumours in adults. Clin Radiol. 64:1214–30.
1022. Holley DG, Martin GR, Brenner JI, et al. (1995). Diagnosis and management of fetal cardiac tumors: a multicenter experience and review of published reports. J Am Coll Cardiol. 26:516–20.
1023. Hollingsworth HC, Stetler-Stevenson M, Gagneten D, et al. (1994). Immunodeficiency-associated malignant lymphoma. Three cases showing genotypic evidence of both T- and B-cell lineages. Am J Surg Pathol. 18:1092–101.
1024. Holst VA, Finkelstein S, Colby TV, et al. (1997). p53 and K-ras mutational genotyping in pulmonary carcinosarcoma, spindle cell carcinoma, and pulmonary blastoma: implications for histogenesis. Am J Surg Pathol. 21:801–11.
1025. Honecker F, Stoop H, Mayer F, et al. (2006). Germ cell lineage differentiation in non-seminomatous germ cell tumours. J Pathol. 208:395–400.
1026. Hong HH, Devereux TR, Melnick RL, et al. (2000). Mutations of ras protooncogenes and p53 tumor suppressor gene in cardiac hemangiosarcomas from B6C3F1 mice exposed to 1,3-butadiene for 2 years. Toxicol Pathol. 28:529–34.
1027. Hong JY, Kim HJ, Ko YH, et al. (2014). Clinical features and treatment outcomes of intravascular large B-cell lymphoma: a single-center experience in Korea. Acta Haematol. 131:18–27.
1028. Honicky RE, dePapp EW (1973). Mediastinal teratoma with endocrine function. Am J Dis Child. 126:650–3.
1029. Hoppe RT, Advani RH, Ai WZ, et al. (2011). Hodgkin lymphoma. J Natl Compr Canc Netw. 9:1020–58.
1030. Horenstein MG, Nador RG, Chadburn A, et al. (1997). Epstein-Barr virus latent gene expression in primary effusion lymphomas containing Kaposi's sarcoma-associated herpesvirus/human herpesvirus-8. Blood. 90:1186–91.
1031. Horeweg N, van der Aalst CM, Thunnissen E, et al. (2013). Characteristics of lung cancers detected by computer tomography screening in the randomized NELSON trial. Am J Respir Crit Care Med. 187:848–54.
1032. Hornick JL, Fletcher CD (2003). Myoepithelial tumors of soft tissue: a clinicopathologic and immunohistochemical study of 101 cases with evaluation of prognostic parameters. Am J Surg Pathol. 27:1183–96.
1033. Hornick JL, Jaffe ES, Fletcher CD (2004). Extranodal histiocytic sarcoma: clinicopathologic analysis of 14 cases of a rare epithelioid malignancy. Am J Surg Pathol. 28:1133–44.
1034. Hoshi R, Furuta N, Horai T, et al. (2010). Discriminant model for cytologic distinction of large cell neuroendocrine carcinoma from small cell carcinoma of the lung. J Thorac Oncol. 5:472–8.
1035. Houghton AM (2013). Mechanistic links between COPD and lung cancer. Nat Rev Cancer. 13:233–45.
1036. Howlader N, Noone AM, Krapcho M, et al., eds. SEER Cancer Statistics Review, 1975-2010. http://seer.cancer.gov/csr/1975_2010
1037. Hsia JY, Chen CY, Hsu CP, et al. (1999). Adenosquamous carcinoma of the lung. Surgical results compared with squamous cell and adenocarcinoma. Scand Cardiovasc J. 33:29–32.
1038. Hsieh MS, Wu CT, Chang YL (2013). Unusual presentation of lymphoepithelioma-like carcinoma of lung as a thin-walled cavity. Ann Thorac Surg. 96:1857–9.
1039. Hsu CP, Chen CY, Chen CL, et al. (1994). Thymic carcinoma. Ten years' experience in twenty patients. J Thorac Cardiovasc Surg. 107:615–20.
1040. Hsueh C, Kuo TT, Tsang NM, et al. (2006). Thymic lymphoepitheliomalike carcinoma in children: clinicopathologic features and molecular analysis. J Pediatr Hematol Oncol. 28:785–90.
1041. Hu YH, Liu CY, Chiu CH, et al. (2007). Successful treatment of elderly advanced lymphomatoid granulomatosis with rituximab-CVP combination therapy. Eur J Haematol. 78:176–7.
1042. Huang CC, Collins BT, Flint A, et al. (2013). Pulmonary neuroendocrine tumors: an entity in search of cytologic criteria. Diagn Cytopathol. 41:689–96.
1043. Huang H, Lu ZW, Jiang CG, et al. (2011). Clinical and prognostic characteristics of pulmonary mucosa-associated lymphoid tissue lymphoma: a retrospective analysis of 23 cases in a Chinese population. Chin Med J (Engl). 124:1026–30.
1044. Huang HH, Huang JY, Lung CC, et al. (2013). Cell-type specificity of lung cancer associated with low-dose soil heavy metal contamination in Taiwan: an ecological study. BMC Public Health. 13:330.
1045. Huang SY, Shen SJ, Li XY (2013). Pulmonary sarcomatoid carcinoma: a clinicopathologic study and prognostic analysis of 51 cases. World J Surg Oncol. 11:252.
1046. Huang X, Kushekhar K, Nolte I, et al. (2012). HLA associations in classical Hodgkin lymphoma: EBV status matters. PLoS ONE. 7:e39986.
1047. Hudacko R, Aviv H, Langenfeld J, et al. (2009). Thymolipoma: clues to pathogenesis revealed by cytogenetics. Ann Diagn Pathol. 13:185–8.
1048. McAllister HA Jr, Fenoglio JJ Jr (1978). Tumors of the Cardiovascular System. AFIP Atlas of Tumor Pathology. 2nd ed. Volume 15. Washington, DC: American Registry of Pathology.
1049. Hughes JH, Young NA, Wilbur DC, et al. (2005). Fine-needle aspiration of pulmonary hamartoma: a common source of false-positive diagnoses in the College of American Pathologists Interlaboratory Comparison Program in Nongynecologic Cytology. Arch Pathol Lab Med. 129:19–22.
1050. Hui G, McAllister HA, Angelini P (1987). Left atrial paraganglioma: report of a case and review of the literature. Am Heart J. 113:1230–4.
1051. Hui KS, Green LK, Schmidt WA (1988). Primary cardiac rhabdomyosarcoma: definition of a rare entity. Am J Cardiovasc Pathol. 2:19–29.
1052. Hultberg B, Isaksson A, Agardh E, et al. (1991). The association between plasma beta-hexosaminidase and its isoenzyme patterns and retinopathy in type 1 diabetes mellitus. Clin Chim Acta. 196:177–83.
1053. Hunter ZR, Xu L, Yang G, et al. (2014). The genomic landscape of Waldenstrom macroglobulinemia is characterized by highly recurring MYD88 and WHIM-like CXCR4 mutations, and small somatic deletions associated with B-cell lymphomagenesis. Blood. 123:1637–46.
1054. Huo L, Moran CA, Fuller GN, et al. (2006). Pulmonary artery sarcoma: a clinicopathologic and immunohistochemical study of 12 cases. Am J Clin Pathol. 125:419–24.
1055. Hurt RD, Bruckman JE, Farrow GM, et al. (1982). Primary anterior mediastinal seminoma. Cancer. 49:1658–63.
1056. Husain AN, Colby T, Ordonez N, et al. (2013). Guidelines for pathologic diagnosis of malignant mesothelioma: 2012 update of the consensus statement from the International Mesothelioma Interest Group. Arch Pathol Lab Med. 137:647–67.
1057. Husain K, Thomas E, Demerdash Z, et al. (2011). Mediastinal ganglioneuroblastoma-secreting vasoactive intestinal peptide causing secretory diarrhoea. Arab J Gastroenterol. 12:106–8.
1058. Hwang DH, Szeto DP, Perry AS, et al. (2014). Pulmonary large cell carcinoma lacking squamous differentiation is clinicopathologically indistinguishable from solid-subtype adenocarcinoma. Arch Pathol Lab Med. 138:626–35.
1059. Hwang H, Tse C, Rodriguez S, et al. (2014). p16 FISH deletion in surface epithelial mesothelial proliferations is predictive of underlying invasive mesothelioma. Am J Surg Pathol. 38:681–8.
1060. Hwang HS, Park CS, Yoon DH, et al. (2014). High Concordance of Gene Expression Profiling-correlated Immunohistochemistry Algorithms in Diffuse Large B-cell Lymphoma, Not Otherwise Specified. Am J Surg Pathol. 38:1046–57.
1061. Hysi I, Wattez H, Benhamed L, et al. (2011). Primary pulmonary myoepithelial carcinoma. Interact Cardiovasc Thorac Surg. 13:226–8.
1062. Iacobone M, Mondi I, Viel G, et al. (2010). The results of surgery for mediastinal parathyroid tumors: a comparative study of 63 patients. Langenbecks Arch Surg. 395:947–53.
1063. Ibi T, Hirai K, Takeuchi S, et al. (2013). Mature teratoma of the posterior mediastinum: report of a case. Gen Thorac Cardiovasc Surg. 61:655–8.
1064. Iczkowski KA, Butler SL, Shanks JH, et al. (2008). Trials of new germ cell immunohistochemical stains in 93 extragonadal and metastatic germ cell tumors. Hum Pathol. 39:275–81.
1065. Iezzoni JC, Gaffey MJ, Weiss LM (1995). The role of Epstein-Barr virus in lymphoepithelioma-like carcinomas. Am J Clin Pathol. 103:308–15.
1066. Iezzoni JC, Nass LB (1996). Thymic basaloid carcinoma: a case report and review of the literature. Mod Pathol. 9:21–5.
1067. Ikdahl T, Josefsen D, Jakobsen E, et al. (2008). Concurrent mediastinal germ-cell tumour and haematological malignancy: case report and short review of literature. Acta Oncol. 47:466–9.
1068. Ikeda J, Morii E, Tomita Y, et al. (2007). Mediastinal lymphangiomatosis coexisting with occult thymic carcinoma. Virchows Arch. 450:211–4.
1069. Ilhan I, Kutluk T, Gogus S, et al. (1994). Hypertrophic pulmonary osteoarthropathy in a child with thymic carcinoma: an unusual presentation in childhood. Med Pediatr Oncol. 23:140–3.
1069A. Illei PB, Ladanyi M, Rusch VW, et al. (2003). The use of CDKN2A deletion as a diagnostic marker for malignant mesothelioma in body cavity effusions. Cancer. 99:51–6.
1070. Illei PB, Rosai J, Klimstra DS (2001). Expression of thyroid transcription factor-1 and other markers in sclerosing hemangioma of the lung. Arch Pathol Lab Med. 125:1335–9.
1071. Illei PB, Rusch VW, Zakowski MF, et al. (2003). Homozygous deletion of CDKN2A and codeletion of the methylthioadenosine phosphorylase gene in the majority of pleural mesotheliomas. Clin Cancer Res. 9:2108–13.
1072. Illouz F, Pinaud F, De Brux JL, et al. (2012). Long-delayed localization of a cardiac functional paraganglioma with SDHC mutation. Ann Intern Med. 157:222–3.
1073. Ilowite NT, Fligner CL, Ochs HD, et al. (1986). Pulmonary angiitis with atypical lymphoreticular infiltrates in Wiskott-Aldrich syndrome: possible relationship of lymphomatoid granulomatosis and EBV infection. Clin Immunol Immunopathol. 41:479–84.
1074. Imai H, Sunaga N, Kaira K, et al. (2009). Clinicopathological features of patients with bronchial-associated lymphoid tissue lymphoma. Intern Med. 48:301–6.
1075. Imai K, Saito H, Minamiya Y, et al. (2008). Malignant fibrous histiocytoma originating from the thymus. Gen Thorac Cardiovasc Surg. 56:606–9.
1076. Imielinski M, Berger AH, Hammerman PS, et al. (2012). Mapping the hallmarks of lung adenocarcinoma with massively parallel sequencing. Cell. 150:1107–20.
1077. Imperatori A, De Monte L, Rotolo N, et al. (2011). Hypertension and intrapericardial paraganglioma: an exceptional presentation of multiple endocrine neoplasia type IIA syndrome. Hypertension. 58:e189–90.
1078. Inagaki H, Chan JK, Ng JW, et al. (2002). Primary thymic extranodal marginal-zone B-cell lymphoma of mucosa-associated lymphoid tissue type exhibits distinctive clinicopathological and molecular features. Am J Pathol. 160:1435–43.
1079. Inagaki H, Okabe M, Seto M, et al. (2001). API2-MALT1 fusion transcripts involved in mucosa-associated lymphoid tissue lymphoma: multiplex RT-PCR detection using formalin-fixed paraffin-embedded specimens. Am J Pathol. 158:699–706.
1080. Inamura K, Kumasaka T, Furuta R, et al. (2011). Mixed squamous cell and glandular papilloma of the lung: a case study and literature review. Pathol Int. 61:252–8.
1081. Inamura K, Satoh Y, Okumura S, et al. (2005). Pulmonary adenocarcinomas with enteric differentiation: histologic and immunohistochemical characteristics compared with metastatic colorectal cancers and usual pulmonary adenocarcinomas. Am J Surg Pathol. 29:660–5.
1082. Incarbone M, Ceresoli GL, Di Tommaso L, et al. (2008). Primary pulmonary meningioma: report of a case and review of the literature. Lung Cancer. 62:401–7.
1083. Inci I, Soltermann A, Schneiter D, et al. (2014). Pulmonary malignant peripheral nerve sheath tumour. Eur J Cardiothorac Surg. 46:331–2.
1084. Inhorn RC, Aster JC, Roach SA, et al. (1995). A syndrome of lymphoblastic lymphoma, eosinophilia, and myeloid hyperplasia/malignancy associated with t(8;13)(p11;q11): description of a distinctive clinicopathologic entity. Blood. 85:1881–7.

1085. Inoki K, Corradetti MN, Guan KL (2005). Dysregulation of the TSC-mTOR pathway in human disease. Nat Genet. 37:19–24.

1086. Inoue A, Tomiyama N, Fujimoto K, et al. (2006). MR imaging of thymic epithelial tumors: correlation with World Health Organization classification. Radiat Med. 24:171–81.

1087. Inoue M, Marx A, Zettl A, et al. (2002). Chromosome 6 suffers frequent and multiple aberrations in thymoma. Am J Pathol. 161:1507–13.

1088. Inoue M, Starostik P, Zettl A, et al. (2003). Correlating genetic aberrations with World Health Organization-defined histology and stage across the spectrum of thymomas. Cancer Res. 63:3708–15.

1089. International Germ Cell Cancer Collaborative Group (1997). International Germ Cell Consensus Classification: a prognostic factor-based staging system for metastatic germ cell cancers. J Clin Oncol. 15:594–603.

1090. Ionescu DN, Sasatomi E, Aldeeb D, et al. (2004). Pulmonary meningothelial-like nodules: a genotypic comparison with meningiomas. Am J Surg Pathol. 28:207–14.

1091. Ionescu DN, Treaba D, Gilks CB, et al. (2007). Nonsmall cell lung carcinoma with neuroendocrine differentiation--an entity of no clinical or prognostic significance. Am J Surg Pathol. 31:26–32.

1092. Iqbal J, Greiner TC, Patel K, et al. (2007). Distinctive patterns of BCL6 molecular alterations and their functional consequences in different subgroups of diffuse large B-cell lymphoma. Leukemia. 21:2332–43.

1093. Isaacson PG (1990). Lymphomas of mucosa-associated lymphoid tissue (MALT). Histopathology. 16:617–9.

1094. Isaacson PG, Chan JK, Tang C, et al. (1990). Low-grade B-cell lymphoma of mucosa-associated lymphoid tissue arising in the thymus. A thymic lymphoma mimicking myoepithelial sialadenitis. Am J Surg Pathol. 14:342–51.

1095. Isaka M, Nakagawa K, Maniwa T, et al. (2011). Disseminated calcifying tumor of the pleura: review of the literature and a case report with immunohistochemical study of its histogenesis. Gen Thorac Cardiovasc Surg. 59:579–82.

1096. Isambert N, Ray-Coquard I, Italiano A, et al. (2014). Primary cardiac sarcomas: a retrospective study of the French Sarcoma Group. Eur J Cancer. 50:128–36.

1097. Ishibashi H, Shimoyama T, Akamatsu H, et al. (2002). [A successfully resected case of giant malignant mediastinal germ cell tumor]. Kyobu Geka. 55:815–8.

1098. Ishibashi H, Takahashi S, Tomoko H, et al. (2003). Primary intrapulmonary thymoma successfully resected with vascular reconstruction. Ann Thorac Surg. 76:1735–7.

1099. Ishida M, Hodohara K, Okabe H (2012). Mediastinal seminoma occurring in Down syndrome. J Pediatr Hematol Oncol. 34:387–8.

1100. Ishii H, Kishi K, Kushima H, et al. (2007). [Pulmonary lymphomatoid granulomatosis radiologically mimicking interstitial pneumonia]. Nihon Kokyuki Gakkai Zasshi. 45:483–8.

1101. Ishii Y, Tomita N, Takasaki H, et al. (2012). Clinical features of extranodal marginal zone lymphoma of mucosa-associated lymphoid tissue. Hematol Oncol. 30:186–9.

1102. Ishikawa Y, Kato K, Taniguchi T, et al. (2013). Imaging of a case of metaplastic thymoma on 18F-FDG PET/CT. Clin Nucl Med. 38:e463–4.

1103. Ishikawa Y, Tateyama H, Yoshida M, et al. (2015). Micronodular Thymoma with Lymphoid Stroma: An Immunohistochemical Study of the Distribution of Langerhans Cells and Mature Dendritic Cells in Six Patients. Histopathology. 66:300-7.

1104. Ishizumi T, McWilliams A, MacAulay C, et al. (2010). Natural history of bronchial preinvasive lesions. Cancer Metastasis Rev. 29:5–14.

1105. Isowa N, Kikuchi R, Kunimoto Y, et al.

(2007). Successful resection of posterior mediastinal thyroid cancer by partial sternotomy combined with video-assisted thoracoscopy. Ann Thorac Cardiovasc Surg. 13:47–9.

1106. Italiano A, Cortot AB, Ilie M, et al. (2009). EGFR and KRAS status of primary sarcomatoid carcinomas of the lung: implications for anti-EGFR treatment of a rare lung malignancy. Int J Cancer. 125:2479–82.

1107. Ito I, Nagai S, Kitaichi M, et al. (2005). Pulmonary manifestations of primary Sjogren's syndrome: a clinical, radiologic, and pathologic study. Am J Respir Crit Care Med. 171:632–8.

1108. Itoh K, Matsumura T, Egawa Y, et al. (1998). Primary mitral valve sarcoma in infancy. Pediatr Cardiol. 19:174–7.

1109. Ivanov SV, Miller J, Lucito R, et al. (2009). Genomic events associated with progression of pleural malignant mesothelioma. Int J Cancer. 124:589–99.

1110. Ivanova AV, Goparaju CM, Ivanov SV, et al. (2009). Protumorigenic role of HAPLN1 and its IgV domain in malignant pleural mesothelioma. Clin Cancer Res. 15:2602–11.

1111. Iwa N, Masuda K, Yutani C, et al. (2009). Imprint cytology of primary cardiac sarcomas: a report of 3 cases. Ann Diagn Pathol. 13:239–45.

1112. Iwa N, Yutani C (1993). Cytology of cardiac myxomas: presence of Ulex europaeus agglutinin-I (UEA-I) lectin by immunoperoxidase staining. Diagn Cytopathol. 9:661–4.

1113. Iwamoto N, Ishida M, Yoshida K, et al. (2013). Mediastinal seminoma: a case report with special emphasis on SALL4 as a new immunocytochemical marker. Diagn Cytopathol. 41:821–4.

1114. Iyoda A, Hiroshima K, Toyozaki T, et al. (2001). Clinical characterization of pulmonary large cell neuroendocrine carcinoma and large cell carcinoma with neuroendocrine morphology. Cancer. 91:1992–2000.

1115. Iyoda A, Travis WD, Sarkaria IS, et al. (2011). Expression profiling and identification of potential molecular targets for therapy in pulmonary large-cell neuroendocrine carcinoma. Exp Ther Med. 2:1041–5.

1116. Izumi N, Nishiyama N, Iwata T, et al. (2009). Primary pulmonary meningioma presenting with hemoptysis on exertion. Ann Thorac Surg. 88:647–8.

1117. Jabir S, Al-Hyassat S (2013). Histological diagnosis of cardiac lipoma in an adult with tuberous sclerosis. BMJ Case Rep 2013:

1118. Jackman DM, Miller VA, Cioffredi LA, et al. (2009). Impact of epidermal growth factor receptor and KRAS mutations on clinical outcomes in previously untreated non-small cell lung cancer patients: results of an online tumor registry of clinical trials. Clin Cancer Res. 15:5267–73.

1119. Jackman DM, Yeap BY, Sequist LV, et al. (2006). Exon 19 deletion mutations of epidermal growth factor receptor are associated with prolonged survival in non-small cell lung cancer patients treated with gefitinib or erlotinib. Clin Cancer Res. 12:3908–14.

1120. Jacob AG, Driscoll DJ, Shaughnessy WJ, et al. (1998). Klippel-Trenaunay syndrome: spectrum and management. Mayo Clin Proc. 73:28–36.

1121. Jacobs JP, Konstantakos AK, Holland FW, et al. (1994). Surgical treatment for cardiac rhabdomyomas in children. Ann Thorac Surg. 58:1552–5.

1122. Jaffe ES, Harris NL, Stein H, et al., eds. (2001). WHO Classification of Tumours. Pathology and Genetics of Tumours of Haematopoietic and Lymphoid Tissues. 1st ed. Lyon: IARC.

1123. Jaffe ES, Chan JK, Su IJ, et al. (1996). Report of the Workshop on Nasal and Related Extranodal Angiocentric T/Natural Killer Cell Lymphomas. Definitions, differential diagnosis, and epidemiology. Am J Surg Pathol. 20:103–11.

1124. Jaffe ES, Pittaluga S (2011). Aggressive

B-cell lymphomas: a review of new and old entities in the WHO classification. Hematology (Am Soc Hematol Educ Program). 2011:506–14.

1125. Jaffe ES, Wilson WH (1997). Lymphomatoid granulomatosis: pathogenesis, pathology and clinical implications. Cancer Surv. 30:233–48.

1126. Jaffe R, Weiss LM, Facchetti F (2008). Tumours derived from Langerhans cells. In: Swerdlow SH, Campo E, Harris NL, Jaffe ES, Pileri SA, Stein H et al., eds. WHO Classification of Tumours of Haematopoietic and Lymphoid Tissues. 4th ed. Lyon: IARC; pp 358–360.

1127. Jagirdar J (2008). Application of immunohistochemistry to the diagnosis of primary and metastatic carcinoma to the lung. Arch Pathol Lab Med. 132:384–96.

1128. Jain D, Maleszewski JJ, Halushka MK (2010). Benign cardiac tumors and tumorlike conditions. Ann Diagn Pathol. 14:215–30.

1129. Jain RK, Mehta RJ, Henley JD, et al. (2010). WHO types A and AB thymomas: not always benign. Mod Pathol. 23:1641–9.

1130. Jaiswal R, Rani P, Devenraj V (2014). Asymptomatic posterior mediastinal teratoma diagnosed incidentally. BMJ Case Rep 2014:

1131. Jakel J, Ramaswamy A, Kohler U, et al. (2006). Massive pulmonary tumor microembolism from a hepatocellular carcinoma. Pathol Res Pract. 202:395–9.

1132. Jakubowski W, Graban W, Kazon M, et al. (1979). [Renal angioscintigraphy (author's transl)]. Pol Przegl Radiol Med Nukl. 43:293–5.

1133. Jansson JO, Svensson J, Bengtsson BA, et al. (1998). Acromegaly and Cushing's syndrome due to ectopic production of GHRH and ACTH by a thymic carcinoid tumour: in vitro responses to GHRH and GHRP-6. Clin Endocrinol (Oxf). 48:243–50.

1134. Jasani B, Gibbs A (2012). Mesothelioma not associated with asbestos exposure. Arch Pathol Lab Med. 136:262–7.

1135. Jaso J, Chen L, Li S, et al. (2012). CD5-positive mucosa-associated lymphoid tissue (MALT) lymphoma: a clinicopathologic study of 14 cases. Hum Pathol. 43:1436–43.

1136. Jayaram G, Yaccob R, Liam CK (2003). Mucinous carcinoma (colloid carcinoma) of the lung diagnosed by fine needle aspiration cytology: a case report. Malays J Pathol. 25:63–8.

1137. Jayawardena S, Eisdorfer J, Volozhanina E, et al. (2008). Non Hodgkin's lymphoma presenting with chest pain. Med Sci Monit. 14:CS55–9.

1138. Jean D, Daubriac J, Le Pimpec-Barthes F, et al. (2012). Molecular changes in mesothelioma with an impact on prognosis and treatment. Arch Pathol Lab Med. 136:277–93.

1139. Jean WC, Walski-Easton SM, Nussbaum ES (2001). Multiple intracranial aneurysms as delayed complications of an atrial myxoma: case report. Neurosurgery. 49:200–2.

1140. Jeanmart M, Lantuejoul S, Fievet F, et al. (2003). Value of immunohistochemical markers in preinvasive bronchial lesions in risk assessment of lung cancer. Clin Cancer Res. 9:2195–203.

1141. Jenner RG, Maillard K, Cattini N, et al. (2003). Kaposi's sarcoma-associated herpesvirus-infected primary effusion lymphoma has a plasma cell gene expression profile. Proc Natl Acad Sci USA. 100:10399–404.

1141A. Jennings TA, Axiotis CA, Kress Y, Carter D (1990). Primary malignant melanoma of the lower respiratory tract. Report of a case and literature review. Am J Clin Pathol. 94:649–55.

1142. Jensen MO, Antonenko D (1992). Thyroid and thymic malignancy following childhood irradiation. J Surg Oncol. 50:206–8.

1143. Jeremy George P, Banerjee AK, Read CA, et al. (2007). Surveillance for the detection of early lung cancer in patients with bronchial dysplasia. Thorax. 62:43–50.

1144. Jeudy J, Kirsch J, Tavora F, et al. (2012). From the radiologic pathology archives: cardiac

lymphoma: radiologic-pathologic correlation. Radiographics. 32:1369–80.

1145. Jhun BW, Lee KJ, Jeon K, et al. (2013). Clinical applicability of staging small cell lung cancer according to the seventh edition of the TNM staging system. Lung Cancer 81: 65–70.

1146. Jiang K, Nie J, Wang J, et al. (2011). Multiple calcifying fibrous pseudotumor of the bilateral pleura. Jpn J Clin Oncol. 41:130–3.

1147. Jiang L, Admirand JH, Moran C, et al. (2006). Mediastinal follicular dendritic cell sarcoma involving bone marrow: a case report and review of the literature. Ann Diagn Pathol. 10:357–62.

1148. Jiang SX, Kameya T, Shoji M, et al. (1998). Large cell neuroendocrine carcinoma of the lung: a histologic and immunohistochemical study of 22 cases. Am J Surg Pathol. 22:526–37.

1149. Jibiki I, Yamaguchi N, Matsuda H, et al. (1990). Imaging of propagated sites of epileptic discharges in repeated 123I-IMP SPECT scans. Eur Neurol. 30:274–6.

1150. Jimenez Heffernan JA, Salas C, Tejerina E, et al. (2010). Gamna-Gandy bodies from cardiac myxoma on intraoperative cytology. Cytopathology. 21:203–5.

1151. Jimenez-Heffernan JA, Lopez-Ferrer P, Vicandi B, et al. (2008). Fine-needle aspiration cytology of large cell neuroendocrine carcinoma of the lung: a cytohistologic correlation study of 11 cases. Cancer. 114:180–6.

1152. Jin E, Fujiwara M, Nagashima M, et al. (2001). Aerogenous spread of primary lung adenocarcinoma induces ultrastructural remodeling of the alveolar capillary endothelium. Hum Pathol. 32:1050–8.

1153. John LC, Kingston J, Edmondson SJ (1993). Teratoma associated with endodermal sinus tumor. Pediatr Hematol Oncol. 10:49–54.

1154. Johnson BE, Russell E, Simmons AM, et al. (1996). MYC family DNA amplification in 126 tumor cell lines from patients with small cell lung cancer. J Cell Biochem Suppl. 24:210–7.

1155. Johnson DE, Appelt G, Samuels ML, et al. (1976). Metastases from testicular carcinoma. Study of 78 autopsied cases. Urology. 8:234–9.

1156. Johnson DH, Fehrenbacher L, Novotny WF, et al. (2004). Randomized phase II trial comparing bevacizumab plus carboplatin and paclitaxel with carboplatin and paclitaxel alone in previously untreated locally advanced or metastatic non-small-cell lung cancer. J Clin Oncol. 22:2184–91.

1157. Johnson H, Cohen C, Fatima N, et al. (2012). Thyroid transcription factor 1 and Napsin A double stain: utilizing different vendor antibodies for diagnosing lung adenocarcinoma. Acta Cytol. 56:596–602.

1158. Johnson SR, Whale CI, Hubbard RB, et al. (2004). Survival and disease progression in UK patients with lymphangioleiomyomatosis. Thorax. 59:800–3.

1159. Johnston WW, Elson CE (1991). Respiratory tract. In: Bibbo M, Day L, eds. Comprehensive Cytopathology. Philadelphia: WB Saunders; pp. 325–402.

1160. Jones D, Amin M, Ordonez NG, et al. (2001). Reticulum cell sarcoma of lymph node with mixed dendritic and fibroblastic features. Mod Pathol. 14:1059–67.

1161. Jones LT (1966). The lacrimal secretory system and its treatment. J All India Ophthalmol Soc. 14:191–6.

1162. Joos S, Otano-Joos MI, Ziegler S, et al. (1996). Primary mediastinal (thymic) B-cell lymphoma is characterized by gains of chromosomal material including 9p and amplification of the REL gene. Blood. 87:1571–8.

1163. Jorge C, Almeida AG, Mendes M, et al. (2013). Multiple 'crumbled' cardiac myxomas presenting as gait ataxia. Int J Cardiol. 167:e104–5.

1164. Jozwiak J, Sahin M, Jozwiak S, et al.

(2009). Cardiac rhabdomyoma in tuberous sclerosis: hyperactive Erk signaling. Int J Cardiol. 132:145–7.
1165. Jozwiak S, Kotulska K, Kasprzyk-Obara J, et al. (2006). Clinical and genotype studies of cardiac tumors in 154 patients with tuberous sclerosis complex. Pediatrics. 118:e1146–51.
1166. Ju YS, Lee WC, Shin JY, et al. (2012). A transforming KIF5B and RET gene fusion in lung adenocarcinoma revealed from whole-genome and transcriptome sequencing. Genome Res. 22:436–45.
1167. Junewick JJ, Fitzgerald NE (1999). The thymus in Langerhans' cell histiocytosis. Pediatr Radiol. 29:904–7.
1168. Jung KJ, Lee KS, Han J, et al. (2001). Malignant thymic epithelial tumors: CT-pathologic correlation. AJR Am J Roentgenol. 176:433–9.
1169. Jung SM, Chu PH, Shiu TF, et al. (2006). Expression of OCT4 in the primary germ cell tumors and thymoma in the mediastinum. Appl Immunohistochem Mol Morphol. 14:273–5.
1170. Jyothirmayi R, Jacob R, Nair K, et al. (1995). Primary fibrosarcoma of the right ventricle--a case report. Acta Oncol. 34:972–4.
1171. Kadakia KC, Patel SM, Yi ES, et al. (2013). Diffuse pulmonary lymphangiomatosis. Can Respir J. 20:52–4.
1172. Kadara H, Wistuba II (2014). Molecular Biology of Lung Preneoplasia. In: Roth JA, Hong WK, Komaki RU, Tsao AS, Chang JY, Blackmon SH, eds. Lung Cancer. 4th ed. Hoboken: John Wiley & Sons, Inc.; pp. 110–28.
1173. Kadota K, Haba R, Katsuki N, et al. (2010). Cytological findings of mixed squamous cell and glandular papilloma in the lung. Diagn Cytopathol. 38:913–7.
1174. Kadota K, Nitadori J, Sarkaria IS, et al. (2013). Thyroid transcription factor-1 expression is an independent predictor of recurrence and correlates with the IASLC/ATS/ERS histologic classification in patients with stage I lung adenocarcinoma. Cancer. 119:931–8.
1174A. Kadota K, Nitadori J, Sima C, et al. (2015). Tumor spread through air spaces is an important pattern of invasion and impacts the frequency and location of recurrences following limited resection for small Stage I lung adenocarcinomas. J Thoracic Oncol. Forthcoming.
1175. Kadota K, Nitadori JI, Woo KM, et al. (2014). Comprehensive Pathological Analyses in Lung Squamous Cell Carcinoma: Single Cell Invasion, Nuclear Diameter, and Tumor Budding Are Independent Prognostic Factors for Worse Outcomes. J Thorac Oncol. 9:1126–39.
1176. Kadota K, Suzuki K, Colovos C, et al. (2012). A nuclear grading system is a strong predictor of survival in epitheloid diffuse malignant pleural mesothelioma. Mod Pathol. 25:260–71.
1177. Kadota K, Suzuki K, Kachala SS, et al. (2012). A grading system combining architectural features and mitotic count predicts recurrence in stage I lung adenocarcinoma. Mod Pathol. 25:1117–27.
1178. Kadota K, Suzuki K, Sima CS, et al. (2011). Pleomorphic epithelioid diffuse malignant pleural mesothelioma: a clinicopathological review and conceptual proposal to reclassify as biphasic or sarcomatoid mesothelioma. J Thorac Oncol. 6:896–904.
1179. Kadota K, Villena-Vargas J, Yoshizawa A, et al. (2014). Prognostic significance of adenocarcinoma in situ, minimally invasive adenocarcinoma, and nonmucinous lepidic predominant invasive adenocarcinoma of the lung in patients with stage I disease. Am J Surg Pathol. 38:448–60.
1180. Kadota K, Yeh YC, Sima CS, et al. (2014). The cribriform pattern identifies a subset of acinar predominant tumors with poor prognosis in patients with stage I lung adenocarcinoma: a conceptual proposal to classify cribriform predominant tumors as a distinct histologic subtype. Mod Pathol. 27:690–700.
1181. Kaira K, Endo M, Abe M, et al. (2010). Biologic correlation of 2-[18F]-fluoro-2-deoxy-D-glucose uptake on positron emission tomography in thymic epithelial tumors. J Clin Oncol. 28:3746–53.
1182. Kaira K, Horie Y, Ayabe E, et al. (2010). Pulmonary pleomorphic carcinoma: a clinicopathological study including EGFR mutation analysis. J Thorac Oncol. 5:460–5.
1183. Kaira K, Murakami H, Serizawa M, et al. (2011). MUC1 expression in thymic epithelial tumors: MUC1 may be useful marker as differential diagnosis between type B3 thymoma and thymic carcinoma. Virchows Arch. 458:615–20.
1184. Kaira K, Sunaga N, Ishizuka T, et al. (2011). The role of [(1)(8)F]fluorodeoxyglucose positron emission tomography in thymic epithelial tumors. Cancer Imaging. 11:195–201.
1185. Kakegawa S, Shimizu K, Sugano M, et al. (2011). Clinicopathological features of lung adenocarcinoma with KRAS mutations. Cancer. 117:4257–66.
1186. Kakinuma H, Mikami T, Iwabuchi K, et al. (2003). Diagnostic findings of bronchial brush cytology for pulmonary large cell neuroendocrine carcinomas: comparison with poorly differentiated adenocarcinomas, squamous cell carcinomas, and small cell carcinomas. Cancer. 99:247–54.
1187. Kakkar N, Vasishta RK, Banerjee AK, et al. (1996). Primary pulmonary malignant teratoma with yolk sac element associated with hematologic neoplasia. Respiration. 63:52–4.
1188. Kaku N, Seki M, Doi S, et al. (2010). A case of intravascular large B-cell lymphoma (IVLBCL) with no abnormal findings on chest computed tomography diagnosed by random transbronchial lung biopsy. Intern Med. 49:2697–701.
1189. Kalari S, Jung M, Kernstine KH, et al. (2013). The DNA methylation landscape of small cell lung cancer suggests a differentiation defect of neuroendocrine cells. Oncogene. 32:3559–68.
1190. Kalemkerian GP, Gadgeel SM (2013). Modern staging of small cell lung cancer. J Natl Compr Canc Netw. 11:99–104.
1191. Kalhor N, Staerkel GA, Moran CA (2010). So-called sclerosing hemangioma of lung: current concept. Ann Diagn Pathol. 14:60–7.
1192. Kalhor N, Suster S, Moran CA (2010). Primary sclerosing neuroendocrine carcinomas of the lung: A clinicopathologic and immunohistochemical study of 10 cases. Am J Clin Pathol. 133:618–22.
1193. Kalhor N, Suster S, Moran CA (2011). Spindle cell thymomas (WHO Type A) with prominent papillary and pseudopapillary features: a clinicopathologic and immunohistochemical study of 10 cases. Am J Surg Pathol. 35:372–7.
1194. Kalhor N, Wistuba II (2013). Perfecting the fine-needle aspirate cell block. Cancer Cytopathol. 121:109–10.
1195. Kamby C, Vejborg I, Kristensen B, et al. (1988). Metastatic pattern in recurrent breast cancer. Special reference to intrathoracic recurrences. Cancer. 62:2226–33.
1196. Kamel OW, Gocke CD, Kell DL, et al. (1995). True histiocytic lymphoma: a study of 12 cases based on current definition. Leuk Lymphoma. 18:81–6.
1197. Kamiya H, Yasuda T, Nagamine H, et al. (2001). Surgical treatment of primary cardiac tumors: 28 years' experience in Kanazawa University Hospital. Jpn Circ J. 65:315–9.
1198. Kanavaros P, Gaulard P, Charlotte F, et al. (1995). Discordant expression of immunoglobulin and its associated molecule mb-1/CD79a is frequently found in mediastinal large B cell lymphomas. Am J Pathol. 146:735–41.
1199. Kanda M, Suzumiya J, Ohshima K, et al. (1999). Intravascular large cell lymphoma: clinicopathological, immuno-histochemical and molecular genetic studies. Leuk Lymphoma. 34:569–80.
1200. Kaneko Y, Frizzera G, Maseki N, et al. (1988). A novel translocation, t(9;17)(q34;q23), in aggressive childhood lymphoblastic lymphoma. Leukemia. 2:745–8.
1201. Kang CH, Kim YT, Jheon SH, et al. (2008). Surgical treatment of malignant mediastinal nonseminomatous germ cell tumor. Ann Thorac Surg. 85:379–84.
1202. Kang G, Yoon N, Han J, et al. (2012). Metaplastic thymoma: report of 4 cases. Korean J Pathol. 46:92–5.
1203. Kang SM, Kang HJ, Shin JH, et al. (2007). Identical epidermal growth factor receptor mutations in adenocarcinomatous and squamous cell carcinomatous components of adenosquamous carcinoma of the lung. Cancer. 109:581–7.
1204. Kansal R, Quintanilla-Martinez L, Datta V, et al. (2013). Identification of the V600D mutation in Exon 15 of the BRAF oncogene in congenital, benign langerhans cell histiocytosis. Genes Chromosomes Cancer. 52:99–106.
1205. Kanzaki R, Ikeda N, Okura E, et al. (2012). Thymic carcinoma with adenoid cystic carcinomalike features with distant metastases. Ann Thorac Cardiovasc Surg. 18:544–7.
1206. Kao CS, Idrees MT, Young RH, et al. (2012). Solid pattern yolk sac tumor: a morphologic and immunohistochemical study of 52 cases. Am J Surg Pathol. 36:360–7.
1207. Kapila K, Pathan SK, Amir T, et al. (2009). Mucoepidermoid thymic carcinoma: a challenging mediastinal aspirate. Diagn Cytopathol. 37:433–6.
1208. Kaplan MA, Tazelaar HD, Hayashi T, et al. (1996). Adenomatoid tumors of the pleura. Am J Surg Pathol. 20:1219–23.
1209. Karagoz Ozen DS, Ozturk MA, Selcukbiricik F, et al. (2013). Primary osteosarcoma of the heart: experience of an unusual case. Case Rep Oncol. 6:224–8.
1210. Karangelis D, Tagarakis G, Hevas A, et al. (2010). Benign primary cardiac tumours and Cowden's syndrome. Interact Cardiovasc Thorac Surg. 11:805.
1211. Karavitakis EM, Moschovi M, Stefanaki K, et al. (2007). Desmoplastic small round cell tumor of the pleura. Pediatr Blood Cancer. 49:335–8.
1212. Karbowniczek M, Astrinidis A, Balsara BR, et al. (2003). Recurrent lymphangiomyomatosis after transplantation: genetic analyses reveal a metastatic mechanism. Am J Respir Crit Care Med. 167:976–82.
1213. Kardamakis D, Bouboulis N, Ravazoula P, et al. (1996). Primary hemangiosarcoma of the mediastinum. Lung Cancer. 16:81–6.
1214. Karpathiou G, Sivridis E, Mikroulis D, et al. (2013). Pulmonary mucus gland adenomas: are they always of endobronchial localization? Case Rep Pathol. 2013:239173.
1215. Kasagi Y, Yamazaki K, Nakashima A, et al. (2009). Chondroblastic osteosarcoma arising from the pleura: report of a case. Surg Today. 39:1064–7.
1216. Katano H, Sato Y, Kurata T, et al. (2000). Expression and localization of human herpesvirus 8-encoded proteins in primary effusion lymphoma, Kaposi's sarcoma, and multicentric Castleman's disease. Virology. 269:335–44.
1217. Kathuria S, Jablokow VR (1987). Primary choriocarcinoma of mediastinum with immunohistochemical study and review of the literature. J Surg Oncol. 34:39–42.
1218. Katlic MR, Grillo HC, Wang CA (1985). Substernal goiter. Analysis of 80 patients from Massachusetts General Hospital. Am J Surg. 149:283–7.
1219. Kato H, Okunaka T, Shimatani H (1996). Photodynamic therapy for early stage bronchogenic carcinoma. J Clin Laser Med Surg. 14:235–8.
1220. Katz SL, Das P, Ngan BY, et al. (2005). Remote intrapulmonary spread of recurrent respiratory papillomatosis with malignant transformation. Pediatr Pulmonol. 39:185–8.
1221. Katzenstein AL, Carrington CB, Liebow AA (1979). Lymphomatoid granulomatosis: a clinicopathologic study of 152 cases. Cancer. 43:360–73.
1222. Katzenstein AL, Doxtader E, Narendra S (2010). Lymphomatoid granulomatosis: insights gained over 4 decades. Am J Surg Pathol. 34:e35–48.
1223. Katzenstein AL, Peiper SC (1990). Detection of Epstein-Barr virus genomes in lymphomatoid granulomatosis: analysis of 29 cases by the polymerase chain reaction technique. Mod Pathol. 3:435–41.
1224. Kaufmann O, Dietel M (2000). Expression of thyroid transcription factor-1 in pulmonary and extrapulmonary small cell carcinomas and other neuroendocrine carcinomas of various primary sites. Histopathology. 36:415–20.
1225. Kaul TK, Fields BL, Kahn DR (1994). Primary malignant pericardial mesothelioma: a case report and review. J Cardiovasc Surg (Torino). 35:261–7.
1226. Kawabe M, Sasaki K, Shinoda T, et al. (2005). [Yolk sac tumor of the anterior mediastinum and pulmonary metastases; report of a case]. Kyobu Geka. 58:1102–5.
1227. Kazerooni EA, Bhalla M, Shepard JA, et al. (1994). Adenosquamous carcinoma of the lung: radiologic appearance. AJR Am J Roentgenol. 163:301–6.
1228. Kazmierczak B, Wanschura S, Rosigkeit J, et al. (1995). Molecular characterization of 12q14-15 rearrangements in three pulmonary chondroid hamartomas. Cancer Res. 55:2497–9.
1229. Kearney DL, Titus JL, Hawkins EP, et al. (1987). Pathologic features of myocardial hamartomas causing childhood tachyarrhythmias. Circulation. 75:705–10.
1230. Keel SB, Bacha E, Mark EJ, et al. (1999). Primary pulmonary sarcoma: a clinicopathologic study of 26 cases. Mod Pathol. 12:1124–31.
1231. Keeling IM, Ploner F, Rigler B (2006). Familial cardiac angiosarcoma. Ann Thorac Surg. 82:1576.
1232. Keenan N, Davies S, Sheppard MN, et al. (2006). Angiosarcoma of the right atrium: a diagnostic dilemma. Int J Cardiol. 113:425–6.
1233. Kelly MD, Sheridan BF, Farnsworth AE, et al. (1994). Parathyroid carcinoma in a mediastinal sixth parathyroid gland. Aust N Z J Surg. 64:446–9.
1234. Kelly RJ, Sharon E, Hassan R (2011). Chemotherapy and targeted therapies for unresectable malignant mesothelioma. Lung Cancer. 73:256–63.
1235. Kerr KM (2012). Personalized medicine for lung cancer: new challenges for pathology. Histopathology. 60:531–46.
1236. Kerr KM, Popper HH (2007). The differential diagnosis of pulmonary pre-invasive lesions. In: Timens W, Popper HH, eds. Pathology of the Lung (European Respiratory Monograph). Vol. 39. European Respiratory Society. pp. 37–62.
1237. Kesler KA, Brooks JA, Rieger KM, et al. (2003). Mediastinal metastases from testicular nonseminomatous germ cell tumors: patterns of dissemination and predictors of long-term survival with surgery. J Thorac Cardiovasc Surg. 125:913–23.
1238. Kesler KA, Patel JB, Kruter LE, et al. (2012). The "growing teratoma syndrome" in primary mediastinal nonseminomatous germ cell tumors: criteria based on current practice. J Thorac Cardiovasc Surg. 144:438–43.
1239. Kesler KA, Rieger KM, Ganjoo KN, et al. (1999). Primary mediastinal nonseminomatous germ cell tumors: the influence of postchemotherapy pathology on long-term survival after surgery. J Thorac Cardiovasc Surg. 118:692–700.
1240. Kesler KA, Rieger KM, Hammoud ZT, et

al. (2008). A 25-year single institution experience with surgery for primary mediastinal nonseminomatous germ cell tumors. Ann Thorac Surg. 85:371–8.

1241. Khalidi HS, Brynes RK, Browne P, et al. (1998). Intravascular large B-cell lymphoma: the CD5 antigen is expressed by a subset of cases. Mod Pathol. 11:983–8.

1242. Khan A, Tischler AS, Patwardhan NA, et al. (2003). Calcitonin immunoreactivity in neoplastic and hyperplastic parathyroid glands: an immunohistochemical study. Endocr Pathol. 14:249–55.

1243. Khan MF, Datta S, Chisti MM, et al. (2013). Cardiac paraganglioma: clinical presentation, diagnostic approach and factors affecting short and long-term outcomes. Int J Cardiol. 166:315–20.

1244. Khawaja MR, Nelson RP Jr, Miller N, et al. (2012). Immune-mediated diseases and immunodeficiencies associated with thymic epithelial neoplasms. J Clin Immunol. 32:430–7.

1245. Khoury T, Chandrasekhar R, Wilding G, et al. (2011). Tumour eosinophilia combined with an immunohistochemistry panel is useful in the differentiation of type B3 thymoma from thymic carcinoma. Int J Exp Pathol. 92:87–96.

1246. Kiffer JD, Sandeman TF (1999). Primary malignant mediastinal germ cell tumours: a literature review and a study of 18 cases. Australas Radiol. 43:58–68.

1247. Kilis-Pstrusinska K, Medynska A, Zwolinska D, et al. (2008). Lymphoepithelioma-like thymic carcinoma in a 16-year-old boy with nephrotic syndrome--a case report. Pediatr Nephrol. 23:1001–3.

1248. Kim CH, Dancer JY, Coffey D, et al. (2008). Clinicopathologic study of 24 patients with primary cardiac sarcomas: a 10-year single institution experience. Hum Pathol. 39:933–8.

1249. Kim DJ, Yang WI, Choi SS, et al. (2005). Prognostic and clinical relevance of the World Health Organization schema for the classification of thymic epithelial tumors: a clinicopathologic study of 108 patients and literature review. Chest. 127:755–61.

1250. Kim DM, Hong JH, Kim SY, et al. (2010). Primary cardiac angiosarcoma presenting with cardiac tamponade. Korean Circ J. 40:86–9.

1251. Kim ES, Herbst RS, Wistuba II, et al. (2011). The BATTLE trial: personalizing therapy for lung cancer. Cancer Discov. 1:44–53.

1252. Kim ES, Hirsh V, Mok T, et al. (2008). Gefitinib versus docetaxel in previously treated non-small-cell lung cancer (INTEREST): a randomised phase III trial. Lancet. 372:1809–18.

1253. Kim JH, Cho JH, Park MS, et al. (2002). Pulmonary inflammatory pseudotumor--a report of 28 cases. Korean J Intern Med. 17:252–8.

1254. Kim JH, Lee SH, Park J, et al. (2004). Primary pulmonary non-Hodgkin's lymphoma. Jpn J Clin Oncol. 34:510–4.

1255. Kim JY, Lee CH, Park WY, et al. (2012). Adenocarcinoma with sarcomatous dedifferentiation arising from mature cystic teratoma of the anterior mediastinum. Pathol Res Pract. 208:741–5.

1256. Kim K, Koo BC, Davis JT, et al. (1984). Primary myelolipoma of mediastinum. J Comput Tomogr. 8:119–23.

1257. Kim KH, Sul HJ, Kang DY (2003). Sclerosing hemangioma with lymph node metastasis. Yonsei Med J. 44:150–4.

1258. Kim KI, Flint JD, Muller NL (1997). Pulmonary carcinosarcoma: radiologic and pathologic findings in three patients. AJR Am J Roentgenol. 169:691–4.

1259. Kim MJ, Shin HC, Shin KC, et al. (2013). Best immunohistochemical panel in distinguishing adenocarcinoma from squamous cell carcinoma of lung: tissue microarray assay in resected lung cancer specimens. Ann Diagn Pathol. 17:85–90.

1260. Kim MP, Correa AM, Blackmon S, et al. (2011). Outcomes after right-side heart sarcoma

resection. Ann Thorac Surg. 91:770–6.

1261. Kim NR, Lee JI, Ha SY (2013). Micronodular thymoma with lymphoid stroma in a multilocular thymic cyst: a case study. Korean J Pathol. 47:392–4.

1262. Kim TH, Kim SJ, Ryu YH, et al. (2004). Pleomorphic carcinoma of lung: comparison of CT features and pathologic findings. Radiology. 232:554–9.

1263. Kim WS, Honma K, Karnan S, et al. (2007). Genome-wide array-based comparative genomic hybridization of ocular marginal zone B cell lymphoma: comparison with pulmonary and nodal marginal zone B cell lymphoma. Genes Chromosomes Cancer. 46:776–83.

1264. Kim WY, Kim H, Jeon YK, et al. (2010). Follicular dendritic cell sarcoma with immature T-cell proliferation. Hum Pathol. 41:129–33.

1265. Kim Y, Lee KS, Jung KJ, et al. (1999). Halo sign on high resolution CT: findings in spectrum of pulmonary diseases with pathologic correlation. J Comput Assist Tomogr. 23:622–6.

1266. Kim Y, Leventaki V, Bhaijee F, et al. (2012). Extracavitary/solid variant of primary effusion lymphoma. Ann Diagn Pathol. 16:441–6.

1267. Kim Y, Park HY, Cho J, et al. (2013). Congenital peribronchial myofibroblastic tumor: a case study and literature review. Korean J Pathol. 47:172–6.

1268. Kim YD, Lee CH, Lee MK, et al. (2007). Primary alveolar soft part sarcoma of the lung. J Korean Med Sci. 22:369–72.

1269. Kim YH, Girard L, Giacomini CP, et al. (2006). Combined microarray analysis of small cell lung cancer reveals altered apoptotic balance and distinct expression signatures of MYC family gene amplification. Oncogene. 25:130–8.

1270. Kim YH, Ishii G, Naito Y, et al. (2006). [A resected case of sclerosing thymoma]. Nihon Kokyuki Gakkai Zasshi. 44:420–3.

1271. Kimura N, Watanabe T, Noshiro T, et al. (2005). Histological grading of adrenal and extra-adrenal pheochromocytomas and relationship to prognosis: a clinicopathological analysis of 116 adrenal pheochromocytomas and 30 extra-adrenal sympathetic paragangliomas including 38 malignant tumors. Endocr Pathol. 16:23–32.

1272. King LJ, Padley SP, Wotherspoon AC, et al. (2000). Pulmonary MALT lymphoma: imaging findings in 24 cases. Eur Radiol. 10:1932–8.

1273. Kini SR (2002). Squamous cell carcinoma. In: Kini SR, ed. Color Atlas of Pulmonary Cytopathology. New York: Springer; pp 82–90.

1274. Kitamura H, Kameda Y, Ito T, et al. (1999). Atypical adenomatous hyperplasia of the lung. Implications for the pathogenesis of peripheral lung adenocarcinoma. Am J Clin Pathol. 111:610–22.

1275. Kitamura H, Kameda Y, Ito T, et al. (1997). Cytodifferentiation of atypical adenomatous hyperplasia and bronchioloalveolar lung carcinoma: immunohistochemical and ultrastructural studies. Virchows Arch. 431:415–24.

1276. Kitazawa R, Kitazawa S, Nishimura Y, et al. (2006). Lung carcinosarcoma with liposarcoma element: autopsy case. Pathol Int. 56:449–52.

1277. Klatt EC, Heitz DR (1990). Cardiac metastases. Cancer. 65:1456–9.

1278. Klebe S, Brownlee NA, Mahar A, et al. (2010). Sarcomatoid mesothelioma: a clinical-pathologic correlation of 326 cases. Mod Pathol. 23:470–9.

1279. Klebe S, Mahar A, Henderson DW, et al. (2008). Malignant mesothelioma with heterologous elements: clinicopathological correlation of 27 cases and literature review. Mod Pathol. 21:1084–94.

1280. Klein F, Amin Kotb WF, Petersen I (2009). Incidence of human papilloma virus in lung cancer. Lung Cancer. 65:13–8.

1281. Klein N, Elis A, Radnay J, et al. (2009). Transformation of MALT lymphoma to pure

plasma cell histology: possible association with anti-CD20 antibody treatment. Isr Med Assoc J. 11:703–4.

1282. Klein R, Marx A, Strobel P, et al. (2013). Autoimmune associations and autoantibody screening show focused recognition in patient subgroups with generalized myasthenia gravis. Hum Immunol. 74:1184–93.

1283. Klein U, Gloghini A, Gaidano G, et al. (2003). Gene expression profile analysis of AIDS-related primary effusion lymphoma (PEL) suggests a plasmablastic derivation and identifies PEL-specific transcripts. Blood. 101:4115–21.

1284. Kleist B, Poetsch M, Breitsprecher C, et al. (2003). Epithelial-myoepithelial carcinoma of the parotid gland-evidence of contrasting DNA patterns in two different histological parts. Virchows Arch. 442:585–90.

1285. Klemm KM, Moran CA, Suster S (1999). Pigmented thymic carcinoids: a clinicopathological and immunohistochemical study of two cases. Mod Pathol. 12:946–8.

1286. Kliche S, Kremmer E, Hammerschmidt W, et al. (1998). Persistent infection of Epstein-Barr virus-positive B lymphocytes by human herpesvirus 8. J Virol. 72:8143–9.

1287. Kliment CR, Clemens K, Oury TD (2009). North american erionite-associated mesothelioma with pleural plaques and pulmonary fibrosis: a case report. Int J Clin Exp Pathol. 2:407–10.

1288. Klimstra DS, Moran CA, Perino G, et al. (1995). Liposarcoma of the anterior mediastinum and thymus. A clinicopathologic study of 28 cases. Am J Surg Pathol. 19:782–91.

1289. Kline ME, Patel BU, Agosti SJ (1990). Noninfiltrating angiolipoma of the mediastinum. Radiology. 175:737–8.

1290. Knapp RH, Fritz SR, Reiman HM (1982). Primary embryonal carcinoma and choriocarcinoma of the mediastinum. A case report. Arch Pathol Lab Med. 106:507–9.

1291. Knapp RH, Hurt RD, Payne WS, et al. (1985). Malignant germ cell tumors of the mediastinum. J Thorac Cardiovasc Surg. 89:82–9.

1292. Knobel B, Rosman P, Kishon Y, et al. (1992). Intracardiac primary fibrosarcoma. Case report and literature review. Thorac Cardiovasc Surg. 40:227–30.

1293. Knosel T, Heretsch S, Altendorf-Hofmann A, et al. (2010). TLE1 is a robust diagnostic biomarker for synovial sarcomas and correlates with t(X;18): analysis of 319 cases. Eur J Cancer. 46:1170–6.

1294. Knowles JW, Elliott AB, Brody J (2007). A case of complete heart block reverting to normal sinus rhythm after treatment for cardiac invasive Burkitt's lymphoma. Ann Hematol. 86:687–90.

1295. Ko HM, Geddie WR, Boerner SL, et al. (2013). Cytomorphological and clinicopathological spectrum of pulmonary marginal zone lymphoma: the utility of immunophenotyping, PCR and FISH studies. Cytopathology.25:250–8.

1296. Ko JM, Jung JI, Park SH, et al. (2006). Benign tumors of the tracheobronchial tree: CT-pathologic correlation. AJR Am J Roentgenol. 186:1304–13.

1297. Ko YH, Han JH, Go JH, et al. (1997). Intravascular lymphomatosis: a clinicopathological study of two cases presenting as an interstitial lung disease. Histopathology. 31:555–62.

1298. Kobayashi M, Okabayashi T, Okamoto K, et al. (2005). Clinicopathological study of cardiac tamponade due to pericardial metastasis originating from gastric cancer. World J Gastroenterol. 11:6899–904.

1299. Kobayashi S, Ji H, Yuza Y, et al. (2005). An alternative inhibitor overcomes resistance caused by a mutation of the epidermal growth factor receptor. Cancer Res. 65:7096–101.

1300. Kobayashi T, Ohno H (2011). Intravascular large B-cell lymphoma associated with t(14;19)(q32;q13) translocation. Intern Med. 50:2007–10.

1301. Kobayashi Y, Kamitsuji Y, Kuroda J, et al. (2007). Comparison of human herpes virus 8 related primary effusion lymphoma with human herpes virus 8 unrelated primary effusion lymphoma-like lymphoma on the basis of HIV: report of 2 cases and review of 212 cases in the literature. Acta Haematol. 117:132–44.

1302. Kobayashi Y, Sakao Y, Ito S, et al. (2013). Transformation to sarcomatoid carcinoma in ALK-rearranged adenocarcinoma, which developed acquired resistance to crizotinib and received subsequent chemotherapies. J Thorac Oncol. 8:e75–8.

1303. Kocak Z, Adli M, Erdir O, et al. (2000). Intrathoracic desmoid tumor of the posterior mediastinum with transdiaphragmatic extension. Report of a case. Tumori. 86:489–91.

1304. Kodama H, Hirotani T, Suzuki Y, et al. (2002). Cardiomyogenic differentiation in cardiac myxoma expressing lineage-specific transcription factors. Am J Pathol. 161:381–9.

1305. Koga K, Matsuno Y, Noguchi M, et al. (1994). A review of 79 thymomas: modification of staging system and reappraisal of conventional division into invasive and non-invasive thymoma. Pathol Int. 44:359–67.

1306. Koga T, Hashimoto S, Sugio K, et al. (2002). Lung adenocarcinoma with bronchioloalveolar carcinoma component is frequently associated with foci of high-grade atypical adenomatous hyperplasia. Am J Clin Pathol. 117:464–70.

1307. Kohno H, Amatya VJ, Takeshima Y, et al. (2010). Aberrant promoter methylation of WIF-1 and SFRP1, 2, 4 genes in mesothelioma. Oncol Rep. 24:423–31.

1308. Kohno T, Ichikawa H, Totoki Y, et al. (2012). KIF5B-RET fusions in lung adenocarcinoma. Nat Med. 18:375–7.

1309. Kohno T, Kakinuma R, Iwasaki M, et al. (2010). Association of CYP19A1 polymorphisms with risks for atypical adenomatous hyperplasia and bronchioloalveolar carcinoma in the lungs. Carcinogenesis. 31:1794–9.

1310. Koita H, Suzumiya J, Ohshima K, et al. (1997). Lymphoblastic lymphoma expressing natural killer cell phenotype with involvement of the mediastinum and nasal cavity. Am J Surg Pathol. 21:242–8.

1311. Koivunen JP, Kim J, Lee J, et al. (2008). Mutations in the LKB1 tumour suppressor are frequently detected in tumours from Caucasian but not Asian lung cancer patients. Br J Cancer. 99:245–52.

1312. Koizumi JH, Schron DS (1997). Cytologic features of colonic adenocarcinoma. Differences between primary and metastatic neoplasms. Acta Cytol. 41:419–26.

1313. Koizumi K, Haraguchi S, Mikami I, et al. (2005). Video-assisted thoracic surgery for Ewing's sarcoma of the mediastinum in a 3-year-old girl. Ann Thorac Cardiovasc Surg. 11:117–20.

1314. Kojika M, Ishii G, Yoshida J, et al. (2009). Immunohistochemical differential diagnosis between thymic carcinoma and type B3 thymoma: diagnostic utility of hypoxic marker, GLUT-1, in thymic epithelial neoplasms. Mod Pathol. 22:1341–50.

1315. Kojima Y, Ito H, Hasegawa S, et al. (2006). Resected invasive thymoma with multiple endocrine neoplasia type 1. Jpn J Thorac Cardiovasc Surg. 54:171–3.

1316. Kollmannsberger C, Beyer J, Droz JP, et al. (1998). Secondary leukemia following high cumulative doses of etoposide in patients treated for advanced germ cell tumors. J Clin Oncol. 16:3386–91.

1317. Kominato S, Nakayama T, Sato F, et al. (2012). Characterization of chromosomal aberrations in thymic MALT lymphoma. Pathol Int. 62:93–8.

1317A. Kondo K (2010). Tumor-node metastasis staging system for thymic epithelial tumors. J Thorac Oncol. 5(10) Suppl 4:S352–6.

1318. Kondo K, Monden Y (2003). Therapy for thymic epithelial tumors: a clinical study of 1,320 patients from Japan. Ann Thorac Surg. 76:878–84.
1319. Kondo K, Yoshizawa K, Tsuyuguchi M, et al. (2004). WHO histologic classification is a prognostic indicator in thymoma. Ann Thorac Surg. 77:1183–8.
1319A. Kondo K, van Schil P, Detterbeck F, et al. (2014). The IASLC/ITMIG Thymic Epithelial Tumors Staging Project: Proposals for the N and M Components for the Forthcoming (8th) Edition of the TNM Classification of Malignant Tumors. J Thorac Oncol. 9(9 Suppl 2):S81–7.
1320. Kondo N, Torii I, Hashimoto M, et al. (2011). Alveolar adenoma of the lung: a case report. Ann Thorac Cardiovasc Surg. 17:71–3.
1321. Kondratiev S, Duraisamy S, Unitt CL, et al. (2011). Aberrant expression of the dendritic cell marker TNFAIP2 by the malignant cells of Hodgkin lymphoma and primary mediastinal large B-cell lymphoma distinguishes these tumor types from morphologically and phenotypically similar lymphomas. Am J Surg Pathol. 35:1531–9.
1322. Kondruweit M, Schmid M, Strecker T (2008). Papillary fibroelastoma of the mitral valve: appearance in 64-slice spiral computed tomography, magnetic resonance imaging, and echocardiography. Eur Heart J. 29:831.
1323. Konoplev S, Lin P, Qiu X, et al. (2010). Clonal relationship of extranodal marginal zone lymphomas of mucosa-associated lymphoid tissue involving different sites. Am J Clin Pathol. 134:112–8.
1324. Konstanty-Kalandyk J, Wierzbicki K, Bartus K, et al. (2013). [Acute myocardial infarction due to coronary embolisation as the first manifestation of left atrial myxoma]. Kardiol Pol. 71:403–5.
1325. Kontic M, Stojsic J, Stevic R, et al. (2013). Could spindle cell lung carcinoma be considered and treated as sarcoma, according to its clinical course, morphology, immunophenotype and genetic finding? Pathol Oncol Res. 19:129–33.
1326. Koo CW, Baliff JP, Torigian DA, et al. (2010). Spectrum of pulmonary neuroendocrine cell proliferation: diffuse idiopathic pulmonary neuroendocrine cell hyperplasia, tumorlet, and carcinoids. AJR Am J Roentgenol. 195:661–8.
1327. Kooijman CD (1988). Immature teratomas in children. Histopathology. 12:491–502.
1328. Kopp BT, Rosen KL, O'Donovan JC, et al. (2014). Cardiac fibroma, anomalous pulmonary venous course, and persistent pneumonia in a patient with Gorlin syndrome. Pediatr Pulmonol. 49:E7–9.
1329. Koppula BR, Pipavath S, Lewis DH (2009). Epstein-Barr virus (EBV) associated lymphoepithelioma-like thymic carcinoma associated with paraneoplastic syndrome of polymyositis: a rare tumor with rare association. Clin Nucl Med. 34:686–8.
1330. Kornstein MJ, Rosai J (1998). CD5 labeling of thymic carcinomas and other nonlymphoid neoplasms. Am J Clin Pathol. 109:722–6.
1331. Koshiol J, Rotunno M, Gillison ML, et al. (2011). Assessment of human papillomavirus in lung tumor tissue. J Natl Cancer Inst. 103:501–7.
1332. Koss MN, Hochholzer L, Frommelt RA (1999). Carcinosarcomas of the lung: a clinicopathologic study of 66 patients. Am J Surg Pathol. 23:1514–26.
1333. Koss MN, Hochholzer L, Langloss JM, et al. (1986). Lymphomatoid granulomatosis: a clinicopathologic study of 42 patients. Pathology. 18:283–8.
1334. Koss MN, Hochholzer L, Moran CA (1998). Primary pulmonary glomus tumor: a clinicopathologic and immunohistochemical study of two cases. Mod Pathol. 11:253–8.
1335. Koss MN, Hochholzer L, Nichols PW, et al. (1983). Primary non-Hodgkin's lymphoma and pseudolymphoma of lung: a study of 161 patients. Hum Pathol. 14:1024–38.
1336. Koss MN, Hochholzer L, O'Leary T (1991). Pulmonary blastomas. Cancer. 67:2368–81.
1337. Kossakowski CA, Morresi-Hauf A, Schnabel PA, et al. (2014). Preparation of cell blocks for lung cancer diagnosis and prediction: protocol and experience of a high-volume center. Respiration. 87:432–8.
1338. Kotake T, Kosugi S, Takimoto T, et al. (2010). Intravascular large B-cell lymphoma presenting pulmonary arterial hypertension as an initial manifestation. Intern Med. 49:51–4.
1339. Kourda J, Ismail O, Smati BH, et al. (2010). Benign myoepithelioma of the lung - a case report and review of the literature. Cases J. 3:25.
1340. Kourea HP, Bilsky MH, Leung DH, et al. (1998). Subdiaphragmatic and intrathoracic paraspinal malignant peripheral nerve sheath tumors: a clinicopathologic study of 25 patients and 26 tumors. Cancer. 82:2191–203.
1341. Kowalski DM, Knetki-Wroblewska M, Winiarczyk K, et al. (2014). Analysis of treatment results in primary germ cell tumours with mediastinal location: own experience. Pneumonol Alergol Pol. 82:116–24.
1342. Kozu Y, Maniwa T, Ohde Y, et al. (2014). A Solitary Mixed Squamous Cell and Glandular Papilloma of the Lung. Ann Thorac Cardiovasc Surg. 20 Suppl:625-8.
1343. Kragel PJ, Devaney KO, Meth BM, et al. (1990). Mucinous cystadenoma of the lung. A report of two cases with immunohistochemical and ultrastructural analysis. Arch Pathol Lab Med. 114:1053–6.
1344. Kranioti EF, Vorniotakis N, Galiatsou C, et al. (2009). Sex identification and software development using digital femoral head radiographs. Forensic Sci Int. 189:113–7.
1345. Kratzke RA, Otterson GA, Lincoln CE, et al. (1995). Immunohistochemical analysis of the p16INK4 cyclin-dependent kinase inhibitor in malignant mesothelioma. J Natl Cancer Inst. 87:1870–5.
1346. Krema H, Navajas E, Simpson ER, et al. (2011). Choroidal metastasis from a mediastinal choriocarcinoma in a male. Can J Ophthalmol. 46:551–2.
1347. Krieger D, Moericke A, Oschlies I, et al. (2010). Frequency and clinical relevance of DNA microsatellite alterations of the CDKN2A/B, ATM and p53 gene loci: a comparison between pediatric precursor T-cell lymphoblastic lymphoma and T-cell lymphoblastic leukemia. Haematologica. 95:158–62.
1348. Krismann M, Muller KM, Jaworska M, et al. (2002). Molecular cytogenetic differences between histological subtypes of malignant mesotheliomas: DNA cytometry and comparative genomic hybridization of 90 cases. J Pathol. 197:363–71.
1349. Kristoffersson U, Heim S, Mandahl N, et al. (1989). Multiple clonal chromosome aberrations in two thymomas. Cancer Genet Cytogenet. 41:93–8.
1350. Krober SM, Marx A, Aebert H, et al. (2004). Sarcoma of follicular dendritic cells in the dorsal mediastinum. Hum Pathol. 35:259–63.
1351. Kruczynski A, Delsol G, Laurent C, et al. (2012). Anaplastic lymphoma kinase as a therapeutic target. Expert Opin Ther Targets. 16:1127–38.
1352. Kuhn E, Wistuba II (2008). Molecular pathology of thymic epithelial neoplasms. Hematol Oncol Clin North Am. 22:443–55.
1353. Kukkady A, Upadhyay V, Pease PW, et al. (2000). Pleuropulmonary blastoma: four cases. Pediatr Surg Int. 16:595–8.
1354. Kung IT, Loke SL, So SY, et al. (1985). Intrapulmonary thymoma: report of two cases. Thorax. 40:471–4.
1355. Kuo KT, Hsu WH, Wu YC, et al. (2003). Sclerosing hemangioma of the lung: an analysis of 44 cases. J Chin Med Assoc. 66:33–8.
1356. Kuo T (1994). Sclerosing thymoma--a possible phenomenon of regression. Histopathology. 25:289–91.
1357. Kuo T, Shih LY (2001). Histologic types of thymoma associated with pure red cell aplasia: a study of five cases including a composite tumor of organoid thymoma associated with an unusual lipofibroadenoma. Int J Surg Pathol. 9:29–35.
1358. Kuo TT, Chan JK (1998). Thymic carcinoma arising in thymoma is associated with alterations in immunohistochemical profile. Am J Surg Pathol. 22:1474–81.
1359. Kuo TT, Chang JP, Lin FJ, et al. (1990). Thymic carcinomas: histopathological varieties and immunohistochemical study. Am J Surg Pathol. 14:24–34.
1360. Kuo TT, Lo SK (1993). Thymoma: a study of the pathologic classification of 71 cases with evaluation of the Muller-Hermelink system. Hum Pathol. 24:766–71.
1361. Kuo T (2000). Cytokeratin profiles of the thymus and thymomas: histogenetic correlations and proposal for a histological classification of thymomas. Histopathology. 36:403–14.
1362. Kuppers R (2012). New insights in the biology of Hodgkin lymphoma. Hematology (Am Soc Hematol Educ Program). 2012:328–34.
1363. Kuppers R, Engert A, Hansmann ML (2012). Hodgkin lymphoma. J Clin Invest. 122:3439–47.
1364. Kure K, Lingamfelter D, Taboada E (2011). Large multifocal cardiac myxoma causing the sudden unexpected death of a 2-month-old infant--a rapidly growing, acquired lesion versus a congenital process?: a case report. Am J Forensic Med Pathol. 32:166–8.
1365. Kurie JM, Shin HJ, Lee JS, et al. (1996). Increased epidermal growth factor receptor expression in metaplastic bronchial epithelium. Clin Cancer Res. 2:1787–93.
1366. Kuroda M, Oka T, Horiuchi H, et al. (1994). Giant cell tumor of the lung: an autopsy case report with immunohistochemical observations. Pathol Int. 44:158–63.
1367. Kuroki S, Nasu K, Murakami K, et al. (2004). Thymic MALT lymphoma: MR imaging findings and their correlation with histopathological findings on four cases. Clin Imaging. 28:274–7.
1368. Kurtin PJ, Myers JL, Adlakha H, et al. (2001). Pathologic and clinical features of primary pulmonary extranodal marginal zone B-cell lymphoma of MALT type. Am J Surg Pathol. 25:997–1008.
1369. Kurtz JE, Serra S, Duclos B, et al. (2004). Diffuse primary angiosarcoma of the pleura: a case report and review of the literature. Sarcoma. 8:103–6.
1370. Kurup AN, Tazelaar HD, Edwards WD, et al. (2002). Iatrogenic cardiac papillary fibroelastoma: a study of 12 cases (1990 to 2000). Hum Pathol. 33:1165–9.
1371. Kurzrock EA, Tunuguntla HS, Busby JE, et al. (2002). Klinefelter's syndrome and precocious puberty: a harbinger for tumor. Urology. 60:514.
1372. Kuwahara M, Nagafuchi M, Rikimaru T, et al. (2010). Pulmonary papillary adenoma. Gen Thorac Cardiovasc Surg. 58:542–5.
1373. Kwak EL, Bang YJ, Camidge DR, et al. (2010). Anaplastic lymphoma kinase inhibition in non-small-cell lung cancer. N Engl J Med. 363:1693–703.
1374. Kwon JW, Goo JM, Seo JB, et al. (1999). Mucous gland adenoma of the bronchus: CT findings in two patients. J Comput Assist Tomogr. 23:758–60.
1375. Kycler W, Laski P (2012). Surgical approach to pulmonary metastases from breast cancer. Breast J. 18:52–7.
1376. La Mantia E, Franco R, Cantile M, et al. (2013). Primary intrapulmonary malignant peripheral nerve sheath tumor mimicking lung cancer. J Thorac Dis. 5:E155–7.
1377. La Rosa S, Chiaravalli AM, Placidi C, et al. (2010). TTF1 expression in normal lung neuroendocrine cells and related tumors: immunohistochemical study comparing two different monoclonal antibodies. Virchows Arch. 457:497–507.
1378. Lack E (2007). Tumors of the adrenal glands and extraadrenal paraganglia. AFIP Atlas of Tumor Pathology. 4th ed. Volume 8. Washington, DC: American Registry of Pathology.
1378A. Ladanyi M. (2005). Implications of P16/CDKN2A deletion in pleural mesotheliomas. Lung Cancer.49, Suppl 1:S95-8.
1379. Ladanyi M, Antonescu CR, Leung DH, et al. (2002). Impact of SYT-SSX fusion type on the clinical behavior of synovial sarcoma: a multi-institutional retrospective study of 243 patients. Cancer Res. 62:135–40.
1380. Ladanyi M, Roy I (1988). Mediastinal germ cell tumors and histiocytosis. Hum Pathol. 19:586–90.
1381. Ladanyi M, Samaniego F, Reuter VE, et al. (1990). Cytogenetic and immunohistochemical evidence for the germ cell origin of a subset of acute leukemias associated with mediastinal germ cell tumors. J Natl Cancer Inst. 82:221–7.
1382. Ladanyi M, Zauderer MG, Krug LM, et al. (2012). New strategies in pleural mesothelioma: BAP1 and NF2 as novel targets for therapeutic development and risk assessment. Clin Cancer Res. 18:4485–90.
1383. Laga S, Gewillig MH, Van Schoubroeck D, et al. (2006). Imminent fetal cardiac tamponade by right atrial hemangioma. Pediatr Cardiol. 27:633–5.
1384. Lagana SM, Hanna RF, Borczuk AC (2011). Pleomorphic (spindle and squamous cell) carcinoma arising in a peripheral mixed squamous and glandular papilloma in a 70-year-old man. Arch Pathol Lab Med. 135:1353–6.
1385. Lagrange W, Dahm HH, Karstens J, et al. (1987). Melanocytic neuroendocrine carcinoma of the thymus. Cancer. 59:484–8.
1386. Lajos P, Hasaniya N, Ehrman W, et al. (2004). Spindle cell sarcoma of the pericardium: a case report. J Card Surg. 19:139–41.
1387. Lale SA, Tiscornia-Wasserman PG, Aziz M (2013). Diagnosis of thymic clear cell carcinoma by cytology. Case Rep Pathol. 2013:617810.
1388. Lam C, Ou JC, Billingsley EM (2013). "PTCH"-ing it together: a basal cell nevus syndrome review. Dermatol Surg. 39:1557–72.
1389. Lam KY, Dickens P, Chan AC (1993). Tumors of the heart. A 20-year experience with a review of 12,485 consecutive autopsies. Arch Pathol Lab Med. 117:1027–31.
1390. Lam S, leRiche JC, Zheng Y, et al. (1999). Sex-related differences in bronchial epithelial changes associated with tobacco smoking. J Natl Cancer Inst. 91:691–6.
1391. Lam S, Standish B, Baldwin C, et al. (2008). In vivo optical coherence tomography imaging of preinvasive bronchial lesions. Clin Cancer Res. 14:2006–11.
1392. Lamant L, McCarthy K, d'Amore E, et al. (2011). Prognostic impact of morphologic and phenotypic features of childhood ALK-positive anaplastic large-cell lymphoma: results of the ALCL99 study. J Clin Oncol. 29:4669–76.
1393. Lamba G, Frishman WH (2012). Cardiac and pericardial tumors. Cardiol Rev. 20:237–52.
1394. Lamy A, Sesboue R, Bourguignon J, et al. (2002). Aberrant methylation of the CDKN2a/p16INK4a gene promoter region in preinvasive bronchial lesions: a prospective study in high-risk patients without invasive cancer. Int J Cancer. 100:189–93.
1395. Lancaster KJ, Liang CY, Myers JC, et al. (1997). Goblet cell carcinoid arising in a mature

teratoma of the mediastinum. Am J Surg Pathol. 21:109–13.
1396. Lang TU, Khalbuss WE, Monaco SE, et al. (2011). Solitary Tracheobronchial Papilloma: Cytomorphology and ancillary studies with histologic correlation. Cytojournal. 8:6.
1397. Lanphear BP, Buncher CR (1992). Latent period for malignant mesothelioma of occupational origin. J Occup Med. 34:718–21.
1398. Lantuejoul S, Constantin B, Drabkin H, et al. (2003). Expression of VEGF, semaphorin SEMA3F, and their common receptors neuropilins NP1 and NP2 in preinvasive bronchial lesions, lung tumours, and cell lines. J Pathol. 200:336–47.
1399. Lantuejoul S, Fior-Gozlan M, Ferretti GR, et al. (2013). Large cell carcinoma and adenosquamous carcinoma of the lung. In: Hasleton P, Flieder DB, eds. Spencer's Pathology of the Lung. 6th ed. Cambridge: Cambridge University Press; pp. 1121–3.
1400. Lantuejoul S, Isaac S, Pinel N, et al. (1997). Clear cell tumor of the lung: an immunohistochemical and ultrastructural study supporting a pericytic differentiation. Mod Pathol. 10:1001–8.
1401. Lantuejoul S, Laverriere MH, Sturm N, et al. (2000). NCAM (neural cell adhesion molecules) expression in malignant mesotheliomas. Hum Pathol. 31:415–21.
1402. Lantuejoul S, Moro D, Michalides RJ, et al. (1998). Neural cell adhesion molecules (NCAM) and NCAM-PSA expression in neuroendocrine lung tumors. Am J Surg Pathol. 22:1267–76.
1403. Lantuejoul S, Moulai N, Quetant S, et al. (2007). Unusual cystic presentation of pulmonary nodular amyloidosis associated with MALT-type lymphoma. Eur Respir J. 30:589–92.
1404. Lantuejoul S, Soria JC, Moro-Sibilot D, et al. (2004). Differential expression of telomerase reverse transcriptase (hTERT) in lung tumours. Br J Cancer. 90:1222–9.
1405. Lappas D, Noussios G, Anagnostis P, et al. (2012). Location, number and morphology of parathyroid glands: results from a large anatomical series. Anat Sci Int. 87:160–4.
1406. Larsen B, Markovetz AJ, Galask RP (1976). The bacterial flora of the female rat genital tract. Proc Soc Exp Biol Med. 151:571–4.
1407. Larsen BT, Klein JR, Hornychova H, et al. (2013). Diffuse intrapulmonary malignant mesothelioma masquerading as interstitial lung disease: a distinctive variant of mesothelioma. Am J Surg Pathol. 37:1555–64.
1408. Larsen M, Evans WK, Shepherd FA, et al. (1984). Acute lymphoblastic leukemia. Possible origin from a mediastinal germ cell tumor. Cancer. 53:441–4.
1409. Larson DA, Derkay CS (2010). Epidemiology of recurrent respiratory papillomatosis. APMIS. 118:450–4.
1410. Laszlo T, Lacza A, Toth D, et al. (2014). Pulmonary enteric adenocarcinoma indistinguishable morphologically and immunohistologically from metastatic colorectal carcinoma. Histopathology. 65:283–7.
1411. Lattuada S, Saggia C, Biaggi G, et al. (2005). Pericardial metastases in a long-surviving patient with sigmoid carcinoma. Tumori. 91:101–2.
1412. Latza U, Foss HD, Durkop H, et al. (1995). CD30 antigen in embryonal carcinoma and embryogenesis and release of the soluble molecule. Am J Pathol. 146:463–71.
1413. Lau K, Massad M, Pollak C, et al. (2011). Clinical patterns and outcome in epithelioid hemangioendothelioma with or without pulmonary involvement: insights from an internet registry in the study of a rare cancer. Chest. 140:1312–8.
1414. Lau SK, Desrochers MJ, Luthringer DJ (2002). Expression of thyroid transcription factor-1, cytokeratin 7, and cytokeratin 20 in bronchioloalveolar carcinomas: an immunohistochemical evaluation of 67 cases. Mod Pathol. 15:538–42.
1415. Lau SK, Weiss LM, Chu PG (2007). D2-40 immunohistochemistry in the differential diagnosis of seminoma and embryonal carcinoma: a comparative immunohistochemical study with KIT (CD117) and CD30. Mod Pathol. 20:320–5.
1416. Lauriola L, Erlandson RA, Rosai J (1998). Neuroendocrine differentiation is a common feature of thymic carcinoma. Am J Surg Pathol. 22:1059–66.
1417. Law KB, Feng T, Nair V, et al. (2012). Cystic tumor of the atrioventricular node: rare antemortem diagnosis. Cardiovasc Pathol. 21:120–7.
1418. Lawrence B, Perez-Atayde A, Hibbard MK, et al. (2000). TPM3-ALK and TPM4-ALK oncogenes in inflammatory myofibroblastic tumors. Am J Pathol. 157:377–84.
1419. Lawson K, Maher TM, Hansell DM, et al. (2012). Successful treatment of progressive diffuse PEComatosis. Eur Respir J. 40:1578–80.
1420. Lazaros GA, Matsakas EP, Madas JS, et al. (2008). Primary myxofibrosarcoma of the left atrium: case report and review of the literature. Angiology. 59:632–5.
1421. Lazzarino M, Orlandi E, Paulli M, et al. (1993). Primary mediastinal B-cell lymphoma with sclerosis: an aggressive tumor with distinctive clinical and pathologic features. J Clin Oncol. 11:2306–13.
1422. Lazzarino M, Orlandi E, Paulli M, et al. (1997). Treatment outcome and prognostic factors for primary mediastinal (thymic) B-cell lymphoma: a multicenter study of 106 patients. J Clin Oncol. 15:1646–53.
1423. Le Bescont A, Vitte AL, Debernardi A, et al. (2015). Receptor-Independent Ectopic Activity of Prolactin Predicts Aggressive Lung Tumors and Indicates HDACi-Based Therapeutic Strategies. Antioxid Redox Signal. 23:1-14.
1424. Le Deley MC, Reiter A, Williams D, et al. (2008). Prognostic factors in childhood anaplastic large cell lymphoma: results of a large European intergroup study. Blood. 111:1560–6.
1425. Le Pavec J, Lorillon G, Jais X, et al. (2012). Pulmonary Langerhans cell histiocytosis-associated pulmonary hypertension: clinical characteristics and impact of pulmonary arterial hypertension therapies. Chest. 142:1150–7.
1425A. Le Quesne J, Maurya M, Yancheva SG, et al. (2014). A comparison of immunohistochemical assays and FISH in detecting ALK translocation in diagnostic histological and cytological lung tumor material. J Thoracic Oncol 9:769–74.
1426. Le Stang N, Belot A, Gilg Soit Ilq A, et al. (2010). Evolution of pleural cancers and malignant pleural mesothelioma incidence in France between 1980 and 2005. Int J Cancer. 126:232–8.
1427. Lechapt-Zalcman E, Challine D, Delfau-Larue MH, et al. (2001). Association of primary pleural effusion lymphoma of T-cell origin and human herpesvirus 8 in a human immunodeficiency virus-seronegative man. Arch Pathol Lab Med. 125:1246–8.
1428. Lee AC, Kwong YI, Fu KH, et al. (1993). Disseminated mediastinal carcinoma with chromosomal translocation (15;19). A distinctive clinicopathologic syndrome. Cancer. 72:2273–6.
1429. Lee AY, He B, You L, et al. (2004). Expression of the secreted frizzled-related protein gene family is downregulated in human mesothelioma. Oncogene. 23:6672–6.
1430. Lee B, Sir JJ, Park SW, et al. (2008). Right-sided myxomas with extramedullary hematopoiesis and ossification in Carney complex. Int J Cardiol. 130:e63–5.
1431. Lee BH, George S, Kutok JL (2003). Langerhans cell histiocytosis involving the thymus. A case report and review of the literature. Arch Pathol Lab Med. 127:e294–7.
1432. Lee DH, Jung TE, Lee JH, et al. (2013). Pulmonary artery intimal sarcoma: poor 18F-fluorodeoxyglucose uptake in positron emission computed tomography. J Cardiothorac Surg. 8:40.
1433. Lee GY, Kim WS, Ko YH, et al. (2013). Primary cardiac lymphoma mimicking infiltrative cardiomyopathy. Eur J Heart Fail. 15:589–91.
1434. Lee GY, Yang WI, Jeung HC, et al. (2007). Genome-wide genetic aberrations of thymoma using cDNA microarray based comparative genomic hybridization. BMC Genomics. 8:305.
1435. Lee JM, Song HN, Kang Y, et al. (2011). Isolated mediastinal myeloid sarcoma successfully treated with chemoradiotherapy followed by unrelated allogeneic stem cell transplantation. Intern Med. 50:3003–7.
1436. Lee JR, Chang JM, Lee C, et al. (2003). Undifferentiated sarcoma of the mitral valve with unique clinicopathologic presentation. J Cardiovasc Surg (Torino). 44:621–3.
1437. Lee JS, Tuder R, Lynch DA (2000). Lymphomatoid granulomatosis: radiologic features and pathologic correlations. AJR Am J Roentgenol. 175:1335–9.
1438. Lee KC, Bercovitch L (2013). Update on infantile hemangiomas. Semin Perinatol. 37:49–58.
1439. Lee KJ, Shin JH, Choi JH, et al. (1998). A case of arteriovenous type cardiac hemangioma. Korean J Intern Med. 13:123–6.
1440. Lee MW, Stephens RL (1987). Klinefelter's syndrome and extragonadal germ cell tumors. Cancer. 60:1053–5.
1441. Lee S, Kim Y, Sun JM, et al. (2011). Molecular profiles of EGFR, K-ras, c-met, and FGFR in pulmonary pleomorphic carcinoma, a rare lung malignancy. J Cancer Res Clin Oncol. 137:1203–11.
1442. Lee WJ, Lee DW, Chang SE, et al. (2008). Cutaneous metastasis of extraskeletal osteosarcoma arising in the mediastinum. Am J Dermatopathol. 30:629–31.
1443. Leer-Florin A, Moro-Sibilot D, Melis A, et al. (2012). Dual IHC and FISH testing for ALK gene rearrangement in lung adenocarcinomas in a routine practice: a French study. J Thorac Oncol. 7:348–54.
1444. Legault S, Couture C, Bourgault C, et al. (2009). Primary cardiac Burkitt-like lymphoma of the right atrium. Can J Cardiol. 25:163–5.
1445. Lehrke HD, Johnson CK, Zapolanski A, et al. (2014). Intracardiac juvenile xanthogranuloma with presentation in adulthood. Cardiovasc Pathol. 23:54–6.
1446. Lei Y, Yong D, Jun-Zhong R, et al. (2012). Treatment of 28 patients with sclerosing hemangioma (SH) of the lung. J Cardiothorac Surg. 7:34.
1447. Leithauser F, Bauerle M, Huynh MQ, et al. (2001). Isotype-switched immunoglobulin genes with a high load of somatic hypermutation and lack of ongoing mutational activity are prevalent in mediastinal B-cell lymphoma. Blood. 98:2762–70.
1448. Lemarie E, Assouline PS, Diot P, et al. (1992). Primary mediastinal germ cell tumors. Results of a French retrospective study. Chest. 102:1477–83.
1449. Leng S, Do K, Yingling CM, et al. (2012). Defining a gene promoter methylation signature in sputum for lung cancer risk assessment. Clin Cancer Res. 18:3387–95.
1450. Leng S, Liu Y, Thomas CL, et al. (2013). Native American ancestry affects the risk for gene methylation in the lungs of Hispanic smokers from New Mexico. Am J Respir Crit Care Med. 188:1110–6.
1451. Leo F, Cagini L, Rocmans P, et al. (2000). Lung metastases from melanoma: when is surgical treatment warranted? Br J Cancer. 83:569–72.
1452. Leone A, Graziano P, Gasbarra R, et al. (2011). Identification of EGFR mutations in lung sarcomatoid carcinoma. Int J Cancer. 128:732–5.
1453. Leong AS, Brown JH (1984). Malignant transformation in a thymic cyst. Am J Surg Pathol. 8:471–5.
1454. Leong PP, Rezai B, Koch WM, et al. (1998). Distinguishing second primary tumors from lung metastases in patients with head and neck squamous cell carcinoma. J Natl Cancer Inst. 90:972–7.
1455. Leroy X, Copin MC, Petit S, et al. (2001). [Malignant solitary fibrous tumor of pleura with focal expression of cytokeratin]. Ann Pathol. 21:153–6.
1456. Leslie KO, Wick MR (2005). Practical Pulmonary Pathology: A diagnostic approach. Philadelphia: Churchill Livingstone.
1456A. Lestuzzi C, Miolo G, De Paoli A (2013). Systemic Therapy, Radiotherapy, and Cardiotoxicity. In: Cardiac Tumor Pathology. Basso C, Valente M, Thiene G (Eds). New York: Springer,;pp 165–182, with kind permission from Springer Science + Business Media.
1457. Levine GD, Rosai J (1976). A spindle cell varient of thymic carcinoid tumor. A clinical, histologic, and fine structural study with emphasis on its distinction from spindle cell thymoma. Arch Pathol Lab Med. 100:293–300.
1458. Levine GD, Rosai J (1978). Thymic hyperplasia and neoplasia: a review of current concepts. Hum Pathol. 9:495–515.
1459. Lewis BD, Hurt RD, Payne WS, et al. (1983). Benign teratomas of the mediastinum. J Thorac Cardiovasc Surg. 86:727–31.
1459A. Lewis DR, Check DP, Caporaso NE, et al. (2014). US lung cancer trends by histologic type. Cancer. 120:2883–92.
1460. Lewis JS, Ritter JH, El-Mofty S (2005). Alternative epithelial markers in sarcomatoid carcinomas of the head and neck, lung, and bladder-p63, MOC-31, and TTF-1. Mod Pathol. 18:1471–81.
1461. Lezmi G, Verkarre V, Khen-Dunlop N, et al. (2013). FGF10 Signaling differences between type I pleuropulmonary blastoma and congenital cystic adenomatoid malformation. Orphanet J Rare Dis. 8:130.
1462. Li H, Loehrer PJ Sr, Hisada M, et al. (2004). Absence of human T-cell lymphotropic virus type I and human foamy virus in thymoma. Br J Cancer. 90:2181–5.
1463. Li H, Wang DL, Liu XW, et al. (2013). Computed tomography characterization of neuroendocrine tumors of the thymus can aid identification and treatment. Acta Radiol. 54:175–80.
1464. Li L, Burke A, He J, et al. (2011). Sudden unexpected death due to inflammatory myofibroblastic tumor of the heart: a case report and review of the literature. Int J Legal Med. 125:81–5.
1465. Li T, Kung HJ, Mack PC, et al. (2013). Genotyping and genomic profiling of non-small-cell lung cancer: implications for current and future therapies. J Clin Oncol. 31:1039–49.
1466. Li X, Zhang W, Wu X, et al. (2012). Mucoepidermoid carcinoma of the lung: common findings and unusual appearances on CT. Clin Imaging. 36:8–13.
1467. Li Z, Hsieh T, Salehi A (2013). Recurrent cardiac intimal (spindle cell) sarcoma of the left atrium. J Cardiothorac Vasc Anesth. 27:103–7.
1468. Liang TC, Lu MY, Chen SJ, et al. (2002). Cardiac tamponade caused by intrapericardial yolk sac tumor in a boy. J Formos Med Assoc. 101:355–8.
1469. Liang X, Lovell MA, Capocelli KE, et al. (2010). Thymoma in children: report of 2 cases and review of the literature. Pediatr Dev Pathol. 13:202–8.
1470. Liang Y, Wang L, Zhu Y, et al. (2012). Primary pulmonary lymphoepithelioma-like carcinoma: fifty-two patients with long-term follow-up. Cancer. 118:4748–58.
1471. Lieberman PH, Jones CR, Steinman

RM, et al. (1996). Langerhans cell (eosinophilic) granulomatosis. A clinicopathologic study encompassing 50 years. Am J Surg Pathol. 20:519–52.
1472. Liebow AA, Carrington CR, Friedman PJ (1972). Lymphomatoid granulomatosis. Hum Pathol. 3:457–558.
1473. Lin BT, Colby T, Gown AM, et al. (1996). Malignant vascular tumors of the serous membranes mimicking mesothelioma. A report of 14 cases. Am J Surg Pathol. 20:1431–9.
1474. Lin D, Jiang Y, Wang J, et al. (2013). Pulmonary mixed squamous cell and glandular papilloma mimicking adenocarcinoma: a case study and literature review. J Thorac Dis. 5:E129–32.
1475. Lin D, Zhao Y, Li H, et al. (2013). Pulmonary enteric adenocarcinoma with villin brush border immunoreactivity: a case report and literature review. J Thorac Dis. 5:E17–20.
1476. Lin KL, Chen CY, Hsu HH, et al. (1999). Ectopic ACTH syndrome due to thymic carcinoid tumor in a girl. J Pediatr Endocrinol Metab. 12:573–8.
1477. Lin O, Frizzera G (1997). Angiomyoid and follicular dendritic cell proliferative lesions in Castleman's disease of hyaline-vascular type: a study of 10 cases. Am J Surg Pathol. 21:1295–306.
1478. Lindell MM, Doubleday LC, von Eschenbach AC, et al. (1982). Mediastinal metastases from prostatic carcinoma. J Urol. 128:331–4.
1479. Lindeman NI, Cagle PT, Beasley MB, et al. (2013). Molecular testing guideline for selection of lung cancer patients for EGFR and ALK tyrosine kinase inhibitors: guideline from the College of American Pathologists, International Association for the Study of Lung Cancer, and Association for Molecular Pathology. J Thorac Oncol. 8:823–59.
1480. Lindeman NI, Cagle PT, Beasley MB, et al. (2013). Molecular testing guideline for selection of lung cancer patients for EGFR and ALK tyrosine kinase inhibitors: guideline from the College of American Pathologists, International Association for the Study of Lung Cancer, and Association for Molecular Pathology. J Mol Diagn. 15:415–53.
1481. Lindholm PM, Salmenkivi K, Vauhkonen H, et al. (2007). Gene copy number analysis in malignant pleural mesothelioma using oligonucleotide array CGH. Cytogenet Genome Res. 119:46–52.
1482. Lindskog BI, Malm A (1965). Diagnostic and surgical considerations on mediastinal (intrathoracic) goiter. Dis Chest. 47:201–7.
1483. Lino-Silva LS, Flores-Gutierrez JP, Vilches-Cisneros N, et al. (2011). TLE1 is expressed in the majority of primary pleuropulmonary synovial sarcomas. Virchows Arch. 459:615–21.
1484. Lipford EH Jr, Margolick JB, Longo DL, et al. (1988). Angiocentric immunoproliferative lesions: a clinicopathologic spectrum of post-thymic T-cell proliferations. Blood. 72:1674–81.
1485. Lipson D, Capelletti M, Yelensky R, et al. (2012). Identification of new ALK and RET gene fusions from colorectal and lung cancer biopsies. Nat Med. 18:382–4.
1486. Lister TA, Crowther D, Sutcliffe SB, et al. (1989). Report of a committee convened to discuss the evaluation and staging of patients with Hodgkin's disease: Cotswolds meeting. J Clin Oncol. 7:1630–6.
1487. Liu A, Cheng L, Du J, et al. (2010). Diagnostic utility of novel stem cell markers SALL4, OCT4, NANOG, SOX2, UTF1, and TCL1 in primary mediastinal germ cell tumors. Am J Surg Pathol. 34:697–706.
1488. Liu B, Rao Q, Zhu Y, et al. (2012). Metaplastic thymoma of the mediastinum. A clinicopathologic, immunohistochemical, and genetic analysis. Am J Clin Pathol. 137:261–9.
1489. Liu CH, Peng YJ, Wang HH, et al. (2014). Spontaneous rupture of a cystic mediastinal teratoma complicated by superior vena cava syndrome. Ann Thorac Surg. 97:689–91.
1490. Liu GB, Qu YJ, Liao MY, et al. (2012). Relationship between computed tomography manifestations of thymic epithelial tumors and the WHO pathological classification. Asian Pac J Cancer Prev. 13:5581–5.
1491. Liu HC, Hsu WH, Chen YJ, et al. (2002). Primary thymic carcinoma. Ann Thorac Surg. 73:1076–81.
1492. Liu TZ, Zhang DS, Liang Y, et al. (2011). Treatment strategies and prognostic factors of patients with primary germ cell tumors in the mediastinum. J Cancer Res Clin Oncol. 137:1607–12.
1494. Liu YG, Sun KK, Sui XZ, et al. (2012). Thymic carcinosarcoma consisting of sarcomatous and adenosquamous carcinomatous component. Chin Med J (Engl). 125:4154–5.
1495. Lock K, Zhang J, Lu J, et al. (2004). Expression of CD33-related siglecs on human mononuclear phagocytes, monocyte-derived dendritic cells and plasmacytoid dendritic cells. Immunobiology. 209:199–207.
1496. Lococo F, Cesario A, Meacci E, et al. (2011). Huge primary pericardial liposarcoma. Thorac Cardiovasc Surg. 59:172–3.
1497. Lococo F, Cesario A, Okami J, et al. (2013). Role of combined 18F-FDG-PET/CT for predicting the WHO malignancy grade of thymic epithelial tumors: a multicenter analysis. Lung Cancer. 82:245–51.
1498. Loddenkemper C, Anagnostopoulos I, Hummel M, et al. (2004). Differential Emu enhancer activity and expression of BOB.1/OBF.1, Oct2, PU.1, and immunoglobulin in reactive B-cell populations, B-cell non-Hodgkin lymphomas, and Hodgkin lymphomas. J Pathol. 202:60–9.
1499. Loeffler-Ragg J, Bodner J, Freund M, et al. (2012). Diagnostic and therapeutic challenges of a large pleural inflammatory myofibroblastic tumor. Case Rep Pulmonol. 2012:102196.
1500. Loehrer PJ Sr, Hui S, Clark S, et al. (1986). Teratoma following cisplatin-based combination chemotherapy for nonseminomatous germ cell tumors: a clinicopathological correlation. J Urol. 135:1183–9.
1501. Logothetis CJ, Samuels ML, Trindade A, et al. (1982). The growing teratoma syndrome. Cancer. 50:1629–35.
1502. Loire R, Hellal H (1993). [Neoplastic pericarditis. Study by thoracotomy and biopsy in 80 cases]. Presse Med. 22:244–8.
1503. Lones MA, Heerema NA, Le Beau MM, et al. (2007). Chromosome abnormalities in advanced stage lymphoblastic lymphoma of children and adolescents: a report from CCG-E08. Cancer Genet Cytogenet. 172:1–11.
1504. Loo PS, Thomas SC, Nicolson MC, et al. (2010). Subtyping of undifferentiated non-small cell carcinomas in bronchial biopsy specimens. J Thorac Oncol. 5:442–7.
1505. Looijenga LH, Gillis AJ, Stoop HJ, et al. (2007). Chromosomes and expression in human testicular germ-cell tumors: insight into their cell of origin and pathogenesis. Ann N Y Acad Sci. 1120:187–214.
1506. Looijenga LH, Hersmus R, Gillis AJ, et al. (2006). Genomic and expression profiling of human spermatocytic seminomas: primary spermatocyte as tumorigenic precursor and DMRT1 as candidate chromosome 9 gene. Cancer Res. 66:290–302.
1507. Looijenga LH, Stoop H, de Leeuw HP, et al. (2003). POU5F1 (OCT3/4) identifies cells with pluripotent potential in human germ cell tumors. Cancer Res. 63:2244–50.
1508. Look Hong NJ, Pandalai PK, Hornick JL, et al. (2012). Cardiac angiosarcoma management and outcomes: 20-year single-institution experience. Ann Surg Oncol. 19:2707–15.
1509. Loong F, Chan AC, Ho BC, et al. (2010). Diffuse large B-cell lymphoma associated with chronic inflammation as an incidental finding and new clinical scenarios. Mod Pathol. 23:493–501.
1510. Lopez-Lago MA, Okada T, Murillo MM, et al. (2009). Loss of the tumor suppressor gene NF2, encoding merlin, constitutively activates integrin-dependent mTORC1 signaling. Mol Cell Biol. 29:4235–49.
1511. Lopez-Martin A, Ballestin C, Garcia-Carbonero R, et al. (2007). Prognostic value of KIT expression in small cell lung cancer. Lung Cancer. 56:405–13.
1512. Lopez-Rios F, Chuai S, Flores R, et al. (2006). Global gene expression profiling of pleural mesotheliomas: overexpression of aurora kinases and P16/CDKN2A deletion as prognostic factors and critical evaluation of microarray-based prognostic prediction. Cancer Res. 66:2970–9.
1513. Lopez-Rios F, Illei PB, Rusch V, et al. (2004). Evidence against a role for SV40 infection in human mesotheliomas and high risk of false-positive PCR results owing to presence of SV40 sequences in common laboratory plasmids. Lancet. 364:1157–66.
1514. Lorentziadis M, Sourlas A (2012). Primary de novo angiosarcoma of the pleura. Ann Thorac Surg. 93:996–8.
1515. Lorsbach RB, Pinkus GS, Shahsafaei A, et al. (2000). Primary marginal zone lymphoma of the thymus. Am J Clin Pathol. 113:784–91.
1516. Lorusso R, De Cicco G, Tironi A, et al. (2009). Giant primary paraganglioma of the left ventricle. J Thorac Cardiovasc Surg. 137:499–500.
1516A. Louis DN, Ohgaki H, Wiestler OD, Cavenee WK (Eds.): World Health Organization Classification of Tumours of the Nervous System (4th edition). IARC: Lyon 2007
1517. Lovly CM, Gupta A, Lipson D, et al. (2014). Inflammatory myofibroblastic tumors harbor multiple potentially actionable kinase fusions. Cancer Discovery 4:889–895.
1518. Lozano R, Naghavi M, Foreman K, et al. (2012). Global and regional mortality from 235 causes of death for 20 age groups in 1990 and 2010: a systematic analysis for the Global Burden of Disease Study 2010. Lancet. 380:2095–128.
1519. Lu HS, Gan MF, Zhou T, et al. (2011). Sarcomatoid thymic carcinoma arising in metaplastic thymoma: a case report. Int J Surg Pathol. 19:677–80.
1520. Luan SL, Boulanger E, Ye H, et al. (2010). Primary effusion lymphoma: genomic profiling revealed amplification of SELPLG and CORO1C encoding for proteins important for cell migration. J Pathol. 222:166–79.
1521. Lucchi M, Ambrogi MC, Duranti L, et al. (2005). Advanced stage thymomas and thymic carcinomas: results of multimodality treatments. Ann Thorac Surg. 79:1840–4.
1522. Luciano C, Francesco A, Giovanni V, et al. (2010). CT signs, patterns and differential diagnosis of solitary fibrous tumors of the pleura. J Thorac Dis. 2:21–5.
1523. Lumadue JA, Askin FB, Perlman EJ (1994). MIC2 analysis of small cell carcinoma. Am J Clin Pathol. 102:692–4.
1524. Lundkvist L, Erntell H (2002). [A case report of two siblings. Cardiac angiosarcoma--rare tumor with non-specific symptoms and poor prognosis]. Lakartidningen. 99:4165–7.
1525. Luppi M, Trovato R, Barozzi P, et al. (2005). Treatment of herpesvirus associated primary effusion lymphoma with intracavity cidofovir. Leukemia. 19:473–6.
1526. Lurito KJ, Martin T, Cordes T (2002). Right atrial primary cardiac osteosarcoma. Pediatr Cardiol. 23:462–5.
1527. Luthra S, Gallo A, Anthony S, et al. (2012). Primary pulmonary artery sarcoma presenting as right heart failure. Eur J Cardiothorac Surg. 42:591.
1528. Luzzi L, Campione A, Gorla A, et al. (2009). Role of fluorine-flurodeoxyglucose positron emission tomography/computed tomography in preoperative assessment of anterior mediastinal masses. Eur J Cardiothorac Surg. 36:475–9.
1529. Lynch DA, Hay T, Newell JD Jr, et al. (1999). Pediatric diffuse lung disease: diagnosis and classification using high-resolution CT. AJR Am J Roentgenol. 173:713–8.
1530. Lynch TJ, Bell DW, Sordella R, et al. (2004). Activating mutations in the epidermal growth factor receptor underlying responsiveness of non-small-cell lung cancer to gefitinib. N Engl J Med. 350:2129–39.
1531. Ma Y, Li Q, Cui W, et al. (2012). Expression of c-Jun, p73, Casp9, and N-ras in thymic epithelial tumors: relationship with the current WHO classification systems. Diagn Pathol. 7:120.
1532. Ma YQ, Miao N, Abulajiang G, et al. (2010). [Clinicopathologic analysis of 52 cases of thymic epithelial tumor]. Zhonghua Bing Li Xue Za Zhi. 39:249–54.
1533. Mabuchi T, Shimizu M, Ino H, et al. (2005). PRKAR1A gene mutation in patients with cardiac myxoma. Int J Cardiol. 102:273–7.
1534. Macarenco RS, Uphoff TS, Gilmer HF, et al. (2008). Salivary gland-type lung carcinomas: an EGFR immunohistochemical, molecular genetic, and mutational analysis study. Mod Pathol. 21:1168–75.
1535. Machado I, Navarro S, Lopez-Guerrero JA, et al. (2011). Epithelial marker expression does not rule out a diagnosis of Ewing's sarcoma family of tumours. Virchows Arch. 459:409–14.
1536. Macher-Goeppinger S, Penzel R, Roth W, et al. (2011). Expression and mutation analysis of EGFR, c-KIT, and beta-catenin in pulmonary blastoma. J Clin Pathol. 64:349–53.
1537. Machin T, Mashiyama ET, Henderson JA, et al. (1988). Bony metastases in desmoplastic pleural mesothelioma. Thorax. 43:155–6.
1538. Macht M, Mitchell JD, Cool C, et al. (2010). A 31-year-old woman with hemoptysis and an intrathoracic mass. Chest. 138:213–9.
1539. Mack AA, Sugden B (2008). EBV is necessary for proliferation of dually infected primary effusion lymphoma cells. Cancer Res. 68:6963–8.
1540. MacKenzie S, Loken S, Kalia N, et al. (2005). Intrapericardial teratoma in the perinatal period. Case report and review of the literature. J Pediatr Surg. 40:e13–8.
1541. Mackie AS, Kozakewich HP, Geva T, et al. (2005). Vascular tumors of the heart in infants and children: case series and review of the literature. Pediatr Cardiol. 26:344–9.
1542. MacLennan KA, Bennett MH, Tu A, et al. (1989). Relationship of histopathologic features to survival and relapse in nodular sclerosing Hodgkin's disease. A study of 1659 patients. Cancer. 64:1686–93.
1543. MacSweeney F, Papagiannopoulos K, Goldstraw P, et al. (2003). An assessment of the expanded classification of congenital cystic adenomatoid malformations and their relationship to malignant transformation. Am J Surg Pathol. 27:1139–46.
1544. Madani A, Spicer J, Alcindor T, et al. (2014). Clinical significance of incidental pulmonary nodules in esophageal cancer patients. J Gastrointest Surg. 18:226–32.
1545. Mader MT, Poulton TB, White RD (1997). Malignant tumors of the heart and great vessels: MR imaging appearance. Radiographics. 17:145–53.
1546. Maeda H, Matsumura A, Kawabata T, et al. (2012). Adenosquamous carcinoma of the lung: surgical results as compared with squamous cell and adenocarcinoma cases. Eur J Cardiothorac Surg. 41:357–61.
1547. Maeda S, Takahashi S, Koike K, et al. (2011). Primary ependymoma in the posterior mediastinum. Ann Thorac Cardiovasc Surg. 17:494–7.

1548. Maemondo M, Inoue A, Kobayashi K, et al. (2010). Gefitinib or chemotherapy for non-small-cell lung cancer with mutated EGFR. N Engl J Med. 362:2380–8.
1549. Maeshima AM, Tochigi N, Yoshida A, et al. (2010). Histological scoring for small lung adenocarcinomas 2 cm or less in diameter: a reliable prognostic indicator. J Thorac Oncol. 5:333–9.
1550. Maghbool M, Ramzi M, Nagel I, et al. (2013). Primary adenocarcinoma of the thymus: an immunohistochemical and molecular study with review of the literature. BMC Clin Pathol. 13:17.
1551. Magnuson WJ, Halligan JB (2010). Successful treatment of melanoma metastatic to the left atrium using external beam radiation therapy. Oncology (Williston Park). 24:650–3.
1552. Mahon BM, Placido JB, Gattuso P (2010). Fine-needle aspiration of classic biphasic pulmonary blastoma. Diagn Cytopathol. 38:427–9.
1553. Maisch B, Ristic A, Pankuweit S (2010). Evaluation and management of pericardial effusion in patients with neoplastic disease. Prog Cardiovasc Dis. 53:157–63.
1554. Majak BM, Bock G (2003). Pulmonary sclerosing haemangioma diagnosed by frozen section. Histopathology. 42:621–2.
1555. Makimoto Y, Nabeshima K, Iwasaki H, et al. (2005). Inflammatory myofibroblastic tumor of the posterior mediastinum: an older adult case with anaplastic lymphoma kinase abnormalities determined using immunohistochemistry and fluorescence in situ hybridization. Virchows Arch. 446:451–5.
1556. Malagon HD, Valdez AM, Moran CA, et al. (2007). Germ cell tumors with sarcomatous components: a clinicopathologic and immunohistochemical study of 46 cases. Am J Surg Pathol. 31:1356–62.
1557. Maleki Z (2011). Diagnostic issues with cytopathologic interpretation of lung neoplasms displaying high-grade basaloid or neuroendocrine morphology. Diagn Cytopathol. 39:159–67.
1558. Maleszewski JJ, Larsen BT, Kip NS, et al. (2014). PRKAR1A in the development of cardiac myxoma: a study of 110 cases including isolated and syndromic tumors. Am J Surg Pathol. 38:1079–87.
1559. Maleszewski JJ, Hristov AC, Halushka MK, et al. (2010). Extranodal Rosai-Dorfman disease involving the heart: report of two cases. Cardiovasc Pathol. 19:380–4.
1560. Maleszewski JJ, Larsen BT, Kip NS, et al. (2014). PRKAR1A in the Development of Cardiac Myxoma: A Study of 110 Cases Including Isolated and Syndromic Tumors. Am J Surg Pathol. 38:1079–87.
1560A. Maleszewski JJ, Tavora F, Burke AP. (2014). Do "intimal" sarcomas of the heart exist? Am J Surg Pathol. 38:1158–9.
1561. Malpeli G, Barbi S, Moore PS, et al. (2004). Primary mediastinal B-cell lymphoma: hypermutation of the BCL6 gene targets motifs different from those in diffuse large B-cell and follicular lymphomas. Haematologica. 89:1091–9.
1562. Manfredi JJ, Dong J, Liu WJ, et al. (2005). Evidence against a role for SV40 in human mesothelioma. Cancer Res. 65:2602–9.
1563. Mangano WE, Cagle PT, Churg A, et al. (1998). The diagnosis of desmoplastic malignant mesothelioma and its distinction from fibrous pleurisy: a histologic and immunohistochemical analysis of 31 cases including p53 immunostaining. Am J Clin Pathol. 110:191–9.
1564. Mani H, Jaffe ES (2009). Hodgkin lymphoma: an update on its biology with new insights into classification. Clin Lymphoma Myeloma. 9:206–16.
1565. Mani H, Zander DS (2012). Immunohistochemistry: applications to the evaluation of lung and pleural neoplasms: part 2. Chest. 142:1324–33.
1566. Manivel C, Wick MR, Abenoza P, et al. (1986). The occurrence of sarcomatous components in primary mediastinal germ cell tumors. Am J Surg Pathol. 10:711–7.
1567. Manivel JC, Priest JR, Watterson J, et al. (1988). Pleuropulmonary blastoma. The so-called pulmonary blastoma of childhood. Cancer. 62:1516–26.
1568. Mann BD, Sparkes RS, Kern DH, et al. (1983). Chromosomal abnormalities of a mediastinal embryonal cell carcinoma in a patient with 47,XXY Klinefelter syndrome: evidence for the premeiotic origin of a germ cell tumor. Cancer Genet Cytogenet. 8:191–6.
1569. Mann JR, Raafat F, Robinson K, et al. (1998). UKCCSG's germ cell tumour (GCT) studies: improving outcome for children with malignant extracranial non-gonadal tumours--carboplatin, etoposide, and bleomycin are effective and less toxic than previous regimens. United Kingdom Children's Cancer Study Group. Med Pediatr Oncol. 30:217–27.
1570. Manning JT Jr, Ordonez NG, Rosenberg HS, et al. (1985). Pulmonary endodermal tumor resembling fetal lung. Report of a case with immunohistochemical studies. Arch Pathol Lab Med. 109:48–50.
1571. Mansencal N, Revault-d'Allonnes L, Pelage JP, et al. (2009). Usefulness of contrast echocardiography for assessment of intracardiac masses. Arch Cardiovasc Dis. 102:177–83.
1572. Mantovani G, Bondioni S, Corbetta S, et al. (2009). Analysis of GNAS1 and PRKAR1A gene mutations in human cardiac myxomas not associated with multiple endocrine disorders. J Endocrinol Invest. 32:501–4.
1573. Mao C, Qiu LX, Liao RY, et al. (2010). KRAS mutations and resistance to EGFR-TKIs treatment in patients with non-small cell lung cancer: a meta-analysis of 22 studies. Lung Cancer. 69:272–8.
1574. Mao L, Lee JS, Kurie JM, et al. (1997). Clonal genetic alterations in the lungs of current and former smokers. J Natl Cancer Inst. 89:857–62.
1575. Marchevsky AM (1999). Mediastinal tumors of peripheral nervous system origin. Semin Diagn Pathol. 16:65–78.
1576. Marchevsky AM, Gal AA, Shah S, et al. (2001). Morphometry confirms the presence of considerable nuclear size overlap between "small cells" and "large cells" in high-grade pulmonary neuroendocrine neoplasms. Am J Clin Pathol. 116:466–72.
1577. Marchevsky AM, Gupta R, Balzer B (2010). Diagnosis of metastatic neoplasms: a clinicopathologic and morphologic approach. Arch Pathol Lab Med. 134:194–206.
1578. Marchevsky AM, Gupta R, Casadio C, et al. (2010). World Health Organization classification of thymomas provides significant prognostic information for selected stage III patients: evidence from an international thymoma study group. Hum Pathol. 41:1413–21.
1579. Marchevsky AM, Gupta R, McKenna RJ, et al. (2008). Evidence-based pathology and the pathologic evaluation of thymomas: the World Health Organization classification can be simplified into only 3 categories other than thymic carcinoma. Cancer. 112:2780–8.
1580. Marchevsky AM, McKenna RJ Jr, Gupta R (2008). Thymic epithelial neoplasms: a review of current concepts using an evidence-based pathology approach. Hematol Oncol Clin North Am. 22:543–62.
1581. Marchevsky AM, Wick MR (2014). Pathology of the Mediastinum. Cambridge: Cambridge University Press.
1582. Margolin K, Traweek T (1992). The unique association of malignant histiocytosis and a primary gonadal germ cell tumor. Med Pediatr Oncol. 20:162–4.
1583. Marina NM, Cushing B, Giller R, et al. (1999). Complete surgical excision is effective treatment for children with immature teratomas with or without malignant elements: A Pediatric Oncology Group/Children's Cancer Group Intergroup Study. J Clin Oncol. 17:2137–43.
1584. Mariusdottir E, Nikulasson S, Bjornsson J, et al. (2010). Thymic epithelial tumours in Iceland: incidence and histopathology, a population-based study. APMIS. 118:927–33.
1585. Marom EM, Milito MA, Moran CA, et al. (2011). Computed tomography findings predicting invasiveness of thymoma. J Thorac Oncol. 6:1274–81.
1586. Martel M, Sarli D, Colecchia M, et al. (2003). Fibroblastic reticular cell tumor of the spleen: report of a case and review of the entity. Hum Pathol. 34:954–7.
1587. Marti A, Culine S, Carde P, et al. (2004). Familial primary mediastinal nonseminomatous germ-cell tumors. Urol Oncol. 22:421–4.
1588. Martignoni G, Pea M, Reghellin D, et al. (2010). Molecular pathology of lymphangioleiomyomatosis and other perivascular epithelioid cell tumors. Arch Pathol Lab Med. 134:33–40.
1589. Martin B, Verdebout JM, Mascaux C, et al. (2002). Expression of p53 in preneoplastic and early neoplastic bronchial lesions. Oncol Rep. 9:223–9.
1590. Martinet N, Alla F, Farre G, et al. (2000). Retinoic acid receptor and retinoid X receptor alterations in lung cancer precursor lesions. Cancer Res. 60:2869–75.
1591. Martinez VD, Buys TP, Adonis M, et al. (2010). Arsenic-related DNA copy-number alterations in lung squamous cell carcinomas. Br J Cancer. 103:1277–83.
1592. Martusewicz-Boros M, Wiatr E, Radzikowska E, et al. (2007). Pulmonary intravascular large B-cell lymphoma as a cause of severe hypoxemia. J Clin Oncol. 25:2137–9.
1593. Maruyama H, Seyama K, Sobajima J, et al. (2001). Multifocal micronodular pneumocyte hyperplasia and lymphangioleiomyomatosis in tuberous sclerosis with a TSC2 gene. Mod Pathol. 14:609–14.
1594. Marx A, Pfister F, Schalke B, et al. (2013). The different roles of the thymus in the pathogenesis of the various myasthenia gravis subtypes. Autoimmun Rev. 12:875–84.
1595. Marx A, Strobel P, Badve SS, et al. (2014). ITMIG consensus statement on the use of the WHO histological classification of thymoma and thymic carcinoma: refined definitions, histological criteria, and reporting. J Thorac Oncol. 9:596–611.
1596. Marx A, Willcox N, Leite MI, et al. (2010). Thymoma and paraneoplastic myasthenia gravis. Autoimmunity. 43:413–27.
1597. Mas C, Penny DJ, Menahem S (2000). Pre-excitation syndrome secondary to cardiac rhabdomyomas in tuberous sclerosis. J Paediatr Child Health. 36:84–6.
1598. Masai K, Tsuta K, Kawago M, et al. (2013). Expression of squamous cell carcinoma markers and adenocarcinoma markers in primary pulmonary neuroendocrine carcinomas. Appl Immunohistochem Mol Morphol. 21:292–7.
1599. Maschek H, Werner M, Busche G, et al. (1992). [Congenital rhabdoid tumor in the mediastinum and liver. Case report and review of the literature]. Pathologe. 13:172–8.
1600. Masood R, Kundra A, Zhu S, et al. (2003). Malignant mesothelioma growth inhibition by agents that target the VEGF and VEGF-C autocrine loops. Int J Cancer. 104:603–10.
1601. Massard G, Eichler F, Gasser B, et al. (1998). Recurrence of the mediastinal growing teratoma syndrome. Ann Thorac Surg. 66:605–6.
1602. Masunaga A, Nagashio R, Iwamoto S, et al. (2012). A case of pulmonary papillary adenoma: possible relationship between tumor histogenesis/tumorigenesis and fibroblast growth factor receptor 2 IIIb. Pathol Int. 62:640–5.
1603. Masuya D, Haba R, Huang CL, et al. (2005). Myoepithelial carcinoma of the lung. Eur J Cardiothorac Surg. 28:775–7.
1604. Matolcsy A, Nador RG, Cesarman E, et al. (1998). Immunoglobulin VH gene mutational analysis suggests that primary effusion lymphomas derive from different stages of B cell maturation. Am J Pathol. 153:1609–14.
1605. Matsubara O, Tan-Liu NS, Kenney RM, et al. (1988). Inflammatory pseudotumors of the lung: progression from organizing pneumonia to fibrous histiocytoma or to plasma cell granuloma in 32 cases. Hum Pathol. 19:807–14.
1606. Matsubayashi J, Sato E, Nomura M, et al. (2012). A case of paravertebral mediastinal chordoma without bone destruction. Skeletal Radiol. 41:1641–4.
1607. Matsudaira N, Hirano H, Itou S, et al. (1994). MR imaging of thymolipoma. Magn Reson Imaging. 12:959–61.
1608. Matsukuma S, Hisaoka M, Obara K, et al. (2012). Primary pulmonary myxoid sarcoma with EWSR1-CREB1 fusion, resembling extraskeletal myxoid chondrosarcoma: Case report with a review of Literature. Pathol Int. 62:817–22.
1609. Matsuno Y, Morozumi N, Hirohashi S, et al. (1998). Papillary carcinoma of the thymus: report of four cases of a new microscopic type of thymic carcinoma. Am J Surg Pathol. 22:873–80.
1610. Matsuno Y, Rosai J, Shimosato Y (2004). Papillary adenocarcinoma. In: Travis WD, Brambilla E, Muller-Hermelink HK, Harris CC, eds. WHO Classification of Tumours. Pathology and Genetics of Tumours of the Lung, Pleura, Thymus and Heart. 3rd ed. Lyon: IARC; pp. 183–183.
1611. Matsushita T, Huynh AT, Singh T, et al. (2007). Aortic valve lipoma. Ann Thorac Surg. 83:2220–2.
1612. Matsuura N, Yokota N, Go T, et al. (2011). Bronchoplastic operation using a continuous anastomosis for mucous gland adenoma. Ann Thorac Surg. 92:2272–4.
1613. Matsuyama A, Hisaoka M, Iwasaki M, et al. (2010). TLE1 expression in malignant mesothelioma. Virchows Arch. 457:577–83.
1614. Mattoo A, Fedullo PF, Kapelanski D, et al. (2002). Pulmonary artery sarcoma: a case report of surgical cure and 5-year follow-up. Chest. 122:745–7.
1615. Matyakhina L, Pack S, Kirschner LS, et al. (2003). Chromosome 2 (2p16) abnormalities in Carney complex tumours. J Med Genet. 40:268–77.
1616. Mavragani CP, Moutsopoulos HM (2014). Sjogren's syndrome. Annu Rev Pathol. 9:273–85.
1617. Mayall FG, Gibbs AR (1992). The histology and immunohistochemistry of small cell mesothelioma. Histopathology. 20:47–51.
1618. Maziak DE, Todd TR, Keshavjee SH, et al. (1996). Adenoid cystic carcinoma of the airway: thirty-two-year experience. J Thorac Cardiovasc Surg. 112:1522–31.
1619. Mazumdar M, Bajorin DF, Bacik J, et al. (2001). Predicting outcome to chemotherapy in patients with germ cell tumors: the value of the rate of decline of human chorionic gonadotrophin and alpha-fetoprotein during therapy. J Clin Oncol. 19:2534–41.
1620. Mazzola A, Spano JP, Valente M, et al. (2006). Leiomyosarcoma of the left atrium mimicking a left atrial myxoma. J Thorac Cardiovasc Surg. 131:224–6.
1621. McCaughan F, Pole JC, Bankier AT, et al. (2010). Progressive 3q amplification consistently targets SOX2 in preinvasive squamous lung cancer. Am J Respir Crit Care Med. 182:83–91.
1622. McClain KL, Leach CT, Jenson HB, et al. (1995). Association of Epstein-Barr virus with leiomyosarcomas in children with AIDS. N Engl J Med. 332:12–8.
1623. McCloskey P, Balduyck B, Van Schil PE,

et al. (2013). Radical treatment of non-small cell lung cancer during the last 5 years. Eur J Cancer. 49:1555–64.

1624. McCormack FX, Inoue Y, Moss J, et al. (2011). Efficacy and safety of sirolimus in lymphangioleiomyomatosis. N Engl J Med. 364:1595–606.

1625. McCormack FX, Travis WD, Colby TV, et al. (2012). Lymphangioleiomyomatosis: calling it what it is: a low-grade, destructive, metastasizing neoplasm. Am J Respir Crit Care Med. 186:1210–2.

1626. McDonald JC (2010). Epidemiology of malignant mesothelioma--an outline. Ann Occup Hyg. 54:851–7.

1627. McDonald JC, Harris J, Armstrong B (2004). Mortality in a cohort of vermiculite miners exposed to fibrous amphibole in Libby, Montana. Occup Environ Med. 61:363–6.

1628. McDonald JC, McDonald AD (1997). Chrysotile, tremolite and carcinogenicity. Ann Occup Hyg. 41:699–705.

1629. McElhinney DB, Carpentieri DF, Bridges ND, et al. (2001). Sarcoma of the mitral valve causing coronary arterial occlusion in children. Cardiol Young. 11:539–42.

1630. McFadden DG, Papagiannakopoulos T, Taylor-Weiner A, et al. (2014). Genetic and clonal dissection of murine small cell lung carcinoma progression by genome sequencing. Cell. 156:1298–311.

1631. McGinnis M, Jacobs G, el-Naggar A, et al. (1993). Congenital peribronchial myofibroblastic tumor (so-called "congenital leiomyosarcoma"). A distinct neonatal lung lesion associated with nonimmune hydrops fetalis. Mod Pathol. 6:487–92.

1632. McGregor CG, Gibson A, Caves P (1984). Infantile cardiomyopathy with histiocytoid change in cardiac muscle cells: successful surgical intervention and prolonged survival. Am J Cardiol. 53:982–3.

1633. McKenney JK, Heerema-McKenney A, Rouse RV (2007). Extragonadal germ cell tumors: a review with emphasis on pathologic features, clinical prognostic variables, and differential diagnostic considerations. Adv Anat Pathol. 14:69–92.

1634. McLoud TC, Kalisher L, Stark P, et al. (1978). Intrathoracic lymph node metastases from extrathoracic neoplasms. AJR Am J Roentgenol. 131:403–7.

1635. McNamee CJ, Lien D, Puttagunta L, et al. (2003). Solitary squamous papillomas of the bronchus: a case report and literature review. J Thorac Cardiovasc Surg. 126:861–3.

1636. McNeil MM, Leong AS, Sage RE (1981). Primary mediastinal embryonal carcinoma in association with Klinefelter's syndrome. Cancer. 47:343–5.

1637. McNiff JM, Cooper D, Howe G, et al. (1996). Lymphomatoid granulomatosis of the skin and lung. An angiocentric T-cell-rich B-cell lymphoproliferative disorder. Arch Dermatol. 132:1464–70.

1638. McWilliams A, Shaipanich T, Lam S (2013). Fluorescence and navigational bronchoscopy. Thorac Surg Clin. 23:153–61.

1639. Medeiros LJ, Peiper SC, Elwood L, et al. (1991). Angiocentric immunoproliferative lesions: a molecular analysis of eight cases. Hum Pathol. 22:1150–7.

1640. Meert AP, Feoli F, Martin B, et al. (2004). Ki67 expression in bronchial preneoplastic lesions and carcinoma in situ defined according to the new 1999 WHO/IASLC criteria: a preliminary study. Histopathology. 44:47–53.

1641. Mega S, Oguri M, Kawasaki R, et al. (2008). Large-cell neuroendocrine carcinoma in the thymus. Gen Thorac Cardiovasc Surg. 56:566–9.

1642. Mei B, Lai YL, He GJ, et al. (2013). Giant primary mesenchymal chondrosarcoma of the lung: case report and review of literature. Ann Thorac Cardiovasc Surg. 19:481–4.

1643. Mei K, Liu A, Allan RW, et al. (2009). Diagnostic utility of SALL4 in primary germ cell tumors of the central nervous system: a study of 77 cases. Mod Pathol. 22:1628–36.

1644. Meir K, Maly A, Doviner V, et al. (2004). Intraoperative cytologic diagnosis of unsuspected cardiac myxoma: a case report. Acta Cytol. 48:565–8.

1645. Meiri E, Mueller WC, Rosenwald S, et al. (2012). A second-generation microRNA-based assay for diagnosing tumor tissue origin. Oncologist. 17:801–12.

1646. Meis-Kindblom JM, Kindblom LG (1998). Angiosarcoma of soft tissue: a study of 80 cases. Am J Surg Pathol. 22:683–97.

1647. Meisinger QC, Klein JS, Butnor KJ, et al. (2011). CT features of peripheral pulmonary carcinoid tumors. AJR Am J Roentgenol. 197:1073–80.

1648. Meissner A, Kirch W, Regensburger D, et al. (1988). Intrapericardial teratoma in an adult. Am J Med. 84:1089–90.

1649. Meister M, Schirmacher P, Dienemann H, et al. (2007). Mutational status of the epidermal growth factor receptor (EGFR) gene in thymomas and thymic carcinomas. Cancer Lett. 248:186–91.

1650. Melloni G, Carretta A, Ciriaco P, et al. (2005). Inflammatory pseudotumor of the lung in adults. Ann Thorac Surg. 79:426–32.

1651. Melzner I, Bucur AJ, Bruderlein S, et al. (2005). Biallelic mutation of SOCS-1 impairs JAK2 degradation and sustains phospho-JAK2 action in the MedB-1 mediastinal lymphoma line. Blood. 105:2535–42.

1652. Mendlick MR, Nelson M, Pickering D, et al. (2001). Translocation t(1;3)(p36.3;q25) is a nonrandom aberration in epithelioid hemangioendothelioma. Am J Surg Pathol. 25:684–7.

1653. Menestrina F, Chilosi M, Bonetti F, et al. (1986). Mediastinal large-cell lymphoma of B-type, with sclerosis: histopathological and immunohistochemical study of eight cases. Histopathology. 10:589–600.

1654. Mensi C, Giacomini S, Sieno C, et al. (2011). Pericardial mesothelioma and asbestos exposure. Int J Hyg Environ Health. 214:276–9.

1655. Mentzel T, Beham A, Calonje E, et al. (1997). Epithelioid hemangioendothelioma of skin and soft tissues: clinicopathologic and immunohistochemical study of 30 cases. Am J Surg Pathol. 21:363–74.

1656. Merchant AM, Hedrick HL, Johnson MP, et al. (2005). Management of fetal mediastinal teratoma. J Pediatr Surg. 40:228–31.

1657. Merrick DT, Kittelson J, Winterhalder R, et al. (2006). Analysis of c-ErbB1/epidermal growth factor receptor and c-ErbB2/HER-2 expression in bronchial dysplasia: evaluation of potential targets for chemoprevention of lung cancer. Clin Cancer Res. 12:2281–8.

1658. Mesri EA, Cesarman E, Boshoff C (2010). Kaposi's sarcoma and its associated herpesvirus. Nat Rev Cancer. 10:707–19.

1659. Metaxa-Mariatou V, Papaioannou D, Loli A, et al. (2005). Subtype C1 persistent infection of HHV-8 in a PEL patient. Leuk Lymphoma. 46:1507–12.

1660. Meuwissen R, Linn SC, Linnoila RI, et al. (2003). Induction of small cell lung cancer by somatic inactivation of both Trp53 and Rb1 in a conditional mouse model. Cancer Cell. 4:181–9.

1661. Meyers DG, Meyers RE, Prendergast TW (1997). The usefulness of diagnostic tests on pericardial fluid. Chest. 111:1213–21.

1662. Michal M, Havlicek F (1993). Immunohistochemical phenotypes of histioeosinophilic granulomas of thymus and reactive eosinophilic pleuritis. Acta Histochem. 94:97–101.

1663. Michaud J, Banerjee D, Kaufmann JC (1983). Lymphomatoid granulomatosis involving the central nervous system: complication of a renal transplant with terminal monoclonal B-cell proliferation. Acta Neuropathol. 61:141–7.

1664. Michel M, Pratt JW (2004). Anterior mediastinal nonseminomatous germ cell tumor with malignant transformation: a case report. Curr Surg. 61:576–9.

1665. Middleton G (1966). Involvement of the thymus by metastic neoplasms. Br J Cancer. 20:41–6.

1666. Miettinen M (2010). Modern Soft Tissue Pathology. Cambridge: Cambridge University Press.

1667. Miettinen M, Fletcher CD, Lasota J (1993). True histiocytic lymphoma of small intestine. Analysis of two S-100 protein-positive cases with features of interdigitating reticulum cell sarcoma. Am J Clin Pathol. 100:285–92.

1668. Miettinen M, McCue PA, Sarlomo-Rikala M, et al. (2014). GATA3: a multispecific but potentially useful marker in surgical pathology: a systematic analysis of 2500 epithelial and nonepithelial tumors. Am J Surg Pathol. 38:13–22.

1669. Miettinen M, Virtanen I (1984). Synovial sarcoma--a misnomer. Am J Pathol. 117:18–25.

1670. Miettinen M, Wang ZF, Paetau A, et al. (2011). ERG transcription factor as an immunohistochemical marker for vascular endothelial tumors and prostatic carcinoma. Am J Surg Pathol. 35:432–41.

1671. Mihal V, Dusek J, Jarosova M, et al. (1989). Mediastinal teratoma and acute megakaryoblastic leukemia. Neoplasma. 36:739–47.

1672. Miki M, Ball DW, Linnoila RI (2012). Insights into the achaete-scute homolog-1 gene (hASH1) in normal and neoplastic human lung. Lung Cancer. 75:58–65.

1673. Mikolaenko I, Listinsky CM (2009). Systemic CD5+ MALT lymphoma: presentation with Waldenstrom syndrome. Ann Diagn Pathol. 13:272–7.

1674. Miller A, Hu B (1995). A molecular model of low-voltage-activated calcium conductance. J Neurophysiol. 73:2349–56.

1675. Miller DV, Tazelaar HD, Handy JR, et al. (2005). Thymoma arising within cardiac myxoma. Am J Surg Pathol. 29:1208–13.

1676. Miller R, Kurtz SM, Powers JM (1978). Mediastinal rhabdomyoma. Cancer. 42:1983–8.

1677. Mills SE (2012). Histology for Pathologists. 4th ed. Philadelphia: Lippincott Williams & Wilkins.

1678. Min KW (2013). Two different types of carcinoid tumors of the lung: immunohistochemical and ultrastructural investigation and their histogenetic consideration. Ultrastruct Pathol. 37:23–35.

1679. Minami Y, Matsuno Y, Iijima T, et al. (2005). Prognostication of small-sized primary pulmonary adenocarcinomas by histopathological and karyometric analysis. Lung Cancer. 48:339–48.

1680. Minami Y, Morishita Y, Yamamoto T, et al. (2004). Cytologic characteristics of pulmonary papillary adenoma. A case report. Acta Cytol. 48:243–8.

1681. Minato H, Nojima T, Kurose N, et al. (2009). Adenomatoid tumor of the pleura. Pathol Int. 59:567–71.

1682. Miniati DN, Chintagumpala M, Langston C, et al. (2006). Prenatal presentation and outcome of children with pleuropulmonary blastoma. J Pediatr Surg. 41:66–71.

1683. Mirza I, Kazimi SN, Ligi R, et al. (2000). Cytogenetic profile of a thymoma. A case report and review of the literature. Arch Pathol Lab Med. 124:1714–6.

1684. Mishriki YY, Lane BP, Lozowski MS, et al. (1983). Hurthle-cell tumor arising in the mediastinal ectopic thyroid and diagnosed by fine needle aspiration. Light microscopic and ultrastructural features. Acta Cytol. 27:188–92.

1685. Mitani Y, Rao PH, Futreal PA, et al. (2011). Novel chromosomal rearrangements and break points at the t(6;9) in salivary adenoid cystic carcinoma: association with MYB-NFIB chimeric fusion, MYB expression, and clinical outcome. Clin Cancer Res. 17:7003–14.

1686. Mitchell A, Meunier C, Ouellette D, et al. (2006). Extranodal marginal zone lymphoma of mucosa-associated lymphoid tissue with initial presentation in the pleura. Chest. 129:791–4.

1687. Mito K, Kashima K, Daa T, et al. (2005). Multiple calcifying fibrous tumors of the pleura. Virchows Arch. 446:78–81.

1688. Mitry E, Guiu B, Cosconea S, et al. (2010). Epidemiology, management and prognosis of colorectal cancer with lung metastases: a 30-year population-based study. Gut. 59:1383–8.

1689. Mitsudomi T, Morita S, Yatabe Y, et al. (2010). Gefitinib versus cisplatin plus docetaxel in patients with non-small-cell lung cancer harbouring mutations of the epidermal growth factor receptor (WJTOG3405): an open label, randomised phase 3 trial. Lancet Oncol. 11:121–8.

1690. Mittal K, Neri A, Feiner H, et al. (1990). Lymphomatoid granulomatosis in the acquired immunodeficiency syndrome. Evidence of Epstein-Barr virus infection and B-cell clonal selection without myc rearrangement. Cancer. 65:1345–9.

1691. Miwa H, Takakuwa T, Nakatsuka S, et al. (2002). DNA sequences of the immunoglobulin heavy chain variable region gene in pyothorax-associated lymphoma. Oncology. 62:241–50.

1692. Miyagawa-Hayashino A, Tazelaar HD, Langel DJ, et al. (2003). Pulmonary sclerosing hemangioma with lymph node metastases: report of 4 cases. Arch Pathol Lab Med. 127:321–5.

1693. Mizuno T, Murakami H, Fujii M, et al. (2012). YAP induces malignant mesothelioma cell proliferation by upregulating transcription of cell cycle-promoting genes. Oncogene. 31:5117–22.

1694. Moavero R, Coniglio A, Garaci F, et al. (2013). Is mTOR inhibition a systemic treatment for tuberous sclerosis? Ital J Pediatr. 39:57.

1695. Mochizuki T, Ishii G, Nagai K, et al. (2008). Pleomorphic carcinoma of the lung: clinicopathologic characteristics of 70 cases. Am J Surg Pathol. 32:1727–35.

1696. Moeller KH, Rosado-de-Christenson ML, Templeton PA (1997). Mediastinal mature teratoma: imaging features. AJR Am J Roentgenol. 169:985–90.

1697. Mogi A, Hirato J, Kosaka T, et al. (2012). Primary mediastinal atypical meningioma: report of a case and literature review. World J Surg Oncol. 10:17.

1698. Mohamed S, Pruna L, Kaminsky P (2013). [Increasing risk of tumors in myotonic dystrophy type 1]. Presse Med. 42:e281–4.

1699. Mohan Rao PS, Moorthy N, Shankarappa RK, et al. (2009). Giant mediastinal thymolipoma simulating cardiomegaly. J Cardiol. 54:326–9.

1700. Mok TS, Wu YL, Thongprasert S, et al. (2009). Gefitinib or carboplatin-paclitaxel in pulmonary adenocarcinoma. N Engl J Med. 361:947–57.

1701. Molajo AO, McWilliam L, Ward C, et al. (1987). Cardiac lymphoma: an unusual case of myocardial perforation--clinical, echocardiographic, haemodynamic and pathological features. Eur Heart J. 8:549–52.

1702. Moldenhauer G, Popov SW, Wotschke B, et al. (2006). AID expression identifies interfollicular large B cells as putative precursors of mature B-cell malignancies. Blood. 107:2470–3.

1703. Molenaar JC (1976). [Phimosis and pseudophimosis in children]. Ned Tijdschr Geneeskd. 120:1006–7.

1704. Molina JR, Aubry MC, Lewis JE, et al. (2007). Primary salivary gland-type lung cancer: spectrum of clinical presentation, histopathologic and prognostic factors. Cancer. 110:2253–9.

1705. Molina JR, Yang P, Cassivi SD, et al. (2008). Non-small cell lung cancer:

epidemiology, risk factors, treatment, and survivorship. Mayo Clin Proc. 83:584–94.
1706. Moller P, Lammler B, Herrmann B, et al. (1986). The primary mediastinal clear cell lymphoma of B-cell type has variable defects in MHC antigen expression. Immunology. 59:411–7.
1707. Moller P, Moldenhauer G, Momburg F, et al. (1987). Mediastinal lymphoma of clear cell type is a tumor corresponding to terminal steps of B cell differentiation. Blood. 69:1087–95.
1708. Monaco SE, Shuai Y, Bansal M, et al. (2011). The diagnostic utility of p16 FISH and GLUT-1 immunohistochemical analysis in mesothelial proliferations. Am J Clin Pathol. 135:619–27.
1709. Monica V, Ceppi P, Righi L, et al. (2009). Desmocollin-3: a new marker of squamous differentiation in undifferentiated large-cell carcinoma of the lung. Mod Pathol. 22:709–17.
1710. Montanaro F, Bray F, Gennaro V, et al. (2003). Pleural mesothelioma incidence in Europe: evidence of some deceleration in the increasing trends. Cancer Causes Control. 14:791–803.
1711. Montani D, Jais X, Sitbon O, et al. (2012). EBUS-TBNA in the differential diagnosis of pulmonary artery sarcoma and thromboembolism. Eur Respir J. 39:1549–50.
1712. Moonim MT, Breen R, Gill-Barman B, et al. (2012). Diagnosis and subclassification of thymoma by minimally invasive fine needle aspiration directed by endobronchial ultrasound: a review and discussion of four cases. Cytopathology. 23:220–8.
1713. Morales M, Trujillo M, del Carmen Maeso M, et al. (2007). Thymoma and progressive T-cell lymphocytosis. Ann Oncol. 18:603–4.
1714. Moran CA (1999). Germ cell tumors of the mediastinum. Pathol Res Pract. 195:583–7.
1715. Moran CA, Hochholzer L, Rush W, et al. (1996). Primary intrapulmonary meningiomas. A clinicopathologic and immunohistochemical study of ten cases. Cancer. 78:2328–33.
1716. Moran CA, Rosado-de-Christenson M, Suster S (1995). Thymolipoma: clinicopathologic review of 33 cases. Mod Pathol. 8:741–4.
1717. Moran CA, Suster S (1995). Mediastinal hemangiomas: a study of 18 cases with emphasis on the spectrum of morphological features. Hum Pathol. 26:416–21.
1718. Moran CA, Suster S (1995). Mediastinal seminomas with prominent cystic changes. A clinicopathologic study of 10 cases. Am J Surg Pathol. 19:1047–53.
1719. Moran CA, Suster S (1995). Mucoepidermoid carcinomas of the thymus. A clinicopathologic study of six cases. Am J Surg Pathol. 19:826–34.
1720. Moran CA, Suster S (1997). Hepatoid yolk sac tumors of the mediastinum: a clinicopathologic and immunohistochemical study of four cases. Am J Surg Pathol. 21:1210–4.
1721. Moran CA, Suster S (1997). Mediastinal yolk sac tumors associated with prominent multilocular cystic changes of thymic epithelium: a clinicopathologic and immunohistochemical study of five cases. Mod Pathol. 10:800–3.
1722. Moran CA, Suster S (1997). Primary germ cell tumors of the mediastinum: I. Analysis of 322 cases with special emphasis on teratomatous lesions and a proposal for histopathologic classification and clinical staging. Cancer. 80:681–90.
1723. Moran CA, Suster S (1997). Primary mediastinal choriocarcinomas: a clinicopathologic and immunohistochemical study of eight cases. Am J Surg Pathol. 21:1007–12.
1724. Moran CA, Suster S (1998). Germ-cell tumors of the mediastinum. Adv Anat Pathol. 5:1–15.
1725. Moran CA, Suster S (1999). Angiomatoid neuroendocrine carcinoma of the thymus: report of a distinctive morphological variant of neuroendocrine tumor of the thymus resembling a vascular neoplasm. Hum Pathol. 30:635–9.
1726. Moran CA, Suster S (1999). Spindle-cell neuroendocrine carcinomas of the thymus (spindle-cell thymic carcinoid): a clinicopathologic and immunohistochemical study of seven cases. Mod Pathol. 12:587–91.
1727. Moran CA, Suster S (2000). Neuroendocrine carcinomas (carcinoid tumor) of the thymus. A clinicopathologic analysis of 80 cases. Am J Clin Pathol. 114:100–10.
1728. Moran CA, Suster S (2000). Primary neuroendocrine carcinoma (thymic carcinoid) of the thymus with prominent oncocytic features: a clinicopathologic study of 22 cases. Mod Pathol. 13:489–94.
1729. Moran CA, Suster S (2000). Thymic neuroendocrine carcinomas with combined features ranging from well-differentiated (carcinoid) to small cell carcinoma. A clinicopathologic and immunohistochemical study of 11 cases. Am J Clin Pathol. 113:345–50.
1730. Moran CA, Suster S (2001). Thymoma with prominent cystic and hemorrhagic changes and areas of necrosis and infarction: a clinicopathologic study of 25 cases. Am J Surg Pathol. 25:1086–90.
1731. Moran CA, Suster S (2004). "Ancient" (sclerosing) thymomas: a clinicopathologic study of 10 cases. Am J Clin Pathol. 121:867–71.
1732. Moran CA, Suster S (2005). Primary parathyroid tumors of the mediastinum: a clinicopathologic and immunohistochemical study of 17 cases. Am J Clin Pathol. 124:749–54.
1733. Moran CA, Suster S, Askin FB, et al. (1994). Benign and malignant salivary gland-type mixed tumors of the lung. Clinicopathologic and immunohistochemical study of eight cases. Cancer. 73:2481–90.
1734. Moran CA, Suster S, Fishback NF, et al. (1995). Primary intrapulmonary thymoma. A clinicopathologic and immunohistochemical study of eight cases. Am J Surg Pathol. 19:304–12.
1735. Moran CA, Suster S, Koss MN (1994). Primary adenoid cystic carcinoma of the lung. A clinicopathologic and immunohistochemical study of 16 cases. Cancer. 73:1390–7.
1736. Moran CA, Suster S, Koss MN (1997). Primary germ cell tumors of the mediastinum: III. Yolk sac tumor, embryonal carcinoma, choriocarcinoma, and combined nonteratomatous germ cell tumors of the mediastinum--a clinicopathologic and immunohistochemical study of 64 cases. Cancer. 80:699–707.
1737. Moran CA, Suster S, Przygodzki RM, et al. (1997). Primary germ cell tumors of the mediastinum: II. Mediastinal seminomas--a clinicopathologic and immunohistochemical study of 120 cases. Cancer. 80:691–8.
1738. Moran CA, Weissferdt A, Kalhor N, et al. (2012). Thymomas I: a clinicopathologic correlation of 250 cases with emphasis on the World Health Organization schema. Am J Clin Pathol. 137:444–50.
1739. Moreira AL, Joubert P, Downey RJ, et al. (2014). Cribriform and fused glands are patterns of high-grade pulmonary adenocarcinoma. Hum Pathol. 45:213–20.
1740. Morency E, Rodriguez Urrego PA, Szporn AH, et al. (2013). The "drunken honeycomb" feature of pulmonary mucinous adenocarcinoma: a diagnostic pitfall of bronchial brushing cytology. Diagn Cytopathol. 41:63–6.
1741. Morgan DE, Sanders C, McElvein RB, et al. (1992). Intrapulmonary teratoma: a case report and review of the literature. J Thorac Imaging. 7:70–7.
1742. Mori K, Cho H, Som M (1977). Primary "flat" melanoma of the trachea. J Pathol. 121:101–5.
1743. Mori M, Chiba R, Tezuka F, et al. (1996). Papillary adenoma of type II pneumocytes might have malignant potential. Virchows Arch. 428:195–200.
1744. Mori M, Rao SK, Popper HH, et al. (2001). Atypical adenomatous hyperplasia of the lung: a probable forerunner in the development of adenocarcinoma of the lung. Mod Pathol. 14:72–84.
1745. Mori T, Nomori H, Ikeda K, et al. (2007). Microscopic-sized "microthymoma" in patients with myasthenia gravis. Chest. 131:847–9.
1746. Mori T, Nomori H, Ikeda K, et al. (2007). Three cases of multiple thymoma with a review of the literature. Jpn J Clin Oncol. 37:146–9.
1747. Mori T, Nomori H, Yoshioka M, et al. (2009). A case of primary mediastinal ependymoma. Ann Thorac Cardiovasc Surg. 15:332–5.
1748. Morin MJ, Hopkins RA, Ferguson WS, et al. (2004). Intracardiac yolk sac tumor and dysrhythmia as an etiology of pediatric syncope. Pediatrics. 113:e374–6.
1749. Morinaga S, Nomori H, Kobayashi R, et al. (1994). Well-differentiated adenocarcinoma arising from mature cystic teratoma of the mediastinum (teratoma with malignant transformation). Report of a surgical case. Am J Clin Pathol. 101:531–4.
1750. Morinaga S, Sato Y, Shimosato Y, et al. (1987). Multiple thymic squamous cell carcinomas associated with mixed type thymoma. Am J Surg Pathol. 11:982–8.
1751. Morita S, Goto A, Sakatani T, et al. (2011). Multicystic mesothelioma of the pericardium. Pathol Int. 61:319–21.
1752. Morita S, Yoshida A, Goto A, et al. (2013). High-grade lung adenocarcinoma with fetal lung-like morphology: clinicopathologic, immunohistochemical, and molecular analyses of 17 cases. Am J Surg Pathol. 37:924–32.
1753. Moritani S, Ichihara S, Mukai K, et al. (2008). Sarcomatoid carcinoma of the thymus arising in metaplastic thymoma. Histopathology. 52:409–11.
1754. Morley JE, Jacobson RJ, Melamed J, et al. (1976). Choriocarcinoma as a cause of thyrotoxicosis. Am J Med. 60:1036–40.
1755. Moro D, Brichon PY, Brambilla E, et al. (1994). Basaloid bronchial carcinoma. A histologic group with a poor prognosis. Cancer. 73:2734–9.
1756. Moro-Sibilot D, Jeanmart M, Lantuejoul S, et al. (2002). Cigarette smoking, preinvasive bronchial lesions, and autofluorescence bronchoscopy. Chest. 122:1902–8.
1757. Moro-Sibilot D, Lantuejoul S, Diab S, et al. (2008). Lung carcinomas with a basaloid pattern: a study of 90 cases focusing on their poor prognosis. Eur Respir J. 31:854–9.
1758. Morris SW, Kirstein MN, Valentine MB, et al. (1994). Fusion of a kinase gene, ALK, to a nucleolar protein gene, NPM, in non-Hodgkin's lymphoma. Science. 263:1281–4.
1759. Motoi N, Szoke J, Riely GJ, et al. (2008). Lung adenocarcinoma: modification of the 2004 WHO mixed subtype to include the major histologic subtype suggests correlations between papillary and micropapillary adenocarcinoma subtypes, EGFR mutations and gene expression analysis. Am J Surg Pathol. 32:810–27.
1760. Motwani M, Kidambi A, Herzog BA, et al. (2013). MR imaging of cardiac tumors and masses: a review of methods and clinical applications. Radiology. 268:26–43.
1761. Motzer RJ, Amsterdam A, Prieto V, et al. (1998). Teratoma with malignant transformation: diverse malignant histologies arising in men with germ cell tumors. J Urol. 159:133–8.
1762. Mueller CM, Hilbert JE, Martens W, et al. (2009). Hypothesis: neoplasms in myotonic dystrophy. Cancer Causes Control. 20:2009–20.
1763. Mukhopadhyay S, Katzenstein AL (2010). Biopsy findings in acute pulmonary histoplasmosis: unusual histologic features in 4 cases mimicking lymphomatoid granulomatosis. Am J Surg Pathol. 34:541–6.
1764. Mukhopadhyay S, Katzenstein AL (2011). Subclassification of non-small cell lung carcinomas lacking morphologic differentiation on biopsy specimens: Utility of an immunohistochemical panel containing TTF-1, napsin A, p63, and CK5/6. Am J Surg Pathol. 35:15–25.
1765. Mukohara T, Civiello G, Davis IJ, et al. (2005). Inhibition of the met receptor in mesothelioma. Clin Cancer Res. 11:8122–30.
1766. Mulamalla K, Truskinovsky AM, Dudek AZ (2007). Pulmonary blastoma with renal metastasis responds to sorafenib. J Thorac Oncol. 2:344–7.
1767. Muller KM, Muller G (1983). The ultrastructure of preneoplastic changes in the bronchial mucosa. Curr Top Pathol. 73:233–63.
1768. Muller-Hermelink HK, Marx A (1999). Pathological aspects of malignant and benign thymic disorders. Ann Med. 31 Suppl 2:5–14.
1769. Muller-Hermelink HK, Strobel PH, Zettl A, et al. (2004). Combined thymic epithelial tumours. In: WHO Classification of Tumours. Pathology and Genetics of Tumours of the Lung, Pleura, Thymus and Heart. Travis WD, Brambilla E, Muller-Hermelink HK, Harris CC, eds. 3rd ed. Lyon: IARC. pp 196–197.
1770. Mulligan S, Hu P, Murphy A, et al. (2011). Variations in MALT1 Gene Disruptions Detected by FISH in 109 MALT Lymphomas Occurring in Different Primary Sites. J Assoc Genet Technol. 37:76–9.
1771. Munoz G, Felipo F, Marquina I, et al. (2011). Epithelial-myoepithelial tumour of the lung: a case report referring to its molecular histogenesis. Diagn Pathol. 6:71.
1772. Murakami H, Mizuno T, Taniguchi T, et al. (2011). LATS2 is a tumor suppressor gene of malignant mesothelioma. Cancer Res. 71:873–83.
1773. Murga Penas EM, Callet-Bauchu E, Ye H, et al. (2007). The translocations t(6;18;11)(q24;q21;q21) and t(11;14;18)(q21;q32;q21) lead to a fusion of the API2 and MALT1 genes and occur in MALT lymphomas. Haematologica. 92:405–9.
1774. Murinello A, Mendonca P, Abreu A, et al. (2007). Cardiac angiosarcoma--a review. Rev Port Cardiol. 26:577–84.
1775. Murphy MC, Sweeney MS, Putnam JB Jr, et al. (1990). Surgical treatment of cardiac tumors: a 25-year experience. Ann Thorac Surg. 49:612–7.
1776. Murphy MN, Glennon PG, Diocee MS, et al. (1986). Nonsecretory parathyroid carcinoma of the mediastinum. Light microscopic, immunocytochemical, and ultrastructural features of a case, and review of the literature. Cancer. 58:2468–76.
1777. Mussot S, Ghigna MR, Mercier O, et al. (2013). Retrospective institutional study of 31 patients treated for pulmonary artery sarcoma. Eur J Cardiothorac Surg. 43:787–93.
1778. Musti M, Kettunen E, Dragonieri S, et al. (2006). Cytogenetic and molecular genetic changes in malignant mesothelioma. Cancer Genet Cytogenet. 170:9–15.
1779. Mut Pons R, Muro V, Sanguesa Nebot C, et al. (2008). [Pleuropulmonary blastoma in children: imaging findings and clinical patterns]. Radiologia. 50:489–94.
1780. Myers JL, Kurtin PJ, Katzenstein AL, et al. (1995). Lymphomatoid granulomatosis. Evidence of immunophenotypic diversity and relationship to Epstein-Barr virus infection. Am J Surg Pathol. 19:1300–12.
1781. Myers PO, Kritikos N, Bongiovanni M, et al. (2007). Primary intrapulmonary thymoma: a systematic review. Eur J Surg Oncol. 33:1137–41.
1782. Naalsund A, Rostad H, Strom EH, et al. (2011). Carcinoid lung tumors--incidence, treatment and outcomes: a population-based study. Eur J Cardiothorac Surg. 39:565–9.
1783. Nador RG, Cesarman E, Chadburn A, et al. (1996). Primary effusion lymphoma: a distinct clinicopathologic entity associated with the Kaposi's sarcoma-associated herpes virus. Blood. 88:645–56.

1784. Nador RG, Milligan LL, Flore O, et al. (2001). Expression of Kaposi's sarcoma-associated herpesvirus G protein-coupled receptor monocistronic and bicistronic transcripts in primary effusion lymphomas. Virology. 287:62–70.

1785. Naffaa LN, Donnelly LF (2005). Imaging findings in pleuropulmonary blastoma. Pediatr Radiol. 35:387–91.

1786. Nagamoto N, Saito Y, Imai T, et al. (1986). Roentgenographically occult bronchogenic squamous cell carcinoma: location in the bronchi, depth of invasion and length of axial involvement of the bronchus. Tohoku J Exp Med. 148:241–56.

1787. Nagata Y, Ohno K, Utsumi T, et al. (2006). Large cell neuroendocrine thymic carcinoma coexisting within large WHO type AB thymoma. Jpn J Thorac Cardiovasc Surg. 54:256–9.

1788. Nagel PD, Feld FM, Weissinger SE, et al. (2014). Absence of BRAF and KRAS hotspot mutations in primary mediastinal B-cell lymphoma. Leuk Lymphoma. 55:2389–90.

1789. Naidich DP, Bankier AA, MacMahon H, et al. (2013). Recommendations for the management of subsolid pulmonary nodules detected at CT: a statement from the Fleischner Society. Radiology. 266:304–17.

1790. Naithani R, Ngan BY, Roifman C, et al. (2012). Thymic mucosa-associated lymphoid tissue lymphoma in an adolescent girl. J Pediatr Hematol Oncol. 34:552–5.

1791. Naka N, Tomita Y, Nakanishi H, et al. (1997). Mutations of p53 tumor-suppressor gene in angiosarcoma. Int J Cancer. 71:952–5.

1792. Nakachi I, Rice JL, Coldren CD, et al. (2014). Application of SNP microarrays to the genome-wide analysis of chromosomal instability in premalignant airway lesions. Cancer Prev Res (Phila). 7:255–65.

1793. Nakagawa K, Matsuno Y, Kunitoh H, et al. (2005). Immunohistochemical KIT (CD117) expression in thymic epithelial tumors. Chest. 128:140–4.

1794. Nakagawa K, Yasumitu T, Fukuhara K, et al. (2003). Poor prognosis after lung resection for patients with adenosquamous carcinoma of the lung. Ann Thorac Surg. 75:1740–4.

1795. Nakagawa M, Hara M, Shibamoto Y, et al. (2008). CT findings of bronchial glandular papilloma. J Thorac Imaging. 23:210–2.

1796. Nakamura S, Fukui T, Taniguchi T, et al. (2013). Prognostic impact of tumor size eliminating the ground glass opacity component: modified clinical T descriptors of the tumor, node, metastasis classification of lung cancer. J Thorac Oncol. 8:1551–7.

1797. Nakamura S, Tateyama H, Taniguchi T, et al. (2012). Multilocular thymic cyst associated with thymoma: a clinicopathologic study of 20 cases with an emphasis on the pathogenesis of cyst formation. Am J Surg Pathol. 36:1857–64.

1798. Nakanishi K (1990). Alveolar epithelial hyperplasia and adenocarcinoma of the lung. Arch Pathol Lab Med. 114:363–8.

1799. Nakanishi K, Kawai T, Kumaki F, et al. (2002). Expression of human telomerase RNA component and telomerase reverse transcriptase mRNA in atypical adenomatous hyperplasia of the lung. Hum Pathol. 33:697–702.

1800. Nakano T, Endo S, Tsubochi H, et al. (2010). Thymic clear cell carcinoma. Gen Thorac Cardiovasc Surg. 58:98–100.

1801. Nakano T, Yokose T, Hasegawa C, et al. (2011). Papillary adenoma of the lung with a peculiar raw macroscopic feature. Pathol Int. 61:475–80.

1802. Nakaoku T, Tsuta K, Ichikawa H, et al. (2014). Druggable oncogene fusions in invasive mucinous lung adenocarcinoma. Clin Cancer Res. 20:3087–93.

1803. Nakas A, Martin-Ucar AE, Edwards JG, et al. (2008). Localised malignant pleural mesothelioma: a separate clinical entity requiring aggressive local surgery. Eur J Cardiothorac Surg. 33:303–6.

1804. Nakatani Y, Dickersin GR, Mark EJ (1990). Pulmonary endodermal tumor resembling fetal lung: a clinicopathologic study of five cases with immunohistochemical and ultrastructural characterization. Hum Pathol. 21:1097–107.

1805. Nakatani Y, Hiroshima H, Mark EJ (2013). Sarcomatoid carcinoma and variants. In: Hasleton P, Flieder DB, eds. Spencer's Pathology of the Lung. 6th ed. Cambridge: Cambridge University Press; pp. 1186–223.

1806. Nakatani Y, Kitamura H, Inayama Y, et al. (1998). Pulmonary adenocarcinomas of the fetal lung type: a clinicopathologic study indicating differences in histology, epidemiology, and natural history of low-grade and high-grade forms. Am J Surg Pathol. 22:399–411.

1807. Nakatani Y, Masudo K, Miyagi Y, et al. (2002). Aberrant nuclear localization and gene mutation of beta-catenin in low-grade adenocarcinoma of fetal lung type: up-regulation of the Wnt signaling pathway may be a common denominator for the development of tumors that form morules. Mod Pathol. 15:617–24.

1808. Nakatani Y, Masudo K, Nozawa A, et al. (2004). Biotin-rich, optically clear nuclei express estrogen receptor-beta: tumors with morules may develop under the influence of estrogen and aberrant beta-catenin expression. Hum Pathol. 35:869–74.

1809. Nakatani Y, Miyagi Y, Takemura T, et al. (2004). Aberrant nuclear/cytoplasmic localization and gene mutation of beta-catenin in classic pulmonary blastoma: beta-catenin immunostaining is useful for distinguishing between classic pulmonary blastoma and a blastomatoid variant of carcinosarcoma. Am J Surg Pathol. 28:921–7.

1810. Nakatsuka S, Yao M, Hoshida Y, et al. (2002). Pyothorax-associated lymphoma: a review of 106 cases. J Clin Oncol. 20:4255–60.

1811. Nakayama H, Noguchi M, Tsuchiya R, et al. (1990). Clonal growth of atypical adenomatous hyperplasia of the lung: cytofluorometric analysis of nuclear DNA content. Mod Pathol. 3:314–20.

1812. Nakayama-Ichiyama S, Yokote T, Kobayashi K, et al. (2011). Primary effusion lymphoma of T-cell origin with t(7;8)(q32;q13) in an HIV-negative patient with HCV-related liver cirrhosis and hepatocellular carcinoma positive for HHV6 and HHV8. Ann Hematol. 90:1229–31.

1813. Nakazato Y, Maeshima AM, Ishikawa Y, et al. (2013). Interobserver agreement in the nuclear grading of primary pulmonary adenocarcinoma. J Thorac Oncol. 8:736–43.

1814. Nam JE, Ryu YH, Cho SH, et al. (2002). Air-trapping zone surrounding sclerosing hemangioma of the lung. J Comput Assist Tomogr. 26:358–61.

1815. Naoki K, Chen TH, Richards WG, et al. (2002). Missense mutations of the BRAF gene in human lung adenocarcinoma. Cancer Res. 62:7001–3.

1816. Nappi O, Glasner SD, Swanson PE, et al. (1994). Biphasic and monophasic sarcomatoid carcinomas of the lung. A reappraisal of 'carcinosarcomas' and 'spindle-cell carcinomas'. Am J Clin Pathol. 102:331–40.

1817. Nascimento AF, Ruiz R, Hornick JL, et al. (2002). Calcifying fibrous 'pseudotumor': clinicopathologic study of 15 cases and analysis of its relationship to inflammatory myofibroblastic tumor. Int J Surg Pathol. 10:189–96.

1818. Nasgashio R, Sato Y, Matsumoto T, et al. (2011). The balance between the expressions of hASH1 and HES1 differs between large cell neuroendocrine carcinoma and small cell carcinoma of the lung. Lung Cancer. 74:405–10.

1819. Nassar AA, Jaroszewski DE, Helmers RA, et al. (2011). Diffuse idiopathic pulmonary neuroendocrine cell hyperplasia: a systematic overview. Am J Respir Crit Care Med. 184:8–16.

1820. Nathaniels EK, Nathaniels AM, Wang CA (1970). Mediastinal parathyroid tumors: a clinical and pathological study of 84 cases. Ann Surg. 171:165–70.

1821. Nayak HK, Vangipuram DR, Sonika U et al. (2011). Mediastinal mass-a rare presentation of desmoplastic small round cell tumour. BMJ Case Rep 2011:

1822. Negron-Soto JM, Cascade PN (1995). Squamous cell carcinoma of the thymus with paraneoplastic hypercalcemia. Clin Imaging. 19:122–4.

1823. Neiman RS, Orazi A (1999). Mediastinal non-seminomatous germ cell tumours: their association with non-germ cell malignancies. Pathol Res Pract. 195:589–94.

1824. Nelson BA, Lee EY, French CA, et al. (2010). BRD4-NUT carcinoma of the mediastinum in a pediatric patient: multidetector computed tomography imaging findings. J Thorac Imaging. 25:W93–6.

1825. Nemolato S, Dettori T, Caria P, et al. (2009). Would a morphomolecular approach help in defining pseudosarcomatous myofibroblastic proliferations? A study of a heart polypoid lesion. J Clin Pathol. 62:377–9.

1826. Nemoto H, Tate G, Kishimoto K, et al. (2012). Heterozygous loss of NF2 is an early molecular alteration in well-differentiated papillary mesothelioma of the peritoneum. Cancer Genet. 205:594–8.

1827. Neragi-Miandoab S, Kim J, Vlahakes GJ (2007). Malignant tumours of the heart: a review of tumour type, diagnosis and therapy. Clin Oncol (R Coll Radiol). 19:748–56.

1828. Neuville A, Collin F, Bruneval P, et al. (2014). Intimal sarcoma is the most frequent primary cardiac sarcoma: clinicopathologic and molecular retrospective analysis of 100 primary cardiac sarcomas. Am J Surg Pathol. 38:461–9.

1829. Ng TL, Gown AM, Barry TS, et al. (2005). Nuclear beta-catenin in mesenchymal tumors. Mod Pathol. 18:68–74.

1830. Ngaage DL, Mullany CJ, Daly RC, et al. (2005). Surgical treatment of cardiac papillary fibroelastoma: a single center experience with eighty-eight patients. Ann Thorac Surg. 80:1712–8.

1831. Nguyen CV, Suster S, Moran CA (2009). Pulmonary epithelial-myoepithelial carcinoma: a clinicopathologic and immunohistochemical study of 5 cases. Hum Pathol. 40:366–73.

1832. Ni YB, Tsang JY, Shao MM, et al. (2014). TTF-1 expression in breast carcinoma: an unusual but real phenomenon. Histopathology. 64:504–11.

1833. Nichols CR (1991). Mediastinal germ cell tumors. Clinical features and biologic correlates. Chest. 99:472–9.

1834. Nichols CR, Heerema NA, Palmer C, et al. (1987). Klinefelter's syndrome associated with mediastinal germ cell neoplasms. J Clin Oncol. 5:1290–4.

1835. Nichols CR, Hoffman R, Einhorn LH, et al. (1985). Hematologic malignancies associated with primary mediastinal germ-cell tumors. Ann Intern Med. 102:603–9.

1836. Nichols CR, Hoffman R, Glant MD, et al. (1986). Malignant disorders of megakaryocytes associated with primary mediastinal germ cell tumors. Prog Clin Biol Res. 215:347–53.

1837. Nichols CR, Roth BJ, Heerema N, et al. (1990). Hematologic neoplasia associated with primary mediastinal germ-cell tumors. N Engl J Med. 322:1425–9.

1838. Nichols CR, Saxman S, Williams SD, et al. (1990). Primary mediastinal nonseminomatous germ cell tumors. A modern single institution experience. Cancer. 65:1641–6.

1839. Nicholson AG, Anderson E, Saha S et al. (2008). Progressive dyspnoea, pleural effusions and lytic bone lesions. Thorax. 63: 492, 554

1840. Nicholson AG, Baandrup U, Florio R, et al. (1999). Malignant myxoid endobronchial tumour: a report of two cases with a unique histological pattern. Histopathology. 35:313–8.

1840A. Nicholson AG, Detterbeck F, Marino M, et al. (2014). The IASLC/ITMIG Thymic Epithelial Tumors Staging Project: Proposals for the T component for the Forthcoming (8th) Edition of the TNM Classification of Malignant Tumors. J Thorac Oncol. 9(9 Suppl 2):S73–80.

1841. Nicholson AG, Gonzalez D, Shah P, et al. (2010). Refining the diagnosis and EGFR status of non-small cell lung carcinoma in biopsy and cytologic material, using a panel of mucin staining, TTF-1, cytokeratin 5/6, and P63, and EGFR mutation analysis. J Thorac Oncol. 5:436–41.

1842. Nicholson AG, Magkou C, Snead D, et al. (2002). Unusual sclerosing haemangiomas and sclerosing haemangioma-like lesions, and the value of TTF-1 in making the diagnosis. Histopathology. 41:404–13.

1843. Nicholson AG, Perry LJ, Cury PM, et al. (2001). Reproducibility of the WHO/IASLC grading system for pre-invasive squamous lesions of the bronchus: a study of inter-observer and intra-observer variation. Histopathology. 38:202–8.

1844. Nicholson AG, Wotherspoon AC, Diss TC, et al. (1995). Pulmonary B-cell non-Hodgkin's lymphomas. The value of immunohistochemistry and gene analysis in diagnosis. Histopathology. 26:395–403.

1845. Nicholson AG, Wotherspoon AC, Diss TC, et al. (1995). Reactive pulmonary lymphoid disorders. Histopathology. 26:405–12.

1846. Nicholson AG, Wotherspoon AC, Diss TC, et al. (1996). Lymphomatoid granulomatosis: evidence that some cases represent Epstein-Barr virus-associated B-cell lymphoma. Histopathology. 29:317–24.

1847. Nicholson AG, Wotherspoon AC, Jones AL, et al. (1996). Pulmonary B-cell non-Hodgkin's lymphoma associated with autoimmune disorders: a clinicopathological review of six cases. Eur Respir J. 9:2022–5.

1848. Nicholson SA, Beasley MB, Brambilla E, et al. (2002). Small cell lung carcinoma (SCLC): a clinicopathologic study of 100 cases with surgical specimens. Am J Surg Pathol. 26:1184–97.

1849. Nicholson SA, Ryan MR (2000). A review of cytologic findings in neuroendocrine carcinomas including carcinoid tumors with histologic correlation. Cancer. 90:148–61.

1850. Nicol KK, Geisinger KR (2000). The cytomorphology of pleuropulmonary blastoma. Arch Pathol Lab Med. 124:416–8.

1851. Nicolini A, Perazzo A, Lanata S (2011). Desmoplastic malignant mesothelioma of the pericardium: Description of a case and review of the literature. Lung India. 28:219–21.

1852. Niederkohr RD, Cameron MJ, French CA (2011). FDG PET/CT imaging of NUT midline carcinoma. Clin Nucl Med. 36:e124–6.

1853. Niehans GA, Manivel JC, Copland GT, et al. (1988). Immunohistochemistry of germ cell and trophoblastic neoplasms. Cancer. 62:1113–23.

1854. Niehues T, Harms D, Jurgens H, et al. (1996). Treatment of pediatric malignant thymoma: long-term remission in a 14-year-old boy with EBV-associated thymic carcinoma by aggressive, combined modality treatment. Med Pediatr Oncol. 26:419–24.

1855. Niho S, Yokose T, Suzuki K, et al. (1999). Monoclonality of atypical adenomatous hyperplasia of the lung. Am J Pathol. 154:249–54.

1856. Ninomiya H, Miyoshi T, Shirakusa T, et al. (2006). Postradiation sarcoma of the chest wall: report of two cases. Surg Today. 36:1101–4.

1857. Nishimura M, Kodama T, Nishiyama H, et al. (1997). A case of sarcomatoid carcinoma of the thymus. Pathol Int. 47:260–3.

1858. Nishiu M, Tomita Y, Nakatsuka S, et al. (2004). Distinct pattern of gene expression in pyothorax-associated lymphoma (PAL), a lymphoma developing in long-standing inflammation. Cancer Sci. 95:828–34.

1859. Nitadori J, Bograd AJ, Kadota K, et al. (2013). Impact of micropapillary histologic subtype in selecting limited resection vs lobectomy for lung adenocarcinoma of 2cm or smaller. J Natl Cancer Inst. 105:1212–20.
1860. Nitadori J, Ishii G, Tsuta K, et al. (2006). Immunohistochemical differential diagnosis between large cell neuroendocrine carcinoma and small cell carcinoma by tissue microarray analysis with a large antibody panel. Am J Clin Pathol. 125:682–92.
1861. Nixon DW, Shlaer SM (1981). Fulminant lung metastases from cancer of the breast. Med Pediatr Oncol. 9:381–5.
1862. Noda T, Higashiyama M, Oda K, et al. (2006). Mucoepidermoid carcinoma of the thymus treated by multimodality therapy: a case report. Ann Thorac Cardiovasc Surg. 12:273–8.
1863. Nogales FF, Quinonez E, Lopez-Marin L, et al. (2014). A diagnostic immunohistochemical panel for yolk sac (primitive endodermal) tumours based on an immunohistochemical comparison with the human yolk sac. Histopathology. 65:51–9.
1864. Noguchi M, Kodama T, Shimosato Y, et al. (1986). Papillary adenoma of type 2 pneumocytes. Am J Surg Pathol. 10:134–9.
1865. Noguchi M, Morikawa A, Kawasaki M, et al. (1995). Small adenocarcinoma of the lung. Histologic characteristics and prognosis. Cancer. 75:2844–52.
1866. Noh TW, Kim SH, Lim BJ, et al. (2001). Thymoma with pseudosarcomatous stroma. Yonsei Med J. 42:571–5.
1867. Nolte I, Gothe R (1982). [Plasma lysozyme activity in tick paralysis of sheep caused by Rhipicephalus evertsi evertsi]. Berl Munch Tierarztl Wochenschr. 95:143–5.
1868. Nomori H, Kobayashi K, Ishihara T, et al. (1990). A case of multiple thymoma: the possibility of intra-thymic metastasis. Jpn J Clin Oncol. 20:209–11.
1869. Nonaka D (2009). Differential expression of SOX2 and SOX17 in testicular germ cell tumors. Am J Clin Pathol. 131:731–6.
1870. Nonaka D (2012). A study of DeltaNp63 expression in lung non-small cell carcinomas. Am J Surg Pathol. 36:895–9.
1871. Nonaka D, Henley JD, Chiriboga L, et al. (2007). Diagnostic utility of thymic epithelial markers CD205 (DEC205) and Foxn1 in thymic epithelial neoplasms. Am J Surg Pathol. 31:1038–44.
1872. Nonaka D, Klimstra D, Rosai J (2004). Thymic mucoepidermoid carcinomas: a clinicopathologic study of 10 cases and review of the literature. Am J Surg Pathol. 28:1526–31.
1873. Nonaka D, Rodriguez J, Rollo JL, et al. (2005). Undifferentiated large cell carcinoma of the thymus associated with Castleman disease-like reaction: a distinctive type of thymic neoplasm characterized by an indolent behavior. Am J Surg Pathol. 29:490–5.
1874. Nonaka D, Rosai J (2012). Is there a spectrum of cytologic atypia in type A thymomas analogous to that seen in type B thymomas? A pilot study of 13 cases. Am J Surg Pathol. 36:889–94.
1875. Nonami Y, Moriki T (2004). Synchronous independent bifocal orthotopic thymomas. A case report. J Cardiovasc Surg (Torino). 45:585–7.
1876. Norkowski E, Ghigna MR, Lacroix L, et al. (2013). Small-cell carcinoma in the setting of pulmonary adenocarcinoma: new insights in the era of molecular pathology. J Thorac Oncol. 8:1265–71.
1877. Nosotti M, Mendogni P, Rosso L, et al. (2012). Alveolar adenoma of the lung: unusual diagnosis of a lesion positive on PET scan. A case report. J Cardiothorac Surg. 7:1.
1878. Notohara K, Hsueh CL, Awai M (1990). Glial fibrillary acidic protein immunoreactivity of chondrocytes in immature and mature teratomas. Acta Pathol Jpn. 40:335–42.
1879. Noussios G, Anagnostis P, Natsis K (2012). Ectopic parathyroid glands and their anatomical, clinical and surgical implications. Exp Clin Endocrinol Diabetes. 120:604–10.
1880. Novak L, Castro CY, Listinsky CM (2003). Multiple Langerhans cell nodules in an incidental thymectomy. Arch Pathol Lab Med. 127:218–20.
1881. Novak R, Dasu S, Agamanolis D, et al. (1997). Trisomy 8 is a characteristic finding in pleuropulmonary blastoma. Pediatr Pathol Lab Med. 17:99–103.
1881A. Oechsle K, Bokemeyer C, Kollmannsberger C, et al. (2012). Bone metastases in germ cell tumor patients. J Cancer Res Clin Oncol. 138:947–52.
1882. O'Mahony D, Debnath I, Janik J, et al. (2008). Cardiac involvement with human T-cell lymphotrophic virus type-1-associated adult T-cell leukemia/lymphoma: The NIH experience. Leuk Lymphoma. 49:439–46.
1883. O'Malley DP, Zuckerberg L, Smith LB, et al. (2014). The genetics of interdigitating dendritic cell sarcoma share some changes with Langerhans cell histiocytosis in select cases. Ann Diagn Pathol. 18:18–20.
1884. O'Neill ID (2009). Gefitinib as targeted therapy for mucoepidermoid carcinoma of the lung: possible significance of CRTC1-MAML2 oncogene. Lung Cancer. 64:129–30.
1885. Odim J, Reehal V, Laks H, et al. (2003). Surgical pathology of cardiac tumors. Two decades at an urban institution. Cardiovasc Pathol. 12:267–70.
1886. Ogawa F, Amano H, Iyoda A, et al. (2009). Thymic neuroblastoma with the syndrome of inappropriate secretion of antidiuretic hormone. Interact Cardiovasc Thorac Surg. 9:903–5.
1887. Ogawa F, Iyoda A, Amano H, et al. (2010). Thymic large cell neuroendocrine carcinoma: report of a resected case - a case report. J Cardiothorac Surg. 5:115.
1888. Ogawa K, Toita T, Uno T, et al. (2002). Treatment and prognosis of thymic carcinoma: a retrospective analysis of 40 cases. Cancer. 94:3115–9.
1889. Ogusa E, Tomita N, Ishii Y, et al. (2013). Clinical manifestations of primary pulmonary extranodal marginal zone lymphoma of mucosa-associated lymphoid tissue in Japanese population. Hematol Oncol. 31:18–21.
1890. Oh SY, Kim WS, Kim JS, et al. (2010). Pulmonary marginal zone B-cell lymphoma of MALT type--what is a prognostic factor and which is the optimal treatment, operation, or chemotherapy?: Consortium for Improving Survival of Lymphoma (CISL) study. Ann Hematol. 89:563–8.
1891. Oh SY, Kim WS, Kim JS, et al. (2010). Multiple mucosa-associated lymphoid tissue organs involving marginal zone B cell lymphoma: organ-specific relationships and the prognostic factors. Consortium for improving survival of lymphoma study. Int J Hematol. 92:510–7.
1892. Ohchi T, Tanaka H, Shibuya Y, et al. (1998). Thymic carcinoid with mucinous stroma: a case report. Respir Med. 92:880–2.
1893. Ohori NP, Santa Maria EL (2004). Cytopathologic diagnosis of bronchioloalveolar carcinoma: does it correlate with the 1999 World Health Organization definition? Am J Clin Pathol. 122:44–50.
1894. Ohtsuka M, Satoh H, Inoue M, et al. (2000). Disseminated metastasis of neuroblastomatous component in immature mediastinal teratoma: a case report. Anticancer Res. 20:527–30.
1895. Okada S, Ohshima K, Mori M (1994). The Cushing syndrome induced by atrial natriuretic peptide-producing thymic carcinoid. Ann Intern Med. 121:75–6.
1896. Okamoto K, Kato S, Katsuki S, et al. (2001). Malignant fibrous histiocytoma of the heart: case report and review of 46 cases in the literature. Intern Med. 40:1222–6.
1897. Okamoto S, Hisaoka M, Daa T, et al. (2004). Primary pulmonary synovial sarcoma: a clinicopathologic, immunohistochemical, and molecular study of 11 cases. Hum Pathol. 35:850–6.
1898. Okamoto T, Miyazaki Y, Sakakibara Y, et al. (2011). Successful diagnosis of a combined thymic epithelial tumor by endobronchial ultrasound-guided transbronchial needle aspiration. J Med Dent Sci. 58:123–6.
1899. Okereke IC, Kesler KA, Freeman RK, et al. (2012). Thymic carcinoma: outcomes after surgical resection. Ann Thorac Surg. 93:1668–72.
1900. Okuda M, Huang CL, Haba R, et al. (2009). Clear cell carcinoma originating from ectopic thymus. Gen Thorac Cardiovasc Surg. 57:269–71.
1901. Okudela K, Nakamura N, Sano J, et al. (2001). Thymic carcinosarcoma consisting of squamous cell carcinomatous and embryonal rhabdomyosarcomatous components. Report of a case and review of the literature. Pathol Res Pract. 197:205–10.
1902. Okudela K, Yazawa T, Tajiri M, et al. (2010). A case of epithelial-myoepithelial carcinoma of the bronchus - a review of reported cases and a comparison with other salivary gland-type carcinomas of the bronchus. Pathol Res Pract. 206:121–9.
1903. Okumura M, Miyoshi S, Fujii Y, et al. (2001). Clinical and functional significance of WHO classification on human thymic epithelial neoplasms: a study of 146 consecutive tumors. Am J Surg Pathol. 25:103–10.
1904. Okumura M, Ohta M, Miyoshi S, et al. (2002). Oncological significance of WHO histological thymoma classification. A clinical study based on 286 patients. Jpn J Thorac Cardiovasc Surg. 50:189–94.
1905. Okumura M, Ohta M, Tateyama H, et al. (2002). The World Health Organization histologic classification system reflects the oncologic behavior of thymoma: a clinical study of 273 patients. Cancer. 94:624–32.
1906. Oliveira AM, Tazelaar HD, Myers JL, et al. (2001). Thyroid transcription factor-1 distinguishes metastatic pulmonary from well-differentiated neuroendocrine tumors of other sites. Am J Surg Pathol. 25:815–9.
1907. Oliveira R, Branco L, Galrinho A, et al. (2010). Cardiac myxoma: a 13-year experience in echocardiographic diagnosis. Rev Port Cardiol. 29:1087–100.
1908. Omezzine N, Khouatra C, Larive S, et al. (2002). Rhabdomyosarcoma arising in mediastinal teratoma in an adult man: a case report. Ann Oncol. 13:323–6.
1909. Onozato ML, Kovach AE, Yeap BY, et al. (2013). Tumor islands in resected early-stage lung adenocarcinomas are associated with unique clinicopathologic and molecular characteristics and worse prognosis. Am J Surg Pathol. 37:287–94.
1910. Onuki N, Wistuba II, Travis WD, et al. (1999). Genetic changes in the spectrum of neuroendocrine lung tumors. Cancer. 85:600–7.
1911. Onuki T, Iguchi K, Inagaki M, et al. (2009). [Lipofibroadenoma of the thymus]. Kyobu Geka. 62:395–8.
1912. Oosterhuis JW, Looijenga LH (2005). Testicular germ-cell tumours in a broader perspective. Nat Rev Cancer. 5:210–22.
1913. Oosterhuis JW, Stoop H, Honecker F, et al. (2007). Why human extragonadal germ cell tumours occur in the midline of the body: old concepts, new perspectives. Int J Androl. 30:256–63.
1914. Opitz I, Soltermann A, Abaecherli M, et al. (2008). PTEN expression is a strong predictor of survival in mesothelioma patients. Eur J Cardiothorac Surg. 33:502–6.
1915. Oprescu N, McCormack FX, Byrnes S, et al. (2013). Clinical predictors of mortality and cause of death in lymphangioleiomyomatosis: a population-based registry. Lung. 191:35–42.
1916. Orazi A, Neiman RS, Ulbright TM, et al. (1993). Hematopoietic precursor cells within the yolk sac tumor component are the source of secondary hematopoietic malignancies in patients with mediastinal germ cell tumors. Cancer. 71:3873–81.
1917. Orazi C, Inserra A, Schingo PM, et al. (2007). Pleuropulmonary blastoma, a distinctive neoplasm of childhood: report of three cases. Pediatr Radiol. 37:337–44.
1918. Ordonez NG (2000). Value of thyroid transcription factor-1 immunostaining in distinguishing small cell lung carcinomas from other small cell carcinomas. Am J Surg Pathol. 24:1217–23.
1919. Ordonez NG (2006). The diagnostic utility of immunohistochemistry in distinguishing between epithelioid mesotheliomas and squamous carcinomas of the lung: a comparative study. Mod Pathol. 19:417–28.
1920. Ordonez NG (2012). A word of caution regarding napsin A expression in squamous cell carcinomas of the lung. Am J Surg Pathol. 36:396–401.
1921. Ordonez NG (2012). Deciduoid mesothelioma: report of 21 cases with review of the literature. Mod Pathol. 25:1481–95.
1922. Ordonez NG (2012). Mesotheliomas with small cell features: report of eight cases. Mod Pathol. 25:689–98.
1923. Ordonez NG (2012). Pleomorphic mesothelioma: report of 10 cases. Mod Pathol. 25:1011–22.
1924. Ordonez NG (2012). Value of PAX 8 immunostaining in tumor diagnosis: a review and update. Adv Anat Pathol. 19:140–51.
1925. Ordonez NG (2013). Application of immunohistochemistry in the diagnosis of epithelioid mesothelioma: a review and update. Hum Pathol. 44:1–19.
1926. Ordonez NG (2013). Value of claudin-4 immunostaining in the diagnosis of mesothelioma. Am J Clin Pathol. 139:611–9.
1927. Ordonez NG (2013). Value of PAX8, PAX2, claudin-4, and h-caldesmon immunostaining in distinguishing peritoneal epithelioid mesotheliomas from serous carcinomas. Mod Pathol. 26:553–62.
1928. Ordonez NG (2013). Value of PAX8, PAX2, napsin A, carbonic anhydrase IX, and claudin-4 immunostaining in distinguishing pleural epithelioid mesothelioma from metastatic renal cell carcinoma. Mod Pathol. 26:1132–43.
1929. Ordonez NG, Sahin AA (2014). Diagnostic utility of immunohistochemistry in distinguishing between epithelioid pleural mesotheliomas and breast carcinomas: a comparative study. Hum Pathol. 45:1529–40.
1930. Orlandi A, Ciucci A, Ferlosio A, et al. (2006). Cardiac myxoma cells exhibit embryonic endocardial stem cell features. J Pathol. 209:231–9.
1931. Orlandi A, Ciucci A, Ferlosio A, et al. (2005). Increased expression and activity of matrix metalloproteinases characterize embolic cardiac myxomas. Am J Pathol. 166:1619–28.
1932. Orlandi A, Ferlosio A, Roselli M, et al. (2010). Cardiac sarcomas: an update. J Thorac Oncol. 5:1483–9.
1933. Orsmond GS, Knight L, Dehner LP, et al. (1976). Alveolar rhabdomyosarcoma involving the heart. An echocardiographic, angiographic and pathologic study. Circulation. 54:837–43.
1934. Osborn M, Mandys V, Beddow E, et al. (2003). Cystic fibrohistiocytic tumours presenting in the lung: primary or metastatic disease? Histopathology. 43:556–62.
1935. Osborne JK, Larsen JE, Shields MD, et al. (2013). NeuroD1 regulates survival and migration of neuroendocrine lung carcinomas via signaling molecules TrkB and NCAM. Proc Natl Acad Sci USA. 110:6524–9.
1936. Oschlies I, Burkhardt B,

Chassagne-Clement C, et al. (2011). Diagnosis and immunophenotype of 188 pediatric lymphoblastic lymphomas treated within a randomized prospective trial: experiences and preliminary recommendations from the European childhood lymphoma pathology panel. Am J Surg Pathol. 35:836–44.
1937. Oshikiri T, Morikawa T, Jinushi E, et al. (2001). Five cases of the lymphangioma of the mediastinum in adult. Ann Thorac Cardiovasc Surg. 7:103–5.
1938. Oshiro Y, Kusumoto M, Matsuno Y, et al. (2004). CT findings of surgically resected large cell neuroendocrine carcinoma of the lung in 38 patients. AJR Am J Roentgenol. 182:87–91.
1939. Ost D, Joseph C, Sogoloff H, et al. (1999). Primary pulmonary melanoma: case report and literature review. Mayo Clin Proc. 74:62–6.
1940. Osterlind K, Andersen PK (1986). Prognostic factors in small cell lung cancer: multivariate model based on 778 patients treated with chemotherapy with or without irradiation. Cancer Res. 46:4189–94.
1941. Otsuka M, Niijima K, Mizuno Y, et al. (1990). Marked decrease of mitochondrial DNA with multiple deletions in a patient with familial mitochondrial myopathy. Biochem Biophys Res Commun. 167:680–5.
1942. Ott G, Katzenberger T, Greiner A, et al. (1997). The t(11;18)(q21;q21) chromosome translocation is a frequent and specific aberration in low-grade but not high-grade malignant non-Hodgkin's lymphomas of the mucosa-associated lymphoid tissue (MALT-) type. Cancer Res. 57:3944–8.
1943. Otto HF, Loning T, Lachenmayer L, et al. (1982). Thymolipoma in association with myasthenia gravis. Cancer. 50:1623–8.
1944. Ou WB, Hubert C, Corson JM, et al. (2011). Targeted inhibition of multiple receptor tyrosine kinases in mesothelioma. Neoplasia. 13:12–22.
1945. Ovrum E, Birkeland S (1979). Mediastinal tumours and cysts. A review of 91 cases. Scand J Thorac Cardiovasc Surg. 13:161–8.
1946. Owe JF, Cvancarova M, Romi F, et al. (2010). Extrathymic malignancies in thymoma patients with and without myasthenia gravis. J Neurol Sci. 290:66–9.
1947. Owens C, Irwin M (2012). Neuroblastoma: the impact of biology and cooperation leading to personalized treatments. Crit Rev Clin Lab Sci. 49:85–115.
1948. Oxnard GR, Miller VA, Robson ME, et al. (2012). Screening for germline EGFR T790M mutations through lung cancer genotyping. J Thorac Oncol. 7:1049–52.
1949. Oyama T, Osaki T, Isse T, et al. (2003). Pleomorphic carcinoma: report of a case with massive pleural effusion and asbestos particles. Ann Thorac Cardiovasc Surg. 9:126–9.
1950. Oyama T, Yamamoto K, Asano N, et al. (2007). Age-related EBV-associated B-cell lymphoproliferative disorders constitute a distinct clinicopathologic group: a study of 96 patients. Clin Cancer Res. 13:5124–32.
1951. Pacini D, Careddu L, Pantaleo A, et al. (2012). Primary benign cardiac tumours: long-term results. Eur J Cardiothorac Surg. 41:812–9.
1952. Padalino MA, Basso C, Milanesi O, et al. (2005). Surgically treated primary cardiac tumors in early infancy and childhood. J Thorac Cardiovasc Surg. 129:1358–63.
1953. Padalino MA, Vida VL, Bhattarai A, et al. (2011). Giant intramural left ventricular rhabdomyoma in a newborn. Circulation. 124:2275–7.
1954. Padalino MA, Vida VL, Boccuzzo G, et al. (2012). Surgery for primary cardiac tumors in children: early and late results in a multicenter European Congenital Heart Surgeons Association study. Circulation. 126:22–30.
1955. Padgett DM, Cathro HP, Wick MR, et al. (2008). Podoplanin is a better immunohistochemical marker for sarcomatoid mesothelioma than calretinin. Am J Surg Pathol. 32:123–7.
1956. Paez JG, Janne PA, Lee JC, et al. (2004). EGFR mutations in lung cancer: correlation with clinical response to gefitinib therapy. Science. 304:1497–500.
1956A. Pacheco-Rodriguez G, Steagall WK, Crooks DM, et al. (2007). TSC2 loss in lymphangioleiomyomatosis cells correlated with expression of CD44v6, a molecular determinant of metastasis. Cancer Res. 67:10573–81.
1957. Paganin F, Prevot M, Noel JB, et al. (2009). A solitary bronchial papilloma with unusual endoscopic presentation: case study and literature review. BMC Pulm Med. 9:40.
1958. Paik PK, Arcila ME, Fara M, et al. (2011). Clinical characteristics of patients with lung adenocarcinomas harboring BRAF mutations. J Clin Oncol. 29:2046–51.
1959. Pairon JC, Laurent F, Rinaldo M, et al. (2013). Pleural plaques and the risk of pleural mesothelioma. J Natl Cancer Inst. 105:293–301.
1960. Palimento D, Picchio M (2006). Meningioma of the mediastinum causing spontaneous hemothorax. Ann Thorac Surg. 81:1903–4.
1961. Paliwal N, Gupta K, Dewan RK, et al. (2013). Adenocarcinoma (somatic-type malignancy) in mature teratoma of anterior mediastinum. Indian J Chest Dis Allied Sci. 55:39–41.
1962. Pallesen G, Hamilton-Dutoit SJ (1988). Ki-1 (CD30) antigen is regularly expressed by tumor cells of embryonal carcinoma. Am J Pathol. 133:446–50.
1963. Palmer RD, Barbosa-Morais NL, Gooding EL, et al. (2008). Pediatric malignant germ cell tumors show characteristic transcriptome profiles. Cancer Res. 68:4239–47.
1964. Palmieri G, Marino M, Buonerba C, et al. (2012). Imatinib mesylate in thymic epithelial malignancies. Cancer Chemother Pharmacol. 69:309–15.
1965. Pan CC, Chen PC, Chiang H (2004). KIT (CD117) is frequently overexpressed in thymic carcinomas but is absent in thymomas. J Pathol. 202:375–81.
1966. Pan CC, Chen PC, Chou TY, et al. (2003). Expression of calretinin and other mesothelioma-related markers in thymic carcinoma and thymoma. Hum Pathol. 34:1155–62.
1967. Pan CC, Chen WY, Chiang H (2001). Spindle cell and mixed spindle/lymphocytic thymomas: an integrated clinicopathologic and immunohistochemical study of 81 cases. Am J Surg Pathol. 25:111–20.
1968. Pan CC, Jong YJ, Chen YJ (2005). Comparative genomic hybridization analysis of thymic neuroendocrine tumors. Mod Pathol. 18:358–64.
1969. Pan CH, Chiang CY, Chen SS (1988). Thymolipoma in patients with myasthenia gravis: report of two cases and review. Acta Neurol Scand. 78:16–21.
1970. Pan Y, Chen JL, Li ZJ, et al. (2012). Cystic tumour of the atrioventricular node: a case report and review of the literature. Chin Med J (Engl). 125:4514–6.
1971. Pan ZG, Zhang QY, Lu ZB, et al. (2012). Extracavitary KSHV-associated large B-Cell lymphoma: a distinct entity or a subtype of primary effusion lymphoma? Study of 9 cases and review of an additional 43 cases. Am J Surg Pathol. 36:1129–40.
1972. Pande M, Wei C, Chen J, et al. (2012). Cancer spectrum in DNA mismatch repair gene mutation carriers: results from a hospital based Lynch syndrome registry. Fam Cancer. 11:441–7.
1973. Paniagua JR, Sadaba JR, Davidson LA, et al. (2000). Cystic tumour of the atrioventricular nodal region: report of a case successfully treated with surgery. Heart. 83:E6.
1974. Pao W, Miller V, Zakowski M, et al. (2004). EGF receptor gene mutations are common in lung cancers from "never smokers" and are associated with sensitivity of tumors to gefitinib and erlotinib. Proc Natl Acad Sci USA. 101:13306–11.
1975. Pao W, Miller VA, Politi KA, et al. (2005). Acquired resistance of lung adenocarcinomas to gefitinib or erlotinib is associated with a second mutation in the EGFR kinase domain. PLoS Med. 2:e73.
1976. Pao W, Wang TY, Riely GJ, et al. (2005). KRAS mutations and primary resistance of lung adenocarcinomas to gefitinib or erlotinib. PLoS Med. 2:e17.
1977. Papagiannopoulos K, Hughes S, Nicholson AG, et al. (2002). Cystic lung lesions in the pediatric and adult population: surgical experience at the Brompton Hospital. Ann Thorac Surg. 73:1594–8.
1978. Papagiannopoulos KA, Sheppard M, Bush AP, et al. (2001). Pleuropulmonary blastoma: is prophylactic resection of congenital lung cysts effective? Ann Thorac Surg. 72:604–5.
1979. Papla B (2009). Papillary adenoma of the lung. Pol J Pathol. 60:49–51.
1980. Paraf F, Bruneval P, Balaton A, et al. (1990). Primary liposarcoma of the heart. Am J Cardiovasc Pathol. 3:175–80.
1981. Paramanathan A, Wright G (2013). Pulmonary metastasectomy for sarcoma of gynaecologic origin. Heart Lung Circ. 22:270–5.
1982. Pardo J, Aisa G, Alava E, et al. (2008). Primary mixed squamous carcinoma and osteosarcoma (carcinosarcomas) of the lung have a CGH mapping similar to primitive squamous carcinomas and osteosarcomas. Diagn Mol Pathol. 17:151–8.
1983. Pardo J, Martinez-Penuela AM, Sola JJ, et al. (2009). Large cell carcinoma of the lung: an endangered species? Appl Immunohistochem Mol Morphol. 17:383–92.
1984. Parish JM, Rosenow ECI, Swensen SJ, et al. (1996). Pulmonary artery sarcoma. Clinical features. Chest. 110:1480–8.
1985. Park IK, Kim YT, Jeon JH, et al. (2013). Importance of lymph node dissection in thymic carcinoma. Ann Thorac Surg. 96:1025–32.
1986. Park IW, Wistuba II, Maitra A, et al. (1999). Multiple clonal abnormalities in the bronchial epithelium of patients with lung cancer. J Natl Cancer Inst. 91:1863–8.
1987. Park J, Song JM, Shin E, et al. (2011). Cystic cardiac mass in the left atrium: hemorrhage in myxoma. Circulation. 123:e368–9.
1988. Park KS, Liang MC, Raiser DM, et al. (2011). Characterization of the cell of origin for small cell lung cancer. Cell Cycle. 10:2806–15.
1989. Park KS, Martelotto LG, Peifer M, et al. (2011). A crucial requirement for Hedgehog signaling in small cell lung cancer. Nat Med. 17:1504–8.
1990. Park KS, Song BG, Ok KS, et al. (2011). Primary cardiac angiosarcoma treated by complete tumor resection with cardiac reconstruction. Heart Lung. 40:e41–3.
1991. Park MS, Chung KY, Kim KD, et al. (2004). Prognosis of thymic epithelial tumors according to the new World Health Organization histologic classification. Ann Thorac Surg. 78:992–7.
1992. Park SH, Kim TJ, Chi JG (1991). Congenital granular cell tumor with systemic involvement. Immunohistochemical and ultrastructural study. Arch Pathol Lab Med. 115:934–8.
1993. Park SK, Cho LY, Yang JJ, et al. (2010). Lung cancer risk and cigarette smoking, lung tuberculosis according to histologic type and gender in a population based case-control study. Lung Cancer. 68:20–6.
1994. Parkash V, Gerald WL, Parma A, et al. (1995). Desmoplastic small round cell tumor of the pleura. Am J Surg Pathol. 19:659–65.
1995. Parravicini C, Chandran B, Corbellino M, et al. (2000). Differential viral protein expression in Kaposi's sarcoma-associated herpesvirus-infected diseases: Kaposi's sarcoma, primary effusion lymphoma, and multicentric Castleman's disease. Am J Pathol. 156:743–9.
1996. Parrens M, Dubus P, Danjoux M, et al. (2002). Mucosa-associated lymphoid tissue of the thymus hyperplasia vs lymphoma. Am J Clin Pathol. 117:51–6.
1997. Parsons A, Daley A, Begh R, et al. (2010). Influence of smoking cessation after diagnosis of early stage lung cancer on prognosis: systematic review of observational studies with meta-analysis. BMJ. 340:b5569.
1998. Parvathy U, Balakrishnan KR, Ranjit MS, et al. (1998). Primary intracardiac yolk sac tumor. Pediatr Cardiol. 19:495–7.
1999. Parwani AV, Esposito N, Rao UN (2008). Primary cardiac osteosarcoma with recurrent episodes and unusual patterns of metastatic spread. Cardiovasc Pathol. 17:413–7.
2000. Parwani AV, Sheth S, Ali SZ (2004). Recurrent respiratory papillomatosis: cytopathological findings in an unusual case. Diagn Cytopathol. 31:407–12.
2001. Pastorino U, McCormack PM, Ginsberg RJ (1998). A new staging proposal for pulmonary metastases. The results of analysis of 5206 cases of resected pulmonary metastases. Chest Surg Clin N Am. 8:197–202.
2002. Pastorino U, Veronesi G, Landoni C, et al. (2003). Fluorodeoxyglucose positron emission tomography improves preoperative staging of resectable lung metastasis. J Thorac Cardiovasc Surg. 126:1906–10.
2003. Patel AS, Murphy KM, Hawkins AL, et al. (2007). RANBP2 and CLTC are involved in ALK rearrangements in inflammatory myofibroblastic tumors. Cancer Genet Cytogenet. 176:107–14.
2004. Patel IJ, Hsiao E, Ahmad AH, et al. (2013). AIRP best cases in radiologic-pathologic correlation: mediastinal mature cystic teratoma. Radiographics. 33:797–801.
2005. Patel J, Sheppard MN (2010). Pathological study of primary cardiac and pericardial tumours in a specialist UK Centre: surgical and autopsy series. Cardiovasc Pathol. 19:343–52.
2006. Patel J, Sheppard MN (2011). Primary malignant mesothelioma of the pericardium. Cardiovasc Pathol. 20:107–9.
2007. Patel R, Lynn KC (2009). Masquerading myxoma. Am J Med Sci. 338:161–3.
2008. Patel S, Macdonald OK, Nagda S, et al. (2012). Evaluation of the role of radiation therapy in the management of malignant thymoma. Int J Radiat Oncol Biol Phys. 82:1797–801.
2009. Paulli M, Strater J, Gianelli U, et al. (1999). Mediastinal B-cell lymphoma: a study of its histomorphologic spectrum based on 109 cases. Hum Pathol. 30:178–87.
2010. Pawlak Cieslik A, Szturmowicz M, Fijalkowska A, et al. (2012). Diagnosis of malignant pericarditis: a single centre experience. Kardiol Pol. 70:1147–53.
2011. Pehrson C, Kock K (2012). [Hydrops foetalis caused by a mediastinal teratoma]. Ugeskr Laeger. 174:2944–5.
2012. Peifer M, Fernandez-Cuesta L, Sos ML, et al. (2012). Integrative genome analyses identify key somatic driver mutations of small-cell lung cancer. Nat Genet. 44:1104–10.
2013. Pellegrino M, Gianotti L, Cassibba S, et al. (2012). Neuroblastoma in the Elderly and SIADH: Case Report and Review of the Literature. Case Rep Med. 2012:952645.
2014. Pelosi G, Fabbri A, Bianchi F, et al. (2012). DeltaNp63 (p40) and thyroid transcription factor-1 immunoreactivity on small biopsies or cellblocks for typing non-small cell lung cancer: a novel two-hit, sparing-material approach. J Thorac Oncol. 7:281–90.
2015. Pelosi G, Fraggetta F, Nappi O, et al. (2003). Pleomorphic carcinomas of the lung show a selective distribution of gene products involved in cell differentiation, cell cycle control, tumor growth, and tumor cell motility: a clinicopathologic and immunohistochemical study of 31 cases. Am J Surg Pathol. 27:1203–15.
2016. Pelosi G, Fumagalli C, Trubia M, et al. (2010). Dual role of RASSF1 as a tumor suppressor and an oncogene in neuroendocrine tumors of the lung. Anticancer Res. 30:4269–81.
2017. Pelosi G, Gasparini P, Cavazza A, et al. (2012). Multiparametric molecular

characterization of pulmonary sarcomatoid carcinoma reveals a nonrandom amplification of anaplastic lymphoma kinase (ALK) gene. Lung Cancer. 77:507–14.
2018. Pelosi G, Masullo M, Leon ME, et al. (2004). CD117 immunoreactivity in high-grade neuroendocrine tumors of the lung: a comparative study of 39 large-cell neuroendocrine carcinomas and 27 surgically resected small-cell carcinomas. Virchows Arch. 445:449–55.
2019. Pelosi G, Pasini F, Olsen Stenholm C, et al. (2002). p63 immunoreactivity in lung cancer: yet another player in the development of squamous cell carcinomas? J Pathol. 198:100–9.
2020. Pelosi G, Rindi G, Travis WD, et al. (2014). Ki-67 antigen in lung neuroendocrine tumors: unraveling a role in clinical practice. J Thorac Oncol. 9:273–84.
2021. Pelosi G, Rodriguez J, Viale G, et al. (2005). Typical and atypical pulmonary carcinoid tumor overdiagnosed as small-cell carcinoma on biopsy specimens: a major pitfall in the management of lung cancer patients. Am J Surg Pathol. 29:179–87.
2022. Pelosi G, Rosai J, Viale G (2006). Immunoreactivity for sex steroid hormone receptors in pulmonary hamartomas. Am J Surg Pathol. 30:819–27.
2023. Pelosi G, Rossi G, Bianchi F, et al. (2011). Immunhistochemistry by means of widely agreed-upon markers (cytokeratins 5/6 and 7, p63, thyroid transcription factor-1, and vimentin) on small biopsies of non-small cell lung cancer effectively parallels the corresponding profiling and eventual diagnoses on surgical specimens. J Thorac Oncol. 6:1039–49.
2024. Pelosi G, Rossi G, Cavazza A, et al. (2013). DeltaNp63 (p40) distribution inside lung cancer: a driver biomarker approach to tumor characterization. Int J Surg Pathol. 21:229–39.
2025. Pelosi G, Scarpa A, Manzotti M, et al. (2004). K-ras gene mutational analysis supports a monoclonal origin of biphasic pleomorphic carcinoma of the lung. Mod Pathol. 17:538–46.
2026. Pelosi G, Sonzogni A, De Pas T, et al. (2010). Review article: pulmonary sarcomatoid carcinomas: a practical overview. Int J Surg Pathol. 18:103–20.
2027. Penzel R, Hoegel J, Schmitz W, et al. (2003). Clusters of chromosomal imbalances in thymic epithelial tumours are associated with the WHO classification and the staging system according to Masaoka. Int J Cancer. 105:494–8.
2028. Percy C, Van Holten V, Muir C (1990). International Classification of Diseases for Oncology. 2nd ed. Geneva: WHO Press.
2029. Perez-Ordonez B, Erlandson RA, Rosai J (1996). Follicular dendritic cell tumor: report of 13 additional cases of a distinctive entity. Am J Surg Pathol. 20:944–55.
2030. Perez-Sirvent C, Garcia-Lorenzo ML, Martinez-Sanchez MJ, et al. (2007). Metal-contaminated soil remediation by using sludges of the marble industry: toxicological evaluation. Environ Int. 33:502–4.
2031. Perkins SM, Shinohara ET (2013). Interdigitating and follicular dendritic cell sarcomas: a SEER analysis. Am J Clin Oncol. 36:395–8.
2032. Perlikos F, Harrington KJ, Syrigos KN (2013). Key molecular mechanisms in lung cancer invasion and metastasis: a comprehensive review. Crit Rev Oncol Hematol. 87:1–11.
2033. Perry AM, Nelson M, Sanger WG, et al. (2013). Cytogenetic abnormalities in follicular dendritic cell sarcoma: report of two cases and literature review. In Vivo. 27:211–4.
2034. Perry L, Florio R, Dewar A, et al. (2000). Giant lamellar bodies as a feature of pulmonary low-grade MALT lymphomas. Histopathology. 36:240–4.
2035. Persson M, Andren Y, Mark J, et al. (2009). Recurrent fusion of MYB and NFIB transcription factor genes in carcinomas of the breast and head and neck. Proc Natl Acad Sci USA. 106:18740–4.
2036. Pertschuk LP, Kim DS, Nayer K, et al. (1990). Immunocytochemical estrogen and progestin receptor assays in breast cancer with monoclonal antibodies. Histopathologic, demographic, and biochemical correlations and relationship to endocrine response and survival. Cancer. 66:1663–70.
2037. Pesatori AC, Carugno M, Consonni D, et al. (2013). Hormone use and risk for lung cancer: a pooled analysis from the International Lung Cancer Consortium (ILCCO). Br J Cancer. 109:1954–64.
2038. Pescarmona E, Rosati S, Pisacane A, et al. (1992). Microscopic thymoma: histological evidence of multifocal cortical and medullary origin. Histopathology. 20:263–6.
2039. Pesch B, Kendzia B, Gustavsson P, et al. (2012). Cigarette smoking and lung cancer--relative risk estimates for the major histological types from a pooled analysis of case-control studies. Int J Cancer. 131:1210–9.
2040. Peters S, Michielin O, Zimmermann S (2013). Dramatic response induced by vemurafenib in a BRAF V600E-mutated lung adenocarcinoma. J Clin Oncol. 31:e341–4.
2041. Petitjean B, Jardin F, Joly B, et al. (2002). Pyothorax-associated lymphoma: a peculiar clinicopathologic entity derived from B cells at late stage of differentiation and with occasional aberrant dual B- and T-cell phenotype. Am J Surg Pathol. 26:724–32.
2042. Peto J, Decarli A, La Vecchia C, et al. (1999). The European mesothelioma epidemic. Br J Cancer. 79:666–72.
2043. Peto J, Seidman H, Selikoff IJ (1982). Mesothelioma mortality in asbestos workers: implications for models of carcinogenesis and risk assessment. Br J Cancer. 45:124–35.
2044. Petrich A, Cho SI, Billett H (2011). Primary cardiac lymphoma: an analysis of presentation, treatment, and outcome patterns. Cancer. 117:581–9.
2044A. Petrini I, Meltzer PS, Kim IK, et al. (2014). A specific missense mutation in GTF2I occurs at high frequency in thymic epithelial tumors. Nat Genet. 46:844–9
2045. Petrini I, Meltzer PS, Zucali PA, et al. (2012). Copy number aberrations of BCL2 and CDKN2A/B identified by array-CGH in thymic epithelial tumors. Cell Death Dis. 3:e351.
2046. Petrini I, Rajan A, Pham T, et al. (2013). Whole genome and transcriptome sequencing of a B3 thymoma. PLoS ONE. 8:e60572.
2046A. Petrini I, Wang Y, Zucali PA, et al. (2013). Copy number aberrations of genes regulating normal thymus development in thymic epithelial tumors. Clin Cancer Res 19:1960–71.
2047. Petrini I, Zucali PA, Lee HS, et al. (2010). Expression and mutational status of c-kit in thymic epithelial tumors. J Thorac Oncol. 5:1447–53.
2048. Petrini P, French CA, Rajan A, et al. (2012). NUT rearrangement is uncommon in human thymic epithelial tumors. J Thorac Oncol. 7:744–50.
2049. Petscavage JM, Richardson ML, Nett M, et al. (2011). Primary chordoid meningioma of the lung. J Thorac Imaging. 26:W14–6.
2050. Pettinato G, Manivel JC, De Rosa N, et al. (1990). Inflammatory myofibroblastic tumor (plasma cell granuloma). Clinicopathologic study of 20 cases with immunohistochemical and ultrastructural observations. Am J Clin Pathol. 94:538–46.
2051. Pfeifer GP, Denissenko MF, Olivier M, et al. (2002). Tobacco smoke carcinogens, DNA damage and p53 mutations in smoking-associated cancers. Oncogene. 21:7435–51.
2052. Piciu D, Piciu A, Irimie A (2012). Papillary thyroid microcarcinoma and ectopic papillary thyroid carcinoma in mediastinum: a case report. Clin Nucl Med. 37:214–5.
2053. Pilarski R, Cebulla CM, Massengill JB, et al. (2014). Expanding the clinical phenotype of hereditary BAP1 cancer predisposition syndrome, reporting three new cases. Genes Chromosomes Cancer. 53:177–82.
2054. Pileri S, Mazza P, Rivano MT, et al. (1985). Malignant histiocytosis (true histiocytic lymphoma) clinicopathological study of 25 cases. Histopathology. 9:905–20.
2055. Pileri SA, Ascani S, Cox MC, et al. (2007). Myeloid sarcoma: clinico-pathologic, phenotypic and cytogenetic analysis of 92 adult patients. Leukemia. 21:340–50.
2056. Pileri SA, Cavazza A, Schiavina M, et al. (2004). Clear-cell proliferation of the lung with lymphangioleiomyomatosis-like change. Histopathology. 44:156–63.
2057. Pileri SA, Gaidano G, Zinzani PL, et al. (2003). Primary mediastinal B-cell lymphoma: high frequency of BCL-6 mutations and consistent expression of the transcription factors OCT-2, BOB.1, and PU.1 in the absence of immunoglobulins. Am J Pathol. 162:243–53.
2058. Pileri SA, Grogan TM, Harris NL, et al. (2002). Tumours of histiocytes and accessory dendritic cells: an immunohistochemical approach to classification from the International Lymphoma Study Group based on 61 cases. Histopathology. 41:1–29.
2059. Pillai R, Deeter R, Rigl CT, et al. (2011). Validation and reproducibility of a microarray-based gene expression test for tumor identification in formalin-fixed, paraffin-embedded specimens. J Mol Diagn. 13:48–56.
2060. Pinede L, Duhaut P, Loire R (2001). Clinical presentation of left atrial cardiac myxoma. A series of 112 consecutive cases. Medicine (Baltimore). 80:159–72.
2061. Pinkard NB, Wilson RW, Lawless N, et al. (1996). Calcifying fibrous pseudotumor of pleura. A report of three cases of a newly described entity involving the pleura. Am J Clin Pathol. 105:189–94.
2062. Pittaluga S, Wilson WH, Jaffe ES (2008). Lymphomatoid granulomatosis. In: Swerdlow SH, Campo E, Harris CC, Jaffe ES, Pileri SA, Stein H, et al., eds. WHO Classification of Tumours of Haematopoietic and Lymphoid Tissues. 4th ed. IARC: Lyon; pp 247–249.
2063. Planchard D, Le Pechoux C (2011). Small cell lung cancer: new clinical recommendations and current status of biomarker assessment. Eur J Cancer. 47 Suppl 3:S272–83.
2064. Plathow C, Staab A, Schmaehl A, et al. (2008). Computed tomography, positron emission tomography, positron emission tomography/computed tomography, and magnetic resonance imaging for staging of limited pleural mesothelioma: initial results. Invest Radiol. 43:737–44.
2065. Pleasance ED, Stephens PJ, O'Meara S, et al. (2010). A small-cell lung cancer genome with complex signatures of tobacco exposure. Nature. 463:184–90.
2066. Policarpio-Nicolas ML, Alasadi R, Nayar R, et al. (2006). Synovial sarcoma of the heart: Report of a case with diagnosis by endoscopic ultrasound-guided fine needle aspiration biopsy. Acta Cytol. 50:683–6.
2067. Polizzotto MN, Uldrick TS, Hu D, et al. (2012). Clinical Manifestations of Kaposi Sarcoma Herpesvirus Lytic Activation: Multicentric Castleman Disease (KSHV-MCD) and the KSHV Inflammatory Cytokine Syndrome. Front Microbiol. 3:73.
2068. Polsani A, Braithwaite KA, Alazraki AL, et al. (2012). NUT midline carcinoma: an imaging case series and review of literature. Pediatr Radiol. 42:205–10.
2069. Pomplun S, Wotherspoon AC, Shah G, et al. (2002). Immunohistochemical markers in the differentiation of thymic and pulmonary neoplasms. Histopathology. 40:152–8.
2070. Ponzoni M, Arrigoni G, Gould VE, et al. (2000). Lack of CD 29 (beta1 integrin) and CD 54 (ICAM-1) adhesion molecules in intravascular lymphomatosis. Hum Pathol. 31:220–6.
2071. Ponzoni M, Ferreri AJ, Campo E, et al. (2007). Definition, diagnosis, and management of intravascular large B-cell lymphoma: proposals and perspectives from an international consensus meeting. J Clin Oncol. 25:3168–73.
2072. Poole-Wilson PA, Farnsworth A, Braimbridge MV, et al. (1976). Angiosarcoma of pericardium. Problems in diagnosis and management. Br Heart J. 38:240–3.
2073. Poorabdollah M, Mehdizadeh E, Mohammadi F, et al. (2009). Metaplastic thymoma: report of an unusual thymic epithelial neoplasm arising in the wall of a thymic cyst. Int J Surg Pathol. 17:51–4.
2074. Popova T, Hebert L, Jacquemin V, et al. (2013). Germline BAP1 mutations predispose to renal cell carcinomas. Am J Hum Genet. 92:974–80.
2075. Popper HH, el-Shabrawi Y, Wockel W, et al. (1994). Prognostic importance of human papilloma virus typing in squamous cell papilloma of the bronchus: comparison of in situ hybridization and the polymerase chain reaction. Hum Pathol. 25:1191–7.
2076. Popper HH, Wirnsberger G, Juttner-Smolle FM, et al. (1992). The predictive value of human papilloma virus (HPV) typing in the prognosis of bronchial squamous cell papillomas. Histopathology. 21:323–30.
2077. Posligua L, Ylagan L (2006). Fine-needle aspiration cytology of thymic basaloid carcinoma: case studies and review of the literature. Diagn Cytopathol. 34:358–66.
2078. Postmus PE, Brambilla E, Chansky K, et al. (2007). The IASLC Lung Cancer Staging Project: proposals for revision of the M descriptors in the forthcoming (seventh) edition of the TNM classification of lung cancer. J Thorac Oncol. 2:686–93.
2079. Povey S, Burley MW, Attwood J, et al. (1994). Two loci for tuberous sclerosis: one on 9q34 and one on 16p13. Ann Hum Genet. 58:107–27.
2080. Poynter JN, Amatruda JF, Ross JA (2010). Trends in incidence and survival of pediatric and adolescent patients with germ cell tumors in the United States, 1975 to 2006. Cancer. 116:4882–91.
2081. Prakash P, Kalra MK, Stone JR, et al. (2010). Imaging findings of pericardial metastasis on chest computed tomography. J Comput Assist Tomogr. 34:554–8.
2082. Prat J, Bhan AK, Dickersin GR, et al. (1982). Hepatoid yolk sac tumor of the ovary (endodermal sinus tumor with hepatoid differentiation): a light microscopic, ultrastructural and immunohistochemical study of seven cases. Cancer. 50:2355–68.
2083. Prayson RA, Farver CF (1999). Primary pulmonary malignant meningioma. Am J Surg Pathol. 23:722–6.
2084. Preusser M, Berghoff AS, Berger W, et al. (2014). High rate of FGFR1 amplifications in brain metastases of squamous and non-squamous lung cancer. Lung Cancer. 83:83–9.
2085. Price B, Ware A (2009). Time trend of mesothelioma incidence in the United States and projection of future cases: an update based on SEER data for 1973 through 2005. Crit Rev Toxicol. 39:576–88.
2086. Priest JR, Andic D, Arbuckle S, et al. (2011). Great vessel/cardiac extension and tumor embolism in pleuropulmonary blastoma: a report from the International Pleuropulmonary Blastoma Registry. Pediatr Blood Cancer. 56:604–9.
2087. Priest JR, Hill DA, Williams GM, et al. (2006). Type I pleuropulmonary blastoma: a report from the International Pleuropulmonary Blastoma Registry. J Clin Oncol. 24:4492–8.

2088. Priest JR, McDermott MB, Bhatia S, et al. (1997). Pleuropulmonary blastoma: a clinicopathologic study of 50 cases. Cancer. 80:147–61.
2089. Priest JR, Williams GM, Hill DA, et al. (2009). Pulmonary cysts in early childhood and the risk of malignancy. Pediatr Pulmonol. 44:14–30.
2090. Prins JB, Williamson KA, Kamp MM, et al. (1998). The gene for the cyclin-dependent-kinase-4 inhibitor, CDKN2A, is preferentially deleted in malignant mesothelioma. Int J Cancer. 75:649–53.
2091. Priola AM, Priola SM, Cataldi A, et al. (2008). CT-guided percutaneous transthoracic biopsy in the diagnosis of mediastinal masses: evaluation of 73 procedures. Radiol Med (Torino). 113:3–15.
2092. Protopapadakis C, Antoniou KM, Nicholson AG, et al. (2009). Erdheim-Chester disease: pulmonary presentation in a case with advanced systemic involvement. Respiration. 77:337–40.
2093. Przygodzki RM, Hubbs AE, Zhao FQ, et al. (2002). Primary mediastinal seminomas: evidence of single and multiple KIT mutations. Lab Invest. 82:1369–75.
2094. Przygodzki RM, Koss MN, Moran CA, et al. (1996). Pleomorphic (giant and spindle cell) carcinoma is genetically distinct from adenocarcinoma and squamous cell carcinoma by K-ras-2 and p53 analysis. Am J Clin Pathol. 106:487–92.
2095. Pucci A, Gagliardotto P, Zanini C, et al. (2000). Histopathologic and clinical characterization of cardiac myxoma: review of 53 cases from a single institution. Am Heart J. 140:134–8.
2096. Puglisi F, Finato N, Mariuzzi L, et al. (1995). Microscopic thymoma and myasthenia gravis. J Clin Pathol. 48:682–3.
2097. Puliyel MM, Mascarenhas L, Zhou S, et al. (2014). Nuclear protein in testis midline carcinoma misdiagnosed as adamantinoma. J Clin Oncol. 32:e57–60.
2098. Puskarz-Thomas S, Dettrick A, Pohlner PG (2012). Cardiac myxoma with oncocytic change--cardiac oncocytoma? Cardiovasc Pathol. 21:e11–3.
2099. Putnam JB Jr, Schantz SP, Pugh WC, et al. (1990). Extended en bloc resection of a primary mediastinal parathyroid carcinoma. Ann Thorac Surg. 50:138–40.
2100. Qi J, Yu J, Zhang M, et al. (2012). Multicentric granular cell tumors with heart involvement: a case report. J Clin Oncol. 30:e79–82.
2101. Qian X, Sun Z, Pan W, et al. (2013). Childhood bronchial mucoepidermoid tumors: A case report and literature review. Oncol Lett. 6:1409–12.
2102. Qian Y, Jiang T, Liu S (2012). Sclerosing hemangioma of the lung manifesting as a cystic lesion with an air-fluid level. Respiration. 84:142–3.
2103. Qin L, Shi JH, Liu HR, et al. (2010). [Non-Hodgkin's lymphoma with diffuse ground-glass opacity on chest CT: a report of 6 cases]. Zhonghua Yi Xue Za Zhi. 90:3283–6.
2104. Qu G, Yu G, Zhang Q, et al. (2013). Lipofibroadenoma of the thymus: a case report. Diagn Pathol. 8:117.
2105. Quaedvlieg PF, Visser O, Lamers CB, et al. (2001). Epidemiology and survival in patients with carcinoid disease in The Netherlands. An epidemiological study with 2391 patients. Ann Oncol. 12:1295–300.
2106. Quail MT (2013). Prekallikrein deficiency. J Pediatr Oncol Nurs. 30:198–204.
2107. Quintanilla-Martinez L, Wilkins EW Jr, Choi N, et al. (1994). Thymoma. Histologic subclassification is an independent prognostic factor. Cancer. 74:606–17.
2108. Quintanilla-Martinez L, Zukerberg LR, Harris NL (1992). Prethymic adult lymphoblastic lymphoma. A clinicopathologic and immunohistochemical analysis. Am J Surg Pathol. 16:1075–84.
2109. Ra SH, Fishbein MC, Baruch-Oren T, et al. (2007). Mucinous adenocarcinomas of the thymus: report of 2 cases and review of the literature. Am J Surg Pathol. 31:1330–6.
2110. Rabkin MS, Kjeldsberg CR, Hammond ME, et al. (1988). Clinical, ultrastructural immunohistochemical and DNA content analysis of lymphomas having features of interdigitating reticulum cells. Cancer. 61:1594–601.
2111. Radhi JM (2000). Immunohistochemical analysis of pleomorphic lobular carcinoma: higher expression of p53 and chromogranin and lower expression of ER and PgR. Histopathology. 36:156–60.
2112. Rady PL, Schnadig VJ, Weiss RL, et al. (1998). Malignant transformation of recurrent respiratory papillomatosis associated with integrated human papillomavirus type 11 DNA and mutation of p53. Laryngoscope. 108:735–40.
2113. Raffa GM, Malvindi PG, Settepani F, et al. (2013). Hamartoma of mature cardiac myocytes in adults and young: case report and literature review. Int J Cardiol. 163:e28–30.
2114. Rajiah P, To AC, Tan CD, et al. (2011). Multimodality imaging of an unusual case of right ventricular lipoma. Circulation. 124:1897–8.
2115. Ramalingam P, Teague D, Reid-Nicholson M (2008). Imprint cytology of high-grade immature ovarian teratoma: a case report, literature review, and distinction from other ovarian small round cell tumors. Diagn Cytopathol. 36:595–9.
2116. Ramasamy K, Lim Z, Pagliuca A, et al. (2007). Acute myeloid leukaemia presenting with mediastinal myeloid sarcoma: report of three cases and review of literature. Leuk Lymphoma. 48:290–4.
2117. Ramirez PT, Ramondetta LM, Burke TW, et al. (2001). Metastatic uterine papillary serous carcinoma to the pericardium. Gynecol Oncol. 83:135–7.
2118. Ramnarine IR, Davidson L, van Doorn CA (2001). Primary cardiac carcinosarcoma: a rare, aggressive tumor. Ann Thorac Surg. 72:927–9.
2119. Rana O, Gonda P, Addis B, et al. (2009). Image in cardiovascular medicine. Intrapericardial paraganglioma presenting as chest pain. Circulation. 119:e373–5.
2120. Rashid A, Molloy S, Lehovsky J, et al. (2008). Metastatic pulmonary intimal sarcoma presenting as cauda equina syndrome: first report of a case. Spine. 33:E516–20.
2121. Rathore KS, Hussenbocus S, Stuklis R, et al. (2008). Novel strategies for recurrent cardiac myxoma. Ann Thorac Surg. 85:2125–6.
2122. Rathore KS, Stuklis R, Allin J, et al. (2010). Spindle cell lipoma of the aortic valve: a rare cardiac finding. Cardiovasc Pathol. 19:e9–11.
2123. Ratschiller D, Heighway J, Gugger M, et al. (2003). Cyclin D1 overexpression in bronchial epithelia of patients with lung cancer is associated with smoking and predicts survival. J Clin Oncol. 21:2085–93.
2124. Ratto GB, Costa R, Alloisio A, et al. (2004). Mediastinal chondrosarcoma. Tumori. 90:151–3.
2125. Ravandi-Kashani F, Cortes J, Giles FJ (2000). Myelodysplasia presenting as granulocytic sarcoma of mediastinum causing superior vena cava syndrome. Leuk Lymphoma. 36:631–7.
2126. Raveglia F, Mezzetti M, Panigalli T, et al. (2004). Personal experience in surgical management of pulmonary pleomorphic carcinoma. Ann Thorac Surg. 78:1742–7.
2127. Reali A, Mortellaro G, Allis S, et al. (2013). A case of primary mediastinal Ewing's sarcoma / primitive neuroectodermal tumor presenting with initial compression of superior vena cava. Ann Thorac Med. 8:121–3.
2128. Regales L, Gong Y, Shen R, et al. (2009). Dual targeting of EGFR can overcome a major drug resistance mutation in mouse models of EGFR mutant lung cancer. J Clin Invest. 119:3000–10.
2129. Regnard JF, Magdeleinat P, Dromer C, et al. (1996). Prognostic factors and long-term results after thymoma resection: a series of 307 patients. J Thorac Cardiovasc Surg. 112:376–84.
2130. Reingold IM, Amromin GD (1971). Extraosseous osteosarcoma of the lung. Cancer. 28:491–8.
2131. Reis-Filho JS, Pope LZ, Milanezi F, et al. (2002). Primary epithelial malignant mesothelioma of the pericardium with deciduoid features: cytohistologic and immunohistochemical study. Diagn Cytopathol. 26:117–22.
2132. Rekhtman N (2010). Neuroendocrine tumors of the lung: an update. Arch Pathol Lab Med. 134:1628–38.
2133. Rekhtman N, Ang DC, Riely GJ, et al. (2013). KRAS mutations are associated with solid growth pattern and tumor-infiltrating leukocytes in lung adenocarcinoma. Mod Pathol. 26:1307–19.
2134. Rekhtman N, Ang DC, Sima CS, et al. (2011). Immunohistochemical algorithm for differentiation of lung adenocarcinoma and squamous cell carcinoma based on large series of whole-tissue sections with validation in small specimens. Mod Pathol. 24:1348–59.
2135. Rekhtman N, Brandt SM, Sigel CS, et al. (2011). Suitability of thoracic cytology for new therapeutic paradigms in non-small cell lung carcinoma: high accuracy of tumor subtyping and feasibility of EGFR and KRAS molecular testing. J Thorac Oncol. 6:451–8.
2136. Rekhtman N, Paik PK, Arcila ME, et al. (2012). Clarifying the spectrum of driver oncogene mutations in biomarker-verified squamous carcinoma of lung: lack of EGFR/KRAS and presence of PIK3CA/AKT1 mutations. Clin Cancer Res. 18:1167–76.
2137. Rekhtman N, Tafe LJ, Chaft JE, et al. (2013). Distinct profile of driver mutations and clinical features in immunomarker-defined subsets of pulmonary large-cell carcinoma. Mod Pathol. 26:511–22.
2138. Remo A, Zanella C, Pancione M, et al. (2013). Lung metastasis from TTF-1 positive sigmoid adenocarcinoma. pitfalls and management. Pathologica. 105:69–72.
2139. Remstein ED, Dogan A, Einerson RR, et al. (2006). The incidence and anatomic site specificity of chromosomal translocations in primary extranodal marginal zone B-cell lymphoma of mucosa-associated lymphoid tissue (MALT lymphoma) in North America. Am J Surg Pathol. 30:1546–53.
2140. Remstein ED, Kurtin PJ, Einerson RR, et al. (2004). Primary pulmonary MALT lymphomas show frequent and heterogeneous cytogenetic abnormalities, including aneuploidy and translocations involving API2 and MALT1 and IGH and MALT1. Leukemia. 18:156–60.
2141. Rena O, Papalia E, Maggi G, et al. (2005). World Health Organization histologic classification: an independent prognostic factor in resected thymomas. Lung Cancer. 50:59–66.
2142. Renshaw AA, Haja J, Lozano RL, et al. (2005). Distinguishing carcinoid tumor from small cell carcinoma of the lung: correlating cytologic features and performance in the College of American Pathologists Non-Gynecologic Cytology Program. Arch Pathol Lab Med. 129:614–8.
2143. Restrepo CS, Largoza A, Lemos DF, et al. (2005). CT and MR imaging findings of malignant cardiac tumors. Curr Probl Diagn Radiol. 34:1–11.
2144. Reuter VE (2002). The pre and post chemotherapy pathologic spectrum of germ cell tumors. Chest Surg Clin N Am. 12:673–94.
2145. Reynen K (1995). Cardiac myxomas. N Engl J Med. 333:1610–7.
2146. Reynen K, Kockeritz U, Strasser RH (2004). Metastases to the heart. Ann Oncol. 15:375–81.
2147. Rezk SA, Spagnolo DV, Brynes RK, et al. (2008). Indeterminate cell tumor: a rare dendritic neoplasm. Am J Surg Pathol. 32:1868–76.
2148. Riaz SP, Luchtenborg M, Coupland VH, et al. (2012). Trends in incidence of small cell lung cancer and all lung cancer. Lung Cancer. 75:280–4.
2149. Ribeiro C, Campelos S, Moura CS, et al. (2013). Well-differentiated papillary mesothelioma: clustering in a Portuguese family with a germline BAP1 mutation. Ann Oncol. 24:2147–50.
2150. Ried M, Neu R, Schalke B, et al. (2013). [Radical pleurectomy and hyperthermic intrathoracic chemotherapy for treatment of thymoma with pleural spread]. Zentralbl Chir. 138 Suppl 1:S52–7.
2151. Ried M, Potzger T, Sziklavari Z, et al. (2014). Extended surgical resections of advanced thymoma Masaoka stages III and IVa facilitate outcome. Thorac Cardiovasc Surg. 62:161–8.
2152. Rieger M, Osterborg A, Pettengell R, et al. (2011). Primary mediastinal B-cell lymphoma treated with CHOP-like chemotherapy with or without rituximab: results of the Mabthera International Trial Group study. Ann Oncol. 22:664–70.
2153. Rieker RJ, Aulmann S, Penzel R, et al. (2005). Chromosomal imbalances in sporadic neuroendocrine tumours of the thymus. Cancer Lett. 223:169–74.
2154. Rieker RJ, Hoegel J, Morresi-Hauf A, et al. (2002). Histologic classification of thymic epithelial tumors: comparison of established classification schemes. Int J Cancer. 98:900–6.
2155. Rieker RJ, Schirmacher P, Schnabel PA, et al. (2010). Thymolipoma. A report of nine cases, with emphasis on its association with myasthenia gravis. Surg Today. 40:132–6.
2156. Riely GJ, Travis WD (2014). Can IASLC/ATS/ERS subtype help predict response to chemotherapy in small biopsies of advanced lung adenocarcinoma? Eur Respir J. 43:1240–2.
2157. Righi L, Volante M, Tavaglione V, et al. (2010). Somatostatin receptor tissue distribution in lung neuroendocrine tumours: a clinicopathologic and immunohistochemical study of 218 'clinically aggressive' cases. Ann Oncol. 21:548–55.
2158. Rikova K, Guo A, Zeng Q, et al. (2007). Global survey of phosphotyrosine signaling identifies oncogenic kinases in lung cancer. Cell. 131:1190–203.
2159. Riles E, Gupta S, Wang DD, et al. (2012). Primary cardiac angiosarcoma: A diagnostic challenge in a young man with recurrent pericardial effusions. Exp Clin Cardiol. 17:39–42.
2160. Rindi G, Klersy C, Inzani F, et al. (2014). Grading the neuroendocrine tumors of the lung: an evidence-based proposal. Endocr Relat Cancer. 21:1–16.
2161. Rios JC, Chavarri F, Morales G, et al. (2013). Cardiac myxoma with prenatal diagnosis. World J Pediatr Congenit Heart Surg. 4:210–2.
2162. Ripamonti D, Marini B, Rambaldi A, et al. (2008). Treatment of primary effusion lymphoma with highly active antiviral therapy in the setting of HIV infection. AIDS. 22:1236–7.
2163. Ritter JH, Wick MR (1999). Primary carcinomas of the thymus gland. Semin Diagn Pathol. 16:18–31.
2164. Ritz O, Guiter C, Castellano F, et al. (2009). Recurrent mutations of the STAT6 DNA binding domain in primary mediastinal B-cell lymphoma. Blood. 114:1236–42.
2165. Ritz O, Rommel K, Dorsch K, et al. (2013). STAT6-mediated BCL6 repression in primary mediastinal B-cell lymphoma (PMBL). Oncotarget. 4:1093–102.
2166. Rivera MP, Detterbeck F, Mehta AC

(2003). Diagnosis of lung cancer: the guidelines. Chest. 123:129S–36S.
2167. Rizvi SM, Goodwill J, Lim E, et al. (2009). The frequency of neuroendocrine cell hyperplasia in patients with pulmonary neuroendocrine tumours and non-neuroendocrine cell carcinomas. Histopathology. 55:332–7.
2168. Rizzo S, Basso C, Buja G, et al. (2014). Multifocal Purkinje-like hamartoma and junctional ectopic tachycardia with a rapidly fatal outcome in a newborn. Heart Rhythm. 11:1264–6.
2169. Rizzoli G, Bottio T, Pittarello D, et al. (2004). Atrial septal mass: transesophageal echocardiographic assessment. J Thorac Cardiovasc Surg. 128:767–9.
2170. Robak T, Kordek R, Urbanska-Rys H, et al. (2006). High activity of rituximab combined with cladribine and cyclophosphamide in a patient with pulmonary lymphomatoid granulomatosis and bone marrow involvement. Leuk Lymphoma. 47:1667–9.
2171. Roberts PJ, Stinchcombe TE (2013). KRAS mutation: should we test for it, and does it matter? J Clin Oncol. 31:1112–21.
2172. Robinson DR, Wu YM, Kalyana-Sundaram S, et al. (2013). Identification of recurrent NAB2-STAT6 gene fusions in solitary fibrous tumor by integrative sequencing. Nat Genet. 45:180–5.
2173. Robinson LA (2006). Solitary fibrous tumor of the pleura. Cancer Contr. 13:264–9.
2174. Roden AC, Erickson-Johnson MR, Yi ES, et al. (2013). Analysis of MAML2 rearrangement in mucoepidermoid carcinoma of the thymus. Hum Pathol. 44:2799–805.
2175. Roden AC, Garcia JJ, Wehrs RN, et al. (2014). Histopathologic, immunophenotypic and cytogenetic features of pulmonary mucoepidermoid carcinoma. Mod Pathol. 27:1479–88.
2176. Roden AC, Hu X, Kip S, et al. (2014). BRAF V600E expression in Langerhans cell histiocytosis: clinical and immunohistochemical study on 25 pulmonary and 54 extrapulmonary cases. Am J Surg Pathol. 38:548–51.
2176A. Roden AC, Yi ES, Cassivi SD, Jenkins SM, Garces YI, Aubry MC (2013). Clinicopathological features of thymic carcinomas and the impact of histopathological agreement on prognostical studies. Eur J Cardiothorac Surg. 43(6):1131–9.
2177. Rodig SJ, Savage KJ, Lacasce AS, et al. (2007). Expression of TRAF1 and nuclear c-Rel distinguishes primary mediastinal large cell lymphoma from other types of diffuse large B-cell lymphoma. Am J Surg Pathol. 31:106–12.
2178. Rodney AJ, Tannir NM, Siefker-Radtke AO, et al. (2012). Survival outcomes for men with mediastinal germ-cell tumors: the University of Texas M. D. Anderson Cancer Center experience. Urol Oncol. 30:879–85.
2179. Rodriguez EF, Monaco SE, Dacic S (2013). Cytologic subtyping of lung adenocarcinoma by using the proposed International Association for the Study of Lung Cancer/American Thoracic Society/European Respiratory Society (IASLC/ATS/ERS) adenocarcinoma classification. Cancer Cytopathol. 121:629–37.
2180. Rodriguez FJ, Aubry MC, Tazelaar HD, et al. (2007). Pulmonary chondroma: a tumor associated with Carney triad and different from pulmonary hamartoma. Am J Surg Pathol. 31:1844–53.
2181. Roeltgen D, Kidwell CS (2014). Neurologic complications of cardiac tumors. Handb Clin Neurol. 119:209–22.
2182. Roeyen G, Van Schil P, Somville J, et al. (1999). Chordoma of the mediastinum. Eur J Surg Oncol. 25:224–5.
2183. Roggli VL (1981). Pericardial mesothelioma after exposure to asbestos. N Engl J Med. 304:1045.
2184. Rohani A, Akbari V (2010). A colossal atrial myxoma. J Cardiovasc Dis Res. 1:158–60.
2185. Rohr UP, Rehfeld N, Pflugfelder L, et al. (2004). Expression of the tyrosine kinase c-kit is an independent prognostic factor in patients with small cell lung cancer. Int J Cancer. 111:259–63.
2186. Roller MB, Manoharan A, Lvoff R (1991). Primary cardiac lymphoma. Acta Haematol. 85:47–8.
2187. Romanos-Sirakis EC, Meyer DB, Chun A, et al. (2010). A primary cardiac sarcoma with features of a desmoplastic small round cell tumor in an adolescent male. J Pediatr Hematol Oncol. 32:236–9.
2188. Roque L, Oliveira P, Martins C, et al. (1996). A nonbalanced translocation (10;16) demonstrated by FISH analysis in a case of alveolar adenoma of the lung. Cancer Genet Cytogenet. 89:34–7.
2189. Rosado-de-Christenson ML, Abbott GF, McAdams HP, et al. (2003). From the archives of the AFIP: Localized fibrous tumor of the pleura. Radiographics. 23:759–83.
2190. Rosado-de-Christenson ML, Pugatch RD, Moran CA, et al. (1994). Thymolipoma: analysis of 27 cases. Radiology. 193:121–6.
2191. Rosado-de-Christenson ML, Strollo DC, Marom EM (2008). Imaging of thymic epithelial neoplasms. Hematol Oncol Clin North Am. 22:409–31.
2192. Rosado-de-Christenson ML, Templeton PA, Moran CA (1992). From the archives of the AFIP. Mediastinal germ cell tumors: radiologic and pathologic correlation. Radiographics. 12:1013–30.
2193. Rosai J, Levine GD (1976). Tumours of the thymus. AFIP Atlas of tumour pathology. 2nd ed. Volume. 13. Washington, DC: American Registry of Pathology:.
2194. Roschewski M, Wilson WH (2012). Lymphomatoid granulomatosis. Cancer J. 18:469–74.
2195. Rose AG (1979). Venous malformations of the heart. Arch Pathol Lab Med. 103:18–20.
2196. Rosell R, Carcereny E, Gervais R, et al. (2012). Erlotinib versus standard chemotherapy as first-line treatment for European patients with advanced EGFR mutation-positive non-small-cell lung cancer (EURTAC): a multicentre, open-label, randomised phase 3 trial. Lancet Oncol. 13:239–46.
2197. Rosenbaum DG, Teruya-Feldstein J, Price AP, et al. (2012). Radiologic features of NUT midline carcinoma in an adolescent. Pediatr Radiol. 42:249–52.
2198. Rosenberg AS, Morgan MB (2001). Cutaneous indeterminate cell histiocytosis: a new spindle cell variant resembling dendritic cell sarcoma. J Cutan Pathol. 28:531–7.
2199. Rosenberger A, Bickeboller H, McCormack V, et al. (2012). Asthma and lung cancer risk: a systematic investigation by the International Lung Cancer Consortium. Carcinogenesis. 33:587–97.
2200. Rosenwald A, Wright G, Leroy K, et al. (2003). Molecular diagnosis of primary mediastinal B cell lymphoma identifies a clinically favorable subgroup of diffuse large B cell lymphoma related to Hodgkin lymphoma. J Exp Med. 198:851–62.
2201. Rossi G, Cadioli A, Mengoli MC, et al. (2012). Napsin A expression in pulmonary sclerosing haemangioma. Histopathology. 60:361–3.
2202. Rossi G, Cavazza A, Marchioni A, et al. (2005). Role of chemotherapy and the receptor tyrosine kinases KIT, PDGFRalpha, PDGFRbeta, and Met in large-cell neuroendocrine carcinoma of the lung. J Clin Oncol. 23:8774–85.
2203. Rossi G, Cavazza A, Sturm N, et al. (2003). Pulmonary carcinomas with pleomorphic, sarcomatoid, or sarcomatous elements: a clinicopathologic and immunohistochemical study of 75 cases. Am J Surg Pathol. 27:311–24.
2204. Rossi G, De Rosa N, Cavazza A, et al. (2013). Localized pleuropulmonary crystal-storing histiocytosis: 5 cases of a rare histiocytic disorder with variable clinicoradiologic features. Am J Surg Pathol. 37:906–12.
2205. Rossi G, Marchioni A, Milani M, et al. (2004). TTF-1, cytokeratin 7, 34betaE12, and CD56/NCAM immunostaining in the subclassification of large cell carcinomas of the lung. Am J Clin Pathol. 122:884–93.
2206. Rossi G, Mengoli MC, Cavazza A, et al. (2014). Large cell carcinoma of the lung: clinically oriented classification integrating immunohistochemistry and molecular biology. Virchows Arch. 464:61–8.
2207. Rossi G, Murer B, Cavazza A, et al. (2004). Primary mucinous (so-called colloid) carcinomas of the lung: a clinicopathologic and immunohistochemical study with special reference to CDX-2 homeobox gene and MUC2 expression. Am J Surg Pathol. 28:442–52.
2208. Rossi G, Papotti M, Barbareschi M, et al. (2009). Morphology and a limited number of immunohistochemical markers may efficiently subtype non-small-cell lung cancer. J Clin Oncol. 27:e141–2.
2209. Rossi V, Donini M, Sergio P, et al. (2013). When a thymic carcinoma "becomes" a GIST. Lung Cancer. 80:106–8.
2210. Rothenbuhler A, Stratakis CA (2010). Clinical and molecular genetics of Carney complex. Best Pract Res Clin Endocrinol Metab. 24:389–99.
2211. Rotstein DL, Bril V (2012). A family with myasthenia gravis with and without thymoma. Can J Neurol Sci. 39:539–40.
2212. Rousseaux S, Debernardi A, Jacquiau B, et al. (2013). Ectopic activation of germline and placental genes identifies aggressive metastasis-prone lung cancers. Sci Transl Med. 5: 186ra66.
2213. Rousselet MC, Francois S, Croue A, et al. (1994). A lymph node interdigitating reticulum cell sarcoma. Arch Pathol Lab Med. 118:183–8.
2214. Roux FJ, Lantuejoul S, Brambilla E, et al. (1995). Mucinous cystadenoma of the lung. Cancer. 76:1540–4.
2215. Rowsell C, Sirbovan J, Rosenblum MK, et al. (2005). Primary chordoid meningioma of lung. Virchows Arch. 446:333–7.
2216. Roy D, Sin SH, Damania B, et al. (2011). Tumor suppressor genes FHIT and WWOX are deleted in primary effusion lymphoma (PEL) cell lines. Blood. 118:e32–9.
2217. Ruan SY, Chen KY, Yang PC (2009). Recurrent respiratory papillomatosis with pulmonary involvement: a case report and review of the literature. Respirology. 14:137–40.
2218. Rubin MA, Snell JA, Tazelaar HD, et al. (1995). Cardiac papillary fibroelastoma: an immunohistochemical investigation and unusual clinical manifestations. Mod Pathol. 8:402–7.
2219. Rudin CM, Durinck S, Stawiski EW, et al. (2012). Comprehensive genomic analysis identifies SOX2 as a frequently amplified gene in small-cell lung cancer. Nat Genet. 44:1111–6.
2220. Rudnicka L, Papla B, Malinowski E (1998). Mature cystic teratoma of the mediastinum containing a carcinoid. A case report. Pol J Pathol. 49:309–12.
2221. Rudomina DE, Lin O, Moreira AL (2009). Cytologic diagnosis of pulmonary adenocarcinoma with micropapillary pattern: does it correlate with the histologic findings? Diagn Cytopathol. 37:333–9.
2222. Rusch V, Klimstra D, Linkov I, et al. (1995). Aberrant expression of p53 or the epidermal growth factor receptor is frequent in early bronchial neoplasia and coexpression precedes squamous cell carcinoma development. Cancer Res. 55:1365–72.
2223. Rusch VW (1995). A proposed new international TNM staging system for malignant pleural mesothelioma. From the International Mesothelioma Interest Group. Chest. 108:1122–8.
2224. Rusch VW (2012). Extrapleural pneumonectomy and extended pleurectomy/decortication for malignant pleural mesothelioma: the Memorial Sloan-Kettering Cancer Center approach. Ann Cardiothorac Surg. 1:523–31.
2225. Rusch VW, Asamura H, Watanabe H, et al. (2009). The IASLC lung cancer staging project: a proposal for a new international lymph node map in the forthcoming seventh edition of the TNM classification for lung cancer. J Thorac Oncol. 4: 568–577.
2226. Rusch VW, Giroux D (2012). Do we need a revised staging system for malignant pleural mesothelioma? Analysis of the IASLC database. Ann Cardiothorac Surg. 1:438–48.
2227. Rusch VW, Giroux D, Kennedy C, et al. (2012). Initial analysis of the international association for the study of lung cancer mesothelioma database. J Thorac Oncol. 7:1631–9.
2228. Rusch VW, Rimner A, Krug LM (2014). The challenge of malignant pleural mesothelioma: new directions. J Thorac Oncol. 9:271–2.
2229. Rush WL, Andriko JA, Galateau-Salle F, et al. (2000). Pulmonary pathology of Erdheim-Chester disease. Mod Pathol. 13:747–54.
2230. Rusner C, Trabert B, Katalinic A, et al. (2013). Incidence patterns and trends of malignant gonadal and extragonadal germ cell tumors in Germany, 1998-2008. Cancer Epidemiol. 37:370–3.
2231. Russell PA, Barnett SA, Walkiewicz M, et al. (2013). Correlation of mutation status and survival with predominant histologic subtype according to the new IASLC/ATS/ERS lung adenocarcinoma classification in stage III (N2) patients. J Thorac Oncol. 8:461–8.
2232. Russell PA, Wainer Z, Wright GM, et al. (2011). Does lung adenocarcinoma subtype predict patient survival?: A clinicopathologic study based on the new International Association for the Study of Lung Cancer/American Thoracic Society/European Respiratory Society international multidisciplinary lung adenocarcinoma classification. J Thorac Oncol. 6:1496–504.
2233. Ruszkiewicz AR, Vernon-Roberts E (1995). Sudden death in an infant due to histiocytoid cardiomyopathy. A light-microscopic, ultrastructural, and immunohistochemical study. Am J Forensic Med Pathol. 16:74–80.
2234. Ryan PE Jr, Obeid AI, Parker FB Jr (1995). Primary cardiac valve tumors. J Heart Valve Dis. 4:222–6.
2235. Ryman NG, Burrow L, Bowen C, et al. (2005). Good's syndrome with primary intrapulmonary thymoma. J R Soc Med. 98:119–20.
2236. Ryu HS, Koh JS, Park S, et al. (2012). Classification of thymoma by fine needle aspiration biopsy according to WHO classification: a cytological algorithm for stepwise analysis in the classification of thymoma. Acta Cytol. 56:487–94.
2237. Ryu JH, Sykes AM, Lee AS, et al. (2012). Cystic lung disease is not uncommon in men with tuberous sclerosis complex. Respir Med. 106:1586–90.
2238. Ryu YJ, Yoo SH, Jung MJ, et al. (2013). Embryonal rhabdomyosarcoma arising from a mediastinal teratoma: an unusual case report. J Korean Med Sci. 28:476–9.
2239. Saarinen S, Kaasinen E, Karjalainen-Lindsberg ML, et al. (2013). Primary mediastinal large B-cell lymphoma segregating in a family: exome sequencing identifies MLL as a candidate predisposition gene. Blood. 121:3428–30.
2240. Saccomanno G, Archer VE, Auerbach O, et al. (1974). Development of carcinoma of the lung as reflected in exfoliated cells. Cancer. 33:256–70.
2241. Saccomanno G, Saunders RP, Archer VE, et al. (1965). Cancer of the lung: the cytology of sputum prior to the development of carcinoma. Acta Cytol. 9:413–23.
2242. Sada E, Shiratsuchi M, Kiyasu J, et al. (2009). Primary mediastinal non-seminomatous germ cell tumor associated with hemophagocytic syndrome. J Clin Exp Hematop. 49:117–20.
2243. Sahm F, Capper D, Preusser M, et al.

(2012). BRAFV600E mutant protein is expressed in cells of variable maturation in Langerhans cell histiocytosis. Blood. 120:e28–34.
2244. Said JW, Shintaku IP, Asou H, et al. (1999). Herpesvirus 8 inclusions in primary effusion lymphoma: report of a unique case with T-cell phenotype. Arch Pathol Lab Med. 123:257–60.
2246. Saito A, Watanabe K, Kusakabe T, et al. (1998). Mediastinal mature teratoma with coexistence of angiosarcoma, granulocytic sarcoma and a hematopoietic region in the tumor: a rare case of association between hematological malignancy and mediastinal germ cell tumor. Pathol Int. 48:749–53.
2247. Saito T, Kimoto M, Nakai S, et al. (2011). Ectopic ACTH syndrome associated with large cell neuroendocrine carcinoma of the thymus. Intern Med. 50:1471–5.
2248. Saitoh Y, Ohsako M, Umemoto M, et al. (1995). [A case of primary mediastinal teratocarcinoma in a young girl]. Nihon Kyobu Geka Gakkai Zasshi. 43:104–8.
2249. Sak SD, Koseoglu RD, Demirag F, et al. (2007). Alveolar adenoma of the lung. Immunohistochemical and flow cytometric characteristics of two new cases and a review of the literature. APMIS. 115:1443–9.
2250. Sakaeda M, Sato H, Ishii J, et al. (2013). Neural lineage-specific homeoprotein BRN2 is directly involved in TTF1 expression in small-cell lung cancer. Lab Invest. 93:408–21.
2251. Sakaguchi M, Minato N, Katayama Y, et al. (2006). Cardiac angiosarcoma with right atrial perforation and cardiac tamponade. Ann Thorac Cardiovasc Surg. 12:145–8.
2252. Sakakibara S, Tosato G (2011). Viral interleukin-6: role in Kaposi's sarcoma-associated herpesvirus: associated malignancies. J Interferon Cytokine Res. 31:791–801.
2253. Sakakura N, Tateyama H, Nakamura S, et al. (2013). Diagnostic reproducibility of thymic epithelial tumors using the World Health Organization classification: note for thoracic clinicians. Gen Thorac Cardiovasc Surg. 61:89–95.
2254. Sakakura N, Tateyama H, Usami N, et al. (2010). Thymic basaloid carcinoma with pleural dissemination that developed after a curative resection: report of a case. Surg Today. 40:1073–8.
2255. Sakamoto H, Sakamaki T, Sumino H, et al. (2004). Production of endothelin-1 and big endothelin-1 by human cardiac myxoma cells--implications of the origin of myxomas--. Circ J. 68:1230–2.
2256. Sakamoto H, Shimizu J, Horio Y, et al. (2007). Disproportionate representation of KRAS gene mutation in atypical adenomatous hyperplasia, but even distribution of EGFR gene mutation from preinvasive to invasive adenocarcinomas. J Pathol. 212:287–94.
2257. Sakamoto I, Tomiyama N, Sugita A, et al. (2004). A case of sclerosing hemangioma surrounded by emphysematous change. Radiat Med. 22:123–5.
2258. Sakurai A, Imai T, Kikumori T, et al. (2013). Thymic neuroendocrine tumour in multiple endocrine neoplasia type 1: female patients are not rare exceptions. Clin Endocrinol (Oxf). 78:248–54.
2259. Sakurai A, Tomii K, Haruna A, et al. (2011). [Two cases of successfully treated intravascular lymphoma presenting with fever and dyspnea]. Nihon Kokyuki Gakkai Zasshi. 49:743–9.
2260. Sakurai H, Hasegawa T, Watanabe S, et al. (2004). Inflammatory myofibroblastic tumor of the lung. Eur J Cardiothorac Surg. 25:155–9.
2261. Sakurai H, Miyashita Y, Oyama T (2008). Adenocarcinoma arising in anterior mediastinal mature cystic teratoma: report of a case. Surg Today. 38:348–51.
2261A. Sale GF, Kulander BG. Benign clear cell tumor of lung with necrosis. Cancer. 1976 May;37(5):2355-8.
2262. Sales LM, Vontz FK (1970). Teratoma and Di Guglielmo syndrome. South Med J. 63:448–50.
2263. Salon C, Merdzhanova G, Brambilla C, et al. (2007). E2F-1, Skp2 and cyclin E oncoproteins are upregulated and directly correlated in high-grade neuroendocrine lung tumors. Oncogene. 26:6927–36.
2264. Salon C, Moro D, Lantuejoul S, et al. (2004). E-cadherin-beta-catenin adhesion complex in neuroendocrine tumors of the lung: a suggested role upon local invasion and metastasis. Hum Pathol. 35:1148–55.
2265. Sambrook Gowar FJ (1978). An unusual mucous cyst of the lung. Thorax. 33:796–9.
2266. Sanchez-Mora N, Parra-Blanco V, Cebollero-Presmanes M, et al. (2007). Mucoepidermoid tumors of the bronchus. Ultrastructural and immunohistochemical study. Histiogenic correlations. Histol Histopathol. 22:9–13.
2267. Sandberg AA, Bridge JA (2002). Updates on the cytogenetics and molecular genetics of bone and soft tissue tumors. Synovial sarcoma. Cancer Genet Cytogenet. 133:1–23.
2268. Sandberg AA, Bridge JA (2002). Updates on the cytogenetics and molecular genetics of bone and soft tissue tumors: congenital (infantile) fibrosarcoma and mesoblastic nephroma. Cancer Genet Cytogenet. 132:1–13.
2269. Sander CA, Medeiros LJ, Weiss LM, et al. (1992). Lymphoproliferative lesions in patients with common variable immunodeficiency syndrome. Am J Surg Pathol. 16:1170–82.
2270. Sane AC, Roggli VL (1995). Curative resection of a well-differentiated papillary mesothelioma of the pericardium. Arch Pathol Lab Med. 119:266–7.
2271. Santagata S, Ligon KL, Hornick JL (2007). Embryonic stem cell transcription factor signatures in the diagnosis of primary and metastatic germ cell tumors. Am J Surg Pathol. 31:836–45.
2272. Santana O, Vivas PH, Ramos A, et al. (1993). Multiple myeloma involving the pericardium associated with cardiac tamponade and constrictive pericarditis. Am Heart J. 126:737–40.
2273. Santangeli P, Pieroni M, Marzo F, et al. (2010). Cardiac myxoma presenting with sensory neuropathy. Int J Cardiol. 143:e14–6.
2274. Santos C, Montesinos J, Castaner E, et al. (2008). Primary pericardial mesothelioma. Lung Cancer. 60:291–3.
2275. Saqi A, Alexis D, Remotti F, et al. (2005). Usefulness of CDX2 and TTF-1 in differentiating gastrointestinal from pulmonary carcinoids. Am J Clin Pathol. 123:394–404.
2276. Sardari Nia P, Colpaert C, Vermeulen P, et al. (2008). Different growth patterns of non-small cell lung cancer represent distinct biologic subtypes. Ann Thorac Surg. 85:395–405.
2277. Sardari Nia P, Van Loo S, Weyler J, et al. (2010). Prognostic value of a biologic classification of non-small-cell lung cancer into the growth patterns along with other clinical, pathological and immunohistochemical factors. Eur J Cardiothorac Surg. 38:628–36.
2278. Sarkaria IS, Bains MS, Sood S, et al. (2011). Resection of primary mediastinal non-seminomatous germ cell tumors: a 28-year experience at memorial sloan-kettering cancer center. J Thorac Oncol. 6:1236–41.
2279. Sarkaria IS, DeLair D, Travis WD, et al. (2011). Primary myoepithelial carcinoma of the lung: a rare entity treated with parenchymal sparing resection. J Cardiothorac Surg. 6:27.
2280. Sarraj A, Duarte J, Dominguez L, et al. (2007). Resection of metastatic pulmonary lesion of ossifying fibromyxoid tumor extending into the left atrium and ventricle via pulmonary vein. Eur J Echocardiogr. 8:384–6.
2281. Sasajima Y, Yamabe H, Kobashi Y, et al. (1993). High expression of the Epstein-Barr virus latent protein EB nuclear antigen-2 on pyothorax-associated lymphomas. Am J Pathol. 143:1280–5.
2282. Satish OS, Aditya MS, Rao MA, et al. (2013). Sporadic cardiac myxoma involving all the cardiac chambers. Circulation. 127:e360–1.
2283. Satoh Y, Ishikawa Y (2010). Primary pulmonary meningioma: Ten-year follow-up findings for a multiple case, implying a benign biological nature. J Thorac Cardiovasc Surg. 139:e39–40.
2284. Satoh Y, Tsuchiya E, Weng SY, et al. (1989). Pulmonary sclerosing hemangioma of the lung. A type II pneumocytoma by immunohistochemical and immunoelectron microscopic studies. Cancer. 64:1310–7.
2285. Savage KJ, Harris NL, Vose JM, et al. (2008). ALK- anaplastic large-cell lymphoma is clinically and immunophenotypically different from both ALK+ ALCL and peripheral T-cell lymphoma, not otherwise specified: report from the International Peripheral T-Cell Lymphoma Project. Blood. 111:5496–504.
2286. Savage KJ, Monti S, Kutok JL, et al. (2003). The molecular signature of mediastinal large B-cell lymphoma differs from that of other diffuse large B-cell lymphomas and shares features with classical Hodgkin lymphoma. Blood. 102:3871–9.
2287. Savci-Heijink CD, Kosari F, Aubry MC, et al. (2009). The role of desmoglein-3 in the diagnosis of squamous cell carcinoma of the lung. Am J Pathol. 174:1629–37.
2288. Sawai T, Inoue Y, Doi S, et al. (2006). Tubular adenocarcinoma of the thymus: case report and review of the literature. Int J Surg Pathol. 14:243–6.
2289. Saygin C, Uzunaslan D, Ozguroglu M, et al. (2013). Dendritic cell sarcoma: a pooled analysis including 462 cases with presentation of our case series. Crit Rev Oncol Hematol. 88:253–71.
2290. Scagliotti GV, Parikh P, von Pawel J, et al. (2008). Phase III study comparing cisplatin plus gemcitabine with cisplatin plus pemetrexed in chemotherapy-naive patients with advanced-stage non-small-cell lung cancer. J Clin Oncol. 26:3543–51.
2291. Scanlan D, Radio SJ, Nelson M, et al. (2008). Loss of the PTCH1 gene locus in cardiac fibroma. Cardiovasc Pathol. 17:93–7.
2292. Schaefer IM, Sahlmann CO, Overbeck T, et al. (2012). Blastomatoid pulmonary carcinosarcoma: report of a case with a review of the literature. BMC Cancer. 12:424.
2293. Schaefer IM, Zardo P, Freermann S, et al. (2013). Neuroendocrine carcinoma in a mediastinal teratoma as a rare variant of somatic-type malignancy. Virchows Arch. 463:731–5.
2294. Scherpereel A, Astoul P, Baas P, et al. (2010). Guidelines of the European Respiratory Society and the European Society of Thoracic Surgeons for the management of malignant pleural mesothelioma. Eur Respir J. 35:479–95.
2295. Schimke RN, Madigan CM, Silver BJ, et al. (1983). Choriocarcinoma, thyrotoxicosis, and the Klinefelter syndrome. Cancer Genet Cytogenet. 9:1–7.
2296. Schirosi L, Nannini N, Nicoli D, et al. (2012). Activating c-KIT mutations in a subset of thymic carcinoma and response to different c-KIT inhibitors. Ann Oncol. 23:2409–14.
2297. Schlick TL, Ding Z, Kovacs EW, et al. (2005). Dual-surface modification of the tobacco mosaic virus. J Am Chem Soc. 127:3718–23.
2298. Schmidt LA, Myers JL, McHugh JB (2012). Napsin A is differentially expressed in sclerosing hemangiomas of the lung. Arch Pathol Lab Med. 136:1580–4.
2299. Schmitz L, Favara BE (1998). Nosology and pathology of Langerhans cell histiocytosis. Hematol Oncol Clin North Am. 12:221–46.
2300. Schmitz R, Hansmann ML, Bohle V, et al. (2009). TNFAIP3 (A20) is a tumor suppressor gene in Hodgkin lymphoma and primary mediastinal B cell lymphoma. J Exp Med. 206:981–9.
2301. Schneider DT, Calaminus G, Koch S, et al. (2004). Epidemiologic analysis of 1,442 children and adolescents registered in the German germ cell tumor protocols. Pediatr Blood Cancer. 42:169–75.
2302. Schneider DT, Calaminus G, Reinhard H, et al. (2000). Primary mediastinal germ cell tumors in children and adolescents: results of the German cooperative protocols MAKEI 83/86, 89, and 96. J Clin Oncol. 18:832–9.
2303. Schneider DT, Schuster AE, Fritsch MK, et al. (2002). Genetic analysis of mediastinal nonseminomatous germ cell tumors in children and adolescents. Genes Chromosomes Cancer. 34:115–25.
2304. Schneider DT, Schuster AE, Fritsch MK, et al. (2001). Multipoint imprinting analysis indicates a common precursor cell for gonadal and nongonadal pediatric germ cell tumors. Cancer Res. 61:7268–76.
2305. Schonfeld N, Dirks K, Costabel U, et al. (2012). A prospective clinical multicentre study on adult pulmonary Langerhans' cell histiocytosis. Sarcoidosis Vasc Diffuse Lung Dis. 29:132–8.
2305A. Schoolmeester JK, Dao LN, Sukov WR, et al. (2015). TFE3 Translocation-associated Perivascular Epithelioid Cell Neoplasm (PEComa) of the Gynecologic Tract: Morphology, Immunophenotype, Differential Diagnosis. Am J Surg Pathol. Forthcoming.
2306. Schoolmeester JK, Sukov WR, Maleszewski JJ, et al. (2013). JAZF1 rearrangement in a mesenchymal tumor of nonendometrial stromal origin: report of an unusual ossifying sarcoma of the heart demonstrating JAZF1/PHF1 fusion. Am J Surg Pathol. 37:938–42.
2307. Schrader KA, Nelson TN, De Luca A, et al. (2009). Multiple granular cell tumors are an associated feature of LEOPARD syndrome caused by mutation in PTPN11. Clin Genet. 75:185–9.
2308. Schuborg C, Mertens F, Rydholm A, et al. (1998). Cytogenetic analysis of four angiosarcomas from deep and superficial soft tissue. Cancer Genet Cytogenet. 100:52–6.
2309. Schuerfeld K, Lazzi S, De Santi MM, et al. (2003). Cytokeratin-positive interstitial cell neoplasm: a case report and classification issues. Histopathology. 43:491–4.
2310. Schuller HM, Jull BA, Sheppard BJ, et al. (2000). Interaction of tobacco-specific toxicants with the neuronal alpha(7) nicotinic acetylcholine receptor and its associated mitogenic signal transduction pathway: potential role in lung carcinogenesis and pediatric lung disorders. Eur J Pharmacol. 393:265–77.
2311. Schulter G (1977). [Effects of conditions of learning and retrieval on recognition memory performance (author's transl)]. Arch Psychol (Frankf). 129:99–109.
2312. Schultz KA, Pacheco MC, Yang J, et al. (2011). Ovarian sex cord-stromal tumors, pleuropulmonary blastoma and DICER1 mutations: a report from the International Pleuropulmonary Blastoma Registry. Gynecol Oncol. 122:246–50.
2313. Schumann C, Kunze M, Kochs M, et al. (2007). Pericardial synovial sarcoma mimicking pericarditis in findings of cardiac magnetic resonance imaging. Int J Cardiol. 118:e83–4.
2314. Schwabe J, Calaminus G, Vorhoff W, et al. (2002). Sexual precocity and recurrent beta-human chorionic gonadotropin upsurges preceding the diagnosis of a malignant mediastinal germ-cell tumor in a 9-year-old boy. Ann Oncol. 13:975–7.
2315. Schwartz BE, Hofer MD, Lemieux ME, et al. (2011). Differentiation of NUT midline carcinoma by epigenomic reprogramming. Cancer Res. 71:2686–96.
2316. Schweigert M, Meyer C, Wolf F, et al. (2011). Peripheral primitive neuroectodermal tumor of the thymus. Interact Cardiovasc Thorac Surg. 12:303–5.
2317. Sciamanna MA, Griesmann GE, Lennon VA (1998). A small cell lung carcinoma line and subclone expressing nicotinic acetylcholine receptors of muscle and neuronal types. Ann N Y Acad Sci. 841:655–8.
2318. Scolyer RA, Thompson JF (2007). Primary melanoma of the lung. Am Surg. 73:937–8.
2319. Segletes LA, Steffee CH, Geisinger KR (1999). Cytology of primary pulmonary

mucoepidermoid and adenoid cystic carcinoma. A report of four cases. Acta Cytol. 43:1091–7.
2320. Seidel D, Zander T, Heukamp LC et al. Clinical Lung Cancer Genome Project (CLCGP) (2013). A genomics-based classification of human lung tumors. Sci Transl Med. 5: 209ra153
2321. Seidemann K, Tiemann M, Schrappe M, et al. (2001). Short-pulse B-non-Hodgkin lymphoma-type chemotherapy is efficacious treatment for pediatric anaplastic large cell lymphoma: a report of the Berlin-Frankfurt-Munster Group Trial NHL-BFM 90. Blood. 97:3699–706.
2322. Sekido Y (2010). Genomic abnormalities and signal transduction dysregulation in malignant mesothelioma cells. Cancer Sci. 101:1–6.
2323. Sekido Y (2011). Inactivation of Merlin in malignant mesothelioma cells and the Hippo signaling cascade dysregulation. Pathol Int. 61:331–44.
2324. Sekido Y, Pass HI, Bader S, et al. (1995). Neurofibromatosis type 2 (NF2) gene is somatically mutated in mesothelioma but not in lung cancer. Cancer Res. 55:1227–31.
2325. Sekimizu M, Sunami S, Nakazawa A, et al. (2011). Chromosome abnormalities in advanced stage T-cell lymphoblastic lymphoma of children and adolescents: a report from Japanese Paediatric Leukaemia/Lymphoma Study Group (JPLSG) and review of the literature. Br J Haematol. 154:612–7.
2326. Sekine S, Shibata T, Matsuno Y, et al. (2003). Beta-catenin mutations in pulmonary blastomas: association with morule formation. J Pathol. 200:214–21.
2327. Selice R, Di Mambro A, Garolla A, et al. (2010). Spermatogenesis in Klinefelter syndrome. J Endocrinol Invest. 33:789–93.
2328. Sensaki K, Aida S, Takagi K, et al. (1993). Coexisting undifferentiated thymic carcinoma and thymic carcinoid tumor. Respiration. 60:247–9.
2329. Seo JB, Im JG, Goo JM, et al. (2001). Atypical pulmonary metastases: spectrum of radiologic findings. Radiographics. 21:403–17.
2330. Seo T, Ando H, Watanabe Y, et al. (1999). Acute respiratory failure associated with intrathoracic masses in neonates. J Pediatr Surg. 34:1633–7.
2331. Seol SH, Kim DI, Jang JS, et al. (2014). Left atrial myxoma presenting as paroxysmal supraventricular tachycardia. Heart Lung Circ. 23:e65–6.
2332. Sequist LV, Waltman BA, Dias-Santagata D, et al. (2011). Genotypic and histological evolution of lung cancers acquiring resistance to EGFR inhibitors. Sci Transl Med. 3:75ra26.
2333. Serezhin BS, Stepanov MI (1990). [A carcinoid tumor in a mature thymic teratoma]. Arkh Patol. 52:59–62.
2334. Seto T, Kiura K, Nishio M, et al. (2013). CH5424802 (RO5424802) for patients with ALK-rearranged advanced non-small-cell lung cancer (AF-001JP study): a single-arm, open-label, phase 1-2 study. Lancet Oncol. 14:590–8.
2335. Sevimli S, Erkut B, Becit N, et al. (2007). Primary benign schwannoma of the left ventricle coursing under the left anterior descending artery. Echocardiography. 24:1093–5.
2336. Shaffer K, Pugatch RD, Sugarbaker DJ (1990). Primary mediastinal leiomyoma. Ann Thorac Surg. 50:301–2.
2337. Shah KV (2007). SV40 and human cancer: a review of recent data. Int J Cancer. 120:215–23.
2338. Shahani L, Beckmann M, Vallurupalli S (2011). Cardiac angiosarcoma-associated membranoproliferative glomerulonephropathy. Case Rep Med. 2011:956089.
2339. Shaher RM, Mintzer J, Farina M, et al. (1972). Clinical presentation of rhabdomyoma of the heart in infancy and childhood. Am J Cardiol. 30:95–103.
2340. Shalini CS, Joseph LD, Abraham G, et al. (2009). Cytologic features of pulmonary blastoma. J Cytol. 26:74–6.
2341. Shames DS, Wistuba II (2014). The evolving genomic classification of lung cancer. J Pathol. 232:121–33.
2342. Shanks JH, Harris M, Banerjee SS, et al. (2000). Mesotheliomas with deciduoid morphology: a morphologic spectrum and a variant not confined to young females. Am J Surg Pathol. 24:285–94.
2343. Shao ZY, Massiani MA, Bazelly B, et al. (2003). [Intrapulmonary rupture of a dermoid cyst: MRI findings]. Rev Pneumol Clin. 59:311–6.
2344. Shapiro B, Sisson J, Kalff V, et al. (1984). The location of middle mediastinal pheochromocytomas. J Thorac Cardiovasc Surg. 87:814–20.
2345. Sharpless SM, Das Gupta TK (1998). Surgery for metastatic melanoma. Semin Surg Oncol. 14:311–8.
2346. Shaw AT, Hsu PP, Awad MM, et al. (2013). Tyrosine kinase gene rearrangements in epithelial malignancies. Nat Rev Cancer. 13:772–87.
2347. Shaw AT, Kim DW, Mehra R, et al. (2014). Ceritinib in ALK-rearranged non-small-cell lung cancer. N Engl J Med. 370:1189–97.
2348. Shaw AT, Solomon B, Kenudson MM (2011). Crizotinib and testing for ALK. J Natl Compr Canc Netw. 9:1335–41.
2349. Shaw AT, Yeap BY, Solomon BJ, et al. (2011). Effect of crizotinib on overall survival in patients with advanced non-small-cell lung cancer harbouring ALK gene rearrangement: a retrospective analysis. Lancet Oncol. 12:1004–12.
2350. Shebib S, Sabbah RS, Sackey K, et al. (1989). Endodermal sinus (yolk sac) tumor in infants and children. A clinical and pathologic study: an 11 year review. Am J Pediatr Hematol Oncol. 11:36–9.
2351. Shehata BM, Bouzyk M, Shulman SC, et al. (2011). Identification of candidate genes for histiocytoid cardiomyopathy (HC) using whole genome expression analysis: analyzing material from the HC registry. Pediatr Dev Pathol. 14:370–7.
2351A Shehata BM, Cundiff CA, Lee K, et al. (2015). Exome sequencing of patients with histiocytoid cardiomyopathy reveals a de novo NDUFB11 mutation that plays a role in the pathogenesis of histiocytoid cardiomyopathy. Am J Med Genet A. 167A:2114-2121
2352. Shehata BM, Patterson K, Thomas JE, et al. (1998). Histiocytoid cardiomyopathy: three new cases and a review of the literature. Pediatr Dev Pathol. 1:56–69.
2353. Shehata BM, Steelman CK, Abramowsky CR, et al. (2010). NUT midline carcinoma in a newborn with multiorgan disseminated tumor and a 2-year-old with a pancreatic/hepatic primary. Pediatr Dev Pathol. 13:481–5.
2354. Sheibani K, Winberg CD, Burke JS, et al. (1987). Lymphoblastic lymphoma expressing natural killer cell-associated antigens: a clinicopathologic study of six cases. Leuk Res. 11:371–7.
2355. Shenoy SS, Barua NR, Patel AR, et al. (1978). Mediastinal lymphangioma. J Surg Oncol. 10:523–8.
2356. Shepherd FA, Crowley J, van Houtte P, et al. (2007). The International Association for the Study of Lung Cancer lung cancer staging project: proposals regarding the clinical staging of small cell lung cancer in the forthcoming (seventh) edition of the tumor, node, metastasis classification for lung cancer. J Thorac Oncol. 2:1067–77.
2357. Sheppard MN, Burke L, Kennedy M (2003). TTF-1 is useful in the diagnosis of pulmonary papillary adenoma. Histopathology. 43:404–5.
2358. Sheridan T, Herawi M, Epstein JI, et al. (2007). The role of P501S and PSA in the diagnosis of metastatic adenocarcinoma of the prostate. Am J Surg Pathol. 31:1351–5.
2360. Shetty Roy AN, Radin M, Sarabi D, et al. (2011). Familial recurrent atrial myxoma: Carney's complex. Clin Cardiol. 34:83–6.
2361. Shia J, Qin J, Erlandson RA, et al. (2005). Malignant mesothelioma with a pronounced myxoid stroma: a clinical and pathological evaluation of 19 cases. Virchows Arch. 447:828–34.
2362. Shibuya K, Nakajima T, Fujiwara T, et al. (2010). Narrow band imaging with high-resolution bronchovideoscopy: a new approach for visualizing angiogenesis in squamous cell carcinoma of the lung. Lung Cancer. 69:194–202.
2363. Shields TW, LoCicero J, Reed CE, et al. (2009). General Thoracic Surgery. 7th ed. Philadelphia: Lippincott Williams & Wilkins.
2364. Shigematsu H, Lin L, Takahashi T, et al. (2005). Clinical and biological features associated with epidermal growth factor receptor gene mutations in lung cancers. J Natl Cancer Inst. 97:339–46.
2365. Shih WJ, McCullough S, Smith M (1993). Diagnostic imagings for primary cardiac fibrosarcoma. Int J Cardiol. 39:157–61.
2366. Shilo K, Foss RD, Franks TJ, et al. (2005). Pulmonary mucoepidermoid carcinoma with prominent tumor-associated lymphoid proliferation. Am J Surg Pathol. 29:407–11.
2367. Shilo K, Miettinen M, Travis WD, et al. (2006). Pulmonary microcystic fibromyxoma: Report of 3 cases. Am J Surg Pathol. 30:1432–5.
2368. Shimada H, Ambros IM, Dehner LP, et al. (1999). The International Neuroblastoma Pathology Classification (the Shimada system). Cancer. 86:364–72.
2369. Shimazaki H, Aida S, Sato M, et al. (2001). Lung carcinoma with rhabdoid cells: a clinicopathological study and survival analysis of 14 cases. Histopathology. 38:425–34.
2370. Shimizu J, Hayashi Y, Morita K, et al. (1994). Primary thymic carcinoma: a clinicopathological and immunohistochemical study. J Surg Oncol. 56:159–64.
2371. Shimizu J, Oda M, Hayashi Y, et al. (1996). A clinicopathologic study of resected cases of adenosquamous carcinoma of the lung. Chest. 109:989–94.
2372. Shimizu K, Ishii G, Nagai K, et al. (2005). Extranodal marginal zone B-cell lymphoma of mucosa-associated lymphoid tissue (MALT lymphoma) in the thymus: report of four cases. Jpn J Clin Oncol. 35:412–6.
2373. Shimizu K, Yoshida J, Kakegawa S, et al. (2010). Primary thymic mucosa-associated lymphoid tissue lymphoma: diagnostic tips. J Thorac Oncol. 5:117–21.
2374. Shimmyo T, Ando K, Mochizuki A, et al. (2014). A Resected Melanoma of the Lung Metastasized from an Occult Skin Lesion: A Case Report. Ann Thorac Cardiovasc Surg. 20 Suppl:554-7.
2375. Shimosato Y, Kameya T, Nagai K, et al. (1977). Squamous cell carcinoma of the thymus. An analysis of eight cases. Am J Surg Pathol. 1:109–21.
2376. Shimosato Y, Mukai K (1997). Tumors of the Mediastinum. AFIP Atlas of tumour pathology. 3rd Edition. Washington: American Registry of Pathology.
2377. Shimosato Y, Mukai K, Matsuno Y (2010). Tumors of the Mediastinum. AFIP Atlas of Tumor Pathology. 4th ed. Volume 11. Washington, DC: American Registry of Pathology.
2378. Shimosato Y, Suzuki A, Hashimoto T, et al. (1980). Prognostic implications of fibrotic focus (scar) in small peripheral lung cancers. Am J Surg Pathol. 4:365–73.
2379. Shin BK, Kim MK, Park SH, et al. (2001). Fine-needle aspiration cytology of pleuropulmonary blastoma: a case report with unusual features. Diagn Cytopathol. 25:397–402.
2380. Shingyoji M, Ikebe D, Itakura M, et al. (2013). Pulmonary artery sarcoma diagnosed by endobronchial ultrasound-guided transbronchial needle aspiration. Ann Thorac Surg. 96:e33–5.
2381. Shinoda H, Yoshida A, Teruya-Feldstein J (2009). Malignant histiocytoses/disseminated histiocytic sarcoma with hemophagocytic syndrome in a patient with mediastinal germ cell tumor. Appl Immunohistochem Mol Morphol. 17:338–44.
2382. Shiozawa T, Ishii G, Goto K, et al. (2013). Clinicopathological characteristics of EGFR mutated adenosquamous carcinoma of the lung. Pathol Int. 63:77–84.
2383. Shoji T, Fushimi H, Takeda S, et al. (2011). Thymic large-cell neuroendocrine carcinoma: a disease neglected in the ESMO guideline? Ann Oncol. 22:2535.
2384. Sholl LM, Yeap BY, Iafrate AJ, et al. (2009). Lung adenocarcinoma with EGFR amplification has distinct clinicopathologic and molecular features in never-smokers. Cancer Res. 69:8341–8.
2385. Shuhaiber J, Cabrera J, Nemeh H (2007). Treatment of a case of primary osteosarcoma of the left heart: a case report. Heart Surg Forum. 10:E30–2.
2386. Sibon D, Fournier M, Briere J, et al. (2012). Long-term outcome of adults with systemic anaplastic large-cell lymphoma treated within the Groupe d'Etude des Lymphomes de l'Adulte trials. J Clin Oncol. 30:3939–46.
2387. Sica G, Wagner PL, Altorki N, et al. (2008). Immunohistochemical expression of estrogen and progesterone receptors in primary pulmonary neuroendocrine tumors. Arch Pathol Lab Med. 132:1889–95.
2388. Sica G, Yoshizawa A, Sima CS, et al. (2010). A grading system of lung adenocarcinomas based on histologic pattern is predictive of disease recurrence in stage I tumors. Am J Surg Pathol. 34:1155–62.
2389. Sickles EA, Belliveau RE, Wiernik PH (1974). Primary mediastinal choriocarcinoma in the male. Cancer. 33:1196–203.
2390. Siddiqui FA, Jain A, Maheshwari V, et al. (2010). FNA diagnosis of teratoma lung: A case report. Diagn Cytopathol. 38:758–60.
2391. Siddiqui MT (2010). Pulmonary neuroendocrine neoplasms: a review of clinicopathologic and cytologic features. Diagn Cytopathol. 38:607–17.
2392. Sidhu JS, Nicolas MM, Taylor W (2002). Mediastinal rhabdomyoma: a case report and review of the literature. Int J Surg Pathol. 10:313–8.
2393. Siegal GP, Dehner LP, Rosai J (1985). Histiocytosis X (Langerhans' cell granulomatosis) of the thymus. A clinicopathologic study of four childhood cases. Am J Surg Pathol. 9:117–24.
2394. Siegel RJ, Bueso-Ramos C, Cohen C, et al. (1991). Pulmonary blastoma with germ cell (yolk sac) differentiation: report of two cases. Mod Pathol. 4:566–70.
2395. Sievers S, Alemazkour K, Zahn S, et al. (2005). IGF2/H19 imprinting analysis of human germ cell tumors (GCTs) using the methylation-sensitive single-nucleotide primer extension method reflects the origin of GCTs in different stages of primordial germ cell development. Genes Chromosomes Cancer. 44:256–64.
2396. Sigel CS, Rudomina DE, Sima CS, et al. (2012). Predicting pulmonary adenocarcinoma outcome based on a cytology grading system. Cancer Cytopathol. 120:35–43.
2397. Sigurjonsson H, Andersen K, Gardarsdottir M, et al. (2011). Cardiac myxoma in Iceland: a case series with an estimation of population incidence. APMIS. 119:611–7.
2398. Silverman JF, Geisinger KR (1996). Fine needle aspiration cytology of the thorax and abdomen. New York: Churchill Livingstone.
2399. Silvestri GA, Gonzalez AV, Jantz MA, et al. (2013). Methods for staging non-small cell lung cancer: Diagnosis and management of lung cancer, 3rd ed: American College of Chest Physicians evidence-based clinical practice guidelines. Chest. 143:e211S–e250S.
2400. Simonelli C, Spina M, Cinelli R, et al. (2003). Clinical features and outcome of primary effusion lymphoma in HIV-infected patients: a single-institution study. J Clin Oncol. 21:3948–54.
2401. Simpson L, Kumar SK, Okuno SH, et al. (2008). Malignant primary cardiac tumors: review of a single institution experience. Cancer. 112:2440–6.
2402. Sinke RJ, van Asseldonk M, de Bruijn D,

et al. (1998). Towards the isolation of a human malignant extragonadal germ cell tumour-associated breakpoint in chromosome 11q13. APMIS. 106:73–8.
2403. Sinke RJ, Weghuis DO, Suijkerbuijk RF, et al. (1994). Molecular characterization of a recurring complex chromosomal translocation in two human extragonadal germ cell tumors. Cancer Genet Cytogenet. 73:11–6.
2404. Sirotkina M, Iwarsson E, Marnerides A, et al. (2012). Fetal mediastinal tumor of neuroepithelial origin in a case of missed abortion. Pediatr Dev Pathol. 15:511–3.
2405. Sirvent N, Coindre JM, Maire G, et al. (2007). Detection of MDM2-CDK4 amplification by fluorescence in situ hybridization in 200 paraffin-embedded tumor samples: utility in diagnosing adipocytic lesions and comparison with immunohistochemistry and real-time PCR. Am J Surg Pathol. 31:1476–89.
2406. Skalidis EI, Parthenakis FI, Zacharis EA, et al. (1999). Pulmonary tumor embolism from primary cardiac B-cell lymphoma. Chest. 116:1489–90.
2407. Skillington PD, Brawn WJ, Edis BD, et al. (1987). Surgical excision of primary cardiac tumours in infancy. Aust N Z J Surg. 57:599–604.
2408. Skodt V, Jacobsen GK, Helsted M (1995). Primary paraganglioma of the lung. Report of two cases and review of the literature. APMIS. 103:597–603.
2409. Skuladottir H, Hirsch FR, Hansen HH, et al. (2002). Pulmonary neuroendocrine tumors: incidence and prognosis of histological subtypes. A population-based study in Denmark. Lung Cancer. 37:127–35.
2410. Slade I, Bacchelli C, Davies H, et al. (2011). DICER1 syndrome: clarifying the diagnosis, clinical features and management implications of a pleiotropic tumour predisposition syndrome. J Med Genet. 48:273–8.
2411. Small EJ, Gordon GJ, Dahms BB (1985). Malignant rhabdoid tumor of the heart in an infant. Cancer. 55:2850–3.
2412. Smith AL, Hung J, Walker L, et al. (1996). Extensive areas of aneuploidy are present in the respiratory epithelium of lung cancer patients. Br J Cancer. 73:203–9.
2413. Smith M, Chaudhry MA, Lozano P, et al. (2012). Cardiac myxoma induced paraneoplastic syndromes: a review of the literature. Eur J Intern Med. 23:669–73.
2414. Smith MA (2007). Multiple synchronous atrial lipomas. Cardiovasc Pathol. 16:187–8.
2415. Smith MD, Christiansen LE, Himes B, et al. (1991). Thymic squamous cell carcinoma. J Am Osteopath Assoc. 91:614–7.
2416. Smith ME, Fisher C, Wilkinson LS, et al. (1995). Synovial sarcoma lack synovial differentiation. Histopathology. 26:279–81.
2417. Snover DC, Levine GD, Rosai J (1982). Thymic carcinoma. Five distinctive histological variants. Am J Surg Pathol. 6:451–70.
2418. Sobin L, Gospodarowicz M, Wittekind C (2009). Pleural Mesothelioma. In: Sobin LH, Gospodarowicz MK, Wittekind C, eds. TNM Classification of Malignant Tumours. 7th ed. Hoboken (NJ): Wiley-Blackwell; pp. 147–50.
2419. Sobin LH, Compton CC (2010). TNM seventh edition: what's new, what's changed: communication from the International Union Against Cancer and the American Joint Committee on Cancer. Cancer. 116: 5336–5339.
2420. Sobin LH, Gospodarowicz MK, Wittekind C, eds. (2009). TNM Classification of Malignant Tumours. 7th ed. Hoboken (NJ): Wiley-Blackwell.
2421. Soda M, Choi YL, Enomoto M, et al. (2007). Identification of the transforming EML4-ALK fusion gene in non-small-cell lung cancer. Nature. 448:561–6.
2422. Soga J, Yakuwa Y (1999). Bronchopulmonary carcinoids: An analysis of 1,875 reported cases with special reference to a comparison between typical carcinoids and atypical varieties. Ann Thorac Cardiovasc Surg. 5:211–9.
2423. Soga J, Yakuwa Y, Osaka M (1999). Evaluation of 342 cases of mediastinal/thymic carcinoids collected from literature: a comparative study between typical carcinoids and atypical varieties. Ann Thorac Cardiovasc Surg. 5:285–92.
2424. Sogabe O, Ohya T (2007). Right ventricular failure due to primary right ventricle osteosarcoma. Gen Thorac Cardiovasc Surg. 55:19–22.
2425. Sogge MR, McDonald SD, Cofold PB (1979). The malignant potential of the dysgenetic germ cell in Klinefelter's syndrome. Am J Med. 66:515–8.
2426. Soh J, Toyooka S, Ichihara S, et al. (2008). Sequential molecular changes during multistage pathogenesis of small peripheral adenocarcinomas of the lung. J Thorac Oncol. 3:340–7.
2427. Sokucu SN, Kocaturk C, Urer N, et al. (2012). Evaluation of six patients with pulmonary carcinosarcoma with a literature review. ScientificWorldJournal. 2012:167317.
2428. Sole F, Bosch F, Woessner S, et al. (1994). Refractory anemia with excess of blasts and isochromosome 12p in a patient with primary mediastinal germ-cell tumor. Cancer Genet Cytogenet. 77:111–3.
2429. Solum AM, Romero SC, Ledford S, et al. (2007). Left atrial hemangioma presenting as cardiac tamponade. Tex Heart Inst J. 34:126–7.
2430. Son C, Choi PJ, Roh MS (2012). Primary Pulmonary Myxoid Liposarcoma with Translocation t(12;16)(q13;p11) in a Young Female Patient: A Brief Case Report. Korean J Pathol. 46:392–4.
2431. Song DH, Choi IH, Ha SY, et al. (2014). Epithelial-myoepthelial carcinoma of the tracheobronchial tree: the prognostic role of myoepithelial cells. Lung Cancer. 83:416–9.
2432. Song JY, Jaffe ES (2013). HHV-8-positive but EBV-negative primary effusion lymphoma. Blood. 122:3712.
2433. Song SY, Ko YH, Ahn G (2005). Mediastinal germ cell tumor associated with histiocytic sarcoma of spleen: case report of an unusual association. Int J Surg Pathol. 13:299–303.
2434. Sonobe H, Ohtsuki Y, Nakayama H, et al. (1998). A thymic squamous cell carcinoma with complex chromosome abnormalities. Cancer Genet Cytogenet. 103:83–5.
2435. Sonobe H, Takeuchi T, Ohtsuki Y, et al. (1999). A thymoma with clonal complex chromosome abnormalities. Cancer Genet Cytogenet. 110:72–4.
2436. Sordillo PP, Epremian B, Koziner B, et al. (1982). Lymphomatoid granulomatosis: an analysis of clinical and immunologic characteristics. Cancer. 49:2070–6.
2437. Sorensen JB (2004). Endobronchial metastases from extrapulmonary solid tumors. Acta Oncol. 43:73–9.
2438. Soudack M, Guralnik L, Ben-Nun A, et al. (2007). Imaging features of posterior mediastinal chordoma in a child. Pediatr Radiol. 37:492–7.
2439. Souhami RL, Bradbury I, Geddes DM, et al. (1985). Prognostic significance of laboratory parameters measured at diagnosis in small cell carcinoma of the lung. Cancer Res. 45:2878–82.
2440. Souza CA, Quan K, Seely J, et al. (2009). Pulmonary intravascular lymphoma. J Thorac Imaging. 24:231–3.
2441. Sozzi G, Pastorino U, Moiraghi L, et al. (1998). Loss of FHIT function in lung cancer and preinvasive bronchial lesions. Cancer Res. 58:5032–7.
2442. Sparrow PJ, Kurian JB, Jones TR, et al. (2005). MR imaging of cardiac tumors. Radiographics. 25:1255–76.
2443. Speights VO Jr, Dobin SM, Truss LM (1998). A cytogenetic study of a cardiac papillary fibroelastoma. Cancer Genet Cytogenet. 103:167–9.
2444. Spencer H (1984). The pulmonary plasma cell/histiocytoma complex. Histopathology. 8:903–16.
2445. Spencer H (1985). Pathology of the Lung. Vol. 4th. Oxford: Pergamon Press.
2446. Spencer H, Dail DH, Arneaud J (1980). Non-invasive bronchial epithelial papillary tumors. Cancer. 45:1486–97.
2447. Spirtas R, Heineman EF, Bernstein L, et al. (1994). Malignant mesothelioma: attributable risk of asbestos exposure. Occup Environ Med. 51:804–11.
2448. Squire JA, Bayani J, Luk C, et al. (2002). Molecular cytogenetic analysis of head and neck squamous cell carcinoma: By comparative genomic hybridization, spectral karyotyping, and expression array analysis. Head Neck. 24:874–87.
2449. Sridhar S, Al-Moallem B, Kamal H, et al. (2013). New insights into the genetics of neuroblastoma. Mol Diagn Ther. 17:63–9.
2450. Srinivasan M, Taioli E, Ragin CC (2009). Human papillomavirus type 16 and 18 in primary lung cancers--a meta-analysis. Carcinogenesis. 30:1722–8.
2451. Staaf J, Isaksson S, Karlsson A, et al. (2013). Landscape of somatic allelic imbalances and copy number alterations in human lung carcinoma. Int J Cancer. 132:2020–31.
2452. Stainback RF, Hamirani YS, Cooley DA, et al. (2007). Tumors of the heart. In: Willerson JT, Cohn JN, Wellens HJJ, Holmes DR, eds. Cardiovascular Medicine. London: Springer-Verlag; pp. 2267–94.
2453. Stefanou D, Goussia AC, Arkoumani E, et al. (2004). Mucoepidermoid carcinoma of the thymus: a case presentation and a literature review. Pathol Res Pract. 200:567–73.
2454. Stefanovic A, Morgensztern D, Fong T, et al. (2008). Pulmonary marginal zone lymphoma: a single centre experience and review of the SEER database. Leuk Lymphoma. 49:1311–20.
2455. Steger C, Steiner HJ, Moser K et al. (2010). A typical thymic carcinoid tumour within a thymolipoma: report of a case and review of combined tumours of the thymus. BMJ Case Rep 2010:
2456. Steger CM, Hager T, Ruttmann E (2012). Primary cardiac tumours: a single-center 41-year experience. ISRN Cardiol. 2012:906109.
2457. Steidl C, Connors JM, Gascoyne RD (2011). Molecular pathogenesis of Hodgkin's lymphoma: increasing evidence of the importance of the microenvironment. J Clin Oncol. 29:1812–26.
2458. Steidl C, Gascoyne RD (2011). The molecular pathogenesis of primary mediastinal large B-cell lymphoma. Blood. 118:2659–69.
2459. Steidl C, Lee T, Shah SP, et al. (2010). Tumor-associated macrophages and survival in classic Hodgkin's lymphoma. N Engl J Med. 362:875–85.
2460. Steidl C, Shah SP, Woolcock BW, et al. (2011). MHC class II transactivator CIITA is a recurrent gene fusion partner in lymphoid cancers. Nature. 471:377–81.
2461. Stein H, Foss HD, Durkop H, et al. (2000). CD30(+) anaplastic large cell lymphoma: a review of its histopathologic, genetic, and clinical features. Blood. 96:3681–95.
2462. Stelow EB (2011). A review of NUT midline carcinoma. Head Neck Pathol. 5:31–5.
2463. Stelow EB, Bellizzi AM, Taneja K, et al. (2008). NUT rearrangement in undifferentiated carcinomas of the upper aerodigestive tract. Am J Surg Pathol. 32:828–34.
2464. Stelow EB, French CA (2009). Carcinomas of the upper aerodigestive tract with rearrangement of the nuclear protein of the testis (NUT) gene (NUT midline carcinomas). Adv Anat Pathol. 16:92–6.
2465. Stenhouse G, Fyfe N, King G, et al. (2004). Thyroid transcription factor 1 in pulmonary adenocarcinoma. J Clin Pathol. 57:383–7.
2466. Stenman G (2013). Fusion oncogenes in salivary gland tumors: molecular and clinical consequences. Head Neck Pathol. 7 Suppl 1:S12–9.
2467. Stephan JL, Galambrun C, Boucheron S, et al. (2000). Epstein-Barr virus--positive undifferentiated thymic carcinoma in a 12-year-old white girl. J Pediatr Hematol Oncol. 22:162–6.
2468. Stephens M, Khalil J, Gibbs AR (1987). Primary clear cell carcinoma of the thymus gland. Histopathology. 11:763–5.
2469. Stephens P, Hunter C, Bignell G, et al. (2004). Lung cancer: intragenic ERBB2 kinase mutations in tumours. Nature. 431:525–6.
2470. Stephens PJ, Davies HR, Mitani Y, et al. (2013). Whole exome sequencing of adenoid cystic carcinoma. J Clin Invest. 123:2965–8.
2471. Sterlacci W, Fiegl M, Hilbe W, et al. (2009). Clinical relevance of neuroendocrine differentiation in non-small cell lung cancer assessed by immunohistochemistry: a retrospective study on 405 surgically resected cases. Virchows Arch. 455:125–32.
2472. Sterner DJ, Mori M, Roggli VL, et al. (1997). Prevalence of pulmonary atypical alveolar cell hyperplasia in an autopsy population: a study of 100 cases. Mod Pathol. 10:469–73.
2473. Stewart BW, Wild CP, eds (2014). World Cancer Report. Lyon: IARC.
2474. Stiller B, Hetzer R, Meyer R, et al. (2001). Primary cardiac tumours: when is surgery necessary? Eur J Cardiothorac Surg. 20:1002–6.
2475. Stolf NA, Santos GG, Sobral ML, et al. (2006). Primary schwannoma of the right atrium: successful surgical resection. Clinics (Sao Paulo). 61:87–8.
2476. Stoppacciaro A, Ferrarini M, Salmaggi C, et al. (2006). Immunohistochemical evidence of a cytokine and chemokine network in three patients with Erdheim-Chester disease: implications for pathogenesis. Arthritis Rheum. 54:4018–22.
2477. Storm PB, Fallon B, Bunge RG (1976). Mediastinal choriocarcinoma in a chromatin-positive boy. J Urol. 116:838–40.
2478. Stratakis CA, Carney JA (2009). The triad of paragangliomas, gastric stromal tumours and pulmonary chondromas (Carney triad), and the dyad of paragangliomas and gastric stromal sarcomas (Carney-Stratakis syndrome): molecular genetics and clinical implications. J Intern Med. 266:43–52.
2479. Stratakis CA, Kirschner LS, Carney JA (2001). Clinical and molecular features of the Carney complex: diagnostic criteria and recommendations for patient evaluation. J Clin Endocrinol Metab. 86:4041–6.
2480. Strecker T, Agaimy A, Marwan M, et al. (2010). Papillary fibroelastoma of the aortic valve: appearance in echocardiography, computed tomography, and histopathology. J Heart Valve Dis. 19:812.
2481. Strecker T, Reimann A, Voigt JU, et al. (2006). A very rare cardiac hibernoma in the right atrium: a case report. Heart Surg Forum. 9:E623–5.
2482. Strecker T, Rosch J, Weyand M, et al. (2012). Primary and metastatic cardiac tumors: imaging characteristics, surgical treatment, and histopathological spectrum: a 10-year-experience at a German heart center. Cardiovasc Pathol. 21:436–43.
2483. Strecker T, Schmid A, Agaimy A, et al. (2011). Giant metastatic alveolar soft part sarcoma in the left ventricle: appearance in echocardiography, magnetic resonance imaging, and histopathology. Clin Cardiol. 34:E6–8.
2484. Strecker T, Schmid A, Zielezinski T, et al. (2011). Left ventricular hemangioma. Heart Surg Forum. 14:E207–9.
2485. Streubel B, Lamprecht A, Dierlamm J, et al. (2003). T(14;18)(q32;q21) involving IGH and MALT1 is a frequent chromosomal aberration in MALT lymphoma. Blood. 101:2335–9.
2486. Strizzi L, Catalano A, Vianale G, et al. (2001). Vascular endothelial growth factor is an autocrine growth factor in human malignant mesothelioma. J Pathol. 193:468–75.

2487. Ströbel P, Bargou R, Wolff A, et al. (2010). Sunitinib in metastatic thymic carcinomas: laboratory findings and initial clinical experience. Br J Cancer. 103:196–200.

2488. Ströbel P, Bauer A, Puppe B, et al. (2004). Tumor recurrence and survival in patients treated for thymomas and thymic squamous cell carcinomas: a retrospective analysis. J Clin Oncol. 22:1501–9.

2489. Ströbel P, Hartmann E, Rosenwald A, et al. (2014). Corticomedullary differentiation and maturational arrest in thymomas. Histopathology. 64:557–66.

2490. Ströbel P, Hartmann M, Jakob A, et al. (2004). Thymic carcinoma with overexpression of mutated KIT and the response to imatinib. N Engl J Med. 350:2625–6.

2491. Ströbel P, Hohenberger P, Marx A (2010). Thymoma and thymic carcinoma: molecular pathology and targeted therapy. J Thorac Oncol. 5:S286–90.

2492. Ströbel P, Marino M, Feuchtenberger M, et al. (2005). Micronodular thymoma: an epithelial tumour with abnormal chemokine expression setting the stage for lymphoma development. J Pathol. 207:72–82.

2493. Ströbel P, Marx A, Zettl A, et al. (2005). Thymoma and thymic carcinoma: an update of the WHO Classification 2004. Surg Today. 35:805–11.

2494. Ströbel P, Murumagi A, Klein R, et al. (2007). Deficiency of the autoimmune regulator AIRE in thymomas is insufficient to elicit autoimmune polyendocrinopathy syndrome type 1 (APS-1). J Pathol. 211:563–71.

2495. Ströbel P, Zettl A, Shilo K, et al. (2014). Tumor genetics and survival of thymic neuroendocrine neoplasms: A multi-institutional clinicopathologic study. Genes Chromosomes Cancer. 59:738–49.

2496. Strollo DC, Dacic S, Ocak I, et al. (2013). Malignancies incidentally detected at lung transplantation: radiologic and pathologic features. AJR Am J Roentgenol. 201:108–16.

2497. Strollo DC, Rosado de Christenson ML, Jett JR (1997). Primary mediastinal tumors. Part 1: tumors of the anterior mediastinum. Chest. 112:511–22.

2498. Strollo DC, Rosado-de-Christenson ML (2002). Primary mediastinal malignant germ cell neoplasms: imaging features. Chest Surg Clin N Am. 12:645–58.

2499. Sturm N, Lantuejoul S, Laverriere MH, et al. (2001). Thyroid transcription factor 1 and cytokeratins 1, 5, 10, 14 (34betaE12) expression in basaloid and large-cell neuroendocrine carcinomas of the lung. Hum Pathol. 32:918–25.

2500. Sturm N, Rossi G, Lantuejoul S, et al. (2003). 34BetaE12 expression along the whole spectrum of neuroendocrine proliferations of the lung, from neuroendocrine cell hyperplasia to small cell carcinoma. Histopathology. 42:156–66.

2501. Sturm N, Rossi G, Lantuejoul S, et al. (2002). Expression of thyroid transcription factor-1 in the spectrum of neuroendocrine cell lung proliferations with special interest in carcinoids. Hum Pathol. 33:175–82.

2502. Su PH, Luh SP, Yieh DM, et al. (2005). Anterior mediastinal immature teratoma with precocious puberty in a child with Klinefelter syndrome. J Formos Med Assoc. 104:601–4.

2503. Subesinghe M, Smith JT, Chowdhury FU (2012). F-18 FDG PET/CT imaging of follicular dendritic cell sarcoma of the mediastinum. Clin Nucl Med. 37:204–5.

2504. Subitha K, Thambi R, Sheeja S, et al. (2013). Role of imprint cytology in intra-operative diagnosis of an unusual variant of teratoma. J Cytol. 30:148–9.

2505. Subramanian J, Govindan R (2007). Lung cancer in never smokers: a review. J Clin Oncol. 25:561–70.

2506. Suemitsu R, Takeo S, Momosaki S, et al. (2011). Thymic basaloid carcinoma with aggressive invasion of the lung and pericardium: report of a case. Surg Today. 41:986–8.

2507. Suenaga M, Matsushita K, Kawamata N, et al. (2006). True malignant histiocytosis with trisomy 9 following primary mediastinal germ cell tumor. Acta Haematol. 116:62–6.

2508. Sugano M, Nagasaka T, Sasaki E, et al. (2013). HNF4alpha as a marker for invasive mucinous adenocarcinoma of the lung. Am J Surg Pathol. 37:211–8.

2509. Sugio K, Kishimoto Y, Virmani AK, et al. (1994). K-ras mutations are a relatively late event in the pathogenesis of lung carcinomas. Cancer Res. 54:5811–5.

2510. Sugio K, Osaki T, Oyama T, et al. (2003). Genetic alteration in carcinoid tumors of the lung. Ann Thorac Cardiovasc Surg. 9:149–54.

2511. Suh JH, Shin OR, Kim YH (2008). Multiple calcifying fibrous pseudotumor of the pleura. J Thorac Oncol. 3:1356–8.

2512. Sumino S, Paterson HS (2005). No regrowth after incomplete papillary fibroelastoma excision. Ann Thorac Surg. 79:e3–4.

2513. Sun S, Schiller JH, Gazdar AF (2007). Lung cancer in never smokers--a different disease. Nat Rev Cancer. 7:778–90.

2514. Sung MT, MacLennan GT, Lopez-Beltran A, et al. (2008). Primary mediastinal seminoma: a comprehensive assessment integrated with histology, immunohistochemistry, and fluorescence in situ hybridization for chromosome 12p abnormalities in 23 cases. Am J Surg Pathol. 32:146–55.

2515. Surdacki A, Kapelak B, Brzozowska-Czarnek A, et al. (2007). Lipoma of the aortic valve in a patient with acute myocardial infarction. Int J Cardiol. 115:e36–8.

2516. Suster S (2005). Thymic carcinoma: update of current diagnostic criteria and histologic types. Semin Diagn Pathol. 22:198–212.

2517. Suster S, Moran CA (1995). Thymic carcinoid with prominent mucinous stroma. Report of a distinctive morphologic variant of thymic neuroendocrine neoplasm. Am J Surg Pathol. 19:1277–85.

2518. Suster S, Moran CA (1996). Primary thymic epithelial neoplasms showing combined features of thymoma and thymic carcinoma. A clinicopathologic study of 22 cases. Am J Surg Pathol. 20:1469–80.

2519. Suster S, Moran CA (1998). Thymic carcinoma: spectrum of differentiation and histologic types. Pathology. 30:111–22.

2520. Suster S, Moran CA (1999). Micronodular thymoma with lymphoid B-cell hyperplasia: clinicopathologic and immunohistochemical study of eighteen cases of a distinctive morphologic variant of thymic epithelial neoplasm. Am J Surg Pathol. 23:955–62.

2521. Suster S, Moran CA (1999). Spindle cell thymic carcinoma: clinicopathologic and immunohistochemical study of a distinctive variant of primary thymic epithelial neoplasm. Am J Surg Pathol. 23:691–700.

2522. Suster S, Moran CA (1999). Thymoma, atypical thymoma, and thymic carcinoma. A novel conceptual approach to the classification of thymic epithelial neoplasms. Am J Clin Pathol. 111:826–33.

2523. Suster S, Moran CA (2001). Neuroendocrine neoplasms of the mediastinum. Am J Clin Pathol. 115 Suppl:S17–27.

2524. Suster S, Moran CA (2005). Primary synovial sarcomas of the mediastinum: a clinicopathologic, immunohistochemical, and ultrastructural study of 15 cases. Am J Surg Pathol. 29:569–78.

2525. Suster S, Moran CA (2005). Problem areas and inconsistencies in the WHO classification of thymoma. Semin Diagn Pathol. 22:188–97.

2526. Suster S, Moran CA, Chan JK (1997). Thymoma with pseudosarcomatous stroma: report of an unusual histologic variant of thymic epithelial neoplasm that may simulate carcinosarcoma. Am J Surg Pathol. 21:1316–23.

2527. Suster S, Moran CA, Dominguez-Malagon H, et al. (1998). Germ cell tumors of the mediastinum and testis: a comparative immunohistochemical study of 120 cases. Hum Pathol. 29:737–42.

2528. Suster S, Moran CA, Koss MN (1994). Epithelioid hemangioendothelioma of the anterior mediastinum. Clinicopathologic, immunohistochemical, and ultrastructural analysis of 12 cases. Am J Surg Pathol. 18:871–81.

2529. Suster S, Moran CA, Koss MN (1994). Rhabdomyosarcomas of the anterior mediastinum: report of four cases unassociated with germ cell, teratomatous, or thymic carcinomatous components. Hum Pathol. 25:349–56.

2530. Suster S, Rosai J (1991). Thymic carcinoma. A clinicopathologic study of 60 cases. Cancer. 67:1025–32.

2531. Sutherland KD, Proost N, Brouns I, et al. (2011). Cell of origin of small cell lung cancer: inactivation of Trp53 and Rb1 in distinct cell types of adult mouse lung. Cancer Cell. 19:754–64.

2532. Suurmeijer AJH, de Bruijn D, Guerts van Kessel A, et al. (2013). Synovial sarcoma. In: Fletcher CDM, Bridge JA, Hogendoorn PCW, Mertens F, eds. WHO Classification of Tumours of Soft Tissue and Bone. Lyon: IARC; pp. 213–5.

2533. Suwatanapongched T, Kiatboonsri S, Visessiri Y, et al. (2011). A 30-year-old woman with intermittent cough and a mass-like opacity in the right upper lobe. Chest. 140:808–13.

2534. Suzuki E, Sasaki H, Kawano O, et al. (2006). Expression and mutation statuses of epidermal growth factor receptor in thymic epithelial tumors. Jpn J Clin Oncol. 36:351–6.

2535. Suzuki H, Saitoh Y, Koh E, et al. (2011). Pulmonary sclerosing hemangioma with pleural dissemination: report of a case. Surg Today. 41:258–61.

2536. Suzuki K, Koike T, Asakawa T, et al. (2011). A prospective radiological study of thin-section computed tomography to predict pathological noninvasiveness in peripheral clinical IA lung cancer (Japan Clinical Oncology Group 0201). J Thorac Oncol. 6:751–6.

2537. Suzuki K, Nagai K, Yoshida J, et al. (1997). The prognosis of resected lung carcinoma associated with atypical adenomatous hyperplasia: a comparison of the prognosis of well-differentiated adenocarcinoma associated with atypical adenomatous hyperplasia and intrapulmonary metastasis. Cancer. 79:1521–6.

2538. Suzuki K, Takahashi K, Yoshida J, et al. (1998). Synchronous double primary lung carcinomas associated with multiple atypical adenomatous hyperplasia. Lung Cancer. 19:131–9.

2539. Suzuki K, Urushihara N, Fukumoto K, et al. (2011). A case of Epstein-Barr virus-associated pulmonary leiomyosarcoma arising five yr after a pediatric renal transplant. Pediatr Transplant. 15:E145–8.

2540. Suzuki K, Yokose T, Yoshida J, et al. (2000). Prognostic significance of the size of central fibrosis in peripheral adenocarcinoma of the lung. Ann Thorac Surg. 69:893–7.

2541. Suzuki Y, Saiga T, Ozeki Y, et al. (1993). [Two cases of intrapulmonary teratoma]. Nihon Kyobu Geka Gakkai Zasshi. 41:498–502.

2542. Svec A, Rangaiah M, Giles M, et al. (2012). EBV+ diffuse large B-cell lymphoma arising within atrial myxoma. An example of a distinct primary cardiac EBV+ DLBCL of immunocompetent patients. Pathol Res Pract. 208:172–6.

2543. Svensson G, Ewers SB, Ohlsson O, et al. (2013). Prognostic factors in lung cancer in a defined geographical area over two decades with a special emphasis on gender. Clin Respir J. 7:91–100.

2544. Swanson PE (1991). Soft tissue neoplasma of the mediastinum. Semin Diagn Pathol. 8:14–34.

2545. Swanton C, Mann DJ, Fleckenstein B, et al. (1997). Herpes viral cyclin/Cdk6 complexes evade inhibition by CDK inhibitor proteins. Nature. 390:184–7.

2546. Swarts DR, Ramaekers FC, Speel EJ (2012). Molecular and cellular biology of neuroendocrine lung tumors: evidence for separate biological entities. Biochim Biophys Acta. 1826:255–71.

2547. Swartz MF, Lutz CJ, Chandan VS, et al. (2006). Atrial myxomas: pathologic types, tumor location, and presenting symptoms. J Card Surg. 21:435–40.

2548. Swerdlow SH, Campo E, Harris NL, et al., eds. (2008). WHO Classification of Tumours of Haematopoietic and Lymphoid Tissues. 4th ed. Lyon: IARC.

2549. Syed IS, Feng D, Harris SR, et al. (2008). MR imaging of cardiac masses. Magn Reson Imaging Clin N Am. 16:137–64. [vii.]

2550. Syed S, Haque AK, Hawkins HK, et al. (2002). Desmoplastic small round cell tumor of the lung. Arch Pathol Lab Med. 126:1226–8.

2551. Szczepanski T, Langerak AW, Willemse MJ, et al. (2000). T cell receptor gamma (TCRG) gene rearrangements in T cell acute lymphoblastic leukemia refelct 'end-stage' recombinations: implications for minimal residual disease monitoring. Leukemia. 14:1208–14.

2552. Szturz P, Rehak Z, Koukalova R, et al. (2012). Measuring diffuse metabolic activity on FDG-PET/CT: new method for evaluating Langerhans cell histiocytosis activity in pulmonary parenchyma. Nucl Med Biol. 39:429–36.

2553. Taeger D, Johnen G, Wiethege T, et al. (2009). Major histopathological patterns of lung cancer related to arsenic exposure in German uranium miners. Int Arch Occup Environ Health. 82:867–75.

2554. Tagawa T, Ohta M, Kuwata T, et al. (2010). S-1 plus cisplatin chemotherapy with concurrent radiation for thymic basaloid carcinoma. J Thorac Oncol. 5:572–3.

2555. Taggart DR, London WB, Schmidt ML, et al. (2011). Prognostic value of the stage 4S metastatic pattern and tumor biology in patients with metastatic neuroblastoma diagnosed between birth and 18 months of age. J Clin Oncol. 29:4358–64.

2556. Tahir M, Noor SJ, Herle A, et al. (2009). Right atrial paraganglioma: a rare primary cardiac neoplasm as a cause of chest pain. Tex Heart Inst J. 36:594–7.

2557. Takagi N, Nakamura S, Yamamoto K, et al. (1992). Malignant lymphoma of mucosa-associated lymphoid tissue arising in the thymus of a patient with Sjogren's syndrome. A morphologic, phenotypic, and genotypic study. Cancer. 69:1347–55.

2558. Takahashi F, Tsuta K, Matsuno Y, et al. (2005). Adenocarcinoma of the thymus: mucinous subtype. Hum Pathol. 36:219–23.

2559. Takahashi H, Tomita N, Yokoyama M, et al. (2012). Prognostic impact of extranodal involvement in diffuse large B-cell lymphoma in the rituximab era. Cancer. 118:4166–72.

2560. Takahashi K, Yoshida J, Nishimura M, et al. (2000). Thymic carcinoma. Outcome of treatment including surgical resection. Jpn J Thorac Cardiovasc Surg. 48:494–8.

2561. Takahashi M, Kanamori Y, Takahashi M, et al. (2014). Detection of a metastatic lesion and tiny yolk sac tumors in two teenage patients by FDG-PET: report of two cases. Surg Today. 44:1962–5.

2562. Takahashi M, Okumura N, Matsuoka T, et al. (2011). Teratoma with naturally occurring malignant transformation in a child. Ann Thorac Cardiovasc Surg. 17:588–90.

2563. Takamochi K, Ogura T, Suzuki K, et al. (2001). Loss of heterozygosity on chromosomes 9q and 16p in atypical adenomatous hyperplasia concomitant with adenocarcinoma of the lung. Am J Pathol. 159:1941–8.

2564. Takamori S, Noguchi M, Morinaga S, et al. (1991). Clinicopathologic characteristics of adenosquamous carcinoma of the lung. Cancer. 67:649–54.

2565. Takeda M, Kasai T, Enomoto Y, et al. (2012). Genomic gains and losses in malignant mesothelioma demonstrated by FISH analysis of paraffin-embedded tissues. J Clin Pathol. 65:77–82.
2566. Takeda S, Miyoshi S, Akashi A, et al. (2003). Clinical spectrum of primary mediastinal tumors: a comparison of adult and pediatric populations at a single Japanese institution. J Surg Oncol. 83:24–30.
2567. Takeda S, Miyoshi S, Ohta M, et al. (2003). Primary germ cell tumors in the mediastinum: a 50-year experience at a single Japanese institution. Cancer. 97:367–76.
2568. Takeda S, Sawabata N, Inoue M, et al. (2004). Thymic carcinoma. Clinical institutional experience with 15 patients. Eur J Cardiothorac Surg. 26:401–6.
2569. Takeda Y, Tsuta K, Shibuki Y, et al. (2008). Analysis of expression patterns of breast cancer-specific markers (mammaglobin and gross cystic disease fluid protein 15) in lung and pleural tumors. Arch Pathol Lab Med. 132:239–43.
2570. Takeshima Y, Amatya VJ, Kushitani K, et al. (2009). Value of immunohistochemistry in the differential diagnosis of pleural sarcomatoid mesothelioma from lung sarcomatoid carcinoma. Histopathology. 54:667–76.
2571. Takeuchi E, Shimizu E, Sano N, et al. (1998). A case of pleomorphic adenoma of the lung with multiple distant metastases--observations on its oncogene and tumor suppressor gene expression. Anticancer Res. 18:2015–20.
2572. Takeuchi I, Kawaguchi T, Kimura Y, et al. (2007). Primary cardiac osteosarcoma in a young man with severe congestive heart failure. Intern Med. 46:649–51.
2573. Takeuchi K, Soda M, Togashi Y, et al. (2011). Pulmonary inflammatory myofibroblastic tumor expressing a novel fusion, PPFIBP1-ALK: reappraisal of anti-ALK immunohistochemistry as a tool for novel ALK fusion identification. Clin Cancer Res. 17:3341–8.
2574. Takeuchi K, Soda M, Togashi Y, et al. (2012). RET, ROS1 and ALK fusions in lung cancer. Nat Med. 18:378–81.
2575. Takeuchi S, Koike M, Park S, et al. (1998). The ATM gene and susceptibility to childhood T-cell acute lymphoblastic leukaemia. Br J Haematol. 103:536–8.
2576. Takeuchi T, Tomida S, Yatabe Y, et al. (2006). Expression profile-defined classification of lung adenocarcinoma shows close relationship with underlying major genetic changes and clinicopathologic behaviors. J Clin Oncol. 24:1679–88.
2577. Takezawa K, Pirazzoli V, Arcila ME, et al. (2012). HER2 amplification: a potential mechanism of acquired resistance to EGFR inhibition in EGFR-mutant lung cancers that lack the second-site EGFRT790M mutation. Cancer Discov. 2:922–33.
2578. Talerman A, Gratama S (1983). Primary ganglioneuroblastoma of the anterior mediastinum in a 61-year-old woman. Histopathology. 7:967–75.
2579. Tallet A, Nault JC, Renier A, et al. (2013). Overexpression and promoter mutation of the TERT gene in malignant pleural mesothelioma. Oncogene. 33:3748–52.
2580. Talukder MQ, Deo SV, Maleszewski JJ, et al. (2010). Late isolated metastasis of renal cell carcinoma in the left ventricular myocardium. Interact Cardiovasc Thorac Surg. 11:814–6.
2581. Tam IY, Chung LP, Suen WS, et al. (2006). Distinct epidermal growth factor receptor and KRAS mutation patterns in non-small cell lung cancer patients with different tobacco exposure and clinicopathologic features. Clin Cancer Res. 12:1647–53.
2582. Tamborini E, Bonadiman L, Negri T, et al. (2004). Detection of overexpressed and phosphorylated wild-type kit receptor in surgical specimens of small cell lung cancer. Clin Cancer Res. 10:8214–9.
2583. Tamenishi A, Matsumura Y, Okamoto H (2012). Malignant fibrous histiocytoma originating from right ventricular outflow tract. Asian Cardiovasc Thorac Ann. 20:702–4.
2584. Tamin SS, Maleszewski JJ, Scott CG, et al. (2015). Prognostic and Bioepidemiologic Implications of Papillary Fibroelastomas. J Am Coll Cardiol. 65:2420–9.
2585. Tampellini M, Alabiso I, Sculli CM, et al. (2006). Stage IB malignant thymoma in a Lynch syndrome patient with multiple cancers: response to incidental administration of oxaliplatin and 5-fluorouracil. J Chemother. 18:433–6.
2586. Tamura T, Jobo T, Watanabe J, et al. (2006). Neuroendocrine features in poorly differentiated endometrioid adenocarcinomas of the endometrium. Int J Gynecol Cancer. 16:821–6.
2587. Tan DF, Huberman JA, Hyland A, et al. (2001). MCM2--a promising marker for premalignant lesions of the lung: a cohort study. BMC Cancer. 1:6.
2588. Tan KL, Scott DW, Hong F, et al. (2012). Tumor-associated macrophages predict inferior outcomes in classic Hodgkin lymphoma: a correlative study from the E2496 Intergroup trial. Blood. 120:3280–7.
2589. Tan TJ, Tan SC (2013). Concomitant early avascular necrosis of the femoral head and acute bacterial arthritis by enteric Gram-negative bacilli in four oncologic patients. Singapore Med J. 54:e108–12.
2590. Tanaka M, Kato K, Gomi K, et al. (2012). NUT midline carcinoma: report of 2 cases suggestive of pulmonary origin. Am J Surg Pathol. 36:381–8.
2591. Tanaka R, Emerson LL, Karwande SV, et al. (2005). Growing pulmonary nodule with increased 18-fluorodeoxyglucose uptake in a former smoker. Chest. 127:1848–51.
2592. Tanas MR, Sboner A, Oliveira AM, et al. (2011). Identification of a disease-defining gene fusion in epithelioid hemangioendothelioma. Sci Transl Med. 3:98ra82.
2593. Tandon S, Kant S, Singh AK, et al. (1999). Primary intrapulmonary teratoma presenting as pyothorax. Indian J Chest Dis Allied Sci. 41:51–5.
2594. Tang D, Kryvenko ON, Mitrache N, et al. (2013). Methylation of the RARB gene increases prostate cancer risk in black Americans. J Urol. 190:317–24.
2595. Tang JY, kay-Wiggan JM, Aszterbaum M, et al. (2012). Inhibiting the hedgehog pathway in patients with the basal-cell nevus syndrome. N Engl J Med. 366:2180–8.
2596. Tangthangtham A, Wongsangiem M, Koanantakool T, et al. (1998). Intrapulmonary teratoma: a report of three cases. J Med Assoc Thai. 81:1028–33.
2597. Taniguchi A, Hashida Y, Nemoto Y, et al. (2013). Pyothorax-associated lymphoma (PAL) with biclonal Epstein-Barr virus infection: characterization of a novel PAL cell line with unique features. Leuk Res. 37:1545–50.
2598. Tanimura S, Tomoyasu H, Kohno T, et al. (2002). [Basaloid carcinoma originated from the wall of thymic cyst presenting as pericardial and thoracic effusion; report of a case]. Kyobu Geka. 55:571–5.
2599. Tateishi U, Muller NL, Johkoh T, et al. (2004). Primary mediastinal lymphoma: characteristic features of the various histological subtypes on CT. J Comput Assist Tomogr. 28:782–9.
2600. Tateyama H, Eimoto T, Tada T, et al. (1999). Immunoreactivity of a new CD5 antibody with normal epithelium and malignant tumors including thymic carcinoma. Am J Clin Pathol. 111:235–40.
2601. Tateyama H, Eimoto T, Tada T, et al. (1995). p53 protein expression and p53 gene mutation in thymic epithelial tumors. An immunohistochemical and DNA sequencing study. Am J Clin Pathol. 104:375–81.
2602. Tateyama H, Saito Y, Fujii Y, et al. (2001). The spectrum of micronodular thymic epithelial tumours with lymphoid B-cell hyperplasia. Histopathology. 38:519–27.
2603. Taube JM, Griffin CA, Yonescu R, et al. (2006). Pleuropulmonary blastoma: cytogenetic and spectral karyotype analysis. Pediatr Dev Pathol. 9:453–61.
2604. Tavora F, Miettinen M, Fanburg-Smith J, et al. (2008). Pulmonary artery sarcoma: a histologic and follow-up study with emphasis on a subset of low-grade myofibroblastic sarcomas with a good long-term follow-up. Am J Surg Pathol. 32:1751–61.
2605. Taylor CA, Barnhart A, Pettenati MJ, et al. (2005). Primary pleuropulmonary synovial sarcoma diagnosed by fine needle aspiration with cytogenetic confirmation: a case report. Acta Cytol. 49:673–6.
2606. Taylor HG, Butler WM, Karcher DS, et al. (1988). Thymic carcinoma: clinical findings in two patients with extrathoracic metastases. South Med J. 81:664–6.
2607. Tazelaar HD, Kerr D, Yousem SA, et al. (1993). Diffuse pulmonary lymphangiomatosis. Hum Pathol. 24:1313–22.
2608. Tazelaar HD, Locke TJ, McGregor CG (1992). Pathology of surgically excised primary cardiac tumors. Mayo Clin Proc. 67:957–65.
2609. Tearney GJ, Brezinski ME, Bouma BE, et al. (1997). In vivo endoscopic optical biopsy with optical coherence tomography. Science. 276:2037–9.
2610. Teh BT (1998). Thymic carcinoids in multiple endocrine neoplasia type 1. J Intern Med. 243:501–4.
2611. Teh BT, Hayward NK, Walters MK, et al. (1994). Genetic studies of thymic carcinoids in multiple endocrine neoplasia type 1. J Med Genet. 31:261–2.
2612. Teh BT, McArdle J, Chan SP, et al. (1997). Clinicopathologic studies of thymic carcinoids in multiple endocrine neoplasia type 1. Medicine (Baltimore). 76:21–9.
2613. Teh BT, Zedenius J, Kytola S, et al. (1998). Thymic carcinoids in multiple endocrine neoplasia type 1. Ann Surg. 228:99–105.
2614. Tehrani OS, Chen EQ, Schaebler DL, et al. (2010). Thymoma associated with malignancies may herald a hereditary cancer syndrome. Fam Cancer. 9:655–7.
2615. TEILUM G (1959). Endodermal sinus tumors of the ovary and testis. Comparative morphogenesis of the so-called mesoephroma ovarii (Schiller) and extraembryonic (yolk sac-allantoic) structures of the rat's placenta. Cancer. 12:1092–105.
2616. Teo M, Crotty P, O'Sullivan M, et al. (2011). NUT midline carcinoma in a young woman. J Clin Oncol. 29:e336–9.
2617. Terada T (2012). Primary sarcomatoid malignant mesothelioma of the pericardium. Med Oncol. 29:1345–6.
2618. Teramoto K, Kawaguchi Y, Hori T, et al. (2012). Thymic papillo-tubular adenocarcinoma containing a cyst: report of a case. Surg Today. 42:988–91.
2619. Terra RM, Fernandez A, Bammann RH, et al. (2008). Pulmonary artery sarcoma mimicking a pulmonary artery aneurysm. Ann Thorac Surg. 86:1354–5.
2620. Terra SB, Aubry MC, Yi ES, et al. (2014). Immunohistochemical study of 36 cases of pulmonary sarcomatoid carcinoma--sensitivity of TTF-1 is superior to napsin. Hum Pathol. 45:294–302.
2621. Terry J, Leung S, Laskin J, et al. (2010). Optimal immunohistochemical markers for distinguishing lung adenocarcinomas from squamous cell carcinomas in small tumor samples. Am J Surg Pathol. 34:1805–11.
2622. Terry J, Saito T, Subramanian S, et al. (2007). TLE1 as a diagnostic immunohistochemical marker for synovial sarcoma emerging from gene expression profiling studies. Am J Surg Pathol. 31:240–6.
2623. Tessema M, Yingling CM, Thomas CL, et al. (2012). SULF2 methylation is prognostic for lung cancer survival and increases sensitivity to topoisomerase-I inhibitors via induction of ISG15. Oncogene. 31:4107–16.
2624. Testa JR, Cheung M, Pei J, et al. (2011). Germline BAP1 mutations predispose to malignant mesothelioma. Nat Genet. 43:1022–5.
2625. Teta MJ, Lau E, Sceurman BK, et al. (2007). Therapeutic radiation for lymphoma: risk of malignant mesothelioma. Cancer. 109:1432–8.
2626. The Cancer Genome Atlas Research Network, Collisson EA et al. (2014). Comprehensive Molecular Profiling of Lung Adenocarcinoma. Nature. 511:543–50.
2627. The Non-Hodgkin's Lymphoma Classification Project (1997). A clinical evaluation of the International Lymphoma Study Group classification of non-Hodgkin's lymphoma. Blood. 89:3909–18.
2628. Basso C, Valente M, Thiene G, eds. (2013). Cardiac Tumor Pathology. New York: Springer.
2628A. Thiene G, Valente M, Basso C (2013). Cardiac Tumors: From Autoptic Observations to Surgical Pathology in the Era of Advanced Cardiac Imaging. In: Cardiac Tumor Pathology. Basso C, Valente M, Thiene G (Eds). New York: Springer; pp 1–22, with kind permission from Springer Science + Business Media.
2629. Thistlethwaite PA, Renner J, Duhamel D, et al. (2011). Surgical management of endobronchial inflammatory myofibroblastic tumors. Ann Thorac Surg. 91:367–72.
2630. Thomas-de-Montpreville V, Ghigna MR, Lacroix L, et al. (2013). Thymic carcinomas: clinicopathologic study of 37 cases from a single institution. Virchows Arch. 462:307–13.
2631. Thomas-de-Montpreville V, Nottin R, Dulmet E, et al. (2007). Heart tumors in children and adults: clinicopathological study of 59 patients from a surgical center. Cardiovasc Pathol. 16:22–8.
2632. Thomas-de-Montpreville V, Zemoura L, Dulmet E (2002). [Thymoma with epithelial micronodules and lymphoid hyperplasia: six cases of a rare and equivocal subtype]. Ann Pathol. 22:177–82.
2633. Thomason R, Schlegel W, Lucca M, et al. (1994). Primary malignant mesothelioma of the pericardium. Case report and literature review. Tex Heart Inst J. 21:170–4.
2634. Thompson L, Chang B, Barsky SH (1996). Monoclonal origins of malignant mixed tumors (carcinosarcomas). Evidence for a divergent histogenesis. Am J Surg Pathol. 20:277–85.
2635. Thun MJ, Hannan LM, Adams-Campbell LL, et al. (2008). Lung cancer occurrence in never-smokers: an analysis of 13 cohorts and 22 cancer registry studies. PLoS Med. 5:e185.
2636. Thunnissen E, Beasley MB, Borczuk AC, et al. (2012). Reproducibility of histopathological subtypes and invasion in pulmonary adenocarcinoma. An international interobserver study. Mod Pathol. 25:1574–83.
2637. Thunnissen E, Boers E, Heideman DA, et al. (2012). Correlation of immunohistochemical staining p63 and TTF-1 with EGFR and K-ras mutational spectrum and diagnostic reproducibility in non small cell lung carcinoma. Virchows Arch. 461:629–38.
2638. Thunnissen E, Kerr KM, Herth FJ, et al. (2012). The challenge of NSCLC diagnosis and predictive analysis on small samples. Practical approach of a working group. Lung Cancer. 76:1–18.
2638A. Thunnissen E, Noguchi M, Aisner S, et al. (2014). Reproducibility of histopathological diagnosis in poorly differentiated NSCLC: an international multiobserver study. J Thorac Oncol. 9:1354–62.
2639. Thunnissen FB, Arends JW, Buchholtz RT, et al. (1989). Fine needle aspiration cytology of inflammatory pseudotumor of the lung

(plasma cell granuloma). Report of four cases. Acta Cytol. 33:917–21.
2640. Thurneysen C, Opitz I, Kurtz S, et al. (2009). Functional inactivation of NF2/merlin in human mesothelioma. Lung Cancer. 64:140–7.
2641. Thway K, Fisher C (2012). Tumors with EWSR1-CREB1 and EWSR1-ATF1 fusions: the current status. Am J Surg Pathol. 36:e1–11.
2642. Thway K, Nicholson AG, Lawson K, et al. (2011). Primary pulmonary myxoid sarcoma with EWSR1-CREB1 fusion: a new tumor entity. Am J Surg Pathol. 35:1722–32.
2643. Thway K, Nicholson AG, Wallace WA, et al. (2012). Endobronchial pulmonary angiomatoid fibrous histiocytoma: two cases with EWSR1-CREB1 and EWSR1-ATF1 fusions. Am J Surg Pathol. 36:883–8.
2644. Tiffet O, Nicholson AG, Ladas G, et al. (2003). A clinicopathologic study of 12 neuroendocrine tumors arising in the thymus. Chest. 124:141–6.
2645. Timoteo AT, Branco LM, Bravio I, et al. (2010). Primary angiosarcoma of the pericardium: case report and review of the literature. Kardiol Pol. 68:802–5.
2646. Tirabosco R, Lang-Lazdunski L, Diss TC, et al. (2009). Clear cell sarcoma of the mediastinum. Ann Diagn Pathol. 13:197–200.
2647. Tochigi N, Attanoos R, Chirieac LR, et al. (2013). p16 Deletion in sarcomatoid tumors of the lung and pleura. Arch Pathol Lab Med. 137:632–6.
2648. Tochigi N, Dacic S, Nikiforova M, et al. (2011). Adenosquamous carcinoma of the lung: a microdissection study of KRAS and EGFR mutational and amplification status in a western patient population. Am J Clin Pathol. 135:783–9.
2649. Tolstrup K, Shiota T, Gurudevan S, et al. (2011). Left atrial myxomas: correlation of two-dimensional and live three-dimensional transesophageal echocardiography with the clinical and pathologic findings. J Am Soc Echocardiogr. 24:618–24.
2650. Tomita M, Matsuzaki Y, Edagawa M, et al. (2002). Clinical and immunohistochemical study of eight cases with thymic carcinoma. BMC Surg. 2:3.
2651. Tomiyama N, Johkoh T, Mihara N, et al. (2002). Using the World Health Organization Classification of thymic epithelial neoplasms to describe CT findings. AJR Am J Roentgenol. 179:881–6.
2652. Tomizawa K, Suda K, Onozato R, et al. (2011). Prognostic and predictive implications of HER2/ERBB2/neu gene mutations in lung cancers. Lung Cancer. 74:139–44.
2653. Tongsong T, Sirichotiyakul S, Sittiwangkul R, et al. (2004). Prenatal sonographic diagnosis of cardiac hemangioma with postnatal spontaneous regression. Ultrasound Obstet Gynecol. 24:207–8.
2654. Tonon G, Modi S, Wu L, et al. (2003). t(11;19)(q21;p13) translocation in mucoepidermoid carcinoma creates a novel fusion product that disrupts a Notch signaling pathway. Nat Genet. 33:208–13.
2655. Tonon G, Wong KK, Maulik G, et al. (2005). High-resolution genomic profiles of human lung cancer. Proc Natl Acad Sci USA. 102:9625–30.
2656. Toomes H, Delphendahl A, Manke HG, et al. (1983). The coin lesion of the lung. A review of 955 resected coin lesions. Cancer. 51:534–7.
2657. Topalian SL, Hodi FS, Brahmer JR, et al. (2012). Safety, activity, and immune correlates of anti-PD-1 antibody in cancer. N Engl J Med. 366:2443–54.
2658. Toprani TH, Tamboli P, Amin MB, et al. (2003). Thymic carcinoma with rhabdoid features. Ann Diagn Pathol. 7:106–11.
2659. Toren A, Ben-Bassat I, Rechavi G (1996). Infectious agents and environmental factors in lymphoid malignancies. Blood Rev. 10:89–94.
2660. Torimitsu S, Nemoto T, Wakayama M, et al. (2012). Literature survey on epidemiology and pathology of cardiac fibroma. Eur J Med Res. 17:5.
2661. Torres-Mora J, Dry S, Li X, et al. (2014). Malignant melanotic schwannian tumor: a clinicopathologic, immunohistochemical, and gene expression profiling study of 40 cases, with a proposal for the reclassification of "melanotic schwannoma". Am J Surg Pathol. 38:94–105.
2662. Toufan M, Jodati A, Safaei N, et al. (2012). Myxomas in All Cardiac Chambers. Echocardiography.29: E270-E272.
2663. Toyokawa G, Takenoyama M, Taguchi K, et al. (2013). The first case of lung carcinosarcoma harboring in-frame deletions at exon19 in the EGFR gene. Lung Cancer. 81:491–4.
2664. Toyooka S, Maruyama R, Toyooka KO, et al. (2003). Smoke exposure, histologic type and geography-related differences in the methylation profiles of non-small cell lung cancer. Int J Cancer. 103:153–60.
2665. Toyooka S, Yatabe Y, Tokumo M, et al. (2006). Mutations of epidermal growth factor receptor and K-ras genes in adenosquamous carcinoma of the lung. Int J Cancer. 118:1588–90.
2666. Traub B (1991). Mucinous cystadenoma of the lung. Arch Pathol Lab Med. 115:740–1.
2667. Traverse-Glehen A, Pittaluga S, Gaulard P, et al. (2005). Mediastinal gray zone lymphoma: the missing link between classic Hodgkin's lymphoma and mediastinal large B-cell lymphoma. Am J Surg Pathol. 29:1411–21.
2668. Travis LB, Fossa SD, Schonfeld SJ, et al. (2005). Second cancers among 40,576 testicular cancer patients: focus on long-term survivors. J Natl Cancer Inst. 97:1354–65.
2669. Travis WD (2010). Advances in neuroendocrine lung tumors. Ann Oncol. 21 Suppl 7:vii65–71.
2670. Travis WD (2010). Sarcomatoid neoplasms of the lung and pleura. Arch Pathol Lab Med. 134:1645–58.
2671. Travis WD (2012). Update on small cell carcinoma and its differentiation from squamous cell carcinoma and other non-small cell carcinomas. Mod Pathol. 25 Suppl 1:S18–30.
2672. Travis WD, Brambilla E, Muller-Hermelink HK, et al., eds. (2004). WHO Classification of Tumours. Pathology and Genetics of Tumours of the Lung, Pleura, Thymus and Heart. 3rd ed. Lyon: IARC.
2673. Travis WD, Brambilla E, Noguchi M, et al. (2013). Diagnosis of lung adenocarcinoma in resected specimens: implications of the 2011 International Association for the Study of Lung Cancer/American Thoracic Society/European Respiratory Society classification. Arch Pathol Lab Med. 137:685–705.
2674. Travis WD, Brambilla E, Noguchi M, et al. (2013). Diagnosis of lung cancer in small biopsies and cytology: implications of the 2011 International Association for the Study of Lung Cancer/American Thoracic Society/European Respiratory Society classification. Arch Pathol Lab Med. 137:668–84.
2675. Travis WD, Brambilla E, Noguchi M, et al. (2011). International Association for the Study of Lung Cancer/American Thoracic Society/European Respiratory Society: international multidisciplinary classification of lung adenocarcinoma: executive summary. Proc Am Thorac Soc. 8:381–5.
2676. Travis WD, Brambilla E, Noguchi M, et al. (2011). International association for the study of lung cancer/american thoracic society/european respiratory society international multidisciplinary classification of lung adenocarcinoma. J Thorac Oncol. 6:244–85.
2677. Travis WD, Brambilla E, Rami-Porta R, et al. (2008). Visceral pleural invasion: pathologic criteria and use of elastic stains: proposal for the 7th edition of the TNM classification for lung cancer. J Thorac Oncol. 3: 1384–1390.
2678. Travis WD, Colby TV, Corrin B, et al. (1999). WHO Histological Classification of Tumours. Histological Typing of Lung and Pleural Tumours. 3rd ed. Berlin: Springer.
2679. Travis WD, Gal AA, Colby TV, et al. (1998). Reproducibility of neuroendocrine lung tumor classification. Hum Pathol. 29:272–9.
2680. Travis WD, Giroux DJ, Chansky K, et al. (2008). The IASLC Lung Cancer Staging Project: proposals for the inclusion of broncho-pulmonary carcinoid tumors in the forthcoming (seventh) edition of the TNM Classification for Lung Cancer. J Thorac Oncol. 3:1213–23.
2681. Travis WD, Linnoila RI, Tsokos MG, et al. (1991). Neuroendocrine tumors of the lung with proposed criteria for large-cell neuroendocrine carcinoma. An ultrastructural, immunohistochemical, and flow cytometric study of 35 cases. Am J Surg Pathol. 15:529–53.
2682. Travis WD, Rekhtman N (2011). Pathological diagnosis and classification of lung cancer in small biopsies and cytology: strategic management of tissue for molecular testing. Semin Respir Crit Care Med. 32:22–31.
2683. Travis WD, Rush W, Flieder DB, et al. (1998). Survival analysis of 200 pulmonary neuroendocrine tumors with clarification of criteria for atypical carcinoid and its separation from typical carcinoid. Am J Surg Pathol. 22:934–44.
2684. Travis WD, Travis LB, Devesa SS (1995). Lung cancer. Cancer. 75:191–202.
2685. Trojani M, Contesso G, Coindre JM, et al. (1984). Soft-tissue sarcomas of adults; study of pathological prognostic variables and definition of a histopathological grading system. Int J Cancer. 33:37–42.
2686. Truini A, Coco S, Alama A, et al. (2014). Role of microRNAs in malignant mesothelioma. Cell Mol Life Sci. 71:2865–78.
2687. Truong LD, Mody DR, Cagle PT, et al. (1990). Thymic carcinoma. A clinicopathologic study of 13 cases. Am J Surg Pathol. 14:151–66.
2688. Tryfon S, Dramba V, Zoglopitis F, et al. (2012). Solitary papillomas of the lower airways: epidemiological, clinical, and therapeutic data during a 22-year period and review of the literature. J Thorac Oncol. 7:643–8.
2689. Tsang P, Cesarman E, Chadburn A, et al. (1996). Molecular characterization of primary mediastinal B cell lymphoma. Am J Pathol. 148:2017–25.
2690. Tsao MS, Fraser RS (1991). Primary pulmonary adenocarcinoma with enteric differentiation. Cancer. 68:1754–7.
2690A. Tsao MS, Marguet S, Le Teuff G, et al. (2015). Subtype classification of lung adenocarcinoma predicts benefit from adjuvant chemotherapy in patients undergoing complete resection. J Clin Oncol. 33:3439-46.
2691. Tsuchida M, Umezu H, Hashimoto T, et al. (2008). Absence of gene mutations in KIT-positive thymic epithelial tumors. Lung Cancer. 62:321–5.
2692. Tsuchida M, Yamato Y, Hashimoto T, et al. (2001). Recurrent thymic carcinoid tumor in the pleural cavity. 2 cases of long-term survivors. Jpn J Thorac Cardiovasc Surg. 49:666–8.
2693. Tsuchiya R, Koga K, Matsuno Y, et al. (1994). Thymic carcinoma: proposal for pathological TNM and staging. Pathol Int. 44:505–12.
2695. Tsukadaira A, Okubo Y, Ogasawara H, et al. (2002). Chromosomal aberrations in intravascular lymphomatosis. Am J Clin Oncol. 25:178–81.
2696. Tsukamoto H, Yoshinari M, Okamura K, et al. (1992). Meningioma developed 25 years after radiation therapy for Cushing's disease. Intern Med. 31:629–32.
2697. Tsunoda Y, Tanaka K, Okada K, et al. (2010). [Thymic basaloid carcinoma]. Kyobu Geka. 63:857–61.
2698. Tsuta K, Ishii G, Nitadori J, et al. (2006). Comparison of the immunophenotypes of signet-ring cell carcinoma, solid adenocarcinoma with mucin production, and mucinous bronchioloalveolar carcinoma of the lung characterized by the presence of cytoplasmic mucin. J Pathol. 209:78–87.
2699. Tsuta K, Kawago M, Inoue E, et al. (2013). The utility of the proposed IASLC/ATS/ERS lung adenocarcinoma subtypes for disease prognosis and correlation of driver gene alterations. Lung Cancer. 81:371–6.
2700. Tsuta K, Kozu Y, Mimae T, et al. (2012). c-MET/phospho-MET protein expression and MET gene copy number in non-small cell lung carcinomas. J Thorac Oncol. 7:331–9.
2701. Tsutani Y, Miyata Y, Yamanaka T, et al. (2013). Solid tumors versus mixed tumors with a ground-glass opacity component in patients with clinical stage IA lung adenocarcinoma: prognostic comparison using high-resolution computed tomography findings. J Thorac Cardiovasc Surg. 146:17–23.
2702. Tsutsumi K, Aida Y, Ohno T, et al. (2005). Primary cardiac rhabdomyosarcoma following a uterine leiomyosarcoma: double primary sarcomas. Jpn J Thorac Cardiovasc Surg. 53:458–62.
2703. Turhan N, Ozguler Z, Cagli K, et al. (2011). Primary cardiac undifferentiated sarcoma: role of intraoperative imprint cytology and frozen section of two cases. Cardiovasc Pathol. 20:232–7.
2704. Turner AR, MacDonald RN, Gilbert JA, et al. (1981). Mediastinal germ cell cancers in Klinefelter's syndrome. Ann Intern Med. 94:279.
2705. Turner BM, Cagle PT, Sainz IM, et al. (2012). Napsin A, a new marker for lung adenocarcinoma, is complementary and more sensitive and specific than thyroid transcription factor 1 in the differential diagnosis of primary pulmonary carcinoma: evaluation of 1674 cases by tissue microarray. Arch Pathol Lab Med. 136:163–71.
2706. Tutak E, Satar M, Ozbarlas N, et al. (2008). A newborn infant with intrapericardial rhabdomyosarcoma: a case report. Turk J Pediatr. 50:179–81.
2707. Twa DD, Chan FC, Ben-Neriah S, et al. (2014). Genomic rearrangements involving programmed death ligands are recurrent in primary mediastinal large B-cell lymphoma. Blood. 123:2062–5.
2708. Uchikov AP, Belovezhdov VT, Uzunova VN, et al. (2009). Primary pulmonary paraganglioma. Folia Med (Plovdiv). 51:74–6.
2709. Ueda Y, Omasa M, Taki T, et al. (2012). Thymic Neuroblastoma within a Thymic Cyst in an Adult. Case Rep Oncol. 5:459–63.
2710. Uerbach O, Stout AP, Hammond EC, et al. (1961). Changes in bronchial epithelium in relation to cigarette smoking and in relation to lung cancer. N Engl J Med. 265:253–67.
2711. Ulbright TM, Clark SA, Einhorn LH (1985). Angiosarcoma associated with germ cell tumors. Hum Pathol. 16:268–72.
2712. Ulbright TM, Loehrer PJ, Roth LM, et al. (1984). The development of non-germ cell malignancies within germ cell tumors. A clinicopathologic study of 11 cases. Cancer. 54:1824–33.
2713. Ulbright TM, Michael H, Loehrer PJ, et al. (1990). Spindle cell tumors resected from male patients with germ cell tumors. A clinicopathologic study of 14 cases. Cancer. 65:148–56.
2714. Ulbright TM, Roth LM (1990). A pathologic analysis of lesions following modern chemotherapy for metastatic germ-cell tumors. Pathol Annu. 25(Pt 1):313–40.
2715. Ulbright TM, Roth LM, Brodhecker CA (1986). Yolk sac differentiation in germ cell tumors. A morphologic study of 50 cases with emphasis on hepatic, enteric, and parietal yolk sac features. Am J Surg Pathol. 10:151–64.
2716. Umsawasdi T, Chong C, Weedn VW, et al. (1986). Squamous cell carcinoma of the thymus: a case report of rapid response to cyclophosphamide, doxorubicin, cisplatin, and prednisone. Med Pediatr Oncol. 14:338–41.
2717. Uner A, Dogan M, Sal E, et al. (2010). Stroke and recurrent peripheral embolism in left atrial myxoma. Acta Cardiol. 65:101–3.
2718. United States Public Health Service Office

of the Surgeon General and National Center for Chronic Disease Prevention and Health Promotion (US) Office on Smoking and Health The health consequences of smoking – 50 years of progress: a report of the Surgeon General.U.S. Department of Health and Human Services, Centers for Disease Control and Prevention, National Center for Chronic Disease Prevention and Health Promotion, Office on Smoking and Health2014

2719. Urban C, Lackner H, Schwinger W, et al. (2003). Fatal hemophagocytic syndrome as initial manifestation of a mediastinal germ cell tumor. Med Pediatr Oncol. 40:247–9.

2720. Urban T, Lazor R, Lacronique J, et al. (1999). Pulmonary lymphangioleiomyomatosis. A study of 69 patients. Groupe d'Etudes et de Recherche sur les Maladies "Orphelines" Pulmonaires (GERM"O"P). Medicine (Baltimore). 78:321–37.

2721. Uruga H, Fujii T, Kurosaki A, et al. (2013). Pulmonary tumor thrombotic microangiopathy: a clinical analysis of 30 autopsy cases. Intern Med. 52:1317–23.

2722. Ustun MO, Demircan A, Paksoy N, et al. (1996). A case of intrapulmonary teratoma presenting with hair expectoration. Thorac Cardiovasc Surg. 44:271–3.

2723. Usuda K, Saito Y, Nagamoto N, et al. (1993). Relation between bronchoscopic findings and tumor size of roentgenographically occult bronchogenic squamous cell carcinoma. J Thorac Cardiovasc Surg. 106:1098–103.

2724. Uto T, Bando M, Yamauchi H, et al. (2011). Primary cardiac angiosarcoma of the right auricle with difficult-to-treat bilateral pleural effusion. Intern Med. 50:2371–4.

2725. Uyttebroeck A, Vanhentenrijk V, Hagemeijer A, et al. (2007). Is there a difference in childhood T-cell acute lymphoblastic leukaemia and T-cell lymphoblastic lymphoma? Leuk Lymphoma. 48:1745–54.

2726. Uzun O, Wilson DG, Vujanic GM, et al. (2007). Cardiac tumours in children. Orphanet J Rare Dis. 2:11.

2727. Vaccaro A, Vierucci F, Dini F, et al. (2013). Anterior mediastinal mature teratoma focally infiltrating pulmonary parenchyma. APSP J Case Rep. 4:50.

2728. Vaideeswar P (2009). Sclerosing hemangioma with lymph nodal metastases. Indian J Pathol Microbiol. 52:392–4.

2729. Vaideeswar P (2011). Microscopic thymoma: a report of four cases with review of literature. Indian J Pathol Microbiol. 54:539–41.

2730. Vaideeswar P, Gupta R, Mishra P, et al. (2012). Atypical cardiac myxomas: a clinicopathologic analysis and their comparison to 64 typical myxomas. Cardiovasc Pathol. 21:180–7.

2731. Vaishnavi A, Capelletti M, Le AT, et al. (2013). Oncogenic and drug-sensitive NTRK1 rearrangements in lung cancer. Nat Med. 19:1469–72.

2732. Val-Bernal JF, Figols J, Gomez-Roman JJ (2002). Incidental localized (solitary) epithelial mesothelioma of the pericardium: case report and literature review. Cardiovasc Pathol. 11:181–5.

2733. Val-Bernal JF, Martino M, Mayorga M, et al. (2007). Prichard's structures of the fossa ovalis are age-related phenomena composed of nonreplicating endothelial cells: the cardiac equivalent of cutaneous senile angioma. APMIS. 115:1234–40.

2734. Vallance HD, Jeven G, Wallace DC, et al. (2004). A case of sporadic infantile histiocytoid cardiomyopathy caused by the A8344G (MERRF) mitochondrial DNA mutation. Pediatr Cardiol. 25:538–40.

2735. Valli M, Fabris GA, Dewar A, et al. (1994). Atypical carcinoid tumour of the thymus: a study of eight cases. Histopathology. 24:371–5.

2736. Valli M, Fabris GA, Dewar A, et al. (1994). Atypical carcinoid tumour of the lung: a study of 33 cases with prognostic features. Histopathology. 24:363–9.

2737. Vallieres E, Shepherd FA, Crowley J, et al. (2009). The IASLC Lung Cancer Staging Project: proposals regarding the relevance of TNM in the pathologic staging of small cell lung cancer in the forthcoming (seventh) edition of the TNM classification for lung cancer. J Thorac Oncol. 4:1049–59.

2738. van Boerdonk RA, Daniels JM, Bloemena E, et al. (2013). High-risk human papillomavirus-positive lung cancer: molecular evidence for a pattern of pulmonary metastasis. J Thorac Oncol. 8:711–8.

2739. van Boerdonk RA, Daniels JM, Snijders PJ, et al. (2014). DNA copy number aberrations in endobronchial lesions: a validated predictor for cancer. Thorax. 69:451–7.

2740. van Boerdonk RA, Sutedja TG, Snijders PJ, et al. (2011). DNA copy number alterations in endobronchial squamous metaplastic lesions predict lung cancer. Am J Respir Crit Care Med. 184:948–56.

2741. Van den Berghe I, Debiec-Rychter M, Proot L, et al. (2002). Ring chromosome 6 may represent a cytogenetic subgroup in benign thymoma. Cancer Genet Cytogenet. 137:75–7.

2742. van den Bosch JM, Wagenaar SS, Corrin B, et al. (1987). Mesenchymoma of the lung (so called hamartoma): a review of 154 parenchymal and endobronchial cases. Thorax. 42:790–3.

2743. van den Oord JJ, De Wolf-Peeters C, de Vos R, et al. (1986). Sarcoma arising from interdigitating reticulum cells: report of a case, studied with light and electron microscopy, and enzyme- and immunohistochemistry. Histopathology. 10:509–23.

2744. van der Meij JJ, Boomars KA, van den Bosch JM, et al. (2005). Primary pulmonary malignant meningioma. Ann Thorac Surg. 80:1523–5.

2745. van der Sijp Jr, van Meerbeeck JP, Maat AP, et al. (2002). Determination of the molecular relationship between multiple tumors within one patient is of clinical importance. J Clin Oncol. 20:1105–14.

2746. van der LC, Klootwijk PJ, van Geuns RJ, et al. (2009). Angiosarcoma of the right atrium presenting as collapse. Int J Cardiol. 132:e17–9.

2747. van Echten J, de Jong B, Sinke RJ, et al. (1995). Definition of a new entity of malignant extragonadal germ cell tumors. Genes Chromosomes Cancer. 12:8–15.

2748. Van Loo S, Boeykens E, Stappaerts I, et al. (2011). Classic biphasic pulmonary blastoma: a case report and review of the literature. Lung Cancer. 73:127–32.

2749. van Meerbeeck JP, Fennell DA, De Ruysscher DK (2011). Small-cell lung cancer. Lancet. 378:1741–55.

2750. van Meerbeeck JP, Gaafar R, Manegold C, et al. (2005). Randomized phase III study of cisplatin with or without raltitrexed in patients with malignant pleural mesothelioma: an intergroup study of the European Organisation for Research and Treatment of Cancer Lung Cancer Group and the National Cancer Institute of Canada. J Clin Oncol. 23:6881–9.

2751. van Muijen GN, Ruiter DJ, Warnaar SO (1985). Intermediate filaments in Merkel cell tumors. Hum Pathol. 16:590–5.

2752. van Noesel J, van der Ven WH, van Os TA, et al. (2013). Activating germline R776H mutation in the epidermal growth factor receptor associated with lung cancer with squamous differentiation. J Clin Oncol. 31:e161–4.

2753. Van Schil PE, Asamura H, Rusch VW, et al. (2012). Surgical implications of the new IASLC/ATS/ERS adenocarcinoma classification. Eur Respir J. 39:478–86.

2754. Van Schil PE, Opitz I, Weder W, et al. (2014). Multimodal management of malignant pleural mesothelioma: where are we today? Eur Respir J. 44:754–64.

2755. van Slegtenhorst M, de Hoogt R, Hermans C, et al. (1997). Identification of the tuberous sclerosis gene TSC1 on chromosome 9q34. Science. 277:805–8.

2756. van Spronsen DJ, Vrints LW, Hofstra G, et al. (1997). Disappearance of prognostic significance of histopathological grading of nodular sclerosing Hodgkin's disease for unselected patients, 1972-92. Br J Haematol. 96:322–7.

2757. Vandermeers F, Neelature Sriramareddy S, Costa C, et al. (2013). The role of epigenetics in malignant pleural mesothelioma. Lung Cancer. 81:311–8.

2758. Vanhentenrijk V, Vanden Bempt I, Dierickx D, et al. (2006). Relationship between classic Hodgkin lymphoma and overlapping large cell lymphoma investigated by comparative expressed sequence hybridization expression profiling. J Pathol. 210:155–62.

2759. Vargas SO, French CA, Faul PN, et al. (2001). Upper respiratory tract carcinoma with chromosomal translocation 15;19: evidence for a distinct disease entity of young patients with a rapidly fatal course. Cancer. 92:1195–203.

2760. Vasey PA, Dunlop DJ, Kaye SB (1994). Primary mediastinal germ cell tumour and acute monocytic leukaemia occurring concurrently in a 15-year-old boy. Ann Oncol. 5:649–52.

2761. Vassallo J, Lamant L, Brugieres L, et al. (2006). ALK-positive anaplastic large cell lymphoma mimicking nodular sclerosis Hodgkin's lymphoma: report of 10 cases. Am J Surg Pathol. 30:223–9.

2762. Vassallo R, Ryu JH, Colby TV, et al. (2000). Pulmonary Langerhans'-cell histiocytosis. N Engl J Med. 342:1969–78.

2763. Vassallo R, Ryu JH, Schroeder DR, et al. (2002). Clinical outcomes of pulmonary Langerhans'-cell histiocytosis in adults. N Engl J Med. 346:484–90.

2764. Vaughan CJ, Veugelers M, Basson CT (2001). Tumors and the heart: molecular genetic advances. Curr Opin Cardiol. 16:195–200.

2765. Vaughan P, Pabla L, Hobin D, et al. (2011). Cardiac paraganglioma and gastrointestinal stromal tumor: a pediatric case of Carney-Stratakis syndrome. Ann Thorac Surg. 92:1877–8.

2766. Vaziri M (2012). Primary mediastinal leiomyosarcoma. Gen Thorac Cardiovasc Surg. 60:522–4.

2767. Vaziri M, Sadeghipour A, Pazooki A, et al. (2008). Primary mediastinal myelolipoma. Ann Thorac Surg. 85:1805–6.

2768. Vazquez MF, Koizumi JH, Henschke CI, et al. (2007). Reliability of cytologic diagnosis of early lung cancer. Cancer. 111:252–8.

2769. Veinot JP (2008). Cardiac tumors of adipocytes and cystic tumor of the atrioventricular node. Semin Diagn Pathol. 25:29–38.

2770. Vencio EF, Jenkins RB, Schiller JL, et al. (2007). Clonal cytogenetic abnormalities in Erdheim-Chester disease. Am J Surg Pathol. 31:319–21.

2771. Venkataraman G, Song JY, Tzankov A, et al. (2013). Aberrant T-cell antigen expression in classical Hodgkin lymphoma is associated with decreased event-free survival and overall survival. Blood. 121:1795–804.

2772. Ventura A, Florean P, Trevisan M, et al. (1987). [Anti-alpha-gliadin antibodies. Sensitivity, specificity and correlation with blood xylose test in the 3 diagnostic stages of celiac disease in children]. Pediatr Med Chir. 9:653–60.

2773. Venuta F, Anile M, Diso D, et al. (2010). Thymoma and thymic carcinoma. Eur J Cardiothorac Surg. 37:13–25.

2774. Vermi W, Giurisato E, Lonardi S, et al. (2013). Ligand-dependent activation of EGFR in follicular dendritic cells sarcoma is sustained by local production of cognate ligands. Clin Cancer Res. 19:5027–38.

2775. Vermi W, Lonardi S, Bosisio D, et al. (2008). Identification of CXCL13 as a new marker for follicular dendritic cell sarcoma. J Pathol. 216:356–64.

2776. Veugelers M, Wilkes D, Burton K, et al. (2004). Comparative PRKAR1A genotype-phenotype analyses in humans with Carney complex and prkar1a haploinsufficient mice. Proc Natl Acad Sci USA. 101:14222–7.

2777. Veyssier-Belot C, Cacoub P, Caparros-Lefebvre D, et al. (1996). Erdheim-Chester disease. Clinical and radiologic characteristics of 59 cases. Medicine (Baltimore). 75:157–69.

2778. Videtic GM, Truong PT, Ash RB, et al. (2005). Does sex influence the impact that smoking, treatment interruption and impaired pulmonary function have on outcomes in limited stage small cell lung cancer treatment? Can Respir J. 12:245–50.

2779. Vigano S, Papini GD, Cotticelli B, et al. (2013). Prevalence of cerebral aneurysms in patients treated for left cardiac myxoma: a prospective study. Clin Radiol. 68:e624–8.

2780. Villacampa VM, Villarreal M, Ros LH, et al. (1999). Cardiac rhabdomyosarcoma: diagnosis by MR imaging. Eur Radiol. 9:634–7.

2781. Viswanathan S, Gibbs JL, Roberts P (2003). Clonal translocation in a cardiac fibroma presenting with incessant ventricular tachycardia in childhood. Cardiol Young. 13:101–2.

2782. Vladislav IT, Gokmen-Polar Y, Kesler KA, et al. (2013). The role of histology in predicting recurrence of type A thymomas: a clinicopathologic correlation of 23 cases. Mod Pathol. 26:1059–64.

2783. Vladislav IT, Gokmen-Polar Y, Kesler KA, et al. (2014). The prognostic value of architectural patterns in a study of 37 type AB thymomas. Mod Pathol. 27:863–8.

2784. Vladislav T, Jain RK, Alvarez R, et al. (2012). Extrathoracic metastases of thymic origin: a review of 35 cases. Mod Pathol. 25:370–7.

2785. Vlasveld LT, Splinter TA, Hagemeijer A, et al. (1994). Acute myeloid leukaemia with +i(12p) shortly after treatment of mediastinal germ cell tumour. Br J Haematol. 88:196–8.

2786. Vogt FM, Hunold P, Ruehm SG (2003). Images in vascular medicine. Angiosarcoma of superior vena cava with extension into right atrium assessed by MD-CT and MRI. Vasc Med. 8:283–4.

2787. Volkl TM, Langer T, Aigner T, et al. (2006). Klinefelter syndrome and mediastinal germ cell tumors. Am J Med Genet A. 140:471–81.

2788. von Ahsen I, Rogalla P, Bullerdiek J (2005). Expression patterns of the LPP-HMGA2 fusion transcript in pulmonary chondroid hamartomas with t(3;12)(q27 approximately 28;q14 approximately 15). Cancer Genet Cytogenet. 163:68–70.

2789. von der Thusen JH, Tham YS, Pattenden H, et al. (2013). Prognostic significance of predominant histologic pattern and nuclear grade in resected adenocarcinoma of the lung: potential parameters for a grading system. J Thorac Oncol. 8:37–44.

2790. Vos JA, Abbondanzo SL, Barekman CL, et al. (2005). Histiocytic sarcoma: a study of five cases including the histiocyte marker CD163. Mod Pathol. 18:693–704.

2791. Vougiouklakis T, Goussia A, Ioachim E, et al. (2001). Cardiac fibroma. A case presentation. Virchows Arch. 438:635–6.

2792. Wage R, Kafka H, Prasad S (2008). Images in cardiovascular medicine. Cardiac rhabdomyoma in an adult with a previous presumptive diagnosis of septal hypertrophy. Circulation. 117:e469–70.

2793. Wagner T, Brechemier D, Dugert E, et al. (2012). Diffuse pulmonary uptake on FDG-PET with normal CT diagnosed as intravascular large B-cell lymphoma: a case report and a discussion of the causes of diffuse FDG uptake in the lungs. Cancer Imaging. 12:7–12.

2794. Wakely PE Jr (2005). Cytopathology of thymic epithelial neoplasms. Semin Diagn Pathol. 22:213–22.

2795. Wakely PE Jr (2008). Fine needle aspiration in the diagnosis of thymic epithelial neoplasms. Hematol Oncol Clin North Am.

22:433–42.
2796. Wakely P Jr, Suster S (2000). Suster S (2000). Langerhans' cell histiocytosis of the thymus associated with multilocular thymic cyst. Hum Pathol. 31:1532–35.
2797. Walter M, Thomson NM, Dowling J, et al. (1979). Lymphomatoid granulomatosis in a renal transplant recipient. Aust N Z J Med. 9:434–6.
2798. Wang C, Mahaffey JE, Axelrod L, et al. (1979). Hyperfunctioning supernumerary parathyroid glands. Surg Gynecol Obstet. 148:711–4.
2799. Wang CX, Liu B, Wang YF, et al. (2014). Pulmonary enteric adenocarcinoma: a study of the clinicopathologic and molecular status of nine cases. Int J Clin Exp Pathol. 7:1266–74.
2800. Wang DY, Kuo SH, Chang DB, et al. (1995). Fine needle aspiration cytology of thymic carcinoid tumor. Acta Cytol. 39:423–7.
2801. Wang F, Liu A, Peng Y, et al. (2009). Diagnostic utility of SALL4 in extragonadal yolk sac tumors: an immunohistochemical study of 59 cases with comparison to placental-like alkaline phosphatase, alpha-fetoprotein, and glypican-3. Am J Surg Pathol. 33:1529–39.
2802. Wang J, Kragel AH, Friedlander ER, et al. (1993). Granular cell tumor of the sinus node. Am J Cardiol. 71:490–2.
2803. Wang JG, Li NN (2013). Primary cardiac synovial sarcoma. Ann Thorac Surg. 95:2202–9.
2804. Wang NS, Seemayer TA, Ahmed MN, et al. (1974). Pulmonary leiomyosarcoma associated with an arteriovenous fistula. Arch Pathol. 98:100–5.
2805. Wang QB, Chen YQ, Shen JJ, et al. (2011). Sixteen cases of pulmonary sclerosing haemangioma: CT findings are not definitive for preoperative diagnosis. Clin Radiol. 66:708–14.
2806. Wang R, Hu H, Pan Y, et al. (2012). RET fusions define a unique molecular and clinicopathologic subtype of non-small-cell lung cancer. J Clin Oncol. 30:4352–9.
2807. Wang XL, Mu YM, Dou JT, et al. (2011). Medullar thyroid carcinoma in mediastinum initially presenting as Ectopic ACTH syndrome. A case report. Neuroendocrinol Lett. 32:421–4.
2808. Wang YL, Yi XH, Chen G, et al. (2009). [Thymoma associated with an lipofibroadenoma: report of a case]. Zhonghua Bing Li Xue Za Zhi. 38:556–7.
2809. Warnke RA, Weiss LM, Chan JKC, et al. (1995). Tumors of the Lymph Nodes and Spleen. AFIP Atlas of Tumor Pathology. 3rd ed. Volume 14. Washington, DC: American Registry of Pathology.
2810. Warth A, Muley T, Meister M, et al. (2012). The novel histologic International Association for the Study of Lung Cancer/American Thoracic Society/European Respiratory Society classification system of lung adenocarcinoma is a stage-independent predictor of survival. J Clin Oncol. 30:1438–46.
2811. Warth A, Stenzinger A, von Brunneck AC, et al. (2012). Interobserver variability in the application of the novel IASLC/ATS/ERS classification for pulmonary adenocarcinomas. Eur Respir J. 40:1221–7.
2812. Watanabe K, Saito N, Sugito M, et al. (2013). Incidence and predictive factors for pulmonary metastases after curative resection of colon cancer. Ann Surg Oncol. 20:1374–80.
2813. Watanabe Y, Tsuta K, Kusumoto M, et al. (2014). Clinicopathologic features and computed tomographic findings of 52 surgically resected adenosquamous carcinomas of the lung. Ann Thorac Surg. 97:245–51.
2814. Watchell M, Heritage DW, Pastore L, et al. (2000). Cytogenetic study of cardiac papillary fibroelastoma. Cancer Genet Cytogenet. 120:174–5.
2815. Watson GH (1991). Cardiac rhabdomyomas in tuberous sclerosis. Ann N Y Acad Sci. 615:50–7.
2816. Weber C, Pautex S, Zulian GB, et al. (2013). Primary pulmonary malignant meningioma with lymph node and liver metastasis in a centenary woman, an autopsy case. Virchows Arch. 462:481–5.
2817. Wei B, Inabnet W, Lee JA, et al. (2011). Optimizing the minimally invasive approach to mediastinal parathyroid adenomas. Ann Thorac Surg. 92:1012–7.
2818. Weichert W, Schewe C, Denkert C, et al. (2009). Molecular HPV typing as a diagnostic tool to discriminate primary from metastatic squamous cell carcinoma of the lung. Am J Surg Pathol. 33:513–20.
2819. Weide LG, Ulbright TM, Loehrer PJ Sr, et al. (1993). Thymic carcinoma. A distinct clinical entity responsive to chemotherapy. Cancer. 71:1219–23.
2820. Weidner N (1999). Germ-cell tumors of the mediastinum. Semin Diagn Pathol. 16:42–50.
2821. Weiler R, Feichtinger H, Schmid KW, et al. (1987). Chromogranin A and B and secretogranin II in bronchial and intestinal carcinoids. Virchows Arch A Pathol Anat Histopathol. 412:103–9.
2822. Weinbreck N, Vignaud JM, Begueret H, et al. (2007). SYT-SSX fusion is absent in sarcomatoid mesothelioma allowing its distinction from synovial sarcoma of the pleura. Mod Pathol. 20:617–21.
2823. Weinstein IB, Joe AK (2006). Mechanisms of disease: Oncogene addiction--a rationale for molecular targeting in cancer therapy. Nat Clin Pract Oncol. 3:448–57.
2824. Weir BA, Woo MS, Getz G, et al. (2007). Characterizing the cancer genome in lung adenocarcinoma. Nature. 450:893–8.
2825. Weirich G, Schneider P, Fellbaum C, et al. (1997). p53 alterations in thymic epithelial tumours. Virchows Arch. 431:17–23.
2826. Weis CA, Yao X, Deng Y, et al. (2015). The Impact of Thymoma Histotype on Prognosis in a Worldwide Database. J Thorac Oncol. 10:367–72.
2827. Weiss SW, Antonescu CR, Bridge JA, et al. (2013). Epitheliod haemangioendothelioma. In: Fletcher CDM, Bridge JA, Hogendoorn PCW, Mertens F, eds. WHO Classification of Tumours of Soft Tissue and Bone. 4th ed. Lyon: IARC; pp. 155–6.
2828. Weiss SW, Ishak KG, Dail DH, et al. (1986). Epithelioid hemangioendothelioma and related lesions. Semin Diagn Pathol. 3:259–87.
2829. Weissferdt A, Kalhor N, Suster S (2011). Malignant mesothelioma with prominent adenomatoid features: a clinicopathologic and immunohistochemical study of 10 cases. Ann Diagn Pathol. 15:25–9.
2830. Weissferdt A, Kalhor N, Suster S, et al. (2010). Primary angiosarcomas of the anterior mediastinum: a clinicopathologic and immunohistochemical study of 9 cases. Hum Pathol. 41:1711–7.
2831. Weissferdt A, Moran CA (2010). Primary vascular tumors of the lungs: a review. Ann Diagn Pathol. 14:296–308.
2832. Weissferdt A, Moran CA (2011). Pax8 expression in thymic epithelial neoplasms: an immunohistochemical analysis. Am J Surg Pathol. 35:1305–10.
2833. Weissferdt A, Moran CA (2011). Primary MALT-type lymphoma of the thymus: a clinicopathological and immunohistochemical study of six cases. Lung. 189:461–6.
2834. Weissferdt A, Moran CA (2011). Pulmonary salivary gland-type tumors with features of malignant mixed tumor (carcinoma ex pleomorphic adenoma): a clinicopathologic study of five cases. Am J Clin Pathol. 136:793–8.
2835. Weissferdt A, Moran CA (2011). Thymic carcinoma associated with multilocular thymic cyst: a clinicopathologic study of 7 cases. Am J Surg Pathol. 35:1074–9.
2836. Weissferdt A, Moran CA (2012). Anaplastic thymic carcinoma: a clinicopathologic and immunohistochemical study of 6 cases. Hum Pathol. 43:874–7.
2837. Weissferdt A, Moran CA (2012). Micronodular thymic carcinoma with lymphoid hyperplasia: a clinicopathological and immunohistochemical study of five cases. Mod Pathol. 25:993–9.
2838. Weissferdt A, Moran CA (2012). Thymic carcinoma, part 1: a clinicopathologic and immunohistochemical study of 65 cases. Am J Clin Pathol. 138:103–14.
2839. Weissferdt A, Moran CA (2012). Thymic carcinoma, part 2: a clinicopathologic correlation of 33 cases with a proposed staging system. Am J Clin Pathol. 138:115–21.
2840. Weissferdt A, Moran CA (2012). Thymomas with prominent signet ring cell-like features: a clinicopathologic and immunohistochemical study of 10 cases. Hum Pathol. 43:1881–6.
2841. Weissferdt A, Moran CA (2013). Staging of primary mediastinal tumors. Adv Anat Pathol. 20:1–9.
2842. Weissferdt A, Moran CA (2013). The impact of neoadjuvant chemotherapy on the histopathological assessment of thymomas: a clinicopathological correlation of 28 cases treated with a similar regimen. Lung. 191:379–83.
2843. Weissferdt A, Moran CA (2013). Thymomas with prominent glandular differentiation: a clinicopathologic and immunohistochemical study of 12 cases. Hum Pathol. 44:1612–6.
2844. Weissferdt A, Suster S, Moran CA (2012). Primary mediastinal "thymic" seminomas. Adv Anat Pathol. 19:75–80.
2845. Weissferdt A, Tang X, Wistuba II, et al. (2013). Comparative immunohistochemical analysis of pulmonary and thymic neuroendocrine carcinomas using PAX8 and TTF-1. Mod Pathol. 26:1554–60.
2846. Weissferdt A, Wistuba II, Moran CA (2012). Molecular aspects of thymic carcinoma. Lung Cancer. 78:127–32.
2847. Weksler B, Dhupar R, Parikh V, et al. (2013). Thymic carcinoma: a multivariate analysis of factors predictive of survival in 290 patients. Ann Thorac Surg. 95:299–303.
2848. Weksler B, Nason KS, Mackey D, et al. (2012). Thymomas and extrathymic cancers. Ann Thorac Surg. 93:884–8.
2849. Wen J, Fu JH, Zhang W, et al. (2011). Lung carcinoma signaling pathways activated by smoking. Chin J Cancer. 30:551–8.
2850. Weniger MA, Gesk S, Ehrlich S, et al. (2007). Gains of REL in primary mediastinal B-cell lymphoma coincide with nuclear accumulation of REL protein. Genes Chromosomes Cancer. 46:406–15.
2851. Weniger MA, Melzner I, Menz CK, et al. (2006). Mutations of the tumor suppressor gene SOCS-1 in classical Hodgkin lymphoma are frequent and associated with nuclear phospho-STAT5 accumulation. Oncogene. 25:2679–84.
2852. Went PT, Dirnhofer S, Stallmach T, et al. (2005). Placental site trophoblastic tumor of the mediastinum. Hum Pathol. 36:581–4.
2853. Wessalowski R, Schneider DT, Gobel U, et al. (2013). Salvage treatment of relapsed or refractory germ-cell tumours - authors' reply. Lancet Oncol. 14:e486–7.
2854. Wessendorf S, Barth TF, Viardot A, et al. (2007). Further delineation of chromosomal consensus regions in primary mediastinal B-cell lymphomas: an analysis of 37 tumor samples using high-resolution genomic profiling (array-CGH). Leukemia. 21:2463–9.
2855. West JA, Viswanathan SR, Yabuuchi A, et al. (2009). A role for Lin28 in primordial germ-cell development and germ-cell malignancy. Nature. 460:909–13.
2856. Wetterskog D, Wilkerson PM, Rodrigues DN, et al. (2013). Mutation profiling of adenoid cystic carcinomas from multiple anatomical sites identifies mutations in the RAS pathway, but no KIT mutations. Histopathology. 62:543–50.
2857. Weynand B, Noel H, Goncette L, et al. (1997). Solitary fibrous tumor of the pleura: a report of five cases diagnosed by transthoracic cutting needle biopsy. Chest. 112:1424–8.
2858. Whang-Peng J, Kao-Shan CS, Lee EC, et al. (1982). Specific chromosome defect associated with human small-cell lung cancer; deletion 3p(14-23). Science. 215:181–2.
2859. Wheler J, Hong D, Swisher SG, et al. (2013). Thymoma patients treated in a phase I clinic at MD Anderson Cancer Center: responses to mTOR inhibitors and molecular analyses. Oncotarget. 4:890–8.
2860. Wheler JJ, Falchook GS, Tsimberidou AM, et al. (2013). Aberrations in the epidermal growth factor receptor gene in 958 patients with diverse advanced tumors: implications for therapy. Ann Oncol. 24:838–42.
2861. White W, Shiu MH, Rosenblum MK, et al. (1990). Cellular schwannoma. A clinicopathologic study of 57 patients and 58 tumors. Cancer. 66:1266–75.
2862. Whitehouse AC, Black CB, Heppe MS, et al. (2008). Environmental exposure to Libby Asbestos and mesotheliomas. Am J Ind Med. 51:877–80.
2863. Whitesell PL, Peters SG (1993). Pulmonary manifestations of extrathoracic malignant lesions. Mayo Clin Proc. 68:483–91.
2864. Whithaus K, Fukuoka J, Prihoda TJ, et al. (2012). Evaluation of napsin A, cytokeratin 5/6, p63, and thyroid transcription factor 1 in adenocarcinoma versus squamous cell carcinoma of the lung. Arch Pathol Lab Med. 136:155–62.
2865. Wiatrowska BA, Krol J, Zakowski MF (2001). Large-cell neuroendocrine carcinoma of the lung: proposed criteria for cytologic diagnosis. Diagn Cytopathol. 24:58–64.
2866. Wick MR (1990). Mediastinal cysts and intrathoracic thyroid tumors. Semin Diagn Pathol. 7:285–94.
2867. Wick MR (2000). Immunohistology of neuroendocrine and neuroectodermal tumors. Semin Diagn Pathol. 17:194–203.
2868. Wick MR, Carney JA, Bernatz PE, et al. (1982). Primary mediastinal carcinoid tumors. Am J Surg Pathol. 6:195–205.
2869. Wick MR, Ritter JH, Humphrey PA (1997). Sarcomatoid carcinomas of the lung: a clinicopathologic review. Am J Clin Pathol. 108:40–53.
2870. Wick MR, Ritter JH, Humphrey PA, et al. (1997). Clear cell neoplasms of the endocrine system and thymus. Semin Diagn Pathol. 14:183–202.
2871. Wick MR, Rosai J (1988). Neuroendocrine neoplasms of the thymus. Pathol Res Pract. 183:188–99.
2872. Wick MR, Rosai J (1991). Neuroendocrine neoplasms of the mediastinum. Semin Diagn Pathol. 8:35–51.
2873. Wick MR, Scheithauer BW, Weiland LH, et al. (1982). Primary thymic carcinomas. Am J Surg Pathol. 6:613–30.
2874. Wick MR, Zettl A, Kuo TT, et al. (2004). Clear cell carcinoma. In: Travis WD, Brambilla E, Muller-Hermelink HK, Harris CC, eds. WHO Classification of Tumours. Pathology and Genetics of Tumours of the Lung, Pleura, Thymus and Heart. 3rd ed. Lyon: IARC; pp. 182–182.
2875. Wiesner T, Fried I, Ulz P, et al. (2012). Toward an improved definition of the tumor spectrum associated with BAP1 germline mutations. J Clin Oncol. 30:e337–40.
2876. Wijesuriya S, Chandratreya L, Medford AR (2013). Chronic pulmonary emboli and radiologic mimics on CT pulmonary angiography: a diagnostic challenge. Chest. 143:1460–71.
2877. Wikstrom AM, Dunkel L (2008). Testicular function in Klinefelter syndrome. Horm Res. 69:317–26.
2878. Wikstrom AM, Hoei-Hansen CE, Dunkel L, et al. (2007). Immunoexpression of androgen receptor and nine markers of maturation in the testes of adolescent boys with Klinefelter syndrome: evidence for degeneration of germ cells at the onset of meiosis. J Clin Endocrinol Metab. 92:714–9.
2879. Wilken JJ, Meier FA, Kornstein MJ (2000).

Kaposiform hemangioendothelioma of the thymus. Arch Pathol Lab Med. 124:1542–4.
2880. Williams DM, Hobson R, Imeson J, et al. (2002). Anaplastic large cell lymphoma in childhood: analysis of 72 patients treated on The United Kingdom Children's Cancer Study Group chemotherapy regimens. Br J Haematol. 117:812–20.
2881. Willis RA (1950). The borderland of embryology and pathology. Bull N Y Acad Med. 26:440–60.
2882. Wilson CI, Inchausti BC, Griffith KM, et al. (1999). Cardiac myxoma with chondroid features. Ann Diagn Pathol. 3:309–14.
2883. Wilson KS, McKenna RW, Kroft SH, et al. (2002). Primary effusion lymphomas exhibit complex and recurrent cytogenetic abnormalities. Br J Haematol. 116:113–21.
2884. Wilson RW, Gallateau-Salle F, Moran CA (1999). Desmoid tumors of the pleura: a clinicopathologic mimic of localized fibrous tumor. Mod Pathol. 12:9–14.
2885. Wilson RW, Moran CA (1997). Primary melanoma of the lung: a clinicopathologic and immunohistochemical study of eight cases. Am J Surg Pathol. 21:1196–202.
2886. Wilson RW, Moran CA (1998). Primary ependymoma of the mediastinum: a clinicopathologic study of three cases. Ann Diagn Pathol. 2:293–300.
2887. Wilson WH, Kingma DW, Raffeld M, et al. (1996). Association of lymphomatoid granulomatosis with Epstein-Barr viral infection of B lymphocytes and response to interferon-alpha 2b. Blood. 87:4531–7.
2887A. Wilson WH, Pittaluga S, Nicolae A, et al. (2014). A prospective study of mediastinal grayzone lymphoma. Blood. 124:1563–9.
2888. Wisnivesky JP, Yung RC, Mathur PN, et al. (2013). Diagnosis and treatment of bronchial intraepithelial neoplasia and early lung cancer of the central airways: Diagnosis and management of lung cancer, 3rd ed: American College of Chest Physicians evidence-based clinical practice guidelines. Chest. 143:e263S–e277S.
2889. Wistuba II, Behrens C, Milchgrub S, et al. (1999). Sequential molecular abnormalities are involved in the multistage development of squamous cell lung carcinoma. Oncogene. 18:643–50.
2890. Wistuba II, Behrens C, Virmani AK, et al. (2000). High resolution chromosome 3p allelotyping of human lung cancer and preneoplastic/preinvasive bronchial epithelium reveals multiple, discontinuous sites of 3p allele loss and three regions of frequent breakpoints. Cancer Res. 60:1949–60.
2891. Wistuba II, Berry J, Behrens C, et al. (2000). Molecular changes in the bronchial epithelium of patients with small cell lung cancer. Clin Cancer Res. 6:2604–10.
2892. Wistuba II, Gazdar AF (2003). Characteristic genetic alterations in lung cancer. Methods Mol Med. 74:3–28.
2893. Wistuba II, Gazdar AF (2006). Lung cancer preneoplasia. Annu Rev Pathol. 1:331–48.
2894. Wistuba II, Gelovani JG, Jacoby JJ, et al. (2011). Methodological and practical challenges for personalized cancer therapies. Nat Rev Clin Oncol. 8:135–41.
2895. Wistuba II, Lam S, Behrens C, et al. (1997). Molecular damage in the bronchial epithelium of current and former smokers. J Natl Cancer Inst. 89:1366–73.
2896. Witherby SM, Butnor KJ, Grunberg SM (2007). Malignant mesothelioma following thoracic radiotherapy for lung cancer. Lung Cancer. 57:410–3.
2897. Witkin GB, Rosai J (1989). Solitary fibrous tumor of the mediastinum. A report of 14 cases. Am J Surg Pathol. 13:547–57.
2897A. Wittekind Ch, Greene F, Henson DE, Hutter RVP, Sobin L, eds. (2003). TNM Supplement. A Commentary on Uniform Use. 3rd ed. Hoboken (NJ): John Wiley & Sons.
2898. Wittenberg KH, Swensen SJ, Myers JL (2000). Pulmonary involvement with Erdheim-Chester disease: radiographic and CT findings. AJR Am J Roentgenol. 174:1327–31.
2899. Woessmann W, Lisfeld J, Burkhardt B (2013). Therapy in primary mediastinal B-cell lymphoma. N Engl J Med. 369:282.
2900. Wolfe JTI, Wick MR, Banks PM, et al. (1983). Clear cell carcinoma of the thymus. Mayo Clin Proc. 58:365–70.
2901. Wolff M, Goodman EN (1980). Functioning lipoadenoma of a supernumerary parathyroid gland in the mediastinum. Head Neck Surg. 2:302–7.
2902. Wolff M, Rosai J, Wright DH (1984). Sebaceous glands within the thymus: report of three cases. Hum Pathol. 15:341–3.
2903. Wong JW, Pitlik D, Abdul-Karim FW (1997). Cytology of pleural, peritoneal and pericardial fluids in children. A 40-year summary. Acta Cytol. 41:467–73.
2904. Wood DE (2000). Mediastinal germ cell tumors. Semin Thorac Cardiovasc Surg. 12:278–89.
2905. World Health Organization (1976). International Classification of Diseases for Oncology. 1st ed. Geneva: WHO Press.
2906. Wright CD, Kesler KA, Nichols CR, et al. (1990). Primary mediastinal nonseminomatous germ cell tumors. Results of a multimodality approach. J Thorac Cardiovasc Surg. 99:210–7.
2907. Wright CD, Wain JC, Wong DR, et al. (2005). Predictors of recurrence in thymic tumors: importance of invasion, World Health Organization histology, and size. J Thorac Cardiovasc Surg. 130:1413–21.
2908. Wright GL Jr, Haley C, Beckett ML, et al. (1995). Expression of prostate-specific membrane antigen in normal, benign, and malignant prostate tissues. Urol Oncol. 1:18–28.
2909. Wu D, Hiroshima K, Matsumoto S, et al. (2013). Diagnostic usefulness of p16/CDKN2A FISH in distinguishing between sarcomatoid mesothelioma and fibrous pleuritis. Am J Clin Pathol. 139:39–46.
2910. Wu J, Chu PG, Jiang Z, et al. (2013). Napsin A expression in primary mucin-producing adenocarcinomas of the lung: an immunohistochemical study. Am J Clin Pathol. 139:160–6.
2911. Wu L, Xu Z, Zhao X, et al. (2009). Surgical treatment of lung cancer invading the left atrium or base of the pulmonary vein. World J Surg. 33:492–6.
2912. Wu M, Sun K, Gil J, et al. (2009). Immunohistochemical detection of p63 and XIAP in thymic hyperplasia and thymomas. Am J Clin Pathol. 131:689–93.
2913. Wu SG, Li Y, Li B, et al. (2014). Unusual combined thymic mucoepidermoid carcinoma and thymoma: a case report and review of literature. Diagn Pathol. 9:8.
2914. Wu TC, Kuo TT (1993). Study of Epstein-Barr virus early RNA 1 (EBER1) expression by in situ hybridization in thymic epithelial tumors of Chinese patients in Taiwan. Hum Pathol. 24:235–8.
2915. Wu W, Youm W, Rezk SA, et al. (2013). Human herpesvirus 8-unrelated primary effusion lymphoma-like lymphoma: report of a rare case and review of 54 cases in the literature. Am J Clin Pathol. 140:258–73.
2916. Wu XQ, Huang C, He X, et al. (2013). Feedback regulation of telomerase reverse transcriptase: new insight into the evolving field of telomerase in cancer. Cell Signal. 25:2462–8.
2917. Wychulis AR, Payne WS, Clagett OT, et al. (1971). Surgical treatment of mediastinal tumors: a 40 year experience. J Thorac Cardiovasc Surg. 62:379–92.
2917A. Wynes MW, Sholl LM, Dietel M, et al. (2014). An international interpretatino study using the ALK IHC antibody D5F3 and a sensitive detection kit demonstrates high concordance between ALK IHC and ALK FISH and between evaluators. J. Thoracic Oncol 9:631–8.
2918. Xio S, Li D, Vijg J, et al. (1995). Codeletion of p15 and p16 in primary malignant mesothelioma. Oncogene. 11:511–5.
2919. Yahng SA, Kang HH, Kim SK, et al. (2009). Erdheim-Chester disease with lung involvement mimicking pulmonary lymphangitic carcinomatosis. Am J Med Sci. 337:302–4.
2920. Yamada S, Noguchi H, Nabeshima A, et al. (2012). Basaloid carcinoma of the lung associated with central cavitation: a unique surgical case focusing on cytological and immunohistochemical findings. Diagn Pathol. 7:175.
2921. Yamada T, Chiba W, Hitomi S (2006). [Thymic basaloid carcinoma]. Kyobu Geka. 59:1154–8.
2922. Yamada Y, Tomaru U, Ishizu A, et al. (2014). Expression of thymoproteasome subunit beta5t in type AB thymoma. J Clin Pathol. 67:276–8.
2923. Yamada Y, Tomaru U, Ishizu A, et al. (2011). Expression of proteasome subunit beta5t in thymic epithelial tumors. Am J Surg Pathol. 35:1296–304.
2924. Yamaguchi H, Soda H, Kitazaki T, et al. (2006). Thymic carcinoma with epidermal growth factor receptor gene mutations. Lung Cancer. 52:261–2.
2925. Yamaji I, Iimura O, Mito T, et al. (1984). An ectopic, ACTH producing, oncocytic carcinoid tumor of the thymus: report of a case. Jpn J Med. 23:62–6.
2926. Yamamoto H, Higasa K, Sakaguchi M, et al. (2014). Novel germline mutation in the transmembrane domain of HER2 in familial lung adenocarcinomas. J Natl Cancer Inst. 106:djt338.
2927. Yamamoto T, Tamura J, Orima S, et al. (1999). Rhabdomyosarcoma in a patient with mosaic Klinefelter syndrome and transformation of immature teratoma. J Int Med Res. 27:196–200.
2928. Yamashita H, Suzuki A, Takahashi Y, et al. (2012). Intravascular large B-cell lymphoma with diffuse FDG uptake in the lung by 18FDG-PET/CT without chest CT findings. Ann Nucl Med. 26:515–21.
2929. Yamashita K, Haga H, Kobashi Y, et al. (2008). Lung involvement in IgG4-related lymphoplasmacytic vasculitis and interstitial fibrosis: report of 3 cases and review of the literature. Am J Surg Pathol. 32:1620–6.
2930. Yamashita S, Nakamura K, Shinozaki H, et al. (2011). Lymphangioleiomyomatosis suspected to be a gynecologic disease. J Obstet Gynaecol Res. 37:267–9.
2931. Yamauchi K, Yasuda M (2002). Comparison in treatments of nonleukemic granulocytic sarcoma: report of two cases and a review of 72 cases in the literature. Cancer. 94:1739–46.
2932. Yamazaki K (2004). Type-II pneumocyte differentiation in pulmonary sclerosing hemangioma: ultrastructural differentiation and immunohistochemical distribution of lineage-specific transcription factors (TTF-1, HNF-3 alpha, and HNF-3 beta) and surfactant proteins. Virchows Arch. 445:45–53.
2933. Yanagawa N, Wang A, Kohler D, et al. (2013). Human papilloma virus genome is rare in North American non-small cell lung carcinoma patients. Lung Cancer. 79:215–20.
2934. Yang CJ, Cheng YJ, Kang WY, et al. (2007). A case of dermoid cyst ruptured into the lung. Respirology. 12:931–3.
2935. Yang GC, Hwang SJ, Yee HT (2002). Fine-needle aspiration cytology of unusual germ cell tumors of the mediastinum: atypical seminoma and parietal yolk sac tumor. Diagn Cytopathol. 27:69–74.
2936. Yang JT, Chang CM, Lee MH, et al. (2010). Thymic squamous cell carcinoma with multiple brain metastases. Acta Neurol Taiwan. 19:41–4.
2937. Yang M, Nonaka D (2010). A study of immunohistochemical differential expression in pulmonary and mammary carcinomas. Mod Pathol. 23:654–61.
2938. Yang X, Gao X, Wang S (2009). Primary mediastinal malignant meningioma. Eur J Cardiothorac Surg. 36:217–8.
2939. Yang X, Sun X (2007). Meta-analysis of several gene lists for distinct types of cancer: a simple way to reveal common prognostic markers. BMC Bioinformatics. 8:118.
2940. Yano M, Sasaki H, Yokoyama T, et al. (2008). Thymic carcinoma: 30 cases at a single institution. J Thorac Oncol. 3:265–9.
2941. Yano M, Yamakawa Y, Kiriyama M, et al. (2002). Sclerosing hemangioma with metastases to multiple nodal stations. Ann Thorac Surg. 73:981–3.
2942. Yao JC, Hassan M, Phan A, et al. (2008). One hundred years after "carcinoid": epidemiology of and prognostic factors for neuroendocrine tumors in 35,825 cases in the United States. J Clin Oncol. 26:3063–72.
2943. Yap CH, Hair C, Foy S, et al. (2007). Resection of right atrial metastatic large-cell neuroendocrine carcinoma. Asian Cardiovasc Thorac Ann. 15:e20–2.
2944. Yaris N, Nas Y, Cobanoglu U, et al. (2006). Thymic carcinoma in children. Pediatr Blood Cancer. 47:224–7.
2945. Yashima K, Litzky LA, Kaiser L, et al. (1997). Telomerase expression in respiratory epithelium during the multistage pathogenesis of lung carcinomas. Cancer Res. 57:2373–7.
2946. Yasuda H, Kobayashi S, Costa DB (2012). EGFR exon 20 insertion mutations in non-small-cell lung cancer: preclinical data and clinical implications. Lancet Oncol. 13:e23–31.
2947. Yasuda H, Park E, Yun CH et al. (2013). Structural, biochemical, and clinical characterization of epidermal growth factor receptor (EGFR) exon 20 insertion mutations in lung cancer. Sci Transl Med 5: 216ra177
2948. Yasuda M, Hanagiri T, Oka S, et al. (2011). Results of a surgical resection for patients with thymic carcinoma. Scand J Surg. 100:159–63.
2949. Yasuda M, Yasukawa T, Ozaki D, et al. (2006). Mucoepidermoid carcinoma of the thymus. Jpn J Thorac Cardiovasc Surg. 54:23–6.
2950. Yatabe Y (2010). EGFR mutations and the terminal respiratory unit. Cancer Metastasis Rev. 29:23–36.
2951. Yatabe Y, Kosaka T, Takahashi T, et al. (2005). EGFR mutation is specific for terminal respiratory unit type adenocarcinoma. Am J Surg Pathol. 29:633–9.
2952. Yatabe Y, Takahashi T, Mitsudomi T (2008). Epidermal growth factor receptor gene amplification is acquired in association with tumor progression of EGFR-mutated lung cancer. Cancer Res. 68:2106–11.
2953. Yates DH, Corrin B, Stidolph PN, et al. (1997). Malignant mesothelioma in south east England: clinicopathological experience of 272 cases. Thorax. 52:507–12.
2954. Ye B, Li W, Liu XY, et al. (2010). Multiple organ metastases of Pulmonary Epithelioid Haemangioendothelioma and a review of the literature. Med Oncol. 27:49–54.
2955. Ye H, Liu H, Attygalle A, et al. (2003). Variable frequencies of t(11;18)(q21;q21) in MALT lymphomas of different sites: significant association with CagA strains of H pylori in gastric MALT lymphoma. Blood. 102:1012–8.
2956. Ye Z, Shi H, Peng T, et al. (2011). Clinical and pathological features of high grade primary cardiac osteosarcoma. Interact Cardiovasc Thorac Surg. 12:94–5.
2957. Yeh YC, Chou TY (2014). Pulmonary neuroendocrine tumors: study of 90 cases focusing on clinicopathological characteristics, immunophenotype, preoperative biopsy, and frozen section diagnoses. J Surg Oncol. 109:280–6.
2958. Yekeler E, Dursun M, Yildirim A, et al. (2005). Diffuse pulmonary lymphangiomatosis: imaging findings. Diagn Interv Radiol. 11:31–4.
2959. Yellin A, Simansky DA, Ben-Avi R, et al. (2013). Resection and heated pleural chemoperfusion in patients with thymic epithelial

malignant disease and pleural spread: a single-institution experience. J Thorac Cardiovasc Surg. 145:83–7.
2960. Yendamuri S, Caty L, Pine M, et al. (2012). Outcomes of sarcomatoid carcinoma of the lung: a Surveillance, Epidemiology, and End Results Database analysis. Surgery. 152:397–402.
2961. Yiakoumis X, Pangalis GA, Kyrtsonis MC, et al. (2010). Primary effusion lymphoma in two HIV-negative patients successfully treated with pleurodesis as first-line therapy. Anticancer Res. 30:271–6.
2962. Yim J, Zhu LC, Chiriboga L, et al. (2007). Histologic features are important prognostic indicators in early stages lung adenocarcinomas. Mod Pathol. 20:233–41.
2963. Yin Z, Kirschner LS (2009). The Carney complex gene PRKAR1A plays an essential role in cardiac development and myxomagenesis. Trends Cardiovasc Med. 19:44–9.
2964. Yoh K, Nishiwaki Y, Ishii G, et al. (2008). Mutational status of EGFR and KIT in thymoma and thymic carcinoma. Lung Cancer. 62:316–20.
2965. Yokose T, Ito Y, Ochiai A (2000). High prevalence of atypical adenomatous hyperplasia of the lung in autopsy specimens from elderly patients with malignant neoplasms. Lung Cancer. 29:125–30.
2966. Yokota K, Sasaki H, Okuda K, et al. (2012). KIF5B/RET fusion gene in surgically-treated adenocarcinoma of the lung. Oncol Rep. 28:1187–92.
2967. Yokoyama T, Osada H, Murakami H, et al. (2008). YAP1 is involved in mesothelioma development and negatively regulated by Merlin through phosphorylation. Carcinogenesis. 29:2139–46.
2968. Yoneda S, Marx A, Heimann S, et al. (1999). Low-grade metaplastic carcinoma of the thymus. Histopathology. 35:19–30.
2969. Yoneda S, Marx A, Muller-Hermelink HK (1999). Low-grade metaplastic carcinomas of the thymus: biphasic thymic epithelial tumors with mesenchymal metaplasia--an update. Pathol Res Pract. 195:555–63.
2970. Yoon DH, Roberts W (2002). Sex distribution in cardiac myxomas. Am J Cardiol. 90:563–5.
2971. Yoon RG, Kim MY, Song JW, et al. (2013). Primary endobronchial marginal zone B-cell lymphoma of bronchus-associated lymphoid tissue: CT findings in 7 patients. Korean J Radiol. 14:366–74.
2972. Yoshida A, Kohno T, Tsuta K, et al. (2013). ROS1-rearranged lung cancer: a clinicopathologic and molecular study of 15 surgical cases. Am J Surg Pathol. 37:554–62.
2973. Yoshida A, Tsuta K, Ohno M, et al. (2014). STAT6 immunohistochemistry is helpful in the diagnosis of solitary fibrous tumors. Am J Surg Pathol. 38:552–9.
2974. Yoshida A, Tsuta K, Wakai S, et al. (2014). Immunohistochemical detection of ROS1 is useful for identifying ROS1 rearrangements in lung cancers. Mod Pathol. 27:711–20.
2975. Yoshida A, Tsuta K, Watanabe S, et al. (2011). Frequent ALK rearrangement and TTF-1/p63 co-expression in lung adenocarcinoma with signet-ring cell component. Lung Cancer. 72:309–15.
2976. Yoshida M, Okabe M, Eimoto T, et al. (2006). Immunoglobulin VH genes in thymic MALT lymphoma are biased toward a restricted repertoire and are frequently unmutated. J Pathol. 208:415–22.
2977. Yoshida Y, Shibata T, Kokubu A, et al. (2005). Mutations of the epidermal growth factor receptor gene in atypical adenomatous hyperplasia and bronchioloalveolar carcinoma of the lung. Lung Cancer. 50:1–8.
2978. Yoshiike F, Koizumi T, Yoneyama A, et al. (2004). Thymic squamous cell carcinoma producing parathyroid hormone-related protein and CYFRA 21-1. Intern Med. 43:493–5.
2979. Yoshikai M, Kamohara K, Fumoto H, et al. (2003). Left ventricular myxoma originating from the papillary muscle. J Heart Valve Dis. 12:177–9.
2980. Yoshikawa T, Noguchi Y, Matsukawa H, et al. (1994). Thymus carcinoid producing parathyroid hormone (PTH)-related protein: report of a case. Surg Today. 24:544–7.
2981. Yoshikawa Y, Sato A, Tsujimura T, et al. (2012). Frequent inactivation of the BAP1 gene in epithelioid-type malignant mesothelioma. Cancer Sci. 103:868–74.
2982. Yoshino M, Sekine Y, Koh E, et al. (2014). Pericardial synovial sarcoma: a case report and review of the literature. Surg Today. 44:2167-73.
2983. Yoshizawa A, Motoi N, Riely GJ, et al. (2011). Impact of proposed IASLC/ATS/ERS classification of lung adenocarcinoma: prognostic subgroups and implications for further revision of staging based on analysis of 514 stage I cases. Mod Pathol. 24:653–64.
2984. Yoshizawa A, Sumiyoshi S, Sonobe M, et al. (2013). Validation of the IASLC/ATS/ERS lung adenocarcinoma classification for prognosis and association with EGFR and KRAS gene mutations: analysis of 440 Japanese patients. J Thorac Oncol. 8:52–61.
2985. Young L, Lee HS, Inoue Y, et al. (2013). Serum VEGF-D a concentration as a biomarker of lymphangioleiomyomatosis severity and treatment response: a prospective analysis of the Multicenter International Lymphangioleiomyomatosis Efficacy of Sirolimus (MILES) trial. Lancet Respir Med. 1:445–52.
2986. Yousem SA (2005). Pulmonary intestinal-type adenocarcinoma does not show enteric differentiation by immunohistochemical study. Mod Pathol. 18:816–21.
2987. Yousem SA, Colby TV, Chen YY, et al. (2001). Pulmonary Langerhans' cell histiocytosis: molecular analysis of clonality. Am J Surg Pathol. 25:630–6.
2988. Yousem SA, Dacic S, Nikiforov YE, et al. (2013). Pulmonary Langerhans cell histiocytosis: profiling of multifocal tumors using next-generation sequencing identifies concordant occurrence of BRAF V600E mutations. Chest. 143:1679–84.
2989. Yousem SA, Hochholzer L (1986). Alveolar adenoma. Hum Pathol. 17:1066–71.
2990. Yousem SA, Hochholzer L (1987). Malignant fibrous histiocytoma of the lung. Cancer. 60:2532–41.
2991. Yousem SA, Hochholzer L (1987). Mucoepidermoid tumors of the lung. Cancer. 60:1346–52.
2992. Yousem SA, Weiss LM, Colby TV (1986). Primary pulmonary Hodgkin's disease. A clinicopathologic study of 15 cases. Cancer. 57:1217–24.
2993. Yousem SA, Weiss LM, Warnke RA (1985). Primary mediastinal non-Hodgkin's lymphomas: a morphologic and immunologic study of 19 cases. Am J Clin Pathol. 83:676–80.
2994. Yousem SA, Wick MR, Randhawa P, et al. (1990). Pulmonary blastoma. An immunohistochemical analysis with comparison with fetal lung in its pseudoglandular stage. Am J Clin Pathol. 93:167–75.
2995. Yu GH, Kussmaul WG, DiSesa VJ, et al. (1993). Adult intracardiac rhabdomyoma resembling the extracardiac variant. Hum Pathol. 24:448–51.
2996. Yu H, Gibson JA, Pinkus GS, et al. (2007). Podoplanin (D2-40) is a novel marker for follicular dendritic cell tumors. Am J Clin Pathol. 128:776–82.
2997. Yu K, Liu Y, Wang H, et al. (2007). Epidemiological and pathological characteristics of cardiac tumors: a clinical study of 242 cases. Interact Cardiovasc Thorac Surg. 6:636–9.
2998. Yu N, Kim HR, Cha YJ, et al. (2011). Development of acute megakaryoblastic leukemia with isochromosome (12p) after a primary mediastinal germ cell tumor in Korea. J Korean Med Sci. 26:1099–102.
2999. Yu W, Chan-On W, Teo M, et al. (2011). First somatic mutation of E2F1 in a critical DNA binding residue discovered in well-differentiated papillary mesothelioma of the peritoneum. Genome Biol. 12:R96.
3000. Yu Y, Song Z, Gao H, et al. (2012). EGFR L861Q mutation is a frequent feature of pulmonary mucoepidermoid carcinoma. J Cancer Res Clin Oncol. 138:1421–5.
3001. Yurick BS, Ottoman RE (1960). Primary mediastinal choriocarcinoma. Radiology. 75:901–7.
3002. Yutaka Y, Omasa M, Shikuma K, et al. (2009). Spontaneous regression of an invasive thymoma. Gen Thorac Cardiovasc Surg. 57:272–4.
3003. Zabarovsky ER, Lerman MI, Minna JD (2002). Tumor suppressor genes on chromosome 3p involved in the pathogenesis of lung and other cancers. Oncogene. 21:6915–35.
3004. Zafar N, Johns CD (2011). Pleomorphic (sarcomatoid) carcinoma of lung--cytohistologic and immunohistochemical features. Diagn Cytopathol. 39:115–6.
3005. Zakowski MF, Huang J, Bramlage MP (2010). The role of fine needle aspiration cytology in the diagnosis and management of thymic neoplasia. J Thorac Oncol. 5:S281–5.
3006. Zaman SS, van Hoeven KH, Slott S, et al. (1997). Distinction between bronchioloalveolar carcinoma and hyperplastic pulmonary proliferations: a cytologic and morphometric analysis. Diagn Cytopathol. 16:396–401.
3007. Zamboni M, Lannes DC, Cordeiro PB, et al. (2009). Transthoracic biopsy with core cutting needle (Trucut) for the diagnosis of mediastinal tumors. Rev Port Pneumol. 15:589–95.
3008. Zamo A, Malpeli G, Scarpa A, et al. (2005). Expression of TP73L is a helpful diagnostic marker of primary mediastinal large B-cell lymphomas. Mod Pathol. 18:1448–53.
3009. Zauderer MG, Bott M, McMillan R, et al. (2013). Clinical characteristics of patients with malignant pleural mesothelioma harboring somatic BAP1 mutations. J Thorac Oncol. 8:1430–3.
3010. Zeren H, Moran CA, Suster S, et al. (1995). Primary pulmonary sarcomas with features of monophasic synovial sarcoma: a clinicopathological, immunohistochemical, and ultrastructural study of 25 cases. Hum Pathol. 26:474–80.
3011. Zettl A, Ströbel P, Wagner K, et al. (2000). Recurrent genetic aberrations in thymoma and thymic carcinoma. Am J Pathol. 157:257–66.
3012. Zhang C, Myers JL (2013). Crystal-storing histiocytosis complicating primary pulmonary marginal zone lymphoma of mucosa-associated lymphoid tissue. Arch Pathol Lab Med. 137:1199–204.
3013. Zhang L, Ellis J, Kumar D, et al. (2008). Primary right ventricular osteosarcoma. Can J Cardiol. 24:225–6.
3014. Zhang M, Ding L, Liu Y, et al. (2014). Cardiac myxoma with glandular elements: a clinicopathological and immunohistochemical study of five new cases with an emphasis on differential diagnosis. Pathol Res Pract. 210:55–8.
3015. Zhang M, Wu QC (2013). Giant cardiac myxoma involving the left atrium, left ventricule, right atrium and superior vena cava. J Card Surg. 28:704.
3016. Zhang PJ, Brooks JS, Goldblum JR, et al. (2008). Primary cardiac sarcomas: a clinicopathologic analysis of a series with follow-up information in 17 patients and emphasis on long-term survival. Hum Pathol. 39:1385–95.
3017. Zhang PJ, Livolsi VA, Brooks JJ (2000). Malignant epithelioid vascular tumors of the pleura: report of a series and literature review. Hum Pathol. 31:29–34.
3018. Zhang WD, Guan YB, Li CX, et al. (2011). Pulmonary mucosa-associated lymphoid tissue lymphoma: computed tomography and (1)(8)F fluorodeoxyglucose-positron emission tomography/computed tomography imaging findings and follow-up. J Comput Assist Tomogr. 35:608–13.
3019. Zhang X, Ren G, Yao H, et al. (2013). Mixed dendritic cell tumours with follicular-fibroblastic dendritic cell features of lymph node. Pathology. 45:704–6.
3020. Zhao GQ, Dowell JE (2012). Hematologic malignancies associated with germ cell tumors. Expert Rev Hematol. 5:427–37.
3021. Zhao XG, Wang H, Wang YL, et al. (2012). Malignant solitary fibrous tumor of the right atrium. Am J Med Sci. 344:422–5.
3022. Zhao Y, Zhao H, Hu D, et al. (2013). Surgical treatment and prognosis of thymic squamous cell carcinoma: a retrospective analysis of 105 cases. Ann Thorac Surg. 96:1019–24.
3023. Zheng Z, Guo F, Pan Y (2011). Primary intrapulmonary thymoma mimicking lung cancer. Am Surg. 77:E222–3.
3024. Zhou Q, Lu G, Liu A, et al. (2012). Extraskeletal myxoid chondrosarcoma in the lung: asymptomatic lung mass with severe anemia. Diagn Pathol. 7:112.
3025. Zhou W, Ercan D, Chen L, et al. (2009). Novel mutant-selective EGFR kinase inhibitors against EGFR T790M. Nature. 462:1070–4.
3026. Zhou Y, Fan X, Routbort M, et al. (2013). Absence of terminal deoxynucleotidyl transferase expression identifies a subset of high-risk adult T-lymphoblastic leukemia/lymphoma. Mod Pathol. 26:1338–45.
3027. Zhou Z, Sehn LH, Rademaker AW, et al. (2014). An enhanced International Prognostic Index (NCCN-IPI) for patients with diffuse large B-cell lymphoma treated in the rituximab era. Blood. 123:837–42.
3028. Zhu B, Laskin W, Chen Y, et al. (2011). NUT midline carcinoma: a neoplasm with diagnostic challenges in cytology. Cytopathology. 22:414–7.
3029. Zinzani PL, Martelli M, Poletti V, et al. (2008). Practice guidelines for the management of extranodal non-Hodgkin's lymphomas of adult non-immunodeficient patients. Part I: primary lung and mediastinal lymphomas. A project of the Italian Society of Hematology, the Italian Society of Experimental Hematology and the Italian Group for Bone Marrow Transplantation. Haematologica. 93:1364–71.
3030. Zinzani PL, Pellegrini C, Gandolfi L, et al. (2013). Extranodal marginal zone B-cell lymphoma of the lung: experience with fludarabine and mitoxantrone-containing regimens. Hematol Oncol. 31:183–8.
3031. Zlotchenko G, Futuri S, Dillon E, et al. (2013). A rare case of lymphoma involving the tricuspid valve. J Cardiovasc Comput Tomogr. 7:207–9.
3032. Zolota V, Tzelepi V, Charoulis N, et al. (2006). Mediastinal rhabdomyoma: case report and review of the literature. Virchows Arch. 449:124–8.
3033. Zon R, Orazi A, Neiman RS, et al. (1994). Benign hematologic neoplasm associated with mediastinal mature teratoma in a patient with Klinefelter's syndrome: a case report. Med Pediatr Oncol. 23:376–9.
3034. Zwiebel BR, Austin JH, Grimes MM (1991). Bronchial carcinoid tumors: assessment with CT of location and intratumoral calcification in 31 patients. Radiology. 179:483–6.
3035. Zynger DL, Dimov ND, Luan C, et al. (2006). Glypican 3: a novel marker in testicular germ cell tumors. Am J Surg Pathol. 30:1570–5.
3036. Zynger DL, Everton MJ, Dimov ND, et al. (2008). Expression of glypican 3 in ovarian and extragonadal germ cell tumors. Am J Clin Pathol. 130:224–30.

Subject index

Symbols

34βE12 82, 87, 93, 227
α-SMA 105, 120
β-catenin 42, 92, 94, 119, 172, 179, 180
βhCG 244, 246–251, 260, 262
ΔNp63 83

A

A20 136, 269, 271
Acinar adenocarcinoma 10, 26, 33, **35**
Acinar predominant adenocarcinoma 26
Adenocarcinoma 18, 82, 115, 184, **26**–37, **226**–228
Adenocarcinoma in situ 10, 39, 47, **48**–50
Adenocarcinoma, NOS 184
Adenochondroma 116
Adenocystic carcinoma 101
Adenoid cystic carcinoma 10, 58, **101**, 102, 227
Adenoma 10, 110
Adenomatoid tumour 154, **171**
Adenomyoepithelioma 103
Adenosquamous carcinoma 10, 15, 17, 19–21, 55, 82, **86**, 87, 91, 98, 99, 184, 219, 224, **233**
Adult cellular rhabdomyoma 300, **310**
Adult intracardiac rhabdomyoma 310
AE1/AE3 66, 76, 93–96, 111, 160, 166, 197, 211, 235, 239, 247, 253, 324
AE3 66, 76, 93–96, 111, 160, 166, 191, 197, 211, 235, 239, 247, 253, 324
AFP 244, 246–248, 251–254, 260, 262
Aggressive fibromatosis 179
Aggressive t(15;19) positive carcinoma 97, 229
AIRE 191, 197
AIS See Adenocarcinoma in situ
ALCL See Anaplastic large cell lymphoma
ALCL, ALK-negative (ALK–) 184
ALCL, ALK-positive (ALK+) 184
ALK 16, 21–24, 36, 37, 83, 87, 90, 122, 151, 167, 184, 275, 276, 279, 281, 294
ALK1 122, 137, 180, 326
ALK-negative anaplastic large cell lymphoma 275
ALK-positive anaplastic large cell lymphoma 275
Alveolar adenoma 10, **112**, 113
Alveolar rhabdomyosarcoma 223, 337
Anaplastic carcinoma 232
Anaplastic large cell lymphoma 184, **275**
Anaplastic large cell lymphoma and other rare mature T- and NK-cell lymphoma 184, 275
Ancient thymoma 210
Angiocentric immunoproliferative lesion 138
Angioendotheliomatosis proliferans syndrome 140

Angioendotheliotropic lymphoma 140
Angiogenic squamous dysplasia 59
Angiosarcoma 150, 154, 161, 165, **177**, 184, 264, **292**, 293, 300, 302, **329**, **344**
APC 61, 164, 180, 192, 195, 215
API2 136
Arachnocytosis of the myocardium 307
ARID1A 76
ASCL1 63
ASCL4 55
ATF1 133
ATM 102, 272, 274
Atrioventricular node mesothelioma 323
ATRX 294
Atypical adenomatous hyperplasia 10, **46**–48
Atypical alveolar cell hyperplasia 46
Atypical alveolar epithelial hyperplasia 46
Atypical alveolar hyperplasia 46
Atypical bronchioloalveolar hyperplasia 46
Atypical carcinoid 10, 67, **73**, 74, 76, 77, 184, 215, 234, **237**
Atypical endocrine tumours of the lung 69
Atypical thymoma 202
Atypical type A thymoma 187, 189
Autoimmune regulator 191, 197

B

BAI3 68
BALT See Bronchus-associated lymphoid tissue (BALT) lymphoma
BALTOMA 134
BAP1 157, 162, 163, 171, 215
Basaloid carcinoma 10, 56–58, 67, 71, 80, 98, 102, 131, 132, 215, **216**, 217
Basaloid squamous cell carcinoma **56**, 184, 216, 217
B-cell lymphoma, unclassifiable, with features intermediate between diffuse large B-cell and classical Hodgkin lymphoma 184, 272, 278–**280**
Bcl2 58, 61, 68, 72, 95, 127, 135, 165, 173, 177, 178, 192, 201, 204, 205, 208, 210, 215, 268–270, 279, 341, 344
Bcl6 135, 136, 173, 268, 269, 278, 279, 281, 341
BCL11A 269
BCLU See B-cell lymphoma, unclassifiable, with features intermediate between diffuse large B-cell and classical Hodgkin lymphoma
Benign mesothelioma 178
Benign mixed tumour 105
BerEP4 97, 160, 168, 227, 230
BET-rearranged carcinoma 97, 229
Biphasic mesothelioma 154, **165**, 166, 169
Biphasic thymoma 207
Biphasic-type synovial sarcoma 94
BOB.1 268, 281, 283
Body cavity-based lymphoma 172

Angioendotheliotropic lymphoma 140

BRAF 22–24, 36, 83, 88, 114, 141–143, 151, 215, 269, 283
BRD3 98, 231
BRD4 98, 230, 231
BRN2 68
Bronchial adenoma 46, 113, 115
Bronchial adenoma arising in mucous glands 115
Bronchial cystadenoma 115
Bronchial premalignancy 59
Bronchiolar carcinoma 26
Bronchioloalveolar carcinoma 18, 26, 32, 38, 39, 44, 48, 50
Bronchoalveolar carcinoma 26, 38
Bronchus-associated lymphoid tissue (BALT) lymphoma 134
BUB1 58, 164

C

Calcifying fibrous pseudotumour 180
Calcifying fibrous tumour 154, **180**
CALM-AF10 274
CAM5.2 66, 109, 111, 120, 166, 235, 239, 253, 308
CAMTA1 124, 176, 293, 330
Capillary haemangioma 292, 300, **318**
Carcinoembryonic (CEA) antigen 97
Carcinoid tumour 10, 71, **73**, 74, 78, 114, 184, 234, 235, 327
Carcinoma of the thymus with clear cell features 222
Carcinoma with t(15;19) translocation 97, 229
Carcinosarcoma 10, 15, 83, 88, **91**, 92, 105, 208, 224, 226, 339
Cardiac angioma 318
Cardiac fibroma 300, 306, **320**, 321, 344
Cardiac fibromatosis 320
Cardiac hamartoma 309
Cardiac lymphoma 300, 340
Cardiac myxoma 300, **311**, 312, 317
Cardiac papilloma 315
Cardiac rhabdomyoma 305, 306
Cardiac vascular malformation 318
Carney-Stratakis syndrome 327
Cavernous haemangioma 300, **318**
CBX6 76
CCN2 68
CCNE1 84
CD1a 142, 143, 197, 201, 205, 273, 282, 283, 285–287
CD2 175, 273
CD3 96, 137, 139, 140, 175, 191, 194, 197, 205, 211, 221, 242, 266, 270, 273, 274, 281
CD4 139, 143, 172, 175, 197, 266, 273, 281, 283, 286
CD7 175, 266, 273
CD8 95, 96, 139, 197, 273
CD10 136, 205, 266, 268, 270, 273, 281, 341

CD13 273, 283
CD14 266, 283, 286
CD15 137, 139, 140, 160, 174, 268, 276, 278, 280, 281, 283
CD19 173, 174, 266, 268, 273, 341
CD20 96, 191, 194, 205, 271
CD21 135, 283–285
CD22 268, 273
CD23 135, 205, 268–270, 285
CD29 140
CD31 20, 90, 121, 123, 129, 161, 165, 176, 177, 293, 314, 316, 329, 330, 345
CD33 266, 273, 283, 288
CD35 135, 283, 285, 287
CD38 173
CD40 191, 194
CD42b 266
CD43 135, 270, 288
CD45 20, 137, 140, 161, 173, 242, 268, 283, 286
CD45RB 67
CD54 140, 268
CD56 20, 57, 58, 65–67, 70, 71, 75, 81, 127, 140, 192, 235, 237, 239, 242, 254, 266, 273
CD57 120, 203
CD61 266, 288
CD68 120, 143, 266, 283, 285–288, 308, 324
CD69 308
CD70 298
CD71 266
CD74 24, 40
CD79 175
CD79a 135, 137, 141, 173, 174, 197, 205, 266, 268, 270, 273, 281, 341
CD99 67, 126, 127, 177, 178, 205, 208, 210, 242, 273, 338, 344
CD123 266
CD138 173, 174
CD163 266, 283
CD205 191, 214, 298
CD207 282, 286, 287
CDK4 290, 291
CDKN2A 54, 55, 72, 84, 85, 102, 162–164, 192, 201, 204, 215, 274, 303
CDKN2B 162, 163
CDX2 20, 40, 43, 150, 160, 228, 253, 254, 298
CEBPA 283
CEBPB 283
Chemodectoma 133, 326
Childhood fibrous tumour with psammoma bodies 180
Chloroma 288
Chondroid hamartoma 116
Chondroma 10, 117
Chondromatous hamartoma 116
Chondrosarcoma 91–93, 117, 126, 128–130, 133, 167, 225, 264, 295, 333, 339
Chorioblastoma 255
Choriocarcinoma 184, 247, 248, 253, 255, 256
Chorioepithelioma 255
Chorionic carcinoma 255
Chromogranin 20, 42, 57, 65–67, 70, 71, 75, 79, 81, 93, 97, 225, 230, 235, 239, 240, 242, 296, 297, 324, 325, 327
CIITA 269, 279

CIRC See Cytokeratin-positive interstitial reticulum cell
Clara cell adenoma 113
Clara cells 34, 38, 44, 45–49, 69, 93, 111, 113
Clear cell carcinoma 184, 222, 223
Clear cell tumour 10, 118, 119
CLTC 122
Colloid adenocarcinoma 10, 18, 40, 41
Columnar cell papilloma 108
Combined large cell neuroendocrine carcinoma 10, 69, 184, 239
Combined small cell carcinoma 10, 63, 65, 66, 68, 184, 234, 241
Combined thymic carcinoma 184, 189, 190, 200, 203, 212, 242
Combined thymic epithelial tumour 212, 242
Composite thymoma-thymic carcinoma 242
Congenital bronchopulmonary leiomyosarcoma 119
Congenital fibrosarcoma 119
Congenital leiomyosarcoma 119, 120
Congenital mesenchymal malformation of lung 119
Congenital peribronchial myofibroblastic tumour 10, 119, 120
Congenital pulmonary myofibroblastic tumour 119
CORO1C 173
Cortical thymoma 199
CREB1 10, 129–131, 133
CREBBP 68, 72
cREL/p65 281
CRTC1 100
CTNNB1 42, 94, 179, 180
CUL3 55
CXCL13 285
CYB 308
Cyclin D1 61, 66, 136, 270
Cyclin E 61, 68, 77
CYLD 102, 215
Cylindroma 101
CYP19A1 46
Cystic tumour 300, 323
Cystic tumour of the atrioventricular node 8, 300, 323
Cytokeratin-positive interstitial reticulum cell tumour 286

D
D2-40 121, 160, 162, 166, 247, 253, 285
DDIT3 133, 291
Dedifferentiated liposarcoma 184, 290, 291
Dendritic reticulum cell tumour 284
der(16)t(1:16)(q12;q12.1) 226
Dermoid cyst 346
Desmocollin 3 18, 89
Desmoid tumour 179
Desmoid-type fibromatosis 154, 179
Desmoplastic mesothelioma 154, 165, 166, 168
Desmoplastic round cell tumour 154, 180
Desmoplastic small round cell tumour 295, 339
DICER1 76, 125, 126
Diffuse idiopathic pulmonary neuroendocrine cell hyperplasia 10, 63, 73, 78, 79, 150

Diffuse large B-cell lymphoma 10, 135, 136, 137, 139, 154
Diffuse large B-cell lymphoma associated with chronic inflammation 154, 174, 175
Diffuse large B-cell non-Hodgkin lymphoma 136
Diffuse malignant mesothelioma 154, 156–158, 170, 345
Diffuse pulmonary lymphangiomatosis 10, 121
DIPNECH See Diffuse idiopathic pulmonary neuroendocrine cell hyperplasia
DLBCL See Diffuse large B-cell lymphoma
DNMT1 58
DNMT3A 58
DSRCT See Desmoplastic small round cell tumour
DUTT1 68
Dysgerminoma 244

E
E2F 58
E2F1 68, 77, 171
E2F2 68
E26 129, 161
EBER1 95, 96
EBNA1 172, 175
EBNA2 175
EBV 83, 95–97, 132, 136–140, 172–175, 209, 220–222, 267, 270, 277–280, 314, 340
Ectopic heterotopia 323
Ectopic parathyroid tumour 185, 296
Ectopic thyroid tumour 185, 296
Ectopic tumours of the thymus 185, 296
EFT See Ewing family of tumours
EIF1AX 76
Embryonal carcinoma 184, 247, 248, 249, 250, 253, 260
Embryonal rhabdomyosarcoma 264, 295, 337
Embryonal rhabdomyosarcoma arising within congenital bronchogenic cyst 124
EML4 21, 22, 24, 37, 90
Endodermal heterotopia/inclusion/cyst 323
Endodermal sinus tumour 251, 327, 346
Endothelioma 323
Enteric adenocarcinoma 10, 18, 42, 43
Eosinophilic granuloma 282
EP300 68, 72, 84
EPHA7 68
Epidermoid carcinoma 51
Epidermoid keratinizing carcinoma 212
Epidermoid non-keratinizing carcinoma 212
Epimyoepithelial carcinoma 103
Epithelial-myoepithelial carcinoma 10, 103, 104, 131
Epithelial-myoepithelial tumour 103
Epithelial-myoepithelial tumour of unproven malignant potential 103
Epithelial thymoma 202
Epithelial-type mesothelioma 156
Epithelioid haemangioendothelioma 10, 90, 123, 124, 161, 176, 292, 293, 330
Epithelioid hemangioendothelioma 154, 184

Epithelioid leiomyosarcoma 336
Epithelioid malignant mesothelioma 156, 159–164, 170
Epithelioid mesothelioma 154, **156**, 159, 165, 168, 169
ERBB2 22–24, 29, 36, 40, 84
ERBB2/HER2 22, 36
Erdheim-Chester disease **142**, 143
ERG 161, 165, 176, 177, 293, 329, 330, 345
ERβ 42
Ewing family of tumours 67, 339
Ewing sarcoma 98, 127, 133, 181, 230, 295, 339, 345
EWSR1 67, 129–132, 180, 181
EWSR1-CREB1 129–131
Exophytic squamous cell papilloma **106**
Extra-adrenal phaeochromocytoma 326
Extramedullary myeloid tumour 288
Extramedullary acute myeloid leukaemia 183, 184, **288**
Extranodal marginal zone lymphoma of mucosa-associated lymphoid tissue (MALT lymphoma) 10, **134**, 184, **270**
Extrarenal rhabdoid tumour 339
Extraskeletal Ewing sarcoma 339
Extraskeletal osteosarcoma 129, 333
EZH2 76

F

FBXW7 274
Fetal adenocarcinoma 10, 18, **41**, 42
Fetal-type adenocarcinoma 94
FEV1 142
FGF3 58
FGF10 126
FGF19 58
FGFR1 22, 55, 68, 72, 85, 87, 273
FGFR2 90, 102, 113, 164
FHIT 61, 68, 85
Fibroblastic dendritic cell tumour 286
Fibroblastic reticular cell tumour 184, **286**
Fibroelastic hamartoma 320
Fibroelastic papilloma 315
Fibrolipoma 322
Fibromyxosarcoma 334
Fibrous hamartoma 320
Fibrous histiocytoma 119, 121, 130, 131, 133, 149, 287, 291, 295, 331, 334
Fibrous mesothelioma 178
Fibroxanthoma 121
FLI1 123, 161, 165, 339, 345
Foamy myocardial transformation 307
Focal lipid cardiomyopathy 307
Folate binding protein 61
Follicular adenoma 296
Follicular carcinoma 296
Follicular dendritic cell sarcoma 184, **284**, 285
Follicular dendritic cell tumour 284
Former pulmonary blastoma 41
FOXN1 191, 214, 298
FOXP1 55
FRA3B 68
FUS 132, 133
FUS1 68

G

Ganglioneuroblastoma 185, **294**
Ganglioneuroma 185, **294**
GATA3 54, 150, 160, 298
GCDFP15 150, 160, 228
Germ cell neoplasms 144
Germ cell tumours 10, 144, 148, 150, 151, 184, 244, 253, 263, 265, 288, 300, 327, 346
Germ cell tumours of the mediastinum 8, 184, 244
Germ cell tumours with associated haematological malignancy 184, **265**
Germ cell tumours with somatic-type malignancy 184, **263**
Germ cell tumours with somatic-type solid malignancy 184, **263**
Germ cell tumour with malignant transformation 263
Germ cell tumour with non-germ cell malignancy 263
Germinoma 244
Giant cell carcinoma 10, **88–90**
Giant Lambl excrescence 315
Glandular papilloma 10, **108**
GLUT1 203, 204, 214, 215, 243, 319
Glypican 3 42, 250, 253, 254, 256
Grade 1 neuroendocrine carcinoma 73
Grade 2 neuroendocrine carcinoma 73
Granular cell myoblastoma 324
Granular cell nerve sheath tumour 324
Granular cell tumour 300, **324**
Granulocytic sarcoma 288
GTF2I 192, 195, 198, 201, 204, 215

H

Haemangioma 184, **292**, 300, 302, 314, **318**
Haemangioma, NOS 300, 318
Haemangiopericytoma 127, 178, 189, 190, 344
Haemangiosarcoma 177
HAM56 308
Hamartochondroma 116
Hamartoma of adult cardiac myocytes 309
Hamartoma of mature cardiac myocytes 8, 300, **309**
Hepatoid carcinoma 184, **233**
HepPar-1 253, 254
HER2 22, 36, 61, 87, 151, 215
Heterologous sarcomatoid carcinoma 91
HHF35 120
HHV8 172, 173
High-grade intraepithelial neoplasia 59
High-grade mucosa-associated lymphoid tissue lymphoma 136
Histiocytic and dendritic cell neoplasms of the mediastinum 184
Histiocytic sarcoma 184, **283**, 284
Histiocytoid cardiomyopathy 300–302, **307**, 308
Histiocytosis X 141, 282
HLA-A, 55
HLA-DR 273, 283
HMB45 103, 119, 121, 146, 150, 161, 286, 321

HMGA2 105, 117, 289
HNF4A 45
Hodgkin disease 277
Hodgkin-like anaplastic large cell lymphoma 280
Hodgkin lymphoma 28, 96, 136, 137, 139, 140, 157, 184, 210, 222, 268, 269, 271, 272, 276, **277–281**, 340
Homologous sarcomatoid carcinoma 91
HRAS 103, 192
Hybrid dendritic cell tumour 287

I

IDH1/2 167
IGF2 179, 344
IGH 136, 271
Indeterminate dendritic cell tumour 184, 287
Infantile cardiomyopathy 307
Infantile cardiomyopathy with histiocytoid changes 307
Infantile xanthomatous cardiomyopathy 307
Inflammatory myofibroblastic tumour 10, 90, **121**, 122, 302, **326**
Inflammatory pseudotumour 121, 326
Interdigitating dendritic cell sarcoma 8, 184, **285**
Interdigitating dendritic cell tumour 285
Intermediate cell type carcinoma 63
Intimal sarcoma 10, 128, 129, 331, 334
Intracardiac endodermal sinus tumour 327
Intracardiac teratoma 327
Intrapulmonary thymoma 10, **145**
Intravascular bronchioloalveolar tumour 123, 176
Intravascular large B-cell lymphoma 10, **140**
Intravascular lymphomatosis 140
Invasive fibrous tumour of the tracheobronchial tree 121
Invasive mucinous adenocarcinoma 10, 18, **38–40**
Inverted squamous cell papilloma **106**
IRF4/MUM1 173, 174, 268, 278, 281, 341
Isolated cardiac lipidosis 307

J

JAK2/PDL2 269, 281
JAK-STAT 269, 279
JAZF1/PHF1 333

K

Kaposi sarcoma 121, 132, 172, 173, 175, 340
Kaposi sarcoma-associated herpesvirus 172, 173, 175, 340
KEAP1 55, 72
Keratinizing squamous cell carcinoma 10, **51–53**
Ki1 lymphoma 275
KIT 66, 68, 102, 103, 151, 192, 195, 201, 204, 215, 218, 244, 247, 253
KL1 166
KRAS 19, 22–25, 36–38, 40, 47, 50, 55, 83–85, 87, 90, 92, 96, 103, 114, 151, 165, 192, 215, 269, 330

KSHV See Kaposi sarcoma-associated herpesvirus

L

LANA 172, 173
Langerhans cell lesions 184, 282, 287
Langerhans cell histiocytosis 141, 184, 282
Langerhans cell sarcoma 184, **282**, 287
Large cell anaplastic carcinoma 80
Large cell carcinoma 10, 17, 18, 33, 35, 53, 69, 71, **80**, 81, 83
Large cell neuroendocrine carcinoma 10, 17, 19, 20, 21, 35, 36, 57, 63, 66, 67, **69**–71, 73, 78, 80, 84, 91, 184, 215, 233, **239**, 240, 242, 243, 297
Large cell neuroendocrine tumour 69
Large cell undifferentiated carcinoma 80
LATS1 163
LATS2 163
LCNEC See Large cell neuroendocrine carcinoma
Leiomyosarcoma 129, 300, **336**
Lepidic adenocarcinoma 10, 26, 30, 31, **34**
Lepidic predominant adenocarcinoma 26, 32
LIN28 247, 253, 254
Lipid (cholesterol) granulomatosis 143
Lipofibroadenoma 184, **210**, 211
Lipogranulomatosis 143
Lipoidgranulomatosis 143
Lipoma 184, 289, **290**, 300, 302, **322**
Liposarcoma 92, 131, 133, 184, 264, 289, **290**, 291, 295, 322, 339
LKB1 87
LMP1 95, 139, 172, 173, 175, 222
LMP2A 172
LN3 308
Localized fibrous tumour 178, 291, 344
Localized malignant mesothelioma 7, 154, **169**
Localized mesothelioma 169, 178
Low-grade malignant myxoid endobronchial tumour 129
Low-grade metaplastic carcinoma 207
LPP 117
Lymphangioendothelioma 323
Lymphangioleiomyomatosis 10, **118**, 119, 121
Lymphangioma 113, 133, 184, **292**, 293, 323
Lymphangiomatosis 121
Lymphatic dysplasia 121
Lymphocyte-rich thymoma 196
Lymphocytic thymoma 196
Lymphoepithelial carcinoma 95, 220
Lymphoepithelial-like carcinoma 220
Lymphoepithelioma 80, 95, 96, 159, 215, 220–222, 224, 232, 243, 285
Lymphoepithelioma-like carcinoma 10, **95**, 96, 184, **220**–222
Lymphomatoid granulomatosis 10, 139
Lymphoproliferative disorders 154, 172

M

MAC387 143, 308
MAD1L1 68
Malignant angioendotheliomatosis 140
Malignant extrarenal rhabdoid tumour 339
Malignant fibrous histiocytoma 331
Malignant haemangioendothelioma 177
Malignant mesothelioma 345
Malignant mixed tumour comprising epithelial and myoepithelial cells 103
Malignant myoepithelial tumour 131
Malignant peripheral nerve sheath tumour 264, 286, 293, 339
Malignant solitary fibrous tumour 154, 178
Malignant synovioma 127, 177
Malignant teratoma intermediate 260
Malignant teratoma undifferentiated 249
MALT1 136, 271
MALT lymphoma See Extranodal marginal zone lymphoma of mucosa-associated lymphoid tissue (MALT lymphoma)
MAML2 87, 99, 100, 219
MAPK 164, 172, 302
MCM2 61
MDM2 94, 102, 129, 279, 290, 291, 303, 332, 335
Mediastinal diffuse large cell lymphoma with sclerosis 267
Mediastinal grey zone lymphoma 269, 280
Medullary thymoma 187
Medullary thyroid carcinoma 296
Melanoma 10, **146**, 149
Melanoma of unknown primary 146
MEN1 63, 68, 73, 76, 234, 235, 237
Meningioma, NOS 10, **147**
Merkel cell carcinoma 67
MERT See Malignant extrarenal rhabdoid tumour
Mesenchymal tumours 10, 116, 132, 147, 154, 176
MET 22–24, 90, 164
Metaplastic carcinoma 207, 224
Metaplastic thymoma 184, 189, **207**, 208, 225
Metastasis to the heart 342
Metastasis to the lung 148
Metastasis to the mediastinum 298
Metastasis to the pericardium 347
Metastasis to the thymus 298
Metastatic tumours 10, 113, 148, 300, 327, 342, 347, 348
MGZL See Mediastinal grey zone lymphoma
MIA See Minimally invasive adenocarcinoma
MIB1 308
Microinvasive adenocarcinoma 44
Micronodular thymoma with lymphoid B cell hyperplasia 205

Micronodular thymoma with lymphoid stroma 184, **205**, 206
Micropapillary adenocarcinoma 10, 26, 33, **35**
Micropapillary predominant adenocarcinoma 26
Microscopic thymoma 184, **209**
Midline carcinoma of children and young adults with NUT rearrangement 97, 229
Midline lethal carcinoma 97, 229
Minimally invasive adenocarcinoma 10, 18, 39, **44**, 45

Mixed epithelial and sarcomatous mesothelioma 165
Mixed epithelioid and sarcomatoid mesothelioma 165
Mixed germ cell tumour 184, 248, **260**, **346**, 300
Mixed invasive mucinous and non-mucinous adenocarcinoma 10
Mixed mesenchymoma 116
Mixed mesothelioma 165
Mixed mucinous and non-mucinous adenocarcinoma 10, 38
Mixed papilloma 108
Mixed polygonal and spindle cell type thymoma 207
Mixed small cell carcinoma 63
Mixed large cell carcinoma 63
Mixed squamous cell and glandular papilloma 10, **108**, 109
Mixed thymoma 193
MKI67 58
MLL 68, 72, 267
MLL2 55
MNF116 66, 135
MOC31 160, 168
Moderately differentiated neuroendocrine carcinoma 73, 237
MPNST See Malignant peripheral nerve sheath tumour
MT-TK 308
MUC1 61, 109, 203, 204, 214, 243
MUC2 40, 218, 228
Mucinous adenocarcinoma 10, 18, 30–34, 36, 38–41, 44–50, 136, 149, 184, 219, 226–228, 314
Mucinous bronchioloalveolar carcinoma 38
Mucinous bronchoalveolar carcinoma 38
Mucinous cystadenocarcinoma 32, 40, 114
Mucinous cystadenoma 10, **114**
Mucinous cystic tumour of borderline malignancy 40
Mucoepidermoid carcinoma 10, **99**, 100, 184, **218**, 219
Mucoepidermoid tumour 99
Mucous cell adenoma polyadenoma 115
Mucous gland adenoma 10, 108, **115**
Müllerian tumour 94
MYB 58, 102
MYC 22, 58, 68, 84, 173, 240, 269, 279
MYCL 68
MYCN 295
MYD88 134, 136
Myeloid sarcoma 184, **288**
Myocardial or conduction system hamartoma 307
MyoD1 90, 166, 181
Myoepithelial carcinoma 10, 103, 104, **131**
Myoepithelial tumour 10, 131
Myoepithelioma 10, **131**, 132
Myogenin 83, 92, 94, 129, 166, 168, 181, 259, 377
Myomelanocytoma 118
Myxofibrosarcoma 300, 331, **334**
Myxoid fibrosarcoma 334
Myxoid liposarcoma 133, 160, 180, 184, 290, 291, 334, 335, 344
Myxoid liposarcoma/round cell liposarcoma 290

Myxoid malignant fibrous histiocytoma 334

N

NAB2 165, 179, 344
NAB2-STAT6 165, 179
NANOG 58, 250, 253
Napsin A 18, 35, 39, 45, 50, 66, 71, 81–83,
        89, 99, 111, 150, 160, 166
NCAM 66, 67, 70, 71, 235
NDUFB11 308, 309
NEF2L2 55
Neonatal pulmonary hamartoma 119
Neurilemmoma 325
Neurinoma 325
Neuroblastoma 185, **294**
NeuroD1 63
Neuroendocrine tumours 10
Neurogenic tumours 185, 293
Neurolemmoma 325
NF2 162, 163, 171
NFE2L2 55
NFIB 102
NF-κB 136, 172, 269, 271, 279
NIPBL 76
Nodular hyperplasia of the thymic
        epithelium 209
Nodular sclerosis classical Hodgkin
        lymphoma 268, 277, 278, 280
Non-keratinizing squamous cell carcinoma
        10, **51**, 53, 54, 82
Non-papillary adenocarcinoma 226
Non-small cell carcinoma 18, 21, 27, 28, 51,
        63, 67, 70, 80–82, 89, 91
Non-small cell lung cancer 16–18, 30
NOTCH1 55, 102, 274
NOTCH2 55
NPM1 275, 276
NR4A3 131
NR4A3-EWSR1 131
NR4A3-TAF15 131
NRAS 215
NRG1 22, 36, 40
NSCC See Non-small cell carcinoma
NSCHL See Nodular sclerosis classical
        Hodgkin lymphoma
NSCLC See Non-small cell lung cancer /
        carcinoma
NSD3 98, 231
NTRK1 22, 36
Nuclear protein in testis (NUT) 58, 97, 230
NUP214-ABL1 274
NUT carcinoma 57, 58, **97**, 98, 184, 215,
        229–233
NUTM1 97, 98, 230
NUT midline carcinoma 97, 98, 229

O

Oat cell carcinoma 63, 241
OCT2 268, 280, 281
OCT3 233, 247, 250
OCT4 58, 233, 247, 250, 251, 253, 254, 256,
        262
Oncocytic cardiomyopathy 307
Oncocytic (Hurthle cell) carcinoma 296
Organoid thymoma 196

OSCAR 166
Osteoblastic osteosarcoma 333
Osteochondroma 117
Osteogenic sarcoma 333
Osteosarcoma 129, 300, **333**
Other rare ectopic tumours 185, 297
Other rare mesenchymal tumours 295
Other rare thymic carcinomas 184, 233
Other rare thymomas 184, 209

P

p14 68, 77, 163, 164
p15INK4b 162, 163
p16 55, 61, 62, 76, 79, 104, 162–164,
        168, 215
p21 103, 172
p27 172
p38 164, 302
p40 18–21, 35, 36, 53, 54, 57, 67, 71, 80–83,
        87, 92, 96, 97, 132, 150, 161, 165,
        166, 230
p53 See TP53
Papanicolaou staining 19, 41, 49, 52, 65, 101
Papillary adenocarcinoma 10, 26, 33, **35**,
        184, **226**–228
Papillary adenoma 10, **113**
Papillary adenoma of type II
        pneumocytes 113
Papillary fibroelastoma 300, 314, **315**, 316
Papillary predominant adenocarcinoma 26
Papilloma 10, 106
Paraganglioma 294, 300, **326**, 327
Parathyroid adenoma 296
Parathyroid carcinoma 296
PARP1 68
PAX2 160
PAX3/7-FKHR 337
PAX5 173, 268, 273, 278, 281
PAX8 42, 71, 150, 160, 191, 197, 203, 214,
        233, 297, 298
PBRM1 215
PCNA 61
PD1 24, 269
PDCD6 46
PDGFRA 129, 303
PDL1 24, 269, 279
PDL2 269, 279, 281
PEComa 10, 117, 118, 223, 295
PEComa, benign 10, **118**
PEComa, malignant **118**
PEComatous tumours 10, 103, **117**, 119
PEL See Primary effusion lymphoma
Pericardial teratoma 346
Peripheral papillary tumour of type II
        pneumocytes 113
PGP9.5 314
Phaeochromocytoma 326
PHOX2B 294
PI3K 164
PICALM-MLLT10 274
PIK3CA 22, 55, 102, 215
PLAG1 105
PLAP 150, 247, 253, 256, 264
Plasma cell granuloma 121
PLCH See Pulmonary Langerhans cell
        granulomatosis
Pleomorphic adenoma 10, 102, **105**, 131

Pleomorphic carcinoma 10, **88**, 89
Pleomorphic liposarcoma 10, 19, 88, 89, 92,
        102, 105, 131, 167, 184, 281,
        290, 291
Pleural fibroma 178
Pleuropulmonary blastoma 10, 93, 94,
        124, 125
Pleuropulmonary blastoma in congenital
        cystic adenomatoid malformation 124
PMBL See Primary mediastinal large B-cell
        lymphoma
Pneumocytic adenomyoepithelioma 103
Polyadenoma 115
Polyostotic sclerosing histiocytosis 143
Polyphenotypic small round cell tumour 180
Poorly differentiated (high-grade)
        neuroendocrine carcinoma 239, 241
PRDM1/BLIMP1 173
Precursor T-ALL/precursor T-LBL 272
Predominantly cortical thymoma 196
Preinvasive squamous lesion 59
Primary bronchopulmonary mesenchymal
        tumours 132
Primary effusion lymphoma 154, **172**, 173
Primary mediastinal clear cell lymphoma of
        B-cell type 267
Primary mediastinal large B-cell lymphoma
        8, 137, 184, **267**–269
Primary pulmonary myxoid sarcoma 129, 130
Primary thymic extranodal marginal zone
        lymphoma 270
Primitive neuroectodermal tumour 125, 181,
        242, 264, 339, 345
PRKAR1A 302, 312, 314
Pseudolymphoma 134
Pseudosarcomatous myofibroblastic
        proliferation 326
Pseudosarcomatous myofibroblastic
        tumour 121
PSP1 76
PTCH1 302, 321
PTEN 55, 68, 104, 215
PTPN1 269
PTPN11 324
PU.1 268, 283
Pulmonary artery intimal sarcoma 10,
        128, 129
Pulmonary artery sarcoma 128
Pulmonary blastoma 10, 92, **93**, 94
Pulmonary blastoma associated with cystic
        lung disease 124
Pulmonary blastoma of childhood 124
Pulmonary endodermal tumour resembling
        fetal lung 41
Pulmonary eosinophilic granuloma 141
Pulmonary hamartoma 10, **116**
Pulmonary histiocytosis X 141
Pulmonary intestinal-type
        adenocarcinoma 42
Pulmonary Langerhans cell
        granulomatosis 141
Pulmonary Langerhans cell histiocytosis
        7, 10, **141**
Pulmonary myxoid sarcoma with EWSR1-
        CREB1 translocation 10, **129**
Pulmonary sarcoma arising in mesenchymal
        cystic hamartoma 124
Pyothorax-associated lymphoma 173, 174

R

RANBP2 122
RARB 61, 164
RAS 24, 102, 204
RASSF1 68, 164
RB 22, 61, 68, 72, 157, 195
RB1 55, 68, 72, 76, 84, 85, 192
REL 268, 269, 279, 281
REL/BCL11A 269
RET 22–24, 36, 87, 215, 327
Rhabdomyoma 300, 302, **305**, 314
Rhabdomyosarcoma 124, 300, **337**
Rhabdomyosarcoma arising in congenital
        cystic adenomatoid malformation 124
Romanowsky staining 19, 41, 52, 81
ROS1 22–24, 36, 87, 151

S

Salivary gland myoepithelial tumour 131
Salivary gland-type tumour 10, 76
SALL4 42, 150, 233, 247, 250, 253, 254,
        256, 262
Sarcoma 92, 132, 342, 344
Sarcomatoid carcinoma 7–10, 83, 88, 165,
        184, 208, **224**, 225
Sarcomatoid, desmoplastic, and biphasic
        mesothelioma 165
Sarcomatoid mesothelioma 154, **165**, 169
Sarcomatous mesothelioma 165
Schwannoma 300, **325**
Sclerosed lipoma 322
Sclerosing haemangioma 110
Sclerosing pneumocytoma 10, **110**, 111,
        113, 114
Sclerosing thymoma 184, 209, **210**
SDHB 327
SELPG 173
Seminoma 184, **244**–248, 253, 260
SF3B1 102
SKP2 68
SLC34A2 24
SLIT2 68
Small cell anaplastic carcinoma 63
Small cell carcinoma **65**–73, **241**–243
SMARCA4 76
SMARCB1 162
SMARCC1 76
SMARCC2 76
Soft tissue tumours of the mediastinum
        8, 184, 289
Solid adenocarcinoma 10, 26, 34, **35**
Solid predominant adenocarcinoma with
        mucin and/or pneumocyte marker
        expression 26
Solitary fibrous tumour 154, 165, 169, **178**,
        179, 184, 208, 210, **291**, 300,
        338, **344**
Solitary fibrous tumour, malignant 344
Solitary malignant mesothelioma 169
SOX 58
SOX2 55, 58, 62, 68, 85, 247, 250, 251, 253
SOX10 146, 161, 286
SPEN 102
Spindle cell carcinoma 10, 63, 66, 69, 70,
        88–90, 127, 224, 225
Spindle cell rhabdomyosarcoma 337

Spindle cell thymoma 187
Spread through air spaces (STAS) 33
Squamoid thymoma 202
Squamous atypia 59
Squamous cell carcinoma **51**–60, **212**–218
Squamous cell papilloma 10, **106**
Squamous cell carcinoma in situ **59**
Squamous dysplasia 59
Squamous papilloma 106
SS18 90, 92, 94, 128, 178, 291, 338, 345
SS18L1-SSX1 128, 178
SS18-SSX 90, 92, 94, 291, 338
SS18-SSX2 128
SSX 90, 92, 94, 165, 291, 338
SSX1 128, 178, 338
SSX2 128, 178
STAT6 165, 178–180, 192, 208, 210, 269,
        291, 344
STK11 72, 85
Submesothelial fibroma 291
SUFU 102
Sugar tumour 118
Synovial cell sarcoma 127
Synovial sarcoma 10, 90, **127**, 128, 154, 161,
        162, 169, **177**, 178, 184, **291**, 292,
        300, **338**, **344**
Synovial sarcoma, biphasic 127, 177,
        184, 291
Synovial sarcoma, epithelioid cell 127, 177,
        184, 291
Synovial sarcoma, NOS 184, 291
Synovial sarcoma, spindle cell 127, 177,
        184, 291
Synovioblastic sarcoma 127, 291
Synoviosarcoma 291
SYT 128, 165, 178, 338, 345

T

t(1;3)(p36.3;q25) 124
t(3;12)(q27-28;q14-15) 117
t(8;10)(p11.2;p15) 120
t(9;17)(q34;q23) 274
t(11;18)(q21;q21) 136
t(12;15)(p13;q2526) 120
t(14;18)(q32;q21) 136
t(14;19)(q32;q13) 141
t(15;19) carcinoma 97, 229
t(15;22)(p11;q11) 192
T790M 23, 36
TCRA/TCRD 274
Tenosynovial sarcoma 177, 291
Teratocarcinoma 260, 283
Teratoma 10, 144, 184, 245, 247, 257, 300,
        302, 346
Teratoma, immature 10, **144**, **257**, 300,
        327, **346**
Teratoma, mature 10, **144**, **257**, 300,
        327, **346**
TERT 46, 168
TET1 58
TGFBR2 46
Thymic carcinoma 184, 214, 226, 227,
        233, 254
Thymic carcinoma, NOS 184, **233**
Thymic carcinoma with adenoid cystic
        carcinoma-like features 184, **226**
Thymic carcinoma with t(15;19) 229

Thymic extranodal marginal zone lymphoma
        of mucosa-associated lymphoid
        tissue (MALT lymphoma) **270**, 271
Thymic Langerhans cell histiocytosis
        184, **282**
Thymic neuroendocrine tumour 184,
        225, 234
Thymic squamous cell carcinoma 192, 204,
        212–215
Thymolipoma 184, 211, **289**
Thymolipomatous hamartoma 289
Thymoma 98, 145, 161, 184, 187, 207,
        210, 214
Thymoma with pseudosarcomatous
        stroma 207
TIMP 61
TLE1 127, 162, 177, 192, 338, 345
T lymphoblastic leukaemia / lymphoma
        8, 184, **272**, 273
TNFa/b/c 136
TNFAIP2 268
TNFAIP3 269, 279
Tobacco smoking 26, 28
TP53 55, 61, 62, 94, 96, 163, 172
TP63 54, 55
TPM3 122
TPM4 122
Transitional cell papilloma 108
True histiocytic lymphoma 283
TSC1 102, 301, 306
TSC2 118, 301, 306
TSQCC See Thymic squamous cell
        carcinoma
t(X;18) 127, 128, 162, 168, 177, 178, 291,
        292, 338
t(X;18)(p11.2;q11.2) 127, 128, 168, 177,
        178, 338
Type AB thymoma 184, 190, 192,
        193–195, 206
Type A thymoma 184, **187**–192, 194, 197,
        200, 203, 205, 207, 208, 213,
        285, 293
Type A thymoma, including atypical variant
        184, 187
Type B1 thymoma 184, 192, **196**–198,
        200, 201
Type B2 thymoma 184, 192, 198, **199**–201
Type B3 thymoma 184, 192, 201,
        202–204, 243
Type C thymoma 212
Type II pneumocyte adenoma 113
Typical carcinoid 10, 67, **73**–76, 184, **234**,
        235, 237

U

Undifferentiated carcinoma 80, 89, 98, 137,
        184, 221, 224, 225, 230, **232**,
        233, 287
Undifferentiated pleomorphic sarcoma
        8, 300, 302, **331**, 332
Undifferentiated sarcoma 129, 331
Undifferentiated small cell carcinoma 63

V

V600D 283

V600E 24, 141–143, 283
Vascular neoplasms 184, 292, 293
VEGF 61, 119, 164
VEGFR 164
vGPCR 172
VH 271
VHL 68, 327
vIL6 172
von Hippel-Lindau disease 327

W

WDPM See Well-differentiated papillary
        mesothelioma
Well-differentiated liposarcoma 52, 170, 171,
        184, 290, 291, 333
Well-differentiated liposarcoma/adipocytic
        liposarcoma 290
Well-differentiated neuroendocrine carcinoma
        73, 234
Well-differentiated papillary mesothelioma
        154, **170**, 171
Well-differentiated thymic carcinoma 202
Wiskott-Aldrich syndrome 138
WT1 71, 160, 162, 166, 180, 181, 298, 339
WWTR1 124, 176, 293, 330
WWTR1-CAMTA1 124, 176, 330

X

X;18 translocation 90, 126
X-linked lymphoproliferative disease 138

Y

YAP1-TFE3 124, 176
Yolk sac tumour 93, 94, 144, 184, 244, 245,
        247, 248, 250, **251**–254, 260–263,
        265, 266, 283, 300, **327**, 328, 346

List of abbreviations

AFP	α-fetoprotein
AIDS	acquired immunodeficiency syndrome
CT	computed tomography
DNA	deoxyribonucleic acid
EBV	Epstein-Barr virus
EGFR	epidermal growth factor receptor
FDG	18F-fluorodeoxyglucose
FISH	fluorescence in situ hybridization
H&E	haematoxylin and eosin
HHV8	human herpesvirus 8
HIV	human immunodeficiency virus
HPV	human papillomavirus
IASLC	International Association for the Study of Lung Cancer
ATS	American Thoracic Society
ERS	European Respiratory Society
ICD-O	International Classification of Diseases for Oncology
ITMIG	International Thymic Malignancy Interest Group
IU/L	international units per litre
MALT	mucosa-associated lymphoid tissue
MEN1	multiple endocrine neoplasia type 1
MRI	magnetic resonance imaging
NK cell	natural killer cell
NOS	not otherwise specified
NUT	nuclear protein in testis
PCR	polymerase chain reaction
PET	positron emission tomography
PNC	pulmonary neuroendocrine cell
RNA	ribonucleic acid
RS cell	Reed-Sternberg cell
SEER	Surveillance, Epidemiology, and End Results
TdT	terminal deoxynucleotidyl transferase
TNM	tumour, node, metastasis
βhCG	β-subunit of human chorionic gonadotropin